A Comprehensive Textbook of

POSTPARTUM HEMORRHAGE

An Essential Clinical Reference
for Effective Management

2nd Edition

Very pleased to present this
to staff, residents and students
of RVH and McGill University

André Lalonde M.D.
Resident RVH 1970-73

A Comprehensive Textbook of

POSTPARTUM HEMORRHAGE

*An Essential Clinical Reference
for Effective Management*

2nd Edition

Edited by

Sir Sabaratnam Arulkumaran MD, PhD, FRCS, FRCOG
St George's, University of London, UK

Mahantesh Karoshi MD, MRCOG, DCRCM
Barnet and Chase Farm Hospitals NHS Trust, Barnet, London, UK

Louis G. Keith MD, PhD, FACOG, FRCOG
Northwestern University, Chicago, USA

André B. Lalonde MD, FRCSC, FRCOG
University of Ottawa and McGill University, Ottawa, Canada

Christopher B-Lynch FRCS, FRCOG, D.Univ
Milton Keynes General Hospital NHS Foundation Trust (Oxford Deanery), UK

Published
on behalf of

The Global Library of Women's Medicine
(www.glowm.com)

by

Sapiens Publishing

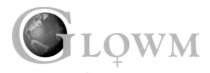

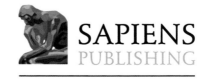

All the authors and editors have contributed to this publication on a strictly charitable basis and have received no remuneration of any kind for their contributions.

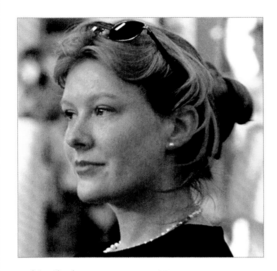

Abigail Bloomer, 1970–2001

This book has been produced and published on a not-for-profit, charitable basis by the Founders of **The Global Library of Women's Medicine** *(and of Sapiens Publishing) in*

loving memory of their daughter ABIGAIL BLOOMER, who worked alongside them in medical publishing for a number of years and who sadly died at the early age of 31 from breast cancer in December 2001. Abigail was especially involved in publishing on women's health issues. She is greatly missed.

Whilst this book is being made available via the normal publishing channels in the Western World, it will be supplied free to selected physicians in less-resourced countries. It is also being made available universally free, and in full, on the website of **The Global Library of Women's Medicine** (www.glowm.com).

A wall chart on this topic, designed to inform and support birth assistants, is also being made available.

Published by
Sapiens Publishing Ltd, 32 Meadowbank, London, NW3 3AY, UK
email: info@sapienspublishing.com
www.sapienspublishing.com

CIP data or a catalogue record for this book is available from the British Library.
ISBN: 978-0-9552282-7-8

Typeset by AMA DataSet Limited, Preston, Lancashire, UK
Printed and bound by Butler Tanner & Dennis, Frome, Somerset, UK

Contents

Section 3: Demographic Considerations

Section 4: Causation

Section 5: Placental Abnormalities

Section 6: Misoprostol

The Editors

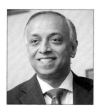

Sir Sabaratnam Arulkumaran, MD, PhD, FRCS, FRCOG
Professor and Head of Obstetrics and Gynaecology
St George's, University of London, UK

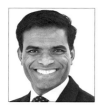

Mahentesh Karoshi, MD, MRCOG, DCRCM
Consultant Obstetrician and Gynaecologist
Department of Obstetrics and Gynaecology
Barnet and Chase Farm Hospitals NHS Trust
Barnet, London, UK

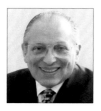

Louis G. Keith, MD, PhD, ScD (Hon), FACOG, FRCOG
Professor Emeritus
Department of Obstetrics and Gynecology
Northwestern University
Former Head, Section of Undergraduate Education and Medical Student Affairs, Chicago, IL, USA

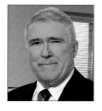

André B. Lalonde, MD, FRCSC, FRCOG
Professor of Obstetrics and Gynaecology
University of Ottawa and McGill University
Ottawa, Canada

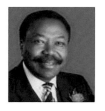

Christopher B-Lynch, MBBS, LRCP, FRCS, FRCOG, MAE, D.Univ, MCIArb QDR
Consultant Obstetrician and Gynaecological Surgeon
Professor (visiting) Cranfield University (Health Faculty);
Consultant Emeritus
Milton Keynes General Hospital NHS Foundation Trust (Oxford Deanery), Milton Keynes, UK

Publishers' Acknowledgments

The Publishers would like to express their sincere thanks to all the Editors and Contributors for their kindness in providing their contributions to this textbook without any remuneration or royalty. It is their generosity that has made this publication possible.

We should also like to express particular thanks to Professor Louis Keith who assumed the primary responsibility for reading and reviewing all the chapters of the book at the both manuscript and proofing stages; his contribution has been a notable one.

In addition to this printed edition, this book is also available *free* online on the website of *The Global Library of Women's Medicine* (www.glowm.com) – and in this version it also incorporates a number of video clips that serve to illustrate and amplify certain elements of the text.

The Contributors

E. T. Abrams, PhD
Department of Anthropology
University of Illinois at Chicago
Chicago, IL, USA

C. E. M. Aiken, MB/BChir, MA, PhD
Department of Obstetrics and Gynaecology
The Rosie Hospital
Addenbrooke's Hospital
Cambridge, UK

D. Armbruster, CNM, MPH, FACNM
Senior Maternal and Newborn Health Advisor
USAID/GH/HIDN/MCH
Washington, DC, USA

Sir S. Arulkumaran, MD, PhD, FRCS, FRCOG
Professor and Head of Obstetrics and Gynaecology
St George's, University of London, UK

R. K. Atalla, MB, ChB, MRCOG
Consultant Obstetrician and Gynaecologist
Queen Elizabeth II Hospital
Welwyn Garden City, UK

J. Barrett, MD, FRCOG, FRSCS
Division Chief of Maternal Fetal Medicine
Program Research Director, Women and Babies Unit
Sunnybrook Health Science Centre
Aubrey and Marla Dan Program
Toronto, ON;
Chief of Obstetrics and Gynaecolgy
Director York Central MFM
York Central Hospital
York, ON, Canada

T. F. Baskett, MB, FRCS(C), FRCS (Ed), FRCOG
Professor Emeritus
Department of Obstetrics and Gynaecology
Dalhousie University
Halifax, Nova Scotia, Canada

C. B-Lynch, MBBS, LRCP, FRCS, FRCOG, MAE,
   D.Univ, MCIArb QDR
Consultant Obstetrician and Gynaecological Surgeon
Professor (visiting) Cranfield University (Health Faculty)
Bedfordshire;
Consultant Emeritus
Milton Keynes General Hospital NHS Foundation Trust
   (Oxford Deanery)
Milton Keynes, UK

M. B. Bellad, MD, FICOG
Professor
Department of Obstetrics and Gynecology
Jawaharlal Nehru Medical College
Nehru Nagar
Belgaum, Karnataka, India

T. C. Bello-Munoz, MD
Servei de Obstetrícia i Ginecologia
Department of Obstetrics and Gynecology
Hospital Vall de Hebron de Barcelona
Universitat Autónoma de Barcelona
Barcelona, Spain

P. Beretta, MD
Fellow
Yale University School of Medicine
New Haven, CT, USA;
Monastery of San Peter and Paul
Buccinasco, Milan, Italy

S. Bewley, MA, MD, FRCOG
Professor of Complex Obstetrics, KCL
Honorary Clinical Director Obstetrics, NHS London
Division of Women's Health, KHL
Women's Health Academic Centre, Kings Health Partners
St Thomas' Hospital
London, UK

L. Bonsignore, MD
Obstetrician Gynecologist
Desio Hospital
Desio, Milan, Italy

M. Boucher, MD, FRCSC, DABOG(MFM)
Professor of Obstetrics and Gynecology
CHU Sainte-Justine and Faculty of Medicine
Université de Montréal
Montréal, Québec, Canada

F. Breathnach, MD, MRCOG, MRCPI, DCH,
   DipGUMed
Consultant Obstetrician Gynaecologist
Senior Lecturer Maternal Fetal Medicine
Royal College of Surgeons in Ireland
Rotunda Hospital
Dublin, Ireland

G. H. Breborowicz, MD, PhD
Director of Perinatology and Gynecology
University of Medical Sciences Poznän
Poznän, Poland

F. Burbank, MD, FSIR
Co-Founder and President
The Salt Creek International Women's Health Foundation
San Clemente, CA, USA

L. Cabero-Roura, MD, PhD, FRCOG
Servei de Obstetrícia i Ginecologia
Department of Obstetrics and Gynecology
Hospital Vall de Hebron de Barcelona
Universitat Autónoma de Barcelona
Barcelona, Spain

D. Cabrol, MD, PhD
Maternité Port-Royal
Hôpital Cochin-Saint-Vincent-de-Paul
Université Paris Descartes
Paris, France

M. J. Cameron, MD, MRCOG
Consultant Obstetrician, Subspecialist in Fetal Medicine
Norfolk and Norwich University Hospital
Norwich, Norfolk, UK

M. Campbell, MD, MSc
Obstetrics and Gynaecology Resident
Department of Obstetrics and Gynaecology
University of Toronto
Toronto, ON, Canada

W. B. Campbell, MS, FRCP, FRCS
Consultant Vascular Surgeon
Royal Devon and Exeter Hospital Peninsula Medical
    School
Exeter, UK

B. Carbonne, MD
Professor
Department of Obstetrics
Hopital Trousseau
Université Pierre et Marie Curie
Paris, France

J. C. A. Carvalho, MD, PhD, FANZCA, FRCPC
Professor of Anesthesia and Obstetrics and Gynecology,
    University of Toronto
Director of Obstetric Anesthesia
Mount Sinai Hospital
Toronto, ON, Canada

S. Catling, BA(Cantab), FRCA
Department of Anaesthesia and Intensive Care
Morriston and Singleton Hospitals
Abertawe Bro Morgannwg University Health Board
Swansea, Wales, UK

M. Chauhan, MBBS, FRCA
Consultant in Anaesthesia
Leicester Royal Infirmary
Leicester, UK

K. Choji, FRCR
Consultant in Interventional Radiology
Milton Keynes General Hospital NHS Foundation Trust
    (Oxford Deanery)
Milton Keynes, Bucks, UK

J. G. L. Cockings, MBBS, FRCA, FANZCA, FCICM,
    FFICM
Consultant Intensive Care Physician
Department of Intensive Care Medicine
Royal Berkshire NHS Foundation Trust
Reading, Berkshire, UK

A. Coker, MBBS, MRCOG
Consultant Obstetrician and Gynaecologist
Queen's Hospital
Romford, Essex, UK

D. Cordovani, MD
Obstetric Anesthesia Fellow
Mount Sinai Hospital
University of Toronto
Toronto, Ontario, Canada

R. Dabash, MPH
Director
Gynuity Health Projects
New York, NY, USA

K. J. Dalton, LLM, PhD, FRCOG, FCLM, DFMS
Department of Obstetrics and Gynaecology
University of Cambridge
Cambridge, UK

D. Danso, MBBS, MRCOG
Milton Keynes General Hospital NHS Foundation Trust
    (Oxford Deanery)
Milton Keynes, Bucks, UK

A. E. Dastur, MD, FICOG, FCPS, DGO, DFP,
    FICMU, ATMF(USA)
Honorary Professor Emeritus and Dean
Seth G S Medical College
and Nowrosjee Wadia Maternity Hospital
Mumbai, India

N. A. Dastur, MD, FICOG, DGO, DFP
Honorary Obstetrician and Gynaecologist
Grant Medical College
Seth G S Medical College
and Nowrosjee Wadia Maternity Hospital
Mumbai, India

S. De Carolis, MD
Research Fellow
Department of Obstetrics and Gynecology
Catholic University of the Sacred Heart
Rome, Italy

J. Dela Merced, MD
Attending Physician
White Memorial Medical Center
Los Angeles, CA, USA

R. J. Derman, MD, MPH, FACOG
Chair, Department of Obstetrics and Gynecology
Christiana Care Health Systems
Director, Center for Women's and Children's Health
    Research
Christiana Care Health Systems
Newark, DE;
Professor, Obstetrics and Gynecology
Thomas Jefferson University
Philadelphia, PA, USA

G. A. Dildy, III, MD
Professor of Obstetrics and Gynecology
Director of Obstetrics and Gynecology Quality and Patient
    Safety
Vice Chair of Clinical Affairs
Baylor College of Medicine
Houston, TX, USA

A. Duncan, MBBS, BSc, FRCS, FRCSE, FRCOG
Consultant Gynaecological Surgeon
Northampton General Hospital
Northampton, Northamptonshire, UK

I. Dzuba, MHS
Program Associate
Gynuity Health Projects
New York, NY, USA

G. S. Eglinton, MD
Associate Professor, Obstetrics and Gynecology
Weill Medical College of Cornell University
Chairman, Department of Obstetrics and Gynecology
New York Hospital Medical Center of Queens
Flushing, NY, USA

E. El Hamamy, MBChB, MSc, FRCOG, MRCPI
Consultant Obstetrician and Gynaecologist
Nevill Hall Hospital
Abergavenny, Monmouthshire, Wales, UK

H. El-Refaey, MD, MRCOG
Consultant and Honorary Senior Lecturer
Imperial College School of Medicine
Department of Academic Obstetrics and Gynaecology
Chelsea and Westminster Hospital
London, UK

J. B. Elterman, MD
Oregon Health and Science University
Portland, OR, USA

S. Engelbrecht, CNM, MPH, MSN
Consultant for International Medicine
Kenmore, WA, USA

E. Evans, FRCA
Consultant Anaesthetist
St George's Healthcare NHS Trust
London, UK

D. Farine, MD, FRCSC
Professor of Obstetrics and Gynaecology
Head of the Division of Maternal/Fetal Medicine
Mount Sinai Hospital, University of Toronto
Toronto, ON, Canada

M. M. F. Fathalla, MB, ChB(Hons), MD, MRCOG
Associate Professor of Obstetrics and Gynecology
Department of Obstetrics and Gynecology
Faculty of Medicine
Assiut University Women's Health Hospital
Assiut, Egypt

S. Ferrazzani, MD
Associate Professor of Medicine and Prenatal Age
Department of Obstetrics and Gynecology
Catholic University of the Sacred Heart
Ospedale Cristo Re
Rome, Italy

E. Ferrazzi
Professor and Chairman of Obstetrics and Gynecology
University of Milan
V. Buzzi Children Hospital
Milan, Italy

D. Fleming, MD, MRCOG
Consultant
Department of Obstetrics and Gynaecology
Kingston Hospitals NHS Turst
Kingston Upon Thames, UK

R. V. Ganchev, MBChB, MRCP
Associate Specialist in Haematology
Department of Clinical and Laboratory Haematology
Royal Infirmary of Edinburgh
Edinburgh, Scotland, UK

R. Gangopadhyay, MBBS, DFFP, MRCOG
Department of Obstetrics and Gynaecology
Barnet General Hospital
Barnet, London, UK

M. Geary, MD, FRCOG, FRCPI, DCH
Consultant Obstetrician Gynaecologist
Royal College of Surgeons in Ireland
Rotunda Hospital
Dublin, Ireland

S. E. Geller, PhD
G. William Arends Professor of Obstetrics and Gynecology
Director, Center for Research on Women and Gender
Director, National Center of Excellence in Women's
    Health
College of Medicine
University of Illinois, Chicago
Chicago, IL, USA

C. Georgiou, BSc, PhD, MBBS, MRCOG,
    FRANZCOG
Consultant Obstetrician and Gynaecologist (Wollongong
    Hospital)
Associate Professor Obstetrics and Gynaecology
Illawarra Health and Medical Research Institute;
Academic Lead in Obstetrics and Gynaecology
Graduate School of Medicine
University of Wollongong
Wollongong Hospital Academic Unit
Wollongong, NSW, Australia

F. Goffinet, MD, PhD
Maternité Port-Royal
Hôpital Cochin-Saint-Vincent-de-Paul
Université Paris Descartes
Paris, France

S. S. Goudar, MD, MHPE
Professor
Department of Physiology
J. N. Medical College
Belgaum, Karnataka, India

G. Grangé
Maternité Port-Royal
Hôpital Cochin-Saint-Vincent-de-Paul
Université Paris Descartes
Paris, France

D. Green, MD, PhD
Division of Hematology Oncology
Feinberg School of Medicine
Northwestern University
Chicago IL, USA

K. Groom, MBBS, BSc, PhD, FRANZCOG
Senior Lecturer
Department of Obstetrics and Gynaecology
University of Auckland
New Zealand

A. Hadar, MD
Department of Obstetrics and Gynecology
Faculty of Health Sciences
Ben Gurion University of the Negev
Soroka University Medical Center
Be'er-Sheva, Israel

K. Hayes, MRCOG
Consultant in Obstetrics and Gynaecology
St George's Hospital
London, UK

R. Hebballi, MD, FRCA, FCARCSI, FFICM
Consultant in Anaesthesia and Critical Care Medicine
Glenfield Hospital
University Hospitals of Leicester NHS Trust
Leicester, UK

A. Hemmerling, MD, PhD, MPH
Project Director
UCSF Bixby Center for Global Reproductive Health
Department of Obstetrics, Gynecology and Reproductive
    Sciences
San Francisco, CA, USA

C. E. Henderson, MPH
Bixby Center for Population, Health and Sustainability
School of Public Health
University of California, Berkeley
Berkeley, CA, USA

P. Hensleigh, MD, PhD (deceased)
Professor Emeritus
Department of Obstetrics and Gynecology
Stanford University
Stanford, CA, USA

T. Ikeda, MD, PhD
Director, Department of Perinatology and Gynecology
National Cerebral and Cardiovascular Center
Osaka, Japan

Y. Imaizumi, Dr of Science
Invited Professor, Department of Health Sciences
Graduate School of Medicine
Osaka University
Osaka, Japan

T. Z. Jacobson, MA, MBBS, FRCOG, FRANZCOG
Staff Specialist
Department of Obstetrics and Gynaecology
Mater Mother's Hospital
Brisbane, Queensland;
Senior Lecturer, University of Queensland, Australia

S. Kapoor, FRCA
Queen's Hospital
Romford, Essex, UK

C. Kapungu, PhD
Assistant Professor in Obstetrics and Gynecology
Center for Research on Women and Gender
University of Illinois at Chicago
Chicago, IL, USA

M. Karoshi, MD, MRCOG, DCRCM
Consultant Obstetrician and Gynaecologist
Department of Obstetrics and Gynaecology
Barnet and Chase Farm Hospitals NHS Trust
Barnet, London, UK

G. Kayem, MD
Service de Gynécologie-Obstétrique
CHI Créteil
Université Paris XII Henri Mondor
Paris, France

L. G. Keith, MD, PhD, ScD (Hon), FACOG, FRCOG
Professor Emeritus
Department of Obstetrics and Gynecology
Northwestern University
Former Head, Section of Undergraduate Education and
    Medical Student Affairs
Chicago, IL, USA

P. Kelehan, FRCPath
Consultant Histopathologist (Retired)
Department of Pathology and Laboratory Medicine
National Maternity Hospital
Dublin;
Pathology Assessor, Maternal Death Enquiry
Ireland

A. Kelkar, FRCS
Queen's Hospital
Romford, Essex, UK

R.-U. Khan, BSc, MBBS, MRCOG
Consultant in Obstetrics and Gynaecology
Barts Health NHS Trust;
Honorary Senior Lecturer in Obstetrics and Gynaecology
Queen Mary University of London
London, UK

A. Koch, MA
Center for Research on Women and Gender
University of Illinois at Chicago
Chicago, IL, USA

B. S. Kodkany, MD, DGO, FICS, FICOG
Professor, Department of Obstetrics and Gynaecology
KLE University's Jawaharlal Nehru Medical College
Belgaum, Kanataka;
Director, KLE University's Research Foundation
KLE University
Belgaum, Kanataka, India

J. C. Konje, MD, FMCOG(Nig), FRCOG
Professor, Reproductive Sciences Section
Department of Cancer Studies and Molecular Medicine
University of Leicester
Leicester Royal Infirmary
Leicester, UK

A. B. Lalonde, MD, FRCSC, FRCOG
Professor of Obstetrics and Gynaecology
University of Ottawa and McGill University
Ottawa, Canada

F. Lester, MD, MS, MPH
Health Sciences Clinical Instructor
Department of Obstetrics, Gynecology and Reproductive
    Sciences
Division of Gynecology, Global Women's Health
University of California, San Francisco, USA

J. Liljestrand, MD, PhD
Associate Professor
University Research Co
Cambodia

E. S. Linn, MD
Cook County Health and Hospital Systems Chair
Department of Obstetrics and Gynecology
John H. Stroger Jr Hospital of Cook County;
Associate Professor
Department of Obstetrics and Gynecology
Feinberg School of Medicine Northwestern University
Chicago, IL, USA

E. Lockhart, MD
Associate Medical Director
Duke University Medical Center Transfusion Service
Assistant Professor of Pathology
Duke University Medical Center
Durham, NC, USA

I. P. Lowenwirt, MD
Clinical Assistant Professor of Anesthesiology
Weill Medical College of Cornell University
Associate Chairman and Director of Obstetric
    Anesthesiology
New York Hospital Medical Center of Queens
Flushing, NY, USA

C. A. Ludlam, PhD, FRCP, FRCPath
Professor of Haematology and Coagulation Medicine
Director of Haemophilia and Thrombosis Centre
Royal Infirmary of Edinburgh
Edinburgh, Scotland, UK

S. Mahmoud, MBChB, MSc
Specialist Registrar
Royal Gwent Hospital
Newport, Wales, UK

R. Majumder, MBBS, MS
Senior Registrar
Bhatia Hospital
Mumbai, India

R. Malapati, MD
Associate Residency Program Director Medical
    Co-Director of Obstetrics
Department of Obstetrics and Gynecology
John H Stroger Jr Hospital of Cook County;
Assistant Professor
Feinberg School of Medicine
Northwestern University
Chicago, IL, USA

M. K. Mehasseb, MD, PhD, MRCOG
Department of Obstetrics and Gynaecology
The Rosie Hospital
Addenbrooke's Hospital
Cambridge, UK

S. Miller, CNM, PhD
Associate Professor
Director, Safe Motherhood Programs
Department of Obstetrics, Gynecology and Reproductive
    Sciences
Bixby Center for Global Reproductive Health and Policy
Center of Expertise, Women's Health and Empowerment
Global Health Institute
University of California, San Francisco (UCSF)
San Francisco, CA, USA

E. E. Mooney, FRCPath
Consultant Histopathologist
Department of Pathology and Laboratory Medicine
National Maternity Hospital
Dublin, Ireland

J. L. Morris, MA
Project Specialist, Safe Motherhood Programs
University of California, San Francisco
San Francisco, CA, USA

M. Mourad-Youssif, MD, MRCOG
Consultant Obstetrician and Gynecologist
El-Galaa Maternity Teaching Hospital
Cairo, Egypt

I. Neuman, MPH
Senior Program Development and Implementation
    Manager
Laerdal Global Health AS
Tanke Svilands
Stavanger, Norway

D. S. Newman, ACP, FCollP, FRGS, ALPI
Chairman
South and West Wales Hospital Liaison Committee for
    Jehovah's Witnesses
Cardiff, UK

M. P. O'Connell, MD, FRCOG, FRCPI, MSc, DCH
Coombe Women and Infants University Hospital
Dublin, Ireland

I. Ohel, MD
Department of Obstetrics and Gynecology
Faculty of Health Sciences
Ben Gurion University of the Negev
Soroka University Medical Center
Beer-Sheva, Israel

O. Ojengbede, BSc(Hons), FMCOG, FWACS, FICS
Professor and Director
Centre for Population and Reproductive Health
College of Medicine
University College Hospital
Ibadan, Nigeria

P. Okong, MMed, PhD
Department of Obstetrics and Gynecology
St Francis Hospital Nsambya
Uganda

R. Oliver, MBBS, MRCOG
Queen's Hospital
Romford, Essex, UK

O. Onwuemene, MD
Division of Hematology Oncology
Feinberg School of Medicine
Northwestern University
Chicago, IL, USA

C. Otigbah, MRCOG
Queen's Hospital
Romford, Essex, UK

M. J. Paidas, MD, FACOG
Professor
Co-Director, Yale Women and Children's Center for
    Blood Disorders
Co- Director, National Hemophilia Foundation- Baxter
    Clinical Fellowship Program at Yale
Division of Maternal Fetal Medicine
Department of Obstetrics, Gynecology and Reproductive
    Sciences
Yale University School of Medicine
New Haven, CT, USA

V. P. Paily, MD, MRCOG, FRCOG
Consultant
Mother Hospital and Raji Nursing Home
Thrissur, Kerala, India

J. M. Palacios-Jaraquemada, MD, PhD
Professor, School of Medicine
University of Buenos Aires
Buenos Aires, Argentina

A. Pankhania, MRCS, FRCR
Queen's Hospital
Romford, Essex, UK

A. Patel, MD, MPH
System Director of Family Planning Services
Division of Family Planning
Department of Obstetrics and Gynecology
John H. Stroger Jr Hospital of Cook County;
Associate Professor
Feinberg School of Medicine, Northwestern University;
Senior Medical Director of Research
Planned Parenthood Federation of America
Chicago, IL, USA

S. Paterson-Brown, FRCS, FRCOG
Consultant Obstetrician and Gynaecologist
Queen Charlotte's Hospital
London, UK

P. Patrizio, MD, MBE
Professor, Department of Obstetrics, Gynecology and
    Reproductive Sciences
Director, Yale Fertility Center
Clinical Practice Director, Yale Fertility Center
Yale University School of Medicine
New Haven, CT, USA

A. Perrelli, MD
Consultant
Department of Obstetrics and Gynecology
Catholic University of the Sacred Heart
Rome, Italy

C. Piscicelli, MD
Medical Assistant
Department of Obstetrics and Gynecology
Ospedale Cristo Re
Rome, Italy

M. Potts, MB, BChir, PhD, FRCOG
Bixby Center for Population, Health and Sustainability
School of Public Health
University of California, Berkeley
Berkeley, CA, USA

N. Prata, MD, MSc
Associate Professor in Residence
Scientific Director, Bixby Center for Population Health
    and Sustainability
School of Public Health, University of California, Berkeley
Berkeley, CA, USA

S. Ricci, PhD
Researcher
Department of Electronics and Telecommunications
University of Florence
Florence, Italy

G. M. Riha, MD
Department of Surgery
Oregon Health and Science University
Portland, OR, USA

P. W. Reginald, MD (London), FRCOG
Heatherwood and Wexham Park NHS Trust
Slough, Berkshire, UK

A. B. Roston, BA
Division on Family Planning
Department of Department of Obstetrics and Gynecology
John H. Stroger, Jr Hospital of Cook County
Chicago, IL, USA

A. L. Roston, MPH
Division on Family Planning
Department of Department of Obstetrics and Gynecology
John H. Stroger, Jr Hospital of Cook County
Chicago, IL, USA

R. Rushwan, MD, FRCOG, FACOG
Chief Executive
International Federation of Gynecology and Obstetrics
London, UK

J. N. Rutherford, PhD
University of Illinois at Chicago
Departments of Oral Biology and Anthropology
Chicago, IL, USA

T. Schmitz, MD
Maternité Port-Royal
Hôpital Cochin-Saint-Vincent-de-Paul
Université Paris Descartes
Paris, France

M. A. Schreiber, MD
Department of Surgery
Oregon Health and Science University
Portland, OR, USA

L. Sentilhes, MD, PhD
Service de Gynécologie-Obstétrique
Centre Hospitalier Universitaire d'Angers
France

M. E. Setchell, CVO, MA, MB, BChir (Cantab),
    FRCSEng, FRCOG
Surgeon-Gynaecologist to HM The Queen
Hon. Consultant Obstetrician and Gynaecologist
St Bartholomew's, Homerton, and Whittington Hospitals
London, UK

H. D. Shah, MBBS (Hons), MA (Cantab)
Department of Obstetrics and Gynaecology
Newham University Hospital
Barts Health NHS Trust
London, UK

E. Sheiner, MD, PhD
Department of Obstetrics and Gynecology
Faculty of Health Sciences
Ben Gurion University of the Negev
Soroka University Medical Center
Beer-Sheva, Israel

T. Shimizu
Department of Radiology
Hokkaido University Hospital
Sapporo, Japan

D. W. Skupski, MD
Professor, Obstetrics and Gynecology
Weill Medical College of Cornell University
Associate Chairman and Director of Maternal Fetal
    Medicine
Department of Obstetrics and Gynecology
New York Hospital Medical Center of Queens
Flushing, NY, USA

N. L. Sloan, DrPH
Senior Clinical Researcher
Center for Women's and Children's Health Research
Christiana Care Health Systems
Newark, DE;
Assistant Professor
Department of Population and Family Health
Mailman School of Public Health, Columbia University
New York, NY, USA

H. Snelgrove, MA, MedED, BA(Hon), Dip Ed
St George's Healthcare NHS Trust
Education and Development Department
London, UK

S. Sobieszczyk, MD, PhD
Internal Medicine Consultant
Consultant in Anesthesiology and Intensive Care
Laboratory Director Cardiovascular and Hemostatic
    Disorders
Department of Perinatology and Gynecology
University of School of Medicine
Poznän, Poland

A. L. Stenson, MD, MPH
David Geffen School of Medicine
Department of Obstetrics and Gynecology
Center for the Health Sciences
Los Angeles, CA, USA

P. D. Tank, MD, DNBE, FCPS, DGO, DFP, MNAMS,
    MRCOG
Honorary Clinical Associate
Seth G S Medical College;
Nowrosjee Wadia Maternity Hospital
Mumbai, India

D. Thomas, MBChB, FRCA
Department of Anaesthesia and Intensive Care Medicine
Morriston and Singleton Hospitals
Abertawe Bro Morgannwg University Health Board
Swansea, Wales, UK

M. O. Thompson, MRCOG, FWACS
Queen's Hospital
Romford, Essex, UK

M. K. Tipples, MRCOG, FRCSEd
Western Sussex Hospital Trust
Chichester, West Sussex, UK

P. Tortoli, PhD
Professor
Department of Electronics and Telecommunications
University of Florence
Florence, Italy

V. Tsatsaris, MD, PhD
Maternité Port-Royal
Hôpital Cochin-Saint-Vincent-de-Paul
Université Paris Descartes
Paris, France

J. Unterscheider, MRCPI, MRCOG
Specialist Registrar in Obstetrics and Gynaecology
Royal College of Surgeons in Ireland
Rotunda Hospital
Dublin, Ireland

G. Urban, MD, PhD
Post-Doctoral Fellow
Yale University School of Medicine
New Haven, CT, USA;
Desio Hospital
Desio, Milan, Italy

A. Vais, MRCOG
Clinical Fellow in Maternal Medicine
St Thomas' Hospital
London, UK

H. Valensise
Associate Professor
University of Rome Tor Vergata
Rome, Italy

P. Vergani, MD
Associate Professor
Department of Obstetrics and Gynecology
University of Milan-Bicocca
San Gerardo Hospital
Monza, Italy

A. Virkud, MD, DGO, FCPS, FICOG
37B Shalan Building
Mumbai, India

C. von Widekind, MD, MRCOG
Consultant Obstetrician and Gynaecologist
Northampton General Hospital
Northampton, Northants, UK

C. S. Waldmann, MA, MB, BChir, FRCA, FFICM,
    EDIC
Consultant Intensive Care Physician
Department of Intensive Care Medicine
Royal Berkshire NHS Foundation Trust
Reading, Berkshire, UK

V. Walvekar, MD, DGO, FCPS, FICOG
62 Suraiya Apartments
Worli
Mumbai, India

A. Ward, RM, RN
Head of Midwifery
Supervisor of Midwives
Mid Yorkshire NHS Trust
Pinderfields Hospital
Wakefield, UK

B. Winikoff, MD, MPH
President
Gynuity Health Projects
New York, NY, USA

C. Wohlmuth, MD
Residency Program Director
Department of Obstetrics and Gynecology
White Memorial Medical Center
Los Angeles, CA, USA

FOREWORD: a FIGO Perspective

The second edition of *A Comprehensive Textbook of Postpartum Hemorrhage* will be launched during the International Federation of Gynecology and Obstetrics (FIGO) World Congress in Rome, Italy in October 2012. For FIGO, this marks another important step in the battle to improve maternal health and to decrease maternal mortality.

The international efforts spearheaded by FIGO and UN agencies to reduce maternal mortality have shown positive results in recent years. Studies in 2010, 2011 and 2012 have reported important decreases in maternal mortality worldwide. However, as these estimates are based on mathematical models and many countries still have poor programs related to vital statistics, these reductions must be appraised cautiously.

In spite of the uncertainty regarding exact numbers, no controversy exists about the need for prevention and treatment of postpartum hemorrhage (PPH). Although recent evidence suggests there is a decline in maternal mortality worldwide, a simultaneous increase in the proportion of maternal deaths due to PPH in Latin America, Africa and South East Asia has been noted. Whereas many countries have made progress, others have stagnated, and a few actually show an increase in maternal mortality. In some countries, maternal mortality is the cause of over 50% of maternal deaths, with Guatemala and Afghanistan serving as prime examples.

The original chapters in this book continue to address issues of vital statistic definitions, accurate measurements of blood loss, hospital management and use of new medications to stem the tremendous burden of PPH. In the revised and new chapters, discussion on the increase in incidence of PPH and maternal mortality due to placenta previa and placenta accreta, most probably due to the higher numbers of cesarean sections in the past 5–10 years worldwide is presented.

The balloon internal uterine tamponade, both as a diagnostic test and as a treatment, is expanded in a number of chapters. Because it would be difficult if not unethical to conduct a randomized control trial on tamponade use or many other therapies for PPH,

clinical practice and a registry would go a long way towards establishing this as a true advance in the treatment of severe PPH.

The update on the Prevention of PPH Initiative (POPPHI) project has shown the positive impact of active management of the third stage of labor, so much so that both FIGO and WHO now recommend this as a routine for all women birthing throughout the world. Further presentations are provided on the use of misoprostol for either prevention or treatment in the absence of other available uterotonic medications. Coagulation disorders are discussed, as well as the use of recombinant factor VIIa and the use of carbetocin for the prevention of PPH at cesarean section.

Many chapters discuss the importance of timing in the diagnosis and early treatment of PPH from the community to the referral level. Examples include discussion on misoprostol use by traditional birth attendants under supervision of a trained birth attendant and the non-pneumatic anti-shock garment (NASG). This technique appears to be lifesaving and it continues to be utilized and clinically evaluated throughout the world where women are suffering massive PPH, are in shock and where immediate treatment is not available.

In several chapters the relatively recent recognition that the ratio of fibrinogen : red blood cells : plasma and the timing of their administration has an important effect on enhancing survival is discussed. This information, obtained from military and trauma surgical registers, will be new to many readers, as will the need to use protocols when massive blood transfusion is being administered.

FIGO began its PPH prevention and treatment campaign in 2003. We have made significant progress, but are still faced with serious challenges in order for health care professionals to be trained under one system with available medications at all times and with a system of referral from the community to the first referral hospital. It is not only important to have training programs in place, but also the implementation of training is now the challenge facing health care professionals and birth attendants throughout the world. Countries which have been successful are those countries with a system in place that ensures that medication is available at all times in all birthing units.

PPH continues to threaten women's lives in low and high resource countries and is the most important cause of maternal mortality in low resource countries. The majority of cases of PPH are due to uterine atony where the treatment is well known but needs to be institutionalized all over the world. It is not well understood that in high-risk situations we can reduce risk significantly by having a continuous training evaluation of near misses and maternal deaths and by using simple low-cost technology such as tamponade or the NASG garment.

FIGO and International Confederation of Midwives (ICM) have supported the training and implementation of active management of the third stage of labor. Now is the time for all countries to embrace the FIGO and WHO guidelines on PPH and make these guidelines available in all of the birthing units in our respective countries. We have proposed wall charts for all birthing units in the PPH guideline chapter. Until we systematically address this issue, PPH will continue to be a death threat to many women in the world.

In closing, we would like to thank Mr David Bloomer and his wife Paula who, as publishers of this volume and *The Global Library of Women's Medicine* (GLOWM), provide unconditional support to make this book available throughout the world in many languages.

Gamal Serour, MD, MCROG, FRCS, FRCOG
President, International Federation of Gynecology and Obstetrics (FIGO)
(2009–2012)

André B. Lalonde, MD, FRCSC, FRCOG
Chair, FIGO Safe Motherhood and Newborn Health Committee, 2006–2012

Editors' Preface

The first edition of *A Textbook of Postpartum Hemorrhage* was launched with fanfare on October 11, 2006 by HRH the Princess Royal at Chandos House, The Royal Society of Medicine, London. The four editors and Mr David Bloomer, the book's publisher who, along with his wife Paula supported its publication, could not have anticipated its enthusiastic reception by the medical profession throughout the world. In all, more than 15,000 copies of this volume were distributed free of charge to doctors practicing obstetrics and gynecology in the most diverse locations and under the most varied circumstances. In addition, the book was widely accessed, and individual chapters downloaded, via the website of *The Global Library of Women's Medicine* (www.glowm.com). Of equal importance, when the editors embarked on a series of postgraduate courses in the UK, Egypt, Ukraine, India, Malaysia and China, among others, practitioners invariably voiced their thankfulness for having the book in their hands, noting over and over how their use of it has saved a patient's life.

Of course, it had been our hope and fervent desire that the efforts that we made to prepare the first edition would do just that, i.e. save women's lives and reduce the scandalous loss of maternal life due to postpartum hemorrhage (PPH). In this regard, we were more than compensated for our efforts, but it soon became obvious that a second edition was necessary. Many things had changed since 2005 when we began planning the first edition, not least of which was an important re-evaluation of the most useful methodology to provide massive transfusion and a far clearer understanding of the uterine anatomy as it pertains to the blood vessels of that organ. This latter subject was under-represented in the first edition, and the former was unknown at the time of its writing.

As was the case in the first edition, the complete book is universally available entirely free on the website of *The Global Library of Women's Medicine*. Once again, neither authors nor editors have received compensation for their time and contribution. Many of the original chapters have been revised and updated, whilst new chapters cover a range of additional topics including the uterine anatomy, the recent changes in transfusion practices, difficulties presented by adherent placentas, intrauterine balloon therapy and the active management of the third stage of labor. Where appropriate, links to video clips are provided.

The editors wish to thank Professor Sir Subaratnam Arulkumaran for joining the editorial team in the position of Senior Editor and for his many insights into the global perspectives of PPH at a time when he is about to become President Elect of FIGO. They also wish to thank Professor Louis Keith for his careful editorial expertise in reviewing each chapter at both the manuscript and the page proof stages. Thanks also are extended to Dorothy Walmsley who served as desk editor for the publication and to Julia Tissington who acted as project manager. Finally, but by no means last in terms of the importance of their contributions, immense gratitude is due to Paula and David Bloomer, founders of *The Global Library of Women's Medicine* (and also of Sapiens Publishing). As was the case with the first edition, this book is produced in grateful and loving memory of their daughter, Abigail Bloomer, who sadly died at the early age of 31 from that other scourge of women, breast cancer, in December 2001.

Sir Sabaratnam Arulkumaran, MD, PhD, FRCS, FRCOG
St George's, University of London, UK

Mahantesh Karoshi, MD, MRCOG, DCRCM
Barnet and Chase Farm Hospitals NHS Trust, Barnet, London, UK

Louis G. Keith, MD, PhD, FACOG, FRCOG
Northwestern University, Chicago, USA

André B. Lalonde, MD, FRCSC, FRCOG
University of Ottawa and McGill University, Ottawa, Canada

Christopher B-Lynch, FRCS, FRCOG, D Univ
Milton Keynes General Hospital NHS Foundation Trust (Oxford Deanery), UK

Section 1

Essential 'Must Read' Chapters

1

Managing the Ten Most Common Life-Threatening Scenarios Associated with Postpartum Hemorrhage

M. Karoshi, J. M. Palacios-Jaraquemada and L. G. Keith

INTRODUCTION

Treatment of postpartum hemorrhage (PPH) is never simple, and many paradigms have been presented for consideration over the past several years. Most advocate straightforward approaches directed toward a specific cause of PPH. Rarely have authors put forward a series of treatment plans in the same document that describe treatment related to a variety of causes. The impetus to prepare this chapter derives from a thorough review of published data relating to specific deaths from PPH as described in the Confidential Enquires of the UK[1], Australia[2] and Canada[3]. American data[4], in contrast, are mostly descriptive and contain statistical elements relating to maternal deaths without individual case analyses.

The recurring theme of these reports is quite simple: TOO LITTLE, TOO LATE. Because PPH is episodic in nature and almost always unexpected, birth attendants are not prepared to deal with it on a regular and recurring basis. This is especially true if the PPH appears at night, on weekends, or on holidays, or if the care provider is alone in the delivery unit at the time of its occurrence and is unwilling or unable to seek competent help in a timely manner or if such help is unavailable. Figure 1 (also shown in Chapter 20 by Gangopadhyay *et al.*) shows a 25-year analysis of deaths in the UK reports in which 60–70% of patients received what was described as substandard care.

After analysis of existing reports, we selected ten common PPH scenarios which might be seen by an average obstetrician in his or her practice. All invariably commence as simple challenges which, when appropriate actions are not taken in a timely manner, may lead to serious morbidity and eventually death.

The late Steve Jobs, founder of Apple Computers, was fond of saying that it was extremely difficult to make complex things simple, whereas it was easy to make simple things complex. This statement applies directly to the therapy of PPH because, as the ten scenarios show, the causes of the PPH vary from simple to complex at their onset, and even simple cases become complex with a very short passage of time. This latter thought was described in various terms by authors in the first edition of this text, but no author made the point illustrated in the following box.

> The passage of time is likely to increase the complexity of any given case because continuous bleeding, not appropriately and adequately controlled on a timely basis, invariably leads to coagulopathy.

Once coagulopathy sets in, the simplest case takes a different path, as the need to treat coagulopathy complicates any other planned interventions. Thus, one hears of cases in which compression sutures, embolizations, the use of factor VIIa or even hysterectomies failed to control PPH. When these cases are analysed retrospectively, however, it becomes clear that the practitioners failed to realize they were attempting to correct bleeding from coagulopathy which had not been recognized or even considered.

Seven of the ten scenarios are preceded by an algorithm, and study of these algorithms in conjunction with the proposed therapy reinforces the need to progress from one step to the next in a logical manner. These algorithms have been prepared in such a manner that the reader understands therapy not only progresses logically, but also does so with one eye on the clock. Stated another way, if medical therapy using three or four uterotonic agents has not worked within 1 hour, there is no logical reason to think that it will work in the next hour. Similarly, if compression sutures are delayed until the onset of coagulopathy,

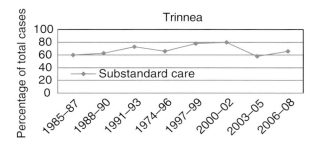

Figure 1 Trends in substandard care (see Chapter 20)

there is no reason to think that they will work unless the coagulopathy has been treated.

It is our earnest hope that this chapter will provide the practitioner with the realization that one specific therapy cannot possibly work for all causes of PPH and that different therapeutic pathways must be chosen depending upon the inherent cause of bleeding. To this end, this chapter makes full use of web links, video clips, illustrations and hyperlinks to other supporting materials, these can be accessed through *The Global Library of Women's Medicine* at www.glowm.com.

SCENARIO 1 – VAGINAL DELIVERY AND PPH

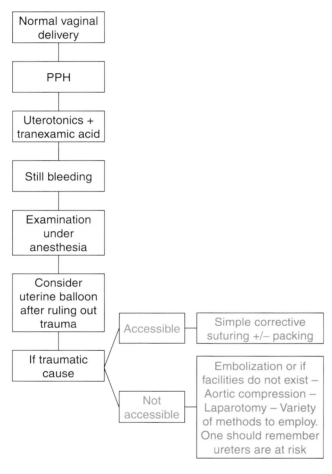

Scenario 1 – Vaginal delivery and PPH

The key to appropriate initiation of therapy in this scenario is to immediately recognize when the patient has lost more than 500 ml of blood or when the hemorrhage has begun to compromise vital signs, as might occur in a woman who entered labor with a hemoglobin of less than 7 g/dl and subsequently loses a mere 200 ml of blood.

At the same time, it is important to recognize that if the woman in the algorithm has had a labor lasting 24 hours or more, her blood loss may be from at least two additional causes besides atony, as both genital tract trauma and associated postlabor dehydration may accentuate the severity and rapid deterioration of clinical parameters.

Because uterine atony is the most logical cause of bleeding in such cases, the use of uterotonic agents represents an appropriate initial therapeutic pathway. Discussions as to which specific uterotonic agent to administer and how to do it are found in other chapters of this book (Section 8). In general oxytocin, Syntocinon®, methergin, prostaglandins and carbetocin are used with similar degrees of success in settings that can provide proper storage of these agents. In contrast oral, vaginal and rectal doses of misoprostol are particularly valuable in areas of the world where standard oxytocics are not available (see Section 6).

The use of tranexamic acid is well characterized in the trauma literature, but not well described in the obstetric literature, although anecdotal reports of its widespread use and success in the treatment of PPH abound. In addition, it is commonly used by cardiothoracic and hepatobiliary surgeons to control bleeding. It does so by stabilizing the clot.

If bleeding continues or even accelerates during the process of medical therapy, it is prudent to conduct a thorough examination of the vaginal walls and vault as well as to examine the cervix for tears whilst using some form of anesthetic. In order to perform such an examination, it is necessary to have at least one assistant, suitable equipment and a light source that illuminates the vaginal vault. Whilst this is taking place, a team member should examine or re-examine the placenta for the missing cotyledons.

Assuming that no obvious vaginal or cervical trauma is recognized and the bleeding continues, any one of the available uterine balloons should be used (for details see Chapters 46–48 and 54).

If vaginal trauma is found to be the principal cause of the bleeding, practitioners may be confronted with one of three different circumstances. In the first, there may be one or two tears of the vagina which are amenable to simple corrective suturing. If, on the other hand, tears are of an explosive nature, i.e. multiple small tears not amenable to individual suturing, or if sutures pull through the edematous tissue thereby causing more bleeding, it is reasonable to inflate a balloon which compresses the entire vaginal wall throughout its circumference. If no balloons are available, packing the vagina with antiseptic impregnated gauge can also be of value. The third variation is the most serious. It is the deep vaginal tear that extends into the abdominal cavity causing either a retroperitoneal hematoma(s) or compromising the urinary tract. An illustration of this variation is found in the Chapter 23 by B-Lynch. It is important to remember that a simple suture of the vaginal wall over what looks to be a deep tear in the posterior or lateral wall may include the rectum, bladder and/or ureter, even though ureteric injury with a tear is most unlikely.

Adequate exposure may be needed and can be achieved by performing an episiotomy (if not present already or if it is too small can be extended) and using a Dever's retractor for the posterior vaginal wall and a Langden or vaginal retractor for the anterolateral vaginal wall. Long Aliss tissue forceps are useful to apply to the vaginal wall near the apex of the tear. It is adequate and better to suture each side of the vaginal wall separately without trying to approximate adjacent walls of the tear to avoid obliterating the view higher up and also causing tension tears of the vagina. The gap left behind will epithelialize rapidly in a few weeks. A suture position as high as possible should be used as a stay suture and traction applied to the suture higher up to arrest bleeding. The consecutive sutures can be held together as stay sutures to prevent tearing of the vaginal wall. Usually bleeding is from an artery that had retracted under the vaginal wall and hence the suture needs to be higher than and lateral to the apex of the tear. Treatment of this variation may involve a combined vaginal–abdominal approach on either side of the trauma (see Chapter 24).

If concerns exist about ureteric injury, immediate cystoscopy can confirm the presence of urinary efflux on both sides of the bladder demonstrating the integrity of the ureters. If cystoscopy cannot be accomplished immediately, an intravenous pyelogram (IVP) can be performed the next day.

In some circumstances, especially those cases being conducted in tertiary centers with full facilities, it may be prudent to correct the coagulopathy and institute embolization before embarking on laparotomy (see Chapters 49 and 50). In other circumstances it is necessary to consider transfer of the bleeding patient to a specialist center with capability for arterial embolization. Two cautionary points are important. First, it is inappropriate to transfer a patient in shock, because the condition will only deteriorate during the transfer process and waiting for the procedure. Second, patients in shock and with coagulopathy are not suitable candidates for embolization. Under such circumstances, the vascular system is in a state of constriction which impedes blood flow in the bleeding vessels. The actual average procedure time for a fully trained interventional radiologist is 1 hour. This does not include transfer and preparation time. One should not forget that fluids and hemostatic support must be provided during the transfer and procedure. Further discussion is found in Chapter 49, in addition, Chapters 38 and 39 describes the use of non-pneumatic antishock garment (NASG) which redistributes blood from the lower extremities to the central circulatory system of the major organs (heart, kidneys, brain).

SCENARIO 2 – INSTRUMENTAL DELIVERY AND PPH

Scenario 2A – ventouse delivery and PPH

When bleeding begins after a ventouse delivery, it is important to distinguish whether it is from a vaginal laceration(s) *per se* or a combination of uterine atony plus vaginal laceration(s). If uterine atony is present, blood will be coming from the cervix in addition to any bleeding that flows from the vaginal walls secondary to trauma. Treatment of the atonic bleeding should follow directions given in Scenario number 1

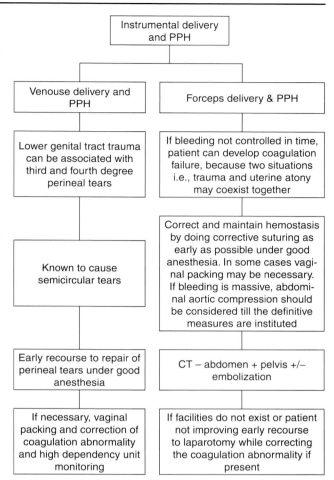

Scenario 2 – Instrumental delivery and PPH

as well as information provided in chapters in Section 8.

Ventouse related lacerations often are circular in nature because of the physical nature of the instrument used. The lacerations are caused by the inadvertent incorporation of vaginal tissue into the ventouse when it slips. Unlike traumatic lacerations which normally take a linear form, these lacerations may actually represent an area of missing vaginal tissue which has been denuded. Because of the friable nature of the vaginal walls, packing is generally advocated using long cotton gauze previously moistened with saline or antiseptic solution. This can remain in place for 24 hours when it can be gently removed. More recently, a specially devised vaginal balloon has been used successfully in these cases (see Chapter 54). Both methodologies provide pressure against the bleeding surfaces.

Rectal and bladder injuries are rare but may occur with instrumental vaginal deliveries (Figure 2). Hence it is important to determine that neither the bladder nor the rectum has been injured after each ventouse delivery. Non-recognition of a bladder or rectal laceration will result in fistula formation and is often followed by litigation issues. Effective anesthesia is paramount for repair efforts. In such cases transfusion may or may not be indicated depending upon the extent of the blood loss and deterioration of vital signs.

Scenario 2B – forceps delivery and PPH

Bleeding after a vaginal delivery with forceps can be complicated by factors that occur prior to delivery. If the woman has had a prolonged labor with or without a prolonged second stage, the likelihood of the coexistence of different causes of PPH is high. For example, such a woman is likely to be dehydrated, uterine atony is more likely to be present, and genital tract trauma may be so severe that its repair by an inexperienced operator would be prolonged, and ineffective in controlling blood loss.

The bleeding from uterine atony appropriately has been described as S1 segment bleeding (Figure 3), a term which is related to the fact that it comes from the upper part of the uterus which is supplied mainly by the ascending branch of the uterine artery (90%) and secondarily by the ovarian artery (10%)[5]. At the same time, bleeding from cervical lacerations or the superior aspect of the vaginal vault is characterized as S2 segment bleeding. Such bleeding mainly derives from two vessels: first, the descending branch of the uterine artery; and second, the vaginal artery which usually arises from the posterior division of internal iliac artery (see Chapter 1).

In such instances, if the patient is taken for an embolization procedure, it is important that the radiologist realize that the vaginal artery is not a branch of the anterior division of the internal iliac artery and that the embolization catheter must enter the posterior internal iliac branch. If the radiologist embolizes the posterior division of the internal iliac to control lower vaginal bleeding, the patient is at risk of having a non-target embolization of the inferior gluteal vessel which supplies the sciatic nerve.

In order to avoid this problem, the bilateral insertion of a balloon into the common iliac arteries is required to provide time (90 min) (Jose Palacios Jaraquemada – personal communication, 31 October 2011) for the surgeon to reach the bleeding field with appropriate instruments or the interventional radiologist to attempt embolization a second time (Figure 4).

The nature and extent of vaginal lacerations cannot be properly assessed in the absence of good light and proper assistance with long retractors. Vaginal lacerations may be simple linear tears or explosive in nature. In addition, they may extend deeply into one or both fornices.

If good assistance is not obtained rapidly and the multiple causes of bleeding are not addressed promptly and adequately, the patient's chance of developing acute coagulation failure and its resultant co-morbidities is extremely high.

Depending upon the extent and quantity of the blood loss, external (and sometimes internal) aortic compression (Videos 1 and 2) may be of great use to gain extra time when the patient is being assessed for the extent of her injuries and early resuscitative measures are being applied. It goes without saying that volume replacement and correction of anemia, acidosis and prevention of hypothermia

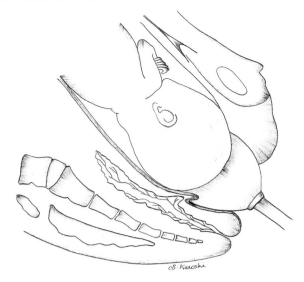

Figure 2 Schematic diagram showing incorrect application of ventouse cup in occiput-posterior position which potentially may cause fourth degree tear causing rectovaginal fistula

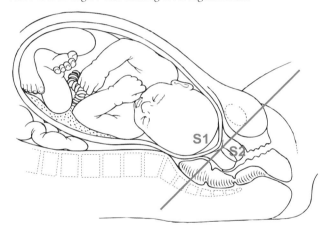

Figure 3 Segment S1 and S2 bleeding: S1, the upper part of the uterus which is supplied mainly by the ascending branch of the uterine artery (90%) and secondarily by the ovarian artery (10%) and S2 the lower part of the uterus supplied by the descending branch of the uterine artery and the vaginal artery. Courtesy of Palacios-Jaraquemada

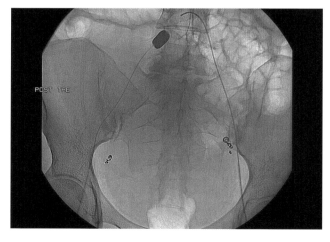

Figure 4 Interventional radiology X-ray image of common iliac balloon. Courtesy of Dr Shih, Jin-Chung, Department of Obstetrics and Gynecology, National Taiwan University Hospital and National Taiwan University College of Medicine, Taipei, Taiwan

must take place while these other interventions are being carried out. In addition, it must be remembered that the continuation of bleeding will precede the onset of coagulopathy. A full discussion of the recent changes in the ratios of fibrinogen to red cells in various transfusion protocols is provided in Chapters 3, 4 and 6.

The present scenario illustrates the concept that PPH cannot be considered solely a uterine problem. Rather, PPH is a condition which affects the entire system and has the potential to have adverse consequences on multiple organs if not treated properly and in a timely manner.

The tendency to perform hysterectomy often is seen in situations such as the one described above. What the practitioner may not realize is that hysterectomy is designed to treat bleeding from the uterine fundus (S1 area) and will not effectively treat bleeding from the lower uterine segment/cervix, parametrium and upper vagina (S2 area), because the bleeding pedicles are different. In fact, performing hysterectomy in such instances may worsen the overall condition of the patient. Moreover, performing hysterectomy will deplete at least 1.5 liters of blood from the already compromised patient's circulation.

SCENARIO 3 – PPH IN THE RECOVERY AREA FOLLOWING ELECTIVE CESAREAN DELIERY

A cesarean section is always major surgery. Therefore, it can cause complications like any other major surgery. PPH following elective cesarean is not an uncommon event. Close vigilance, appropriate monitoring (modified early warning score (MEWS) chart) and seeking help at the appropriate time will avert further serious complications and death.

Patient deterioration can be secondary to revealed PPH or concealed PPH. Concealed PPH is more dangerous than the revealed. Common reasons for the patient to suffer PPH following elective cesarean are atonic uterus, retained fragments of placenta, bleeding uterine angle and rectus sheath hematoma. Detailed examination including checking for vitals signs and

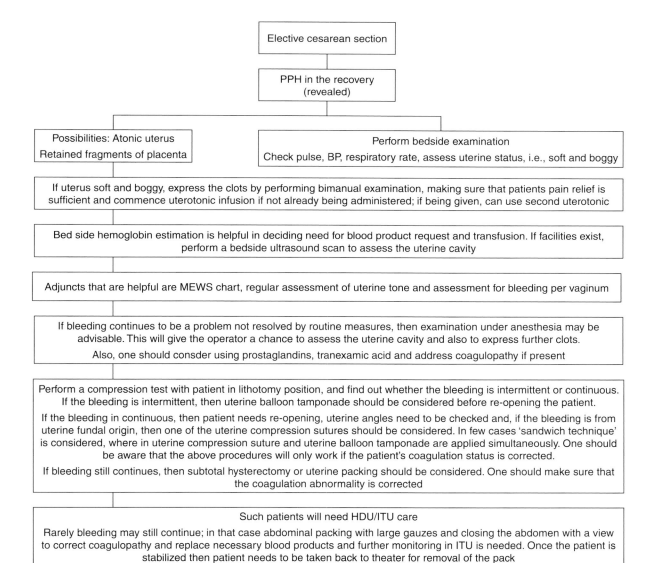

Scenario 3 – PPH in the recovery area following elective cesarean delivery

abdominal and bimanual examination by an experienced professional will usually yield clues as to the origin of the bleeding. If the bleeding is of uterine origin, the uterus is usually soft and markedly enlarged.

If uterine atony is the cause of the PPH, the uterus will be filled with clots, and the patient requires examination under anesthesia, preferably in an operating theater. Clots must be expressed from the uterine cavity and uterine tone sustained or increased by use of an additional uterotonic, assuming that one is already in use.

If bleeding still continues to be a problem and is not relieved by the above measures, then examination under anesthesia should be considered in order to allow assessment of the uterine cavity, expression of further clots and, if necessary, insertion of a uterine balloon tamponade (see Scenario 1).

A uterine compression test should be performed. If bleeding is intermittent, the balloon tamponade should work (see Chapters 45, 47 and 48). If bleeding is continuous, however, the patient will require re-opening. Uterine compression sutures/sandwich technique will only work if there is no coagulopathy.

If bleeding is still not under control, then there should be no hesitation to recourse to subtotal hysterectomy. Following any of the above procedures such patients will need care in a high dependency unit (HDU) or intensive care unit (ITU).

Rarely bleeding may continue from the cervical stump (in the case of subtotal hysterectomy) (see Chapter 55) and, in that case, local sealants may be used if available. In difficult cases abdominal/pelvic packing with larger gauzes and closing the abdomen with a view to correcting the coagulopathy and replacing the necessary blood products, and further monitoring in ITU will be required. Once the patient is stabilized, the patient must be returned to theater for removal of the packing.

SCENARIO 4 – EMERGENCY CESAREAN IN THE FIRST STAGE OF LABOR

Bleeding in emergency cesarean sections in the first stage of labor most commonly occurs from atony or lacerations of the uterine artery at one or both angles of the uterine incision. Therapy of uterine atony is well described in Scenario 1 and chapters in Section 8. The bleeding from incisional angles can be controlled by one of two means, both of which are much more easily accomplished when the uterus is exteriorized and held upwards by an assistant.

The first method is to grasp the angle with a nontraumatic forceps and insert one or more figure-of-8 sutures. The second is to examine the lateral margin of the uterus for the uterine artery itself, because the laceration may be in the ascending, middle or descending branch. If circumstances require ligation of the traumatized artery at the lateral margin of the uterus, it is important to place sutures above and below the level of the lacerated angle and include 1–2 cm of the myometrial tissue. This is because the ascending branch of

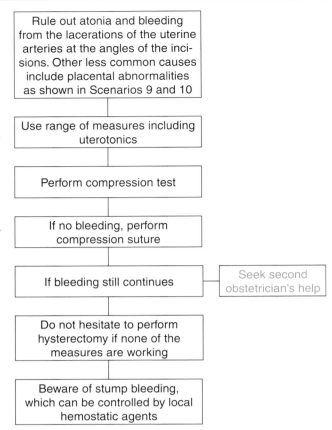

Scenario 4 – Emergency cesarean in the first stage of labor

the uterine artery anastomoses with the descending branch of the ovarian artery, and the descending branch of the uterine artery anastomoses in turn with the ascending branch of the vaginal artery. The ligation of the uterine arteries is totally without consequence to the uterine function because of the rich anastomotic system that exists. A word of caution is necessary, because if the laceration extends laterally and inferiorly, it is possible to inadvertently include the ureter (Figure 5 and Video 3).

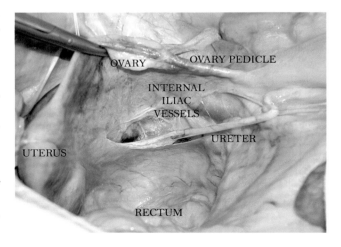

Figure 5 Posterior and right view of female pelvis in a fresh corpse: the image shows the pelvic ureter over the iliac vessels and inside and parallel to the ovary pedicle. Palacios-Jaraquemada, 2012[6], with permission

At the same time as these measures are being carried out, the previously described uterotonic therapy is administered (Scenario 1). Fluid replacement and, if necessary, blood and blood products should also be administered (see Chapters 3–6). If blood is deemed necessary, one should not wait until the laboratory results (hemoglobin, hematocrit, clotting factors, etc.) are present because continued bleeding will lead to coagulopathy[7].

If the uterus appears to be atonic in spite of the uterotonic agents having been administered, bimanual compression of the uterus should be performed with the view to assess the need for placement of compression sutures. It is necessary to be sure that no clotting abnormality is present when the compression test is attempted. Compression should not be performed with the patient in the supine position. Rather, the patient should be placed into the frog-leg position and the uterus should be exteriorized. If the compression test is positive, the operator should place the type of uterine compression suture he/she is most comfortable to perform.

Surgeons competent to perform cesarean sections MUST also be competent to perform one of the available uterine compression sutures in a timely manner (see Chapters 51–53). The advantage of early compression suture is that the hemorrhage has not extended to the point where clotting abnormalities begin. In the recent article by Palacios describing 539 cases, most surgical hemostatic failures that lead to hysterectomy occurred in women with severe hemodynamic deterioration and coagulopathy[7].

If, in the unfortunate event that none of the above-mentioned interventions are effective and the patient continues with bleeding, a second and senior obstetrician should be called to determine whether hysterectomy is warranted. Here too, it is crucial to have stability within the coagulation system.

If a decision is made to perform a hysterectomy, the subtotal type is faster, equally effective and less likely to be associated with surgical complications such as ureteric injuries. Bleeding may occur from the cervical stump, the side walls of the pelvis, or even the ovarian pedicles. Usually this can be controlled with local hemostatic agents (see Chapters 57 and 58) or with a large pelvic pack consisting of a gauze tube filled with laparotomy pads (Figure 6). If a hysterectomy already has been performed, a plastic bag filled with gauze can be placed in the pelvis with the opening of the bag brought out through the vaginal apex which had been left open (see Chapter 54).

Packing can be removed 24 hours later. Patients who have had this intervention should be observed in the intensive care unit for 24–48 hours to monitor for pulmonary edema and diminished urinary output, pain control and restoration of full clotting parameters.

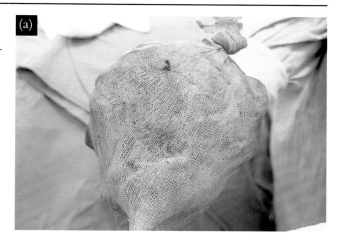

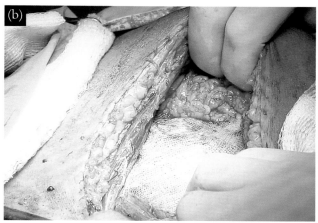

Figure 6 (a) Gauze tube filled with laparotomy pads. (b) Packing with gauze tube filled with laparotomy pads into the pelvis

SCENARIO 5 – FAILED SEQUENTIAL INSTRUMENTAL DELIVERY/EMERGENCY CESAREAN AT SECOND STAGE OF LABOR

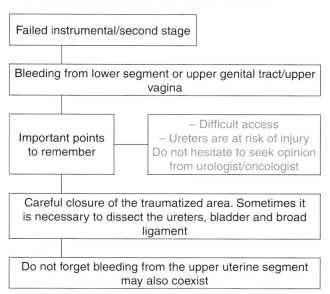

Failed instrumental/second stage

Bleeding from lower segment or upper genital tract/upper vagina

Important points to remember

– Difficult access
– Ureters are at risk of injury
Do not hesitate to seek opinion from urologist/oncologist

Careful closure of the traumatized area. Sometimes it is necessary to dissect the ureters, bladder and broad ligament

Do not forget bleeding from the upper uterine segment may also coexist

Scenario 5 – Failed sequential instrumental delivery/emergency cesarean at second stage of labor

Bleeding from failure of an instrumental delivery followed by a difficult fetal extraction during a cesarean is particularly challenging. This is because the source of bleeding could be from atony or the upper genital tract (S1), the lower uterine segment (trauma with or without obvious evidence) or the upper vagina, cervix and parametrium (S2).

The challenges here are to differentiate rapidly which is the most likely cause and whether more than one cause of bleeding is operating concurrently. Time is required to make this differentiation, and the use of intraoperative aortic compression (Video 2) permits the operator to make careful intraoperative assessment in the presence of the markedly reduced bleeding.

Three causative possibilities must be mentioned. The first is that the operator is able to find the traumatized area and place several simple sutures that control the bleeding. In order to do this, the bladder must have been pushed down to make sure that it is protected from getting accidentally included into a suture.

The second is that the operator is unable to control the bleeding from the lower uterine segment or the upper vagina (Video 4). In this case, it is mandatory to dissect the ureter(s) laterally until it (they) enters the bladder. It is not enough to say the operator visualized the ureter, because the traumatized area may actually involve it (Figure 5 and Video 3). At this point, it is helpful to encircle the lower uterine segment with a wide rubber catheter and secure it tightly with a firm clamp placed at its center (Video 5).

The third option relates to trauma at the middle to lower part of the vagina and the levator ani muscle as described below in Scenario 9.

Comments related to proper fluid and blood replacement as described above also apply here.

SCENARIO 6 – ELECTIVE CESAREAN FOR ADHERENT PLACENTA

Unlike the above-mentioned scenarios, this situation requires advanced planning and numerous preoperative measures that start with proper diagnosis, continue to intensive counseling and end with a detailed surgical plan as arrived at by consensus of a multidisciplinary expert team. This team should involve an obstetrician, sonographer, radiologist, interventional radiologist, hematologist, urologist, intensivist and gynecological oncologist (see Chapters 28–30).

Diagnostic consideration of an adherent placenta starts with a thorough history as obtained at the first visit. Important risk factors include prior cesarean delivery/prior repeat cesareans, surgical termination of pregnancy or illegal abortion, curettage and myomectomy. Ultrasound is the key diagnostic aid. It is available worldwide, cheap and can be performed with great accuracy. Placental magnetic resonance imaging (MRI) is reserved for those cases with doubt regarding the degree of invasion or the extent and topography of the invaded area. It is also the only diagnostic tool which will diagnose or rule out parametrial invasion (see Addendum A and Chapters 28–31).

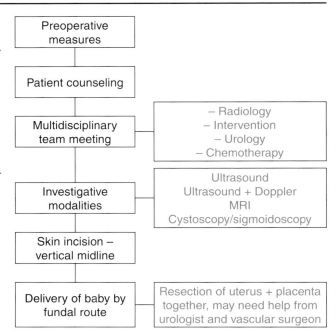

Scenario 6 – Elective cesarean for adherent placenta

Once diagnosis is confirmed, the multidisciplinary team is charged with planning surgery based on the presumed anatomic alterations and the knowledge that the final surgical treatment must be guided by what is found at the time of surgery. Consensus of all team members is optimal, because preoperative diagnosis is invariably less than accurate (see Chapters 28–31).

Controversy exists regarding the proper therapeutic approach when the bladder is invaded. One school of thought proposes leaving the placenta *in situ* even though this may be associated with infectious morbidity; the other advocates performing hysterectomy. Regardless of the decision made, two important factors impinge upon it. The first is whether the woman wants future pregnancies, and the second is the extent of the anatomical abnormalities which can modify any prior decision, i.e., parametrial invasion, bladder invasion, ureteral involvement. Both physicians and patients must recognize that their preconceived plans may not be viewed as realistic during surgery.

Cystoscopy is not useful to determine the extent of bladder invasion; however, it allows insertion of preoperative ureteric catheters.

Providing that the woman has not experienced any antepartum hemorrhage during the present pregnancy, timing of delivery is suggested as follows:

(1) If the placenta is percreta, it is found to involve extensive invasion of the uterine musculature or if parametrial invasion is presumed, then the time of delivery is around 34 completed weeks with antenatal corticosteroids being administered electively.

(2) If the presumed adherent placenta only involves a relatively small area or if invasion through the myometrium is only partial, then elective cesarean delivery is planned around 37 weeks of gestation with steroid coverage.

The time of surgery should be early in the day at the beginning of a week which does not include public holidays. The incision must be midline vertical extending above the umbilicus to the left side so that the baby can be delivered (breech) through a fundal incision (Figure 7).

Once the baby is delivered, the umbilical cord should be cut near to the placental insertion site and the placenta left untouched regardless of whether hysterectomy is planned. One should never try to remove the placenta in such cases, because if bleeding commences, it will be of catastrophic nature within minutes, and circumstances can rapidly become out of control.

If a decision is made to perform hysterectomy, all necessary resources must be on hand. Circumferential suturing is performed around the fundal opening to avoid additional bleeding. Such an operation would require an accurate proximal vascular control such as that provided by aortic or common iliac balloons. This type of vascular control provides hemostasis for both the uterine artery and the lower vascular blood supply (bladder and vagina; S1 and S2 blood supplies) (Figure 8).

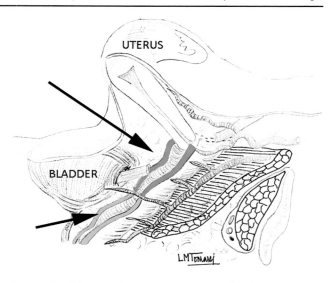

Figure 8   Diagram of access to upper part of vagina

If one decides to perform conservative and restorative surgery as proposed by Palacios-Jaraquemada[8], proceed as described in Chapter 31.

SCENARIO 7 – EMERGENCY CESAREAN SECTION WITH UNEXPECTED DIAGNOSIS OF MORBIDLY ADHERENT PLACENTA

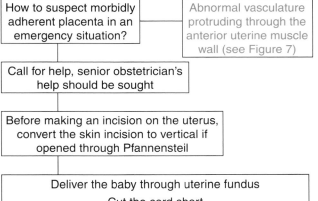

How to suspect morbidly adherent placenta in an emergency situation? — Abnormal vasculature protruding through the anterior uterine muscle wall (see Figure 7)

Call for help, senior obstetrician's help should be sought

Before making an incision on the uterus, convert the skin incision to vertical if opened through Pfannensteil

Deliver the baby through uterine fundus
Cut the cord short
Do not attempt to remove the placenta
Close the uterus in 2–3 layers
Monitor the patient in high dependency unit environment or transfer the patient to tertiary center

Scenario 7 – Emergency cesarean section with unexpected diagnosis of morbidly adherent placenta

Unlike the previous scenario in which the adherent placenta was diagnosed antepartum, the obstetric team must deal with this diagnosis in a state of poor to non-existent preparation when appropriate help is not available or far away. ONCE THE DIAGNOSIS OF ADHERENT PLACENTA IS MADE IN AN EMERGENCY (UNPREPARED) SITUATION, THE OBJECT IS TO DELIVER SAFELY THE BABY THORUGH A FUNDAL INCISION AND LEAVE THE PLACENTA *IN SITU.*

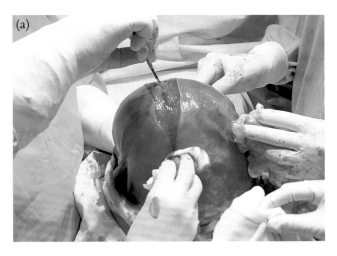

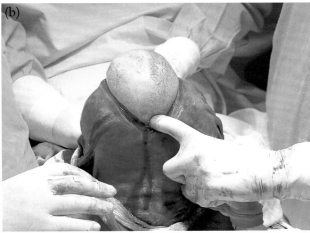

Figure 7   (a) and (b) Fetal delivery through the fundus

The first challenge is to suspect or make the diagnosis. In most instances the visual appearance of the anterior uterine serosa and lower uterine segment at the level of the superior limit of the bladder is sufficient to suggest that something is drastically abnormal. The picture is one of a bulging lower uterine segment with numerous tortuous vessels directly under the serosa or on the peritoneum overlying the bladder (Video 6).

This anatomic distortion is visible immediately upon opening of the peritoneum, especially when a Pfannensteil incision is used. It is important that the obstetrician realize the seriousness of the condition and NOT attempt any manipulations or incisions at this point. Rather, the skin incision should immediately be converted to a vertical incision to the level of the umbilicus or higher in order to have access to the uterine fundus for safe delivery of the baby. Any thoughts of continuing surgery through the Pfannensteil incision should be immediately abandoned, as continuation of surgery will be dangerous and put the mother's life at great risk.

After converting the skin incision and prior to making any uterine incision, help should be requested from the most senior obstetricians and anesthesiologists. In addition, the blood bank should be alerted and samples should be sent for typing and cross-matching.

Delivery of the baby is safest via the fundal route (Figure 7), as this avoids any bleeding complication associated with abnormal placental attachment, especially that which involves the bladder. Once the baby is delivered, the fundal incision can be closed as described in Scenario 6.

Placental delivery should not be attempted in any manner. Similarly, the bladder and its attachments should remain undisturbed, as both can be effectively dealt with at a later time by more experienced personnel with full resources. It is NOT NECESSARY to perform an emergency hysterectomy in this situation.

It is also not necessary to use methotrexate for enhanced placental resorption, because the term placenta has a low level of mitotic activity (less than 1%). However, this statement does not meet with universal agreement.

Even if the patient appears stable after surgery, observation is recommended in a high dependency environment whilst preparations for further care are made.

Additional care at a tertiary center may involve one of three options: first, to leave the placenta *in situ* until spontaneous expulsion or resorption; second, to perform hysterectomy with full resources for the complications that are described in Scenario 6; and third, to perform reconstructive surgery as described in Chapter 31.

SCENARIO 8 – PROGRESSIVE INTERMITTENT PPH

The bleeding in this scenario may follow normal or operative (ventouse, forceps or cesarean) delivery, may commence within a few hours and may last for a few weeks. In other cases, its onset is later (possibly a few days to a week) but its continuation is similar. Because this form of postpartum bleeding is progressive and intermittent, assessment and care may be less than optimal for a number of reasons: (1) failure to keep a running total of the individual episodes of blood loss since delivery or misinterpretation of blood loss as lochia rubra; (2) failure to recognize missing placental cotyledons and/or incompleteness of membranes; and (3) failure to monitor.

The potential gravity of the situation is augmented if the patient's symptoms of dizziness, feeling cold and being weak and tired are ignored or if strict input/output monitoring has not taken place. This latter possibility is more important if the patient has received large quantities of intravenous fluids containing uterotonic agents, and the care givers assume that the situation will correct itself. Other contributing factors include failure to use simple diagnostic aids such as detailed genital examination and/or abdominal and vaginal ultrasound especially after the first 24 hours. The latter may not clearly differentiate between clots and small pieces of retained placental tissue immediately after delivery when the uterus is not fully contracted. Furthermore, the caregiver may underestimate the extent of the blood loss because the patient is hemodynamically stable and her vital signs are well maintained. Finally, if the patient is going to be discharged, she and her family as well as the community health workers or local doctors must be informed about the nature of the small and continuing blood loss. Any patient who leaves the hospital must receive clear and written information about what is considered to be sufficiently abnormal as to require return to the hospital for further care. If she lives a long way from the hospital, she should be given a copy of the discharge summary or some notation as to the nature of the problem and whom to contact with telephone numbers and email addresses if a problem arises.

The following points are provided to ensure optimal follow-up in patients who have intermittent bleeding.

- Intermittent/recurrent bleeding per vaginum following delivery in the first 42 days should be treated as PPH

- Even if the patient's vital signs are stable, it is worthwhile performing an ultrasound scan based on the health center's equipment and resources. If ultrasound is used, it is important to obtain both abdominal and vaginal scans so that the fundal and lower uterine segments can be examined with similar accuracy. If ultrasound scans detect a possible placental segment attachment to a prior cesarean scar, one should be careful with any attempts to remove it manually or by curettage, as such removal may require specialist attention as there is a risk of uterine scar dehiscence, bladder injury or secondary bleeding into the peritoneum

- If possible, the total blood loss from the point of delivery to the current patient encounter should be calculated; do not be afraid to repeat the hemoglobin assessment, if necessary, especially if the patient complains of being tired and weak

- Undocumented blood losses should be carefully assessed, as they may occur with change of bed pans/bed sheets/clothes, or passing of big clots in the toilet pans

- If possible, and if the placenta is still available, it should be re-examined to account for every cotyledon

- If facilities for ultrasound examination do not exist, then examination under anesthesia is required to assess the uterine cavity and remove placental tissue and fragments if they are present. Undetected cervical tears may require simple suturing

- If the operator decides to perform curettage, great care should be exercised to avoid perforation, because the uterine musculature may still be soft and perforations may go unrecognized

- If the bleeding is heavy and intermittent after a few weeks or a month, the most likely diagnosis is not retained placental fragments but PSEUDO-ANEURYSM OF THE UTERINE ARTERY (Figure 9). This condition should be considered when patients have undergone a difficult instrumental delivery, curettage for retained placental fragments, or difficult fetal extraction during a cesarean section. This diagnosis is suspected if the patient has had one, two or more negative ultrasound scans. Diagnostic confirmation is by color Doppler or angiography of the pelvic vessels with the capacity to embolize at the same time. One should not attempt curettage or hysterectomy because the tissues are exceedingly friable and also there is real risk of massive hemorrhage.

SCENARIO 9 – CONCEALED PPH

Concealed PPH is an important cause of maternal death, because either the clinician is not alerted to its presence until late in its course or the obstetrician is unable to control the bleeding at its source. This scenario presents the relevant material in a more traditional manner, as one algorithm would not fit.

Situations which lead to concealed PPH

- Successful but difficult instrumental delivery causing subperitoneal/retroperitoneal/pre-peritoneal space of Retzius hematoma (Figure 10), injury to the puborectal fascicle or to the external muscular covering of the vagina (Figure 11)

- Failed instrumental delivery leading to emergency cesarean section with or without difficult fetal extraction. (Unsuspected broad ligament hematoma, difficult access to the deep uterine angle

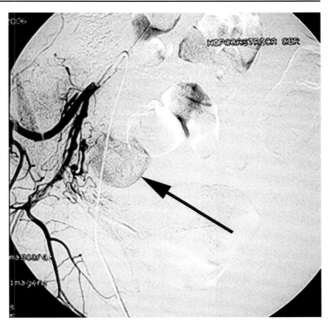
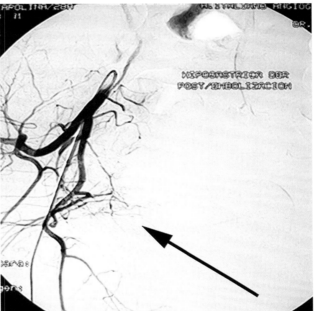
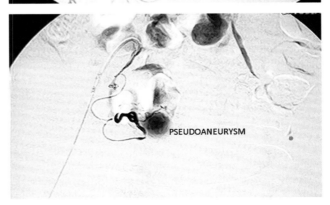

Figure 9 Pseudoaneurysm of the uterine artery – angiography images. Courtesy of Dr Garcio-Mónaco, Buenos Aires, Argentina

extensions, undiagnosed posterior uterine wall injuries, hesitation in closure of uterine angles as the operator is concerned about ureteric ligation and proceeding to close the angles without caution)

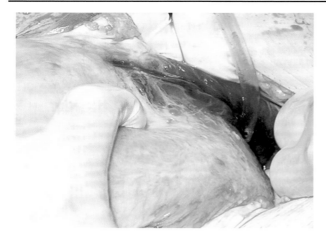

Figure 10 Retroperitoneal hematoma

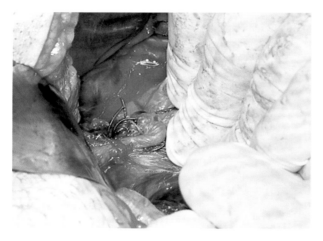

Figure 11 Sutured injury of internal fascicle of levator ani muscle

- If elective cesarean is performed in a woman whose cervix was never dilated in the past, she is particularly at risk of uterine atony with the accumulation of a large amount of intrauterine blood clots before clinical deterioration becomes evident. Detection of clinical deterioration may be so late that the patient succumbs despite emergency measures

- Another contributory factor for accumulation of clots after elective cesarean section followed by atony is the lack of response to oxytocic agents, which although uncommon, must be considered. Therapy consists of restoration of uterine tone and expression of the clots

- Uterine rupture can also be easily missed. Classically, such patients are multiparous and their labors have been augmented with uterotonics, induced with prostaglandins, or were precipitate in nature. It is also possible following a midcavity forceps delivery. Such patients are well for a few minutes following delivery, but bleeding continues intra-abdominally without overt deterioration at first. By the time it is recognized, the clinical picture may be grave and resuscitative measures may be futile

- Rectus sheath hematomas, where blood accumulates above the abdominal cavity without external bleeding, can also cause similar deterioration.

Other contributory factors

- Operator inexperience
- Delivery time of the day with misses more common late at night
- Poor/inexperienced assistant
- Failure to exteriorize uterus to check posterior wall, especially after difficult head extraction
- Operator thinks that small amount of bleeding may diminish over time
- Fast surgery, too much time pressure, too many things to do
- Ignoring clinical signs of deterioration, i.e., worsening tachycardia, falling blood pressure, increasing respiratory rate, increasing abdominal girth, falling urine output and increasing patient demand for analgesic use are all pointers of concealed PPH.

Solutions

- If uterine rupture is suspected, speed and efficiency of the whole team are required. Everyone has a key role starting from the switchboard, to porters, to hematology and blood bank technicians, to midwifery and obstetric and anesthetic teams

- Close monitoring of all patients who need operative intervention is mandatory

- Bedside facilities such as hemoglobin measurement by simple equipment such as Hemacue will aid clinicians rapidly to detect patient deterioration

- Use the modified obstetric early warning scoring system (MOEWS) chart in all at risk patients (see Addendum B of this chapter for a sample chart)

- Education and training of all staff must take place at regular intervals

- Patient counseling must recognize that no cesarean delivery is risk free (either elective or emergency)

- Prompt action by the attending physician is required to establish the cause of a patient's physical deterioration

- From the obstetric point of view, if uterine rupture is suspected and if the patient's situation permits, a bedside ultrasound scan is helpful to diagnose the presence of intraperitoneal bleeding. However, one should also remember not to waste time trying to establish a specific cause, as every second counts in combating situations involving uterine rupture

- If an expanding broad ligament hematoma is suspected, then computed tomography (CT) scanning and embolization of the bleeding vessel has a role. Even if such patients undergo laparotomy, it will be extremely difficult to identify the exact source of bleeding vessel and tissues will be very fragile.

If patient is taken back for re-laparotomy, what necessary steps should be taken?

- Resuscitation and correction of volume deficiency should happen simultaneously

- It is very easy to miss coexisting coagulopathy; hence there is a high possibility that the patient will require replacement of clotting factors (see Chapters 4 and 6 for discussion of controversy regarding the proper ratio of RBC and fibrinogen products during replacement)

- The team should involve a senior obstetrician with support from another senior obstetrician, senior anesthetist, hematologist and occasionally an intensivist and an interventional radiologist

- During re-laparotomy, meticulous attention should be given to each abdominal layer, and the uterus should be exteriorized and its cavity either checked with intraoperative ultrasound or re-opened. If uterine atony was the cause of patient deterioration, then it may be worthwhile inserting a uterine compression suture or uterine tamponade balloon

- If bleeding is from the uterine parametrium, then one should seek help from the urologist or gynecological oncologist, as the ureters are at risk of being injured while achieving hemostasis

- If time and the situation permit, the patient should be counseled about the risks of hysterectomy. Patients also should be counseled that there is a small possibility of not being able to identify the exact source of bleeding and that even if hysterectomy is performed, bleeding may still continue. In such circumstances, the clinician may decide to put several abdominal packs *in situ* and request further monitoring in the intensive care setting (see above). Once the patient's clinical condition improves, usually after 24 hours, the patient would need another laparotomy to remove the abdominal packs. Occasionally, the patient may still require radiological embolization of bleeding pelvic vessels.

SCENARIO 10 – UTERINE INVERSION AND PPH

Usual scenario

Uterine inversion is almost always secondary to strong traction on the umbilical cord which is attached to the placenta when it is implanted in the fundus. The problem here is not that the placenta is abnormally adherent but rather that the traction is too forceful and too early (before the placenta is normally separated). Inversion can be avoided by simple measures: not attempting the forceful cord traction before the signs of placental separation are seen (lengthening of the cord, fresh gush of bleeding, desire to push by the woman) and placement of one hand on the fundus

while the other hand guides the cord. Of those who experience uterine inversion, one in six women will die if appropriate corrective measures are not applied in a timely manner. Always suspect uterine inversion if the patient becomes shocked immediately after birth without an obvious reason.

Inversion of the uterus may be partial or complete. The upper panel illustrates an incomplete inversion in which the most important physical finding is the presence of a dimple in the uterine fundus. The middle panel demonstrates the three degrees of inversion. In stage '3' and '4', the fundus is completely outside of the vulva, and these two variations are the most catastrophic, as any delay in recognition of the inversion and the urgency of correction may be followed by death of the patient.

Symptoms

The initial symptoms depend upon the severity of the uterine inversion. If inversion is only partial, then severe cramping lower abdominal pain and signs of mild shock, i.e., bradycardia and hypotension, may be the initial signs. Massive bleeding will not be present. On the other hand, if the inversion is complete, it is accompanied by a brief period of neurogenic shock shortly followed by massive PPH. Shock is primarily because of parasympathetic activation of the nervous system because of traction on the peritoneum through ligaments supporting the uterus.

Management

It is imperative that the condition be recognized instantaneously and managed promptly and by the person attending the delivery. The uterus (a dark pink/purple fleshy mass) is observed as lying outside the vulva immediately after birth. If the placenta is still *in situ*, manual repositioning should be attempted without removing the placenta. If separation has not occurred and if the situation is ignored, the patient will bleed massively and possibly precipitate further deep shock.

Help should be called for immediately, as the replacement must be performed with the patient in shock. If the birth attendant cannot immediately replace the fundus and the shock continues, a single dose of atropine (one ampoule) should be administered preferably by the intravenous route to address the neurogenic origin of the shock (parasympathetic blockade).

The initial attempt to replace the uterine fundus entails manual replacement through the vagina past the cervical ring. If the patient is receiving a uterotonic (oxytocin) infusion or is about to receive it as a prophylaxis for third stage bleeding, the infusion should be stopped or withheld whichever is appropriate.

The typical maneuver in repositioning the fundus involves the birth attendant's hand being placed inside the vagina (for stage 3) or on the fundus for stage 4, with the cup of the inverted fundus in the palm of the operator's hand and the tips of fingers directed toward the uterosacral ligaments. The fundus is then forcefully

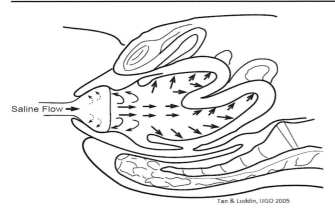

Figure 12 Hydrostatic method of reposition of inverted uterus. From Tan and Luddin, 2005[9], with permission

pushed inside the abdominal cavity above the level of umbilicus and held in that position for 3–5 minutes until the passive action of uterine ligaments corrects the uterine inversion. Care should be taken not to apply so much pressure as to perforate the uterus with the fingertips.

If manual repositioning fails, hydrostatic replacement is the next option. This is carried out using a 6 cm diameter silastic ventouse cup. A good saline seal is crucial for success of hydrostatic reduction. An excellent seal is maintained by pushing the cup to the middle of the vagina and then withdrawing it until it is snugly placed at the vaginal orifice. The accumulating saline will exert pressure backwards to maintain the seal. If necessary, a tocolytic agent can be used to relax any constriction at the level of the cervix. It is important to resist the tendency to push the silastic cup deep inside the vagina (Figure 12).

On occasion, attempts to replace the fundus manually or by hydrostatic pressure fail and the patient must be taken for a laparotomy and surgical correction. A number of measures have been described and are beyond the scope of this chapter. However, one method is found in Chapter 51 by B-Lynch.

Management after successful replacement

As soon as the uterus is restored to its normal position and configuration, it is usual that it remains atonic causing continued massive PPH. Accordingly, a uterotonic infusion is started while the birth attendant maintains the fundus of the uterus in its normal anatomical position. Once this is accomplished, bimanual compression of the uterus aids in control of further hemorrhage until uterine tone is re-established. In some cases, a uterine balloon tamponade may be required. The birth attendant should continue to monitor the uterus vaginally for any evidence of subsequent inversion.

References

1. Confidential Enquires into Maternal Deaths. Saing Mothers Lives (2006–2008). BJOG 2011;118:1–203
2. Sullivan EA, King JF, eds. Maternal Deaths in Austrailia 2000–2002. Sydney, Australia: Australian Institute of Health and Welfare, National Perinatal Statistics Unit, 2006
3. Special Report on Maternal Mortality and Severe Morbidity in Canada: Canadian Perinatal Surveillance System. Canada: Minister of Health, Minister of Public and Government Services, 2004
4. Amnesty International. Deadly Delivery: The Maternal Health Care Crisis in the USA. New York: Amnesty International USA, 2010; http://www.amnestyusa.org/dignity/pdf/Deadly Delivery.pdf
5. Palacios Jaraquemada JM, Mónaco RG, Barbosa NE, et al. Lower uterine blood supply: extrauterine anastomotic system and its application in surgical devascularization techniques. Acta Obstet Gynecol Scand 2007;86:228–34
6. Palacios-Jaraquemada JM. Placental Adhesive Disorders, 1st edn. Berlin, Germany: De Gruyter, 2012;1
7. Palacios-Jaraquemada J, Fiorillo A. Conservative approach in heavy postpartum hemorrhage associated with coagulopathy. Acta Obstet Gynecol Scand 2010;89:1222–5
8. Palacios-Jaraquemada JM. Diagnosis and management of placenta accreta. Best Pract Res Clin Obstet Gynaecol 2008; 22:1133–48
9. Tan KH, Luddin NS. Hydrostatic reduction of acute uterine inversion. Int J Gynaecol Obstet 2005;91:63–4

Addendum A: Guidelines for placental MRIs: technical aspects of MRI scan in morbidly adherent placenta

Like other diagnostic methods placental MRI (pMRI) has certain technical details that can enhance or emphasize its diagnostic accuracy. The main aim of the imaging study is to obtain the best definition of the uterine–placental interphase and its relation to the bladder. Newly formed vessels (NFV) secondary to the development of placenta accreta are underdeveloped in the middle layer. This particularity requires the pMRI study to be performed with a semi-full bladder, to avoid false negatives as a result of overdistension and/or collapse of the NFV, as well as false negatives due to an empty bladder. It is important that the bladder is only partially full; an empty bladder next to the pubic bone would prevent an adequate sign of the uterine–vesical interphase, resulting in diagnostic error. The use of ultrafast techniques that minimize artifacts produced by fetal movement is recommended. T2-weighted imaging highlights urine as a naturally white contrast, thus allowing better delineation of the vesical muscle in relation to the placenta and the underlying myometrium. In the presence of risk factors (multiple D&C, myomectomies or corrective surgery), if there are clinical antecedents for the T2 mode allowing a naturally white contrast and a suspicion of posterior placenta accreta, the use of gadolinium is recommended to improve diagnostic accuracy. Without this, a combination of placenta, myometrium, abdominal viscera and the vertebrae form a complex image, which makes an adequate diagnosis of posterior myometrial placental invasion virtually impossible. So far, gadolinium has not shown any side-effects during pregnancy, and there are no toxicity reports. However, and as a precaution, its use is generally recommended for cases in which diagnosis by other techniques is not possible. It is prudent to use pMRI in all cases with a resulting non-conclusive ultrasound or Doppler examination, when it is important to rule out or confirm the presence of parametrial invasion. Therapeutic options depend on the size of the invasions and exact anatomy of the lesion

Addendum B: Modified obstetric early warning scoring chart

Reproduced, with permission

OBSTETRIC EARLY WARNING CHART. FOR MATERNITY USE ONLY

NAME: _____ DOB: _____

CHI: WARD:

CONTACT DOCTOR FOR EARLY INTERVENTION IF PATIENT TRIGGERS ONE RED OR TWO YELLOW SCORES AT ANY ONE TIME

Date :				
Time :				
RESP (write rate in corresp. box)	>30			>30
	21-30			21-30
	11-20			11-20
	0-10			0-10
Saturations	90-100%			90-100%
	<90%			<90%
O2 Conc.	%			%
Temp	39			39
	38			38
	37			37
	36			36
	35			35
HEART RATE	170			170
	160			160
	150			150
	140			140
	130			130
	120			120
	110			110
	100			100
	90			90
	80			80
	70			70
	60			60
	50			50
	40			40
Systolic blood pressure	200			200
	190			190
	180			180
	170			170
	160			160
	150			150
	140			140
	130			130
	120			120
	110			110
	100			100
	90			90
	80			80
	70			70
	60			60
	50			50
Diastolic blood pressure	130			130
	120			120
	110			110
	100			100
	90			90
	80			80
	70			70
	60			60
	50			50
	40			40
Passed Urine	Y or N			Y or N
Lochia	Normal			Normal
	Heavy / Foul			Heavy / Foul
Proteinuria	2+			2+
	> 2+			>2+
Liquor	Clear / Pink			Clear / Pink
	Green			Green
NEURO RESPONSE (√)	Alert			Alert
	Voice			Voice
	Pain / Unresponsive			Pain / Unresponsive
Pain Score (no.)	2-3			2-3
	0-1			0-1
Nausea (√)	YES (√)			YES (√)
	NO (√)			NO (√)
Looks unwell	YES (√)			YES (√)
Looks unwell	NO (√)			NO (√)
Total Yellow Scores				
Total Red Scores				

18

2

Uterovaginal Blood Supply: the S1 and S2 Segmental Concepts and their Clinical Relevance

J. M. Palacios-Jaraquemada, M. Karoshi and L. G. Keith

ORIGIN OF THE CONCEPT

Recent careful and precise anatomic studies in cadavers demonstrate that the female reproductive system has two separate and completely distinguishable blood supplies. These investigations confirm earlier observations[1] that the blood supplies are anastomotic in nature[2,3]. The distinctive natures of the two areas and their differing blood supplies are shown in the sagittal view of the pelvis as depicted in Figure 1. In practical terms, the two areas can be distinguished by drawing a line perpendicular to the posterior wall of the bladder.

As defined in the writings of Palacios-Jaraquemada, who first used this terminology in 2005, the S1 segment comprises the body of the uterus[2]. In this construct, the S2 segment corresponds to the lower uterine segment, cervix, upper part of the vagina and the respective parametria.

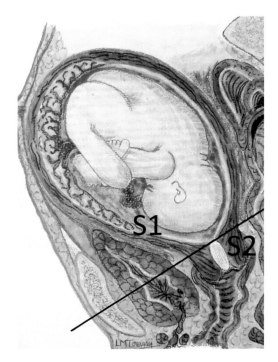

Figure 1 Sagittal line demarcating the S1 and S2 areas of blood supply to the uterus and upper vagina at term.

The S1 segment is supplied by ascending branches of the uterine artery and, to a lesser extent, by the descending branches of the ovarian artery. Rarely, the round ligament artery contributes to the collateral blood supply of the uterus. In contrast, the S2 segment is supplied by branches of the uterine, cervical, upper vesical, vaginal and pudendal arteries. *All of these blood vessels are located subperitoneally.*

A thorough understanding of the differences in the blood supply to both uterine segments (S1 and S2) underlies the proper selection of a therapeutic intervention, be it surgical or radiological, for the treatment of postpartum hemorrhage (PPH). It is possible that the recent increases in maternal mortality in several countries are related to the changes in the rates of PPH, with more severe bleeding related the increased incidence of adherent placentas.

ANATOMIC EVIDENCE

Figure 2 shows a fetal angiographic preparation which facilitates an understanding of the rich arterial anastomotic system between the left uterine artery and the corresponding left lower and middle vaginal arteries[1]. These arteries also anastomose with the descending branches of the uterine artery on the ipsilateral side. In practical terms, this means that the whole of one half of the lower part of the uterus and the upper part of the vagina receives blood from an interconnected system. In this figure, the uterine artery and the middle left vaginal artery are branches of the anterior division of the internal iliac artery, whereas the lower left vaginal artery is a branch of the posterior division of the internal iliac artery. (Note: it could also arise from the internal pudendal artery, which in turn is a branch of the posterior division of internal iliac.)

It is crucial to understand that the system illustrated in this fetal angiogram is fully maintained in the adult and is the system responsible for continuation of uterine blood supply when the uterine arteries are embolized.

The cross anastomoses between the right and the left uterine arteries over the uterine surface shown in

Figure 3 are not evident to the naked eye in either the non-pregnant or the normal pregnant uterus. However, *in the presence of abnormal placentation, they become grossly enlarged and engorged, and are visible on the uterine surface, especially in the lower segment.* This is because the lower segment of pregnant uterus is stretched and thinned.

Figure 4 is a rare adult angiographic preparation showing the features previously described in Figures 2

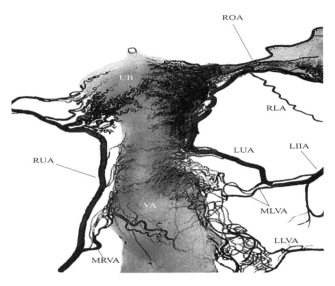

Figure 2 Fetal cadaveric angiographic preparation demonstrating the rich arterial anastomotic system between the left uterine artery and the left lower and middle vaginal arteries. LIIA, left internal iliac artery; LLVA, lower left vaginal artery; LUA, left uterine artery; MLVA, middle left vaginal artery; MRVA, middle right vaginal artery; RLA, round ligament artery; ROA, right ovarian artery; RUA, right uterine artery; UB, uterine body; VA, vagina. From Palacios-Jaraquemada *et al.*, 2007[3], with permission

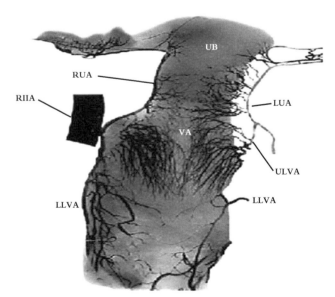

Figure 3 Another view of the preparation shown in Figure 2 but demonstrating cross anastomoses between the right and the left uterine arteries over the uterine surface. LLVA, left lower vaginal artery; LUA, left uterine artery; RIIA, right internal iliac artery; RUA, right uterine artery; UB, uterine body; VA, vagina. From Palacios-Jaraquemada *et al.*, 2007[3], with permission

and 3 which derive from a fetus. First, the anatomy present in the fetus is present and persists through adult life. Second, the bilateral anastomotic flow pathways between the vaginal and uterine arteries remain visible. Third, the side-to-side anastomoses between both uterine arteries are present. This latter point has exceedingly practical implications, because *if one is going to perform stepwise devascularization in cases of major PPH, it must be bilateral (as is the case in bilateral uterine artery embolization) or the procedure will be less than effective as a result of the cross anastomoses.* In contrast, vertical uterine compression sutures (B-Lynch, Hayman) act over both systems.

REASONS FOR FAILURE OF SOME INTERVENTIONAL RADIOLOGICAL PROCEDURES

Figure 4 demonstrates the anatomic basis for the failures of some uterine embolization procedures. It also provides an explanation of why non-target embolizations occur, especially in the bladder where they may cause necrosis. In the majority of instances, the interventional radiologists cannot explain these occurrences, because the embolization material has been injected into the uterine artery and the damage is in the area supplied by the vesical artery.

Under normal circumstances, the connection between the uterine artery and the vesical artery is microscopic; however, in the presence of abnormal placentation and also because of the effect of vascular growth factors, these vessels enlarge and represent neovascularization as they lack a tunica media which in turn allows them to become high flow low resistance reservoirs.

When patients undergo interventional radiological procedures in situations involving abnormal placentation, it is important to be aware of the potential for abnormal connections between uterine and vesical arteries. If the embolization material is injected under pressure and if the particle size is small (usually less than 700 μm), then it is possible to have non-target embolization to the bladder which occasionally becomes necrotic (see Chapter 49 for further reading).

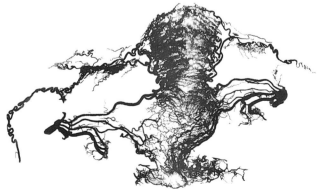

Figure 4 Adult angiographic preparation which shows the features previously described in Figures 2 and 3. From Rohen *et al.*, 2003[5], with permission

The radiograph shown in Figure 5 illustrates the dense anastomotic system present between the vaginal and uterine arteries. In this patient, the catheter was placed at the level of the internal pudendal artery. The contrast material was injected and passed as high as the uterus via intercommunicating anastomoses.

This radiograph can also explain two common clinical scenarios. In the first, where a patient suffers severe PPH following normal vaginal delivery, the interventional radiologist performs embolization of uterine artery and a second embolization attempt is made at the anterior division of internal iliac arteries. Both may fail to produce significant reduction in the intensity of bleeding. This failure can be explained by the presence of rich anastomoses between the internal pudendal anastomotic branches (S2 segment) and the uterine artery (S1) and also by the coexisting uncorrected clotting abnormalities.

In the second clinical scenario, a traumatic instrumental delivery results in deep vaginal tears or causes a retroperitoneal hematoma. When the bleeding cannot be controlled by routine measures, the clinician often elects to perform hysterectomy or uterine artery embolization, either one of which has its main effect on the S1 segment. Both can fail, however, because the origin of the bleeding is from the vessels that arise in the S2 segment shown in Figure 5 (internal pudendal artery).

COMMON PERCEPTIONS AND MISPERCEPTIONS

Students of history are well aware that if one does not learn from the mistakes of the past, one is bound to repeat them. The same is true in anatomy, where 18th century dissections provide important clues to the 21st century dilemmas. Figure 6, to the best of the senior author's (J.P.J.) knowledge, is the first illustration depicting the relationship between the relative diameters of the vaginal and uterine arteries. The common perception is that the diameter of the uterine artery is larger than that of the vaginal artery.

As shown in Figure 6, however, this is not always the case, and the French anatomist's observation[4] has been duplicated by later authors using specialized dissection techniques[3]. In a series of 39 cadaver dissections, the first author demonstrated that the diameter of the inferior vaginal artery was 33% thicker than that of the uterine artery (Table 1).

This important difference between the major blood supplies of the S2 segment and the S1 segment should not be

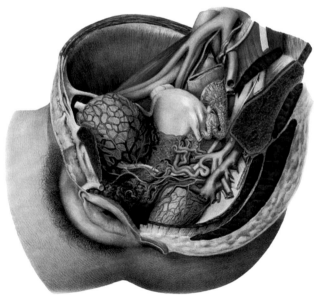

Figure 6 Eighteenth century illustration of the relative diameters of the uterine and vaginal arteries, respectively. From Bourgery, 1833[4]

Table 1 Lower uterine vascular supply. From Palacios-Jaraquemada *et al.*, 2007[3], with permission

Upper pedicle	Uterine artery	100% from IIA
Middle pedicle	Cervical artery	67% from UA
		23% from Vas
		10% from LVeA
Lower pedicle	UVA: 18% from UA	
	MVA: 11% from IIA	
	LVA: 71% from PIA	75% as descending branch
		25% as ascending branch
Sectional diameters	UA: 1.81 mm	MaVA: 1.88 mm

IIA, iliac internal artery; UA, uterine artery; Vas, vaginal arteries; LVeA, lower vesical artery; UVA, upper vaginal artery; MVA, middle vaginal artery; LVA, lower vaginal artery; PIA, pudendal internal artery; MaVA, main vaginal artery

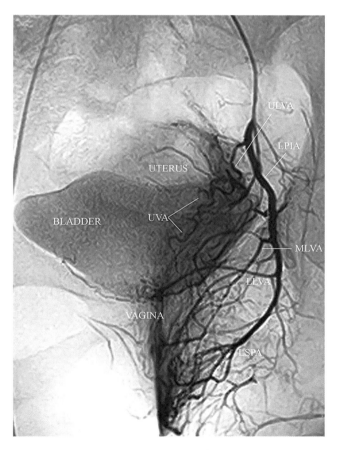

Figure 5 Angiographic illustration of the dense anastomotic system between the vaginal and uterine arteries. From Palacios-Jaraquemada *et al.*, 2007[3], with permission

underestimated. When the obstetrician is trying surgically to correct a PPH involving a traumatic vaginal tear, hysterectomy will not solve the problem. Although it is commonly believed that patients die from uncontrolled uterine arterial tears and do not die from vaginal arterial tears, this misconception is secondary to knowledge gained from reading standard textbooks which fail to explain the differences in the blood supplies of the S1 and S2 segments. Figures 7 and 8 illustrate these anatomic points with cadaver specimens.

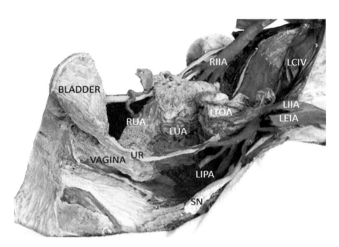

Figure 7 Normal non-pregnant uterine blood supply as commonly appreciated by the general physician. It consists of the uterine artery arising from the anterior division of the internal iliac artery and the ovarian artery which arise directly from the aorta. This is the S1 segmental blood supply area. LIPA, left internal pudendal; LSPA, left superficial perineal; LLVA, lower left vaginal; and LLVeA, lower left vesical artery; LCIA, left common iliac artery; LEIA, left external iliac artery; LIIA, left internal iliac artery; LIPA, left internal pudendal artery; LLVA, lower left vaginal artery; LLVeA, lower left vesical artery; LSPA, left superficial perineal artery; LTOA, left tubo-ovarian artery; LUA, left uterine artery; RIIA, right internal iliac artery; ROA, right ovarian artery; RUA, right uterine artery; SN, schiatic nerve; ULVeA, upper left vesical artery; UR, ureter; URVeA, upper right vesical artery

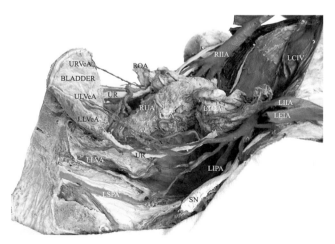

Figure 8 High density and close proximity of the numerous vessels of the S2 segment which comprise branches that mainly arise from the internal pudendal artery. See Figure 7 for abbreviations. From Palacios-Jaraquemada *et al.*, 2007[3], with permission

CLINICAL APPLICATION

Figures 9 and 10 represent initial views of two types of topography associated with abnormal placentation. In Figure 9, the abnormal placentation is located in the S1 segment. The importance of Figure 9 is that the clinician should ensure that there is no abnormal vasculature in the area where the hysterotomy is made to deliver the baby. If PPH supervenes, therapy with subtotal hysterectomy is an appropriate intervention.

In contrast, in Figure 10, the abnormal placentation occupies the S2 segment. The first challenge for the clinician is safely to deliver the baby and safeguard the health of the mother. This can be accomplished by delivering the baby through a uterine fundal incision without any attempt to touch, detach or deliver the placenta. In other words, the placenta will be left *in situ*, the umbilical cord cut short, and the fundus closed. Immediate hysterectomy in this kind of circumstance will precipitate catastrophic hemorrhage putting mother's life at risk.

When the placenta is left *in situ* the following three options may be considered. First is to observe closely the patient in a high dependency environment with the risk of sepsis that could complicate systemic inflammatory response syndrome (SIRS), or hemorrhage and coagulation abnormalities (disseminated

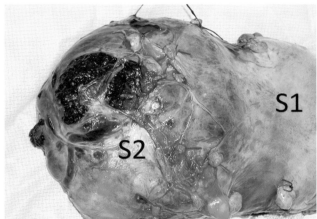

Figure 9 Abnormal placentation in S1 segment

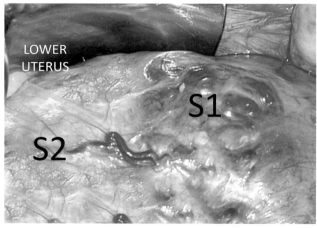

Figure 10 Abnormal placentation in S2 segment

intravascular coagulopathy). Second is to transfer the patient to a tertiary center where hysterectomy can be performed with the full team. Third, embolization may be considered if the patient experiences intermittent hemorrhage with the placenta *in situ* or an adjuvant treatment for a planned hysterectomy.

DISSECTION COURSES AND SELF LEARNING WITH VIDEOS

The challenge for the general obstetrician is to realize that a thorough understanding of the differences between the S1 and S2 segments will be of great value in planning safe, appropriate intervention for PPH. The authors propose that the general obstetrician who regularly performs instrumental deliveries should make every effort to become familiar with the vasculature of the S2 segment and safe access to this area. To gain access to the upper part of the vagina, one should have thorough knowledge of safe dissection of ureters (Video 1) (videos can be viewed via *The Global Library of Women's Medicine* at www.glowm.com). Access to the middle and lower part of the vagina and also to the roof of ischiorectal fossa and internal fascicle of levator ani muscle (pubo rectalis part) is shown in Video 2. This space is accessed by blunt dissection of the retropubic space (space of Retzius, which in the past was used for Burch colposuspension).

One means by which suggested anatomic knowledge and skill can be gained and maintained is by attending fresh cadaver dissection courses (hyperlink: St George's through RCOG at http://www.bgcs.org. uk/events/2012/03/gynaecological-oncology-cadaveric-dissection-course.html). Another way is to access surgical dissection videos on a regular basis. The authors also propose that physicians and their co-workers discuss the case in detail when any surgical intervention has failed.

CONCLUSION

The chapter closes with Video 3 which demonstrates all of the anatomic points discussed above. A major point of the video is to show that after bilateral uterine arterial embolization, the uterine blood flow is compensated by the blood which comes from the inferior vaginal arteries through the anastomotic channels described above.

References

1. Belou P. Anatomic revsion of arterial system. Stereoscopic Atlas of Human Arteries Anatomy 2nd Part. Buenos Aires, Argentina: El Ateneo, 1934;3:115
2. Palacios-Jaraquemada JM, Bruno CH. Magnetic resonance imaging in 300 cases of placenta accreta: surgical correlation of new findings. Acta Obstet Gynecol Scand 2005;84:716–24
3. Palacios-Jaraquemada JM, García Mónaco R, Barbosa NE, Ferle L, Iriarte H, Conesa HA. Lower uterine blood supply: extrauterine anastomotic system and its application in surgical devascularization techniques. Acta Obstet Gynecol Scand 2007;86:228–34
4. Bourgery MJ. Traité Complet de l'Anatomie de l'Homme. Paris, France: Delauney, 1833
5. Rohen JW, Yokochi C, Lütjen-Drecoll E. Atlas de Anatomía Humana, 5th edn. Madrid, Spain: Elsevier España, 2003:348 ©Schattauer GMBH, Stutgart, Alemania

3

Management of Exsanguinating Patients in Trauma: a Model for Postpartum Hemorrhage

J. B. Elterman, G. M. Riha and M. A. Schreiber

INTRODUCTION

Definitive management of the exsanguinating patient challenges providers in multiple specialties. Significant hemorrhage may be encountered in a variety of circumstances including elective or emergent surgical procedures, trauma, gastrointestinal bleeding and major obstetric or postpartum blood loss. Over the past two decades, the vast majority of data and evidence regarding transfusion in the exsanguinating patient has described patients with traumatic injuries. Hemorrhage remains the leading cause of death in the first hour after traumatic injury. It also represents the most frequent potentially preventable cause of early death secondary to trauma[1,2]. The data from such patients can be extrapolated to the treatment of all patients undergoing transfusion for major hemorrhage.

The ultimate goal in the management of exsanguinating patients is to achieve hemostasis and restore circulating blood volume without induction of significant pathologic events such as deep venous thrombosis, cerebrovascular accident, or myocardial infarction[3]. Achieving this goal requires early recognition of the extent of the hemorrhage, control of bleeding which can be accomplished with direct surgical intervention and hemostatic resuscitation with utilization of massive transfusion protocols.

THE LETHAL TRIAD

The 'lethal triad' is presently recognized as playing a major role in the morbidity and mortality of severely injured or bleeding patients[4,5]. Components of the lethal triad consist of hypothermia, acidosis and coagulopathy. This concept was first described by Kashuk and associates in the early 1980s. These authors depicted a 'bloody vicious cycle' in which hemorrhage, cellular shock and tissue injury contribute to the formation of the lethal triad which ultimately resulted in the exacerbation of ongoing hemorrhage[6].

Hypothermia is a common finding in patients with profound blood loss, as patients in hemorrhagic shock have uncoupling of the normal metabolic and thermoregulatory pathways, which results in reduced heat production[7]. The process of resuscitation frequently involves infusion of hypothermic blood and crystalloid, a factor which further contributes to hypothermia[8]. Moreover, patients are often exposed for examination or during surgery and experience ongoing conductive, convective and evaporative heat loss. This is significant, because hypothermia greatly affects platelet activation and the clotting cascade. Indeed, platelet aggregation fails in the majority of patients when the core body temperature falls below 30°C[9]. *Severe hypothermia, defined as a core temperature below 32°C, has been associated with a near 100% mortality in trauma patients with hemorrhagic shock*[10].

The second well-described aspect of the lethal triad is acidosis. By definition hemorrhagic shock results in decreased tissue perfusion. This leads to the build up of the products of anaerobic metabolism, mainly lactic acid. At a lower pH, coagulation is affected by reduced activity of both the intrinsic and extrinsic coagulation pathways as well as alterations in platelet function[11,12]. In addition to a decrease in clot formation, an acidotic state has also been associated with an increase in fibrinolysis in animal models[13].

The third component of the lethal triad is coagulopathy. Multiple factors contribute to coagulopathy in bleeding patients. In addition to the hypothermia and acidosis already discussed, other factors include the consumption of limited clotting factors and fibrinolysis[14–16]. Studies have identified the combination of tissue injury and shock as a primary cause of coagulopathy. Brohi and associates hypothesize that release of activated protein C initiates this coagulopathy after tissue hypoperfusion and have demonstrated that coagulopathy exists very early after injury and before any resuscitative efforts[17–19].

Early recognition of hemorrhagic shock followed by addressing each aspect of the lethal triad is of the utmost importance. Early recognition of significant hemorrhage remains a formidable challenge in obstetrics as hemodynamic changes are often delayed until profound blood loss has already occurred. Therefore, in all patients hypothermia should be avoided by elevating room temperatures and heat-loss prevention strategies should be instituted. Cold, wet, or damp clothing or bedding in contact with the patient should be removed. Heating blankets, solar blankets and other body heating devices can be used to lessen conductive and evaporative heat loss. Additionally, intravenous fluid should be warmed to body temperature or given through an infuser capable of warming the intravenous fluids prior to administration.

Acidosis, the second part of the lethal triad, is addressed by prevention and treatment of shock. This is achieved by restoring the circulating blood volume and therefore global tissue perfusion. The two most common isotonic fluids used in immediate resuscitation are normal saline (NS) and lactated Ringer's solution (LR). The pH of NS ranges between 4 and 6, while the pH of LR ranges between 5.5 and 7[7]. Resuscitation with NS alone has been shown to contribute to acidosis. This is likely related to the excess chloride in normal saline leading to a hyperchloremic metabolic acidosis. In fact, rapid saline infusion in patients undergoing gynecologic surgery has been shown to produce a hyperchloremic acidosis not seen with LR[20]. Animal models of uncontrolled hemorrhage have demonstrated LR to be superior to NS for resuscitation[21–24]. Animals receiving NS required nearly twice the volume of fluid to achieve and maintain their baseline blood pressure and they experienced increased blood loss[22]. Other adjuncts to treat acidosis, such as bicarbonate, have not been shown to reverse acidosis-induced changes in coagulation and are currently recommended only as a temporary measure in those patients with renal dysfunction in which acidosis clearance or compensation is ineffective[8,25].

Coagulopathy represents the third treatable aspect of the lethal triad. Over the past two decades, research in this area has laid the foundation for the concept of 'hemostatic resuscitation' and has been the focus for management of coagulopathy in the hemorrhaging patient.

HEMOSTATIC RESUSCITATION

Hemostatic resuscitation is a dynamic model which incorporates 'damage control surgery', while emphasizing the *early and aggressive utilization of blood components to correct coagulopathy with massive transfusion protocols*. The term damage control surgery has become synonymous with the management of hemorrhaging patients. This technique emphasizes the principle of life-saving hemorrhage control followed by a period of physiologic correction prior to definitive therapies[26,27]. This requires minimal time spent in the operating room with the major resuscitation occurring in the intensive care unit. Operating room time is minimized by planning staged operations and utilization of temporary dressings (Figure 1). This technique has proven essential in the management of traumatic hemorrhage, and it can be extrapolated to the obstetric patient in two specific scenarios. First, for patients who

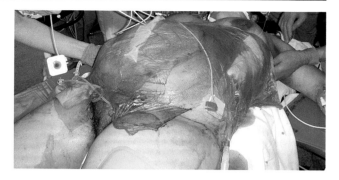

Figure 1 Temporary abdominal closure as part of damage control resuscitation

require operative intervention to manage surgical blood loss, abdominal closure should be delayed. Second, this technique may be required for patients who develop abdominal compartment syndrome as a complication of massive resuscitation and require decompressive laparotomy.

Definitive control of surgical bleeding involves several techniques including vessel ligation, embolization via an endovascular approach or utilization of pressure and packing for local hemorrhage control. The techniques of vessel ligation, embolization and packing are discussed in detail elsewhere in this textbook (see Chapters 49 and 52–54); however, one additional adjunct to packing includes the use of topical hemostatic agents (see Chapter 58). Advances in biotechnology have led to the development of these agents in the local control of hemorrhage. Examples of topical hemostatic dressings include Quick Clot (Z-Medica, Newington, CT) a zeolite-based dressing and HemCon (HemCon, Inc., Portland, OR) a chitosan-based dressing. QuickClot Combat Gauze (Z-Medica, Newington, CT) is gauze impregnated with the hemostatically active clay kaolin. These agents have proved effective in stopping hemorrhage in animal-based studies[28,29], as well as in civilian and military trauma[30–32]. Combat Gauze is the current dressing that is used by the US military. These agents also have been used for vaginal packing to treat PPH in a patient who required emergency cesarean section (Figure 2). A comprehensive review of the subject has been completed by Achneck and associates and includes an evaluation of efficacy and recent recommendations[33].

Aggressive utilization of blood components during hemostatic resuscitation entails delivery of packed red blood cells (PRBC), fresh frozen plasma (FFP) and platelets in a fixed ratio during a massive transfusion. Massive transfusion in the current literature is defined as transfusion of 10 or more units of PRBC within a 24-hour time period[34–39] (see also Chapter 4). *The ratio of 1 unit of FFP and 1 unit of platelets for each unit of PRBC has evolved over the past two decades.* Support for this concept has come through the development of mathematical models, retrospective studies in both the military and civilian settings as well as through multicenter prospective cohort studies. *The basic concept is closely to re-approximate whole blood utilizing component therapy.*

In 2003, a computer model was developed based on trauma patients receiving a massive transfusion at a major trauma center in the United States. This computer model predicted the optimal ratio of PRBC to FFP was 3 : 2 and the optimal ratio of PRBC to platelets was 10 : 8 in order to prevent early coagulopathy[40]. In 2007, Borgman and associates reviewed 246 military trauma patients who underwent massive transfusion. They divided the patients into three groups based on the ratio of FFP to PRBC transfused. A low ratio of FFP to PRBC was defined as 1 : 8, medium ratio was 1 : 2.5 and a high ratio of FFP to PRBC was defined as 1 : 1.4. The mortality decreased from 65% in the low ratio group to 34% in the medium and 19% in the high ratio group[41]. *Studies in civilian trauma patients yielded similar results and concluded that an FFP to packed red blood cell ratio of 1 : 1 confers a survival advantage in patients undergoing massive transfusion*[42,43].

This concept has been expanded to include the use of platelets. Holcomb and associates reviewed the records of 466 trauma patients undergoing massive transfusion and divided them into groups based on FFP and platelet ratios to PRBC. They demonstrated that when high platelet and high FFP to PRBC ratios are combined there was a decrease in hemorrhage and increase in 6 hour, 24 hour and 30 day survival[44]. An additional multicenter retrospective study reviewed transfusion ratios during the first 6 hours after admission. Compared with a platelet to PRBC ratio of more than 1 : 4 versus 1 : 1, 6 hour mortality decreased from 22.8% to 3.2%[45]. While these studies show strong support for the use of high ratios of FFP and platelets to PRBC, it should be noted that not all studies support improved outcomes[46,47].

Retrospective studies showing a benefit of hemostatic resuscitation are potentially confounded by survival bias. Due to the fact that blood components are not administered in a uniform fashion, enhanced survival rates could be due to the fact that patients who received a higher ratio of FFP to PRBC simply live long enough to receive the FFP transfusions, which take time to prepare. Early massive transfusion is dominated by the use of PRBCs because of immediate availability in most centers. Later in the massive transfusion other products become available. Therefore, patients who die early will have received a low ratio of platelets and plasma to PRBCs.

Snyder and associates analysed 134 trauma patients who underwent massive transfusion. Similar to other studies, they found a 63% lower risk of death for patients who received high ratio (1 : 1.3) compared with patients who received a low ratio (1 : 3.7). However, the survival benefit was no longer seen when they treated the FFP : PRBC ratio as a time-dependent co-variate[35]. *Although controversy in opinions exists, the vast majority of authors agree transfusion of a high ratio of FFP and platelets to PRBCs confers a survival advantage in patients undergoing massive transfusion*[7,34,38, 40,41,43,47–55]. *Many trauma centers in the United States presently have adopted a 1 : 1 : 1 ratio of PRBC to FFP to*

platelets as the standard during a massive transfusion and recommend this as a goal ratio in hemostatic resuscitation[7,15, 38,41,42,49–51,55,56] (Figure 3). The ability to transfuse high ratios is facilitated by maintaining a quantity of thawed plasma at all times. In resource poor environments when component therapy is not available, fresh whole blood is superior to high ratio component therapy[57–59]. In order to effectively achieve the goal of a 1 : 1 : 1 ratio, however, massive transfusion protocols should be in place.

MASSIVE TRANSFUSION PROTOCOLS

Massive transfusion protocols (MTPs) vary considerably from institution to institution and no internationally accepted protocol exists. Nevertheless, they should be considered an integral part of hemostatic resuscitation. The goal of these protocols is to produce an algorithmic, proactive, ratio-based approach to facilitate timely blood product release and mitigate blood bank delays[19,51]. Retrospective analyses have compared the mortality rates for trauma patients requiring massive transfusion before and after implementation of a MTP. In addition to a decrease in mortality, these studies have

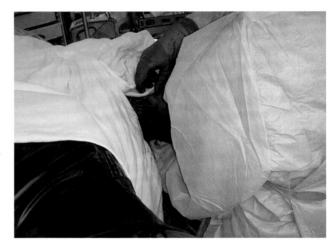

Figure 2 Vaginal packing with Combat Gauze to treat postpartum hemorrhage

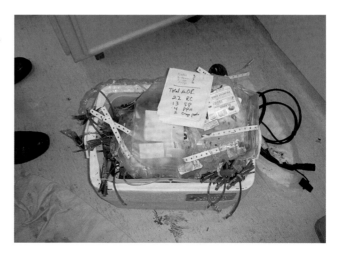

Figure 3 Example of massive transfusion protocol ratios

also demonstrated a decrease usage of crystalloids and an increased FFP : PRBC ratio[60,61].

Cotton and associates developed a trauma exsanguination protocol (TEP) which involved immediate and continued release of blood bank products in a predefined ratio. All TEP activations were retrospectively evaluated with a comparison cohort of patients who received more than 10 units of PRBCs in the 2 year time period prior to TEP initiation at their center. A multivariate analysis was performed which demonstrated a 74% reduction in mortality among patients in the TEP group ($p = 0.001$). Additionally, overall blood product consumption was significantly reduced in the TEP group[62].

COMPLICATIONS OF MASSIVE TRANSFUSION

The transfusion of blood in humans is never devoid of the possibility of complications. This statement has always been true but is more important for clinicians to be aware of as traditional transfusion practices change and patients receive higher ratios of FFP and platelets to PRBCs. A comprehensive review of complications associated with massive transfusion was recently completed by Sihler and Napolitano[8]. Acute complications consist of allergic hemolytic and non-hemolytic transfusion reactions, transfusion related acute lung injury (TRALI), transfusion-associated circulatory overload (TACO) and electrolyte derangements such as hypocalcemia, hypokalemia and hyperkalemia. Delayed complications include transfusion-related immunomodulation (TRIM), transfusion-associated graft versus host disease (TA-GVHD), post-transfusion purpura (PTP), microchimerism, alloimmunization and iron overload[63].

Specifically, TRALI has emerged as the leading cause of transfusion-related morbidity and mortality[64,65]. TRALI is defined as acute lung injury (bilateral pulmonary infiltrates, PaO2/FiO2 ratio of 300 mmHg or less and absence of left atrial hypertension) presenting within 6 hours of transfusion and not clearly related to other risk factors for acute lung injury or acute respiratory distress[66]. FFP and platelets have been the most commonly implicated products[45,67–70], and multiple mechanisms have been proposed including the theory of an immune antibody-mediated process[71,72]. Multiparous females are the highest risk donors for TRALI events when using FFP, and many blood banks now only use FFP from male donors[65]. According to the United States Food and Drug Administration (US FDA), since the implementation of this policy, there has been a marked reduction in the incidence of TRALI from FFP and now PRBCs are the leading cause (Figure 4).

TRANSFUSION AFTER MASSIVE RESUSCITATION

Controversies exist as to what the optimal hemoglobin level should be, and different clinicians also vary on what should be the end points of resuscitation. It should be noted, however, that studies continue to

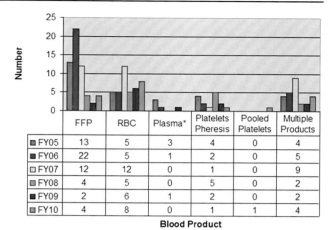

	FFP	RBC	Plasma*	Platelets Pheresis	Pooled Platelets	Multiple Products
FY05	13	5	3	4	0	4
FY06	22	5	1	2	0	5
FY07	12	12	0	1	0	9
FY08	4	5	0	5	0	2
FY09	2	6	1	2	0	2
FY10	4	8	0	1	1	4

Figure 4 Incidence of transfusion related acute lung injury per blood product given in the US 2005–2010. FY, fiscal year

demonstrate blood transfusion as an independent risk factor for infection, multiple organ failure, systemic inflammatory response syndrome and mortality. Furthermore, this increase occurs in a dose dependent manner[73–75]. In the well know Canadian transfusion trial (TRICC), younger patients and patients with a lower APACHE score were shown to have a higher mortality when a liberal transfusion strategy (hemoglobin goal of 10–12 g/dl) was followed compared with a restrictive policy (hemoglobin goal >7.0 g/dl)[75]. Subgroup analysis failed to show a benefit of liberal transfusion in patients with cardiovascular disease. Acutely hemorrhaging patients and patients with active coronary ischemia were excluded from this study[76]. Once definitive hemorrhage control is confirmed, unnecessary transfusions should be avoided to lessen the risk of additional adverse consequences.

PRACTICE POINTS

- Identification and treatment of the components of the 'lethal triad' is critical to the management of the exsanguinating patient

- Transfusion of a high ratio of FFP and platelets to PRBCs confers a survival advantage in patients undergoing massive transfusion

- Massive transfusion protocols (MTP) should be considered an integral part of damage control and hemostatic resuscitation

- Once control of hemorrhage has been established, a restrictive policy regarding blood transfusion should be instituted.

References

1. Sauaia A, Moore FA, Moore EE, Read RA, et al. Epidemiology of trauma deaths: a reassessment. J Trauma 1995;38: 185–93
2. Peng R, Chang C, Gilmore D, Bongard F. Epidemiology of immediate and early trauma deaths at an urban level I Trauma Center. Am Surg 1998;64:950–4

3. Levy JH, Dutton RP, Hemphill JC 3rd, et al. Multi-disciplinary approach to the challenge of hemostasis. Anesthes Analges 2010;110:354–64

4. McLaughlin DF, Niles SE, Salinas J, et al. A predictive model for massive transfusion in combat casualty patients. J Trauma 2008;64(2 Suppl):S57–63

5. Moore EE. Thomas G. Orr Memorial Lecture. Staged laparotomy for the hypothermia, acidosis, and coagulopathy syndrome. Am J Surg 1996;172:405–10

6. Kashuk JL, Moore EE, Millikan JS, Moore JB. Major abdominal vascular trauma – a unified approach. J Trauma 1982;22: 672–9

7. Beekley ACFACS. Damage control resuscitation: A sensible approach to the exsanguinating surgical patient. Critical Care Medicine. The Evolution of Military Trauma and Critical Care Medicine: Applications for Civilian Medical Care Systems 2008;36(Suppl):S267–74

8. Sihler KC, Napolitano LM. Complications of massive transfusion. Chest 2010;137:209–20

9. Kermode JC, Zheng Q, Milner EP. Marked temperature dependence of the platelet calcium signal induced by human von Willebrand factor. Blood 1999;94:199–207

10. Jurkovich GJ, Greiser WB, Luterman A, Curreri PW. Hypothermia in trauma victims: an ominous predictor of survival. J Trauma 1987;27:1019–24

11. Djaldetti M, Fishman P, Bessler H, Chaimoff C. pH-induced platelet ultrastructural alterations. A possible mechanism for impaired platelet aggregation. Arch Surg 1979;114:707–10

12. Meng ZH, Wolberg AS, Monroe DM, 3rd, Hoffman M. The effect of temperature and pH on the activity of factor VIIa: implications for the efficacy of high-dose factor VIIa in hypothermic and acidotic patients. J Trauma 2003;55: 886–91

13. Martini WZ, Holcomb JB. Acidosis and coagulopathy: The differential effects on fibrinogen synthesis and breakdown in pigs. Ann Surg 2007;246:831–5

14. Hess JR. Blood and coagulation support in trauma care. Hematology Am Soc Hematol Educ Program 2007;187–91

15. Hess JR, Holcomb JBMC, Hoyt DB. Damage control resuscitation: the need for specific blood products to treat the coagulopathy of trauma. Transfusion 2006;46:685–6

16. Ganter MT, Brohi K, Cohen MJ, et al. Role of the alternative pathway in the early complement activation following major trauma. Shock 2007;28:29–34

17. Brohi K, Singh J, Heron M, Coats T. Acute traumatic coagulopathy. J Trauma 2003;54:1127–30

18. Brohi K, Cohen MJ, Ganter MT, Matthay MA, Mackersie RC, Pittet JF. Acute traumatic coagulopathy: initiated by hypoperfusion: modulated through the protein C pathway?. Ann Surg 2007;245:812–8

19. Griffee MJ, Deloughery TG, Thorborg PA. Coagulation management in massive bleeding. Curr Opin Anaesthesiol 2010;23:263–8

20. Scheingraber S, Rehm M, Sehmisch C, Finsterer U. Rapid saline infusion produces hyperchloremic acidosis in patients undergoing gynecologic surgery. Anesthesiology 1999;90: 1265–70

21. Todd SR, Malinoski D, Muller PJ, Schreiber MA. Lactated Ringer's is superior to normal saline in the resuscitation of uncontrolled hemorrhagic shock. J Trauma 2007;62:636–9

22. Kiraly LN, Differding JA, Enomoto TM, et al. Resuscitation with normal saline (NS) vs. lactated ringers (LR) modulates hypercoagulability and leads to increased blood loss in an uncontrolled hemorrhagic shock swine model. J Trauma 2006;61:57–64

23. Watters JM, Brundage SI, Todd SR, et al. Resuscitation with lactated ringer's does not increase inflammatory response in a Swine model of uncontrolled hemorrhagic shock. Shock 2004;22:283–7

24. Healey MA, Davis RE, Liu FC, Loomis WH, Hoyt DB. Lactated ringer's is superior to normal saline in a model of massive hemorrhage and resuscitation. J Trauma 1998;45: 894–9

25. Martini WZ, Dubick MA, Pusateri AE, Park MS, Ryan KL, Holcomb JB. Does bicarbonate correct coagulation function impaired by acidosis in swine? J Trauma 2006;61:99–106

26. Rotondo MF, Schwab CW, McGonigal MD, et al. 'Damage control': an approach for improved survival in exsanguinating penetrating abdominal injury. J Trauma 1993;35:375–82

27. Hirshberg A, Mattox KL. Planned reoperation for severe trauma. Ann Surg 1995;222:3–8

28. Alam HB, Chen Z, Jaskille A, et al. Application of a zeolite hemostatic agent achieves 100% survival in a lethal model of complex groin injury in swine. J Trauma 2004;56:974–83

29. Pusateri AE, McCarthy SJ, Gregory KW, et al. Effect of a chitosan-based hemostatic dressing on blood loss and survival in a model of severe venous hemorrhage and hepatic injury in swine. J Trauma 2003;54:177–82

30. Cox ED, Schreiber MA, McManus J, Wade CE, Holcomb JB. New hemostatic agents in the combat setting. Transfusion 2009;49(Suppl 5):248S–55S

31. Rhee P, Brown C, Martin M, et al. QuikClot use in trauma for hemorrhage control: case series of 103 documented uses. J Trauma 2008;64:1093–9

32. Wedmore I, McManus JG, Pusateri AE, Holcomb JB. A special report on the chitosan-based hemostatic dressing: experience in current combat operations. J Trauma 2006;60:655–8

33. Achneck HE, Sileshi B, Jamiolkowski RM, Albala DM, Shapiro ML, Lawson JH. A comprehensive review of topical hemostatic agents: efficacy and recommendations for use. Ann Surg 2010;251:217–28

34. Teixeira PG, Inaba K, Shulman I, et al. Impact of plasma transfusion in massively transfused trauma patients. J Trauma 2009;66:693–7

35. Snyder CW, Weinberg JA, McGwin G Jr, et al. The relationship of blood product ratio to mortality: survival benefit or survival bias? J Trauma 2009;66:358–62

36. Niles SE, McLaughlin DF, Perkins JG, et al. Increased mortality associated with the early coagulopathy of trauma in combat casualties. J Trauma 2008;64:1459–63

37. Cancio LC, Wade CE, West SA, Holcomb JB. Prediction of mortality and of the need for massive transfusion in casualties arriving at combat support hospitals in Iraq. J Trauma 2008; 64(2 Suppl):S51–5

38. Sihler KC, Napolitano LM. Massive transfusion: new insights. Chest 2009;136:1654–67

39. Schreiber MA, Perkins J, Kiraly L, Underwood S, Wade C, Holcomb JB. Early predictors of massive transfusion in combat casualties. J Am Coll Surg 2007;205:541–5

40. Hirshberg A, Dugas MDO, Banez EI, Scott BG, Wall MJJ, Mattox KL. Minimizing dilutional coagulopathy in exsanguinating hemorrhage: a computer simulation. J Trauma 2003;54:454–63

41. Borgman MA, Spinella PC, Perkins JG, et al. The Ratio of Blood Products Transfused Affects Mortality in Patients Receiving Massive Transfusions at a Combat Support Hospital. J Trauma-Injury Infect Crit Care 2007;63:805–813

42. Duchesne JC, Hunt JP, Wahl GNREMTP, et al. Review of current blood transfusions strategies in a mature level i trauma center: were we wrong for the last 60 years? J Trauma 2008;65:272–78

43. Maegele M, Lefering R, Paffrath T, et al. Working Group on Polytrauma of the German Society of Trauma Surgery (DGU). Red-blood-cell to plasma ratios transfused during massive transfusion are associated with mortality in severe multiple injury: a retrospective analysis from the Trauma Registry of the Deutsche Gesellschaft fur Unfallchirurgie. Vox Sang 2008;95:112–9

44. Holcomb JB, Wade CE, Michalek JE, et al. Increased plasma and platelet to red blood cell ratios improves outcome in 466 massively transfused civilian trauma patients. Ann Surg 2008; 248:447–458

45. Silliman CC, Boshkov LK, Mehdizadehkashi Z, et al. Transfusion-related acute lung injury: epidemiology and a prospective analysis of etiologic factors. Blood 2003;101: 454–62

46. Kashuk JL, Moore EE, Johnson JL, et al. Postinjury life threatening coagulopathy: is 1:1 fresh frozen plasma:packed red blood cells the answer? J Trauma 2008;65:261–70

47. Scalea TM, Bochicchio KM, Lumpkins K, et al. Early aggressive use of fresh frozen plasma does not improve outcome in critically injured trauma patients. Ann Surg 2008;248:578–84

48. Hess JR, Holcomb JB. Transfusion practice in military trauma. Transfus Med 2008;18:143–50

49. Gonzalez EA, Moore FA, Holcomb JB, et al. Fresh frozen plasma should be given earlier to patients requiring massive transfusion. J Trauma 2007;62:112–9

50. Ho AMH, Dion PW, Cheng CAY, et al. A mathematical model for fresh frozen plasma transfusion strategies during major trauma resuscitation with ongoing hemorrhage. Can J Surg 2005;48:470–8

51. Greer SE, Rhynhart KK, Gupta R, Corwin HL. New developments in massive transfusion in trauma. Curr Opin Anaesthesiol 2010;23:246–50

52. Sperry JL, Ochoa JB, Gunn SR, et al. An FFP:PRBC transfusion ratio >/=1:1.5 is associated with a lower risk of mortality after massive transfusion. J Trauma 2008;65:986–93

53. Zink KA, Sambasivan CN, Holcomb JB, Chisholm G, Schreiber MA. A high ratio of plasma and platelets to packed red blood cells in the first 6 hours of massive transfusion improves outcomes in a large multicenter study. Am J Surg 2009;197:565–70

54. Gunter OL, Jr Au BK, Isbell JM, Mowery NT, Young PP, Cotton BA. Optimizing outcomes in damage control resuscitation: identifying blood product ratios associated with improved survival. J Trauma 2008;65:527–34

55. Johansson PI, Stensballe J. Hemostatic resuscitation for massive bleeding: the paradigm of plasma and platelets—a review of the current literature. Transfusion 2010;50:701–10

56. Holcomb JBFACS, Jenkins DFACS, Rhee PFACS, et al. Damage control resuscitation: directly addressing the early coagulopathy of trauma. J Trauma 2007;62:307–10

57. Repine TB, Perkins JG, Kauvar DS, Blackborne L. The use of fresh whole blood in massive transfusion. Early Massive Trauma Transfusion: Current State of the Art. J Trauma 2006;60(Suppl):S59–S69

58. Spinella PC, Perkins JG, Grathwohl KW, Beekley AC, Holcomb JB. Warm fresh whole blood is independently associated with improved survival for patients with combat-related traumatic injuries. J Trauma 2009;66(4 Suppl):S69–76

59. Kauvar DS, Holcomb JB, Norris GC, Hess JR. Fresh whole blood transfusion: a controversial military practice. J Trauma 2006;61:181–84

60. Dente CJ, Shaz BH, Nicholas JM, et al. Improvements in early mortality and coagulopathy are sustained better in patients with blunt trauma after institution of a massive transfusion protocol in a civilian level I trauma center. J Trauma 2009;66:1616–24

61. Johansson PI, Stensballe J. Effect of haemostatic control resuscitation on mortality in massively bleeding patients: a before and after study. Vox Sang 2009;96:111–18

62. Cotton BA, Gunter OL, Isbell J, et al. Damage control hematology: the impact of a trauma exsanguination protocol on survival and blood product utilization. J Trauma 2008;64:1177–82

63. Hendrickson JE, Hillyer CD. Noninfectious serious hazards of transfusion. Anesthes Analges 2009;108:759–69

64. Goldman M, Webert KE, Arnold DM, et al. Proceedings of a consensus conference: towards an understanding of TRALI. Transfus Med Rev 2005;19:2–31

65. Triulzi DJ. Transfusion-related acute lung injury: current concepts for the clinician. Anesthes Analges 2009;108:770–6

66. Toy P, Popovsky MA, Abraham E, et al. National Heart, Lung and Blood Institute Working Group on TRALI. Transfusion-related acute lung injury: definition and review. Crit Care Med 2005;33:721–6

67. Gajic O, Dzik WH, Toy P. Fresh frozen plasma and platelet transfusion for nonbleeding patients in the intensive care unit: benefit or harm? Crit Care Med 2006;34(5 Suppl):S170–3

68. Holness L, Knippen MA, Simmons L, Lachenbruch PA. Fatalities caused by TRALI. Transfus Med Rev 2004;18:184–8

69. Gajic O, Rana R, Mendez JL, et al. Acute lung injury after blood transfusion in mechanically ventilated patients. Transfusion 2004;44:1468–74

70. Khan H, Belsher J, Yilmaz M, et al. Fresh-frozen plasma and platelet transfusions are associated with development of acute lung injury in critically ill medical patients. Chest 2007;131:1308–14

71. Bux J, Sachs UJ. The pathogenesis of transfusion-related acute lung injury (TRALI). Br J Haematol 2007;136:788–99

72. Sachs UJ. Pathophysiology of TRALI: current concepts. Intens Care Med 2007;33(Suppl 1):S3–S11

73. Moore FA, Moore EE, Sauaia A. Blood transfusion. An independent risk factor for postinjury multiple organ failure. Arch Surg 1997;132:620–5

74. Dunne JR, Malone DL, Tracy JK, Napolitano LM. Allogenic blood transfusion in the first 24 hours after trauma is associated with increased systemic inflammatory response syndrome (SIRS) and death. Surg Infect 2004;5:395–404

75. Hébert PC, Wells G, Blajchman MA, et al. A multicenter, randomized, controlled clinical trial of transfusion requirements in critical care. Transfusion Requirements in Critical Care Investigators, Canadian Critical Care Trials Group. N Engl J Med 1999;340:409–17

76. Hebert PC, Yetisir E, Martin C, et al. Is a low transfusion threshold safe in critically ill patients with cardiovascular diseases? Crit Care Med 2001;29:227–34

4

Transfusion Management of Obstetric Hemorrhage

E. Lockhart

INTRODUCTION

The importance of transfusion medicine in the management of postpartum hemorrhage (PPH) cannot be overstated and is reflected in the historical record with the first series of successful human-to-human transfusions being performed by James Blundell in 1818, a London obstetrician treating patients with PPH[1]. Blundell wrote the following[2]:

> '. . . if you have under care a patient in whom the flooding has been copious, in whom, further, the womb has been emptied, and the haemorrhages been stopped; should this woman, as I have myself on several occasions seen, be sinking gradually into the grave, so that even to those who have seen much of floodings the case appears to be without hope: under such circumstances, I affirm that it is highly proper to have recourse to the operation of transfusion, provided we are competent to perform it.'

Such prescriptions remain valid today. Without the timely availability of blood products to treat life-threatening anemia and correct the resulting coagulopathy, the morbidity and mortality from obstetric hemorrhage would surely be higher than the current estimates of 100,000–140,000 annually[3,4]. Indeed, the countries with the worst mortality rates from obstetric hemorrhage have significant disadvantages with respect to available medical care[5], including the presence of an adequate and safe blood supply[6,7].

Even in developed countries with sophisticated systems of providing medical care, delayed or improperly executed transfusion contributes to morbidity and mortality associated with obstetric hemorrhage[8]. Compared to other medical disciplines such as emergency medicine and cardiothoracic surgery, hemorrhage requiring transfusion is a relatively rare event in daily obstetric practice. Estimates for PPH incidence vary in the literature but range from 3 to 5%, with less than 1% of obstetric patients being transfused, often in the direst of emergency situations[9,10]. This circumstance results in a lack of familiarity among obstetricians regarding the indications for the use of specific blood components, requesting appropriate laboratory assessment of coagulopathies, and, of equal importance, the mechanisms for ordering blood products emergently. The recently observed increases in PPH incidence in the US and other high resource countries underscore the importance of increasing knowledge of transfusion practice among obstetricians[10,11]. The goal of this chapter is to provide a concise review of blood products and their use in obstetric hemorrhage, with emphasis on transfusion management of massive obstetric hemorrhage. *[Editor's note: This chapter comprises two major sections: a thorough discussion of the various components of blood transfusion products and an exceptional section on management of major obstetric hemorrhage. Readers have the option to continue as their specific interests direct them. L.G.K.]*

BLOOD TRANSFUSION PRODUCTS

Red blood cells

Product description and selection for transfusion

Erythrocytes are the primary delivery system of oxygen to tissues, and play a secondary role for transport of carbon dioxide and nitric oxide as well as in the minor regulation of vascular tone[12]. Erythrocytes are most commonly transfused as packed red blood cells (pRBC), a source of concentrated erythrocytes obtained from either citrated whole blood by centrifugation or the sedimentation of red cells; apheresis (the extracorporeal separation of blood components by centrifugation) is an alternative method of preparation. pRBC units are stored with citrate anticoagulant and a preservative solution to allow extension of storage up to 42 days. Volumes of pRBC units after addition of preservative solution normally range between 300 and 400 ml[13]. These pRBC products are hemoconcentrated relative to circulating blood, with typical pRBC unit hematocrits ranging from 55 to 65%[14], although flow properties remain similar to whole blood. Storage of pRBC units is maintained at 1–6°C, and units must be transfused within 4 hours after issue from the blood bank if not kept under refrigeration.

Because hemolytic transfusion reactions are a significant risk of red cell transfusion, prevention of this potentially fatal occurrence is of primary importance in the selection of pRBC units for transfusion. A pre-transfusion type and screen test achieves this in two manners: first, identifying the patient's ABO group and RhD type and, second, screening the patient's serum for clinically significant red cell alloantibodies to other non-ABO blood group antigens. Identification of non-ABO alloimmunization is of particular importance in obstetric transfusion, as fetomaternal hemorrhage with maternal exposure to foreign RBC antigens occurs in virtually all pregnancies[15]. Red cell units selected for transfusion must not only be ABO compatible with the recipient's plasma (see Table 1), but also antigen negative for any RBC alloantibody specificity. Compatibility between donor and recipient must be determined prior to transfusion by either serologic or computer crossmatching[16]. Provision of ABO-group specific blood is typically possible within 10–15 minutes once type and screen is complete; on the other hand, identification of additional RBC alloantibodies requires serologic crossmatching which can take 45 minutes or longer, depending on compatible pRBC unit availability. When the delay in issuing type-specific or antigen-negative blood would potentially be life threatening, emergency uncrossmatched (most often group O) blood may be administered prior to completion of compatibility testing. Whenever possible, however, emergency uncrossmatched blood provided to women of childbearing age should be RhD negative to avoid the risk of RhD alloimmunization[16].

The need for large volumes of pRBC units during a massive transfusion may necessitate giving antigen-positive units to antigen-negative or previously sensitized patients. For patients who are not previously sensitized (i.e. giving RhD positive units to an RhD negative patient), this may increase the likelihood of alloimmunization, putting future pregnancies at increased risk for hemolytic disease of the fetus and newborn (HDFN). Estimations for RhD alloimmunization after transfusion range from 30 to 80%[17], with lower alloimmunization rates noted for other clinically significant RBC antigens. If under such circumstances the patient receives one RhD-positive pRBC unit, dosing of anti-RhD immunoglobulin depends on the total volume of RhD-positive red cells administered[18]. Should the patient receive two or more RhD-positive units, exchange transfusion can reduce the total circulating RhD antigen burden as well as reduce the amount of anti-RhD immunoglobulin needed for prophylaxis[19]. Regardless

of the amount transfused, consultation with a transfusion medicine physician is recommended for advice regarding management.

Increased vigilance for RBC alloantibody detection should be in place for pregnancies occurring after massive transfusion. For women receiving anti-RhD immunoglobulin as prophylaxis after receiving RhD-positive RBC units, serologic testing for anti-RhD formation may not be conclusive for several months after dosing[19]. Clinicians transfusing uncrossmatched blood in the context of obstetric hemorrhage also should be aware of the increased risk of hemolytic transfusion reactions due to the risk of an undetected clinically significant recipient antibody directed against the recipient's red cells (see section on Acute hemolytic transfusion reactions below). In a patient with life-threatening hemorrhage, not uncommon in the course of PPH, the risk of hemolysis in antigen-positive transfusions to alloimmunized patients must be balanced against the risk of exsanguination.

Indications and contraindications

The only widely accepted criterion for pRBC transfusion is for treatment of symptomatic anemia. Signs and symptoms of blood loss such as diaphoresis, dizziness and tachycardia correlate with blood volume loss up to 15% of a patient's total blood volume, a volume typically lost during a normal vaginal or uncomplicated cesarean delivery[20]. These early clinical signs of hemorrhagic shock may be somewhat masked, however, by the parturient's presentation at delivery. Progression of hypovolemic shock with blood loss greater than 25–30% total blood volume will present with hypotension, agitation, tachypnea, oliguria progressing to anuria and, finally, collapse and cardiac arrest. The time duration between the early and later signs of shock is not rigid, and therefore careful attention to the patient's blood loss at time of delivery (including occult blood loss under drapes or intra-abdominally), vital signs and symptoms is critical in preventing the progression of irreversible shock by providing timely RBC transfusion[21].

Transfusion guidelines for red cells often reference specific levels as triggers in patients without active hemorrhage. For example, the American Society of Anesthesiology Task Force on Blood Product Replacement states that pRBC transfusion is rarely indicated with a hemoglobin level of more than

Table 1 ABO compatibility of blood products for adult transfusion

Recipient blood group	Recipient alloantibodies	ABO Compatible blood products			
		Packed red blood cells	*Plasma*	*Platelets**	*Cryoprecipitate*
O	Anti-A, anti-B	O	A, B, AB, O	A, B, AB, O	A, B, AB, O
A	Anti-B	A or O	A, AB	A, B, AB, O	A, B, AB, O
B	Anti-A	B or O	B, AB	A, B, AB, O	A, B, AB, O
AB	None	A, B, AB, O	AB	A, B, AB, O	A, B, AB, O

*ABO-incompatible platelet transfusions should be avoided if possible to prevent recipient hemolysis from high-titer donor ABO isoagglutinins as well as decreased platelet survival

10 g/dl and virtually always indicated with a hemoglobin less than 6 g/dl[22]. The American Association of Blood Banks (AABB) has recommended that, in stable hospitalized patients without cardiovascular disease, a restrictive RBC transfusion trigger of a hemoglobin level 7–8 g/dl be employed[23]. However, in patients with brisk hemorrhage, target hemoglobin levels (such as 8 g/dl) are often cited, but no consensus on this point exists[24].

A growing number of observational studies suggest that erythrocytes undergo significant alterations during prolonged storage that result in several adverse patient outcomes, including infection, prolonged hospital admission and a higher risk of morbidity and mortality[25]. Considering the widely recognized risks of allogeneic transfusion (infectious disease exposure, transfusion reactions and alloimmunization to RBC antigens, among others) and potential risks from RBC storage, a conservative approach to red cell transfusions may be prudent in the patient who is not experiencing acute and/or massive blood loss. Transfusion decisions between those thresholds should be driven by alterations in the physical exam and vital signs, co-morbidities and the potential for continued blood loss[26]. Stated another way, red cell transfusion should not be administered as a panacea to correct anemias when circumstances permit correction with pharmacologic or nutritional therapies, such as erythropoietin or iron supplementation.

Dose and therapeutic effects

In a 70 kg adult with normal blood volume, a single pRBC unit can be expected to increase the recipient's hemoglobin by 1 g/dl or the hematocrit by 3%. In obstetric patients, however, whose blood volume at term can be as high as 50% above baseline, the expected hemoglobin increase post-transfusion could potentially be substantially less. The accurate assessment of transfusion responses is particularly difficult in patients with active hemorrhage, so replacement of red blood cell mass may be in part driven by clinical judgment and the use of massive transfusion protocols (see below).

Plasma

Product description and selection for transfusion

Plasma is the acellular fraction of blood, separated from the cellular blood components by either centrifugation of citrated whole blood or donor apheresis, with typical units averaging just under 300 ml volume. Currently, multiple forms of plasma are in use worldwide for replacement of all coagulation factors, including the labile factors FV and FVIII. The most widely recognized form is fresh frozen plasma (FFP), so named because of the regulatory requirement for freezing at −18°C or below within 8 hours of collection[13]. Plasma frozen within 24 hours after phlebotomy (FP24) is a product with growing usage; it is similar to FFP in its preparation from whole blood

except that it is frozen at or below −18°C within 24 hours after collection[13]. The preparation of plasma products for transfusion requires thawing at 30–37°C and typically requires approximately 30 minutes. If the prepared plasma is not transfused within the initial 24-hour post-thaw period, it can be relabeled as 'thawed plasma' for use within 5 days after the initial thaw[27]. The use of thawed plasma not only extends the available plasma inventory, but also provides rapidly available plasma products for management of massive hemorrhage, particularly emergency uncross-matched AB plasma for use when the patient's blood type is unknown[28]. Solvent/detergent-treated plasma (SD-P) is an additional pooled plasma product which undergoes a pathogen inactivation treatment, most frequently with 1% tri-(n-butyl)phosphate and 1% Triton-X 100. This treatment significantly inactivates lipid-enveloped viruses such as HIV[29], but is ineffective against non-lipid enveloped viruses such as hepatitis A. Although SD-P retains clotting factor levels close to those in other licensed plasma products, some reductions in protein C, protein S and antitrypsin activity have been noted[30,31]. Currently this product is not approved for use in the US, but is available in Europe and other jurisdictions.

Plasma contains ABO isoagglutinins, the naturally occurring antibodies directed against ABO antigens, and therefore must be ABO-compatible with the recipient's red cells (see Table 1). Group AB plasma, which lacks the isoagglutinins directed against A and B antigens, is compatible with all blood types and is used as emergency release plasma when there is insufficient time for determining the recipient's blood type. RhD compatibility between donor and recipient is not required for plasma transfusion.

Indications

Notable variation exists in published guidelines for plasma transfusion[32], although agreement is present on its indication for replacement of coagulation factors in bleeding or surgical patients, particularly those suffering from disseminated intravascular coagulation (DIC) or undergoing massive transfusion. Consensus on laboratory values for transfusion 'triggers' is lacking, but many guidelines recommend use of the international normalized ratio (INR) at or greater than 1.5 as a range which would indicate the need for plasma transfusion[33]. For massive hemorrhage, empiric transfusion of plasma in set ratios to RBC units is widely practiced (as discussed in the section on massive transfusion), although definitive data for accepting this practice as standard of care are lacking[34].

Plasma is indicated for coagulation factor replacement in patients with congenital factor deficiencies (such as factors II, V, X and XI), but should not be used for factor replacement in congenital factor deficiencies if a specific factor concentrate is available (e.g. FVIII in hemophilia A patients). Additional indications include rapid reversal of warfarin in an actively bleeding patient, but considering the contraindication for use of warfarin in pregnancy, such use should virtually never be seen in routine obstetric practice. Contraindications for plasma include its use as a colloid blood volume expander, a nutritional supplement, or as a source of immunoglobulin.

Dose and therapeutic effect

A volume of 1 ml of plasma in a non-pregnant individual contains approximately 1 unit of coagulation factor activity; plasma products contain slightly less than 1 U/ml clotting factors due to the approximately 10% dilution from the anticoagulant solution[35] and the biological variability in factor levels between individual donors[36]. Administration of a 10–20 ml/kg dose of plasma typically increases circulating coagulation factor levels by 20–30%[37]. This dosage would be appropriate for FFP and FP24, as well as for thawed plasma; these three products are considered essentially equivalent for almost all clotting factors except for FV and FVIII, despite slight variations between clotting factors existing between these products[38–40]. Higher plasma doses present increasing risks for volume overload in the recipient unless given in the context of ongoing blood loss or therapeutic plasmapheresis.

Cryoprecipitate and plasma, cryoprecipitate reduced

Product description and selection for transfusion

Cryoprecipitate, also known as cryoprecipitated anti-hemophilic factor or 'cryo', is a blood fraction derived from frozen plasma by thawing at 1–6°C and collection of the cold-precipitated proteins, typically yielding 10–15 ml per plasma unit derived from whole blood. This fraction contains enriched amounts of factor VIII, von Willebrand factor (vWF), fibrinogen, fibronectin and factor XIII[13]. Cryoprecipitate is stored frozen at −18°C or below, and preparation time for this product also takes 30 minutes or more for thawing and pooling individual units into one dose. Unlike plasma, cryoprecipitate cannot be stored in a thawed form, and it is the blood product which routinely takes the longest time to prepare when used in massive transfusion. After thawing, cryoprecipitate must be kept at room temperature prior to transfusion. Cryoprecipitate administration in adults does not need to be ABO compatible, although the use of large volumes of ABO-incompatible cryoprecipitate may result in positive direct antiglobulin test results in recipients and, rarely, mild hemolysis[41]. Rh compatibility does not need to be considered for pre-transfusion product selection.

The remaining plasma supernatant after the preparation of cryoprecipitate is termed plasma, cryoprecipitate-reduced, also known as 'cryo-poor plasma' or cryosupernatant. This blood fraction is depleted in vWF, FVIII, FXIII and fibrinogen as compared to other plasma products. However, many other remaining clotting factors are found at levels similar to those in FFP or FP24, including factors II, V, VII, IX, X and XI[13,35].

Indications, dosage and therapeutic effect

Cryoprecipitate was originally used as a source of FVIII in patients with hemophilia A; however, the availability of safer and more concentrated FVIII sources has largely superseded its use in these patients. The primary indication for cryoprecipitate in modern transfusion practice is as a fibrinogen concentrate[41]. Cryoprecipitate remains the only widely available fibrinogen concentrate in the US, whereas purified pharmacologic fibrinogen concentrates are available in Europe[42]. Each unit of cryoprecipitate is expected (according to FDA requirement) to contain at least more than 80 IU FVIII and more than 150 mg fibrinogen, with typical adult doses ranging from 6 to 10 pooled units. The 2009 Circular of Information jointly issued by the FDA, the Red Cross, the AABB and other responsible organizations recommends the following formula for calculating cryoprecipitate dosage: body weight (in kg) × 0.02 = number of cryoprecipitate units to raise fibrinogen by 50–100 mg/dl[13]. Recovery of transfused fibrinogen from cryoprecipitate can be impacted by thrombosis or fibrinolysis. A recent retrospective review of plasma fibrinogen increments following cryoprecipitate transfusion in the setting of trauma found a mean increase of 55 mg/dl after an average of 8.7 units (±1.7) transfused[43].

The depletion of FVIII, fibrinogen, vWF and FXIII in cryosupernatant limits its utility for use as a plasma product, and it is not an equivalent substitute for FFP, FP24, or thawed plasma. The primary use for cryosupernatant is as a replacement fluid during therapeutic apheresis for treatment of thrombotic thrombocytopenic purpura[13]. However, it has potential utility for treating acquired coagulation factor deficiency in Jehovah's Witness patients. Whereas many Jehovah's Witness patients refuse transfusion, the Jehovah's Witness community leadership has allowed for individuals to consider accepting processed fractions of blood products[44]. Cryoprecipitate, as a fraction of plasma, has been accepted by some Jehovah's Witness patients in treating coagulopathy associated with cardiopulmonary bypass[45]. Similarly, some Jehovah's Witness patients may accept cryosupernatant (after informed consent) for treating other sources of acquired clotting factor deficiencies[46], such as obstetric hemorrhage (see Chapter 72 for a full discussion of PPH in Jehovah's Witness patients).

Platelets

Product description

Platelets are small (2–3 μm in diameter) anucleate cell fragments which not only bind to injury sites, providing a phospholipid scaffold upon which coagulation enzymes assemble for thrombin generation, but also contribute key protein and molecular elements for fibrin clot formation[47]. Platelets for transfusion are obtained from preparation of platelet concentrates, whole blood or donor platelet apheresis. Platelet concentrates contain greater than 5.5×10^{10} platelets per unit derived from a single 450–500 ml whole blood collection, with a typical adult dose formed by pooling four to six concentrates[13]. Apheresis platelets contain greater than 3×10^{11} platelets per unit, and have the advantage over platelet concentrates in that they represent only a single donor exposure per transfusion, reducing the risk of transfusion-transmitted infections[48]. Some *in vitro* differences have been observed between platelets derived from the different collection methods[49], although differences regarding their *in vivo* properties remain uncertain. Most blood banks and transfusion services use these products interchangeably, driven in part by cost and individual product availability[50].

Platelet concentrates have several properties which make them unique among the blood products discussed in this chapter. First, platelets are cold intolerant. Exposure of platelet concentrates to refrigeration temperatures of 4°C results in platelet shape changes, functional defects and increased circulatory clearance rates[51–53]. Second, platelets have the shortest shelf life of any transfused product: the time from the point of collection to expiration is a mere 5 days. This is due in part to the relatively short functional life of platelets (7–10 days in the circulation), but also to the risks of storing platelets at room temperature which allows for ongoing bacterial proliferation of potentially contaminated units[54]. Platelets, whether in the form of platelet concentrate or apheresis platelets, are a plasma-rich product. In ideal circumstances, this product should be ABO compatible with the recipient to avoid the infusion of ABO isoagglutinins. However, inventory shortages may prompt the use of ABO-incompatible platelets at times. Whereas the vast majority of ABO-incompatible platelet transfusion recipients suffer no ill effects, hemolytic transfusion reactions have been reported in rare instances after such transfusions[55,56]. The ABO-incompatible platelet transfusions at highest risk are those from group O single donor products administered to group A or B recipients, due to the tendency of group O individuals to form high titer anti-A and anti-B[57]. Finally, although platelets do not bear RhD antigens, trace red blood cell content in platelet products support the practice of transfusing RhD-negative donor platelets to RhD-negative recipients to avoid alloimmunization. Should inventory shortages necessitate transfusion of RhD-positive platelets to RhD-negative recipients, treatment with an anti-RhD immunoglobulin product can be considered to avoid RhD alloimmunization[56]. The British Committee for Standards in Haematology recommend 250 IU anti-RhD immunoglobulin for prophylaxis of up to five adult-sized doses of RhD-positive platelets given in a 6 week period[19].

Indication, dose and therapeutic effect

Platelet transfusion serves two purposes: (1) as prophylaxis against hemorrhage in severely thrombocytopenic patients (most widely defined as less than 10,000/µl platelets); and (2) for treatment of bleeding in patients with thrombocytopenia or platelet dysfunction[13,48,58]. Circumstances necessitating prophylactic platelet transfusion are rarely encountered in parturients, and the less than 10,000/µl platelet transfusion trigger was established primarily in patients with hematologic malignancy and/or stem cell transplant recipients with hypoproliferative thrombocytopenia[48]. For obstetric patients, on the other hand, a higher prophylactic transfusion threshold may be considered in light of the large vascular uteroplacental interface, but to date no studies specifically address this clinical question. Therapeutic platelet transfusion in the context of massive transfusions or DIC should be administered with the aim of keeping the recipient's platelet count at more than $50 \times 10^9/l$[59].

MASSIVE TRANSFUSION IN POSTPARTUM HEMORRHAGE

Timely recognition of excessive blood loss of PPH is critical for successful transfusion management. Such recognition is challenging, not only because of difficulties in assessing volume of blood loss at the time of delivery, but also because of variability in the definitions of massive hemorrhage. Although the definition of excessive hemorrhage in obstetric patients at time of delivery has been widely accepted as blood loss of greater than 500 ml for vaginal deliveries and 1000 ml for cesarean deliveries, as discussed in other chapters of the text, obstetricians' estimations of blood loss at time of delivery generally are erroneous and skewed towards underestimations of these volumes[60] (see Chapters 9 and 41). Moreover, the reported literature uses a variety of definitions when clinicians are assessing hemorrhage.

Hemoglobin levels showing a 10 g/dl decrease or greater from antepartum levels have been suggested as a measure of severe PPH, but this construct has very limited practical utility during acute management[61]. Definitions of what constitutes massive hemorrhage in non-obstetric patients (primarily civilian trauma or military casualties) have shown even greater variability, and have been cited as transfusion of more than 10 pRBC units within 24 hours, a loss of more than one entire blood volume within 24 hours, or a loss of more than 50% of the total blood volume within 3 hours[35,62]. Meta-analysis of retrospective massive transfusion studies suggests that these massive hemorrhage definitions under count patients who suffer mortality due to hemorrhage and who may benefit from management with massive transfusion protocols[63]. Clinicians, in general, and obstetricians, in particular, are therefore left to balance multiple considerations at the bedside when determining whether a parturient has crossed the threshold into the zone of what will retrospectively be regarded as excessive blood loss.

Massive transfusion in trauma

Equally daunting to obstetricians is determining the appropriate transfusion management in massive PPH, particularly as no published studies at the time of this writing describe results and outcomes from this specific population on which to base decisions[64]. Rather, the vast majority of data regarding massive transfusion is derived from military and trauma settings and/or databases. Uncontrolled hemorrhage in trauma patients is often complicated by coagulopathy arising from tissue damage, hypothermia, under perfusion and acidosis. Further complicating this self-perpetuating 'bloody vicious cycle'[65] was the adoption of resuscitation protocols first derived from casualty management in the Korean and the Vietnam Wars. These protocols promoted aggressive crystalloid infusion first to support blood pressure and cardiac output, followed by red cell transfusion to replace oxygen-carrying capacity; and only then were plasma and platelet transfusions recommended to correct coagulopathy observed in laboratory testing, a factor which required time and expertise, and clearly delays treatment in obstetric patients[66]. Although worldwide expert opinion embraced these protocols in the 1980s and early 1990s[67–69], they were never subject to randomized controlled trials. Eventually it became apparent that high volume crystalloid resuscitation not only increased coagulopathy in patients with hemorrhagic shock, but also increased adverse outcomes such as acute respiratory distress syndrome and cardiac dysfunction[70].

A retrospective review of Iraq military casualties drew attention to the potential for the preemptive use of plasma, showing a striking difference between mortality rates in patients receiving low and high ratio plasma : RBC concentrations (1 : 8 plasma : RBC, 69% mortality versus 1 : 1.4 plasma : RBC ratio, 19% mortality)[71]. Similar findings have been found in controlled observational studies of trauma patients requiring massive transfusion, with improved survival noted in patients who received higher plasma : RBC transfusion ratios[66,72,73]. Pooled analysis of 10 observational studies where the plasma : RBC ratios ranged from 1 : 2.5 to 1 : 1 showed an association with significantly reduced mortality (odds ratio 0.38, 95% confidence interval 0.24–0.60)[74].

Platelet transfusion in trauma-related coagulopathy has similarly been examined, with both military[75] and civilian data[76,77] showing improved survival with higher platelet : RBC transfusion ratios. Based on the data emerging from recent military experiences, the Surgeon General of the United States Army issued guidelines for use of massive transfusion in combat as follows: plasma : RBC : platelet transfusions in a 1 : 1 : 1 ratio, with a single platelet unit equaling a platelet concentrate derived from whole blood collection[78].

Fibrinogen

The early coagulopathy seen in trauma not only results in coagulation factor and platelet consumption, but also hypofibrinogenemia. Observational studies performed during the early 21st century suggest that early transfusion of cryoprecipitate may convey a survival advantage in trauma patients. A retrospective review of 252 massively transfused military casualties showed a high fibrinogen : RBC ratio, defined as 0.2 g fibrinogen or more (totaled from all transfused blood products) per RBC unit, was significantly associated with improved survival (24% mortality in high fibrinogen : RBC versus 52% mortality in low fibrinogen : RBC ratios, $p < 0.001$) and decreased deaths due to hemorrhage (44% incidence in high fibrinogen : RBC group versus 85% incidence in low fibrinogen : RBC group, $p < 0.001$)[79]. Civilian trauma data comparing a prospective cohort ($n = 132$) to historic controls ($n = 84$) showed a similar association, with those receiving more than 1 : 1 cryoprecipitate : RBC units having a significantly higher 24-hour and 30-day survival as compared to those receiving less than 1 : 2 cryoprecipitate : RBC (84% versus 57% and 66% versus 41% survivals, respectively; $p < 0.01$ for both)[76].

These findings regarding the role of fibrinogen in massive transfusion may be of particular importance for obstetric hemorrhage management, as pregnant women between 35 and 42 weeks' gestation show a marked elevation in fibrinogen levels, with reference ranges reported from 350 to 650 mg/dl as compared to 197–401 mg/dl in non-pregnant individuals[80]. Clinical observation by obstetricians suggests that the fibrinogen level decreases more rapidly in the obstetric patient undergoing massive hemorrhage compared to individuals with war-induced or civilian trauma, but this possibility has not been subject to verification (personal communication from Cynthia Wong to Louis Keith February 22, 2012). Charbit and colleagues examined 128 women suffering from PPH, defined as either severe or non-severe, to determine whether routine coagulation laboratory testing abnormalities were predictive of PPH severity[81]. In multivariate analysis, fibrinogen levels less than 2 g/dl were the only marker associated with PPH severity, with a positive predictive value of 100%. [*Editor's note: This study is seminal and has not yet been replicated in the published literature. However, a personal discussion with Dr Anne-Sophie Ducloy-Bouthors in London on February 25, 2012 confirmed that this was her experience as well, when asked specifically about the Charbit reference. L.G.K.*]

There is biologic plausibility in considering that, similar to massive transfusion in trauma, patients with obstetric hemorrhage may benefit from more aggressive fibrinogen replacement. Indeed, fibrinogen concentrates such as Haemocomplettan® or RiaSTAP® (both CSL Behring, Marberg, Germany), have been used in obstetric hemorrhage management in Europe, with salutary patient outcomes presented as correction of hypofibrinogenemia or reduced blood product transfusion[82–84]. A randomized controlled trial in Denmark is currently enrolling subjects, comparing 2 g of fibrinogen concentrate versus saline early in the course of PPH with the primary outcome examining the incidence of allogeneic blood product transfusion[85]. This study should provide insight into the utility of fibrinogen concentrates in PPH management.

Massive transfusion protocols for postpartum hemorrhage

The potential for applying these emerging massive transfusion data from trauma and military cohorts to patients with PPH is slowly becoming more appreciated by the obstetric community[86]. However, not all institutions have specific protocols for obstetric massive transfusion[87], and fewer still have published these protocols. In 2007, Burtelow and colleagues from Stanford University Medical Center described applying a trauma massive transfusion protocol to obstetric patients suffering PPH[88]. In this protocol, an emergency release package of six pRBC, four thawed plasma and one apheresis platelet are rapidly prepared and delivered in less than 15 minutes. The protocol also describes reflexive laboratory assessment of coagulopathy, with initial values for PT/aPTT, fibrinogen, D-dimer and a complete blood count drawn at the time of protocol activation. Additional blood product administration was given algorithmically based on abnormal lab values in the context of ongoing hemorrhage, with additional massive transfusion protocol (MTP) packages delivered as needed. The California Maternal Quality Care Collaborative Task Force collated best practices from nine maternal hemorrhage protocols derived from expert opinion in obstetrics and hematology[89]. Common elements between these protocols included: (1) partnership between obstetric teams and transfusion services for rapid release of 'obstetrical hemorrhage packs' to include RBC, platelets, plasma and cryoprecipitate; (2) availability of a local expert (hematologist or transfusion medicine physician) for consultation as needed; and (3) a scripted protocol for maternal hemorrhage response which is periodically practiced and assessed. In addition, laboratory assessment of hemoglobin, platelet count, PT/aPTT and fibrinogen is recommended to be performed every 30 minutes until the patient is stabilized.

These published obstetric hemorrhage MTPs bear similarities to trauma MTPs in their higher plasma : RBC ratios (both published protocols having no lower than a 2 : 3 ratio) and early incorporation of platelets and cryoprecipitate. Despite this, creation of obstetric transfusion protocols based on the current trauma data should be approached with a sense of caution for several reasons. Current data on the use of high plasma : RBC ratios in trauma settings are entirely derived from observational studies. Numerous potential sources of bias have been identified in these studies, such as survivor bias, failure to include other pro-hemostatic therapies (such as recombinant factor VIIa) in data interpretation, and lack of standardization between treatment groups[66,72]. Moreover, the majority of trauma data are collected from male patients, particularly those data from military settings. Significant baseline hematologic differences exist between this mostly male cohort and pregnant females, particularly in the coagulation system where pregnant women have significantly higher levels of fibrinogen, factors VII, VIII and IX, and protein S[80] as well as significant expansion of plasma volume. Additionally, higher plasma doses during massive transfusion could potentially be associated with a greater risk of acute respiratory distress syndrome, as suggested by a prospective study of over 1100 adults with blunt trauma[90].

A collaborative review of observational studies to date by the AABB Clinical Transfusion Medicine Committee and subject matter experts recommends neither for nor against use of plasma : RBC transfusion ratios of 1 : 3 or more[91]. Nevertheless, the panel noted that both the death rate and the risk of multiorgan failure were both reduced by 60% as compared to controls, and strongly urged that the question of high plasma : RBC transfusion ratios be addressed in randomized controlled trials. However, until such studies are performed in patients suffering from obstetric hemorrhage, questions will remain regarding the fundamental pathophysiologic difference between trauma and obstetric massive transfusion[64].

Antifibrinolytic therapy

Pharmacologic therapy has shown promise in serving as an adjunct to transfusion in PPH management. Antifibrinolytics may be a particularly useful therapy in light of the increased fibrinolysis which occurs during the third stage of labor and persists for several hours after delivery[92]. Tranexamic acid (TXA), a lysine analogue which competitively blocks plasminogen binding to fibrin, has garnered attention for its use in both preventing and treating PPH[93,94]. A recent multicentered randomized trial examined use of high-dose TXA in treating acute PPH as defined by blood loss exceeding 800 ml within 2 hours after vaginal delivery[95]. Women were randomized to receive either placebo or 4 g TXA given over 1 hour followed with 1 g infused over 6 hours, with transfusion limited to pRBC units until blood loss exceeded 2500 ml ($n = 72$ for each group). Blood loss in the 6 hours following delivery was significantly lower in the TXA group than in the control group (median 170 ml; first to third quartiles, 58–323 ml) than in controls (221 ml; first to third quartiles 110–543 ml) ($p = 0.041$). Additionally, the duration of severe PPH was significantly shorter (median 30 minutes (first to third quartile, 15–40 minutes) compared to median 30 minutes (first to third quartile, 20–93 minutes) ($p = 0.001$), and the overall amount of either plasma transfusion or fibrinogen concentrate administration was significantly less in the TXA group as compared to controls ($n = 1$ versus $n = 7$, $p < 0.001$).

A further large-scale investigation of TXA is currently enrolling subjects: the World Maternal Antifibrinolytic (WOMAN) trial, sponsored by the London School of Hygiene and Tropical Medicine[96,97]. This 15,000 subject multicenter randomized controlled trial will be investigating whether TXA reduces mortality, rate of hysterectomy and other morbidities in PPH following vaginal or cesarean delivery, as well as examining critical safety issues such as thromboembolic events after its use in the setting of PPH. The impact of maternal treatment with TXA on the rate of thromboembolism in breastfed babies will also be monitored. The current literature is encouraging for use of TXA to reduce PPH severity and the overall exposure to allogeneic transfusion. The results of the WOMAN trial will help provide definitive evidence regarding incorporation of tranexamic acid in PPH protocols.

COMPLICATIONS OF TRANSFUSION

Transfusion complications are similar to the potential deleterious effects of organ transplantation in that they often derive from immunologic complications or contamination with infectious agents. A comprehensive review of all adverse transfusion reactions is beyond the scope of this chapter, but transfusion management of obstetric hemorrhages requires familiarity with acute transfusion reactions which may complicate therapy and require rapid intervention (Table 2).

Acute hemolytic transfusion reaction

Acute hemolytic transfusion reactions are one of the most serious complications of transfusion and remain one of the leading causes of transfusion-related mortality worldwide[98]. They result from RBC lysis or accelerated clearance by the reticuloendothelial system resulting from RBC transfusion into a recipient with pre-formed antibodies directed against donor erythrocytes. Only rarely have plasma-rich blood products been implicated in hemolytic reactions directed against recipient erythrocytes[55,56]. Antibodies directed against ABO antigens are the most frequent source of incompatibility, but occasionally alloimmunization against other antigens such as RhD, Duffy, Kidd and Kell is also implicated. The most frequent causes of hemolytic transfusion reactions are clerical errors in

patient identification (either at the time of pretransfusion sample collection or at the point of transfusion) or laboratory errors during compatibility testing[99].

Signs and symptoms of acute hemolysis are not specific, and may include one or more of the following: fever, hypotension, chills/rigors, pain at the infusion site, flank/back/chest pain and coagulopathic bleeding. While these findings are potentially confounded in patients suffering from PPH, hemoglobinemia and hemoglobinuria are the most reliable clues that intravascular hemolysis has transpired. Complement cascade activation by hemolytic antibodies precipitates the lysis of erythrocytes, as well as generating bradykinin, histamines and anaphylatoxins, which may result in shock and DIC[99]. As hemolytic transfusion reactions have been reported after transfusion volumes as small as 30 ml[100], clinicians must maintain constant vigilance for early indicators and immediately terminate any transfusion when such a reaction is first suspected. Rapid notification of the blood bank is essential for serologic compatibility investigation as well as for confirming accuracy of patient identification. Patients may develop hemolytic transfusion reactions after receiving pRBC units having undergone mechanical or osmotic hemolysis due to mishandling, infusion through small-bore IV needles, or co-infusion through IV lines containing incompatible patient support should be directed towards early treatment of hypotension and maintenance of urine output with intravenous fluids, diuretics, inotropes and vasopressors. Patients should also be assessed for the development of DIC with clotting factor replacement as required with platelet, plasma and either cryoprecipitate or fibrinogen concentrate administration (see Blood component administration box below).

Septic transfusion reaction

In most countries, bacterial contamination of blood products remains the leading infectious complication of transfusion. Sources of bacterial contamination most commonly are the donor's skin and blood, but loss of blood product sterility can occur at any step from the point of collection to the moment of bedside infusion. Gram-positive skin commensal organisms such as *Staphylococcus epidermidis* are the most frequent contaminants, but Gram-negative bacteria are also implicated, particularly in severe reactions resulting from endotoxin accumulation in the contaminated blood products[105]. The most commonly affected products are platelet concentrates due to their requirement for storage at room temperature, occurring in up to 1 : 2000 platelet units[106]. While 1 : 2000 platelets are contaminated, the incidence of septic reactions is much lower (around 1 : 12,000 units). Incidence of reactions is dependent upon the bacterial burden in the unit at the time of transfusion and the immune state of the recipient. Many countries, including the US, have culture-based bacterial screening of platelet concentrates. Such procedures have significantly decreased, but not entirely eliminated, the risk of

Table 2 Acute versus delayed adverse transfusion reactions

Acute (onset <24 h post-transfusion)	Delayed (onset >24 h post-transfusion)
Acute hemolysis	Delayed hemolysis
Febrile non-hemolytic	Post-transfusion purpura
Bacterial contamination	Iron overload
Transfusion-related acute lung injury (TRALI)	Graft-versus-host disease
Allergic/anaphylactic	Transfusion-related immunomodulation
Volume overload	Infectious disease*
Metabolic derangement	HIV
Hypocalcemia/citrate toxicity	Viral hepatitis
Hyperkalemia	HTLV
Hypothermia	Cytomegalovirus
Acidosis	Syphilis
	West Nile virus
	Trypanosoma cruzi
	Creutzfeld-Jacob disease
	Malaria

*Note: This is a partial list of transfusion-transmitted infections. Potentially, a multitude of infectious diseases may be transfusion transmissible
HTLV, human T-cell lymphotropic virus

BLOOD COMPONENT ADMINISTRATION

Protocols and procedures for blood administration are the last line of defense in preventing errors which can lead to potentially fatal transfusion reactions. The following list describes critical steps in bedside safety; failure to ensure any of these should prompt withholding of transfusion and return of the blood product to the blood bank[101,102]:

(1) *Positive patient identification* Confirmation of at least two independent patient identifiers (such as full name and date of birth or medical record number) should be performed at the bedside with a second health care provider or barcoding system.

(2) *Component identification* The compatibility tag attached to the unit must be compared to the patient's identification to confirm the unit has been crossmatched to the patient. Spelling discrepancies or omissions in identifier data are contraindications for proceeding with transfusion.

(3) *Medical order* Verify that the patient has a transfusion order by a licensed medical professional for the specific component. Also confirm ordered modifications of the blood product have been performed by inspecting the label (i.e. leukoreduction or irradiation).

(4) *Blood type* Confirm compatibility of the component's ABO group and Rh type with that of the recipient.

(5) *Visual inspection* Blood components should not be transfused if there are visible abnormalities, such as discoloration, clots, or loss of bag integrity.

(6) *Blood product expiration* The expiration date of the component must be confirmed. In addition, blood components should be infused within 4 hours of time of dispense from the blood bank.

Filters and infusion sets

Blood components are administered through IV tubing sets with filters designed to remove harmful clots and debris. Standard sets contain filters with pore sizes between 170 and 260 μm, while micro-aggregate filters (most frequently used during cardiac bypass blood recirculation) have pore sizes of 20–40 μm. Separate filters specifically designed for leukocyte removal are required for bedside leukoreduction of blood components, if pre-storage leukoreduced blood products are not available and leukoreduction is indicated. Manufacturer's instructions should be followed for proper use.

Intravenous solutions and medications

With the exception of 0.9% normal saline (USP), no medications or solutions should be administered simultaneously with blood components through the same tubing[101]. Co-infusion of non-approved solutions or medications may results in reversal of blood component anticoagulation (resulting in clotting) or hemolysis.

Rapid infusion and blood warmer devices

Non-emergent transfusions of single units in adults are typically completed in between 30 and 120 minutes. In patients with massive PPH, significantly faster transfusion rates may be required. A combination of pressure infusion devices and large bore intravenous tubing designed for rapid infusion can achieve transfusion rates as fast as 1500 ml/min[102]. Such flow rates require appropriate filters, as filters with small pore size can significantly slow transfusion rates or cause hemolysis. Since rapid transfusion of chilled blood components has been associated with hypothermia and cardiac arrest[102], the use of rapid infusers has been coupled to the use of blood warmers, devices which safely warm blood components. Indications for use of blood warmers include massive transfusion and an administration rate of more than 50 ml/ min for 30 minutes or more[103]. Blood warmers should be used and maintained according to manufacturer's instructions, with validation of protocols derived from these instructions, and warming of blood components should only be performed in equipment specifically licensed for such use[103]. Non-approved devices for blood warming (such as microwave ovens or immersion in hot water) may result in thermal hemolysis with resultant severe hemolytic transfusion reactions and should not be used. Most rapid infusion devices do not induce significant mechanical hemolysis, but manufacturer inserts should be reviewed to confirm approval for use with specific blood products. Hyperkalemic cardiac arrest has been associated with use of rapid infusion devices, and patients with hemorrhagic shock may have metabolic disturbances (such as acidosis, hypocalcemia and hyperglycemia) which exacerbate hyperkalemia[104].

septic transfusion reactions in either platelets or unscreened blood products such as pRBC units[105,107].

Unlike other transfusion-transmitted infectious diseases, bacterial contamination of blood products can result in rapid and potentially fatal reactions. Signs and symptoms of septic shock (such as fever, rigors, dyspnea and hypotension) can develop within minutes of starting a transfusion, or can manifest hours or days later[107]. Initial clinical suspicion of a septic transfusion reaction should prompt immediate cessation of the transfusion, along with aggressive supportive therapy and immediate administration of broad-spectrum antibiotics. The suspected blood product should be returned to the blood bank immediately for investigation, including inspection for visible abnormalities such as discoloration or hemolysis as well as Gram stain and culture of the implicated product.

Febrile non-hemolytic transfusion reaction

Febrile non-hemolytic transfusion reactions (FNHTR) represent an essentially benign, albeit unpleasant, transfusion reaction most notable for development of fever, defined as a temperature elevation of more than 1°C or 2°F above pre-transfusion temperature. Such patients may also experience chills, rigors, nausea and vomiting, and occasionally manifest these signs and symptoms in the absence of fever. The underlying pathophysiology is believed to be primarily caused by pyrogenic cytokines, such as interleukin (IL-1), IL-6, or tumor necrosis factor (TNF)-α, which accumulate in blood products during storage[108]. Onset of symptoms can occur during transfusion, typically toward the end of transfusion due to the increasing level of cytokine exposure; rarely they will present up to 1–2 hours after transfusion due to the increasing level of cytokine exposure. Diagnosis of FNHTR is one of exclusion, having ruled out other causes of febrile reactions such as hemolytic transfusion reactions, septic reactions or contributions from co-morbidities or medications. It is important to note that FNHTR and acute hemolytic or septic reactions cannot be distinguished by clinical presentation alone; therefore, every febrile transfusion reaction should be acted upon with immediate cessation of transfusion and swift investigation. Treatment for FNHTR is supportive, including antipyretics such as acetaminophen.

Transfusion-related acute lung injury (TRALI)

Transfusion of plasma-containing blood products – which would account for all blood products except washed cellular blood products – may result in a syndrome of non-cardiogenic pulmonary edema and acute respiratory distress. Clinical findings that define this transfusion-related acute lung injury (TRALI) include: (1) onset during or within 6 hours of transfusion; (2) severe hypoxemia, such as less than 90% oxygen saturation of room air; (3) diffuse bilateral pulmonary infiltrates on chest X-ray; (4) absence of evidence suggesting volume overload; and (5) no pre-existing acute lung injury[109]. TRALI may also manifest with fever, chills, hypotension and transient leukopenia. TRALI is the leading cause of transfusion related mortality in the US as well as in Western Europe, with incidences reported as high as one in every 5000 transfusions[110].

The primary suspected pathophysiology of TRALI is believed to be a reaction between donor antileukocyte antibodies and recipient leukocytes resulting in leukocyte activation, sequestration and infiltration into the pulmonary capillary bed. Granulocyte activation results in pulmonary microvascular injury and capillary leakage with influx of proteinaceous fluid into the alveolar space[111]. Female donors sensitized to human leukocyte antigens (HLA) by pregnancy are most frequently implicated as the source of blood products which have been linked to TRALI cases. As a result, many blood collection agencies in the US and Europe limit or prohibit collection of plasma-rich blood products from female donors[112].

The diagnosis of TRALI is clinical and not based on the results of laboratory investigations for the presence of anti-leukocyte antibodies in the donor[109]. Although cognate leukocyte antibody–antigen matches are often seen in TRALI cases, their absence does not rule out TRALI[113–115]. Careful patient evaluation must be undertaken by the clinical team and transfusion service in the wake of a suspected TRALI, including post-transfusion chest X-rays, measures of oxygenation and evaluation for volume overload. Treatment is supportive and includes supplemental oxygen or mechanical ventilation. The pulmonary pathology of TRALI is not responsive to diuretics, and the role of corticosteroids remains unclear. The majority of patients recover with supportive care[109].

Allergic/anaphylaxis

Allergic reactions to blood products are one of the most common adverse complications of transfusion, with incidence rates estimated between 1 and 3%[116]. The spectrum of presentation varies widely, with the majority manifesting with solely cutaneous symptoms, such as pruritis, urticaria, erythema and angioedema[117]. These minor allergic reactions are thought to be most often mediated by recipient IgG or IgE directed against plasma proteins[99]. It is therefore not surprising to find that allergic reactions occur most frequently with plasma-rich products (including platelets), but reactions can also occur in plasma-deplete products such as red cell units. Treatment for minor allergic reactions includes cessation of transfusion and administration of an antihistamine such as diphenhydramine.

Rarely, patients present with moderate or severe allergic reactions with the potential to escalate to anaphylactic shock within minutes after symptom onset. These reactions are characterized by their systemic impact, including wheezing, bronchospasm, hypotension, nausea and vomiting, chest pain and tachycardia[116]. IgA-deficient patients who have developed class-specific anti-IgA are at risk for such severe allergic reactions; however, this group only represents a fraction of anaphylactic transfusion reactions[118]. Causative agents vary widely from anti-haptoglobin antibodies to passive transfer of allergens to which a patient is already sensitized, such as recently ingested foods (i.e. peanuts)[116,119]. Ultimately, anaphylaxis is a mostly unpredictable and potentially fatal transfusion outcome, and clinicians should be aware of this risk and act swiftly should it be encountered. Severe allergic reactions or anaphylaxis should be managed in a similar fashion to anaphylaxis from other causes, with administration of epinephrine (with or without other vasopressors), maintenance of a patent airway and crystalloid infusion to support blood pressure.

Volume overload

Transfusion-associated circulatory overload (TACO) occurs when the rate of transfusion exceeds the recipient's cardiovascular system adaption to the additional workload[99]. The rapid infusion of excessive volume can result in dyspnea, hypoxemia, elevated central venous pressure and pulmonary edema – and in the worst case scenario, congestive heart failure. The initial presentation has significant overlap with TRALI, including similar chest X-ray findings of bilateral infiltrates. Unlike TRALI, however, TACO shows symptomatic improvement with dieresis. Patients at highest risk for TACO are those with diminished cardiovascular function, relatively small intravascular volumes as compared to transfused volumes (e.g. the elderly and young pediatric patients), and severe compensated anemia such as seen in patients with chronic hemolytic anemias. Patients with suspected TACO should have any ongoing transfusion paused to establish the diagnosis, with supportive care and diuretics administered as indicated before attempting further transfusion. Resumption of transfusion should be approached with a slower infusion rate and careful vigilance for recurrent symptoms.

Metabolic complications and hypothermia

As all blood products are collected and stored in citrate-based anticoagulants, large volume transfusions have the potential to be complicated by hypocalcemia. Citrate binds divalent cations such as calcium and magnesium, and is rapidly metabolized by the liver. Whereas citrate is easily cleared during non-urgent transfusions, citrate load during massive transfusion may overwhelm this clearance mechanism. Parturients with liver dysfunction, such as acute fatty liver of pregnancy or hemolysis, elevated liver enzymes, and low platelet (HELLP) syndrome, may be particularly vulnerable to this complication. Hypocalcemia presents initially with chills, tingling, dizziness and tetany; continued progression of citrate toxicity can lead to prolonged QT interval, decreased left ventricular function and cardiac arrhythmias[120]. Typically, hypocalcemia can be managed by slowing the rate of transfusion[99]. However, in ongoing massive transfusion or in patients with liver dysfunction, calcium replacement therapy as guided by the patient's ionized calcium concentration may be required[120].

The occurrence of hypocalcemia during massive transfusion can exacerbate another potential complication: hyperkalemia. During pRBC unit storage, potassium accumulates in the supernatant secondary to impaired function of the transmembrane sodium–potassium ATP pump[120]. This potassium accumulation rarely increases to a clinically significant level. However, large volume transfusions, particularly those complicated by use of malfunctioning blood warmer or rapid infusion devices (see text box above), can rarely result in fatal hyperkalemia in adult recipients. Patients with underlying cardiac, hepatic, or renal dysfunction are especially vulnerable and should be closely monitored during massive transfusion.

Rapid infusion of refrigerated blood products may lead to hypothermia, and can worsen existing hypothermia in obstetric patients undergoing cesarean section or hysterectomy during management of PPH. Hypothermia can lead to multiple systemic derangements, including peripheral vasoconstriction, cardiac dysfunction, acidosis and coagulopathy[120]. The effects of hypothermia and acidosis on coagulation have been observed both clinically and *in vitro*. Decreases in core temperature to less than 34°C and pH less than 7.1 after massive transfusion are predictive for development of coagulopathy[117]. Activity of factor VII–tissue factor and factor Xa–Va (prothrombinase) complexes is directly dependent on temperature, with both showing a 1.1-fold loss of activity at 33°C as compared to 37°C[118]. Even more dramatically, FVIIa–tissue factor and FXa–FVa show sharp decreases in activity in acidic environments, with activity decreasing by 55% and 70% at pH 7.0, respectively[122].

The most effective treatment for hypothermia is also the best prevention: warming the room, warming the patient with blankets and heating lamps, and use of approved blood and fluid warming devices (see text box above). Restoration of tissue perfusion is the definitive therapy for acidosis in massive transfusion, but alkalinizing agents such as sodium bicarbonate can assist in increasing the blood pH during the resuscitation to improve hemostasis[120].

CONCLUSION

Following Blundell's first experiments in the 19th century, the use of blood products has become a life-saving strategy in management of obstetric hemorrhage in general and PPH in particular. Continued advances in blood banking procedures and technology in the second half of the 20th century, including component therapy, infectious disease screening and careful pre-transfusion compatibility testing, have resulted in enormous improvements in safe transfusion practices. Having acknowledged this, transfusion remains associated with numerous risks, and clinicians should be aware of them.

As we progress further into the 21st century, many questions about proper transfusion management remain unanswered. These include but are not limited to: 'What are the risks in transfusing red blood cells or platelets which may have functional changes induced by storage conditions?' and 'What is the best approach for blood product administration during massive hemorrhage?' Such questions remain highly debated among those who practice transfusion medicine, and are even more debatable with regard to obstetric transfusion because of a virtual absence of reliable data for this unique patient population.

An exception to the latter generality is the near consensus of the benefits of having and using an obstetric hemorrhage protocol which is known and available to the entire hospital staff[8,123]. These protocols effectively reduce maternal morbidity and mortality from PPH[124] and are recommended by the American College of Obstetrics and Gynecology[125], the UK Confidential Enquiry into Maternal and Child Health (CEMACH)[8] and the Joint Commission in the United States[126]. CEMACH and other academic bodies recommended that massive hemorrhage protocols should be rehearsed in conjunction with transfusion services[8]. Transfusion protocols not only provide more rapid blood product delivery and laboratory assessment of coagulopathies, but also greatly reduce clinician anxiety by creating a predictable framework for obstetric hemorrhage management[127]. Clinical laboratories and hospital blood banks are critical partners in the care of obstetric hemorrhages, and should be included in the establishment of management protocols or alerted regarding high risk obstetric patients. Active partnership and communication between obstetricians and transfusion medicine experts can help protect mothers' lives and well-being.

PRACTICE POINTS

- Transfusion is a life-saving strategy in the management of obstetric hemorrhage

- Separation of whole blood into components allows for transfusion to treat specific hematologic deficiencies in patients

- Massive transfusion in PPH may benefit from higher ratios of pro-coagulant components (such as plasma, platelets and cryoprecipitate or fibrinogen concentrates) to red blood cell components, but definitive data are lacking for obstetric patients and benefits have been extrapolated from military or civilian trauma data

- Transfusion carries risk; clinicians should be aware of how acute transfusion reactions present and be prepared rapidly to assess and treat these reactions

- All transfusion reactions should be reported to the blood bank or transfusion service at the point of recognition to allow for rapid laboratory investigation

- Multidisciplinary protocols for PPH management should actively include local transfusion medicine experts.

References

1. Baskett TF. James Blundell: the first transfusion of human blood. Resuscitation 2002 52:229–33
2. Blundell J. The principles and practice of obstetricy. London: E. Cox, 1834:349
3. Hogan MC, Foreman KJ, Maghavi M, et al. Maternal mortality for 181 countries, 1980–2008: a systematic analysis of progress towards Millennium Development Goal 5. Lancet 2010;375:1609–23
4. World Health Organization. The World Health Report 2005: Make Every Mother and Child Count. Geneva: World Health Organization, 2005
5. Geller SE, Adams MG, Kelly PJ, Kodkany BS, Derman RJ. Postpartum hemorrhage in resource-poor settings. Int J Gynaecol Obstet 2006;92:202–11
6. Improving blood safety worldwide [Editorial]. Lancet 2007; 370:361
7. World Health Organization. Blood Safety: Key Global Facts and Figures in 2011 (fact sheet #279). Geneva: World Health Organization, 2011 http://www.who.int/world blooddonorday/media/who_blood_safety_factsheet_2011.pdf
8. Lewis G, ed. The Confidential Enquiry into Maternal and Child Health (CEMACH). Why Mothers Die 2000–2002. The Sixth Report on Confidential Enquiries into Maternal Deaths in the United Kingdom. London: CEMACH, 2004
9. James AH, Paglia MJ, Gernsheimer T, et al. Blood component therapy in postpartum hemorrhage. Transfusion 2009; 49:2430–3
10. Callaghan WM, Kuklina EV, Berg CJ. Trends in postpartum hemorrhage: United States 1994–2006. Am J Obstet Gynecol 2010; 202:353e1–6
11. Knight M, Callaghan WM, Berg C, et al. Trends in postpartum hemorrhage in high resource countries: a review and recommendations from the International Postpartum Hemorrhage Collaborative Group. BMC Pregnancy and Childbirth 2009;9:55–65
12. Dzik WH. The air we breathe: three vital respiratory gases and the red blood cell: oxygen, nitric oxide, and carbon dioxide. Transfusion 2011;51:676–85
13. AABB, American Red Cross, America's Blood Centers. Circular of information for the use of human blood and blood components. Bethesda, MD: AABB, 2009
14. Kakaiya R, Aronson CA, Julleis J. Whole blood collection and component processing at blood collection centers. In: Roback JD, Grossman BJ, Harris T, Hillyer CD, eds., Technical Manual, 17th edn. Bethesda, MD: AABB, 2011: 187–226
15. Moise Jr KJ. Management of red cell alloimmunization in pregnancy. In: Sacher RA, Brecher ME, eds., Obstetric Transfusion Practice. Bethesda, MD: AABB Press, 1993: 21–47
16. Downes KA, Schulman IA. Pretransfusion testing. In: Roback JD, Grossman BJ, Harris T, Hillyer CD, eds., Technical Manual, 17th edn. Bethesda, MD: AABB, 2011: 437–62
17. Hendrickson JE, Hillyer CD. Noninfectious serious hazards of transfusion. Anesth Analg 2009;108:759–69
18. Mintz PM. Rh Immune globulin. In: Mintz PM, ed., Transfusion Therapy: Clinical Principles and Practice 3rd edn. Bethesda, MD: AABB Press, 2011:493–510
19. British Committee for Standards in Haematology. Guidelines for the use of prophylactic anti-D immunoglobulin. www.bcshguidelines.com/documents/Anti-D_bcsh_07062006.pdf
20. Bonnar J. Massive obstetric haemmorhage. Bailliere Clin Obstet Gynaecol 2000;14:1–18
21. Cohen WR. Hemorrhagic shock in obstetrics. J Perinat Med 2006;34:263–71
22. American Society of Anesthesiologists Task Force on Perioperative Blood Transfusion and Adjuvant Therapies. Practice guidelines for perioperative blood transfusion and adjuvant therapies: an updated report by the American Society of Anesthesiologists Task Force on Perioperative Blood Transfusion and Adjuvant Therapies. Anesthesiology 2006; 105:198–208
23. Carson JL, Grossman BJ, Kleinman S, et al. Red blood cell transfusion: a clinical practice guideline from the AABB. Ann Intern Med 2012 Mar 26 [Epub ahead of print]

24. So-Osman C, Cicillia J, Brand A, Schipperus M, Berning B, Scherjon S. Triggers and appropriateness of red blood cell transfusions in the post-partum patient—a retrospective audit. Vox Sanguinins 2010;98:65–9

25. Isbister JP, Shander A, Spahn DR, Erhard J, Farmer SL, Hofmann A. Adverse blood transfusion outcomes: establishing causation. Transfus Med Rev 2011;25:89–101

26. Fuller AJ, Bucklin BA. Blood Product Replacement for Postpartum Hemorrhage. Clin Obstet Gynecol 2010;53:196–208

27. Eder AF, Sebok MA. Plasma components: FFP, FP24, and thawed plasma. Immunohematology 2007;23:150–7

28. Wehrli G, Taylor NE, Haines AL, et al. Instituting a thawed plasma procedure: It just makes sense and saves cents. Transfusion 2009;49:2625–30

29. Horowitz B, Bonomo R, Prince AM, Chin SN, Brotman B, Shulman RW. Solvent/detergent-treated plasma: a virus-inactivation substitute for fresh frozen plasma. Blood 1992;79:826–31

30. Solheim BG, Seghatchian J. Update on pathogen reduction technology for therapeutic plasma: An overview. Transfus Apher Sci 2006;35:83–90

31. Gilcher RO, Smith JW. Apheresis: Principles and technology of hemapheresis. In: Simon TL, Snyder EL, Solheim BG, Stowell CP, Strauss RG, Petrides M, eds., Rossi's Principles of Transfusion Medicine, 4th edn. Oxford, UK: Wiley-Blackwell, 2009:617–28

32. Iorio A, Basileo M, Marchesini E, et al. The good use of plasma. A critical analysis of five international guidelines. Blood Transfusion 2008;6:18–24

33. O'Shaughnessy DF, Atterbury C, Bolton MP. Guidelines for the use of fresh-frozen plasma, cryoprecipitate and cryosupernatant. Br J Haematol 2004;126:11–28

34. Dzik WH, Blajchman MA, Fergusson D, et al. Clinical review: Canadian National Advisory Committee on Blood and Blood Products Massive Transfusion Consensus Conference 2011: report of the panel. Critical Care 2001;15:242

35. Ortel TO, Lockhart EL, Humphries JE. Treatment of acquired disorders of hemostasis. In: Mintz PD, ed., Transfusion Therapy: Clinical Principles and Practice, 3rd edn. Bethesda, MD: AABB Press 2010:127–66

36. Stanworth S. The evidence-based use of FFP and cryoprecipitate for abnormalities of coagulation tests and clinical coagulopathy. Hematology Am Soc Hematol Educational Program 2007:179–86

37. Spector I, Corn M, Ticktin HE. Effect of plasma transfusions on the prothrombin time and clotting factors in liver disease. N Engl J Med 1996;275:1032–7

38. Downes KA, Wilson E, Yomtovian R, Sarode R. Serial measurement of clotting factors in thawed plasma stored for 5 days [letter]. Transfusion 2001;41:570

39. Sidhu RS, Le T, Brimhall B, Thompson H. Study of coagulation factor activities in aphered thawed fresh frozen plasma at 1–6 C for five days. J. Clin Apher 2006;21:224–6

40. Yazer MH, Cortese-Hassett A, Triulzi DJ. Coagulation factor levels in plasma frozen within 24 hours of phlebotomy over 5 days of storage at 1 to 6 C. Transfusion 2008;48:2525–30

41. Callum JL, Karkouti K, Lin Y. Cryoprecipitate: the current state of knowledge. Transfus Med Rev 2009;23:177–88

42. Kreuz W, Meili E, Peter-Salonen K, et al. Efficacy and tolerability of a pasteurised human fibrinogen concentrate in patients with congenital fibrinogen deficiency. Transfus Apheres Sci 2005;32:247–53

43. Nascimento B, Rizoli S, Rubenfeld G, et al. Cryoprecipitate transfusion: assessing appropriateness and dosing in trauma. Transfus Med 2011;21:394–401

44. Hughes DB, Ullery BW, Barie PS. The contemporary approach to the care of Jehovah's witnesses. J Trauma 2008;65:237–47

45. Sniecinski RM, Chen EP, Levy JH, et al. Coagulopathy after cardiopulmonary bypass in Jehovah's Witness patients: management of two cases using fractionated components and factor VIIa. Anesth Analg 2007;104:763–5

46. West J. "Informed refusal—the Jehovah's Witness patient", Clinical Ethics in Anesthesiology: A Case-Based Textbook. Cambridge University Press, 2011:19–26

47. Hoffman M, Monroe D. A cell based model of hemostasis. Thromb Haemost 2001;85:958–65

48. Slichter SJ. Platelet transfusion therapy. Hematol Oncol Clin North Am 2007;21:697–729

49. Vasconcelos, E, Figueredo AC, and Seghatchian J. Quality of platelet concentrates derived by platelet rich plasma, buffy coat and apheresis. Transf Apher Sci 2003;29:13–16

50. Chambers L, Herman J. Considerations in the selection of a platelet component: apheresis versus whole blood-derived. Transf Med Rev 1999;13:311–22

51. Rao AK, Murphy S. Secretion defects in platelets stored at 4 degrees C. Thromb Haemost 1982;47:221–25

52. White JG, Rao GH. Microtubule coils versus the surface membrane cytoskeleton in maintenance and restoration of platelet discoid shape. Am J Pathol 1998;152:597–609

53. Hoffmeister KM, Felbinger TW, Falet H, et al. The clearance mechanism of chilled blood platelets. Cell 2003;112:87–97

54. Palavecino EL, Yomtovian RA, Jacobs MR. Bacterial contamination of platelets. Transfus Apheres Sci 2010;42:71–82

55. Fung MK, Downes KA, Shulman IA. Transfusion of platelets containing ABO-incompatible plasma: a survey of 3156 North American laboratories. Arch Pathol Lab Med 2007;131:909–16

56. Holland L. Role of ABO and Rh Type in Platelet Transfusion. Lab Medicine 2006;37:758–60

57. Josephson CD, Castillejo M-I, Grima K, Hillyer CD. ABO-mismatched platelet transfusions: Strategies to mitigate patient exposure to naturally occurring hemolytic antibodies. Transfus Apheres Sci 2010;42:83–8

58. Speiss BD. Platelet transfusions: the science behind safety, risks, and appropriate applications. Best Pract Res Clin Anaesthesiol 2010;24:65–83

59. British Committee for Standards in Haematology. Guidelines for the Use of Platelet Transfusions. Br J Haematol 2003;122:10–23

60. Bose P, Regan F, Paterson-Brown S. Improving the accuracy of estimated blood loss at obstetric haemorrhage using clinical reconstructions. BJOG 2006;113:919–24

61. Padmanabhan A, Schwartz J, Spialnik SL. Transfusion Therapy in Postpartum Hemorrhage. Semin Perinatol 2009;33:124–7

62. Holcomb J. Optimal use of blood products in severely injured trauma patients. Hematology Am Soc Hematol Educ Program 2010;2010:465–9

63. Stanworth SJ, Morris TP, Gaarder C, Goslings JC, et al. Reappraising the concept of massive transfusion in trauma. Crit Care 2010;14:R239

64. McLintock C, James AH. Obstetric hemorrhage. J Thromb Haemost 2011;9:1441–51

65. Kashuk JL, Moore EE, Millikan JS, Moore JB. Major abdominal vascular trauma—a unified approach. J Trauma 1982;22:672–9

66. Stansbury LG, Dutton RP, Stein DM, et al. Controversy in trauma resuscitation: do ratios of plasma to red blood cells matter? Transfus Med Rev 2009;23:255–65

67. Collins JA. Recent developments in the area of massive transfusion. World J Surg 1987;11:75–81

68. Hewitt PE, Machin SJ. ABC of transfusion: Massive blood transfusion. BMJ 1990;300:107–9

69. Hanf CD, Pesola G, Kvetan V. Fluid therapy in shock. In: Dutcher JP, ed., Modern Transfusion Therapy. Boca Raton, FL: CRC Press, 1990;1:177–98

70. Cotton BA, Guy JS, Morris Jr JA, Abumrad NN. The cellular, metabolic, and systemic consequences of aggressive fluid resuscitation strategies. Shock 2006;26:115–21

71. Borgman MA, Spinella PC, Perkins JG, et al. The ratio of blood products transfused affects mortality in patients

receiving massive transfusions at a combat support hospital. J Trauma 2007;63:805–13

72. Spinella PC, Holcomb JB. Resuscitation and transfusion principles for traumatic hemorrhagic shock. Blood Rev 2009;23:231–40

73. Johansson PI, Stensballe J. Hemostatic resuscitation for massive bleeding: the paradigm of plasma and platelets – a review of the current literature. Transfusion 2010;50: 701–10

74. Murad MH, Stubbs JR, Gandhi MJ, Wang AT, et al., The effect of plasma transfusion on morbidity and mortality: a systematic review and meta-analysis. Transfusion 2010;50: 1370–83

75. Perkins JG, Andrew CP, Spinella PC, et al. An evaluation of the impact of apheresis platelets used in the setting of massively transfused trauma patients. J Trauma 2009;66: S77–85

76. Shaz BH, Dente CJ, Nicholas J, et al. Increased number of coagulation products in relationship to red blood cell products transfused improves mortality in trauma patients. Transfusion 2010;50:493–500

77. Holcomb JB, Zarzabal LA, Michalek, et al. Increased platelet: RBC ratios are associated with improved survival after massive transfusion. J Trauma 2011;71:S318–28

78. The United States Army Institute of Surgical Research. Joint Theater Trauma System Damage Control Resuscitation Guideline. Available at: http://www.usaisr.amedd. army.mil/cpgs/Damage_Control_Resuscitation_10_Aug_ 11.pdf

79. Stinger HK, Spinella PC, Perkins JG, et al. The Ratio of Fibrinogen to Red Cells Transfused Affects Survival in Casualties Receiving Massive Transfusions at an Army Combat Support Hospital. J Trauma 2008;64:S79–85

80. Szecsi PB, Jorgensen M, Klajnbard A, et al. Haemostatic reference intervals in pregnancy. Thromb Haemost 2010; 103:718–27

81. Charbit B, Mandelbrot L, Samain E, et al. The decrease of fibrinogen is an early predictor of the severity of post partum hemorrhage. J Thromb Haemost 2007;5:266–73

82. Bell SF, Rayment R, Collins PW, et al. The use of fibrinogen concentrate to correct hypofibrinogenaemia rapidly during obstetric haemorrhage. Int J Obstet Anesth 2010;19: 218–23

83. Fenger-Eriksen C, Lindberg-Larsen M, Christensen AQ, et al. Fibrinogen concentrate substitution therapy in patients with massive haemorrhage and low plasma fibrinogen concentrations. Br J Anaesth 2008;101:769–73

84. Glover NJ, Collis RE, Collins P. Fibrinogen concentrate use during major obstetric haemorrhage. Anaesthesia 2010; 65:1229–30

85. US National Institutes of Health. Fibrinogen Concentrate as Initial Treatment for Postpartum Haemorrhage: A Randomised Clinically Controlled Trial (FIB-PPH). US National Institute of Health, 2012. http://clinicaltrials.gov/ ct2/show/NCT01359878?term=fibrinogen+concentrate& rank=2

86. Barbieri RL. Control of massive hemorrhage: Lessons from Iraq reach the US labor and delivery suite. OBG Management 2007;19:8–16

87. Goodnough LT, Daniels K, Wong AE, Viele M, Fontaine MF, Butwick AJ. How we treat: transfusion medicine support of obstetric services. Transfusion 2011;51:2540–8

88. Burtelow M, Riley E, Druzin M, Fontaine M, Viele M, Goodnough LT. How we treat: management of life-threatening primary postpartum hemorrhage with a standardized massive transfusion protocol. Transfusion 2007; 47:1564–72

89. Lagrew D, Lyndon A, Main E, et al. Obstetric Hemorrhage Toolkit: Improving Health Care Response to Obstetric Hemorrhage. California Maternal Quality Care Collaborative, June 2010. www.cmqcc.org

90. Watson GA, Sperry JL, Rosengart MR, et al. Fresh frozen plasma is independently associated with a higher risk of

multiple organ failure and acute respiratory distress syndrome. J Trauma 2009;67:221–7

91. Roback JD, Caldwell S, Carson J, et al. Evidence-based guidelines for plasma transfusion. Transfusion 2010;50: 1227–39

92. Hellgren M. Hemostasis during normal pregnancy and puerperium. Semin Thromb Hemost 2003;29:125–30

93. Novikova N, Hofmeyr GJ. Tranexamic acid for preventing postpartum haemorrhage. Cochrane Database Syst Rev 2010;(7):CD007872.

94. Ferrer P, Roberts I, Sydenham E, et al. Anti-fibrinolytic agents in post partum haemorrhage: a systematic review. BMC Pregnancy Childbirth 2009;9:29

95. Ducloy-Bouthors AS, Jude B, Duhamel A, et al. High-dose tranexamic acid reduces blood loss in postpartum haemorrhage. Crit Care 2011;15:R117

96. US National Institutes of Health. World Maternal Antifibrinolytic Trial (WOMAN). US National Institutes of Health, 2012. http://clinicaltrials.gov/ct2/show/ NCT00872469

97. Shakur H, Elbourne D, Gulmezoglu M, et al. The WOMAN Trial (World maternal Antifibrinolytic Trial): tranexamic acid for the treatment of postpartum haemorrhage: an international randomized, double blind placebo controlled trial. Trials 2010;11:40

98. Vamvakas EC, Blajchman MA. Blood still kills: six strategies to further reduce allogeneic blood transfusion-related mortality. Transfus Med Rev 2010;24:77–124

99. Eder AF, Chambers LA. Noninfectious complications of blood transfusion. Arch Pathol Lab Med 2007;131:708–18

100. Sazama K. Reports of 355 transfusion-associated deaths: 1976 through 1985. Transfusion 1990;30:583–90

101. Carson TH, ed. Standards for Blood Banks and Transfusion Services, 27th edn. Bethesda, MD: AABB, 2011

102. Sink BLS, Administration of Blood Components. In: Roback JD, Grossman BJ, Harris T, Hillyer CD, eds. Technical Manual, 17th edn. Bethesda, MD: AABB, 2011: 617–29

103. Hrovat TM, Passwater M, Palmer RN. Guidelines for the Use of Blood Warming Devices. Bethesda, MD: AABB, 2002

104. Smith HM, Farrow SJ, Ackerman JD, Stubbs JR and Sprung J. Cardiac arrests associated with hyperkalemia during red blood cell transfusion: a case series. Anesth Analg 2008;106:1062–9

105. Eder AF, Kennedy JM, Dy BA, et al. Bacterial screening of apheresis platelets and the residual risk of septic transfusion reactions: the American Red Cross experience (2004–2006). Transfusion 2007;47:1134–42

106. Goodnough LT. Risks of blood transfusion. Anesthesiol Clin North America 2005;23:241–52

107. Ramirez-Arcos S, Goldman M, Blajchman MA. Bacterial contamination. In: Popovsky MA, ed., Transfusion Reactions, 3rd edn. Bethesda, MD: AABB Press, 2007: 163–206

108. Heddle NM. Febrile nonhemolytic transfusion reactions. In: Popovsky MA, ed., Transfusion Reactions, 3rd edn. Bethesda, MD: AABB Press, 2007:57–103

109. Triulzi DJ. Transfusion-related acute lung injury: current concepts for the clinician. Anesth Analg 2009;108:770–6

110. Popovsky MA, Moore SB. Diagnostic and pathogenic considerations in transfusion-associated acute lung injury. Transfusion 1985;25:573–7

111. Fung YL, Silliman CC. The role of neutrophils in the pathogenesis of transfusion-related acute lung injury. Transf Med Rev 2009;23:266–83

112. Stafford-Smith M, Lockhart E, Bandarenko N, Welsby I. Many, but not all, outcome studies support exclusion of female plasma from the blood supply. Expert Rev Hematol 2010;3:551–8

113. Kopko PM, Marshall CS, Mackenzie MR, et al. Transfusion-related acute lung injury: report of a clinical lookback investigation. JAMA 2002;287:1968–71

114. Toy P, Hollis-Perry KM, Jun J, et al. Recipients of blood from a donor with multiple HLA antibodies: a lookback study of transfusion-related acute lung injury. Transfusion 2004;44:1683–8

115. Kopko PM, Paglieroni TG, Popovsky MA, et al. TRALI: correlation of antigen-antibody and monocyte activation in donor recipient pairs. Transfusion 2003;43:177–84

116. Vamvakas EC. Allergic and anaphylactic reactions. In: Popovsky MA, ed., Transfusion Reactions, 3rd edn. Bethesda, MD: AABB Press, 2007:105–56

117. Domen RE, Hoeltge GA. Allergic transfusion reactions: an evaluation of 273 consecutive reactions. Arch Path Lab Med 2003;127:316–320

118. Sandler SG, Mallory D, Malamut D, Eckrich R. IgA anaphylactic transfusion reactions. Transf Med Rev 1995;9:1–8

119. Jacobs JF, Baumert JL, Brons PP, et al. Anaphylaxis from passive transfer of peanut allergen in a blood product. N Engl J Med 2011;364:1981–2

120. Sihler KC, Napolitano LM. Complications of massive transfusion. Chest 2010;137:209–20

121. Cosgriff N, Moore EE, Sauaia A, et al. Predicting life-threatening coagulopathy in the massively transfused trauma patient: hypothermia and acidoses revisited. J Trauma 1997; 42:857–61

122. Meng ZH, Wolberg AS, Monroe DM, Hoffman M. The effect of temperature and pH on the activity of factor VIIa: implications for the efficacy of high-dose factor VIIa in hypothermic and acidotic patients. J Trauma 2003;55: S86–91

123. Joint Commission on Accreditation of Healthcare Organizations, USA. Preventing Maternal Death. Sentinel Event Alert, January 26, 2010;44:1–4

124. Skupski DW, Lowenwirt IP, Weinbaum FI, et al. Improving hospital systems for the care of women with major obstetric hemorrhage. Obstet Gynecol 2006;107: 977–83

125. American College of Obstetrics and Gynecology, ACOG Practice Bulletin: Clinical Management Guidelines for Obstetrician-Gynecologists Number 76, October 2006: postpartum Hemorrhage. Obstet Gynecol 2006;108: 1039–47

126. Joint Commission on Accreditation of Healthcare Organizations, USA. Preventing Maternal Death. Sentinel Event Alert, January 26, 2010;44:1–4

127. Benedetti TJ. Obstetric hemorrhage. In: Gabbe SG, Niebyl JR, Simpson JL, eds. Obstetrics: Normal and Problem Pregnancies, 4th edn. New York: Churchill-Livingstone, 2002: 503–38

5

Early Use of Fibrinogen in the Treatment of Postpartum Hemorrhage

O. Onwuemene, D. Green and L. G. Keith

CURRENT CONCEPTS IN THE MANAGEMENT OF POSTPARTUM HEMORRHAGE

The management of PPH has evolved over the years. Whereas the initial focus was on volume resuscitation with crystalloids followed by transfusion of red cells, attention to coagulation deficits came later, and waited until the first two processes were finished or nearly so[1]. The impetus for this triad of interventions came from the military experiences in the Vietnam War[2,3]. This treatment approach was subsequently adopted by trauma centers in the United States and Europe, but to our knowledge has never been subject to a randomized controlled trial. Recent data from military combat casualties in Afghanistan and Iraq indicate that survival after massive hemorrhage is significantly improved by the introduction of fibrinogen-containing products early in the course of resuscitation efforts[4,5], and early adoption of this approach in the management of PPH has been cautiously reported in the obstetrics literature[6,7]. However, the concept of early use of fibrinogen has not yet been widely adopted by obstetricians.

PATHOPHYSIOLOGY OF COAGULOPATHY

In the normal hemostatic response to tissue injury, thrombin generation, mediated by tissue factor and activated factor VII, is localized to the site of injury. This localization of thrombin to the site of injury leads to formation of a hemostatic plug composed of platelets and cross-linked fibrin[8]. In massive uterine hemorrhage, however, bleeding is associated with extensive clot formation and consumption of fibrinogen. As bleeding continues, these newly formed clots are fibrinogen-poor, and thrombin is able to leak from them and gain access to the systemic circulation where it binds to and depletes antithrombin. The decrease in antithrombin is exacerbated by infusions of crystalloids (Figure 1)[8,9]. The direct consequence of circulating thrombin, unopposed by antithrombin, is disseminated intravascular coagulation (DIC).

DIC is characterized by the intravascular deposition of fibrin. Plasminogen, the precursor molecule of the fibrinolytic system, is bound to fibrin and converted to plasmin, the principle fibrinolytic enzyme. Plasmin attacks circulating fibrinogen as well as fibrin, resulting in hypofibrinogenemia. In addition, the ongoing fibrinolysis generates fibrin and fibrinogen degradation products, which inhibit platelet aggregation as well as fibrin formation. The resulting consumptive coagulopathy is manifest by the depletion of fibrinogen, prothrombin, factors V and VIII, and platelets[9] which invariably results in worsening of bleeding.

Volume resuscitation

In the initial resuscitative efforts of PPH, volume resuscitation with crystalloid and colloid is the easiest and quickest supportive measure to implement and helps rapidly to improve hypovolemia. However, *in vitro* as well as *in vivo* studies show that the degree of dilutional coagulopathy and accompanying decrease in antifibrinolytic factors is proportional to the infused volume[10]. Thrombin generation is also decreased by dilution to a greater extent by crystalloid than by fresh frozen plasma (Figure 1)[8,11]. Data from a German Trauma Registry in 2006 with over 8700 patients (about 30% female) revealed that up to 34% of patients

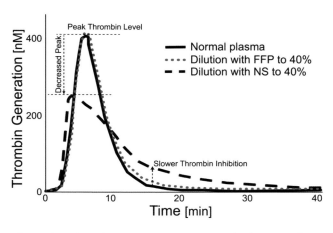

Figure 1 Thrombin generation patterns in platelet-poor plasma before and after dilution to about 40% of baseline. The patterns are similar between baseline and dilution with fresh frozen plasma (FFP). The peak thrombin level is lower (downward arrow) after dilution with normal saline (NS) because of a reduced concentration of procoagulant clotting factor. A concomitant reduction in antithrombin results in sustained thrombin activity (upward arrow). Reproduced from Bolliger *et al.*, 2010[8], with permission

presenting to the emergency room after a traumatic event were coagulopathic at the time of their presentation. Coagulopathy was associated with the extent of prior crystalloid resuscitation; however, up to 10% of patients were already coagulopathic after having received 500 ml or less of IV fluids[12]. Thus, crystalloid resuscitation may exacerbate pre-existing coagulopathy in patients with PPH.

Management of the coagulopathy

Given the circumstances outlined above, most patients with severe PPH have declining levels of fibrinogen as well as other procoagulant factors *early* in the course of bleeding. This has been clearly demonstrated in patients undergoing major surgery[12]. Therefore, as efforts are being made to control the underlying source of bleeding and restore tissue oxygenation by transfusion of red blood cells, the early introduction of fibrinogen and other procoagulants should logically be considered in obstetrics, in accord with it having been advocated so strongly by the military surgeons in today's battlefields.

Why fibrinogen first?

From the information presented above, one can appreciate that a *significant decrease in procoagulant factors and fibrinogen is present early in the course of PPH*. Furthermore, the data suggest that a decrease in fibrinogen is an early predictor of the severity of PPH[13]. Assessing this information together, the early use of fibrinogen-containing products should be prioritized in the current management of PPH. Bolliger *et al.*[9] recommend a fibrinogen target of at least 200 mg/dl. This is particularly important when one considers the normal lag time between receipt of the request for and delivery of blood products from the blood bank or fibrinogen concentrate from the pharmacy. *Waiting until fibrinogen levels are less than 100 mg/dl prior to transfusing fails to take this delay into account and runs the risk of jeopardizing patient survival.*

Fibrinogen replacement: cryoprecipitate or fibrinogen concentrate?

While both cryoprecipitate and fibrinogen concentrate are capable of correcting hypofibrinogenemia, the choice of product requires careful consideration, based on patient characteristics and availability of material. Table 1 examines a number of features of each product. RiaSTAP® is a fibrinogen concentrate which is currently approved in the US for the treatment of bleeding in congenital fibrinogen deficiency. Compared to cryoprecipitate, this fibrinogen concentrate is more potent, has less risk of infection transmission and is easier to administer. On the other hand, it is more expensive, might be more thrombogenic and is not FDA-approved for the management of PPH. However, it might be preferred over cryoprecipitate in a massively bleeding patient because it is capable of

Table 1 Comparison of cryoprecipitate and fibrinogen concentrate (RiaSTAP®)

Characteristic	Cryoprecipitate	Fibrinogen concentrate
Fibrinogen content	≥150 mg in 1 bag	900–1300 mg in 1 vial
Fibrinogen concentration	Variable from bag to bag; usual dose up to 10 bags	Indicated on label; predictable response
Viral inactivation/ removal	None	Enveloped and non-enveloped viruses*
Administration	Requires thawing, slow IV infusion	Rapid reconstitution and IV infusion
Storage	Bags must be kept frozen	Room temperature with shelf-life of 30 months
Allergy	Chills, fever, pruritus, anaphylaxis	Chills, fever, pruritus, anaphylaxis
Thrombosis	Yes	Yes

*HIV, West Nile virus, herpes simplex virus-1, hepatitis A virus, surrogates for hepatitis C virus and B19 parvovirus

rapidly and predictably increasing the fibrinogen level. A randomized, controlled trial that will examine the safety and efficacy of fibrinogen concentrate for PPH is underway in Denmark[14].

Monitoring therapy

As previously noted, waiting for the results of coagulation tests prior to infusing blood products might jeopardize the survival of a patient with severe PPH. Recent work indicates that the thromboelastograph (TEG) can assist in the selection of blood products for massively bleeding patients[15,16]. The TEG can be acquired in the emergency room, operating room, or intensive care unit to guide the selection of blood products. De Loughery suggests that fresh frozen plasma (FFP) is indicated if the TEG reaction time is prolonged, fibrinogen if the kinetics are impaired, platelets if the maximum amplitude is reduced, and inhibitors of fibrinolysis if the lysis index is increased[17]. Whether the TEG will improve the management of PPH awaits prospective studies.

Battlefield evidence

Retrospective data from casualties in army combat support hospitals in Iraq show a significant survival advantage with the introduction of fibrinogen-containing products – FFP or cryoprecipitate – early in the course of a massive transfusion protocol. A review of 246, predominantly male, battlefield-injured patients treated at a combat support hospital in Iraq revealed that patients who received a higher ratio of plasma to red blood cell transfusions had a significantly higher rate of survival. In the group with the lowest plasma to red blood cell transfusion, mortality was 65% compared to 19% ($p < 0.001$) in the group with the highest plasma to red blood cell transfusion.[18] Evaluation of a similar population looking at the ratio of fibrinogen to red cells transfused noted a comparable improvement in survival in those having received a higher ratio of fibrinogen to red cells transfused[5].

Additionally, in patients who did not receive massive transfusion (defined as ≤10 units of red blood cells), transfusion of FFP was independently associated with increased survival[19]. Findings that replicate these results have also been described in transfused civilian trauma patients[20]. It is important to note, however, that although none of these data are from prospective trials, their findings are nevertheless compelling and require attention from the obstetric community as well as the development of trials to evaluate these protocols prospectively in patients with PPH.

A need for a change from tradition

As with many things in medicine, change is slow and difficult. Nevertheless, there is an urgent need for a change in the tradition of late use of fibrinogen in management of PPH. Such changes ideally should be generated on the basis of investigations which concern themselves with patients who have PPH. Although some authors have recently recognized the importance of addressing coagulopathy and incorporating some of the findings from military data into their recommendations[21,22], the numbers are small. It is hoped that this chapter and others in this volume will spur readers to re-examine the management of severe PPH.

References

1. Watson P. Postpartum hemorrhage and shock. Clin Obstet Gynecol 1980;23:985–1001
2. Miller RD, Robbins TO, Tong MJ, Barton SL. Coagulation defects associated with massive blood transfusions. Ann Surg 1971;174:794–801
3. Miller RD. Massive blood transfusions: the impact of Vietnam military data on modern civilian transfusion medicine. Anesthesiology 2009;110:1412–6
4. Holcomb JB, Jenkins D, Rhee P, et al. Damage control resuscitation: directly addressing the early coagulopathy of trauma. J Trauma 2007;62:307–10
5. Stinger HK, Spinella PC, Perkins JG, et al. The ratio of fibrinogen to red cells transfused affects survival in casualties receiving massive transfusions at an army combat support hospital. J Trauma 2008;64(2 Suppl):S79–85
6. James AH, Paglia MJ, Gernsheimer T, Grotegut C, Thames B. Blood component therapy in postpartum hemorrhage. Transfusion 2009;49:2430–3
7. Bell SF, Rayment R, Collins PW, Collis RE. The use of fibrinogen concentrate to correct hypofibrinogenaemia rapidly during obstetric haemorrhage. Int J Obstet Anesth 2010; 19:218–23
8. Bolliger D, Gorlinger K, Tanaka KA. Pathophysiology and treatment of coagulopathy in massive hemorrhage and hemodilution. Anesthesiology 2010;113:1205–19
9. Bolliger D, Szlam F, Levy JH, Molinaro RJ, Tanaka KA. Haemodilution-induced profibrinolytic state is mitigated by fresh-frozen plasma: implications for early haemostatic intervention in massive haemorrhage. Br J Anaesth 2010;104: 318–25
10. Tanaka KA, Szlam F. Treatment of massive bleeding with prothrombin complex concentrate: argument for. J Thromb Haemost 2010;8:2589–91
11. Bolliger D, Szlam F, Molinaro RJ, Rahe-Meyer N, Levy JH, Tanaka KA. Finding the optimal concentration range for fibrinogen replacement after severe haemodilution: an in vitro model. Br J Anaesth 2009;102:793–9
12. Maegele M, Lefering R, Yucel N, et al. Early coagulopathy in multiple injury: an analysis from the German Trauma Registry on 8724 patients. Injury 2007;38:298–304
13. Charbit B, Mandelbrot L, Samain E, et al. The decrease of fibrinogen is an early predictor of the severity of postpartum hemorrhage. J Thromb Haemost 2007;5:266–73
14. Fibrinogen Concentrate as Initial Treatment for Postpartum Haemorrhage: A Randomized Clinically Controlled Trial (FIB-PPH). In: Clinical Trials.gov, ed. US National Institute of Health, 2012
15. Walsh M, Thomas SG, Howard JC, et al. Blood component therapy in trauma guided with the utilization of the perfusionist and thromboelastography. J Extra Corpor Technol 2011;43:162–7
16. DeLoughery TG. Management of acquired bleeding problems in cancer patients. Emerg Med Clin North Am 2009;27: 423–44
17. DeLoughery TG. Logistics of massive transfusions. Hematology Am Soc Hematol Educ Program 2010;2010:470–3
18. Borgman MA, Spinella PC, Perkins JG, et al. The ratio of blood products transfused affects mortality in patients receiving massive transfusions at a combat support hospital. J Trauma 2007;63:805–13
19. Spinella PC, Perkins JG, Grathwohl KW, et al. Effect of plasma and red blood cell transfusions on survival in patients with combat related traumatic injuries. J Trauma 2008;64 (2 Suppl):S69–77
20. Holcomb JB, Wade CE, Michalek JE, et al. Increased plasma and platelet to red blood cell ratios improves outcome in 466 massively transfused civilian trauma patients. Ann Surg 2008; 248:447–58
21. Pacheco LD, Saade GR, Gei AF, Hankins GD. Cutting-edge advances in the medical management of obstetrical hemorrhage. Am J Obstet Gynecol 2011;205:526–32
22. McLintock C, James AH. Obstetric hemorrhage. J Thromb Haemost 2011;9:1441–51

6

New Approaches to Transfusion Therapy for Postpartum Hemorrhage

M. J. Paidas

INTRODUCTION

Blood product replacement, first introduced in 1818, remains the mainstay of life-saving interventions for hemorrhage and in particular postpartum hemorrhage (PPH). Numerous refinements in transfusion therapy have occurred over the past several decades, whereas similar breakthrough advances in blood product replacement have not been forthcoming until quite recently and then prompted initially by the reports of surgeons practicing in battlefields.

Given the alarmingly high rate of maternal mortality, particularly in developing countries, where the maternal mortality rate associated with PPH is 34% and facilities for blood storage are often scarce to non-existent, attempts to simplify blood storage prior to its use are indeed appealing. For example, interest in lyophilization of plasma, essentially creating 'freeze dried plasma' is considerable, and this technique is actively being investigated[1]. If techniques such as these are successful, delivery of critical blood components without the need of present day storage requirements such as refrigeration may prove to be a key intervention in reducing maternal mortality globally. Unlike the futuristic approaches of storage component therapy, one intervention currently receiving intense scrutiny has the potential for transforming transfusion algorithms addressing PPH, namely fibrinogen replacement.

FIBRINOGEN AND POSTPARTUM HEMORRHAGE

Fibrinogen is an acute phase reactant, produced in the liver, and having a plasma concentration of 2.0–3.5 g/l in non-pregnant individuals[2]. In pregnancy, circulating plasma concentrations increase to 5 g/l in the third trimester. Fibrinogen has a half life of 3–5 days in plasma, and is acknowledged to play a fundamental role in hemostasis. Fibrinogen is a precursor of fibrin, which is cross linked to form blood clotting, and is a mediator of platelet aggregation. In normal pregnancy, delivery is characterized by marked increases in the clotting system and fibrinolytic activities[3].

Of relevance to PPH, however, tissue trauma and hypoperfusion both lead to acidosis, which increases fibrinogen consumption and impaired clotting. In particular, hypoperfusion triggers endothelial activation of thrombomodulin, and results in hyperfibrinolysis[4]. Severe PPH is characterized in a variety of manners including transfusion requiring four or more units of blood; estimated blood loss of 50% of circulating blood volume in under 3 h; estimated blood loss of greater than 150 ml/min within 20 min (≥50% blood volume); peripartum decrease in hemoglobin concentration of 4 g/l or more; sudden blood loss of more than 1500 ml (25% of blood volume)[5]. One landmark prospective study with 128 patients comparing severe versus non-severe PPH demonstrated the utility of measuring fibrinogen levels[6]. Univariate analysis revealed significantly lower levels of coagulation parameters fibrinogen, factor V, antithrombin and protein C antigen; and significantly elevated levels of prothrombin time, d-dimer and thrombin–antithrombin complexes. However, when multivariate analysis was performed, only the fibrinogen level remained significant as a marker of severe PPH (defined as a decrease of hemoglobin ≥4 g/l, transfusion ≥4 U packed red blood cells (pRBC), hemostatic intervention, or maternal death). In fact, the risk of severe PPH was 2.63-fold higher for each 1 g/l decrease of fibrinogen. Equally important, the negative predictive value of a fibrinogen concentration greater than 4 g/l was 79% and the positive predictive value of a fibrinogen level of 2 g/l or less was 100%.

In another, albeit retrospective review of 18,501 deliveries with 456 cases of PPH (2.5% of deliveries) with blood loss of at least 1500 ml, fibrinogen levels were found to be the best coagulation parameter correlated with blood loss ($r = 0.48$, $p < 0.01$); moreover, they fell progressively as the volume of PPH increased[7] (Figure 1). The presence of hypofibrinogenemia can be accurately, and rapidly, predicted using thromboelastometry, as demonstrated by the prospective observational study of Huissoud and colleagues[8]. Thrombelastography (TEG) and thrombelastometry (ROTEM) are viscoelastic whole-blood assays evaluating the hemostatic capacity of blood. In the Huissoud study in 37 women with PPH and 54 women without abnormal bleeding, the clotting times at 5 min (CA_5) and 15 min CA_{15}), and the maximum clot firmness were significantly lower in the PPH group than in controls (*p* <0.0001). These parameters were strongly correlated with fibrinogen levels in both groups (*r* = 0.84–0.87, *p* <0.0001) (Figure 2, Table 1). A recent Cochrane systematic review concerning the use of thrombelastography or thromboelastometry to guide transfusion therapy, although not specific to pregnancy, found a significant reduction in blood loss favoring the use of TEG/ROTEM (85 ml; 95% CI 29.4–140.7) and in the proportion of patients receiving freshly frozen plasma and platelets (relative risk (RR) 0.39, 95% CI 0.27–0.57)[9]. Table 2 lists the classification of thrombelastography and thrombelastometry parameters[10].

FIBRINOGEN REPLACEMENT THERAPY

Fibrinogen concentrate has been used to correct hypofibrinogenemia in the setting of obstetric hemorrhage. Bell and colleagues reported the use of fibrinogen concentrate to treat six cases of obstetric hemorrhage in conjunction with other blood components including platelets, fresh frozen plasma and pRBC[11]. In their experience, coagulation parameters normalized rapidly and hemorrhage improved. Table 3 highlights the differences in the volume of fibrinogen replacement products[11]. Table 4 provides characteristics of the available fibrinogen replacement products[2].

A randomized, double blind, placebo controlled trial is underway to assess the utility of fibrinogen replacement in the setting of PPH (Fibrinogen Concentrate as Initial Treatment for PPH: A Randomised Clinically Controlled Trial (FIB-PPH, Copenhagen, Denmark, ClinicalTrials.gov Identifier: NCT01359878). The aim of the study is to determine

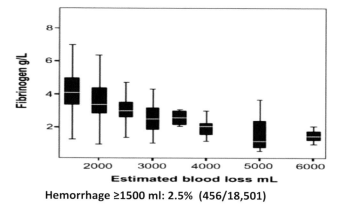

Hemorrhage ≥1500 ml: 2.5% (456/18,501)

Figure 1 Fibrinogen levels in postpartum hemorrhage. From de Lloyd *et al.*, 2011[7], with permission

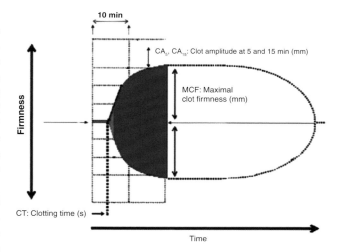

Figure 2 Assessment of fibrinogen level in PPH by thromboelastography: fib-tem® test. From Huissoud *et al.*, 2009[8], with permission

Table 1 Cut off values for CA$_5$ fib-tem® in PPH. From Huissoud *et al.*, 2009[9], with permission

Fibrinogen levels (g/l)	Fib-tem cut-off values (mm)	Sensitivity % (95% CI)	Specificity % (95% CI)	PPV % (95% CI)	NPV % (95% CI)	AUC
Fibrinogen <2	CA$_5$ = 6	100 (100–100)	87 (77–96)	50 (36–64)	100 (100–100)	0.97
Fibrinogen <1.5	CA$_5$ = 5	100 (100–100)	85 (76–95)	30 (17–43)	100 (100–100)	0.96
Fibrinogen <1	CA$_5$ = 4	100 (100–100)	86 (76–96)	13 (3–22)	100 (100–100)	0.96
Fibrinogen <2	CA$_{15}$ = 8	100 (100–100)	84 (75–94)	46 (32–60)	100 (100–100)	0.96
Fibrinogen <1.5	CA$_{15}$ = 6	100 (100–100)	88 (78–97)	33 (20–46)	100 (100–100)	0.97
Fibrinogen <1	CA$_{15}$ = 5	100 (100–100)	88 (79–97)	14 (5–24)	100 (100–100)	0.97

AUC, area under curve; CI, confidence interval; NPV, negative predictive value; PPV, positive predictive value

Table 2 Classification of thromboelastometry (TEG) and thromboelastography (ROTEM). From Armstrong *et al.*, 2011[10], with permission

Curve parameter	Definition	ROTEM® abbreviation	TEG® abbreviation	Clinical application
Clotting time (s)	Time from start of test until the start of clot formation (2 mm amplitude of deflection)	CT	r	Assesses activation of coagulation – primarily clotting factors
Clot formation time (s)	Time from beginning of clot formation to amplitude of 20 mm	CFT	k	Assesses rate of clot development
Alpha angle (°)	The angle of a tangent to the curve at 2 mm amplitude		α	Assesses both rate and strength of clot formation
Maximum clot firmness (mm)	Maximal amplitude of the curve	MCF	MA	Assesses contribution of fibrinogen and platelets to the clot
Amplitude at set times (mm)	Amplitude of the curve at 5, 10, 15 and 20 min	A5,A10	A30,60	Assesses of rate of clot formation

whether early treatment with fibrinogen concentrate (Haemocomplettan®, CSL Behring 2 g IV) compared to saline (100 ml) can reduce the incidence of blood transfusion in PPH. The study is planned to finish October 2013, after evaluating 245 patients from four hospitals in Denmark over a 2 year period. The primary outcome of the study is the incidence of transfusion with allogenic transfusion blood products during hospitalization or until 6 weeks postintervention. The secondary outcomes include the following:

(1) Severe PPH as shiown by decrease in hemoglobin more than 2.5 mmol/l, transfusion of 4 pRBC or more, or hemostatic intervention (embolization, surgical arterial ligation or hysterectomy, death);

(2) Estimated blood loss during hospitalization or until 6 weeks postintervention;

(3) Total amount of transfused blood products during hospitalization or until 6 weeks postintervention;

(4) Rebleeding during hospitalization or until 6 weeks postintervention (bleeding reoccurring after primary hemostasis) and requiring surgical procedures or intervention;

(5) Hemoglobin less than 3.6 mmol/l during hospitalization or until 6 weeks postintervention;

(6) Side-effects: including thromboembolic complications (safety measures/potential known side-effects) or until 6 weeks postintervention.

Inclusion criteria for the trial consist of informed consent from patient; women who develop PPH as bleeding from uterus and/or the birth canal within 24 h postpartum; age 18 years or older; if vaginal birth indication of either estimated blood loss of 500 ml or more and indication of manual removal of placenta or indication of manual exploration of uterus due to continuous bleeding after birth of placenta in the operating theater with anesthetic assistance; and if birth by cesarean section, perioperative blood loss of 1000 ml or more. The study exclusion criteria consist of patients with known inherited deficiencies of coagulation; patients in antithrombotic treatment antepartum due to increased risk of thrombosis; pregnancy with pre-pregnancy weight less than 45 kg; and patients who refuse to receive blood transfusion. Thromboelastography will be evaluated in the trial using the TEG/Functional Fibrinogen/Rapid-TEG, at baseline; immediately after intervention, and 4 hours and 24 hours after intervention. The baseline test is blinded to the providers, while the remainder are clinically available to the care providers. Fibrinogen levels, d-dimer, international normalized ratio (INR), platelet count, and antithrombin will be assessed as well. This trial will provide necessary data to formulate clinical guidelines regarding the use of fibrinogen replacement in the setting of PPH.

Fibrinogen therapy is a promising intervention for PPH. Key questions which remain unanswered regarding PPH are outlined below. What is the trigger for fibrinogen replacement? Will it be used for prophylaxis or treatment, or both? Where does fibrinogen fit in postpartum prevention and/or treatment

Table 3 Comparison of cost and quantity of fresh frozen plasma (FFP), fibrinogen concentrate and cryoprecipitate required to raise plasma fibrinogen concentration by 1 g/l in a 70-kg adult. From Bell et al., 2010[11], with permission

Blood product	Predicted quantity required to increase plasma fibrinogen concentration by 1 g/l (ml)	Cost to increase plasma fibrinogen concentration by 1 g/l
FFP[6]	4 units (1000 ml)	£384
Cryoprecipitate[6]	13 units (260 ml)	£478
Fibrinogen concentrate[8]	2 g (100 ml)	£440

Quantities may vary according to ongoing consumption or dilution of fibrinogen. Prices obtained from the University Hospital of Wales Blood Bank, 2008

Table 4 Comparison of attributes of fresh frozen plasma (FFP), cryoprecipitate and fibrinogen concentrate. From Rahe-Meyer and Sørensen, 2011[2], with permission

Attribute	Fibrinogen concentrate	Cryoprecipitate	Human plasma
Constituents	Pure preparation of fibrinogen (few other constituents)	Contains clotting factors VIII and XIII as well as fibrinogen Also contains von Willebrand factor	Contains all clotting factors and numerous other proteins
Safety and transmission of pathogens	Viral inactivation, therefore minimal risk of pathogen transmission No unwanted clotting factors Low thombogenic potential	No viral inactivation, therefore potential risk of pathogen transmission Transfusion of large quantities can raise levels of several coagulation factors Thrombotic risk established	No viral inactivation (except commercially produced plasma products), therefore potential risk of pathogen transmission Risk of transfusion-related reactions (e.g. TRALI) and hypervolemia
Dosing: control and consistency	Well-defined quantity of fibrinogen Accurate and consistent dosing Low infusion volume	Variable fibrinogen levels, which are donor dependent Accurate dosing not possible Low infusion volume, albeit larger than fibrinogen concentrate	Variable fibrinogen levels, which are donor dependent Accurate dosing not possible Only modest increase in fibrinogen is possible High infusion volume
Administration	Rapidly reconstituted – administered with minimal delay (5 min) No cross-matching required	Must first be thawed, delaying administration (45 min) Cross-matching is required	Must first be thawed, delaying administration (45 min) High volume: time-consuming infusion Donor-recipient AB compatibility is required

TRALI, transfusion-related lung injury

algorithm? What is the optimal dose? Should fibrinogen replacement be given before severe PPH, for example, based upon evidence of hypofibrinogenemia? The safety of fibrinogen therapy must be established, specifically related to risks of infection, thrombosis and risks with concomitant agents.

Finally, antifibrinolytic therapy has been well described in the setting of PPH prevention, as summarized in the Cochrane systematic review, which included two randomized controlled trials[12]. Blood loss greater than 400 ml was less common in women who received tranexamic acid after vaginal birth or cesarean section in the dosage of 1 g or 0.5 g intravenously (two studies, 453 women, RR 0.51, 95% CI 0.36–0.72). There were no serious side-effects reported in women who received tranexamic acid. Tranexamic acid is currently being evaluated in a very large, multicenter, international, randomized controlled trial, called the World Maternal Antifibrinolytic Trial, or WOMAN Trial. This trial is sponsored by the London School of Hygiene and Tropical Medicine will enroll 15,000 women who will be randomized to 1–2 g of tranexamic acid intravenously versus saline. The inclusion criteria are an estimated blood loss of 500 ml or more after vaginal delivery or 1000 ml or more after cesarean delivery. The primary outcome is hysterectomy or death. Secondary outcome measures are other surgical interventions, transfusions, thromboembolism and other relevant medical events[13].

CONCLUSION

In summary, soon obstetric care providers will no longer need to rely solely on the experience of clinical trials involving transfusion therapy in other specialties to guide management and tailor treatments according to the unique needs of our patients. This fact in itself represents a breakthrough in PPH management. Advances in blood component storage offer the opportunity ultimately to provide more patients with life-saving therapies in catastrophic PPH.

References

1. Inaba K. Freeze-dried plasma. J Trauma 2011;70(5 Suppl): S57–8
2. Rahe-Meyer N, Sørensen B Fibrinogen concentrate for management of bleeding. J Thromb Haemost 2011;9:1–5
3. Bremme KA. Haemostatic changes in pregnancy. Best Pract Res Clin Haematol 2003;16:153–68
4. Lier H, Böttiger BW, Hinkelbein J, Krep H, Bernhard M. Coagulation management in multiple trauma: a systematic review. Intensive Care Med 2011;37:572–82
5. Rath WH. Postpartum hemorrhage—update on problems of definitions and diagnosis. Acta Obstet Gynecol Scand 2011; 90:421–8
6. Charbit B, Mandelbrot L, Samain E, et al.; PPH Study Group. The decrease of fibrinogen is an early predictor of the severity of postpartum hemorrhage. J Thromb Haemost 2007;5:266–73
7. de Lloyd L, Bovington R, Kaye A, et al. Standard haemostatic tests following major obstetric haemorrhage. Int J Obstet Anesth 2011;20:135–41
8. Huissoud C, Carrabin N, Audibert F, et al. Bedside assessment of fibrinogen level in postpartum haemorrhage by thrombelastometry. BJOG 2009;116:1097–102
9. Gurusamy KS, Pissanou T, Pikhart H, et al. Methods to decrease blood loss and transfusion requirements for liver transplantation. Cochrane Database Syst Rev 2011;(12): CD009052
10. Armstrong S, Fernando R, Ashpole K, Simons R, Columb M. Assessment of coagulation in the obstetric population using ROTEM® thromboelastometry. Int J Obstet Anesth 2011;20:293–8
11. Bell SF, Rayment R, Collins PW, Collis RE. The use of fibrinogen concentrate to correct hypofibrinogenaemia rapidly during obstetric haemorrhage. Int J Obstet Anesth 2010;19:218–23
12. Novikova N, Hofmeyr GJ. Tranexamic acid for preventing postpartum haemorrhage. Cochrane Database Syst Rev 2010; (7):CD007872
13. Shakur H, Elbourne D, Gülmezoglu M, et al. The WOMAN Trial (World Maternal Antifibrinolytic Trial): tranexamic acid for the treatment of postpartum haemorrhage: an international randomised, double blind placebo controlled trial. Trials 2010;11:40

Section 2

Introduction

7

Is Postpartum Hemorrhage a Legacy of our Evolutionary Past?

E. T. Abrams and J. N. Rutherford

INTRODUCTION

From an evolutionary perspective, postpartum hemorrhage (PPH) is an enigma: why is something with such a high risk of death so common? This chapter suggests that the increased risk of PPH in humans compared with non-human primates is an unfortunate side-effect of natural selection for larger brains. The complementary increase in neonatal brain size over the course of human evolution was enabled by the extremely invasive pattern of human placentation, which led to an increase in complications of placental separation from the uterine wall at delivery.

Each year, approximately 350,000 maternal deaths occur worldwide. The majority take place in developing countries[1]. Worldwide, one woman in 74 will die of maternal causes; in sub-Saharan Africa, however, the risk of maternal mortality can be as high as one in six[2]. Estimates from historical data and religious groups that decline medical treatment suggest that without intervention maternal mortality rates (MMRs) would be very high, perhaps 1000–1500 maternal deaths per 100,000 live births[3]. This rate approximates the current MMR in the sub-Saharan countries with the highest rates of maternal mortality, i.e. Chad, Malawi and the Central African Republic ($n = 1065$, 1140 and 1570, respectively)[1]. Because medical interventions such as cesarean sections are a relatively recent development in the course of human history, MMRs have very likely been as high or higher in the past.

The high rate of maternal mortality in humans stems in part from two unique human adaptations: bipedalism, which emerged at the origin of the human lineage around 7 million years ago; and enlarged brains, first seen at the emergence of our genus, *Homo*, around 2 million years ago. The development of bipedalism is thought to have allowed the earliest humans to respond to climate (and therefore habitat) change by permitting more efficient terrestrial locomotion, improved evaporative heat loss, and/or the ability to carry objects while traveling. Anatomically, however, the adoption of bipedal locomotion involved numerous changes to the bony pelvis, including the lateral widening of the pelvic girdle, a feature which led to significant shifts in the mechanism of birth[4–6]. In monkeys, the long axes of the inlet, midplane and outlet of the birth canal line up in the anterior–posterior dimension, thereby allowing the widest portion of the neonatal skull (also the anterior–posterior dimension) to navigate the birth canal without rotation, despite a relatively close correspondence between the maternal pelvic dimensions and neonatal head size[4–6]. In contrast, due to the changes in the human pelvic dimensions secondary to bipedalism, the long axes of the inlet and outlet of the modern human pelvis are perpendicular[4–6]. To navigate the tortuous birth canal, the human neonate rotates twice, once to accommodate aligning the widest portion of the fetal skull with the widest dimensions of the maternal pelvis and again so the shoulders can follow, a pattern that is thought to have originated relatively early in human history[5,6]. The process of human birth became even riskier when brain size began to enlarge dramatically with the origin of the genus *Homo* around 2 million years ago. The timing of this dramatic encephalization approximately coincided with the further narrowing of the obstetric dimensions of the pelvis, an adaptation that is thought to have greatly increased the efficiency of bipedal locomotion. The resulting incompatibility between the size and shape of the bipedal pelvis and the enlarged fetal brain, also known as cephalopelvic disproportion, is an important factor in explaining the prevalence of obstructed labor in modern humans, which accounts for 8% of maternal mortality[4,5,7].

The leading cause of maternal mortality worldwide is PPH, accounting for up to 35% of maternal deaths[8]. PPH is estimated to affect 10.5% of human births worldwide[9], but, despite its ubiquity, the underlying reasons why humans are so vulnerable to this condition remain unclear. From an evolutionary perspective, PPH is an enigma: why is something with such a high risk of death so common? Most disorders with high mortality risks are uncommon, such as Tay-Sachs disease, or more common after the completion of reproduction, as is the case with many cancers. An evolutionary approach to answering this question may therefore offer a fresh perspective on the ultimate causes of PPH in humans and, thus, on the costs and the benefits of specific features of human anatomy and physiology.

This chapter explores a novel, evolutionarily driven hypothesis regarding PPH, arguing that as adult (and therefore fetal) brain and body size increased over the course of human evolution, existing primate patterns of invasive placentation were modified to allow for increased maternal nutrient transfer *in utero*[10,11]. Unfortunately, the resultant pattern of placentation came at an unfortunate cost: uteroplacental separation at birth is more likely to be hindered, thereby leading to high rates of PPH. To support these arguments, this chapter discusses some of the key features of invasive human placentation, reviews suggestions that overly aggressive placental invasion may be critical to the etiology of PPH, and examines the comparative evidence for placental disorders related to trophoblast invasion. The chapter concludes with a consideration of the causes, timing and effects of PPH over the course of human evolution.

THE INVASIVE PATTERN OF HUMAN PLACENTATION

The existing pattern of human placentation has recently been argued to be a modification of existing patterns of primate placentation to increase nutrient transport *in utero* and support the increase in fetal brain size over time. A brief description of the development and functional morphology of the placenta is thus central to this argument[12–17]. The primate placenta forms within a few days of fertilization from trophoblastic cells of fetal origin. The trophoblasts comprise the outer cell mass (OCM) of the early blastocyst, a hollow ball of cells derived from the fertilized egg[12,13], while the inner cell mass of the blastocyst gives rise to the fetus. Because of its shared origin with the fetus, the placenta can be viewed as an extrasomatic fetal organ, which acts as a sensor of nutrient availability in the maternal circulation and thus a calibrator of fetal growth[18].

Placentas show striking variations in invasiveness, exhibiting three main phenotypes[19]. The *epitheliochorial* placenta, found in ruminants, horses and swine, is the least invasive form; it adheres to the epithelial lining of the uterine wall without penetrating it, thereby providing no contact with the underlying maternal vasculature. Nutrient transport into the fetal circulation occurs via diffusion through several layers of tissue: the walls of the maternal vessels, the surrounding endometrial stroma, the uterine epithelium and finally the chorion, which is comprised of trophoblasts from the OCM and of fetal mesoderm, a tissue deriving from one of the main three cell layers of the early embryo. In order of invasiveness, the next mode is *endotheliochorial* (as seen in dogs and cats), whereby the chorion penetrates the endometrial surface and is in contact with the endothelium of maternal vessels but is not immediately adjacent to maternal blood. The most invasive placental form is the *hemochorial* placenta (as seen in rodents and primates), in which the chorion penetrates the endometrial epithelium and the deeper endometrial stroma to arrive in direct contact with maternal vessels, the walls of which are

subsequently penetrated, so that placental tissue is in direct contact with maternal blood.

Further differentiation occurs within hemochorial placentation in terms of depth of implantation. In monkeys, implantation is superficial, with only moderate penetration of the uterine wall by the chorion[17]. Trophoblast cells surround maternal vessels within the endometrium and cause them to lose some of their muscularity, which, in turn, lowers vascular resistance and increases blood flow to the developing embryo[20]. The monkey placenta thus forms a trophoblast shell, which is a mostly continuous layer of trophoblast cells within the endometrium that largely limits trophoblast invasion into the myometrium[21,22]. In contrast, the human placenta is much more invasive, lacking a trophoblast shell and deeply penetrating the uterine epithelium, even migrating through the endometrial stroma beneath into the upper third of the myometrium in a process called interstitial implantation[13,23,24]. The human trophoblasts extensively remodel the maternal spiral arterioles to nourish the rich endometrium[25]. Less is known about placentation in the other hominoids than in modern humans, but recent reports suggest that more invasive interstitial placentation also occurs in the African great apes, although the currently available data are drawn from only two chimpanzee placentas[26].

To accomplish the extraordinary feat of deeply invading the uterus and remodeling its vessels, trophoblast cells develop an invasive phenotype (Figure 1). Some become the villous cytotrophoblasts (VCT) that cover mesoderm cores to become the chorionic villi. These villi are in direct contact with maternal blood pulsating throughout the placenta. As gestation progresses, most of the cytotrophoblasts fuse to form a continuous multinucleated layer called the syncytiotrophoblast (SCT), across which nutrient, gas and waste transport takes place. Other trophoblast cells mediate the placental adherence to the uterine wall as

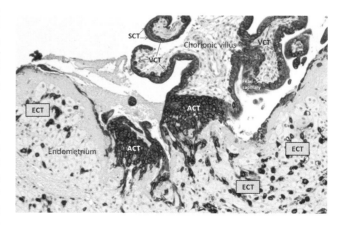

Figure 1 Human placenta. Section through chorionic villus (fetal mesoderm core covered in trophoblast) and underlying endometrium. Dark staining cells are various trophoblast phenotypes: SCT, syncytiotrophoblast; VCT, villous cytotrophoblast; ACT, anchoring cytotrophoblast; ECT, extravillous invasive cytotrophoblast. Courtesy of Harvey Kliman, MD, PhD, Yale University

anchoring columns (ACT)[27]. A final group of cytotrophoblast cells develops a highly invasive phenotype. These extravillous invasive cytotrophoblasts break free from the other trophoblast cells and migrate deeper into the uterus. They surround the maternal spiral arterioles and initiate a breakdown of their internal muscular layer (the tunica media) (Figure 2). This replaces the muscular and elastic tissue of the arteriole wall with a thick layer of non-contractile fibrinoid material, which in turn reduces vascular resistance. The shape of the vessel is also converted in such a way that its diameter increases, while its distal portion opens into a funnel-like outlet into the growing placenta[28,29]. Such changes combine to maximize blood flow, increase hemodynamic efficiency, and reduce the potential impact of vasoconstrictors[28]. The invasion and subsequent conversion of the deeper vessels of the human uterus takes place early in the second trimester, around 15 weeks[30]. In summary, these transformations increase maternal syncytiotrophoblast surface area and render maternal vasculature relatively powerless to limit physically blood flow to the placenta; these strategies channel large quantities of nutrients and oxygen to the large-for-maternal-body-size newborns of hominoids, including humans[31–34].

THE LINK BETWEEN PLACENTATION AND POSTPARTUM HEMORRHAGE

The processes of trophoblast differentiation, invasion and vascular conversion are normal components of human gestation, but all carry potentially significant risks. Pre-eclampsia, characterized by shallow trophoblast invasion and insufficient remodeling of maternal vessels, is a prime example of the disruption of the delicate balance *in utero*. In pre-eclampsia, rather than being transformed into the wide, straight funnels that easily conduct maternal blood to the placenta and in turn the fetus, the maternal spiral arterioles remain coiled, their muscular walls intact and operable, thus

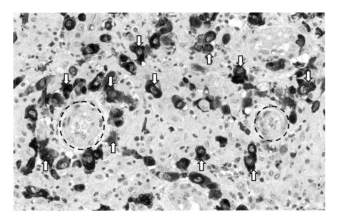

Figure 2 Darkly staining invasive extravillous cytotrophoblasts (ECT, some indicated by white arrows) surrounding maternal uterine arterioles (outlined in dashed black circles). Arteriole on the left is completely surrounded by ECT and further along the conversion process than the arteriole on the right. Courtesy of Harvey Kliman, MD, PhD, Yale University

restricting blood flow to the placenta[35]. The resultant placental insufficiency may induce symptoms that include hypertension, proteinuria and renal pathologies, and, in the case of eclampsia, convulsions and death. Pre-eclampsia has been frequently described as a disorder unique to humans because of the role of trophoblast invasion and vascular remodeling[36–39]. Carter and Martin[40] recently critiqued the conventional thinking of pre-eclampsia being a uniquely human condition, suggesting that this assumption has not been exposed to extensive inquiry. They cite examples of physiological changes in pregnant primates that may indicate a deeper evolutionary timeline for pre-eclampsia. For example, in a study of five pregnant baboons who underwent uterine artery ligation (a treatment that effectively limits blood flow to the placenta and increases maternal blood pressure), symptoms consistent with pre-eclampsia were observed, namely, changes to the microscopic kidney morphology, proteinuria and increased blood pressure[41]. Hennessy *et al.*[42] described similar renal and hypertensive symptoms in a baboon pregnant with twins. Comparable changes to the kidney were reported in a single chimpanzee[43], and symptoms tentatively described as eclamptic convulsions were reported in two matrilineally related gorillas[44].

Although this small dataset ($n = 9$ across three genera) points to the possibility that pre-eclamptic symptoms may not be limited to humans, none of these studies described any morphological features of the placenta corresponding to the well described alteration of invasive events that characterizes pre-eclampsia in humans[35]. What is consistent in these examples, however, is the induction of a hypertensive environment, either through the mechanical restriction of blood flow to the uterus or via the demands of multiple pregnancy. Further, as Carter and Martin also note, the invasive extravillous trophoblasts responsible for the extensive remodeling of the human uterine vasculature appear to be absent in baboons and macaques, the monkey species in which placentation has been most studied[40]. Taken together, the available observations suggest that while the *hypertensive* symptoms of pre-eclampsia may be inducible within the primate order, the underlying placental causation – blocking of the characteristically deep invasion and extensive vascular remodeling – is unique to humans, or at least has not yet been definitively shown to be a component of the etiology of gestational hypertension in non-human primates.

In addition to pre-eclampsia, a number of disorders in humans represent the range of placental invasiveness. At one end of the spectrum is placental abruption, in which the placenta prematurely separates from the uterine wall, suggestive of shallow implantation[45]. On the other is the cluster of highly invasive disorders comprising placental accreta, whereby trophoblast invasion is severely dysregulated and the placenta implants far beyond its normal limits[46]. The most invasive of these is placenta percreta, in which the placenta completely penetrates the myometrium, in some cases migrating out onto organs outside the reproductive tract, such as the rectum or kidneys[47]. Placenta percreta, which can lead to spontaneous uterine rupture[48], is often localized to areas of prior uterine scarring, as the non-vascular fibrous scar tissue that replaces the muscle may allow overimplantation[49]. The highly invasive nature of human trophoblasts can also give rise to gestational trophoblastic diseases such as choriocarcinoma, a neoplasm that can metastasize to the lungs and cause death years after pregnancy[50,51].

Just as pre-eclampsia is a gestational disorder arising from impaired placentation and the resultant under-remodeling of uterine vasculature, PPH may have its roots in overly aggressive placental invasion and vascular remodeling[10]. In support of this hypothesis (and in direct contrast to pre-eclampsia), one of the clinical risk factors for PPH is macrosomia[52], which is suggestive of a high rate of nutrient delivery to the fetus, as would be expected if the vessels supplying the placenta were expanded in size, number, or power. A number of factors may contribute to this over-remodeling. For example, the maternal immune system could respond inadequately to counter the activity of invasive trophoblasts on the arterioles, leaving these vessels vulnerable to excessive remodeling and therefore overly conductive of maternal blood to the fetoplacental unit[51]. Alternatively or concomitantly, more arterioles than usual may be remodeled or even recruited to form *de novo* by the invasive cells. Indeed, invasive trophoblast cells are capable of attracting and increasing neighboring maternal blood flow through the production of factors that promote vessel dilation and discourage clot formation[53–55]. These invasive cells can also completely displace the maternal cells lining the remodeled vessels, essentially forming new blood vessels of placental origin within the uterus[55]. In addition to the great advantage of directly soliciting and facilitating increased maternal blood flow to the placenta and fetus, these mechanisms, when unchecked, may also have the effect of replacing or handicapping uterine muscle cells, thus diminishing the effective ratio of contractile to non-contractile tissue in the myometrium and dampening the ability of the uterus to contract immediately postpartum. In addition, a high rate of vascular turnover and inflammation could be accompanied by an accumulation of subclinical uterine trauma and scarring, which could also hamper contractility when it is urgently needed.

What has been laid forth above strongly suggests that the human pattern of trophoblast invasion and/or the extensive vascular remodeling of the uterus may impede the normal processes of myometrial contraction and clot formation after delivery. In a typical delivery, the placenta begins to separate from the uterine wall even before the delivery of the baby[49]. Any resulting uterine bleeding at the site of placental separation is normally stopped by 'the mechanical constriction of the blood vessels due to the uterine muscle contraction and retraction and by clots sealing off the raw surface in the placental bed'[56]. When uterine bleeding during labor or immediately after the delivery is not stopped by these mechanisms, the threat of maternal death from catastrophic hemorrhage is very real. The two major risk factors for PPH, uterine atony and a prolonged third phase of labor, together account for 93% of PPH-related deaths[57]. Uterine atony, the absence of adequate uterine contractions to sufficiently clamp the uterine vessels and stop bleeding from the 20 cm diameter wound that remains on the uterine wall when the placenta does separate, is the leading risk factor for PPH, accounting for 70% of the cases[49]. The underlying causes of uterine atony, however, are unclear. Uterine atony is often associated with retained or incomplete placenta delivery[49], but the directionality of this link is not clear. It is possible that a retained placenta and its vascular attachments may present a physical barrier to uterine muscle contraction. Conversely, uterine atony could hinder placental separation and expulsion. In addition to the physical and physiological factors that may interfere with uterine contraction, risk factors that overstretch the uterus, including multiple pregnancy, macrosomia and polyhydramnios, are also associated with atony[49]. Considering the importance of reproduction to the process of evolution by natural selection, the integration of clinical medicine and evolutionary biology is a logical avenue to pursue, despite our incomplete knowledge of the ultimate causes of PPH.

HUMAN VULNERABILITY TO POSTPARTUM HEMORRHAGE IN AN EVOLUTIONARY CONTEXT

PPH is rare in domestic animals for which data are available[58]. Noakes *et al.* report that because many domesticated animals (e.g. swine, horses, cattle) have non-invasive epitheliochorial placentas, bleeding at the time of delivery is only likely if excessive force is used to deliver the placenta[59]. In these animals, trauma followed by hemorrhage is paramount: 'the usual cause of serious hemorrhage is laceration of a uterine blood vessel by a fetal appendage, obstetric instrument, or hand of the obstetrician'[58]. In fact, Rooney[58] reports ten fatal cases of PPH in aging mares, all related to lacerations of arteries. In carnivores such as the house cat, moderately invasive endotheliochorial placentas allow for an increased risk of blood loss at delivery, which often occurs when the placenta is precipitously removed during cesarean sections[58]. These data, albeit minimal, suggest that blood loss at delivery has a direct connection to the degree of placental invasiveness, such that animals with minimally invasive epitheliochorial placentas are unlikely to bleed at delivery except in the case of induced vascular trauma, whereas those with moderately invasive endotheliochorial placentas may bleed if the placenta is prematurely separated from the uterine wall.

If indeed broad categories of placental invasiveness predict the probability and/or volume of blood loss at delivery, then primates with hemochorial placentation, which involves remodeling of at least the endometrial vasculature, should be expected to lose a small volume of blood postpartum. Unfortunately, data available on postpartum bleeding or its risk factors in non-human primates are scant at best, save two published reports of retained placenta[60,61]. At the same time, however, few other primates approach the extreme level of cephalopelvic disproportion exhibited by humans, indicating that overall, labor in non-human primates is a simpler, less potentially traumatic event. Considering the importance of pregnancy and labor in zoos as well as captive research and breeding facilities, the lack of an anecdotal literature on PPH in non-human primates can be viewed as tentative support for the hypothesis that the elevated incidence of PPH is unique to humans, although more systematic study is clearly required, particularly among the great apes.

If PPH is not a common feature of mammalian or even primate pregnancy, when did this vulnerability arise in human history? Rockwell *et al.* suggest that the shift toward bipedal locomotion approximately seven million years ago and its attendant consequences for pelvic anatomy may have spurred changes in patterns of placental invasiveness and vascular remodeling to counteract gravitational effects[29]. A shift to habitually erect posture and bipedal locomotion places the major abdominal vasculature (e.g. abdominal aorta, inferior vena cava) at risk of compression by the gravid uterus[62]. This in turn constrains blood flow and thus oxygen to the uteroplacental unit, with potentially deleterious consequences for the developing fetus. In response, the human placenta could have modified the pre-existing primate pattern of placentation, implanting even more extensively into the myometrium and actively altering the maternal vasculature to improve placental perfusion, thereby protecting the fetus from the vascular effects of gravity[29]. Because increases in invasiveness expand the placental surface area available for transport of nutrients from the maternal to the fetal circulation[63,64], it is reasonable to suggest that changes in placental anatomy allowed an increase in intra-uterine nutrition for the developing hominin fetus[11].

INCREASED FETAL NUTRIENT REQUIREMENTS IN THE GENUS *HOMO*

The origin of the genus *Homo* around 2 million years ago was marked by a number of key changes in hominin morphology, the most significant of which, from an energetic standpoint, were a significant increase in body size and a tripling of brain size, from approximately 400 cc in the earliest human ancestors to approximately 1400 cc in modern humans. This latter volume is three times larger than would be expected for a commensurately sized great ape[33,34]. Such shifts in adult body proportions would have also been associated with similar shifts in offspring proportions, such that energetic investment in fetuses and neonates in the genus *Homo* would have increased substantially as well. Modern human infants are the largest of all primate neonates[65], even though humans are not the largest primates. Corrected for maternal body size, the relationship of neonatal mass to maternal mass is still larger in humans than in almost all other

primates[32–34]. Modeling by DeSilva and Lesnik[66] suggests that neonatal brain size increased 25–50% from australopithecines (~180 cc) 3 million years ago to members of the genus *Homo* (~225–270 cc) 2 million years ago. If the cost of fetal brain metabolism approximates that of the neonatal period (60–74% of energy intake compared to 20% in the adult)[33,67], then increases in absolute neonatal brain size and metabolism meant increases in the amount of energy needed during pregnancy to support a fetus. Furthermore, modern human newborns appear to be fatter than most other mammalian newborns, with the exception of guinea pigs and some aquatic mammals[32,68,69]. It is highly likely that significant changes in dietary quality, most probably increases in animal product intake (e.g. meat) relative to other foods, accompanied the origin of the genus *Homo*[70–72]. Taken together, the enhanced metabolic requirements of pregnancy due to increased human neonatal weight, adiposity and especially brain size suggest that the origin of the genus *Homo* was accompanied by a significant increase in the energetic cost of bringing a fetus to term[11].

Skeletal anatomy related to habitual bipedalism applies a constraint on this investment and resultant *in utero* brain growth, in that it 'determines rigidity and arrangement of the bones in the pelvis, affects the size of the birth canal, and thus determines the maximum fetal size at birth'[7]. A number of human adaptations maximize the deliverable neonatal head size, including an expandable pubic symphysis[73,74] and compressible fetal skull[75]. In addition, traditional labor positions, such as squatting, take advantage of gravity and allow the pelvis to open to its maximum width[7]. Furthermore, the uniquely human pattern of assistance during labor permits manual rotation and/or maneuvering of the fetus during parturition[7].

Human parturition occurs at the point beyond which fetal and potentially maternal demise would be far too likely to be favored by selection, as too large a fetal head simply would not be able to exit the pelvis. As a result of this constraint, the human fetus has often been characterized as being born at a far more immature developmental stage than the other primates[33,76,77], yet nonetheless it has the biggest absolute brain size. The large size of the human neonatal brain relative to maternal mass[78] suggests that additional energy is being channeled to the fetus.

In particular, maternal fatty acids such as docosa-hexaenoic acid (DHA) are key nutrients for intrauterine and postnatal brain development[71,79], especially for the production of myelin, the fatty sheath encasing axons and enhancing cognitive function. The fatty acid concentration in placental circulation is dependent on two main factors: the maternal concentration of fatty acids and their efficient transfer across the placenta[80,81]. Although long chain poly-unsaturated fatty acids (LCPUFA) can be transported passively across the maternal–fetal concentration gradient, recent research emphasizes the importance of plasma membrane-located transport/binding proteins in this process[82,83]. The transport proteins existing on the placental interface are saturable, so that the rate of LCPUFA transport is maximized when all the binding sites are filled. Because the rates of both passive transport by diffusion, which is directly correlated to surface area, and active transport via transport proteins, which increases in number as the area of the membrane increases, are related to surface area, increased placental surface area might thus allow for increased transfer of fatty acids across the placenta. An expansion of placental surface area would be one way to increase the efficiency of intrauterine nutrient transport in hominins without the need for qualitatively altering caloric intake relative to other primates. Rutherford and Tardif demonstrated that the placentas of marmoset monkey triplet litters had a significantly expanded transport surface area compared with those of twin litters, despite a reduction in the ratio of maternal to fetal mass, suggesting that increasing the area available for transport is an efficient strategy to support greater fetal growth in primates[84]. Taken together with the hypothesized shifts in early hominin diets to include more animal products[70,71], which in turn would be expected to increase maternal fatty acid and ketone concentrations[85] and thus the supply available to the developing fetus, increases in placental fatty acid transport to the fetus were very likely critical to the evolutionary trajectory of hominin brain development. It has been proposed recently that without changes in hominin placentation that both intensify invasion into the uterine wall and expand the surface area in contact with maternal blood, combined with changes in diet quality, growing a large and highly myelinized fetal brain would have represented so large a portion of maternal energy expenditure as to render increases in fetal brain growth prohibitively costly, aside from any mechanical constraints of the abdominal and pelvic anatomy on parturition[11].

EVIDENCE FOR THE LONGSTANDING HISTORY OF POSTPARTUM HEMORRHAGE IN HUMANS

Genetic and ethnographic evidence offer more clues to a longstanding human history of PPH. Lindqvist and colleagues[86,87] argue that thrombophilias, polymorphisms that promote coagulation, have been selected for their ability to counterbalance the risk of PPH. Factor V Leiden (FVL), one of the best characterized procoagulatory mutations, causes a resistance to the anticoagulatory activity of activated protein C (APC)[88], which allows individuals with the FVL mutation to clot faster. Approximately 5% of Europeans carry the FVL gene, and frequencies can reach as high as 10–15% in northern Europe, where the mutation likely arose[88] approximately 21,000 years ago[89]. In a retrospective Swedish study, Lindqvist et al. found that women who were homozygous or heterozygous for the FVL mutation lost significantly less blood at delivery (an average of 60 ml less blood lost; $p = 0.001$) and were significantly less likely to hemorrhage than individuals without the mutation (defined in this study as 600 ml blood loss or more; 2% of those

with the mutation versus 14% of those without it; $p = 0.01$)[86]. Even if thrombophilias offer protection against PPH, carriers may incur other potentially significant costs. The most significant of these costs is an increased risk of thromboembolism in pregnancy, which accounts for approximately 15% of maternal deaths[8]. A recent systematic literature review and meta-analysis of the risk of thrombosis in pregnancy for FVL carriers determined that homozygotes have a relative risk as high as 34.4% compared with the 8.3% risk of heterozygotes, although this does not translate to an exceptionally high absolute risk (3.4% in homozygotes and 0.8% in heterozygotes), given the rarity of thrombosis in the overall population (1:1000)[90]. The costs of FVL, which accounts for over 40% of all thromboses, are also suggested by its virtual absence among natives of Africa and Asia[88], parts of the world where the mortality rate due to PPH is especially high. Lindqvist and colleagues[86,87] argue that the maintenance of the FVL allele at such a high frequency despite its associated risks is indicative of strong balancing selection for protection against PPH.

In addition to genetic factors, humans have developed multiple behavioral interventions for PPH and its risk factors. Lefeber and Voorhoeve extensively reviewed child birth customs and discussed a number of interventions used by traditional birth attendants (TBAs) that appear to replicate the effects of active management of the third phase of labor[91]. First, if the placenta is delayed, TBAs may administer substances or perform actions that will cause the delivering woman to sneeze, gag, or vomit, thus tensing her abdominal muscles and potentially contracting the uterus. For example, TBAs may insert garlic or hair into the woman's mouth or administer salted water to induce gagging or vomiting[91]. In Jamaica, the woman may be encouraged to inhale deeply followed by exhaling forcefully into a bottle; this maneuver applies internal pressure to the uterus and can stimulate contractions[92]. Second, abdominal pressure and uterine massage, pressing and rubbing are widely reported[91]. In West Melanesia, a hot compress made of wood may be applied to the vulva and abdomen to stop the flow of blood[93]. Third, while it is not precisely 'controlled cord traction', Lefeber and Voorhoeve present examples from India, Malaysia, Ghana and Indonesia of TBAs pulling on the umbilical cord and manually removing the placenta[91]. Such examples demonstrate that TBAs may attend to cues of possible PPH and possibly intervene in manners that may replicate WHO's mechanisms of active management of the third phase of labor. The cross-cultural variations in these interventions suggest these traditions have longstanding cultural roots, and the minimal materials required suggest that these sorts of interventions could have been performed by earlier hominins[94].

CONCLUSION

PPH is the leading cause of maternal mortality worldwide. The condition exacts huge tolls on human capital, particularly where women do not have ready access to medical care. Research on PPH traditionally has focused on treatments and risk factors, whereas comparatively little work has been performed to explore the underlying mechanisms of this potentially fatal disorder. As argued here, the high risk of PPH-related mortality in humans is potentially a consequence of placental adaptations toward intense invasiveness and radical remodeling of maternal vasculature, driven by the energetic demands of the large-bodied and large-brained hominin fetus. However, the transformative activity of the human trophoblast cells carries with it significant risk of gestational complications for both mother and offspring. The example of pre-eclampsia – a serious hypertensive complication of pregnancy caused by inadequate vascular remodeling of the uteroplacental unit – serves as a corollary for the etiology of PPH reviewed here and illustrates the delicate balance between investment and risk. If adequate uterine vascular remodeling is not achieved, then the mother is placed at risk of hypertension and death, and the fetus may experience growth restriction and its cascade of lifelong health consequences. If the target of vascular remodeling is exceeded, on the other hand, the resultant excessive remodeling, hyperperfusion of the placenta, and over nourishment of the fetus, may lead to catastrophic maternal bleeding and maternal and fetal death.

Although the human placenta shares deep phylogenetic roots with the primate hemochorial placenta, the morphology of the modern human placenta appears to be distinct from that of other primates, as indicated by available histological and physiological studies of the placenta, comparative data on pregnancy outcomes, and the time depth of PPH suggested by coagulation factor polymorphism distribution and ethnographic consilience in birth practices[10,11]. Because more than 50% of PPH cases currently have no identifiable risk factors[95], understanding the underlying cause of the increased risk of PPH in humans is an important step toward discovering new modes of treatment and eventually prevention on a global scale. Interdisciplinary collaborations based on an understanding of the evolutionary biology and physiological mechanisms of placentation and uterine vascular remodeling may hold the best hope for aiding women and health care providers to make evidence-based, pragmatic choices about place of delivery.

PRACTICE POINTS

- The pattern of human placentation is highly invasive, which is likely an adaptation to support intense brain growth *in utero*

- The deeply invasive nature of the human placenta may impede the process of uteroplacental separation at birth, thereby leading to high rates of PPH

- Based on available data, the frequency of PPH in humans is much higher than in our closest relatives, the non-human primates, which generally have less invasive placentas and less brain growth *in utero*

- The high prevalence of PPH in humans may have begun 2 million years ago, when human brain size expanded; this longstanding history is reflected in genetic and cultural adaptations to PPH.

ACKNOWLEDGMENTS

Thanks are due to Drs Louis Keith and Christopher Jones for first bringing the evolutionary enigma of PPH to our attention. We are grateful to Drs Crystal Patil, Alison Doubleday, Harvey Kliman and Robert Martin for their thoughtful comments on previous versions of our manuscript. Drs Michelle Kominiarek and Stacie Geller, both of the UIC Department of Obstetrics and Gynecology, offered important perspectives on the clinical treatment and global scope of PPH. Discussions with Drs Anthony Carter and Steven Ross provided important information regarding birth outcomes in non-human primates. We thank Fiona Lynch for preliminary research on this topic and Victoria deMartelly for her help with bibliographical matters. Final perspectives and errors remain ours alone. Significant financial support was provided by Wenner-Gren (Elizabeth Abrams and Crystal Patil) and by a University of Illinois at Chicago Building Interdisciplinary Research Careers in Women's Health (BIRCWH) faculty scholarship to Julienne Rutherford from the National Institute of Child Health and Human Development and the National Institutes of Health Office of Research on Women's Health (K12HD055892). The content is solely the responsibility of the authors and does not necessarily represent the official views of the National Institute of Child Health and Human Development or the National Institutes of Health.

References

1. Hogan MC, Foreman KJ, Naghavi M, et al. Maternal mortality for 181 countries, 1980–2008: a systematic analysis of progress towards Millennium Development Goal 5. Lancet 2010;375:1609–23
2. Ronsmans C, Graham WJ. Maternal mortality: who, when, where, and why. Lancet 2006;368:1189–200
3. Van Lerberghe W, De Brouwere V. Of blind alleys and things that have worked: History's lessons on reducing maternal mortality. Stud Health Serv Org Policy 2001;17:7–34
4. Rosenberg K. The evolution of modern human childbirth. Yearbook Physical Anthropol 1992;35:89–124
5. Rosenberg K, Trevathan W. Bipedalism and human birth: the obstetrical dilemma revisited. Evol Anthropol 1996;4:161–8
6. Rosenberg K, Trevathan W. Birth, obstetrics and human evolution. Br J Obstet Gynaecol 2002;109:1199–206
7. Trevathan W. Human Birth: An Evolutionary Perspective. New York, NY: Aldine de Gruyter, 1987
8. Khan KS, Wojdyla D, Say L, Gulmezoglu AM, Van Look PF. WHO analysis of causes of maternal death: A systematic review. Lancet 2006;367:1066–74
9. WHO. The World health report: 2005: make every mother and child count. Geneva, Switzerland: World Health Organization, 2005

10. Abrams E, Rutherford J. Framing postpartum hemorrhage as a consequence of human placental biology: an evolutionary and comparative perspective. Am Anthropol 2011;113:417–30

11. Rutherford J, Abrams E, Said SJ. Developing the brain: a potential role for the placenta in hominin brain evolution. American Association of Physical Anthropologists, Portland, OR, Oral Presentation, 13 April 2012

12. Mossman HW. Comparative morphogenesis of the fetal membranes and accessory uterine structures. Carnegie Inst Contrib Embryol 1937;26:129–246

13. Mossman HW. Vertebrate Fetal Membranes. New Brunswick, NJ: Rutgers University Press, 1987

14. Luckett WP. Comparative development and evolution of the placenta in primates. Contrib Primatol 1974;3:142–234

15. Wislocki GB. On the placentation of primates, with a consideration of the phylogeny of the placenta. Contrib Embryol 1929;20:51–80

16. Benirshcke K, Kaufmann P. Anatomical and functional differences in the placenta of primates. Biol Reprod 1982;26:29–53

17. Luckett WP. Cladistic relationships among primate higher categories: evidence of the fetal membranes and placenta. Folia Primatol (Basel) 1976;25:245–76

18. Jansson T, Powell TL. IFPA 2005 Award in Placentology Lecture. Human placental transport in altered fetal growth: does the placenta function as a nutrient sensor? — a review. Placenta 2006;27 (Suppl A):S91–7

19. Grosser O. Vergleichende Anatomie und Entwicklungsgeschichte der Eihäute und der Placenta. Vienna, Austria: Wilhelm Braumüller, 1909

20. Kaufmann P, Black S, Huppertz B. Endovascular trophoblast invasion: implications for the pathogenesis of intrauterine growth retardation and preeclampsia. Biol Reprod 2003;69:1–7

21. Blankenship TN, Enders AC. Modification of uterine vasculature during pregnancy in macaques. Microsc Res Tech 2003;60:390–401

22. Ramsey EM, Houston ML, Harris JW. Interactions of the trophoblast and maternal tissues in three closely related primate species. Am J Obstet Gynecol 1976;124:647–52

23. Enders AC, Lantz KC, Schlafke S. Preference of invasive cytotrophoblast for maternal vessels in early implantation in the macaque. Acta Anatomica (Basel) 1996;155:145–62

24. Pijnenborg R, D'Hooghe T, Vercruysse L, Bambra C. Evaluation of trophoblast invasion in placental bed biopsies of the baboon, with immunohistochemical localisation of cytokeratin, fibronectin, and laminin. J Med Primatol 1996;25:272–81

25. Robillard P-Y, Dekker GA, Hulsey TC. Evolutionary adaptations to pre-eclampsia/eclampsia in humans: low fecundability rate, loss of oestrus, prohibitions of incest and systematic polyandry. Am J Reprod Immunol 2002;47:104–11

26. Carter AM, Pijnenborg R. Evolution of invasive placentation with special reference to non-human primates. Best Pract Res Clin Obstet Gynaecol 2010;24:I1–I2

27. Kliman HJ. Uteroplacental Blood Flow: The story of decidualization, menstruation, and trophoblast invasion. Am J Pathol 2000;157:1759–68

28. Espinoza J, Romero R, Mee Kim Y, et al. Normal and abnormal transformation of the spiral arteries during pregnancy. J Perinat Med 2006;34:447–58

29. Rockwell LC, Vargas E, Moore LG. Human physiological adaptation to pregnancy: inter- and intraspecific perspectives. Am J Hum Biol 2003;15:330–41

30. Robillard P, Dekker G. Evolutionary adaptations to pre-eclampsia/eclampsia in humans: low fecundability rate, loss of oestrus, prohibitions of incest and systematic polyandry. Am J Reprod Immunol 2002;47:104–14

31. Chaline J. Increased cranial capacity in hominid evolution and preeclampsia. J Reprod Immunol 2003;59:137–52

32. Dufour DL, Sauther ML. Comparative and evolutionary dimensions of the energetics of human pregnancy and lactation. Am J Hum Biol 2002;14:584–602

33. Martin RD. Human brain evolution in an ecological context. Fifty-second James Arthur Lecture on the Evolution of the Human Brain; American Museum of Natural History, New York, 1983

34. Martin RD. Human reproduction: a comparative background for medical hypotheses. J Reprod Immunol 2003;59:111–35

35. Fisher SJ. The placental problem: linking abnormal cytotrophoblast differentiation to the maternal symptoms of pre-eclampsia. Reprod Biol Endocrinol 2004;2:53

36. Jauniaux E, Poston L, Burton GJ. Placental-related diseases of pregnancy: involvement of oxidative stress and implications in human evolution. Hum Reprod Update 2006;12:747–55

37. Chez RA. Nonhuman primate models of toxemia of pregnancy. In: Lindheimer M, Katz A, Zuspan F, editors. Hypertension in Pregnancy. New York: John Wiley & Sons, 1976

38. Pijnenborg R, Vercruysse L, Hanssens M. The uterine spiral arteries in human pregnancy: facts and controversies. Placenta 2006;27:939–58

39. Rosenberg K, Trevathan W. An anthropological perspective on the evolutionary context of preeclampsia in humans. J Reprod Immunol 2007;76:91–7

40. Carter AM, Martin RD. Comparative anatomy and placental evolution. In: Pijnenborg R, Brosens I, Romero R, eds. Placental Bed Disorders: Basic Science and its Translation to Obstetrics. Cambridge: Cambridge University Press, 2010:109–26

41. Makris A, Thornton C, Thompson J, et al. Uteroplacental ischemia results in proteinuric hypertension and elevated sFLT-1. Kidney Int 2007;71:977–84

42. Hennessy A, Gillin AG, Painter DM, Kirwan PJ, Thompson JF, Horvath JS. Evidence for preeclampsia in a baboon pregnancy with twins. Hypertens Preg 1997;16:223–8

43. Stout C, Lemmon WC. Glomerular capillary endothelial swelling in a pregnant chimpanzee. Am J Obstet Gynecol 1969;105:212–5

44. Thornton JG, Onwude JL. Convulsions in pregnancy in related gorillas. Am J Obstet Gynecol 1992;167:240–1

45. Tikkanen M. Etiology, clinical manifestations, and prediction of placental abruption. Acta Obstet Gynecol Scand 2010;89:732–40

46. Angstmann T, Gard G, Harrington T, Ward E, Thomson A, Giles W. Surgical management of placenta accreta: a cohort series and suggested approach. Am J Obstet Gynecol 2010;202:38 e1–9

47. Moore LE, Gonzalez I. Placenta percreta with bladder invasion diagnosed with sonography: images and clinical correlation. J Diagn Med Sonograph 2008;24:238–41

48. Esmans A, Gerris J, Corthout E, Verdonk P, Declercq S. Placenta percreta causing rupture of an unscarred uterus at the end of the first trimester of pregnancy: case report. Hum Reprod 2004;19:2401–3

49. Khan RU, El-Refaey H. Pathophysiology of postpartum hemorrhage and third stage of labor. In: B-Lynch C, Keith LG, Lalonde AB, Karoshi M, eds. A Textbook of Postpartum Hemorrhage. Duncow, UK: Sapiens Publishing, 2006:62–9

50. Shintaku M, Hwang MH, Amitani R. Primary choriocarcinoma of the lung manifesting as diffuse alveolar hemorrhage. Arch Pathol Lab Med 2006;130:540–3

51. Smith HO, Kohorn EI, Cole LA. Choriocarcinoma and gestational trophoblastic disease. Obstet Gynecol Clin North Am 2005;32:661–84

52. Sacks DA, Chen W. Estimating fetal weight in the management of macrosomia. Obstet Gynecol Surg 2000;55:229–39

53. Athanassiades A, Lala PK. Role of placenta growth factor (PIGF) in human extravillous trophoblast proliferation, migration and invasiveness. Placenta 1998;19:465–73

54. Cross JC, Hemberger M, Lu Y, et al. Trophoblast functions, angiogenesis and remodeling of the maternal vasculature in the placenta. Mol Cell Endocrinol 2002;187:207–12

55. Hemberger M, Nozaki T, Masutani M, Cross JC. Differential expression of angiogenic and vasodilatory factors by invasive trophoblast giant cells depending on depth of invasion. Dev Dynam 2003;227:185–91

56. Choo WL, Chua S, Chong YS, et al. Correlation of change in uterine activity to blood loss in the third stage of labour. Gynecol Obstet Invest 1998;46:178–80

57. Carroli G, Cuesta C, Abalos E, Gulmezoglu AM. Epidemiology of postpartum haemorrhage: a systematic review. Best Pract Res Clin Obstet Gynaecol 2008;22:999–1012

58. Rooney JR. Internal hemorrhage related to gestation in the mare. Cornell Vet 1964;54:11–17

59. Noakes DE, Parkinson TJ, England GCW, Arthur GH. Arthur's Veterinary Reproduction and Obstetrics, 8th edn. Philadelphia, PA: WB Saunders, 2001

60. Bronson E, Deem SL, Sanchez C, Murray S. Placental retention in a golden lion tamarin (Leontopithecus rosalia). J Zoo Wildlife Med 2005;36:716–8

61. Halbwax M, Mahamba CK, Ngalula A-M, Andre C. Placental retention in a bonobo (Pan paniscus). J Med Primatol 2009;38:171–4

62. Abitbol MM. Growth of the fetus in the abdominal cavity. Am J Physic Anthropol 1993;91:367–78

63. Baur R. Morphometric data and questions concerning placental transfer. Placenta 1981;2(Suppl):S35–S44

64. Baur R. Morphometry of the placental exchange area. Adv Anat Embryol Cell Biol 1977;53:3–65

65. Smith R, Leigh S. Sexual dimorphism in primate neonatal body mass. J Hum Evol. 1998;34:173–201

66. DeSilva JM, Lesnik JJ. Brain size at birth throughout human evolution: A new method for estimating neonatal brain size in hominins. J Hum Evolut 2008;55:1064–74

67. Holliday MA. Metabolic rate and organ size during growth from infancy to maturity and during late gestation and early infancy. Pediatrics 1971;47:169

68. Kuzawa CW. Adipose tissue in human infancy and childhood: an evolutionary perspective. Yearbook Physical Anthropol 1998;41:177–209

69. Garn SM. Fat thickness and growth process during infancy. Hum Biol 1956;28:232–50

70. Aiello LC, Wheeler P. The expensive-tissue hypothesis: the brain and the digestive system in human and primate evolution. Curr Anthropol 1995;36:199–221

71. Cunnane SC, Crawford MA. Survival of the fattest: fat babies were the key to evolution of the large human brain. Comp Biochem Physiol A Mol Integr Physiol 2003;136:17–26

72. Leonard WR, Robertson ML. Evolutionary perspectives on human nutrition: The influence of brain and body size on diet and metabolism. Am J Hum Biol 1994;6:77–88

73. Putschar WGJ. The structure of the human symphysis pubis with special consideration of parturition and its sequelae. Am J Phys Anthropol 1976;45:589–94

74. Hisaw FL, Zarrow MX. The physiology of relaxin. In: Harris RS, Thimann KV, eds. Vitamins and Hormones: Advances in Research and Applications. New York: Academic Press Inc, 1951

75. Lapeer RJ, Prager RW. Fetal head moulding: finite element analysis of a fetal skull subjected to uterine pressures during the first stage of labour. J Biomechan 2001;34:1125–33

76. Dienske H. A Comparative approach to the question of why human infants develop so slowly. In: Else JG, Lee PC, eds. Primate Ontogeny, Cognition and Social Behaviour. Cambridge, UK: Cambridge University Press, 1986:145–54

77. Martin RD. The evolution of human reproduction: a primatological perspective. Am J Phys Anthropol 2007;(Suppl 45):59–84

78. Zihlman A. The natural history of apes: Life history features of females and males. In: Morbeck M, Galloway A, Zihlman A, eds. The Evolving Female A Life History Perspective. Princeton, NJ: Princeton University Press, 1997:86–103

79. Innis SM. Dietary (n-3) fatty acids and brain development. J Nutrit 2007;137:855–9

80. Cetin I, Alvino G, Cardellicchio M. Long chain fatty acids and dietary fats in fetal nutrition. J Physiol 2009;587:3441–51

81. Haggarty P, Ashton J, Joynson M, Abramovich DR, Page K. Effect of maternal polyunsaturated fatty acid concentration on transport by the human placenta. Biol Neonate 1999;75:350–9

82. Duttaroy AK. Transport of fatty acids across the human placenta: A review. Prog Lipid Res 2009;48:52–61

83. Hanebutt FL, Demmelmair H, Schiessl B, Larque E, Koletzko B. Long-chain polyunsaturated fatty acid (LC-PUFA) transfer across the placenta. Clin Nutrit 2008;27:685–93

84. Rutherford JN, Tardif SD. Developmental plasticity of the microscopic placental architecture in relation to litter size variation in the common marmoset monkey (Callithrix jacchus). Placenta 2009;30:105–10

85. Adam-Perrot A, Clifton FB. Low-carbohydrate diets: nutritional and physiological aspects. Obesity Rev 2006;7:49–58

86. Lindqvist PG, Svensson PJ, Dahlback B, Marsal K. Factor V Q506 mutation (activated protein c resistance) associated with reduced intrapartum blood loss — a possible evolutionary selection mechanism. Thromb Haemost 1998;79:69–73

87. Lindqvist PG, Dahlback B. Carriership of factor V Leiden and evolutionary selection advantage. Curr Med Chem 2008;15:1541–4

88. Spina V, Aleandri V, Morini F. The impact of the factor V Leiden mutation on pregnancy. Hum Reprod Update 2000;6:301–6

89. Zivelin A, Mor-Cohen R, Kovalsky V, et al. Prothrombin 20210G>A is an ancestral prothrombotic mutation that occurred in whites approximately 24 000 years ago. Blood 2006;107:4666–8

90. Robertson L, Wu O, Langhorne P, et al. Thrombophilia in pregnancy: a systematic review. Br J Haematol 2006;132:171–96

91. Lefeber Y, Voorhoeve HWA. Indigeous Customs in Childbirth and Child Care. Assen, The Netherlands: Van Gorcum & Comp, 1998

92. Kitzinger S. The Social Context of Birth: Some comparisons between childbirth in Jamaica and Britain. In: MacCormack C, ed. Ethnography of Fertility and Birth. London: Academic Press, 1982

93. Kuntner L. Die Gebarhaltung der Frau. Munich: Hans Marseille Verlag, 1988

94. Lynch FG, Abrams ET. Obligate Midwifery as a Strategy to Minimize Postpartum Hemorrhage. 34th Annual Meeting of the Human Biology Association; Chicago, IL, 2009

95. Kominiarek MA. Postpartum hemorrhage. Hospital Phys Obstet Gynecol Board Rev Manual 2008;11:1–12

8

Postpartum Hemorrhage Today: Living in the Shadow of the Taj Mahal

A. B. Lalonde, J. Liljestrand, H. Rushwan and P. Okong

'Women are not dying because of a disease we cannot treat. They are dying because societies have yet to make the decision that their lives are worth saving.'
Mahmoud F. Fathalla, President of the International Federation of Gynecology and Obstetrics (FIGO), World Congress, Copenhagen, 1997

INTRODUCTION

The wife of the Shah Jahan of India, the Empress Mumtaz, had 14 children and died after her last childbirth of a postpartum hemorrhage (PPH) in 1630. So great was the Shah Jahan's love for his wife that he built the world's most beautiful tomb in her memory – the Taj Mahal[1]. Far away to the north another country was taking a different approach: in 1663, the Swedish Collegium Medicum was established. The Swedish clergy created an information system that by 1749 provided the first national vital statistics registry in Europe; by 1757, a national training was approved by Queen Eleonora of Sweden for midwives in all parishes. In the 1860s, parliament legislated that all Swedish parishes must have a midwife, and in the next three decades, maternal mortality fell abruptly. The resulting infrastructure – a comprehensive community midwifery system, with physician back-up expertise and an outcome reporting system – is today considered responsible for reducing the maternal mortality rate (MMR) in Sweden from 900 to 230 per 100,000 livebirths in the years between 1751 and 1900[2]. It is noteworthy that an MMR of 230 per 100,000 livebirths was thus reached in an era before cesarean sections, blood transfusions and antibiotics existed. To this day, Sweden enjoys the lowest maternal mortalities in the world, and midwifery remains strong even though birthing care has long since moved to hospitals[2].

In 2012, each nation must decide whether it is going to build monuments to hardship and suffering or take the steps to avoid it. Three years remain until the target date of 2015, and it is already predicted that the Millennium Development Goal (MDG) number 5 to reduce maternal mortality by 75% will only be reached by few low resource countries. Maternal mortality is currently estimated, in three different studies[3–5], to be between 291,000 and 340,000 deaths per year, a number that translates into a global ratio of 200–250 maternal deaths per 100,000. Another way to characterize these deaths is to say that one woman dies every minute of every hour of every day. There needs to be a 5.5% decline in MMR to reach MDG 5, 2.6% for sub-Saharan Africa; however, the overall decline has been 3.1%. Only 13 developing countries will reach MDG 5 by 2015, nine countries of these will achieve both MDG 4 and 5[3].

Most of the deaths and disabilities attributed to childbirth are avoidable, because the medical solutions are well known. Indeed, 99% of maternal deaths occur in developing countries that have an inadequate transport system, limited access to skilled care-givers and poor emergency obstetric services[6]. It is axiomatic that each and every mother and newborn require care that is close to where they live, respectful of their culture and provided by persons with enough skill to act immediately should an unpredictable complication occur. The challenges that remain internationally are not technological but strategic and organizational[6].

PPH is the most common cause of maternal mortality and accounts for 35% of the maternal deaths worldwide. In some countries, it can be up to 55%. The optimal solution for the vast majority, if not all, of these tragedies is prevention, before the birth, by ensuring that women are sufficiently healthy to withstand PPH should it occur and by prevention and treatment of anemia. At the time of the birth, the systematic use of active management of the third stage of labor is promoted, a management strategy that unfortunately is dependent on circumstances and the availability of oxytocics. To their credit, the International Confederation of Midwives (ICM) as well as the International Federation of Gynecology and Obstetrics (FIGO) have engaged their membership in a worldwide campaign since 2003 to address this travesty.

POSTPARTUM HEMORRHAGE: WHEN, WHY AND WHERE

Postpartum hemorrhage definition

PPH has been defined as blood loss in excess of 500 ml in a vaginal birth and in excess of 1000 ml in a cesarean delivery. For clinical purposes, any blood loss that has the potential to produce hemodynamic instability should be considered a PPH. Clinical estimates of blood loss are often inaccurate (see Chapter 9).

Primary postpartum hemorrhage

Primary (immediate) PPH occurs within the first 24 hours after delivery. Approximately 70% of immediate PPH cases are due to uterine atony. Atony of the uterus is defined as the failure of the uterus to contract adequately after the child is born.

Secondary postpartum hemorrhage

Secondary (late) PPH occurs between 24 hours after delivery of the infant and 6 weeks postpartum. Most late PPH is due to retained products of conception, infection, or both.

Etiology

It may be helpful to think of the causes of PPH in terms of the four 'T's:

- Tone: uterine atony, distended bladder
- Trauma: uterine, cervical, or vaginal injury
- Tissue: retained placenta or clots
- Thrombin: pre-existing or acquired coagulopathy.

The World Health Organization (WHO) has examined studies on PPH published between 1997 and 2002 in order to arrive at more precise definitions of PPH and its incidence[7]. Available resources – data from 50 countries, 116 studies and 155 unique data sets – were reported to be poor in quality. Definitions of PPH were lacking in 58% of the published studies and, in the population-based surveys of medium quality, the prevalence ranged from a low of 0.55% of deliveries in Qatar to a high of 17.5% in Honduras.

A systematic review of 120 data sets on the prevalence of PPH published in *Best Practice and Research* reported approximately 6.6% incidence of PPH and 1.86% of severe PPH[8].

A recent nationwide study in the USA reported 2.9% of all deliveries to be complicated by PPH[9]. Very severe PPH was recently reported in a study covering all hospital births in the UK to be at 2.2/10,000 births[7]; it can be expected to be at least four times this level in low income countries.

One of the major problems plaguing the field is how to measure PPH with accuracy. Published data are scant, and an adequate and accurate gold-standard method is lacking. Clinical visual estimation of blood loss is not reliable[10]. As is often the case, necessity becomes the mother of invention. In the rural areas of Tanzania, the use of a 'kanga' has been adopted as a valid measurement tool[11]. Convenient because it is produced and sold locally, the pre-cut kanga is a standard-sized rectangle (100 cm × 155 cm) of local cotton fabric. When three to four soaked kangas are

observed at a delivery, the trained traditional birth attendant (TBA) is entrusted to transfer patients to a health center.

Even when a good measurement methodology is in place, there is still difficulty in defining PPH simply as blood loss greater than 500 ml because it fails to take into account predisposing health factors that are reflected in such a definition. Since the quantity of blood loss is less often important than the actual effect that it has on the laboring woman, it has been suggested that the definition take into account any blood loss that causes a major physiological change, such as low blood pressure, which threatens the woman's life. These issues are discussed in greater detail in Chapter 11.

About 87% of maternal deaths in 2011 were equally distributed between Asia and sub-Saharan Africa[5] but the risks are higher in Africa because it has a smaller population than Asia. For decades, sub-Saharan Africa has been the region with the highest MMR in the world, at over 500/100,000 livebirths. In this region, the numbers of births attended by skilled health personnel and life expectancy at birth strongly correlate with maternal mortality. As an example, the increased ability to measure maternal mortality in Afghanistan has revealed a heretofore suspected but unconfirmed reality. The Center for Disease Control and Prevention's retrospective cohort study of women of reproductive age in four selected districts in four provinces reported an astounding maternal mortality of 1900 per 100,000 live births[12]. Another group of authors, working in the same country, described the reasons for such a high MMR ratio in the Province of Herat:

'. . . conditions for individual and community health often depend on the protection and promotion of human rights. The findings of this study identify a number of human rights factors that contribute to preventable maternal deaths in Herat Province. These include access to and quality of health services, adequate food, shelter, and clean water, and denial of individual freedoms such as freely entering into marriage, access to birth control methods and possibly control over the number and spacing of one's children.'[13]

Sixty per cent of all pregnancy-related maternal deaths occur during the postpartum period and one source suggests 45% of them occur in the first 24 h after delivery[14].

Compared with the other four main causes of direct maternal deaths – hypertensive disease, obstructed or prolonged labor, unsafe abortion and severe infection – PPH is very swift to kill. It is also mostly unexpected and sudden. This means that in a setting where skilled birth attendance is increasing, and many births take place in health centers, the other causes can be effectively dealt with while PPH soon will stand out as a predominant cause of maternal death. Other deaths are easier to prevent through an effective referral system. In low resource settings, PPH needs extra attention in order to reduce MMR. The introduction of appropriate measures to manage PPH at non-hospital level (see Chapter 67) should be seen in this light.

The risk of dying from PPH depends not only on the amount and rate of blood loss, but also the health status of the woman[15]. Poverty, lifestyle, malnutrition and women's lack of decision-making power to control their own reproductive health are some of the broad issues that have unfortunately come to be accepted as inevitable and unchangeable. Despite policy statements by FIGO on task shifting[16,17], there are still many areas of the world where midwives, nurses and other trained health workers cannot use medications on their own volition to prevent and/or treat PPH. The insidious reality about having a PPH is that two-thirds of the women who experience it have no identifiable clinical risk factors such as multiple births or fibroids. In this regard PPH is a veritable equal-opportunity occurrence. However, it is not an equal-opportunity killer because it is the poor, malnourished, unhealthy woman who delivers away from medical care who will die from it, whereas those who are fortunate enough to deliver in a well-supplied and staffed medical facility most likely will survive three delays at the actual time of birth: delay in the decision to recognize a complication and seek help; delay in accessing transportation to reach a medical facility; and, finally, delay in receiving adequate and comprehensive care upon arrival.

Maternal death is closely linked to the access to family planning. A woman who has gone through many births is older, and in many countries often poor. She may also be living in a remote or underserved area. Since the uterus in a grand multiparous woman (usually defined as having gone through six births or more) is thinner and weaker, and this often is combined with anemia and malnutrition, a grand multiparous woman runs much higher risk of PPH, and thereby risk of maternal death in a low resource setting.

In many other countries, hemorrhage accounts for more than half of the maternal deaths, rather than the 33% of maternal mortality usually cited worldwide. For example, in Indonesia it has been reported at 43%, in the Philippines at 53% and in Guatemala at 53%[6].

Within given countries, certain populations are also at increased risk. In Latin America, for example, the Pan American Health Organization (PAHO) has identified reasons why maternal mortality is higher among the indigenous populations:

(1) The professional teams in charge of maternity care underrate or are ignorant of traditional cultural practices;

(2) The health team and pregnant women often communicate poorly, a principal factor behind the low maternity coverage;

(3) Public policies for consensus building and intercultural dialogue on maternal health are in conflict over objectives and goals and the allocation of resources[18].

EXISTING EVIDENCE FOR PREVENTION OF HEMORRHAGE

See the FIGO guidelines on the prevention and treatment of PPH in low resource countries Appendix.

Active management of the third stage of labor[19]

Data support the routine use of active management of the third stage of labor (AMTSL) by all skilled birth attendants, regardless of where they practice; AMTSL reduces the incidence of PPH, the quantity of blood loss and the need for blood transfusion, and thus should be included in any program of intervention aimed at reducing death from PPH (see Chapters 14 and 15).

The usual components of AMTSL include[19]:

(1) Administration of oxytocin (the preferred storage of oxytocin is refrigeration but it may be stored at temperatures up to 30°C for up to 3 months without significant loss of potency) or another uterotonic drug within 1 minute after birth of the infant. Alternatively, a combination of oxytocin 5 IU and ergometrine 0.5 mg per ampoule IM, or misoprostol 600 μg orally. Uterotonics require proper storage:

(a) Ergometrine or methylergometrine: 2–8°C and protect from light and from freezing;

(b) Misoprostol: in aluminum blister pack, room temperature, in a closed container;

(c) Oxytocin: 15–30°C, protect from freezing.

(2) Controlled cord traction.

(3) Uterine massage after delivery of the placenta.

(4) Counseling on the adverse effects and contraindications of these drugs should be given.

Warning! *Do not give ergometrine, methylergometrine, or syntometrine (because they contain ergot alkaloids) to women with heart disease, pre-eclampsia, eclampsia, or high blood pressure.*

Misoprostol and the prevention of postpartum hemorrhage

The 18th Expert Committee on the Selection and Use of Essential Medicines met in March 2011, and approved the addition of misoprostol for the prevention of PPH to the WHO model list of essential medicines[20]. It reported that misoprostol 600 μg orally can be used for the prevention of PPH where oxytocin is not available or cannot be safely used. Misoprostol should be administered by health care workers trained in its use during the third stage of labor, soon after birth of the infant, to reduce the occurrence of PPH[21]. The most common adverse effects are transient shivering and pyrexia. Education of women and birth attendants in the proper use of misoprostol is essential. Recent studies in Afghanistan and Nepal demonstrate that community-based distribution of misoprostol can be successfully implemented under government health services in a low-resource setting, and, accompanied by education can be a safe, acceptable, feasible and effective way to prevent PPH[22,23].

The usual components of management of the third stage of labor with misoprostol include[21]:

- A single dose of 600 μg administered orally (data from two trials comparing misoprostol with placebo show that misoprostol 600 μg given orally reduces PPH with or without controlled cord traction or use of uterine massage

- Controlled cord traction **only** when a skilled attendant is present at the birth

- Uterine massage after delivery of the placenta, as appropriate.

An even more promising alternative method to deal with PPH was undertaken in Indonesia, where 1811 women were offered counseling about the prevention of PPH and use of misoprostol by trained and supervised volunteers. This study demonstrated that misoprostol was safely used in a self-directed manner among study participants who had home deliveries in the intervention area.[24]

A recent study, not yet published, has questioned the need for massage and control cord traction. It would appear that the oxytocic is the most important factor in AMTSL. However, teaching staff and patients about uterine massage has huge benefits in preventing unsuspected PPH especially in delivery units with inadequate staff.

Misoprostol is available in many countries (see Addendum A). There are, however, restrictions to its use in many countries resulting from the fear that it will be used as an abortifacient. Given the potential benefits of misoprostol to the major goal of the MDG 5 (maternal mortality), and the fact that WHO has added it to its list of 'essential medicines' there appears to be a role for FIGO, ICM and the research community in closing the gaps on research as well as the barriers to availability of this medication.

ONGOING INITIATIVES TO PREVENT POSTPARTUM HEMORRHAGE

Every childbearing woman is potentially at risk for PPH, but biological/physiological considerations are only a part of the picture. Broader issues suggest that health care workers should assume more of an attitude of service and responsibility in the larger public health issues, empowering women to seek help because the health care culture is acceptable to them. With respect to indigenous populations and minority groups forgotten or subjugated by a dominant culture, more sensitive approaches that respect pregnancy and birth as a social and cultural rather than a medical act and incorporating traditional practitioners, e.g. the 'partera' in Central America, into the health care team, are an important step forward. It is crucial that physicians,

midwives, and nurses work with communities and women's groups to bridge existing gaps in care.

An international group including the ICM, FIGO members, researchers and experts met in Ottawa, Canada, in August 2003 to craft the Ottawa Statement on prevention of PPH[25] and offer new options for its treatment. At the World Congress of FIGO in Chile in 2003, President Arnaldo Acosta announced that FIGO, in partnership with ICM, would launch an initiative that would promote AMTSL to prevent PPH and increase the knowledge of nurses, midwives and physicians in the medical and surgical treatment of PPH. Both FIGO and ICM collaborated with the Program for Appropriate Technology for Health (PATH) to conduct a project: Prevention of PPH Initiative (POPPHI), 2005–2010[26]. The program has created tool kits and educational modules for implementation of the AMTSL. POPPHI provided small grants to countries for FIGO and ICM members to collaborate on scaling up the use of AMTSL. The results of this initiative are discussed in more detail in Chapter 15. These initiatives have been prompted in large part by the fact that past efforts have not decreased maternal mortality and morbidity substantially. PPH prevention and treatment procedures are well known and are proven to be scientifically beneficial but not readily available to health workers and pregnant women.

FIGO 2012 postpartum hemorrhage guideline for low resource countries[27] (see Appendix on PPH Guidelines)

Management of third-stage labor should be offered to women since it reduces the incidence of PPH due to uterine atony.

Protocols on management of PPH in general and the use of medications for prevention and treatment are provided in the FIGO guideline. New therapies such as balloon tamponade (see Chapters 47 and 48) and conservative surgical therapies are now the mainstay of severe PPH treatment[28] (see Chapters 51 and 52).

THE ROLE OF NATIONAL PROFESSIONAL ORGANIZATIONS

Key actions to reduce postpartum hemorrhage

(1) Disseminate the FIGO 2012 clinical guideline on prevention and management of PPH in low resource countries to all national associations of midwives, nurses, medical officers and obstetrician–gynecologists, and ask them to implement the guideline at the national, district and community level.

(2) Obtain support for this statement from agencies in the field of maternal and neonatal health care, such as UN agencies, donors, governments and others.

(3) Recommend that this guideline become a Global Initiative to be adopted by health policy makers and politicians in all countries.

(4) Recommend that this Global Initiative on the prevention of PPH be integrated into the curricula of midwifery, medical and nursing schools.

(5) Advocacy for public education about the right of every woman to have skilled attendants at birth and the need for early prevention and treatment of PPH.

FIGO will work toward ensuring that:

(1) Every mother giving birth anywhere in the world will be offered AMTSL for the prevention of PPH.

(2) Every skilled attendant will have training in AMTSL and in techniques for the treatment of PPH.

(3) Every health facility where births take place will have adequate supplies of uterotonic drugs, equipment and protocols for both the prevention and the treatment of PPH.

(4) PPH emergency trays and wall mounted protocols will be available in all birthing units.

(5) Blood transfusion facilities are available in centers that provide comprehensive health care (secondary and tertiary levels of care). Primary level centers need access to blood supplies quickly or be prepared for quick effective transfers when basic treatment appears to be unsuccessful (see Chapter 67).

(6) Physicians and midwives are trained in simple conservative techniques such as intravenous infusions, aortic compression, bimanual massage of the uterus, removal of retained placenta and uterine tamponade.

(7) Every doctor who can perform a laparotomy and basic clinical officers who are responsible for the surgical management at the peripheral hospital level are provided with surgical training to perform 'simple conservative surgery', including compression sutures and sequential devascularization as well as repairs of cervical lacerations, deep vaginal lacerations and subtotal hysterectomy.

(8) The study of promising new drugs and technologies to prevent and treat PPH is supported by donors and governments.

(9) Member countries are surveyed regularly to evaluate the uptake of these recommendations.

Key steps for success in reducing maternal mortality and morbidity due to PPH

(1) Ensure pre- and in-service training to health care providers in early diagnosis, prevention and treatment of PPH. Promote and reinforce the value and effectiveness of AMTSL as a best practice standard.

(2) All health care providers/professionals and/or birth attendants need to continue advocating at community, district and regional and national health facilities for a secure continuous supply of oxytocics, basic equipment for diagnosis and treatment of PPH.

(3) Health care professionals need to be knowledgeable about physiologic management because they may practice in an environment where AMTSL may not be feasible. Training of all health care providers/professionals and/or birth attendants in the practice of physiologic management, AMTSL, diagnosis and management of PPH.

(4) Prepare and disseminate PPH prevention and treatment protocols.

(5) Monitor the incidence of PPH and ensure quality assurance of treatment at local, regional and national levels.

CONCLUSION

Tourists flock to the Taj Mahal, largely unaware how often around the world the event symbolized by this monument still occurs in the shadows of a woman's blood-soaked dirt floor, or when a desperate husband's rough cart is dragged over poor roads and fails to arrive in time, or in the sad eyes of a basic health-unit nurse. Governments have been slow to prioritize women's health and donor countries have not shown sufficient commitment to dealing with maternal mortality.

The recent Muskoka initiative in Canada by the G-8–G-20 countries in 2010–2011 has shown tremendous leadership in addressing this issue as part of MDG 4 and 5[29]. The secretary general of the UN, Ban Ki-Mon, further launched a funding commitment of all UN countries. This is in a context in which there is supposed recognition that poverty reduction and education are the keys to good health – that there is no health without education and no education without health[30].

To address the issue of PPH, ICM and FIGO have launched a worldwide initiative to promote the offer of active management to all women. Recent advances in the past 20 years have produced new techniques such as balloon tamponade, shock garment (refer to Chapters 38, 39, 47, 48 and 58) and other non-invasive techniques to treat PPH. Both organizations need the support of governments, donors and the public to support the campaign that will lead to addressing MDG 5.

We respectfully request that professional associations implement FIGO guidelines to prevent and treat PPH, and work with government leaders and civil society on the broader issues of poverty, nutrition, status of women and access to heath and education for all girls in the country. Health care professionals can be part of the solution to attain MDG 5. The time is right to act upon the answers that have been staring us in the face for some time. The Taj Mahal monument serves as a reminder that all women deserve a safe birth.

References

1. Taj Mahal History and Pictures. http://www.indianchild.com/taj_mahal.htm
2. Hogberg U. The decline in maternal mortality in Sweden: the role of community midwifery. Am J Pub Health 2004; 94:1312–9
3. Lozanso R, Wang H, Foreman KJ, et al. Progress towards MDG 4 and 5 on maternal and child mortality: An updated systematic analysis. Lancet 2011;378;1139–65
4. Hogan MC, Foreman KJ, Naghavi M, et al. Maternal mortality for 181 countries 1980–2008. A systematic analysis of progress towards Millennium Development Goal 5. Lancet 2010;375:1609–23
5. WHO. Trends in Maternal Mortality 1990–2008. Estimates developed by WHO, UNICEF, UNFPA and the World Bank. www.who.int/reproductivehealth/publications/.../en/index.html
6. Abou Zahr C. Antepartum and postpartum haemorrhage. In: Murray CJL, Lopez AD, eds. Health Dimensions of Sex and Reproduction. Boston: Harvard University Press, 1998: 172–81
7. Gulmezoglu AM. Postpartum haemorrhage (1997–2002). Monitoring and Evaluation Department of Reproductive Health and Research, 25–26 May 2004. Geneva: WHO, 2004
8. Carroli G, Cuesta C, Abalos E, Gulmezoglu AM. Epidemiology of post partum haemorrhage: a systematic review. Best Pract Res Clin Obstet Gynaecol 2008;22:999–1012
9. Bateman BT, Berman MF, Riley LE, Leffert LR. The epidemiology of postpartum hemorrhage in a large, nationwide sample of deliveries. Anesth Analg 2010;110:1368–73
10. Razvi K, Chua S, Arulkumaran S, Ratnam SS. A comparison between visual estimation and laboratory determination of blood loss during the 3rd stage of labour. Aust N Z J Obstet Gynaecol 1996;36:152–4
11. Prata N, Mbaruku G, Campbell M. Using the kanga to measure postpartum blood loss. Int J Gynaecol Obstet 2005;89: 49–50
12. Bartlett LA, Mawji S, Whitehead S, et al. Where giving birth is a forecast of death: maternal mortality in four districts of Afghanistan, 1999–2002. Lancet 2005;365:864–70
13. Physicians for Human Rights. Maternal Mortality in Heart Province, Afghanistan, 2002. www.phrusa.org/research/afghanistan/maternal_mortality
14. Li XF, Fortney JA, Kotelchuck M, Glover LH. The postpartum period: the key to maternal mortality. Int J Gynaecol Obstet 1996;52:1–10
15. Coombs CA, Murphy EZ, Laros RK. Factors associated with postpartum hemorrhage with vaginal birth. Obstet Gynecol 1991;77:69–76
16. Lalonde A, FIGO SMNH Committee. Human resources for health in low resource world: Collaborative practice and task shifting in maternal and neonatal care. Int J Obstet Gynecol 2009;105:74–6
17. Gessessew A, Barnabas GA, Prata N, Weidert K. Task shifting and sharing in Tigray, Ethiopia to achieve comprehensive emergency obstetrical care. Int J Obstet Gynecol 2011;113: 28–31
18. Maxine S, Rojas R, PAHO/WHO. Maternal and child mortality among the indigenous peoples of the Americas. Healing our Spirit Worldwide 2004;2:1–3
19. Prendiville W, Elbourne D, McDonald S, Active versus expectant management in the third stage of labour. Cochrane Database Syst Rev 2009;(3):CD000007
20. World Health Organization. Unedited Report of the 18th Committee on the Selection and Use of Essential Medicines. 2011 (cited 9th May 2011). Available at: http://www.who.int/selection_medicines/complete_unedited_TRS_18th.pdf
21. Mobeen N, Durocher J, Zuberi N, et al. Administration of misoprostol by trained traditional birth attendants to prevent postpartum haemorrhage in homebirths in Paskistan: A randomised placebo-controlled trial. BJOG 2011;118:353–61
22. Sanghvi H, Ansari N, Prata NJ, Gibson H, Ehsan AT, Smith JM. Prevention of postpartum hemorrhage at home births in Afghanistan. Int J Gynecol Obstet 2010;108:276–81
23. Rajbhandari S, Hodgins S, Sanghvi H, McPherson R, Pradhan YV, Baqui AH. Expanding uterotonic protection following childbirth through community-based distribution of misoprostol: Operations research study in Nepal. Int J Gynecol Obstet 2010;108:282–8
24. Sanghvi H, Wiknjosastro G, Chanpong G, Fishel J, Ahmed S, Zulkarnain M. Prevention of postpartum hemorrhage in West Java, Indonesia. Baltimore: JHPIEGO Brown's Wharf, 2004
25. Lalonde A, Daviss BA, Acosta A, Herschderfer K. Post partum hemorrhage today: ICM/FIGO initiative 2004–2006. Int J Obstet Gynecol 2006:94:243–53
26. Program for Appropriate Technology for Health (PATH). Maternal and child health: Safe birth and newborn care: Preventing postpartum hemorrhage. Available at: www.path.org/projects/preventing_postpartum_hemorrhage.php. Accessed on January 3, 2012
27. Lalonde A, Okong P, Zulfigar Bhutta S, et al. FIGO Guidelines: Prevention and treatment of postpartum hemorrhage in low-resource settings. Submitted for publication in FIGO Journal, February 2012
28. Kayem G, Kurinczuk JJ, Alfirevic S, Spark P, Brocklehurst P, Knight M. Specific second-line treatments for postpartum hemorrhage: A national cohort study. BJOG 2011;118: 856–64
29. United Nations Development Program (UNDP). The Millennium development goals: Eight goals for 2015. Available at: www.beta.undp.org/content/undp/en/home/mdgoverview.html. Accessed on January 8, 2012
30. Sachs JD. Macroeconomics and Health: Investing in Health for Economic Development. Geneva: World Health Organization, 2001

Addendum A: Countries in which misoprostol is approved

Reproduced from Gynuity, with permission

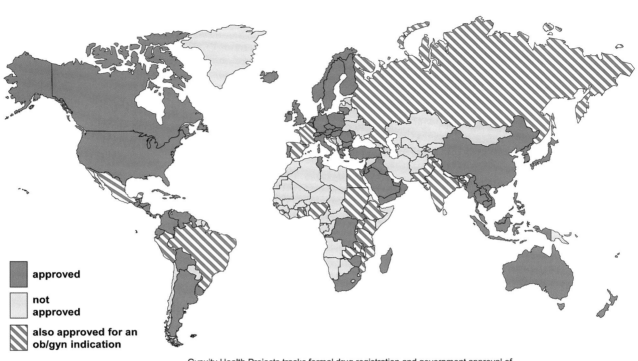

approved

not approved

also approved for an ob/gyn indication

© 2011 Gynuity Health Projects
Updated July 2011

Gynuity Health Projects tracks formal drug registration and government approval of misoprostol throughout the world. This map reflects our latest information. If you become aware of registration or approval in new countries, please write to pubinfo@gynuity.org.

9

Blood Loss: Accuracy of Visual Estimation

A. B. Roston, A. L. Roston and A. Patel

As discussed repeatedly in other chapters of this text-book, clinical estimation of blood loss is notoriously inaccurate, although the degree of inaccuracy varies greatly. While some studies have indicated over-estimates as high as 500%[1], others have reported underestimates as low as 30–50%[2–5] of actual losses. Despite conflicting observations, it is likely that overestimation of blood loss occurs at low volumes and underestimation at high volumes. Clearly, the volume of loss affects the degree of accuracy of visual estimates[1,3,5,6].

When translated into clinical practice, overestimation may result in unnecessary and costly interventions, and, perhaps more importantly, underestimation may delay or deter identification and diagnosis of what is truly a hemorrhage. This latter circumstance may result in an unplanned obstetric emergency with catastrophic outcome. To mitigate these potential negative sequelae, multidisciplinary drills to highlight the nature of the problem are mandatory, particularly in training programs (see Chapters 36 and 40).

A labor ward drill conducted at the John H. Stroger Jr Hospital of Cook County provided obstetric care teams with an opportunity to assess their skills at determining blood loss. A multi-station blood loss simulation was designed with seven stations which created opportunities to assess predetermined simulated blood losses. Grape jelly and pomegranate juice were used to simulate clots and blood. Each station had a measured amount, ranging from 50 to 4000 ml. Simulated blood quantities were placed on sanitary pads, delivery pads, basins, drapes and on the floor. This study was approved by the Institution Review Board.

A total of 49 participants (medical students, physician assistants, nurses, obstetric and gynecologic residents and attending staff) completed the skills session. Study results are depicted in Figure 1. The findings clearly document the inaccuracy of blood estimation, as well as the fact that the accuracy of the estimate decreased with an increase in blood volume. This was particularly true above 1000 ml. Of interest, the under buttocks absorbent delivery pad was most deceptive for estimating. In general, underestimates were similar for liquid and clots, but the 4000 ml station consisted entirely of 'clots' and was most underestimated by the vast majority of participants.

This training program was enlightening for participants to understand the limitations of the visual assessment of blood loss. Repetitive interval sessions may aid individuals to increase their accuracy and/or develop a personal blood loss assessment coefficient to anticipate levels of underestimation. Such a coefficient would be comparable to a golf handicap and of great use to individuals who regularly are called upon to assess blood loss in a variety of situations. Future studies could expand on this experiment with larger numbers and under more varied conditions, of which the quality and quantity of atmospheric lighting is most important. This information may be informative in the ongoing education of labor and delivery room staff in drills and other attempts to simulate real-time emergency situations.

Visual estimates provide a quick and inexpensive method of assessing blood loss without technical limitations. However, issues of inaccuracy must be overcome to enhance the reliability of such estimations. The implementation of standardized visual estimation and training programs has the potential to improve accuracy[6]. In addition, as opposed to unaided visual estimates, the use of simple tools such as the collection drape with a calibrated collection pouch has shown great potential for producing more accurate blood loss estimates[5,7]. Accurate detection of blood loss is crucial to reduce the morbidity and mortality of postpartum hemorrhage.

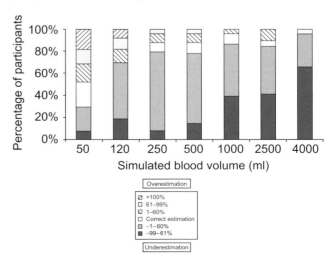

Figure 1 Accuracy of blood volume estimate

References

1. Yoong W, Karavolos S, Damodaram M, et al. Observer accuracy and reproducibility of visual estimation of blood loss in obstetrics: how accurate and consistent are health-care professionals? Arch Gynecol Obstet 2010;281:207–13
2. Chua S, Ho LM, Vanaja K, Nordstrom L, Roy AC, Arulkumaran S. Validation of a laboratory method of measuring postpartum blood loss. Gynecol Obstet Invest 1998;46:31–3
3. Duthie SJ, Ven D, Yung GL, Guang DZ, Chan SY, Ma HK. Discrepancy between laboratory determination and visual estimation of blood loss during normal delivery. Eur J Obstet Gynecol Reprod Biol 1991;38:119–24
4. Razvi K, Chua S, Arulkumaran S, Ratnam SS. A comparison between visual estimation and laboratory determination of blood loss during the third stage of labor. Aust N Z J Obstet Gynaecol 1996;36:152–4
5. Toledo P, McCarthy RJ, Hewlett BJ, Fitzgerald PC, Wong CA. The accuracy of blood loss estimation after simulated vaginal delivery. Anesth Analg 2007;105:1736–40
6. Dildy GA 3rd, Paine AR, George NC, Velasco C. Estimating blood loss: can teaching significantly improve visual estimation? Obstet Gynecol 2004;104:601–6
7. Patel A, Goudar SS, Geller SE, et al. Drape estimation vs. visual assessment for estimating postpartum hemorrhage. Int J Gynaecol Obstet 2006;93:220–4

10

Assessing and Replenishing Lost Volume

J. G. L. Cockings and C. S. Waldmann

INTRODUCTION

Classically, shock is defined as a state of inadequate tissue perfusion in relation to the metabolic needs of a given patient. Inadequate blood flow may manifest clinically as tachycardia, pallor, oliguria, altered mental status, the development of lactic acidosis, or a combination of these changes.

From a physiological point of view, shock is hypovolemic, cardiogenic, anaphylactic or cytotoxic. Hypovolemic shock is classically associated with postpartum hemorrhage (PPH) and due to loss of circulating blood volume. Hypotension is often present in severe cases, but is a late sign and is a poor guide to the volume of blood lost, as pregnancy is accompanied by an alteration of cardiovascular physiology, and the response to blood loss and its management may differ from the non-pregnant situation.

In the UK today, massive PPH accounts for 35% of obstetric admissions to intensive care[1-3]. The 2006–2008 Confidential Enquiry into Maternal Deaths[1] shows that PPH continues to be a significant cause of peripartum maternal deaths, despite the relative luxury of equipment, staffing and other resources. It is axiomatic that bleeding patients demand rapid assessment and judicious replenishment of lost circulating volume, albeit within the context of the compensatory effects of hypovolemic shock and the physiological changes that occur in late pregnancy.

PHYSIOLOGY

The normal circulating blood volume for a healthy non-pregnant adult is 70 ml/kg, or 7.5% of body weight. Cardiac output is 4–6 l/min, and the non-pregnant adult systemic vascular resistance is 10–15 mmHg/l/min (900–1200 dyne.s/cm[5]). Maternal blood volume increases during pregnancy to 40% above baseline by the 30th week, with an accompanying but smaller (20–30%) increase in red cell volume. Cardiac output increases to 50% above pre-pregnancy levels by the 24th week. Systemic blood pressure is more variable in healthy uncomplicated pregnancy, with a small fall in the first and second trimesters, but return to pre-pregnancy levels by the third. Resting heart rate increases progressively in the first and second trimesters to 15–20 bpm above pre-pregnant levels. In addition to these changes, others take place in the autoregulation of intravascular volume and the circulation, both of which affect the body's response to blood loss. Examples include a blunted response to angiotensin II, which in part may be due to an increased production of nitric oxide[4], a decreased tolerance to postural changes and an increased cardiac noradrenaline turnover[5,6].

Circulating volume, clinical signs of hypovolemia and the body's ability to compensate for volume loss are also all affected by pregnancy related diseases and their treatment, the effects of which continue on into the early postpartum period. Pre-eclampsia, for example, causes a contracted effective arterial blood volume compared with the normal peripartum state. Vascular reactivity is increased, and widely used drugs such as hydralazine and magnesium compromise the body's ability to produce compensatory vasoconstriction in the face of hemorrhage. Indeed, it appears that there is a failure to increase plasma volume and reduce systemic vascular resistance in pre-eclampsia due to inadequate trophoblastic invasion into the spiral arteries of the uterus[6]. Pre-eclamptic patients thus have an increased tendency to develop pulmonary edema during volume replacement due to many factors, including increased capillary permeability, hypoalbuminemia and left ventricular dysfunction[6].

Normal delivery results in predictable blood losses which range from 300–500 ml for vaginal deliveries to 750–1000 ml for cesarean section births, although these numbers are variously described not only in this text, but also in the literature published in the past 5 years (see Chapter 11). Regardless, in addition to blood lost from the body, a substantial amount of blood is also redirected into the systemic circulation, often referred to as the autotransfusion effect. This results in an increase in cardiac output by as much as 80% (see Chapter 22). The effect persists in uncomplicated patients, gradually returning to non-pregnant levels at 2–3 weeks[6].

ASSESSMENT OF CIRCULATING BLOOD VOLUME

Young healthy adults can compensate for the loss of large volumes from the circulation with few initially obvious external signs. To say that accurate assessment of blood loss is difficult for the experienced as well as the inexperienced examiner is not only correct but also represents an important theme that is re-echoed in numerous chapters of this book.

In cases of hemorrhage, symptoms often precede signs. These include unexplained anxiety and restlessness, the feeling of breathlessness (with or without an increased respiratory rate), and a sensation of being cold or generally unwell. For healthy, non-pregnant adults, hypovolemia and associated signs can be divided into four stages (Table 1). These range from the largely undetectable stage 1 with less than 15% loss of volume, to the severe life-threatening stage 4 when more than 40% has been lost. Unfortunately, comparable tables for early and late pregnancy and the immediate postpartum period have not been compiled, but the signs follow a similar pattern.

As helpful as such tables may be, the most important clinical principle in the treatment of PPH is early recognition and prompt correction of lost circulating volume, together with simultaneous medical and/or surgical intervention to prevent further loss. Early recognition of life-threatening physiological derangements can be improved by the use of early-warning scoring systems.

Recording physiological observations at regular intervals has long been routine practice in hospitals. Early-warning scores derived from simple routine physiological recordings can identify those patients with greater risk of critical illness and mortality. In recognition of the normal physiological changes in pregnancy, specialized scores have been developed for use in the obstetric population. These Modified Early Obstetric Warning Scores (MEOWS) are increasingly used in obstetric units throughout the UK and other jurisdictions. Their real value is that they can flag the early but sometimes subtle signs of concealed and largely compensated hemorrhage in the early postpartum patient. These scores use the physiological parameters most likely to detect impending life-threatening compromise. They are based on simple physiological observations which do not demand special skills, thus allowing them to be used across all health care systems, rich or poor. The variables usually comprise respiratory rate, heart rate, systolic blood pressure, temperature and mental awareness, each being assigned a weighted score while the total score is the sum of these. Such systems are reproducible and effective at predicting the likelihood of progression to critical illness. They also are well suited to the early detection of the often subtle signs of unappreciated blood loss. Their use allows a trigger value for ward staff to call for assistance from intensive care or other senior staff. An example of an early warning score for the obstetric population used in the UK is given in Table 2.

Once the possibility of intravascular depletion has been raised, a prompt clinical assessment is urgent, as the clinical condition of the patient can change rapidly. Clinical assessment, in association with non-invasive and invasive monitoring where appropriate, must be made by senior clinicians (if available), with special attention to repeated assessment at frequent intervals to detect the problem as early as possible. If senior clinicians are not available, they should be notified as described in the protocols in Chapters 40 and 41.

Clinical examination is performed simultaneously with incident-related history taking. This history may elicit obvious features associated with shock such as overt blood loss and pain, but may also elicit more subtle features such as general malaise, anxiety and restlessness, a poorly defined sense of doom and breathlessness. Physical examination is directed to the fundamental areas of vital function, the conscious state and airway protection, the adequacy of respiratory function, oxygenation and circulation. In particular, the following should be assessed and documented:

(1) Early stages of shock are associated with restlessness and agitation, sometimes with a heightened sense of thirst, but these progress to drowsiness when around 30% of blood volume is lost. Loss of consciousness is a very late sign, with significant risk of imminent death.

(2) Tachypnea is an early sign, partly driven initially by the anxiety, but is an independent sign, and the respiratory rate increases with progressive blood loss and will usually exceed 20 breaths/min when 30% of blood volume is lost.

(3) Oxygenation becomes harder to assess clinically as peripheral pallor becomes more marked, and the pulse oximeter becomes less reliable as peripheral perfusion becomes weaker.

(4) A fall in the jugular venous pressure occurs reasonably early, but is partly compensated for by a

Table 1 Stages of shock

Classification	Stage 1	Stage 2	Stage 3	Stage 4
Blood loss (% volume lost)	10–15	15–30	30–40	>40
Conscious state	Alert, mild thirst	Anxious and restless	Agitated or confused	Drowsy, confused or unconscious
Respiratory rate	Normal	Mildly elevated	Raised	Raised
Complexion	Normal	Pale	Pale	Marked pallor or gray
Extremities	Normal	Cool	Pale and cool	Cold
Capillary refill	Normal	Slow (>2 s)	Slow (>2 s)	Minimal or absent
Pulse rate	Normal	Normal	Elevated	Fast but thready
Systolic blood pressure	Normal	Normal	Normal or slightly low	Hypotensive
Urine output	Normal	Reduced	Reduced	Oligoanuric

Modified from Baskett, 1990[7]

Table 2 Modified early obstetric warning score. Reproduced with permission by Dr R. Jones, Consultant Anaesthetist, Royal Berkshire Hospital, UK

	Score						
	3	*2*	*1*	*0*	*1*	*2*	*3*
Respiratory rate (bpm)		<8		9–18	19–25	26–30	>30
Pulse rate (bpm)		<40	40–50	51–100	101–110	111–129	>129
Systolic blood pressure (mmHg)	<70	71–80	81–100	101–164	165–200	>200	
Diastolic blood pressure (mmHg)				<95	95–104	>105	
Conscious level	Unresponsive	Responds to pain	Responds to voice	Alert	Irritated		
Urine hourly (ml/h) or in 24 h	0	<30 (<720 ml)	<45 (<1000 ml)	>45 (>1000 ml)			

Final score = sum of individual scores at any one time
Action:
Score 0 or 1 Repeat observations when appropriate for clinical scenario
Score 2 Inform midwife in charge, repeat in 15 min
Score 3 Inform midwife in charge, obstetric registrar and duty anesthetist
Score ≥4 As above but the consultant obstetrician should be informed
Consider informing duty consultant anesthetist and intensive care team*
*The timing of involvement of the most senior obstetrician and anesthetist, as well as the timing of intensive care involvement will be highly dependent on the staffing structure, seniority and operating principles in the particular institution. Each institution, if introducing an Early Warning Score system, should define the callout thresholds appropriate for their own particular organizational structure

reduction in venous capacitance. However, the jugular veins can be hard to visualize reliably in postpartum women.

(5) A more reliable indication of hypovolemia from the central venous pressure is the poor increase observed following volume administration.

(6) The pulse rate increases after around 15–20% of blood volume has been lost, but this sign can be unreliable as a sinus tachycardia is physiological in late pregnancy and in the early postpartum period.

(7) Capillary refill is slowed after 15% of blood volume is lost and is almost completely absent when 40% of volume is lost.

(8) Blood pressure is well maintained, despite a falling cardiac output and tissue perfusion, until over 30–40% of circulating volume is lost.

MANAGEMENT

When the compensating mechanisms directed toward maintaining the blood pressure are exhausted, pressure readings fall dramatically. At this point, shock is advanced and the risk of imminent death is significant. If the patient is under competent medical care, however, by this same point in time, the significant blood loss will have been recognized, volume and, in the majority of instances, blood replacement begun via large-bore peripheral access and medical therapies and surgical intervention organized. Clinical signs alone, even by experienced clinicians, are often unreliable in estimating the volume deficit and the degree of shock when well compensated. Therefore, other methods to assess more accurately volume status and circulatory adequacy must be used to aid clinical assessment.

The first and simplest of these is invasive measurement of central venous pressure. A central venous catheter can be placed in any central vein, but it should be remembered that, once the patient is in actual hypovolemia, identification of a central vein may be difficult without the use of ultrasound. The internal jugular vein is the preferred site in this situation, as the femoral vein is relatively inaccessible, and the subclavian route may have a higher risk of complications in late pregnancy and the early postpartum period, especially if inserted under urgent conditions.

The National Institute for Clinical Excellence (NICE) suggests that cannulation of central veins using two-dimensional ultrasound imaging is the preferred method, with the evidence strongest for the internal jugular route[8]. In the healthy, non-pregnant adult, the systemic venous capacity is 3–4 liters, or 75% of circulating volume. If the tone of the venous capacitance vessels did not change as volume was lost from the circulation, the central venous pressure would fall quickly and early, with early compromise of the cardiac output. However, as blood volume is lost, the tone in these venous capacitance vessels increases, moving blood centrally, and maintaining central venous pressure.

Confusion surrounding the concept of venous return can be dispelled if it is thought of in terms of right atrial pressure rather than an increased flow of blood to the right atrium. As blood is lost, the volume in the venous capacitance vessels is reduced and the tone in these vessels increases. The central venous pressure falls progressively, but to a lesser degree due to the compensatory increase in this venous tone. Figure 1 shows the relationship between venous capacitance and central venous pressure during acute blood loss and immediate replacement. As blood is lost from the circulation, the patient follows the line A to B (Figure 1). The central venous pressure falls slowly at first, then more steeply as the extent of blood loss increases. As volume is returned to the circulation, the patient will follow first the line B to C and then C to D, rather than simply returning from B to A. This is

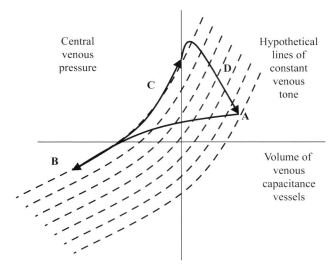

Figure 1 Central venous pressure and venous capacitance during blood loss and replacement. Modified from Bradley, 1977[9]

due to a number of factors and is addressed in a later section in this chapter.

The ability to palpate a peripheral pulse is a good sign, but correlates poorly to any specific arterial pressure. Loss of peripheral pulses is a late preterminal sign of hypovolemic shock. Arterial pressure is most simply measured using a sphygmomanometer. This is familiar to all clinicians and uses a Riva Rocci cuff placed around the upper arm. The correct size of cuff must be chosen, however, because if the arm is too large for the chosen cuff, the estimated reading will be falsely high.

Frequently, arterial blood pressure is measured non-invasively by means of an automated version of this technique. Unfortunately, such methods become inaccurate and unreliable when the blood pressure deviates significantly from normal, especially in times of poor peripheral perfusion and hypotension[10], which are the very conditions seen in marked hypovolemia due to PPH. Automated non-invasive blood pressure devices tend to over-estimate hypotension and under-estimate hypertension. They can repeatedly cycle in an attempt to measure when marked hypotension is present, which can delay its early recognition. Finally, they can sometimes give a totally erroneous reading suggesting an adequate blood pressure when, in reality, the blood pressure is absent or unmeasurable due to marked hypovolemic shock, thereby giving a false sense of security[10].

The most reliable method of arterial blood pressure measurement under abnormal or rapidly changing conditions is by means of an intra-arterial cannula and direct measurement via a transducer. This method has the added advantage of providing easy access for blood samples for arterial blood gas analysis and other blood tests. Although such systems commonly use heparinized saline, the use of heparin is unnecessary[11], and the use of plain saline allows samples to be taken for coagulation tests without fear of contamination and erroneous results.

Hemoglobin estimates indicate the concentration of hemoglobin in the sample. The simplicity of this statement only reinforces the point that the concentration of hemoglobin following acute blood loss reflects either medical intervention or the patient's compensation to blood loss. Acute blood loss alone will not change the concentration of hemoglobin in the blood left in the system. The concentration is reduced only when the lost volume is replaced by internal fluid shifts or external fluids are added to the system that are low in hemoglobin. If left untreated, however, acute blood loss results in a fall in hemoglobin concentration after about 4–6 h due to internal compensatory fluid shifts. In contrast, intravenous administration of fluid will dilute the hemoglobin more quickly.

Further information regarding the status of the circulation can be gained by more invasive or complex techniques. These include the pulmonary artery catheter, pulse contour analysis and the esophageal Doppler technique. The measurement of cardiac output by means of the thermodilution technique using a pulmonary artery catheter was first described by Bradley and Branthwaite in 1968[12] and subsequently popularized by Swann, Ganz and co-workers[13]. Despite being the gold standard for invasive assessment of cardiac output and left atrial pressure for several decades, some evidence suggests that the risks of this technique may outweigh its benefits in many circumstances[14]. The benefit of the pulmonary artery catheter is that it provides reliable measurements even in the face of changing body position and is equally effective in the awake, conscious patient as well as the sedated or anesthetized patient receiving artificial ventilation. The risks include those associated with the insertion of a large-bore cannula into a central vein, which is higher risk in the volume-depleted patient suffering massive blood loss, even with the aid of the two-dimensional ultrasound technique. Risks also relate to infection, cardiac arrhythmias, pulmonary artery damage and lung injury. To date, experience with the pulmonary artery catheter in the obstetric population[15] has been in patients with pre-eclampsia and eclampsia rather than massive PPH.

Fortunately, pulse contour analysis is a realistic alternative to the pulmonary artery catheter[16]. This system requires only standard peripheral arterial and central venous cannulae. A common example of this technique uses cardiac output estimated initially and periodically thereafter by the lithium dilution technique (LiDCO Ltd., Cambridge, UK)[17]. The pressure waveform is analysed using this static cardiac output measurement as a reference to estimate a stroke volume. Changes to the pulse waveform and heart rate from this point are used to estimate stroke volume and cardiac output on a continuous display. Calibration is performed by periodic re-assessment of the cardiac output using the lithium dilution technique. Limitations relate to issues of non-linearity or aortic compliance, how closely the radial arterial pulse waveform resonance relates to the proximal aortic waveform and, therefore, stroke volume, the common problems of damped arterial waveforms, drift between static measurements of cardiac output, and problems associated with poor transmission of pulse waves in severe arrhythmias[18]. Despite these concerns, this technique can provide a continuous idea of cardiac output, systemic blood pressure and vascular resistance in any patient with central venous and peripheral arterial access and is well suited for monitoring the postpartum patient who has undergone massive hemorrhage and is undergoing resuscitation. Other commercially available pulse contour analysis systems use alternative methods for measurement of the reference cardiac output. An example is the PiCCO system (Pulsion Medical Systems, Munich, Germany) which employs a transpulmonary thermodilution measurement from an axillary or femoral artery.

REPLENISHING LOST VOLUME

[Editor's Note: This topic is under intense debate on an international basis. A thorough discussion is provided by Lockhart in Chapter 4 and Paidas in Chapter 6. L.G.K.]

Replacing lost circulating volume should commence as soon as significant bleeding is recognized and, ideally, before the signs of significant hypovolemia have developed. Important initial measures are to simultaneously provide supplemental oxygen, ensure multiple large-bore peripheral intravenous access, undertake an initial rapid clinical assessment and summon senior members from anesthesia, intensive care, surgical and hematology departments for assistance when these individuals are available. Each institution should have a rapid response protocol in place for the management of massive hemorrhage and PPH in particular. This protocol should be familiar to all, easily accessible and followed (see Chapters 36 and 40).

The principal underlying aim of volume replacement during and following massive PPH is restoration and maintenance of tissue perfusion to all body organs in order to maintain cellular function and viability. Although the initial focus should be on restoration of the common clinical indicators of shock, the clinician must proceed further. Even if all conventionally used criteria resolve, shock may still be present on a cellular, tissue or organ basis[19]. Compensated shock is the term often used to describe the state where conventional hemodynamic parameters have been returned to normal, despite persisting occult tissue hypoperfusion, typically in the splanchnic bed. In spite of adequate volume replacement, patients may develop multiple organ dysfunction with its associated morbidity and mortality.

Replenishing the lost blood volume must take place simultaneously with control of the bleeding. *Medical and surgical attempts to control bleeding must not be delayed by prolonged volume resuscitation in the face of ongoing blood loss.* Volume resuscitation should be aimed at restoration of circulating blood volume as well as returning the oxygen-carrying capacity and hemostatic functions to an effective, albeit subnormal, level.

Initial volume replacement enhances right atrial filling and improves cardiac output. As shock develops with blood loss, venous tone increases as described above. Volume administration should be rapid, but titrated to the right atrial filling pressure. Initially, right atrial filling pressure may be restored by a smaller volume than that lost due to the reduced capacity in the venous capacitance vessels. Indeed, immediate rapid re-infusion of the entire volume lost may provoke fluid overload if the tone in the capacitance vessels did not decrease as rapidly. This can be appreciated from Figure 1; here, rapid volume replacement occurs along the line B to C. Central venous pressure rises despite the intravascular compartment remaining depleted. As the venous tone relaxes following resuscitation, further volume administration can occur with a central venous pressure falling toward normal as the volume in the venous capacitance becomes replete (line C to D). Thus, volume administration should be rapid but infused in discrete volume challenges, with the effect on the right atrial filling pressure, systemic blood pressure and other hemodynamic variables being monitored. Commonly, 250–500 ml of either a crystalloid or a colloid is administered over a period of 10–20 min as the urgency dictates and while blood is being obtained (a patient with life-threatening stage 4 shock will receive 2–3 liters more quickly, but, even then, the principles of monitoring the hemodynamic variables during the infusion of fluid remain). Simple measures of tissue underperfusion, which may persist after apparent restoration of global hemodynamics, include the base deficit and serum lactate. Efforts to measure and enhance tissue perfusion should continue until all such parameters return to normal. More specific measures to monitor tissue perfusion, including tissue oxygen tension devices[20] and gastric tonometry[21], are not widely used.

The best fluid to use for volume expansion in hemorrhagic shock remains a matter of debate. Both crystalloid and colloid are effective, but each has advantages and disadvantages[22,23] (Table 3).

One recent large study showed no difference in mortality in intensive care patients requiring volume expansion whether this expansion was made with saline or albumin[24]. Colloids expand the intravascular space preferentially, whereas crystalloids quickly become distributed throughout the extracellular space. Saline has the disadvantage of hyperchloremia, which causes a dilutional or hyperchloremic acidosis[25,26]. The use of crystalloids is not associated with anaphylaxis, whereas colloids such as the gelatins can produce severe life-threatening reactions, although this is less common with hydroxyethyl starch[27]. Crystalloids have minimal effect on coagulation other than a dilutional effect, although saline infusions may have a procoagulant effect[28]. Overall, crystalloids have a lower cost and lower incidence of side-effects, but the colloids have several theoretical advantages regarding tissue edema and oxygen delivery to the tissues. Despite intense debate and research interest, neither crystalloids nor colloids have been shown to be

Table 3 Intravenous fluids

Type of fluid	Advantages	Disadvantages
Crystalloids		
Saline	Cheap; easily available; long history of use	Produces a hyperchloremic acidosis; small procoagulant effect
Hartmann's	No risk of anaphylaxis; minimal direct effect on the base deficit; easily available	Mildly hypotonic
5% Dextrose	No place in acute expansion of the intravascular space	Hypotonic; no significant expansion of the vascular space; rapid distribution to intracellular and extracellular spaces
Hypertonic saline	Rapid expansion of the intravascular space in excess of the volume infused; possible beneficial effects on red cell and endothelial edema and capillary blood flow	Insufficient data; uncertainty regarding possible adverse effects such as on the immune system
Colloids		
Gelatins	Largely remains in the intravascular space for 2–4 h	Risk of anaphylaxis; no clear survival advantage over crystalloids
4% Human albumin	More physiological than gelatins; remains predominantly in the intravascular space for 12 h	Expensive; no clear survival advantage over crystalloids
Hydroxyethyl starch	Remains in the intravascular space for 12–24 h	Risk of coagulopathy, renal injury and reticulo-endothelial accumulation

superior to one another regarding survival outcome from hemorrhagic shock.

Regardless of which substance is selected for volume expansion at the start of therapy, it is essential that blood be administered and that a protocol be available for the use of blood products in instances of massive bleeding. In the UK, the responsibility for maintaining such a protocol lies with the hospital blood transfusion committee, a multidisciplinary committee that all hospitals must by law ensure is in place and answerable to the hospital executive. *It is unacceptable to have situations where the laboratory insists on blood samples being sent for blood count and coagulation studies before any blood products are issued; the on-call hematology consultant should be actively involved and aid with the use of blood, fresh frozen plasma, platelets, cryoprecipitate and the use of recombinant activated factor VII.*

The Trendelenburg position is often used in the management of the hypotensive patient, but its benefit has been questioned. The concept is to displace blood from the lower limbs centrally, to increase preload and enhance cardiac output as a temporary measure until adequate blood volume can be restored. However, little proof exists that this theoretical benefit occurs in practice. Sibbald and colleagues in 1979[29] showed that, in hypotensive patients, the Trendelenburg position did not significantly increase preload, but did increase afterload and blood pressure at the expense of cardiac output. A review of available data concludes that the Trendelenburg position 'is probably not a good position for resuscitation of patients who are hypotensive'[30].

The conventional approach to severe hemorrhage, where the endpoint is euvolemia with restoration of a normal blood pressure, heart rate and cardiac output, has been questioned in the out-of-hospital trauma setting[31]. Although not based on evidence from the obstetric population, the physiological rationale may still be applicable. Falling blood pressure and cardiac output, together with increased sympathetic tone and release of endogenous catecholamines, reduce the rate of blood loss. Restoration of these parameters without

control of the bleeding will increase the total volume of blood loss, increasing the degree of coagulopathy, reducing oxygen-carrying capacity and ensuing multiple organ dysfunction[32]. Low-volume fluid resuscitation for hemorrhagic shock may be a possibility[33] and the evidence suggests that volume resuscitation should be deliberately limited to the minimum required to sustain vital organ function until the bleeding has been arrested, such as by surgery[31,34].

Small-volume hypertonic resuscitation also has been advocated for hemorrhagic shock. Here too, the target population was not obstetric, and the shock was not from PPH. The concept is that a relatively small infused volume will cause much larger expansion of the circulation by drawing water into the intravascular compartment. There is evidence that there may be beneficial effects of endothelial and red cell edema and capillary flow, but concerns are present regarding other potentially adverse effects such as that on the immune system[35]. This latter concern has not been shown to be a problem in clinical practice[36].

Maintenance of the hemoglobin concentration is essential for oxygen-carrying capacity and delivery to the tissues. Titration of fluid and blood products to an exact hemoglobin level in a rapidly bleeding patient is difficult. A hemoglobin level of 7–8 g/dl appears an appropriate threshold for transfusion in the intensive-care population, with possible benefit for a higher level of 9 g/dl for those with ischemic heart disease[37]. It is logical to aim at the high end of the target range when resuscitating from hemorrhagic shock as there is a tendency to drift down. A target of 10 g/dl has been suggested as a reasonable goal in the actively bleeding patient[38]. In the case of PPH, however, the goal is two-fold cessation of the hemorrhage as well as restoration of the hemoglobin level.

Coagulation disorders are both predisposing factors for, and consequences of, massive PPH. A bleeding diathesis from a coagulopathy, thrombocytopenia or platelet dysfunction may result from pre-existing disease, a pregnancy-acquired disorder, such as eclampsia, or treatment, such as aspirin. Massive blood loss also creates both a coagulopathy and thrombocytopenia through dilution and consumption. These issues and their management are discussed in detail in Chapters 25 and 50.

SUMMARY

Rapid assessment of the presence of occult bleeding or intravascular volume depletion is essential. The body can compensate for blood loss such that, by the time obvious clinical signs are present, a significant volume can already be lost and tissues already in a state of hypoperfusion. Normal physiological adaptations in late pregnancy that persist into the postpartum period can make recognition and quantification of intravascular loss difficult, and can render the body less capable of withstanding massive blood loss. This can be further complicated by pregnancy-related disease such as pre-eclampsia and its treatment, and modalities such as hydralazine and magnesium.

Assessment of both the degree of loss and the response to volume replacement require clinical skills, invasive hemodynamic monitoring and the early involvement of senior clinicians. The use of Modified Obstetric Early Warning Scores in all patients to aid the early detection of concealed hemorrhage and serious acute illness is to be strongly encouraged. A simple system such as this based on easy to measure physiological variables is easy to implement, does not rely on extensive training or experience and does not need to be limited to the developed world.

There is no one correct fluid to use. It is usual to use a combination of crystalloids or colloids and blood products to maintain a hemoglobin concentration of near 10 g/dl during the actively bleeding period (7–9 g/dl is probably safe once the active bleeding has been stopped). Coagulopathies and thrombocytopenia also need to be corrected with appropriate transfusion products and with active involvement of the hematologists. There may be a place for limited volume expansion before the bleeding has been stopped surgically to reduce the volume lost, but this must not be at the cost of demonstrable organ ischemia.

Prompt recognition, close monitoring of volume status, rapid arrest of the bleeding and adequate volume resuscitation are all required but when used together can reduce mortality from PPH.

References

1. Lewis G. ed. Saving Mothers' Lives: Reviewing Maternal Deaths to Make Motherhood Safer – 2006–2008. The Eighth Report on Confidential Enquiries into Maternal Deaths in the United Kingdom. London: CMACE, 2011
2. Umo-Etuk J, Jumley J, Holdcroft A. Critically ill parturient women and admissions to intensive care: a 5-year review. Int J Obstet Anesth 1996;5:79–84
3. Schofield H, et al. Providing Equity of Critical and Maternity Care for the Critically Ill Pregnant or Recently Pregnant Woman. Maternity Critical Care Working Group, July 2011
4. Wong AYH, Kulandavelu S, Whiteley KH, Qu D, Lowell-Langille B. Maternal cardiovascular changes during pregnancy and postpartum in mice. Am J Physiol Heart Circ Physiol 2002;282:H918–25
5. Cohen WR, Galen LH, Vega-Rich M, Young JB. Cardiac sympathetic activity during rat pregnancy. Metabolism 1988; 37:771–7
6. Fujitani S, Baldisseri MR. Hemodynamic assessment in a pregnant and peripartum patient. Crit Care Med 2005;33 (Suppl):S354–61
7. Baskett PJF. ABC of major trauma. Management of hypovolemic shock. BMJ 1990;300:1453–7
8. National Institute for Clinical Excellence. Guidance on the use of ultrasound locating devices for placing central venous catheters. Technology Appraisal Guidance 49. London: NHS Publishers, 2002
9. Bradley RD. Studies in Acute Heart Failure. London: Edward Arnold, 1977:11
10. Cockings JGL. The Australian Incident Monitoring Study. Blood pressure monitoring – applications and limitations: an analysis of 2000 incident reports. Anaesth Intensive Care 1993;21:565–9
11. Gamby A, Bennett J. A feasibility study of the use of non-heparinised 0.9% sodium chloride for transduced arterial and venous lines. Intensive Critical Care Nursing 1995;11:148–50
12. Branthwaite MA, Bradley RD. Measurement of cardiac output by thermal dilution in man. J Applied Physiol 1968; 24:434
13. Swan HJ, Ganz W, Forrester J, Marcu H, Diamond G, Chonette D. Catheterization of the heart in man with use of a flow-directed balloon-tipped catheter. N Engl J Med 1970; 283:447–51
14. Harvey S, Harrison DA, Singer M, et al. Assessment of the clinical effectiveness of pulmonary artery catheters in management of patients in intensive care (PAC-Man): a randomised controlled trial. Lancet 2005;366:472–7
15. Nolan TE, Wakefield ML, Devoe LD. Invasive hemodynamic monitoring in obstetrics. A critical review of its indications, benefits, complications, and alternatives. Chest 1992;101:1429–33
16. Godje O, Hoke K, Goetz AE. Reliability of a new algorithm for continuous cardiac output determination by pulse-contour analysis during hemodynamic instability. Crit Care Med 2002;30:52–8
17. Linton RA, Band DM, Haire KM. A new method of measuring cardiac output in man using lithium dilution. Br J Anaesth 1993;71:262–6
18. Van Lieshout JJ, Wesseling KH. Editorial II: Continuous cardiac output by pulse contour analysis. Br J Anaesth 2001; 86:467–8
19. Dabrowski GP, Steinberg SM, Ferrara JJ, Flint LM. A critical assessment of endpoints of shock resuscitation. Surg Clin North Am 2000;80:825–44
20. Huang YC. Monitoring oxygen delivery in the critically ill. Chest 2005;128(5 Suppl 2):554–60S
21. Totapally BR, Fakioglu H, Torbati D, Wolfsdorf J. Esophageal capnography during hemorrhagic shock and after resuscitation in rats. Crit Care 2003;7:19–20
22. Perel P, Roberts I. Colloids versus crystalloids for fluid resuscitation in critically ill patients. Cochrane Database Syst Rev 2011;(3):CD000567
23. Finfer S, Liu B, Taylor C, et al., SAFE TRIPS Investigators Resuscitation fluid use in critically ill adults: an international cross-sectional study in 391 intensive care units. Crit Care 2010;14:R185
24. Finfer S, The SAFE Study Investigators. A comparison of albumin and saline for fluid resuscitation in the intensive care unit. N Engl J Med 2004;350:2247–56
25. Walters JH, Gottlieb A, Schoenwald P, Popovich MJ, Sprung J, Nelson DR. Normal saline versus lactated Ringer's solution for intraoperative fluid management in patients undergoing abdominal aortic aneurysm repair: an outcome study. Anesth Analg 2001;93:817–22
26. Scheingraber S, Rehm M, Sehmisch C, Finsterer U. Rapid saline infusion produces hyperchloraemic acidosis in patients

undergoing gynaecological surgery. Anesthesiology 1999;90: 1265–70

27. Laxenaire MC, Charpentier C, Feldman L.Anaphylactoid reactions to colloid plasma substitutes: incidence, risk factors, mechanisms. A French multicenter prospective study. Ann Fr Anesth Reanim 1994;13:301–10

28. Ruttmann TG, James MF, Aronson I. In vivo investigation into the effects of haemodilution with hydroxyethyl starch (200/0.5) and normal saline on coagulation. Br J Anaesth 1998;80:612–6

29. Sibbald WJ, Paterson NA, Holliday RL, Baskerville J. The Trendelenburg position: hemodynamic effects in hypotensive and normotensive patients. Crit Care Med 1979;7:218–24

30. Bridges N, Jarquin-Valdivia AA. Use of the trendelenburg position as the resuscitiation position: to T or not to T? Am J Crit Care 2005;14:364–8

31. National Institute for Clinical Excellence. Prehospital initiation of fluid replacement therapy in trauma: Technology appraisal guidance 74. London: NHS Publishers, 2004

32. American College of Surgeons. Advanced Trauma Life Support. 2011 www.facs.org/trauma/atls/index.html

33. Stern SA. Low-volume fluid resuscitation for presumed hemorrhagic shock: helpful or harmful. Curr Opin Crit Care 2001;7:422–30

34. Kreimeier U, Prueckner S, Peter K. Permissive hypotension. Schweiz Med Wochenschr 2000;130:1516–24

35. Rocha-e-Silva. Small volume hypertonic resuscitation of circulatory shock. Clinics 2005;60:159–72

36. Kolsen-Petersen JA. Immune effect of hypertonic saline: fact or fiction? Acta Anaesthesiol Scand 2004;48:667–78

37. Herbert PC, Wells G, Blajchman MA, et al. A multicenter, randomized, controlled clinical trial of transfusion requirements in critical care. Transfusion Requirements in Critical Care Investigators, Canadian Critical Care Trials Group. N Engl J Med 1999;340:409–17

38. Gutierrez G, Reines HD, Wulf-Gutierrez ME. Clinical review: hemorrhagic shock. Crit Care 2004;8:373–81

11

Pitfalls in Assessing Blood Loss and Decision to Transfer

B. S. Kodkany, R. J. Derman and N. L. Sloan

INTRODUCTION

It is axiomatic that most postpartum hemorrhage (PPH) occurs unpredictably, and no parturient is immune from its risk. Unlike uterine rupture which can precede death by 24 h and antepartum hemorrhage may lead to death in half that time, PPH most often occurs within 2 h of delivery and can be lethal within that time period[1]. Women who voluntarily present for delivery in health care facilities that can promptly and effectively manage PPH have a far lower chance of death from hemorrhage[2]. Most maternal deaths continue to occur in developing countries in women delivering at home or in health care facilities that do not efficiently manage obstetric complications including PPH[3].

Our understanding of the definitions of PPH is evolving, as most women experiencing a loss of 500 ml of blood, the common definition of PPH, do not receive clinical intervention or experience serious consequences[4,5]. These definitions are described in Chapter 16. Traditionally, blood loss after delivery is visually estimated. The birth attendant makes a gross quantitative estimate; however, there is wide variation and inaccuracy in such estimates. The importance of accurately measuring vaginal blood loss at delivery was stressed by Williams as early as 1919[6]. In the past, various mechanisms have been advocated to estimate postpartum blood loss. These include the acid hematin method, by which blood in the sponges and pads was mixed with a solution that converted hemoglobin to acid hematin or cyanmethemoglobin, which in turn was measured by a colorimeter. Other methods were plasma volume determinations before and after delivery using radioactive tracer elements, determination of changes in other blood indices before and after delivery, and use of ^{51}Cr-labeled erythrocytes[7]. Quantitative methods for estimating vaginal blood loss include direct collection of blood into bedpans or plastic bags and gravimetric methods wherein pads are weighed before and after use, the difference in the weight being used to determine the amount of blood lost[8].

Numerous studies of carefully quantified postpartum blood loss indicate that clinical visual assessment is unreliable and generally underestimates measured postpartum blood loss, with an average underestimation of 100–150 ml; of equal importance, using visual estimation is accompanied by greater inaccuracy with higher volume blood loss, which may underestimate the incidence of PPH by 30–50%[7–13]. For example, the prevalence of PPH and severe PPH (loss of 1000 ml or more) is 6.1% and 1.7%, respectively, when visually estimated, and 10.6% and 3.0%, respectively, when quantitatively measured[4]. The prevalence of PPH is also much lower in observational studies (6.0% in 31) than in clinical trials (13.9% in 24) that place greater priority on accurately evaluating blood loss[7]. As a result, numerous authorities advocate a more objective approach to the diagnosis of PPH.

The accurate measurement of blood loss by an ideal method remains a gray area. While measurement of postpartum vaginal blood loss is critical in research, the methods described above have not been adopted in clinical practice because of their complexity, expense and the time required to obtain results before being able to act upon them. Given these circumstances, visual (clinical) estimation, inaccurate as it may be, remains the norm. To facilitate accurate and timely measurement, the BRASSS-V drape™ (discussed below), an elongated, V-shaped calibrated plastic pouch, sometimes tied around the woman's waist, with a funnel portion hanging between her legs (Excellent Fixable Drapes, Madurai, Tamil Nadu, India) was developed in 2002 and costs less than 3 US dollars each[12].

NORMAL BLOOD LOSS DURING DELIVERY

The range of average blood loss during vaginal delivery is uncertain, being variously reported at the low end as 343 ml in 1000 consecutive term vaginal deliveries, as 339 ml and 490 ml in two separate albeit small studies of 100 and 123 patients, respectively, using the acid hematin spectrophotometric method and as 450 ml in 123 deliveries using chromium-labeled erythrocytes[8,14–16]. Despite these variations, it is generally accepted that blood loss during vaginal delivery varies from 400 to 500 ml[17], whereas most cesarean births are associated with 500–800 ml loss[18,19]. Unfortunately, these values are mostly reflective of hospital based data, primarily obtained among women in the developed world, most of whom receive prophylactic uterotonics to prevent PPH. A recent meta-analysis of measured loss indicates that median postpartum loss without prophylactic uterotonics ranges from 450 to 500 ml compared with 200 to 300 ml in women receiving prophylactic uterotonics[17].

PHYSIOLOGICAL ADAPTATIONS IN PREGNANCY

Antepartum adaptations for physiologic blood loss at delivery include a 51% increase in plasma volume and a 21% increase in red blood cell volume by the third trimester[20]. Women who develop pre-eclampsia either experience little or no expansion over non-pregnant levels or lose whatever gain had been accrued early in gestation during the third trimester[21]. In severe pre-eclampsia, on the other hand, the blood volume frequently fails to expand and may remain similar to that in a non-pregnant woman[22]. One of the hallmarks of eclampsia is hemoconcentration with increased sensitivity to even a normal blood loss at delivery[23]. Women so afflicted are less prepared to withstand blood loss and may experience life threatening hypovolemia with smaller amounts of hemorrhage[21]. Women with hypertension/HELLP (hemolysis, elevated liver enzymes, low platelets) syndrome are 39% more likely to receive blood transfusions and 157% more likely to receive intensive care than women experiencing PPH[24].

Progressively more complicated deliveries are usually accompanied by greater degrees of blood loss: vaginal delivery (500 ml), cesarean section (1000 ml), repeat cesarean section plus hysterectomy (1500 ml) and emergency hysterectomy (3500 ml)[25,26]. Factors associated with increased blood loss in the third stage of labor include multiple gestation, forceps delivery and episiotomy, particularly when accompanied by laceration[27–30]. By itself, episiotomy increases postpartum blood loss and the risk of PPH by 70%[31], whereas forceps delivery does not appear to contribute to blood loss *per se*. Any excess bleeding in this instance is due to the required episiotomy.

DIAGNOSIS OF POSTPARTUM HEMORRHAGE

Over the years, different methods have been used for estimation of blood loss; these can be classified as clinical or quantitative.

Clinical methods

Clinical estimation remains the primary means of diagnosing the extent of bleeding and directing interventional therapy in obstetric practice. Examples include internal hemorrhage due to ruptured tubal pregnancy, ruptured uterus and the concealed variety of abruptio placentae. The classification of hemorrhage can be based on a graded physiological response to the loss of circulating blood volume (Table 1)[21,32,33].

This scheme has worked well in the initial management of trauma patients in clinical settings. Knowing that the blood volume of a pregnant woman is 8.5–9%

of her weight, one is able to quickly approximate blood loss based on changes in pulse, systolic blood pressure and mean arterial pressure. Thus, the failure to respond to the initial administration of 3000 ml of crystalloid would suggest a class II hemorrhage with loss greater than 20–30% of the total blood volume or acute ongoing bleeding[21,32,34]. A systolic blood pressure below 100 mmHg and a pulse rate above 100 beats/min are late signs of depleted blood volume and indicate commencing failure of compensatory mechanisms[34], whereas acute blood loss might not be reflected by a decrease in hematocrit or hemoglobin level for 4 h or more[21,32,33]. Significant cardiovascular changes occur immediately postpartum. The cardiac output remains elevated for 24 h, blood pressure declines initially and then stabilizes on postpartum day 2. Maternal physiological changes of hemodilution lead to reduced hemoglobin and hematocrit values, reflecting the importance of timing of the measurement[35]. In the majority of patients[36], no single timed hemoglobin or hematocrit determination in the first 24 h postpartum will detect the peak. The importance of arriving at a diagnosis when the patient is at the class I stage cannot be too strongly emphasized, as women can progress into class II rapidly. At level III, without prompt, appropriate intervention, women can progress to shock.

Quantitative methods
Visual assessment

The standard observational method for the measurement of blood loss is straightforward and requires no expenditure[1]. In medical emergencies, however, the estimation of blood loss in simulated situations (albeit, not PPH) was found to be so poor that use of vital signs, symptoms of shock and co-morbidities was recommended to determine response[38,39]. Given inaccuracy and interobserver variation, most visual assessments underestimate blood loss, and may be indicative that women require clinical intervention at higher levels (more than 500 ml) of blood loss, to avert serious sequelae[40–42].

The major advantage of direct measurement is that it provides a real-time assessment and enables the birth attendant to correlate findings, on an individualized

Table 1 Classes of hemorrhage[37]

| Class | Blood loss | | Blood pressure (mmHg) | Signs and symptoms |
	ml	%		
I	500–1000	10–15	Normal	Palpitations, dizziness, tachycardia
II	1000–1500	15–25	Slightly low	Weakness, sweating, tachycardia
III	1500–2000	25–35	70–80	Restlessness, pallor, oliguria
IV	2000–3000	35–45*	50–70	Collapse, air hunger, anuria

*> 2500 ml blood loss – 50% mortality if not managed urgently and appropriately

basis, with the clinical presentation. However, the significant differences between clinical estimates and actual measurements are demonstrated in several studies and commented upon in other chapters of this book[17,35]. The most common error is underestimation of blood lost, with an average error of 35–50% when estimates at the time of delivery are compared with those of more precise methodology. As might be expected, observers tend to give median or average estimate of blood loss (called 'heaping' whereby amounts are aggregated at round or common values, i.e. 100 ml, 250 ml and 500 ml). When losses are large, they are far more likely to be underestimated; on the other hand, when losses are less than average, they are often overestimated[7,15,43].

The accuracy of visual estimation can be improved by training and standardization[7,42]. One simple approach is to train the observer to determine the blood loss using a single collecting container and fixed-sized gauze pads of size 10×10 cm, using simulated scenarios with known measured blood volumes (Figure 1)[36,44]. This methodology is useful and can be routinely practiced in low or high resource settings, albeit differing somewhat based on training the providers and standardization of the pads (size and quality) used during delivery[7,39]. Still, visual estimation is more accurate when blood is collected in containers rather than pads or cloth[42]. The accuracy of estimated blood loss has not been shown to be dependent upon the age or the clinical experience of the observer[17,38,45,46]. Of particular clinical importance is a reduction in underestimation of blood loss in the face of greater degrees of measured blood loss; correction of this practice has the strongest potential to reduce hemorrhage–related morbidity and mortality[47].

Direct collection of blood into fixed containers or cloth

Another method of calculation is to allow blood to drain into a fixed collecting container (Figure 2) for estimation at the end of 1 h. Blood losses on the delivery table, garments and floor should also be assessed[39]. At the end of 1 h, the total amount of blood lost is estimated by totaling up the blood in the container, in the sponges and secondary blood spillage on the delivery table, garments and floor. How often such calculation is utilized is unknown, but failure to do so contributes to underestimation[42].

In Tanzania, traditional birth attendants (TBA) have used a method to identify excess postpartum blood loss in home births by placing standard size kangas (100 cm × 155 cm cotton cloth, similar to a sarong in Asia or cotton skirt wrap elsewhere), under women during, and after delivery[48]. A small validation trial found two soaked kangas predicted an average blood loss of 500 ml. Interestingly, the TBAs had typically qualified postpartum blood loss as excessive when three to four kangas were soaked, indicating that, as in the case of trained clinicians, experienced TBAs are prompted to intervene at levels of blood loss higher

than 500 ml. A consistent size and weight of cloth is critical to widespread use of this method.

Direct collection of blood into bedpan or plastic bags

This approach was used in the World Health Organization (WHO) multicenter, randomized trial of misoprostol in the management of the third stage of labor[2]. In this trial, blood loss was measured from the time of delivery until the mother was transferred to postnatal care. Immediately after the cord was clamped and cut, the blood collection was started by passing a flat bedpan under the buttocks of a woman delivering in a bed or placing an unsoiled sheet for a woman delivering on a delivery table.

Blood collection and measurement continued until cessation of the third stage of the labor when the woman was transferred to the postnatal ward. This period was generally 1 h postpartum. At that time, the collected blood was poured into a standard measuring jar provided by WHO and its volume measured. To simplify the procedure for measurement of total blood loss, any small gauze swabs soaked with blood were put into the measuring jar and included in the measurement together with the blood and clots. A validity study was performed before the trial to assess the effect of adding the gauze swabs; this process increased the blood loss measurements by approximately 10%.

The errors associated with collection of blood by any of the methods described thus far are numerous; moreover, they are compounded by ignoring maternal

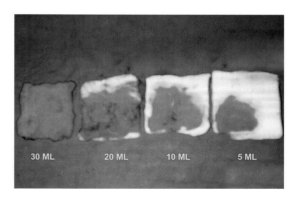

Figure 1 Soakage characteristics of 10×10 cm pads

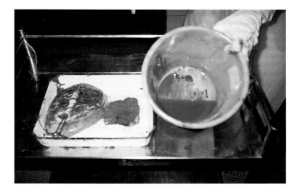

Figure 2 Blood drained into a fixed collecting container

blood within the placenta (approximately 150 ml) and spillage, confusion related to the mixing of blood contaminated with amniotic fluid and urine, and technical inaccuracies associated with transfer of the collection to a measuring device[39]. In non-clinical settings in tropical climates, care must be taken to minimize evaporation before retrieval and measurement of blood directly collected or transferred into containers or plastic bags[49].

Gravimetric method

The gravimetric method requires the weighing of materials such as soaked sponges on a scale and subtracting the known dry weights of these materials to determine the blood loss[50]. The difference in weight provides a rough estimate of blood loss. This method has been used most to assess blood loss associated with surgery, and is sometimes used in combination with other methods to calculate blood loss[51–53]. Inaccuracies can arise at several steps in this procedure, including lack of international standardization of size and weight of gauze, sponges and pads[53].

Determination of changes in hematocrit and hemoglobin

Changes in the hematocrit and hemoglobin values before and after delivery provide quantitative measurements of blood loss, as depicted in Figure 3[54–56]. The American College of Obstetricians and Gynecologists cites a 10% post-delivery decline in hematocrit compared with pre-delivery as a secondary definition of PPH, but notes that postpartum hemoglobin and hematocrit concentrations do not always directly reflect hematologic status[53]. Routine hematocrit determination is possible where equipment is available. However, routine postpartum hematocrits are unnecessary in clinically stable patients with an estimated blood loss of less than 500 ml. After delivery associated with an average blood loss, the hematocrit drops moderately for 3–4 days, followed by an increase. The peak drop may be appreciated on day 2 or day 3 postpartum[57]. By days 5–7, the postpartum hematocrit will be similar to the pre-labor hematocrit[20]. Should the postpartum hematocrit be lower than the pre-labor hematocrit, it is an indication that blood loss may have been larger than appreciated[25].

Acid hematin method

This method is based on collected blood being mixed with a standardized solution which converts hemoglobin to acid hematin or cyanmethemoglobin. This in turn can be measured by a spectrophotometer or colorimeter. Spectrophotometric analyses are described by Chua et al.[58], Brant et al.[34], and Wallace[59]. Photometric analyses are described in Duthie et al.[8], Duthie et al.[18], Larsson et al.[60] and Wilcox et al.[61]. Razvi et al.[11] describe the colorimetric approach. The first study reporting measurement of blood loss during surgical procedures employed the colorimetric technique, which required that hemoglobin be washed from surgical materials in a blender and measured in a colorimeter[62]. Clearly, use of the acid hematin method of calculating blood loss is impractical in obstetric care.

Plasma volume changes

The plasma volume can be determined before and after delivery using radioactive tracer elements. Stafford et al.[19] found visual assessment underestimates calculated measurements of postpartum blood loss based on maternal blood volume by a third in vaginal and by over half in cesarean births. Blood volume estimation using dye- or radioisotope dilution techniques is more difficult and requires special equipment and serial measurements[63,64]. Measurement of erythrocytes appears to be more consistent than estimates of plasma volume in pregnancy[12,65]. As is the case with acid hematin, this method is impractical for use in a bleeding patient.

BRASSS-V DRAPE: BLOOD LOSS COLLECTION TOOL

A randomized, placebo-controlled trial to test the effectiveness of oral misoprostol to reduce the incidence of acute PPH and hence maternal morbidity and mortality was conducted in women delivering in rural villages (away from major hospitals) in Belgaum District, Karnataka, India. The intervention was delivered by local health care workers. A critical component of this trial was the development of a specially designed low-cost 'calibrated plastic blood collection drape' that would objectively measure the amount of blood collected in the immediate postpartum period. The BRASSS-V drape was developed by the NICHD-funded Global Network UMKC/JNMC/UIC collaborative team specifically to estimate postpartum blood loss[66,67]. (The name 'BRASSS-V' was coined by adding the first letter of the names of the seven collaborators who developed the drape.) The drape has a calibrated and funneled collecting pouch, incorporated within a plastic sheet that is placed under

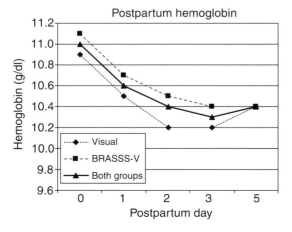

Figure 3 Postpartum hemoglobin changes

the buttocks of the patient immediately after the delivery of the baby. The upper end of the sheet has a belt, which is loosely tied around the woman's abdomen to optimize blood collection, particularly for deliveries performed on the floor or on a flat surface at homes or in rural primitive health posts. This simple tool not only has the potential for more accurate detection of postpartum blood loss, but also may improve timely response with the ultimate goal of decreasing maternal morbidity and mortality associated with PPH. Since most developing countries use some form of under-buttock sheet, either at home, in the health center or in hospitals, drape substitution is acceptable and relatively simple. The BRASSS-V calibrated drape used for objective estimation of blood loss is shown in Figure 4.

Results of three studies conducted at JNMC, Belgaum, Karnataka, India[12,68,69] strongly suggest that the BRASSS-V drape is an accurate and practical tool to measure blood loss in the third stage of labor. Although the ranges of blood loss were similar in both visual and drape assessment among women with little blood loss, the actual visual assessment amount was considerably lower compared with the calibrated drape values (Table 2 and Figure 5). This observation further attests to the inaccuracy of the visual estimation method as described in the literature; in contrast, differences between the drape and spectrophotometry values were found to be 37.15 ml, with the drape having the higher value (an average error of 16.1%). The drape measured blood loss equally efficiently as gold-standard spectrophotometry (Pearson' correlation coefficient of 0.928; $p = 0.01$, Table 3).

Use of the drape diagnosed postpartum blood loss of 500 ml or more four times as often as the visual estimate (Figure 6). The drape has been used in a number of international settings including India[12,70], Tibet, Vietnam, Egypt, Ecuador, Brazil and Argentina, and has been most recently employed in randomized controlled trials of treatment for PPH in Burkina Faso, Ecuador, Egypt, Turkey and Vietnam[71,72].

Based on the initial Indian experience, the drape appears to have great potential for training delivery attendants to determine postpartum blood loss in an accurate and timely manner. Apart from being an objective tool for measurement of postpartum blood loss, it also provided a hygienic delivery surface while permitting early management and referral. Residents and nurses in hospital settings and the nurse midwives who used the BRASSS-V drape during home delivery all found it to be a very useful tool that often led to earlier transfer from rural areas to a higher level facility[70]. At the same time, women who delivered at home and their family members appreciated the ease with which body fluids could be disposed of after birth[68].

In home deliveries or facilities in resource poor areas that do not have the capability to manage acute PPH, accurate measurement of blood loss at delivery as a means of early detection of PPH may improve care and outcome for several reasons. Uterotonics,

while an important component for addressing the third stage of labor, do not address all factors related to PPH. Trauma of the birth canal during delivery and retained placental fragments are also important causes

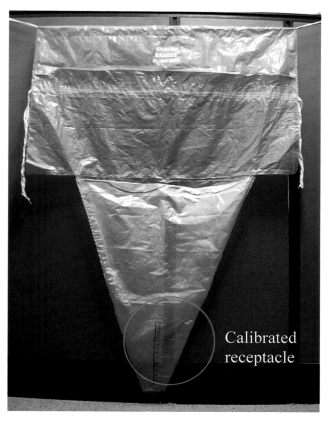

Figure 4 BRASSS-V blood collection drape with calibrated receptacle

Table 2 Distribution of blood loss

	Blood loss (ml)		
	Visual (n = 61)	Drape (n = 62)	All cases (n = 123)
Mean ± SD (range)	203.1 ± 147.5 (50–950)	302.8 ± 173.3 (50–975)	253.4 ± 168.9 (50–975)

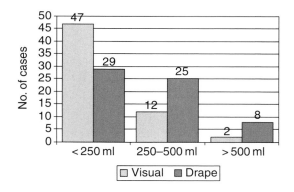

Figure 5 Number of cases detected for specific blood loss (*p* <0.01). The calibrated drape more accurately determined true blood loss when ≥250 ml and more accurately estimated overall levels

Table 3 Comparison between drape-measured and spectrometrically analysed blood loss

	Blood loss (ml)	
	Drape-measured	Spectrometry
Mean ± SD (range)	225.0 ± 96.1 (100–350)	187.8 ± 61.8 (93.2–286.0)

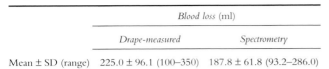

Figure 6 Number of cases of postpartum hemorrhage (PPH) detected for specific blood loss ($p < 0.01$). The calibrated drape diagnosed PPH at a rate four times that of the visual estimate method

of PPH and may occur more often than previously reported. Visual assessment of blood loss in the presence of a contracted uterus may diagnose traumatic PPH late and therefore result in delayed referrals.

In India and many other developing nations, a large percentage of all births take place in rural areas. Most of these deliveries are conducted by indigenous health care providers such as dais (traditional birth attendants) or auxiliary nurse midwives who have varying levels of training. Blood loss appears to be commonly underestimated, as visual assessment is the only means available to the birth attendant to diagnose PPH. The clinical symptoms of blood loss (low blood pressure, fast pulse, pallor and sweating, signs of hypovolemia and impending shock) are often the primary indicators for intervention. However, relying on the onset of such symptoms may lead to delayed intervention, resulting in increased rates of morbidity and mortality. As other quantitative methods employed have practical as well as technical limitations, the employment of simple tools, such as the BRASSS-V drape with a calibrated receptacle can be effectively employed for objectively assessing the blood loss.

ACKNOWLEDGMENTS

Our sincere thanks to Dr Shivaprasad S. Goudar, Professor of Physiology and Research, Coordinator Global Network for Women's and Children's Health Research Site 8, and Dr Kamal Patil, Associate Professor of Obstetrics and Gynecology, JNMC, for invaluable assistance in the preparation of this manuscript. We also acknowledge the contribution of Dr Kuldeep Wagh and Dr B. V. Laxmi, residents in the Department of Obstetrics and Gynecology, JNMC for participating in the validation study and to Dr A. Patel for her contributions to the design of the BRASSS-V drape.

References

1. Maine D. Safe Motherhood Programs: Options and Issues. Columbia University: Center for Population & Family Health, 1993:42
2. Gülmezoglu AM, Villar J, Ngoc NT, et al. WHO Multi-centre randomized trial of misoprostol in the management of the third stage of labour. Lancet 2001;358:689–95
3. WHO, UNICEF, UNFPA. The World Bank. Maternal mortality in 2005: estimates developed by WHO, UNICEF, UNFPA, and the World Bank. Geneva: World Health Organization, 2005:16–17, 23–27, 29–38
4. Carroli G, Cuesta C, Abalos E, Gulmezoglu AM. Epidemiology of postpartum hemorrhage: a systematic review. Best Pract Res Clin Obstet Gynaecol 2008;22:999–1012
5. Selo-Ojeme DO. Primary postpartum hemorrhage. J Obstet Gynaecol 2002;22:463–9
6. Williams JW. The tolerance of freshly delivered women to excessive loss of blood. Am J Obstet Gynecol 1919;90:1
7. Schorn MN. Measurement of blood loss: Review of the literature. J Midwifery Women's Health. 2010;55:20–7
8. Duthie SJ, Ven D, Yung GL, Guang DZ, Chan SY, Ma HK. Discrepancy between laboratory determination and visual estimation of blood loss during normal delivery. Eur J Obstet Gynecol Reprod Biol 1990;38:119–24
9. Prasertcharoensuk W, Swadpanich U, Lumbiganon P. Accuracy of the blood loss estimation in the third stage of labor. Int J Gynecol Obstet 2000;71:69–70
10. Glover P. Blood loss at delivery: how accurate is your estimation? Aust J Midwifery 2003;16:21–4
11. Razvi K, Chua S, Arulkumaran S, Ratnam SS. A comparison between visual estimation and laboratory determination of blood loss during the third stage of labour. Aust NZ J Obstet Gynaecol 1996;36:152–4
12. Patel A, Goudar SS, Geller SE, et al. Drape estimation vs. visual assessment for estimating postpartum hemorrhage. Int J Gynaecol Obstet 2006;93:220–4
13. Pritchard J. Changes in the blood volume during pregnancy and delivery. Anesthesiology 1965;26:393–9
14. Newton M, Mosey IM, Egli GE, Gifford WB, Hull CT. Blood loss during and immediately after delivery. Obstet Gynecol 1961;17:9–18
15. Newton M. Postpartum hemorrhage. Am J Obstet Gynecol 1966;94:711–16
16. Gahres EE, Albert SN, Dodek SM. Intrapartum blood loss measured with Cr51-tagged erythrocytes. Obstet Gynecol 1962;19:455–62
17. Sloan NL Durocher J, Aldrich T, Blum J, Winikoff B. What measured blood loss tells us about postpartum bleeding: a systematic review. Br J Obstet Gynaecol 2010; DOI: 10.1111/j.1471-0528.2010.02567.x.
18. Duthie SJ, Ghosh A, Ng A, Ho PC. Intra-operative blood loss during elective lower segment caesarean section. Br J Obstet Gynaecol 1992;99:364–7
19. Stafford I, Dildy GA, Clark SL, Belfort MA. Visually estimated and calculated blood loss in vaginal and cesarean delivery. Am J Obstet Gynecol 2008;199:519.e1–e7
20. Whittaker PG, Macphail S, Lind T. Serial hematologic changes and pregnancy outcome. Obstet Gynecol 1996;88:33–9
21. Knuppel RA, Hatangadi SB. Acute hypertension related to hemorrhage in obstetric patients. Obstet Gynecol Clin North Am 1995;22:111–29

22. Francois KE, Foley MR. Antepartum and postpartum hemorrhage. In Gabbe SG, Niebyl JR, Simpson JL, eds. Obstetrics Normal and Problem Pregnancies, 5th edn. Philadelphia: Churchill-Livingston, 2007

23. Cunningham FG, Gilstrap LC, Gant NF, et al., eds. Williams Obstetrics, 21st edn. New York: McGraw-Hill, 2001

24. Baskett TF, O' Connell CM. Severe obstetric maternal morbidity: A 15-year population-based study. J Obstet Gynecol 2005;25:7–9

25. Pritchard JA, Baldwin RM, Dickey JC, et al. Blood volume changes in pregnancy and the puerperium. II. Red blood cell loss and change in apparent blood volume during and following vaginal delivery, cesarean section, and caesarean section plus total hysterectomy. Am J Obstet Gynecol 1962;84:1272–82

26. Clark SL, Yeh SY, Phelan JP, et al. Emergency hysterectomy for obstetric hemorrhage. Obstet Gynecol 1984;64:376–80

27. Waters EG. Surgical management of postpartum hemorrhage with particular reference to ligation of uterine arteries. Am J Obstet Gynecol 1952;64:1143–8

28. Combs CA, Murphy EL, Laros RK Jr. Factors associated with hemorrhage in cesarean deliveries. Obstet Gynecol 1991;77:77–82

29. Calkins LA. Factors governing blood loss in the third stage of labor. Am J Obstet Gynecol 1929;17:578

30. Hill JA, Fadel HE, Nelson MC, Nelson RM, Nelson GH. Blood loss at vaginal delivery. South Med J 1986;79:188–92

31. Sosa CG. Althabe F. Belizan JM. Buekens P. Risk factors for postpartum hemorrhage in. vaginal deliveries in a Latin-American population. Obstet Gynecol 2009;113:1313–9

32. Arulkumaran S, Symonds IB, Fowlie A. Massive obstetric hemorrhage. In Oxford Handbook of Obstetrics and Gynaecology. Oxford: Oxford University Press, 2003:399

33. Spoerel WE, Heagy FC. The use of blood volume determination for the evaluation of blood loss during operation. Can J Surg 1962;5:25–32

34. Brant HA. Precise estimation of postpartum haemorrhage: difficulties and importance. Br Med J 1967;1:398–400

35. Robson SC, Boys RJ, Hunter S, Dunlop W. Maternal hemodynamics after normal delivery and delivery complicated by postpartum hemorrhage. Obstet Gynecol 1989;74:234–9

36. Nelson GH. Consideration of blood loss at delivery as a percentage of estimated blood volume. Am J Obstet Gynecol 1980;138:1117

37. ACOG. Teaching module on postpartum hemorrhage. 2010. www.acog.org/ACOG_Districts/dist1jf/teachingmodulepostpartumhemorrhage.ppt - 2010-01-20

38. Tall G, Wise D, Grove P, Wilkinson C. The accuracy of external blood loss estimation by ambulance and hospital personnel. Emerg Med (Fremantle) 2003;15:318–21

39. Patton K, Funk DL, McErlean M, Bartfield JM. Accuracy of estimation of external blood loss by EMS personnel. J Trauma 2001;50:13–20

40. Bose P, Regan F, Paterson-Brown S. Improving the accuracy of estimated blood loss at obstetric haemorrhage using clinical reconstructions. Br J Obstet Gynaecol 2006;113:919–24

41. Prendiville WJ, Harding JE, Elbourne DR, Stirrat GM. The Bristol third stage trial: active versus physiological management of third stage of labour. Br Med J 1988;297:1295–300

42. Hofmeyr JG, Nikodem V, de Jager M, Gelbart BR. A randomized placebo controlled study of oral misoprostol in the third stage of labour. Br J Obstet Gynaecol 1998;105:971–5

43. Buckland SS, Homer CSE. Estimating blood loss after birth: Using simulated clinical examples. Women Birth 2007;20:85–8

44. Maslovitz S, Barkai G, Lessing JB, Ziv A, Many A. Improved accuracy of postpartum blood loss estimation as assessed by simulation. Acta Obstet Gynecol Scand 2008;87:929–34

45. Dildy GA, Paine AR, George NC, Velasco C. Estimating blood loss: can teaching significantly improve visual estimation? Obstet Gynecol 2004;104:601–6

46. Grant JM. Treating postpartum haemorrhage. Br J Obstet Gynaecol 1997;104:vii

47. Luegenbiehl DL, Debra L. Improving visual estimation of blood volume on peripads. MCN Am J Matern Child Nurs 1997;22:294–8

48. Prata N, Mbaruku G, Campbell M. Using the kanga to measure postpartum blood loss. Int J Obstet Gynecol 2005;89:49–50

49. Walraven G, Blum J, Dampha Y, Sowe M, Morison L, Winikoff B, Sloan N. Misoprostol in the management of the third stage of labour in the home delivery setting in rural Gambia; a randomised controlled trial. Br J Obstet Gynaecol 2005;112:1277–83

50. Buchman MI. Blood loss during gynaecological operations. Am J Obstet Gynecol 1953;65:53–64

51. Lee MH, Ingvertsen BT, Kirpensteign J, Jensen AL, Kristensen AT. Quantification of surgical blood loss. Vet Surg 2006;35:388–93

52. Johar RS, Smith RP. Assessing gravimetric estimation of intraoperative blood loss. J Gynecol Surg 1993;9:151–4

53. Walsh CA, Manias T, Brockelsby J. Relationship between haemoglobin change and estimated blood loss after delivery. Br J Obstet Gynaecol 2007;114:1447–8

54. American College of Obstetricians and Gynecologists. Postpartum hemorrhage. ACOG Practice Bulletin No. 76. Obstet Gynecol 2006;108:1039–47

55. Jansen AJ, leNoble PJ, Steegers EA, van Rhenen DJ, Duvekot JJ. Relationship between haemoglobin change and estimated blood loss after delivery. Br J Obstet Gynaecol 2007;114:657

56. Budny PG, Regan PJ, Roberts AHN. The estimation of blood loss during burns surgery. Burns 1993;19:134–7

57. Maruta S. The observation of the maternal haemodynamics during labour and caesarean section. Nippon Sanka Fujionka Gakkai Zasshi 1982;34:776–84

58. Chua S, Ho LM, Vanaja K, Nordstrom L, Roy AC, Arulkumaran S. Validation of a laboratory method of measuring postpartum blood loss. Gynecol Obstet Invest 1998;46:31–3

59. Wallace G. Blood loss in obstetrics using a haemoglobin dilution technique. J Obstet Gynaecol Br Commonw 1967;74:64–7

60. Larsson C, Saltvedt S, Wilkund I, Pahlen S, Andolf E. Estimation of blood loss after cesarean section and vaginal delivery has low validity with a tendency to exaggeration. Acta Obstet Gynecol Scand 2006;85:1448–52

61. Wilcox CF, Hunt AB, Owen CA. The measurement of blood lost during cesarean section. Am J Obstet Gynecol 1959; 77:772–9

62. Gatch WD, Little WD. Amount of blood lost during some of the more common operations. JAMA 1924;83:1075–6

63. Quinlivan WLG, Brock JA, Sullivan H. Blood volume changes and blood loss associated with labor. Correlation of changes in blood volume measured by 131I-albumin and Evans blue dye, with measured blood loss. Am J Obstet Gynecol 1970;6:843–9

64. Ueland K. Maternal cardiovascular dynamics. VII. Intrapartum blood volume changes. Am J Obstet Gynecol 1976; 126:671–7

65. Nelson GH, Ashford CB, Williamson R. Method for calculating blood loss at vaginal delivery. South Med J 1981;74:550–2

66. Kodkany BS, Derman RJ, Goudar SS, et al. Initiating a novel therapy in preventing postpartum hemorrhage in rural India: a joint collaboration between the United States and India. Int J Fertil Women Med 2004;49:91–6

67. Geller SE, Patel A, Naik VA, et al. Conducting international collaborative research in developing nations. Int J Gynaecol Obstet 2004;87:267–71

68. Derman RJ, Kodkany BS, Goudar SS, et al. Oral misoprostol in preventing postpartum hemorrhage in resource-poor communities: a randomized controlled trial. Lancet 2006; 368:1248–53

69. Tourne G, Collet F, Lasnier P, Seffert P. Usefulness of a collecting bag for the diagnosis of post-partum hemorrhage. J Gynecol Obstet Biol Reprod (Paris) 2004;33:229–34

70. Ambardekar S, Coyaji K, Otiv S, Bracken H, Winikoff B. A comparison of drape estimation and a standardized weight method for the measurement of postpartum blood loss. Int J Gynaecol Obstet 2009;107(Suppl 2):S10

71. Winikoff B, Dabash R, Durocher J, et al. Treatment of post-partum haemorrhage with sublingual misoprostol versus oxytocin in women not exposed to oxytocin during labour: a double-blind, randomised, non-inferiority trial. Lancet 2010;375:210–6

72. Blum J, Winikoff B, Raghavan S, et al. Treatment of post-partum haemorrhage with sublingual misoprostol versus oxytocin in women receiving prophylactic oxytocin: a double-blind, randomised, non-inferiority trial. Lancet 2010; 375:217–23

12

Doppler Evaluation of Hemodynamic Changes in Uterine Blood Flow

G. Urban, H. Valensise, E. Ferrazzi, P. Beretta, P. Tortoli, L. Bonsignore, S. Ricci, P. Vergani, P. Patrizio and M. J. Paidas

INTRODUCTION

The main uterine artery and its branches are derivatives of the hypogastric artery. At the level of the internal cervical os, the uterine artery bifurcates into the descending (cervical) and ascending (to the body) branches. At the uterotubal junction, the ascending branch turns laterally and upward toward the ovary where it establishes anastomoses with the ovarian artery, forming an arterial arcade that provides perfusion to the upper aspect of the uterine corpus (see Chapter 22). Blood flow takes a linear course in the hypogastric artery, then turns in a serpentine course in the uterine artery, and finally regains a linear course throughout the gestation, as the uterus gradually increases in size.

Approximately eight to ten arcuate arteries originate from each uterine branch and envelope both the anterior and the posterior walls of the uterus for about one-third of the thickness of the myometrium[1]. These arteries take a tortuous course and establish anastomoses with the corresponding arteries from the contralateral side in the midline of uterine myometrium (see Chapter 22).

The radial arteries arise from the arcuate arteries and are directed inward toward the uterine mucosa. The total number is undefined and most likely is dependent on parity and human biodiversity.

In the past, unsuccessful attempts were made to use conventional Doppler techniques to study uterine hemodynamic patterns to provide diagnostic clues for the management of postpartum hemorrhage (PPH). However, advances in signal acquisition and processing have facilitated precise and reproducible analyses of velocity profile patterns and other variables such as wall distension and shear rates at specific sites of the uterine circulation.

Several studies have shown a progressive decline in impedance in all compartments of the uterine circulation, from the main arteries to the spiral arteries, as pregnancy advances[2–4]. The impedance of the spiral arteries decreases and blood flow velocities increase between the 5th and 7th weeks of gestation. During that period, the hemodynamic status of the uterine and arcuate arteries remains unchanged; it is only after the 8th week of gestation that a decrease in impedance and an increase in absolute flow velocities are detectable. This delay between the changes in the spiral and uterine arteries may represent the magnitude of the increase of placental volume and spiral arterial involvement, both of which are needed to effect appropriate and supportive uterine hemodynamics[5].

INTRAPARTUM DOPPLER VELOCIMETRY

Fleischer et al.[6] assessed 12 normal parturients throughout labor with a continuous wave Doppler unit to assess intrapartum changes in uterine and umbilical artery waveforms during labor. Each patient served as her own control. No significant changes were noted in umbilical artery systolic/diastolic (S/D) ratios before, during or after a uterine contraction in the latent phase of labor and with intact membranes, as well as in the active phase after rupture of membranes or during oxytocin stimulation. The uterine artery end-diastolic flow velocity fell progressively during uterine contractions, reaching 0 when the uterine pressure exceeded 35 mmHg. Despite intrauterine pressure of more than 60 mmHg, the diastolic notch did not appear. This study demonstrated that, at term, umbilical artery velocity waveforms do not change over a wide range of uterine pressures. Changes seen in uterine artery waveforms, on the other hand, suggested that the end-diastolic component is primarily determined by changes in the arcuate and spiral arteries, both of which are affected during uterine contractions.

MULTIGATE SPECTRAL DOPPLER ANALYSIS

In our studies, we used multigate spectral Doppler analysis (MSDA) to investigate blood flow. The MSDA overcomes the limitations related to the use of a single sample volume[7–11]. With this method, 256 small sample volumes are aligned along an ultrasound scan line that intercepts the blood vessel, and the Doppler data from each sample volume are independently analysed to produce a high-resolution flow profile. This non-standard method has been implemented in a system based on a proprietary electronic board connected to a commercial ultrasound machine (Aloka SSD1400) and a personal computer. The board, installed on a PCI slot of a host PC, samples the I/Q signals and processes the data in an on-board digital signal processor (DSP) to carry out the velocity profile. The profile is finally transferred in real-time to the PC to be displayed on the monitor.

The hypogastric, uterine and arcuate arteries were investigated in women in labor before epidural anesthesia, after at least 1 h postpartum, and in women before pregnancy. To our knowledge, no group of investigators had previously considered flow rates in terms of the capacity to sustain a life-threatening PPH.

This Doppler evaluation shows essentially how we define the bidimensional Doppler or '2-DD' quality Doppler profile (QDP). Multi-sample volumes from multigate acquisitions along the scan line depict a bidimensional dynamic representation of the blood flow, where the horizontal axis is the depth and the longitudinal axis is the velocity. Actually, this is the best estimation in real-time of the blood flow throughout the vessels, showing an areal flow (cm^2/s) [from depth (cm) × velocity (cm/s)]. Our experience shows that, during menses, areal flow through the arcuate artery is one-eighth (or perhaps one-tenth, depending on the anatomic variants) of the flow in the uterine artery, which is three-quarters of the flow in the hypogastric artery at the start of the menstrual cycle. This flow increases by one-third until ovulation (Figure 1) and remains constant until menstruation. By way of comparison, after conception and in early gestation, this flow increases until the end of the second trimester, after which it remains stable throughout

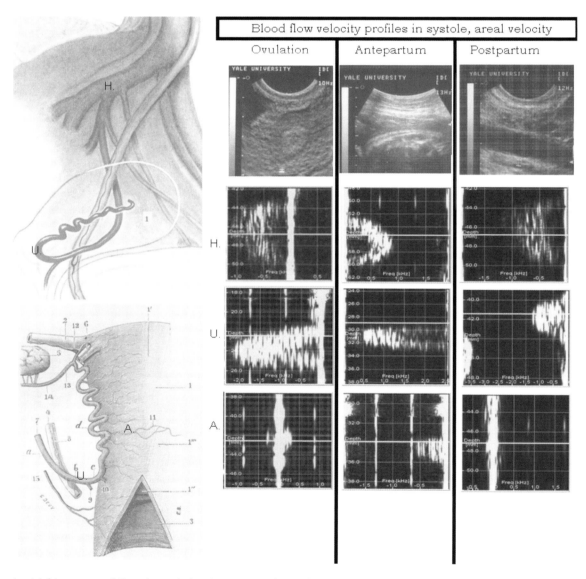

Figure 1 Multigate spectral Doppler analysis using GASP software for areal velocity in women at the ovulation phase of the normal menstrual cycle, in the antepartum phase of labor and at 1 h postpartum, respectively. In each column, the first image is the conventional bidimensional image of the area of interest during multigate acquisition, the following from top to bottom are hypogastric (H) artery velocity profile (areal flow), uterine (U) artery velocity profile (areal flow), and arcuate (A) artery velocity profile (areal flow). All images are frozen in systolic peak

labor, at which time the arcuate artery flow is one-fifth of the uterine, or almost double the flow before pregnancy. In the first and second stages of labor, this flow is markedly reduced, if not totally discontinued, by compressive action of the uterine contractions. During uterine contractions, the myometrial fibers also obliterate the flow in the radial arteries, reflecting the fact that they are tributaries of the arcuate arteries (see above), wherein flow stops until the end of contraction and then rises to reach a steady-state flow until the next contraction ensues. During each contraction, the placental lacunar space is compressed, thus pumping the blood to the fetal circulation throughout the umbilical vein. The compression of the radial arteries during each contraction acts as a valvular mechanism, avoiding reverse flow in the uterine circulation while, at the same time, directing the flow to the fetus. After delivery of the placenta, the resistance in the radial and spiral arteries decreases abruptly, being close to '0'. *As a consequence, there is an open flow of blood in the uterine cavity, which is contained by the compression caused by the prolonged uterine contractions. At this stage, the arcuate and radial flow is almost absent. The absence of flow through the radial and spiral arteries facilitates the clotting mechanism in the endometrial bed.*

Inefficiency of uterine contractions for whatever reason is an important risk factor for PPH. Likewise, an increase in the areal flow of the arcuate arteries, i.e. higher than one-fifth of the flow in the uterine arteries, is also a potential risk for PPH. The differences of areal flow between the hypogastric, uterine and arcuate arteries, in various physiologic conditions, including postpartum, are shown in Figure 1.

DIAGNOSTIC APPLICATION

After 10 years of our experimental work, the ultrasound industry has integrated this new Doppler signal processing made on MyLab from ESAOTE® (Florence, Italy) in a portable ultrasound machine. The velocity profile has been synthesized in a quality Doppler profile (QDP) function; this tool has the option DIR (direction) to indicate the mean interpolation of velocity profile in real time.

QDP is brand new technology developed by Esaote in collaboration with the University of Florence. QDP technology enables the acquisition of the signals of a large number of sample volumes placed across one or more blood flows. These sample volumes show the frequency content of each one of the related signals.

Studying the DIR shape of uterine artery immediately after delivery, we described the morphology of the uterine flow profile, comparing it with the postpartum quantity of blood loss.

Study design

We enrolled 236 consecutive women in labor. Within 15 min of placental delivery, both uterine arteries where investigated with approximately 60° of incidence using the QDP tool with the DIR activated at a

distance of twice the vessel diameter. After acquisition, the frame was frozen at the systolic peak in both arteries and the profile shape shown with DIR. Using the turbulence index (TI) classification, both arteries

Table 1 Data on 236 women in labor evaluated between October 7 2010 and December 27 2010. Data are expressed as numbers and percentages unless otherwise stated

	n	*%*
Parity		
0	135	57.2
1	81	34.3
2	16	6.8
3	2	0.8
4	2	0.8
Gestational week		39 ± 1.4
Previous cesarean section	9	3.8
Maternal age (years)		31.5 ± 1.5
Induction		
Vaginal dinoprostone 2 mg	57	24.2
1 dose	25	10.6
2 doses	21	8.9
3 doses	8	3.4
4 doses	3	1.3
Oxytocin	83	35.2
Dilating time at the admission (min)		120 ± 90
Expulsive time (min)		28.5 ± 21.2
Birth weight (g)		3360 ± 423
Blood loss (ml)		200 ± 233
PPH (blood loss >1000 ml)	17	7
Bakri balloon insertion	7	3

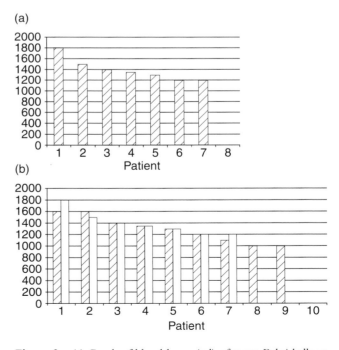

Figure 2 (a) Graph of blood losses (ml) of seven Bakri balloon patients. (b) Graph blood losses (ml) in PPH patients with Bakri balloon insertion (hollow bars) and without insertion (hatched bars)

where assigned a value between 0 and 3 (0 with maximum convexity and 3 maximum turbulence). Parity, gestational age, maternal age, previous cesarean section, dosage and mode of induction, labor duration, operative or spontaneous vaginal delivery, and blood loss, where recorded and analysed using non-parametric Spearman r^s.

Results

We evaluated 236 women in labor between October 7 2010 and December 27 2010, at a mean gestational age of 39 weeks. Of these, 24% underwent induction of labor, 87% had vaginal delivery and 12% vacuum operative delivery. Birth weight ranged between 1790 and 4330 g. Postpartum blood losses ranged between 50 and 1800 ml. In 17 cases, patients were determined to have PPH (blood loss of 1000 ml or more); seven cases required Bakri balloon insertion (Figure 2).

When patients were divided into three classes by quantity of blood loss (<500 ml, between 500 and 1000 ml, and >1000 ml), we found an inverse correlation between the turbulence index (TI) and blood loss (r^s −0.651; p <0.0001); the correlation was similar for birth weight (r^s −0.156; p <0.017). In contrast, no correlation was present between induction and blood loss. Interestingly, in the seven cases of Bakri insertion the TI was 1 before insertion, whereas it became 3 after inflation of 250 ml.

CONCLUSIONS

We found a strict correlation between the TI and blood loss, in PPH and non-PPH, as well as before and

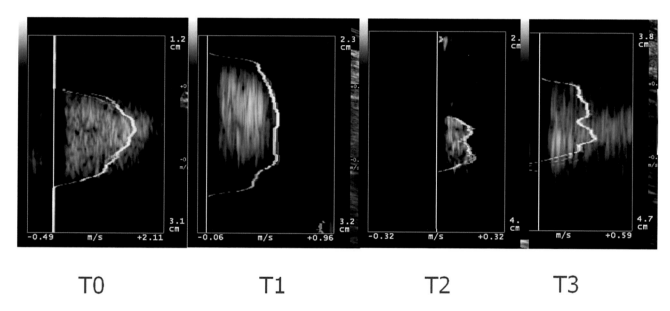

Figure 3 Quality Doppler profile (QDP) example of each profile in peak systolic in uterine artery at postpartum according to the turbulence index classification

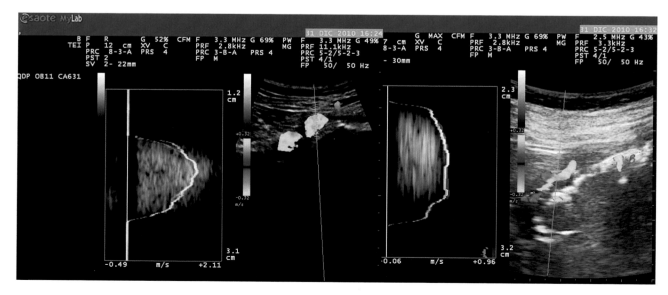

Figure 4 Sequence shows the mutation of flow profile from pseudolaminar flow during a PPH into the turbulent flow 8 min after the final of inflation of 250 ml of water into the Bakri balloon

after insertion of Bakri balloon, even if in a small series. Figure 3 shows examples of different classes of TI from 0 to 3. Figure 4 shows an example of the effect on the QDP of the inflation of Bakri balloon. The routine use of ultrasound in labor in our study was also useful in seven cases for contextual diagnosis of retained material individuation, as recently remarked in a retrospective study[12]. The combination of portable ultrasound system and the integration of QDP is now a new diagnostic tool to monitor bleeding and risks for PPH.

ACKNOWLEDGMENTS

Our thanks go to Dr Lorenzo Battiato and Giorgio Pardi Foundation for non-profit funding support and to Esaote Research and Development for their industrial support.

References

1. Ramsey EM, Donner MW. Placental Vasculature and Circulation. Stuttgart: Georg Thieme, 1980
2. Jurkovic D, Jananiaux E, Kurjak A, et al. Transvaginal color Doppler assessment of the uteroplacental circulation in early pregnancy. Obstet Gynecol 1991;77:365–9
3. Jauniaux E, Jurkovic D, Campbell S, et al. Doppler ultrasonographic features of the developing placental circulation; correlation with anatomic findings. Am J Obstet Gynecol 1992;166:585–7
4. Arduini D, Rizzo G, Romanini C. Doppler Ultrasonography in early pregnancy does not predict adverse pregnancy outcome. Ultrasound Obstet Gynecol 1991;1:180–5
5. Makikallio K, Tekay A, Jouppila P. Uteroplacental hemodynamics during early human pregnancy: a longitudinal study. Gynecol Obstet Invest 2004;58:49–54
6. Fleischer A, Anyagebunam A, Schulman H, et al. Uterine and umbilical artery velocimetry during normal labor. Am J Obstet Gynecol 1987;157:40–3
7. Bambi G, Morganti T, Ricci S, et al. A novel ultrasound instrument for investigation of arterial mechanics. Ultrasonics 2004;42:731–7
8. Tortoli P, Guidi G, Berti P, Guidi F, Righi D. An FFT-based flow profiler for high-resolution in vivo investigations. Ultrasound Med Biol 1997;23:899–910
9. Tortoli P, Michelassi V, Bambi G, Guidi F, Righi D. Interaction between secondary velocities, flow pulsation and vessel morphology in the common carotid artery. Ultrasound Med Biol 2003;29:407–15
10. Urban G, Paidas MJ, Bambi G, et al. Multigate spectral Doppler analysis,new application in maternal-foetal science. Ultrasound Obstet Gynecol 2004;24:217–8
11. Morganti T, Ricci S, Vittone F, Palombo C, Tortoli P. Clinical validation of common carotid artery wall distension assessment based on multigate Doppler processing. Ultrasound Med Biol 2005;31:937–45
12. Lousquy R, Morel O, Soyer P, Malartic C, Gayat E, Barranger E. Routine use of abdominopelvic ultrasonography in severe postpartum hemorrhage: retrospective evaluation in 125 patients. Am J Obstet Gynecol 2011;204:232

13

Pathophysiology of Postpartum Hemorrhage and Third Stage of Labor

R.-U. Khan and H. El-Refaey

INTRODUCTION

The physiology of postpartum hemostasis depends primarily upon mechanical events, mediated by hormones, which induce strong uterine muscular contractions. Virtually all recent studies focus on the latter activity rather than the former, but the phenomenon cannot be understood without examining why uterine contraction stops bleeding. Broadly speaking, myometrium and decidua are arranged such that powerful muscular contractions after delivery favor hemostasis (Figure 1)[1–3]. Spiral arteries 'fan out' to create a low-resistance vascular bed in the intervillous space,

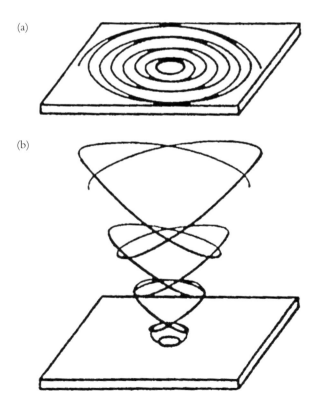

Figure 1 (a) Circular uterine muscle at rest: two sets of crossing spirals; (b) at term: stretching of the spirals[1]. The innermost part of the muscular layer has been described as superficially 'circular' musculature, which is in fact two sets of crossing spirals[2]. An alternative description of muscle fibers traveling in all directions has been described[3]. Both descriptions suggest that blood vessels are compressed during contraction of muscle cells

which facilitates placental blood flow (see also Chapter 22). This flow decreases with muscular activity[4]. Third-stage contractions are powerful and prolonged: they act to stop placental blood flow and to separate the placenta and membranes.

PLACENTAL SEPARATION AND UTERINE ACTIVITY

Mechanical events

The biomechanical events which lead to delivery of the placenta and its membranes begin even before the onset of the second stage of labor when membrane detachment starts during the first stage and slowly spreads upwards from the internal os[5].

As the trunk of the baby is delivered, the uterine muscle fibers undergo a very powerful contraction. Muscle fibers shorten, and the uterus is reduced in size and volume, a process characterized as retraction. These events are probably facilitated by the spiral arrangement of uterine muscle fibers, whereby the reduction in uterine volume leads to a reduction in placental site surface area. As the placenta is a relatively rigid and inelastic structure, the surface area of its attachment site decreases when it is tightly compressed.

According to Brandt, compression of the placenta forces placental blood back into the sinuses in the decidua basalis[6]. These sinuses become blocked by the action of the strong myometrial contraction, and thus the compressed placenta attempts to force blood back into a high-resistance system. Ultimately, the sinuses become so congested that they rupture. The blood from the ruptured sinuses tears the fine septae of the spongy layer of the decidua basalis, and ultimately the placenta is sheared off[7]. Dieckmann and colleagues implied that this 'retroplacental hematoma' has no functional value, and a subsequent investigation suggested that it is the contraction and retraction of the uterine wall itself that cause it to rend itself apart from the placenta[7,8]. *[Editor's note: the reader should be aware that both the Brandt and the Dieckmann references were published more than 50 years ago and reflect, to a certain extent, the relative lack interest among the obstetric community in updating older concepts on practical points that they dealt with on a daily basis. L.G.K.]*

Ultrasonographic investigations more recently corroborated that the Dieckmann theory is correct. Herman and colleagues conducted real-time ultrasonographic imaging of the third stage of labor and identified a 'detachment phase', wherein the placenta completes its separation[9]. This detachment is preceded by a 'contraction phase', in which the placental site uterine wall undergoes thickening. However, the 'latent phase' before this thickening occurs varies between patients and was thought to determine the overall length of the third stage. Of interest, neither the latent phase nor the contraction phase was associated with ultrasound evidence of retroplacental hematoma formation.

The two classical methods of placental delivery result in different bleeding patterns. In the Schultze method, separation begins in the center of the placenta (the fetal surface), and this part descends first, with the remainder following. The Matthew Duncan separation method involves detachment of the leading edge of the placenta, and the entire organ slips down and out of the uterus sideways. The latter method is much less common (20% of the total), but is supposed to result in more bleeding for two possible reasons. First, in the Schultze method, any extravasated blood is trapped within the membranes which follow the placenta and may form a retroplacental clot, whereas this blood escapes immediately in the Matthew Duncan method. Second, placental separation is slower in the Matthew Duncan method, allowing more time for bleeding[10]. As clinicians are able to neither predict nor alter the method of placental separation, the distinction between the Schultze and Matthew Duncan methods is most probably clinically irrelevant *[although it was noted in every delivery conducted by this editor in the 1960s. L.G.K.]*

Control of postpartum bleeding results from contraction and retraction of the interlacing myometrial fibers surrounding maternal spiral arteries of the placental bed. Myometrial contraction compresses the spiral arteries and veins, thereby obliterating their lumina. It is for this reason that these specific myometrial fibers are often referred to as 'living ligatures'[10]. In addition, it is thought that some hemostasis occurs by means of direct pressure as the uterine walls are forced firmly to oppose one another as a result of myometrial contraction (see Chapter 22).

It is worth noting the physiological effect of early cord clamping, a common intervention in the active management of the third stage of labor, is to retain blood in the placenta, which prevents it from being so tightly compressed by the uterus. This, in turn, reduces the amount of myometrial retraction and contraction, leading to more, not less, bleeding. However, this blood is thought to form a retroplacental clot, which speeds up the shearing off of the placenta. Ultimately, the consequent speedy delivery of the placenta should lead to quicker hemostasis, but the intervention of cord clamping is a paradox in that it involves causing increased initial bleeding to reduce ultimate total bleeding.

Unfortunately, apart from the recent ultrasound studies mentioned above, there is a decided paucity of information about the physical changes which lead to hemostasis and placental separation.

Endocrine mechanisms leading to mechanical events

Like all muscular activity, uterine contractility depends on both electrical and hormonal stimuli. 'Intrinsic' activity may be mediated by stretch receptors, although it is unclear whether such mechanisms are neural or neurohormonal. Two classes of hormones have been implicated in third-stage uterine contractility, namely oxytocin and prostaglandins.

Oxytocin

Interest in the role of oxytocin in the third stage has been partly motivated by the long-standing experience with the therapeutic use oxytocin to prevent postpartum hemorrhage (PPH). Broadly speaking, oxytocin causes increased uterine contractions by acting on myometrial oxytocin receptors. However, research has failed to show a clear and simple relationship between physiological oxytocin action and third-stage events for a number of reasons. Oxytocin assays are notoriously unreliable, because the decidua synthesizes its own oxytocin. As a result, plasma levels do not reflect oxytocin concentrations at the myometrial level. Moreover, plasma oxytocin levels take no account of the density of myometrial oxytocin receptors, which has been shown to participate in a complex control mechanism with oxytocin itself and other factors. Finally, oxytocinase, a plasma enzyme, denatures oxytocin before it reaches its site of action[11].

During labor, oxytocin is released in a pulsatile manner, and both the pulse frequency and duration increase[12]. Exactly what triggers the pulsatile oxytocin release is currently unclear. Ferguson speculated that uterine stretching of the rabbit cervix stimulates oxytocin release, leading to uterine contractions[13]. This phenomenon so far has not been demonstrated in humans, but there may be significant pressure changes on adjacent pelvic organs and the vagina which result in neurological stimulation.

A pulse of oxytocin does not necessarily correspond to a uterine contraction, and some women do not experience a rise in plasma oxytocin after the delivery of the baby[14]. Moreover, it is not necessary to have an oxytocin pulse in order to deliver the placenta and achieve hemostasis. Additional methods of control must be involved. Whereas it is known that myometrial oxytocin receptor density increases during pregnancy and labor, the precise controls of this up-regulation are unknown[15].

For many years, synthetic oxytocic agents have been successfully used in the third stage both to prevent and to treat PPH. At the same time, however, therapeutic oxytocic agents used to augment labor are sometimes associated with uterine atony in the third stage. In this latter circumstance, the non-pulsatile administration of these agents may lead to down-regulation of oxytocin receptors, as has been demonstrated in *in vitro* studies[15]. Despite the acknowledged therapeutic role of oxytocic agents in the third stage of labor, the true physiological role of oxytocin in the third stage remains unclear. It appears to have an inconsistent or paradoxical relationship with the third stage.

Prostaglandins

Prostaglandins are potent stimulators of myometrial contractility, acting via cyclic AMP-mediated calcium release. The therapeutic usefulness of prostaglandin agents in PPH lends credence to the possibility of a physiological role for prostaglandins in the third stage of labor. The prostaglandins involved in uterine contraction are produced in decidual tissue, placental tissue and fetal membranes[16]. The uterotonic action of prostaglandins does not depend on gestation. There are many classes of prostaglandin; the two classes implicated in uterine contraction are PGE2 and PGF2α.

Several observers have noted that large amounts of prostaglandin are released in the third stage of labor. In an elegant experiment, Noort and colleagues measured plasma levels of prostaglandin metabolites during and up to 48 h after labor[17]. PGF2α levels reached their maximum and started to decline within 10 min after placental separation (Figure 2). The subsequent rapid decline in these levels suggested that the prostaglandins arise from necrosis/cellular disruption either at the placental site or the fetal membranes. The latter are known to be a major source of prostaglandins. *In vitro* experiments have shown that intrapartum amniotic fluid triggers prostaglandin synthesis in fetal membranes. The 'active agent' in the amniotic fluid remains unknown[16]; however, these observations are thought to reflect the active role of prostaglandins in securing hemostasis by way of myometrial contraction in the third stage.

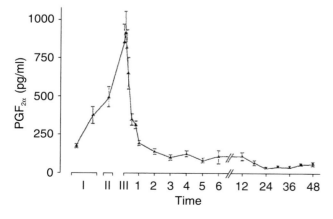

Figure 2 Plasma PGF2α levels (pg/ml; mean ± standard equivalent of the mean). (I) In early labor and at full dilatation; (II) at delivery of the fetal head; (III) at placental separation and up to 48 h after placental separation[17]

The interaction between prostaglandins and endogenous or therapeutic oxytocin in the third stage is not well understood. Numerous animal experiments have demonstrated interactions between prostaglandins and oxytocin at luteolysis, initiation and maintenance of pregnancy, and possibly at onset of labor[18]. However, therapeutic oxytocic agents used in the third stage do not appear to have a significant effect on prostaglandin metabolite concentrations[19]. Further studies are required better to understand from where these prostaglandins arise, and what controls their release.

In the past few years, misoprostol, a prostaglandin E1 analogue with uterotonic properties, has played an increasing role in the management of the third stage, as it is both cheaper and more thermostable than existing agents. Its uses are discussed in detail in several other chapters in this volume (see Chapters 32–35).

Coagulation

Many standard obstetric textbooks provide only the vaguest of suggestions that coagulation at the placental site represents an important hemostatic mechanism. Whilst this is certainly true, the exact pathway(s) involved are unclear (see Chapters 4 and 22). Before and after delivery, subtle changes take place in both coagulation factors and fibrinolysis agents. Plasma concentrations of clotting factors increase not only during pregnancy but also after delivery, which suggests a hypercoagulable state[20]. However, after placental separation, the fibrinolytic potential of the maternal blood also increases, and this tends to reduce the potential of blood to clot[21].

These conflicting changes are difficult to reconcile and are further complicated by changes in platelet activity before and after delivery. Perhaps of greater importance, they are poorly appreciated by many clinicians who are alone in a delivery room when what appears to be unusual bleeding commences. In addition to the changes in platelet activity, there are indications that an inflammatory response arises at the placental bed after placental delivery[22]. Such a response would promote local coagulation. This finding is important in terms of evolutionary advantage, because it allows prevention of hemorrhage at the placental site, while elsewhere (particularly in deep pelvic and leg veins) thrombi are less likely to persist, due to the increased fibrinolysis.

von Willebrand disease (factor VIII deficiency) is an important example of a coagulopathy which can result in increased risk of PPH. This is especially true in the disease variant featuring factor VIIIc deficiency. In many ways, von Willebrand disease mimics a platelet adhesion dysfunction, and indeed the only aspect of hematological hemostasis after placental delivery which can be emphasized with any certainty is the formation of platelet plugs at arterioles. PPH rates in von Willebrand's disease are in excess of 15%, and it has been suggested that this hemorrhage is largely preventable by minimizing maternal trauma at delivery and giving prophylactic treatment with desmopressin (DDAVP)[23].

In summary, the hemostatic mechanisms during and after placental separation probably involve the contraction of muscle sheaths around the spiral arteries, leading to platelet plug formation, retraction of the uterus causing mechanical occlusion of arterioles facilitating platelet plug formation, and the activation of both the clotting cascade and fibrinolysis. Many of these events are vague assumptions rather than demonstrated facts, as research into many aspects of third-stage physiology has been grossly neglected. Indeed, the fact that for decades effective treatments have been available for PPH in the developed world has acted as a true disincentive for novel work and ideas. It is tragic that the third stage of labor, the most dangerous moment of pregnancy, is so poorly understood.

PATHOPHYSIOLOGY OF POSTPARTUM HEMORRHAGE

Although most of the physiological processes in the third stage of labor remain unclear, they broadly help to explain the etiology of atonic PPH. In this section, the etiology and accompanying pathophysiology are discussed.

Uterine atony

The most common cause of PPH is uterine atony, i.e. failure of the uterus to contract. Primary PPH due to uterine atony occurs when the relaxed myometrium fails to constrict the blood vessels that traverse its fibers, thereby allowing hemorrhage. Since up to one-fifth of maternal cardiac output, or 1000 ml/min, enters the uteroplacental circulation at term, PPH can lead to exsanguination within a short time.

Whilst uterine atony is responsible for 75–90% of primary PPH, traumatic causes of primary PPH (including obstetric lacerations, uterine inversion and uterine rupture) comprise about 20% of all primary PPH. Significant but less common causes of PPH include congenital and acquired clotting abnormalities, which comprise around 3% of the total[24]. Uterine atony is responsible for the majority of primary PPH originating from the placental bed. Although the most important risk factor is a previous history of atonic PPH (relative risk 3.3)[25], many other important risk factors are often found in combination.

Failure of the uterus to contract may be associated with retained placenta or placental fragments, either as disrupted portions or, more rarely, as a succenturiate lobe. The retained material acts as a physical block against strong the uterine contraction which is needed to constrict placental bed vessels. In most cases, however, dysfunctional postpartum contraction is the primary reason for placental retention. It is more likely for the placenta to be retained in cases of atonic PPH, and so the contraction failure often becomes self-perpetuating. The reasons for this contractile dysfunction are unknown. The exception is uterine

fibroids, where the source of distension cannot be removed by uterine contraction, and must therefore cause the atony. However, the uterus does not even have to be distended during the third stage for contractile dysfunction to occur. Distension prior to delivery, which occurs with multiple pregnancy and polyhydramnios, also affects the ability of the uterus to contract efficiently after delivery, and is thus another risk factor for atonic PPH.

When PPH occurs following an antepartum hemorrhage, the scenario is particularly difficult since there have been two episodes of blood loss. A rare but serious complication of abruption is extravasation of blood into the myometrium, known as a Couvelaire uterus, which impairs the physiological uterine contraction/retraction hemostatic process. However, the relationship between the extravasation process and uterine dysfunction is not fully understood. Chorioamnionitis has a similar effect for unknown reasons. Both antepartum hemorrhage and chorioamnionitis also impair uterine contraction during the first two stages of labor, and prolonged labor in general is a risk factor for PPH. Conventional wisdom suggests that delay in the first two stages leads to uterine atony, but it is more logical to suggest that uterine dysfunction before onset of labor results in delay in all three stages, and thus causes PPH. As far as we are aware, there is no ongoing research into this 'universal uterine dysfunction'.

The lower segment as an implantation site

[Editor's note: The three sections that follow can be supplemented by reading the chapters by Palacios-Jaraquemada and co-workers in Section 1 of this volume, which describe the differences in the blood supply to the upper and the lower segments. L.G.K.]

Classic teaching suggests that the lower segment arises from the cervical isthmus. The isthmus is the region joining the muscle fibers of the corpus uteri to the dense connective tissue of the cervix. Thus, the major part of the lower segment arises from the cervix, with an uncertain smaller portion coming from the corpus uteri.

In both placenta previa and placenta previa accreta, the placental bed (and thus the postpartum bleeding site) is in the lower segment. The presence of lower segment implantation makes hemorrhage and placental retention much more likely. Although existing evidence is scanty, there are indications that the etiology of pathological bleeding is inextricably linked with the anatomical and physiological limitations of the lower segment.

At term the lower segment is continuous with the upper segment. Goerttler's original studies from the 1930s suggested that muscle fibers of the lower segment are more vertical than those of the upper segment, and run down like a spiral staircase[1]. The classical (and perhaps rather simplistic) interpretation of this arrangement suggests that, whereas upper segment fibers allow contraction and retraction in the third stage, lower segment fibers merely allow dilatation in parallel with the cervix.

There are large gaps of knowledge regarding the histology of the lower segment. Traditional teaching describes only gross differences in the amounts of muscle between upper and lower segments, and in the patterns of muscle fibers as already described[1,26]. More recently, some studies have investigated lower segment implantation, but the researchers have focused on parameters measuring placental invasion, usually with a view to explaining the etiology of pre-eclampsia[27].

A pregnancy sac implanted in a scarred myometrial area, with a deficient endometrium and blood supply, results in a cascade of poorly understood reactions with variable outcomes. These range from miscarriage to placenta accreta. The outcome probably depends on the nature and degree of the deficient endometrium, and where the blastocyst was implanted within it.

Placenta previa

In placenta previa, the placental site is located in an abnormally low position. Atonic PPH is a recognized complication and, even if cesarean section is performed, severe intraoperative bleeding is a significant risk[28]. The usual pharmacological methods used to stem hemorrhage are often less effective. Surgical methods, such as oversewing of bleeding sinuses and the B-Lynch suture (see Chapter 51), are sometimes also ineffective so that hysterectomy (see Chapter 55) proves necessary. Hemorrhage is often not stopped unless the entire lower segment is removed; a subtotal hysterectomy is often inadequate, and many surgeons perform total abdominal hysterectomy as the operation of choice. Thus, the involvement of the lower segment makes it more likely not only that hemorrhage will occur, but also that standard treatment modalities will fail (see Chapter 1).

Authors in conventional texts often suggest that, in lower segment implantation, the muscle surrounding the placental bed is inadequate to the task of postpartum contraction/retraction, and thus hemorrhage ensues[28]. As contraction and/or retraction are considered essential prerequisites for both placental detachment and postpartum hemostasis, the inference is that physiological hemostasis from a lower segment placental bed is difficult if not impossible. This is obviously not the case, however, as clearly not all cases of grade IV placenta previa necessitate hysterectomy. The only possible conclusion is that there are qualitative and quantitative differences in the musculature of the lower segment in different patients. A literature search on this topic confirms that neither the nature nor the origin of these differences have been investigated.

Biswas and colleagues have compared placental bed biopsy changes in placenta previa and normally implanted placenta, showing that previa is associated with significantly higher trophoblastic giant cell infiltration and physiological changes of the myometrial

spiral arterioles[29]. This work is typical of modern obstetric research in that it concentrates on antenatal events while ignoring postpartum events. However, the findings are interesting because they suggest that the seeds of potential placenta accreta are sown in most cases of placenta previa. Nonetheless, no knowledge regarding the qualitative features of lower segment myometrium exists.

Placenta accreta

Placenta accreta is morbid adherence of placenta such that it invades the myometrium. It is rare; in 1990, the quoted incidence was around 1 in 2000 to 1 in 3500 pregnant women in North America[30]. This number may be increasing, however, not only in North America, but also worldwide for reasons discussed below. Placental adherence is also associated with a deficiency of decidua in the lower segment, the most common cause of which is endometrial scarring secondary to previous history of cesarean section or myomectomy, endometritis, evacuation of retained products of conception or uterine abnormalities (see also Chapter 28).

It is widely held in the recent literature that uterine surgery is a major risk factor for placenta previa and placenta accreta[31]. There is an increased tendency for placental implantation in the vicinity of the uterine scar with secondary trophoblast invasion of the myometrium. *[Editorial note: This is the most common reason to implicate prior cesarean sections, of which the numbers are rising worldwide, but it does not take into account the fact that this operation was performed regularly prior to the recent epidemic and accreta was an extraordinarily rare occurrence. L.G.K.]* Uterine scarring is also known to be associated with an increased risk of scar dehiscence, febrile morbidity and other factors[32]. Thus the scar is classically considered to be a 'weak area'. Scarring of muscle results in the normal tissue being replaced by fibrous tissue. Intrauterine retraction forces induced during labor tend to thin out the lower segment, and these forces stretch the scar to the point of rupture. Uterine rupture is not considered predictable[33], but is more likely with each cesarean section. Although poorly described in the literature, our personal clinical experience suggests that, with each ensuing cesarean section, the entire lower segment often seems to become thinner. Indeed, the lower segment may take on a translucent quality. This appearance is not limited to the scar itself. It is possible that the 'weak scar' in fact represents a generalized lower segment weakness induced by previous surgery.

Clinical experience also suggests that it is not enough to assume that PPH is more common with lower segment implantation purely because lower segment muscle is inadequate to the task. In cases of placenta previa and placenta accreta, the lower segment looks even thinner than normal. We hypothesize that the contractile nature of lower segment muscle, which is already less than that of the upper segment, is further lowered by the presence of the placenta. This would mean that implantation itself has an adverse effect on lower segment myometrium. Furthermore, there is a body of anecdotal evidence which implies that placental size and trophoblast invasion are greater in areas of limited decidual tissue, including implantation on scars and in ectopic pregnancies. We hypothesize that trophoblast would invade more readily into the poorly decidualized lower uterine segment, increasing the likelihood that placenta accreta will develop.

In terms of the previous discussion, it is unfortunate that a dramatic and remorseless rise in the cesarean section rate is being observed throughout the developed world. This phenomenon will inevitably give rise to an increase in the complications associated with placenta previa, placenta accreta and scar rupture. These complications are particularly important because they tend to be relatively less amenable to medical treatment and sometimes necessitate radical surgical intervention, such as hysterectomy; while such operations are readily available in many areas of the world with organized medical systems, they are not available in other parts of the world, a discrepancy which contributes heavily to the disparities seen in death rates.

Whereas knowledge of the ultrastructure of placental bed musculature is at best 'lacking' with regards to the upper segment, it is virtually non-existent for the lower segment. New research into this area is urgently needed, because all non-surgical therapeutic modalities for atonic PPH involve enhancement of uterotonicity and, in the absence of sufficient myometrium, they will simply not work. We hypothesize that lower segment placentation/surgery leads to structural and thus functional changes in the muscle histology. Thus, we envisage a new, clinically important class of PPH, 'lower segment PPH'. This new subclass will be best managed by new protocols which address the features specific to lower segment involvement (see Chapter 1).

References

1. Goerttler K. Die Architektur der Muskelwand des menschlichen Uterus ind ihre funktionelle Bedeutung. [The architecture of the muscle bonds of the human uterus and their functional behavior.] Gegenbaurs morphologisches Jahrbuch 1931;45–128
2. Fuchs A, Fuchs F. Physiology of parturition. In: Gabbe S, Niebyl J, Simpson J, eds. Obstetrics: Normal and Problem Pregnancies, 2nd edn. New York: Churchill Livingstone, 1991:147–74
3. Renn K. Untersuchungen ueber die raeumliche Anordnung der Muskelbuendel im Corpus bereich des menschilichen Uterus. Z Anat Entwicklungsgesch 1970;132:75–106
4. Lees M, Hill J, Ochsner A, et al. Maternal placental and myometrial blood flow of the rhesus monkey during uterine contractions. Am J Obstet Gynecol 1971;110:68–81
5. de Groot A. Safe motherhood – the role of oral (methyl)ergometrine in the prevention of postpartum hemorrhage. MD Thesis, University of Nijmegen, 1995
6. Brandt M. The mechanism and management of the third stage of labor. Am J Obstet Gynecol 1933;25:662–7
7. Dieckmann W, Odell L, Williger V, et al. The placental stage and postpartum hemorrhage. Am J Obstet Gynecol 1947;54:415–27
8. Inch S. Management of the third stage of labour – another cascade of intervention? Midwifery 1985;1:114–22
9. Herman A, Weinrauth Z, Bukovsky I, et al. Dynamic ultrasonographic imaging of the third stage of labor. New perspectives into third stage mechanisms. Am J Obstet Gynecol 1993;168:1496–9
10. Sweet D, Kiran B. Mayes' Midwifery. London: Balliere Tindall, 1997
11. Hirst J, Chibbar R, Mitchell B. Role of oxytocin in the regulation of uterine activity during pregnancy and in the initiation of labour. Semin Reprod Endocrinol 1993;11:219–33
12. Fuchs A, Romero R, Keefe D, et al. Oxytocin secretion and human parturition: pulse frequency and duration increase during spontaneous labour in women. Obstet Gynecol 1991;165:1515–23
13. Ferguson J. A study of the motility of the intact uterus of the rabbit at term. Surg Gynecol Obstet 1941;73:359–66
14. Thornton S, Davison J, Baylis P. Plasma oxytocin during third stage of labour: comparison of natural and active management. Br Med J 1988;297:167–9
15. Phaneuf S, Asboth G, Carrasco M, et al. Desensitisation of oxytocin receptors in human myometrium. Hum Reprod Update 1998;4:625–33
16. Brennand J, Leask R, Kelly R, et al. The influence of amniotic fluid on prostaglandin synthesis and metabolism in human fetal membranes. Acta Obstet Gynecol Scand 1998;77:142–50
17. Noort W, van Buick B, Vereecken A, et al. Changes in prostaglandin levels of $PGF_2\alpha$ and PGI_2 metabolites at and after delivery at term. Prostaglandins 1989;37:3–12
18. Jenkin G. Oxytocin and prostaglandin interactions in pregnancy and at parturition. J Reprod Fertil 1992;45(Suppl):97–111
19. Ilancheran A, Ratnam S. Effect of oxytocics on prostaglandin levels in the third stage of labour. Gynecol Obstet Invest 1990;29:177–80
20. Wallenburg H. Changes in the coagulation system and platelets in pregnancy-induced hypertension and pre-eclampsia. In Sharp F, Symonds E, eds. Hypertension in Pregnancy. Ithaca: Perinatology Press, 1987:227–48
21. Shimada H, Takshima E, Soma M, et al. Source of increased plasminogen activators during pregnancy and puerperium. Thromb Res 1989;54:91–8
22. Louden K, Broughton Pipkin F, Symonds F, et al. A randomised placebo-controlled study of the effect of low dose aspirin on platelet reactivit and serum thromboxane B2 production in nonpregnant women, in normal pregnancy, and in gestational hypertension. Br J Obstet Gynaecol 1992;99:371–6
23. Kadir R, Lee C, Sabin C, et al. Pregnancy in women with von Willebrand's disease or factor XI deficiency. Br J Obstet Gynaecol 1998;105:314–21
24. Prendiville W, Elbourne D. Care during the third stage of labour. In: Chambers I, Enkin M, Keirse M, eds. Effective Care in Pregnancy and Childbirth. Oxford: Oxford University Press, 1989;2:1145–70
25. Stones R, Paterson C, Saunders N. Risk factors for major obstetric hemorrhage. Eur J Obstet Gynecol Reprod Biol 1993;48:15–18
26. Davey D. Normal Pregnancy: Anatomy, Endocrinology and Physiology. Dewhurst's Textbook of Obstetrics and Gynaecology for Postgraduates. Oxford: Blackwell Science, 1995:87–108
27. Roberston WB, Khong TY, Brosens I, De Wolf F, Sheppard BL, Bonnar J. The placental bed biopsy: review from three European centres. Am J Obstet Gynecol 1986;155:401–12
28. Konje J, Whalley R. Bleeding in late pregnancy. In: James D, Steer P, Weiner C, Gonik B, eds. High-risk Pregnancy Management Options. London: Saunders, 1994:119–36
29. Biswas R, Sawhney H, Dass R, Saran R, Vasishta K. Histopathological study of placental bed biopsy in placenta previa. Acta Obstet Gynecol Scand 1999;78:173–9
30. Zahan C, Yeomans E. Postpartum hemorrhage: placenta accreta, uterine inversion and puerperal hematomas. Clin Obstet Gynecol 1990;33:422–31

31. Dickinson J. Previous Caesarean section. In James D, Steer P, Weiner C, Gonik B, eds. High-risk Pregnancy Management Options. London: Saunders, 1994:207–16

32. Enkin M, Wilkinson C. Manual removal of placenta at caesarean section (Cochrane review). In: Keirse MJNC, Renfrew MJ, Neilson JP, Crowther C, eds. Pregnancy and Childbirth Module. The Cochrane Pregnancy and Childbirth Database [database on disk and CDROM]. The Cochrane Collaboration; Issue 2, Oxford: Update Software, 1999. Available from BMJ Publishing Group, London

33. Beasley J. Complications of the third stage of labour. In: Whitfield C, ed. Dewhurst's Textbook of Obstetrics and Gynaecology for Postgraduates, 5th edn. Oxford: Blackwall Science, 1995:368–76

14

Active Management of the Third Stage of Labor

M. P. O'Connell

THE EVIDENCE

Traditionally, the third stage of labor is defined as that time between the delivery of the baby and the delivery of the placenta. Separation of the placenta from the uterine wall results from a combination of capillary hemorrhage and uterine muscular contraction. The length of the third stage of labor, and its subsequent complications, depends on a combination of the lengths of time it takes for placental separation and for the uterine muscle to contract.

Clinical management of the third stage of labor varies from the purely expectant to an active approach, or some variation thereof. The expectant ('pure' physiological) approach involves waiting for clinical signs of placental separation (alteration of the form and size of the uterus, descent and lengthening of the umbilical cord and a modest gush of blood) and allowing the placenta to deliver either unaided using gravity or with the aid of nipple stimulation, as described in most maternity books[1,2]. In contrast, the full active approach involves administration of an oxytocic agent, early umbilical cord clamping and division and controlled cord traction for delivery of the umbilical cord[3–6].

In daily practice, the term 'active management' does not mean the same thing to all health care professionals, and marked variations in practice regularly occur. A recent survey of management of the third stage of labor in 14 European countries confirmed such variations[7]. Whereas all units professed to practice active management of the third stage of labor, prophylactic uterotonics were infrequently employed in units in Austria and Denmark. Controlled cord traction was almost universally practiced in Ireland and the UK, but took place in less than 50% of units in the other 12 countries surveyed. Policies with respect to clamping and cutting the umbilical cord also varied widely, with most practitioners clamping and cutting immediately. However, this was not the case in many units in Austria, Denmark, Finland, Hungary and Norway, where health care personnel waited until the cord stopped pulsating[7]. *[Editor's note: To add to this confusion, there is some concern that early clamping may deprive the neonate of an important amount of blood and its associated hemoglobin, a factor of great importance in many countries of the world. The components of active management of the third stage of labor (AMTSL), as outlined in the November 2003 Joint Statement of the International Confederation of Midwives (ICM) and the International Federation of Gynecology and Obstetrics (FIGO), include administration of a uterotonic agent (oxytocin is the drug of choice), controlled cord traction and uterine massage, after delivery of the placenta. See further discussion below. L.G.K.]*

Given these circumstances, we reiterate the definition of the combined approach as using three component interventions: (1) a prophylactic uterotonic agent; (2) early clamping and division of the umbilical cord; and (3) controlled cord traction.

UTEROTONIC AGENTS

The commonly used uterotonic agents are divided into three groups: oxytocin and oxytocin agonists, ergot alkaloids and prostaglandins.

Oxytocin

Oxytocin (Syntocinon®) is a cyclic nonapeptide that is obtained by chemical synthesis. This synthetic form is identical to the natural hormone that is stored in the posterior pituitary and released into the systemic circulation in response to suckling and labor. Oxytocin stimulates the smooth muscle of the uterus, more powerfully towards the end of pregnancy, during labor and immediately postpartum. At these times, the oxytocin receptors in the myometrium are increased[8,9]. The oxytocin receptor is coupled via G9q proteins to phospholipase C. The resultant activation triggers release of calcium from intracellular stores and thus leads to myometrial contraction[10].

Low-dose intravenous infusion of oxytocin elicits rhythmic uterine contractions similar in frequency, force and duration to those observed during labor. Higher-dose infusions, on the other hand, can cause sustained uterine contractions. A transient relaxation of smooth muscle, with an associated brief episode of hypotension, flushing and reflex tachycardia, has been observed with rapidly administered intravenous bolus injections[11].

Oxytocin acts rapidly, with a latency period of less than 1 min after intravenous injection and 2–4 min after intramuscular injection. When oxytocin is administered by a continuous intravenous infusion, the uterine response begins gradually and reaches a steady state within 20–40 min. Removal of oxytocin from plasma is accomplished mainly by the liver and kidneys, with less than 1% excreted unchanged in urine. The metabolic clearance rate amounts to 20 ml/kg/min in the pregnant woman[12,13]. The prophylactic use of oxytocin in the third stage of labor has been described in a Cochrane review, where oxytocin alone was compared to no uterotonic and also compared to ergot alkaloids[14].

Oxytocin vs. no uterotonics

Seven trials including more than 3000 women have been described[15–21]. Variations were noted, not only in sample size and administered dose of oxytocin, but also in mode of administration, with the intramuscular route preferred in three trials[15–17] and the intravenous route four[18–21]. Those who received prophylactic oxytocin had clear benefit in terms of PPH (Figures 1 and 2). Although debate surrounds the precise definition of PPH, this benefit was present whether the cut-off was taken as blood loss of more than 500 ml (relative risk (RR) 0.5, 95% confidence interval (CI) 0.43–0.59) or more than 1000 ml (RR 0.61, 95% CI 0.44–0.87). A trend towards a decreased need for therapeutic oxytocin was also found (RR 0.50, CI 0.39–0.64) in those who received prophylactic oxytocin. It is not feasible to comment on a possible relationship with manual removal of the placenta or the need for a blood transfusion from the data in this review (Figures 1 and 2).

Oxytocin vs. ergot alkaloids

Six trials including over 2800 women were described in this comparison[15,18,19,22–24]. Variation was present, not only in sample size, dose of oxytocin and preparation of ergot alkaloid, but also in the mode of administration, with the intramuscular route being used in one trial[15], the intravenous route in four[18,19,22,23] and both intravenous and intramuscular routes in a single trial[24]. Few differential effects were demonstrated between these two oxytocics (Figures 3 and 4). Ergometrine was associated with more manual removal of the placenta (RR 0.57, 95% CI 0.41–0.79) and a statistically insignificant tendency towards hypertension (RR 0.53, 95% CI 0.19–1.58).

Oxytocin agonists

Carbetocin appears to be the most promising of these agents in preventing PPH[25]. Carbetocin is a long-acting synthetic octapepetide analogue of oxytocin, with agonist properties and similar clinical and pharmacological properties to naturally occurring oxytocin. It binds to oxytocin receptors and causes rhythmic contractions of uterine smooth muscle, increases the frequency of contractions and increases uterine tone. Intramuscular injections of carbetocin provide similar responses to tetanic contractions (in approximately 2 min) as does intravenous administration, but with a longer duration of activity[26].

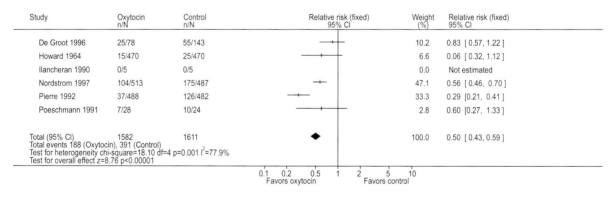

Figure 1 Comparison of oxytocin vs. no uterotonics (all trials), with outcome of PPH (clinically estimated blood loss ≥500 ml). Cochrane review[14]

Figure 2 Comparison of oxytocin vs. no uterotonics (all trials), with outcome of severe PPH (clinically estimated blood loss ≥1000 ml). Cochrane review[14]

Study	Oxytocin n/N	Ergot alkaloids n/N	Relative risk (fixed) 95% CI	Weight (%)	Relative risk (fixed) 95% CI
De Groot 1996	1/78	2/146		1.7	0.94 [0.09, 10.16]
Fugo 1958	55/324	36/149		60.5	0.70 [0.48, 1.02]
Sorbe 1978	10/508	32/543		37.8	0.34 [0.17, 0.68]
Total (95% CI)	908	838		100.0	0.57 [0.41, 0.79]

Total events: 66 (Oxytocin), 70 (Erot alkaloids)
Test for heterogeneity chi-square=3.60 df=2 p=0.17 I^2=44.5%
Test for overall effect z=3.39 p<0.0007

0.001 0.01 0.1 1 10 100 1000
Favors oxytocin   Favors ergots

Figure 3 Comparison of oxytocin vs. ergot alkaloids (all trials), with outcome of manual removal of the placenta. Cochrane review[14]

Study	Oxytocin n/N	Ergot alkaloids n/N	Relative risk (fixed) 95% CI	Weight (%)	Relative risk (fixed) 95% CI
McGinty 1958	4/50	15/100		100.0	0.53 [0.19, 1.52]
Total (95% CI)	50	100		100.0	0.53 [0.19, 1.52]

Total events: 4 (Oxytocin), 15 (Ergot alkaloids)
Test for heterogeneity: not applicable
Test for overall effect z=1.17 p<0.2

0.1 0.2 0.5 1 2 5 10
Favors oxytocin   Favors ergot

Figure 4 Comparison of oxytocin vs. ergot alkaloids (all trials), with outcome of diastolic blood pressure of more than 100 mmHg between delivery of the baby and discharge from labor ward. Cochrane review[14]

Oxytocin agonists have been compared to conventional uterotonics in a Cochrane review[27]. Three trials[28–30] compared the use of carbetocin and oxytocin for a total of 876 women who received either oxytocin or carbetocin. One trial[31] compared carbetocin with placebo (saline). Here, the use of carbetocin resulted in a statistically significant reduction in the need for therapeutic uterotonic agent (RR 0.44, 95% CI 0.25–0.78) compared to oxytocin for those who underwent cesarean section, but not for vaginal delivery. However, currently there is insufficient evidence to suggest that carbetocin is as effective as oxytocin to prevent postpartum hemorrhage (PPH).

Syntometrine

Syntometrine is a mixture of 5 IU oxytocin (Syntocinon) and 500 μg ergometrine maleate. Ergometrine is a naturally occurring ergot alkaloid which stimulates contractions of uterine and vascular smooth muscle. Following administration, it increases the amplitude and frequency of uterine contractions and tone, thus impeding uterine blood flow. Intense contractions are produced and are usually followed by periods of relaxation. Hemostasis is caused by contractions of the uterine wall around bleeding vessels at the placental site.

The vasoconstriction caused by ergometrine involves mainly capacitance vessels, leading to an increase in central venous pressure and blood pressure. Ergometrine produces arterial vasoconstriction by stimulation of the α-adrenergic and serotonin receptors and inhibition of endothelial-derived relaxation factor release. Uterine contractions are initiated within 1 min of intravenous injection and last for up to 45 min, whilst, with the intramuscular injection, contractions are initiated within 2–3 min and last for 3 h or longer[31–34].

The prophylactic use of ergometrine–oxytocin in the third stage of labor has also been the subject of a Cochrane review, where ergometrine-oxytocin was compared to oxytocin[35].

Ergometrine–oxytocin vs. oxytocin

Six trials including 9332 women were described in this comparison[36–41]. Variations were noted in sample size and in outcomes measured. Maternal outcomes in terms of nausea and vomiting, the need for blood transfusion and blood pressure changes were considered in four trials[36–41], as was manual removal of the placenta in two trials[37,40]. All six addressed the issue of PPH, but variations were seen in quantification of blood lost[36–41].

In terms of PPH, all six trials[36–41] demonstrated a significantly lower rate with ergometrine–oxytocin regardless of the dose of oxytocin used (odds ratio (OR) 0.82, 95% CI 0.71–0.95). Four trials examined the effects of uterotonics on diastolic blood pressure[36–39]. Whilst there was a marked difference in the criteria used to ascertain the changes in diastolic blood pressure, a consistent picture nevertheless emerges demonstrating an elevation of diastolic blood pressure with ergometrine–oxytocin or oxytocin administration. However, the use of ergometrine–oxytocin was associated with a greater increase in blood pressure than oxytocin alone (OR 2.40, 95% CI 1.58–3.64).

The incidence of nausea and/or vomiting was addressed in four trials[36–39]. A greater incidence of these side-effects was noted with ergometrine–oxytocin use compared to oxytocin alone (vomiting: OR 4.92, 95% CI 4.03–6.00; nausea: OR 4.07, 95% CI 3.43–4.84; vomiting and nausea: OR 5.71, 95% CI 4.97–6.57). In terms of the need for blood transfusion, the same trials found no difference (OR 1.37, 95% CI

0.89–2.10). The two trials that addressed the issue of manual removal of the placenta found no significant differences (OR 1.03, 95% CI 0.80–1.33)[37,40].

Prophylactic use of ergot alkaloids in the third stage of labor

Ergot alkaloids are amide derivatives of the tetracyclic compound lysergic acid and include three categories: (1) the ergotamine group: ergotamine, ergosine and isomers; (2) the regotoxine group: ergocornine, ergocristine, ergokryptine and isomers; and (3) the ergotamine and isomers.

The ergot alkaloids act as partial agonists or antagonists at adrenergic, dopaminergic and tryptaminergic receptors. All the ergot alkaloids significantly increase the motor activity of the uterus producing persistent contractions in the inner zone of myometrium through calcium channel mechanism and actin–myosin interaction that lead to the shearing effect on placental separation. The gravid uterus is very sensitive to ergot alkaloids, whereby small doses administered immediately postpartum result in a marked uterine response. The different preparations and routes of administration have been the subject of a number of investigations, both for therapeutic and prophylactic use[15,42–45]. All ergot alkaloids have the same qualitative effect on the uterus; ergometrine is the most active and is also less toxic than ergotamine. For this reason, ergometrine and its semi-synthetic derivative methylergometrine have replaced other ergot preparations as uterine-stimulating agents in obstetrics. Unfortunately, the injectable forms of both preparations are unstable when stored unrefrigerated and at high temperatures. Similarly, the oral forms deteriorate within weeks when stored in increased temperatures. These latter qualities are crucial in determining whether these agents can be used in many parts of the world and are perhaps more important than the pharmacological properties. Methylergometrine differs little from ergometrine in its pharmacokinetics.

Clinical trials have been conducted on the use of ergot alkaloids in the third stage of labor for prevention of PPH[15,23,42]. The use of ergot alkaloids in the third stage of labor compared with no uterotonic drugs and with different routes of administration is the subject of a Cochrane review[46]. The authors of this review conclude that prophylactic intramuscular or intravenous injections of ergot alkaloids are effective in reducing blood loss, PPH and the use of therapeutic uterotonics, but adverse effects include elevated blood pressure and pain after birth requiring analgesia, particularly with the intravenous route of administration.

Prostaglandins

Prostaglandins ripen the cervix by altering the extracellular ground substance, increasing the activity of collagenase and increasing the elastase, glycoaminoglycans, dermatan sulfate and hyaluronic acid levels in the cervix[47,48]. These agents allow for cervical smooth muscle relaxation and increase intracellular calcium, thus facilitating contraction of the myometrium.

Misoprostol is a synthetic analogue of naturally occurring prostaglandin E1. It is rapidly absorbed following oral administration and its bioavailability exceeds 80%. Peak plasma levels are reached in 30–60 min, and it is converted to active misoprostol acid, which has a half-life of 30–60 min. It is metabolized in the liver, and less than 1% of the active metabolite is excreted in the urine. In pregnancy, it is absorbed across the vaginal mucosa. After oral administration, the plasma concentration increases rapidly to reach a peak in 30 min and rapidly declines, whereas with vaginal administration the peak is reached in 1.5 h before steadily declining. Moreover, the area under the misoprostol concentration vs. time curve is increased, implying greater exposure time[49].

The prophylactic use of prostaglandins in the management of the third stage of labor is the subject of a Cochrane review wherein misoprostol was compared[50] to: (1) either placebo or no uterotonic; (2) conventional injectable uterotonic; or (3) injectable prostaglandin vs. injectable uterotonic.

Misoprostol vs. placebo/no uterotonic

Six trials were included in this comparison. Misoprostol 400 μg was the dose in three trials[51–53], a dose of 600 μg was used in an additional three trials[54–56], and one trial compared doses of 600 μg and 400 μg with placebo/no uterotonic[57].

At both doses (400 or 600 μg), misoprostol was either equal or less effective than placebo/no treatment for blood loss of 1000 ml or more; it also appeared to have a protective effect on the use of additional uterotonics, although this effect did not reach statistical significance. However, misoprostol was, associated with a triad of non-lethal side effects (more vomiting, shivering and pyrexia than placebo), and this observation was dose-related and occurred across the trials.

Rectal misoprostol was compared to placebo in one trial[53]. No statistically significant reduction in blood loss of at least 1000 ml (RR 0.69, 95% CI 0.35–1.37) or need to use additional uterotonic agents (RR 0.70, 95% CI 0.31–1.62) was observed.

Misoprostol vs. conventional injectable uterotonics

Fourteen trials were included in this comparison[55,58–73]. The trials are heterogeneous in terms of dose of misoprostol administered, route of administration and type of injectable uterotonic. Overall, the risk of PPH of at least 1000 ml was higher for the misoprostol group (RR 1.32, 95% CI 1.16–1.51) compared to either intravenous or intramuscular injections of oxytocin[74].

Injectable prostaglandins vs. injectable uterotonics

Seven trials compared injectable prostaglandins with conventional injectable uterotonics[17,45,77–81]. The trials were heterogeneous, and reliable estimates of outcomes were not possible. The injectable prostaglandins were associated with less blood loss, a shorter duration of the third stage of labor, more vomiting, diarrhea and abdominal pain than conventional uterotonics. *[Editor's note: Interested readers should see also Section 6. L.G.K.]*

EARLY CORD CLAMPING AND DIVISION

The timing of umbilical cord clamping is variable[82]. In the active management of the third stage of labor, early cord clamping is generally carried out in the first 30 seconds after birth, regardless of the presence or absence of cord pulsations[83]. Late cord clamping constitutes expectant management, whereby clamping is deferred until cord pulsations have ceased. A precise definition of early or late cord clamping is not currently available[84].

Delayed clamping of the cord facilitates placental transfusion and results in an increase in infant blood volume by 30%, and an increase in hematocrit and hemoglobin levels, with a resultant increase in iron stores and less anemia in infancy[84–86]. The benefits associated with this increase in infant blood volume are short-lived, however, lasting no longer than 3 months[85]. In Rhesus-negative women, early clamping of the cord may increase the likelihood of fetomaternal transfusion and thus exacerbate the risk of iso-immunization[84]. Early clamping of the cord has also been associated with a higher risk of respiratory distress syndrome in pre-term infants[87]. The recent Cochrane review concludes that delayed cord clamping is not associated with an increase in PPH. However, in neonatal terms, delayed cord clamping is associated with an increase in iron store, albeit with an increase in risk of neonatal jaundice requiring phototherapy[88].

COMPARISON OF ACTIVE VERSUS EXPECTANT MANAGEMENT

As noted above, the active management of the third stage of labor consists of three interlocking interventions: a prophylactic uterotonic agent, early clamping and division of the umbilical cord, and controlled cord traction.

This management package has been compared to expectant management of the third stage of labor in a Cochrane review[89]. Five trials were included in the analysis[90–94]. Active management was routinely practiced in the first four, and both active and expectant management were practiced in the fifth trial. The oxytocics used included oxytocin alone, ergometrine alone and a combination of oxytocin and ergometrine.

The incidence of PPH both at the 500 ml (RR 0.34, 95% CI 0.27–0.044) and 1000 ml (0.34, 95% CI 0.14–0.87) levels was significantly decreased in the actively managed group compared to the expectantly managed group (Figures 5 and 6). More importantly, the need for blood transfusion was also significantly less in the actively managed group (RR 0.35, 95% CI 0.22–0.55), and the duration of the third stage of labor was not unexpectedly shorter in the actively managed group (RR 0.15, 95% CI 0.12–0.19).

The authors conclude that active management is superior to expectant management in terms of blood loss and other serious complications of the third stage of labor, and that active management should be

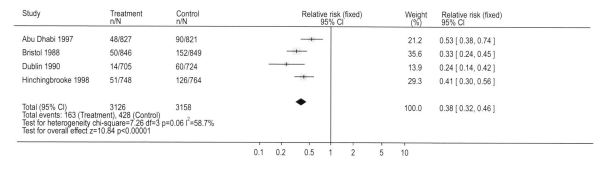

Figure 5 Comparison of active vs. expectant management (all women), with outcome of postpartum hemorrhage (clinically estimated blood loss ≥500 ml)

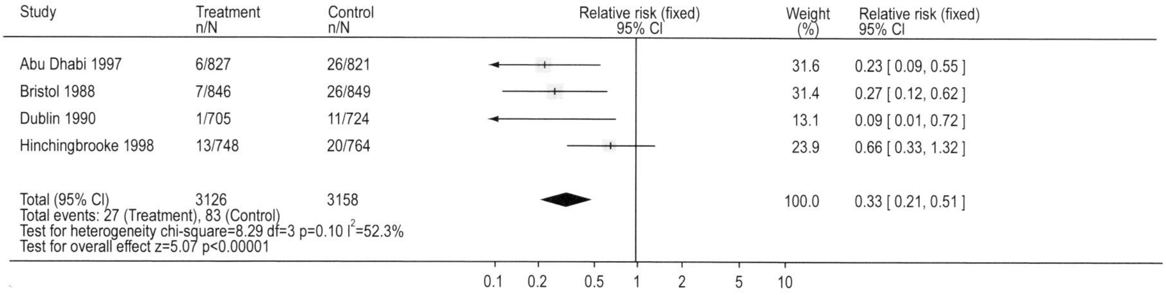

Figure 6 Comparison of active vs. expectant management (all women), with outcome of postpartum hemorrhage (clinically estimated blood loss ≥1000 ml)

routine for women expecting a vaginal delivery in a maternity hospital. *[Editor's note: At the International Conference on the Prevention of Post Partum Hemorrhage held in Goa on July 12–15, 2006, there was considerable discussion on the appropriateness of this intervention to be performed in the hands of skilled birth attendants who were working in a domiciliary delivery, although it was recognized that all such individuals would not have access to an injectable uterotonic for logistic reasons. L.G.K.]*

The European 5th Framework has funded an expert group from 14 European Union (EU) countries to address PPH in the EU. The group reviewed the literature, surveyed participants with respect to current protocols, devised a consensus document[95], and clarified the definition of active management of the third stage of labor. The consensus document has received wide support from a large number of international authorities and forms the basis for future comparative research and audit. It is reproduced in full as Addendum A to this chapter.

References

1. Sweet D. Mayes Midwifery, 12th edn. London: WB Saunders Co, 1997
2. Stables D. Physiology in Childbearing with Anatomy and Related Biosciences. London: Balliere Tindall, 1999
3. Prendiville WJ, Harding JE, Elbourne DR, Stirrat GM. The Bristol third stage trial: active vs physiological management of the third stage of labour. Br Med J 1988;297:1295–1300
4. Den Hertog CE, DeGroot AN, VanDongen PW. History and use of oxytocics. Eur J Obstet Gynaecol Reprod Med 2001;94:8–12
5. McCormick ML, Sanghvi HC, Kinzie B, McIntosh N. Preventing postpartum haemorrhage in low-resource settings. Int J Gynaecol Obstet 2002;77:267–75
6. World Health Organization. Pregnancy, Childbirth, Postpartum and Newborn Care: a Guide for Essential Practice. Geneva: World Health Organization, 2003
7. Winter C, Macfarlane A, Deneux C, et al. Policies for management of the third stage of labour and the immediate management of postpartum haemorrhage in Europe: what is the role of evidence? BJOG 2007;114:845–54
8. Alexandrova M, Soloff MA. Oxytocin receptors and parturition. I. Control of oxytocin receptor concentration in the rat myometrium at term. Endocrinology 1980;106:730–5
9. Fuchs AR, Fuchs F, Hurstein P, Soloff MS, Fernstrom MJ. Oxytocin receptors and human parturition: a dual role for oxytocin in the initiation of labor. Science (New York) 1982;215:1396–8
10. Sanborn BM, Dodge K, Monga M, Qian A, Wang W, Yue C. Molecular mechanisms regulating the effects of oxytocin on myometrial intercellular calcium. Adv Exp Med Biol 1998;449:277–86
11. Parker SL, Schimmer BP. Pituitary hormones and their hypothalamic releasing hormones. In Goodman and Gilman, eds. The Pharmacological Basis of Therapeutics, 11th edn. New York: McGraw Hill, 2006:1489–510
12. Amico JA, Seitchik J, Robinson AG. Studies of oxytocin in plasma of women during hypocontractile labor. J Clin Endocrinol Metab 1984;58:274–9
13. De Groot AN, Vree TB, Hekster YA, et al. Bioavailability and pharmacokinetics of sublingual oxytocin in male volunteers. J Pharm Pharmacol 1995;47:571–5
14. Cotter AM, Amen Ness A, Tolosa JE Prophylactic oxytocin for the third stage of labour. Cochrane Database Syst Rev 2010;(4):CD001808
15. De Groot ANJA, Van Roosmalen J, Van Dongen PWJ, Borm GF. A placebo-controlled trial of oral ergometrine to reduce postpartum haemorrhage. Acta Obstet Gynecol Scand 1996;75:464–8
16. Newton M, Mosey LM, Egli GE, Gifford WB, Hull CT. Blood loss during and immediately after delivery. Obstet Gynecol 1961;17:9–18
17. Poeschmann RP, Doesburg WH, Eskes TKAB. A randomised comparison of oxytocin, sulprostone and placebo in the management of the third stage of labour. Br J Obstet Gynaecol 1991;98:528–30
18. Howard WF, McFadden PR, Keetek WC. Oxytocic drugs in the fourth stage of labor. JAMA 1964;189:411–13
19. Ilancheran A, Ratnam SS. Effect of oxytocin on prostaglandin levels in the third stage of labour. Gynecol Obstet Invest 1990;29:177–80
20. Nordstrom L, Fogelstam K, Friedman G, Larsson A, Rydhstroem H. Routine oxytocin in the third stage of labour: a placebo controlled randomised trial. Br J Obstet Gynaecol 1997;104:781–6
21. Pierre F, Mesnard L, Body G. For a systematic policy of iv oxytocin where a fairly active management of third stage of labour is yet applied: results of a controlled trial. Eur J Obstet Gynaecol Reprod Med 1992;43:131–5
22. Fugo NW, Dieckmann WJ. A comparison of oxytocic drugs in the management of the placental stage. Am J Obstet Gynecol 1958;76:141–6
23. Sorbe B. Active pharmacological management of the third stage of labor. A comparison of oxytocin and ergometrine. Obstet Gynecol 1978;52:694–7
24. McGinty LB. A study of the vasopressor effects of oxytocics when used intravenously in the third stage of labour. Western J Surg 1956;64:22–8
25. Chong YS, Su LL, Arulkumaran S. Current strategies for the prevention of postpartum haemorrhage in the third stage of labour. Curr Opin Obstet Gynecol 2004;16:143–50
26. Hunter DJ, Schulz P, Wassenaar W. Effects of carbetocin, a long acting oxytocin analog on the postpartum uterus. Clin Pharm Therapeu 1992;52:60–7
27. Su LL, Chong YS, Samuel M. Carbetocin for preventing postpartum haemorrhage. Cochrane Database Syst Rev 2012; (4):CD005457
28. Boucher M, Horbay GL, Griffin P, et al. Double-blind, randomized comparison of the effect of carbetocin and oxytocin on intraoperative blood loss and uterine tone of patients undergoing caesarean section. J Perinatol 1998;18: 202–7
29. Boucher M, Nimrod CA, Tawagi GF, Meeker TA, Rennicks White RE, Varin, J. Comparison of carbetocin and oxytocin for the prevention of postpartum haemorrhage following vaginal delivery: a double-blind randomized trial. J Obstet Gynaecol Canada JOGC 2004;26:481–8
30. Dansereau J, Joshi AK, Helewa ME, et al. Double-blind comparison of carbetocin versus oxytocin in prevention of uterine atony after caesarean section. Am J Obstet Gynecol 1999;180: 670–6
31. Barton SR, Jackson A. The safety and efficiency of carbetocin to control uterine bleeding following caesarean section. Prenat Neonat Med 1996;1:185
32. Rall TW. Oxytocin, prostaglandins, ergot alkaloids, and other drugs; tocolytic agents. In: Goodman, Gilman A, Rall TW, Nies AS, Taylor P, eds. Goodman and Gilman's The Pharmacological Basis of Therapeutics. Toronto: Pergamon Press, 1990:933–53
33. Berde E, Stürmer E. Introduction to the pharmacology of ergot alkaloids and related compounds as a basis to their therapeutic application. In: Berde B, Schild HO, eds. Ergot Alkaloids and Related Compounds. New York: Springer Verlag, 1978:1–28
34. Müller-Schweinitzer E, Weidmann H. Basic pharmacological propertes. In: Berde B, Schild HO, eds. Ergot Alkaloids and Related Compounds. New York: Springer Verlag, 1978: 87–232

35. McDonald S, Abbott JM, Higgins SP. Prophylactic ergometrine-oxytocin versus oxytocin for the third stage of labour. Cochrane Database Syst Rev 2004;(1):CD000201

36. Choy CMY, Lau WC, Tam WH, Yuen PM. A randomised controlled trial of intramuscular syntometrine and intravenous oxytocin in the management of the third stage of labour. Br JObstet Gynaecol 2002;109:173–7

37. Khan GQ, John LS, Chan T, Wani S, Hughes AO, Stirrat GM. Abu Dhabi third stage trial: Oxytocin versus syntometrine in the active management of the third stage of labour. Eur J Obstet Gynaecol Reprod Med 1995;58:147–51

38. McDonald SJ, Prendiville W, Blair E. Randomised controlled trial of oxytocin alone versus oxytocin and ergometrine in the active management of the third stage of labour. Br Med J 1993;307:1167–71

39. Yuen PM, Chan NST, Yim SF, Chang AMZ. A randomised double blind comparison of syntometrine and syntocinon in the management of the third stage of labour. Br J Obstet Gynaecol 1995;102:377–80

40. Nieminen U, Jarvinen PA. A comparative study of different medical treatments of the third stage of labour. Ann Chirurig Gynaecol Fenniae 1963;53:424–9

41. Mitchell GG, Elbourne DR. The Salford third stage trial: oxytocin plus ergometrine versus oxytocin alone in the active management of the third stage of labour. Online J Curr Clin Trials 1993;2:Doc 83

42. Andersen B, Andersen LL, Sorensen T. ethylergometrine during the early puerperium; a prospective randomized double blind study. Acta Obstet Gynecol Scand 1998;77:54–7

43. Borri P, Gerli P, Antignani FL, et al. Methylergonovine maleate: a proposal for its more specific use. Biol Res Preg Perinatol 1986;7:128–30

44. Moir DD, Amoa AB. Ergometrine or oxytocin? Blood loss and side effects at spontaneous vertex delivery. Br J Anaes 1979;51:113–17

45. Van Selm M, Kanhai HH, Keirse MJ. Preventing the recurrence of atonic postpartum hemorrhage: a double blind trial. Acta Obstet Gynecol Scand 1995;74:270–4

46. Liabsuetrakul T, Choobun T, Peeyananjarassri K, Islam QM. Antibiotic prophylaxis for operative vaginal delivery. Cochrane Database Syst Rev 2009;(2):CD004455

47. Uldbjerg N, Ekman G, Malmstrom A, Sporrong B, Ulmstein U, Wingerup L. Biochemical and morphological changes of human cervix after local application of prostaglandin E2 in pregnancy. Lancet 1981;1:267–8

48. Uldbjerg N, Ekman G, Malmstrom A, Olsson K, Ulmstein U. Ripening of the human uterine cervix related to changes in collagen, glycosaminoglycans, and collagenolytic activity. Am J Obstet Gynecol 1983;147:662–6

49. More B. Misoprostol: an old drug, new indications. J Postgrad Med 2002;48:336–9

50. Gülmezoglu AM, Forna F, Villar J, Hofmeyr GJ. Prostaglandins for preventing postpartum haemorrhage. Cochrane Database Syst Rev 2007;(3):CD000494

51. Hofmeyr GJ, Nikodem VC, deJager M, Gelbart BR. A randomised placebo controlled trial of oral misoprostol in the third stage of labour. Br J Obstet Gynaecol 1998;105:971–5

52. Hofmeyr GJ, Nikodem VC, deJager M, Drakely A, Gelbart B. Oral misoprostol for labour third stage management: randomised assessment of side effects (part 2). Proceedings of the 17th Conference on Priorities in Perinatal care; 1998, South Africa, 1998:53–4

53. Bamigboye AA, Hofmeyr GJ, Merrell DA. Rectal misoprostol in the prevention of postpartum hemorrhage: a placebo controlled trial. Am J Obstet Gynecol 1998;179:1043–6

54. Surbek DV, Fehr P, Hoesli I, Holzgreve W. Oral misoprostol for third stage of labor: a randomised placebo-controlled trial. Obstet Gynecol 1999;94:255–8

55. Benchimol M, Gondry J, Mention J, Gagneur O, Boulanger J. Role of misoprostol in controlled delivery [Place du misoprostol dans la direction de la deliverance]. J Gynecol Obstet Biol Reprod 2001;30:576–83

56. Hofmeyr GJ, Nikodem VC, deJager M, Drakely A. Side effects of oral misoprostol in the third stage of labour: a randomised placebo controlled trial. South Afr Med J 2001; 91:432–5

57. Hofmeyr GJ, Nikodem VC, de Jager M, Gelbart BR. A randomized placebo-controlled trial of oral misoprostol in the third stage of labour. Br J Obstet Gynaecol 1998;105:971–5

58. Caliskan E, Dilbaz B, Meydanli M, Ozturk N, Narin MA, Haberal P. Oral misoprostol for the third stage of labor: a randomized controlled trial. Obstet Gynecol 2003;101:921–8

59. Cook C, Spurrett B, Murray H. A randomized clinical trial comparing oral misoprostol with synthetic oxytocin or syntometrine in the third stage of labour. Aust N Z J Obstet Gynaecol 1999;39:414–19

60. Amant F, Spitz B, Timmerman D, Corremans A, Van Assche FA. Misoprostol compared with methylergometrine for the prevention of postpartum haemorrhage: a double-blind randomised trial. Br J Obstet Gynaecol 1999;106:1066–70

61. Lumbiganon P, Hofmeyr J, Gulmezoglu AM, Villar J. Misoprostol dose related shivering and pyrexia in the third stage of labour. Br J Obstet Gynaecol 1999;106:304–8

62. Whalley RL, Wilson JB, Crane JM, Matthews K, Sawyer E, Hutchens D. A double-blind placebo controlled randomised trial of misoprostol and oxytocin in the management of the third stage of labour. Br J Obstet Gynaecol 2000;107:1111–15

63. El-Refaey H, Nooh R, O'Brien P, Abdalla M, Geary M, Walder J, Rodeck C. The misoprostol third stage of labour study: a randomised controlled comparison between orally administered misoprostol and standard treatment. Br J Obstet Gynaecol 2000;107:1104–10

64. Ng PS, Chan ASM, Sin WK, Tang LCH, Cheung KB, Yuen PM. A multicentre randomized trial of oral misoprostol and i.m syntometrine in the management of the third stage of labour. Hum Reprod 2001;16:31–5

65. Bugalho A, Daniel A, Faundes A, Cunha M. Misoprostol for prevention of postpartum haemorrhage. Int J Gynaecol Obstet 2001;73:1–6

66. Lokugamage A, Paine M, Bassaw-Balroop K, et al. Active management of the third stage at Cesarean section: a randomized controlled trial of misoprostol versus syntocinon. Aust N Z Obstet Gynaecol 2001;41:411–14

67. Gerstenfeld TS, WingDA. Rectal misoprostol versus intravenous oxytocin for the prevention of postpartum hemorrhage after vaginal delivery. Am J Obstet Gynecol 2001;185:878–82

68. Gulmezoglu AM, Villar J, Ngoc NT, et al. The WHO multicentre double-blind randomized trial to evaluate the use of misoprostol in the management of the third stage of labour. Lancet 2001;358:689–95

69. Kundodyiwa TW, Majoko F, Rusakaniko S. Misoprostol versus oxytocin in the third stage of labor. Int J Obstet Gynaecol 2001;75:235–41

70. Karkanis SG, Caloia D, Salenieks ME, et al. Randomized controlled trial of rectal misoprostol versus oxytocin in third stage management. J Obstet Gynecol Can 2002;24:149–54

71. Penaranda W, Arrieta O, Yances B. Active management of the childbirth with sublingual misoprostol: a clinical controlled trial in the Hospital de Maternidad Rafeal Calvo. Revista Colomb Obstet Ginecol 2002;53:87–92

72. Caliskan E, Meydanli M, Dilbaz B, Aykan B, Sonmezer M, Haberal A. Is rectal misoprostol really effective in the treatment of third stage of labor? A randomized controlled trial. Am J Obstet Gynecol 2002;187:1038–45

73. Caliskan E, Dilbaz B, Meydanli M, Ozturk N, Narin M, Haberal A. Oral misoprostol for the third stage of labor: a randomized controlled trial. Obstet Gynecol 2003;101:921–8

74. Parsons S, Walley RL, Crane JMG, Matthews K, Hutchens D. Oral misoprostol versus oxytocin in the management of the third stage of labour. J Obstet Gynaecol Canada JOGC 2006;28:20–6

75. Lam H, Tang OS, Lee CP, Ho PC. A pilot-randomized comparison of sublingual misoprostol with syntometrine on the blood loss in third stage of labor. Acta Obstet Gynecol Scand 2004;83:647–50

76. Gulmezoglu AM, Villar J, Ngov NT, et al. WHO multi-centre randomized controlled trial of misoprostol in the management of the third stage of labour. Lancet 2001;358:689–95

77. Abdel-Aleem H, Abol-Oyoun EM,Moustafa SAM, Kamel HS, Abdel-Wahab HA. Carboprost trometamol in the management of the third stage of labor. Int J Obstet Gynaecol 1993;42:247–50

78. Bhattacharya P, Devi PK, Jain S, Kanthamani CR, Raghavan KS. Prophylactic use of 15(S) 15 methyl PGF2 alpha by intramuscular route for control of postpartum bleeding – a comparative trial with methylergometrine. Acta Obstet Gynecol Scand 1998;(Suppl 145):13–15

79. Chua S, Chew SL, Yeoh CL, et al. A randomized controlled study of prostaglandin 15-methyl F2 alpha compared with syntometrine for prophylactic use in the third stage of labour. Aust N Z J Obstet Gynaecol 1995;35:413–16

80. Catanzarite VA. Prophylactic intramyometrial carboprost tromethamine does not substantially reduce blood loss relative to intramyometrial oxytocin at routine caesarean section. Am J Perinatol 1990;7:39–42

81. Chou MM, MacKenzie IZ. A prospective, double blind, randomized comparison of prophylactic intramyometrial 15-methyl prostaglandin F2 alpha, 125 micrograms, and intravenous oxytocin, 20 units, for the control of blood loss at elective caesarean section. Am J Obstet Gynecol 1994;171:1356–60

82. Inch S. Management of the third stage of labour: another cascade of intervention? Midwifery 1991;7:64–70

83. McDonald SJ. Management in the Third Stage of Labour. Western Australia: University of Western Australia, 1996

84. Prendiville WJ, Elbourne D. Care during the third stage of labour. In Chalmers I, Enkin M, Keirse MJNC, eds. Effective Care in Pregnancy and Childbirth. Oxford: Oxford University Press, 1989:1145–69

85. World Health Organisation. Care of the umbilical cord: a review of the evidence. Geneva: World Health Organisation, 1998

86. Mercer JS. Current best evidence: a review of the literature on umbilical cord clamping. J Midwifery Women's Health 2001;46:402–14

87. Rabe H, Reynolds G, Diaz-Rossello J. Early versus delayed umbilical cord clamping in preterm infants. Cochrane Database Syst Rev 2004;(3):CD003248

88. McDonald SJ, Middleton P. Effect of timing of umbilical cord clamping of term infants on maternal and neonatal outcomes. Cochrane Database Syst Rev 2008;(2):CD004074

89. Begley CM, Gyte GM, Murphy DJ, Devane D, McDonald SJ, McGuire W. Active versus expectant management for women in the third stage of labour. Cochrane Database Syst Rev 2010;(7):CD007412

90. Khan GQ, John LS, Wani S, Doherty T, Sibai BM. Controlled cord traction versus minimal intervention techniques in delivery of the placenta: a randomized controlled trial. Am J Obstet Gynecol 1997;177:770–4

91. Thilaganathan B, Cutner A, Latimer J, Beard R. Management of the third stage of labour in women at low risk of postpartum haemorrhage. Eur J Obstet Gynaecol Reprod Biol 1993;48:19–22

92. Prendiville WJ, Harding JE, Elbourne D, Stirrat GM. The Bristol Third Stage Trial: active vs. physiological management of third stage of labour. BMJ 1988;297:1295–300

93. Begley CM. A comparison of active and physiological management of the third stage of labour. Midwifery 1990;6:3–17

94. Rogers J, Wood J, McCandlish R, Ayers S, Truesdale A, Elbourne D. Active vs expectant management of the third stage of labour: the Hitchingbrooke randomised controlled trial. Lancet 1998;351:693–9

95. EUPHRATES group. European consensus on prevention and management of postpartum haemorrhage. 2005. www.euphrates.inserm.fr/inserm/euphrates.nsf/AllDocumentsBy UNID/95A14F46F31A5246C125707400485AED?Open Document&l = 3.1

Addendum A: European Consensus on Prevention and Management of Postpartum Hemorrhage

*The EUPHRATES group (**EU**ropean **P**roject on obstetric **H**aemorrhage **R**eduction: **A**ttitudes, **T**rial, and **E**arly warning **S**ystem), European Union 5th Framework*

INTRODUCTION

The EUPHRATES study comprises five parts, the second of these being 'the development of a minimal European core consensus on prevention and management of post partum hemorrhage'. This consensus is not a protocol or guideline. It represents a European consensus on what could be agreed on by all. Each maternity unit should have its own written protocol concerning prevention and treatment of postpartum hemorrhage (PPH).

Method

This consensus is based on three pillars: (a) review of literature, (b) survey of present protocols and practice, (c) consensus by experts gathered in a special board (see list of members at the end of this Addendum). he following principle was followed. Where solid evidence was available (level of evidence = 1), a consensus process was not necessary. Consensus was necessary in two circumstances: disagreement as to the clinical relevance of an outcome measure clearly shown to be affected by an intervention (e.g. active management of third stage) and situations where action has to be taken but no high-level evidence is available (e.g. medications in presence of continuing PPH).

STATEMENTS

1. General considerations

1(a) *Definition of PPH in terms on milliliters lost*

Evaluation of blood loss is unreliable.

Action is often taken following maternal signs (e.g. hypotension, malaise) rather than on estimated blood loss.

Blood loss at cesarean section is generally greater than at vaginal delivery.

Despite these three caveats, our group endorses the following classical definitions:

- ≥500 ml = PPH
- >1000 ml = severe PPH
- ≤24 h = primary, or early, PPH
- >24 h = secondary, or late, PPH

In regions and in groups where anemia of pregnancy is revalent, the recognition of lesser amounts is clinically important.

1(b) *Communication*

Substandard care is often related to lack of communication within the team and between the team and other professionals. Managing difficult cases as a team may make the difference between life and death. Identified communication problems include the following:

- Failure by the first-line care providers to call senior colleagues in time
- Reluctance of senior colleagues to come, when informed of problem
- Failure by the obstetrical team to inform on time other specialists, e.g. intensive care, anesthesiology, hematology.
- In theater, failure of anesthesists and obstetricians to keep each other informed of relevant events, such as rapid blood loss, tachycardia, blood pressure support interventions (fluid replacement and/or vasopressor use), etc.
- Failure to obtain blood, because of lack of perception by the laboratory/blood transfusion staff of the severity of the case

1(c) *Implementing local policies to ensure rapid availability of blood products at all times*

It is mandatory that appropriate blood products be available easily and rapidly in units where women deliver. Different European countries achieve this through different systems and there is no evidence that one system should prevail.

There should be a written document, detailing how this is to be implemented and including practical information such as transfusion department phone number, etc. This document should be widely disseminated.

1(d) *Audits and enquiries*

The impact of existing guidelines/consensus statements on severe maternal hemorrhage should be monitored by audit and/or confidential enquiries.

2. Prevention of PPH at vaginal birth

2(a) Active management of the third stage of labor

- Active management of the third stage of labor is usually defined as a three-component intervention: (1) prophylactic uterotonic, (2) early (or less early) clamping of cord, and (3) controlled cord traction. Active management in the third stage of labor has been proven to be effective in reducing blood loss in all women[1]. The evidence that active routine management reduces severe maternal adverse effects (morbidity) resulting from PPH is less convincing.

The full package of active management is certainly a valid (and validated) option.

- Isolated uterotonics may also be a useful option[2].

Our group concludes:

- Caregivers should be trained to be proficient in active third-stage management, and to offer it to all women.

- It is acknowledged, however, that, provided the woman and caregiver are fully informed, a decision not to use active management in some individual cases and/or settings should not be considered substandard care.

2(b) Type, dosage, route, speed and timing of administration of prophylactic uterotonic drugs

There is a lack of randomized trials addressing the questions of dosage, route and timing of prophylactic uterotonic drug administration, because most trials have compared the full package made up of three interventions to no intervention.

(i) Type of drug

- Oxytocin is the most frequently used drug for active management in Europe.

- In the United Kingdom and Ireland, Syntometrine is widely used. This is a combination of oxytocin and ergometrine. Syntometrine is more effective but is associated with more side-effects than oxytocin[3]. Syntometrine is not suitable for all women, e.g. in hypertension.

- Ergometrine has been reported in the European survey as additional prophylaxis (following the administration of oxytocin), after the placenta has been delivered in women with risk factors such as multiple pregnancy or grand multiparae. This has never been assessed in a randomized trial.

- Misoprostol is less effective than injectable uterotonics in reducing postpartum blood loss; however, its superiority over placebo as part of the active management of the third stage of labor remains uncertain[4].

Our group concludes:

- Oxytocin is the first drug of choice for all women in the third stage of labor.

- Syntometrine may be preferred by some clinicians but is contraindicated in hypertension and pre-eclampsia.

- Additional ergometrine (following the administration of oxytocin) in selected cases is considered acceptable practice.

- Misoprostol, although less effective, may be considered in situations where injectable uterotonics are not available.

(ii) Dosage

- Oxytocin: most trials have used intramuscular (IM) or intravenous (IV) administration of 5 or 10 IU of oxytocin. The European survey shows this dosage to be widely practiced. Particular dosages have been reported in various settings, e.g. 20 IU in 500 ml IV bolus 5 or lower doses such as 1 IU in 10 min ('turning up the drip').

- For Syntometrine, there is only one dosage: ergometrine 500 μg with oxytocin 5 units (Syntometrine® 1 ml contained in one ampoule).

- Misoprostol: most trials have used 400–600 μg when administered orally, and 400 μg per rectum.

(iii) Route of administration

- Oxytocin: If an IV line is in situ, the intravenous route is the route of choice. 'Turning up the drip' delivers low quantities, e.g. 1–2 IU (1000–2000 mU) in 10 min. If no IV line, IM administration is preferable.

- Syntometrine/ergometrine: Intramuscular administration.

- Misoprostol can be administered orally or intrarectally.

(iv) Speed of administration

A case of maternal death in the 1997–1999 UK Confidential Enquiry was attributed to severe hypotension following rapid administration of 10 IU oxytocin IV. A key recommendation was made that the administration should be 'slow'. However, no definition of 'slow' is available.

(v) Timing of administration

A recommendation often made, among others in the Bristish National Formulary, is to administer prophylactic oxytocic therapy 'on (= just after) delivery of the anterior shoulder', and that is also the timing in use in many randomized trials. In practice, it is reported in our survey that it is usually administered after delivery of the baby. Two randomized, controlled trials[5,6] compared oxytocin given before and after the placenta had delivered, and found no benefit in providing the uterotonic as early as possible. Further research is needed.

Our group concludes:

- The best time to administer prophylactic oxytocic therapy is just after birth.

- Whether it is administered before or after cord pulsation has ceased seems relatively unimportant.

2(c) *Manual removal of the placenta*

- Should be performed without delay in presence of hemorrhage.

- No European consensus could be obtained as to when this should be performed in the absence of bleeding. Some would act after 20 min while others would wait for more than 1 hour. Evidence is lacking and further research is needed.

2(d) *Other*

Nipple stimulation or early breastfeeding have been advocated for prevention of PPH, as simple and physiological, in particular in low-resource settings. The available evidence from two randomized controlled trials[7,8] is insufficient to reach a conclusion.

3. Prevention of PPH at cesarean section

- For women undergoing delivery by cesarean section, there is an increased risk that blood transfusion may be necessary.

- It is reasonable to advise routine administration of an uterotonic drug immediately after the baby has been born by cesarean section.

- Accurate blood loss assessment at cesarean section is difficult. Measuring both vaginal as well as abdominal blood loss may increase accuracy.

- For cesarean sections that are considered to be at greater risk of hemorrhage (e.g. placenta previa, especially in the presence of uterine scar), it is recommended that a senior obstetrician be present.

4. Management of PPH

4(a) *PPH after vaginal delivery*

We divided the event into three stages:
(i) concern about possible excessive bleeding,
(ii) early management of hemorrhage, and
(iii) continuing hemorrhage.

(i) *Concern about possible excessive bleeding*

- If relevant, remove placenta

- Empty bladder, massage uterus until it is well contracted, give additional uterotonics

- Look for any obvious bleeding in episiotomy or tear, and act on findings.

(ii) *Immediate management in case of hemorrhage*

- Call for help

- Measure blood loss, blood pressure, and pulse rate, insert large gauge intravenous infusion if not yet in place and take blood samples

- Check the placenta for completeness

(iii) *If bleeding continues*

- Circulatory support as necessary with crystalloids, colloids and/or blood products

- Ensure appropriate care with sufficient staff or appropriate referral

- Administer additional uterotonic drugs (injectable prostaglandins)

- Perform bimanual compression (time awareness)

- Explore under anesthesia the genital tract for retained placenta or part thereof, or traumatic damage and act on findings.

Whether an anesthetist is available immediately and whether the woman has got an effective epidural will determine the order in which the above and the following occur.

- Keep communication open with the anesthetist and the rest of the team.

(iv) *If bleeding still not controlled*

- Circulatory support as necessary with colloids and/or blood products, and vasopressors if needed

- Ensure appropriate oxygenation

- Monitor for coagulation abnormalities

- Uterine packing or intrauterine balloon

- Uterine artery embolization

4(b) *Hemorrhage at cesarean section*

(i) *Immediate management*

- Ensure bladder is empty.

- Explore the uterine cavity and remove the placenta and/or clots

- Massage uterus until well contracted, give additional uterotonics

- Look for and repair trauma, consider exteriorization of uterus

- Measure blood loss

(ii) *Hemorrhage not controlled*

- Continue circulatory support as necessary with colloids and/or blood products and vasopressors if needed

- Ensure appropriate oxygenation and consider mechanical ventilation when needed

- Ensure appropriate care with sufficient staff

- Additional uterotonic drugs (injectable prostaglandins)

- Appropriate surgery

4(c) *Factor VII*

Recombinant activated factor VII (Novo-Seven®) may be a future option in catastrophic hemorrhage, permitting sometimes to avoid hysterectomy. At present, NovoSeven is very expensive and its safety has not yet been adequately evaluated. Therefore, the use of this drug should be limited to units with adequate expertise and resources, and participating in ongoing registers of use.

Consensus Special Board

The Special Board was made up of experts from 14 European countries:

Austria: Mathias Klein (Obstetrician), Heinz Leipold (Obstetrician);
Belgium: Sophie Alexander (Obstetrician, Epidemiologist), Paul Defoort (Obstetrician), Corinne Hubinont
(Obstetrician), Wei hong Zhang (Epidemiologist);
Denmark: Jens Langhoff-Roos (Obstetrician), Desiree Rosenborg (Anesthetist);
Finland: Risto Erkkola (Obstetrician), Vedran Stefanovic (Obstetrician), Jukka Uotila (Obstetrician);
France: Marie-Hélène Bouvier-Colle (Epidemiologist), Gérard Breart (Epidemiologist), Catherine Deneux (Epidemiologist), Thierry Harvey (Obstetrician), Frédéric Mercier (anesthetist);
Hungary: Istvan Berbik (Obstetrician), Jeno Egyed (Obstetrician), Janos Herczeg (Obstetrician);
Ireland: Mikael O'Connell (Obstetrician), Walter Prendiville (Obstetrician);
Italy: Anna Maria Marconi (Obstetrician), Graziella Sacchetti (Obstetrician);

Nederlands: Kathy Herschderfer (Midwife), Jos Van Roosmalen (Obstetrician);
Norway: Bente Ronnes (Midwife), Babill Stray-Pedersen (Obstetrician);
Portugal: Diogo Ayres-de-Campos (Obstetrician), Nuno Clode (Obstetrician), Teresa Rodrigues (Obstetrician);
Spain: Enrique Barrau (Obstetrician), Vicenç Cararach (Obstetrician), Dolores Gomez (Obstetrician);
Switzerland: Olivier Irion (Obstetrician), Carolyn Troeger (Obstetrician);
United Kingdom: Zarko Alfirevic (Obstetrician), Peter Brocklehurst (Obstetrician, Epidemiologist), Alison MacFarlane (Epidemiologist), Jane Rogers (Midwife), Clare Winter (Midwife).

References

1. Prendiville WJ, Elbourne D, MacDonald S. Active versus expectant management in the third stage of labour (Cochrane Review). Cochrane Library, Issue 2, 2004. Chichester, UK: John Wiley & Sons, Ltd
2. Elbourne DR, Prendiville WJ, Carroli G, Wood J, MacDonald S. Prophylactic use of oxytocin in the third stage of labour (Cochrane Review). Cochrane Library, Issue 2, 2004. Chichester, UK: John Wiley & Sons, Ltd
3. MacDonald S, Abbott JM, Higgins SP. Prophylactic ergometrine-oxytocin versus oxytocin for the third stage of labour (Cochrane Review). Cochrane Library, Issue 2, 2004. Chichester, UK: John Wiley & Sons, Ltd
4. Villar J, Gülmezoglu AM, Hofmeyr J, Forna F. Systematic review of randomized controlled trials of misoprostol to prevent postpartum hemorrhage. Obstet Gynecol 2002;100: 1301–12
5. Jackson KW Jr, Allbert JR, Schemmer GK, Elliot M, Humphrey A, Taylor J. A randomized controlled trial comparing oxytocin administration before and after placental delivery in the prevention of postpartum hemorrhage. Am J Obstet Gynecol 2001;185:873–7
6. Huh WK, Chelmow D, Malone FD. A double blinded, randomized controlled trial of oxytocin at the beginning versus the end of the third stage of labor for prevention of postpartum hemorrhage. Gynecol Obstet Invest 2004;58:72–6
7. Bullough C, Msuku R, Karonde L. Early sucking and post partum haemorrhage: controlled trial in deliveries by traditional birth attendants. Lancet 1989;334:522–5
8. Irons D, Sriskandabalan, Bullough C. A simple alternative to parenteral oxytocic for the third stage of labour. Int J Gynaecol Obstet 2004;46:15–18

15

Active Management of the Third Stage of Labor: Current Evidence, Instructions for Use and Global Programmatic Activities

D. Armbruster, A. Lalonde, S. Engelbrecht and B. Carbonne

INTRODUCTION AND BACKGROUND

Third stage of labor defined

The third stage of labor has traditionally been defined as the time between the birth of the baby and the delivery of the placenta and membranes. It is the third stage that is the most perilous for the woman because of the risk of postpartum hemorrhage (PPH). The third stage of labor typically lasts between 10 and 30 minutes; if the placenta fails to separate within 30 minutes after childbirth, the third stage is considered to be prolonged[1]. If the third stage of labor lasts longer that 18 minutes, it is associated with a significant risk of PPH; and there is a six-fold increase in PPH when the third stage of labor lasts longer than 30 minutes[2].

Management of the third stage of labor

The third stage of labor may be managed expectantly or actively (see Addendum A for a comparison of expectant and active management of the third stage of labor). In expectant (physiological) management, uterotonic drugs are not given prophylactically, the cord may or may not be clamped early, and the placenta is delivered by maternal effort. In active management, uterotonic drugs are given before delivery of the placenta, the cord is usually cut 2–3 minutes after birth, and the placenta is delivered by controlled cord traction (CCT).

Active management of the third stage labor (AMTSL) was challenged because critics felt that (1) there was not a scientific basis for its routine use and (2) it interfered with physiologic processes to the detriment of both the woman and her baby. Criticism of AMTSL led to the seminal Bristol[3] (1988) randomized controlled trial that set out to determine whether, in terms of maternal and fetal morbidity, continuing with routine active rather than physiological management of the third stage of labor was justified. The conclusions of the study team were that AMTSL reduced the incidence of PPH, shortened the third stage of labor and resulted in reduced neonatal packed cell volumes.

In 1998, the Hinchingbrooke[4] randomized controlled trial compared the effects of active and expectant management of the third stage of labor on maternal and neonatal morbidity, and attempted to address the following three issues raised about the results of previous randomized controlled trials, including the Bristol trial:

(1) Since active management was the norm in hospitals involved in the controlled trials on AMTSL vs. expectant management, women assigned expectant management might have been at a disadvantage because midwives were less experienced in this approach;

(2) Many women who choose expectant management of the third stage are encouraged to expel the placenta by adopting an upright posture, and differences in blood loss between active and expectant management could be due to position rather than other factors;

(3) Hazards of expectant management in the short term may be outweighed by physical and psychological advantages for the mother in the months after childbirth.

The conclusion of the study team was that AMTSL reduces the risk of PPH, whatever the woman's posture, even when midwives are familiar with both approaches.

These two trials showed that active management prevents up to 60% of PPH and provides several benefits for the woman compared to expectant management. Table 1 provides detailed results from these two important studies comparing active and expectant management of the third stage of labor.

These results indicate:

(1) That for every 12 patients receiving active rather than physiological management, one case of PPH is prevented;

(2) For every 67 patients so managed, one woman would avoid transfusion with blood products.

Table 1 Bristol and Hinchingbrooke study results comparing active and physiologic management of the third stage of labor

Factors	Bristol			Hinchingbrooke		
	Active	Physiologic	OR and 95% CI	Active	Physiologic	OR and 95% CI
PPH (blood loss = 500 ml?)	5.9%	79.9%	3.13 (2.3–4.2)	6.8%	16.5%	2.42 (1.78–3.3)
Average length of the third stage of labor	5 min	15 min	Not performed	8 min	15 min	Not performed
Third stage of labor longer than 30 min	2.9%	26%	6.42 (4.9–8.41)	3.3%	16.4%	4.9 (3.22–7.43)
Blood transfusion required	2.1%	5.6%	2.56 (1.57–4.19)	0.5%	2.6%	4.9 (1.68–14.25)
Additional uterotonic drugs needed to manage PPH	6.4%	29.7%	4.83 (3.77–6.18)	3.2%	21.1%	6.25 (4.33–9.96)

In addition, these studies also confirm that **AMTSL decreases**:

- Incidence of PPH

- Length of third stage of labor

- Percentage of third stage of labor lasting longer than 30 minutes

- Need for blood transfusion

- Need for uterotonic drugs to manage PPH.

Many researchers have since replicated these findings in a variety of settings in different regions of the world. These studies collectively provide a strong evidence base in support of the use of AMTSL as an evidence-based, cost-effective intervention that provides dramatic results to address the single most important cause of maternal mortality globally – PPH.

DISCUSSION OF COMPONENTS OF ACTIVE MANAGEMENT OF THE THIRD STAGE OF LABOR

AMTSL was defined by the Bristol and Hinchingbrooke trials as:

(1) Uterotonic drug was administered with the birth of the anterior shoulder;

(2) Immediate cord clamping;

(3) CCT with the first contraction.

More recently, the steps of AMTSL have been integrated into routine care for the woman AND her newborn and have been refined to include the following:

(1) Administration of a uterotonic drug within 1 minute after the baby's birth and after ruling out the presence of another baby;

(2) Clamping and cutting the cord after cord pulsations have ceased or approximately 2–3 minutes after birth of the baby, whichever comes first;

(3) CCT during a contraction with counter traction to support the uterus, including gently turning the placenta as it is delivered to prevent tearing of the membranes;

(4) Massaging the uterus immediately after delivery of the placenta.

Clinical guidelines for management of the third stage of labor will generally also include careful inspection of the placenta and genitalia to rule out retained placenta/placental fragments and genital lacerations, and careful monitoring of the woman and her newborn for at least the first 6 hours postpartum.

Administration of a uterotonic drug

Administering a uterotonic drug within 1 minute after the baby's birth promotes strong uterine contractions and leads to faster retraction and placental delivery. This decreases the amount of maternal blood loss. More effective uterine activity also leads to a reduction in the incidence of retained placenta. Based on results of efficacy studies, WHO[5] recommends oxytocin (10 IU by IM injection) as the uterotonic drug of choice for prevention of PPH during the third stage of labor because it is effective 2–3 minutes after injection, has minimal side-effects and can be used in all women. However, if oxytocin is not available:

- Syntometrine® (fixed drug combination of 0.5 mg of ergometrine with 5 IU of oxytocin by IM injection) and ergometrine (0.2 mg by IM injection) should be the uterotonic drugs of choice when oxytocin is not available and there are no contraindications to their use

- Misoprostol (400–600 μg by mouth) should be used if the person administering the drug is not authorized or trained to give injections, or if the woman has contraindications to the use of ergometrine or the fixed drug combination of ergometrine and oxytocin.

When choosing a uterotonic drug, the following issues should also be considered:

- Ergometrine (and the fixed drug combination of oxytocin and ergometrine) is contraindicated in women with a history of hypertension, heart disease, pre-eclampsia or eclampsia. The provider must be able to ascertain that these conditions do not exist before administering ergometrine. Therefore, safely to use ergometrine or the fixed drug combination of oxytocin and ergometrine, the birth attendant must have a functional blood pressure (BP) apparatus and stethoscope, be able to measure BP competently, and be able to ascertain whether there are contraindications to its use before administering it

- Both ergometrine (and the fixed drug combination of ergometrine and oxytocin) and misoprostol have side-effects. Oxytocin has no known side-effects if administered postpartum

  - Major side-effects for ergometrine include nausea, vomiting, headache, elevated blood pressure (diastolic BP >100 mmHg) and tonic–clonic uterine contractions

  - Side-effects for misoprostol include shivering and elevated temperature; in regimens using higher doses, nausea, vomiting and diarrhea occur more frequently

  - If ergometrine or misoprostol is used, then counseling on the side-effects of these drugs should be given

- **Administration costs** of oxytocin in ampoules, ergometrine and the fixed drug combination of oxytocin and ergometrine are likely to be generally equivalent. Administration costs of misoprostol will be less because it does not require a syringe and needle or consumables and supplies to ensure safe injection and infection prevention practices

- **Storage costs** may be higher for **ergometrine** (and the fixed drug combination of oxytocin and ergometrine) because it requires temperature-controlled transport and storage, and protection from light. Oxytocin is more stable and storage costs may be less than ergometrine[6]. Costs for storage of misoprostol are minimal because it is the most stable of the three uterotonic drugs and can be stored at room temperature, provided that it is protected from humidity

- **Access** to **injectable** uterotonic drugs is limited to points of care where a skilled birth attendant is trained and authorized to administer injections. Misoprostol is administered orally and does not require refrigeration; therefore it has the potential to increase access in the community level and in births not attended by a skilled birth attendant[7]. Several studies have demonstrated the safety and efficacy of introducing use of misoprostol by health workers[8], traditional birth attendants[9], or pregnant women themselves[10] trained in its use.

A theoretical risk of a trapped twin exists if providers administer a uterotonic drug with an undiagnosed twin pregnancy. However, quality clinical assessment in labor and following delivery of the first baby can establish the diagnosis before giving a uterotonic drug.

Cord clamping

Current recommendations for cord clamping are to wait to clamp and cut the cord until 2–3 minutes after the baby's birth[11], even if oxytocin is given within 1 minute after birth of the baby.

Immediate cord clamping can decrease the red blood cells an infant receives at birth by more than 50%[12]. Studies show that delaying clamping and cutting of the umbilical cord is helpful to both full-term and preterm babies. In full-term babies, there were fewer cases of anemia at 2 months of age and increased duration of early breastfeeding when cord clamping and cutting was delayed[13]. In high-risk situations (e.g. low birth weight or premature infant), delaying clamping by as little as a few minutes is helpful. In situations where cord clamping and cutting was delayed for preterm babies, these infants had higher hematocrit and hemoglobin levels and a lesser need for transfusions in the first 4–6 weeks of life than preterm babies whose cords were clamped and cut immediately after birth.

Giving oxytocin before cord clamping has no known harmful effects. Mothers naturally produce some oxytocin during labor which is transmitted to the infants. Oxytocin given either IM or IV at delivery supplements this natural process. Administering a uterotonic drug immediately after birth also can speed the transfer of blood into the baby from the placenta, thus increasing the infant's red cell mass[10].

Controlled cord traction

CCT assists with rapid delivery of the placenta. It is important that the placenta be removed quickly once it has separated from the uterine wall because the uterus cannot contract efficiently if the placenta remains inside. CCT includes supporting the uterus by applying pressure on the lower segment of the uterus in an upward direction towards the woman's head, while at the same time pulling with a firm, steady tension on the cord in a downward direction during contractions. Supporting or guarding the uterus ('counter pressure' or 'counter traction') helps prevent uterine inversion. CCT should only be performed during a contraction and if counter traction is being applied.

Advocates of CCT argue that when expectant management is used, the placenta may be detached but remain at the level of the internal os. If this occurs, blood trapped behind the placenta in this position can distend the uterus, preventing further retraction and increasing the likelihood of PPH. CCT, however, requires the presence of a birth attendant trained in its use, thus severely limiting access to the life-saving effects of AMTSL. This has led international researchers to study the effects of managing the third stage of labor with a uterotonic drug in the absence of CCT. In 2006, WHO, the International Federation of Gynecology and Obstetrics (FIGO) and the International Confederation of Midwives (ICM) recommended that in the absence of AMTSL (that is active management without CCT), a uterotonic drug (oxytocin or misoprostol) be offered by a health worker trained in its use for prevention of PPH[14]. This was based on two randomized trials that reported the use of oxytocin in the absence of active management[15] and one trial with misoprostol[8]. More recently (2011), WHO conducted a hospital-based, multicenter, individually randomized controlled trial to assess the 'non-inferiority' of a 'simplified package' for actively managing the third stage of labor (use of uterotonic *without* CCT) compared to the 'full package' for actively managing the third stage of labor (use of uterotonic *and* CCT). Based on findings of this study, the investigators made the following two inferences from the trial: '1. CCT is safe and in settings where it is routinely practised it can be continued; and 2. the main component of active management is the uterotonic and in settings where it is not possible to employ the full package one can safely focus on the uterotonic component'[16]. Study results give strength to earlier WHO, FIGO and ICM recommendations and, by avoiding the need for a manual procedure that requires training, the third stage management can be implemented in a more widespread and cost-effective manner around the world even at the most peripheral levels of the health care system.

Some authors advocate the use of uterine massage and CCT if a uterotonic agent is not available for prophylactic use. No good evidence supports this recommendation. The risks of cord traction when the uterus is not well contracted are substantial, including uterine inversion and ruptured cord.

Uterine massage

Once the placenta is delivered, the uterus may have a tendency to relax slightly which could result in heavy bleeding. Although the prophylactic use of a uterotonic drug helps ensure that the uterus continues to contract and retract, the provider must continue to palpate the abdomen to assess and monitor uterine tone and size, and massage the uterus as needed. Massaging the uterus stimulates uterine contractions and may help expel blood and clots that might prevent contraction. As uterine massage can be uncomfortable; it is important to explain the rationale to the patient. Teaching the woman how to assess and massage her own uterus will prevent finding the woman in a 'pool' of her own blood during routine monitoring.

ACTIVE MANAGEMENT OF THE THIRD STAGE OF LABOR WITHOUT CONTROLLED CORD TRACTION

Numerous research trials and studies have shown the clinical efficacy of AMTSL in preventing PPH, but the evidence supported a package of interventions with few data on the contribution of each of the components of AMTSL. Little was known about the contribution of controlled cord traction. In 2007, WHO initiated a randomized non-inferiority controlled trial with the primary objective being to determine whether the simplified package of oxytocin 10 IU IM/IV, without CCT, is not less effective than the full AMTSL package with regard to reducing blood loss of 1000 ml or more in the third stage of labor. If the 'simplified package' was not worse than the 'full package' by more than the margin in terms of efficacy, the 'simplified package' would be valuable and could be implemented in settings without the manual skills needed for CCT.

Recruitment began in June 2009 and the trial ran to November 2010. The multicenter trial was conducted in 16 hospitals and two primary health care centers in eight countries: Argentina, Egypt, India, Kenya, the Philippines, South Africa, Thailand and Uganda. A total of 24,390 women (36,131 assessed for eligibility with 11,741 excluded) enrolled in the trial.

Based on agreed assumptions, a trial of 22,908 women would have 80% power to show non-inferiority of the simplified package within 0.45% of the full AMTSL package's PPH rate (i.e. $(1 - 0.70) \times (3.0 - 1.5)$, with a two-sided CI of 95%, and an alpha of 2.5%. In relative terms, this gives a margin of non-inferiority of 1.3, i.e. $(1.5 + 0.45)/1.5 = 1.95/1.5$).

The main findings of the study are:

- The policy of the simplified package was on the borderline of non-inferiority (2.06% vs. 1.88%, RR 1.09, 95% CI 0.91–1.31) for severe hemorrhage

- There was more blood loss of 500 ml or more (13.75% vs. 12.85%, RR 1.07, CI 1.00–1.14) and manual removal (1.30% vs. 0.89%, RR 1.45, CI 1.14–1.86) with the simplified package.

- In sensitivity analyses excluding Philippine data, severe hemorrhage (1.63% vs. 1.49%, RR 1.9, CI 0.87–1.37) was still borderline, while hemorrhage (10.5% vs. 9.84%, RR 1.07, CI 0.98–1.16) and manual removal (0.65% vs. 0.68%, RR 0.97, CI 0.68–1.37) were clinically similar

- Overall, one woman (full package) had uterine inversion.

The findings confirm the key role the uterotonic plays in PPH prevention and suggest that the omission of CCT results in little increased risk of severe PPH. In calculating the numbers needed to harm, for every 581 women who receive the simplified package, there would be only one additional woman who would have a severe PPH than if all received the full AMTSL package. While borderline for non-inferiority and the experts agreeing with the above stated results, the fact that the study results crossed the pre-stated upper limit of the confidence interval of 1.30 with a risk ratio of 1.09 (95% CI 0.91–1.31) must be acknowledged as leaving a very small possibility of chance results. Another issue for the trial was with the quality of the data from one of the Philippine sites which required a sensitivity analysis. The sensitivity analysis was performed after the protocol was written but before the outcome data were analysed. In addition to frequent closures during the study period, one of the

Philippine sites continued their routine policy of using ergometrine as part of third stage management during the study. For these reasons and the association of ergometrine with placental retention identified earlier in the literature, the trial steering committee decided that the sensitivity analyses were justified.

The investigators make the following two inferences from the trial: '1. CCT is safe and in settings where it is routinely practised it can be continued; and 2. the main component of active management is the uterotonic and in settings where it is not possible to employ the full package one can safely focus on the uterotonic component'[16].

STEPS IN ACTIVE MANAGEMENT OF THE THIRD STAGE OF LABOR

The three main components or steps of AMTSL – administering a uterotonic drug, CCT and massaging the uterus – should be implemented along with the provision of immediate newborn care.

(1) Thoroughly dry the baby, assess its breathing and perform resuscitation if needed, and then place the baby in skin-to-skin contact with the mother:

(a) After birth of the baby, immediately dry the infant and assess its breathing. If the baby requires resuscitation you may need to cut the cord immediately to care for the baby.

(b) Then place the reactive infant, prone, in skin-to-skin contact, on the mother. If the umbilical cord is long enough, place the baby directly on the mother's chest. If the umbilical cord is short, place the baby on the mother's abdomen until after cutting the cord. Be careful to leave some slack on the umbilical cord and do not unduly stretch the cord.

Note: If the baby has poor color or needs resuscitation, the cord may be cut immediately so that adequate resuscitation can be performed immediately.

(c) Remove the cloth used to dry the baby.

(d) Cover both the mother and infant with a dry, warm cloth or towel to prevent heat loss.

(e) Cover the baby's head with a cap or cloth (Figure 1).

(2) Administer a uterotonic drug within 1 minute of the baby's birth:

(a) Before performing AMTSL, gently palpate the woman's abdomen to rule out the presence of another baby. At this point, do not massage the uterus.

(b) If another baby is not present, begin the procedure by giving the woman 10 IU of oxytocin by IM injection in the upper thigh. This should be done within 1 minute of childbirth. If available, a qualified assistant should give the injection.

(c) In patients with intravenous access in place, 10–20 IU may be placed in 500–1000 ml of crystalloid and run quickly or 5 IU may be administered as an intravenous bolus, followed by a similar infusion.

Note: Ergometrine should not be used in the absence of CCT because of the risk of retained placenta associated with tonic–clonic contractions induced by ergometrine (Figure 2).

(3) Clamp and cut the umbilical cord:

(a) Place one clamp 4 cm from the baby's abdomen after cord pulsations have ceased or approximately 2–3 minutes after birth of the baby, whichever comes first.

Note: If national guidelines for newborn interventions to prevent/reduce the risk of maternal-to-child transmission of HIV/AIDS include early clamping of the cord, then the protocol for AMTSL may have to be revised.

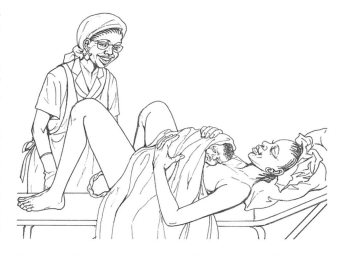

Figure 1 Place the baby in skin-to-skin contact with the mother. From POPPHI. Managing the third stage of labor in peripheral health care settings: a guide to train auxillary midwives. Seattle, WA: PATH, with permission

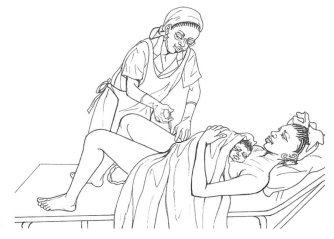

Figure 2 Administer a uterotonic within 1 minute of the baby's birth. From POPPHI. Managing the third stage of labor in peripheral health care settings: a guide to train auxillary midwives. Seattle, WA: PATH, with permission

(b) Gently milk the cord towards the woman's perineum and place a second clamp on the cord approximately 2 cm from the first clamp.

(c) Cut the cord using sterile scissors under cover of a gauze swab to prevent blood spatter. After mother and baby are safely cared for, tie the cord (Figure 3).

Note: Delaying cord clamping allows for transfer of red blood cells from the placenta to the baby that can decrease the incidence of anemia during infancy.

(d) Place the baby on the woman's chest, in skin-to-skin contact, and encourage breastfeeding (Figure 4).

(4) Perform CCT:

WHO, FIGO and ICM recommend that in the absence of a skilled provider, third stage should be managed by administering a uterotonic drug (oxytocin or misoprostol) without CCT for the prevention of PPH.

(a) Place the clamp near the woman's perineum to make CCT easier.

(b) Hold the cord close to the perineum using a clamp.

(c) Place the palm of the other hand on the lower abdomen just above the woman's pubic bone to assess for uterine contractions. If a clamp is not available, CCT can be applied by encircling the cord around the hand.

(d) Wait for a uterine contraction. Only perform CCT when there is a contraction (Figure 5)

(e) When there is a contraction, apply external pressure on the uterus in an upward direction

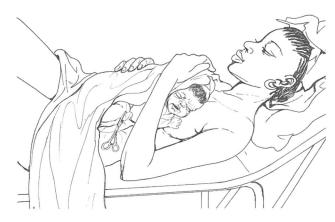

Figure 4 Place the baby on the woman's chest and encourage breastfeeding. From POPPHI. Managing the third stage of labor in peripheral health care settings: a guide to train auxillary midwives. Seattle, WA: PATH, with permission

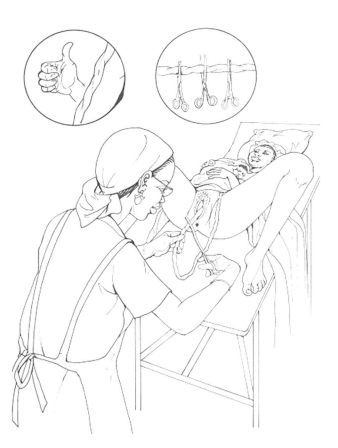

Figure 3 Clamp and cut the umbilical cord. From POPPHI. Managing the third stage of labor in peripheral health care settings: a guide to train auxillary midwives. Seattle, WA: PATH, with permission

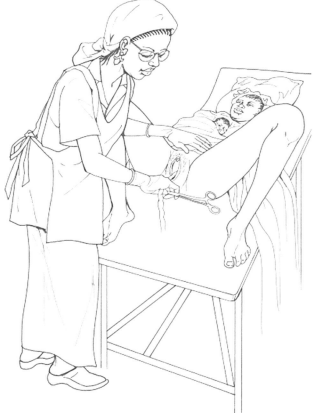

Figure 5 Place the palm on the lower abdomen to assess for a uterine contraction. From POPPHI. Managing the third stage of labor in peripheral health care settings: a guide to train auxillary midwives. Seattle, WA: PATH, with permission

(toward the woman's head) with the hand just above the pubic bone.

(f) At the same time with your other hand, pull with firm, steady tension on the cord in a downward direction (follow the direction of the birth canal). Avoid jerky or forceful pulling (Figure 6).

Note: If the placenta does not descend during 30–40 seconds of CCT (i.e. there are no signs of placental separation), do not continue to pull on the cord:

(g) Gently hold the cord and wait until the uterus is well contracted again. If necessary, use a sponge forceps to clamp the cord closer to the perineum as it lengthens.

(h) With the next contraction, repeat CCT with counter traction.

(i) Do not release support on the uterus until the placenta is visible at the vulva. Deliver the

placenta slowly and support it with both hands (Figure 7).

(j) As the placenta is delivered, hold and gently turn it with both hands until the membranes are twisted.

(k) Slowly pull to complete the delivery. Gently move membranes up and down until delivered (Figure 8).

Note: If the membranes tear, gently examine the upper vagina and cervix wearing high-level disinfected or sterile gloves and use a sponge forceps to remove any pieces of remaining membrane.

(5) Massage the uterus:

(a) Massage the uterus immediately after delivery of the placenta and membranes until it is firm.

(b) After stopping massage, it is important that the uterus does not relax again.

(c) Palpate for a contracted uterus every 15 minutes and repeat uterine massage as needed during at least the first 2 hours after childbirth (Figure 9).

(d) Instruct the woman how to massage her own uterus, and ask her to call if her uterus becomes soft (Figure 10).

(6) Examine the placenta and membranes for completeness.

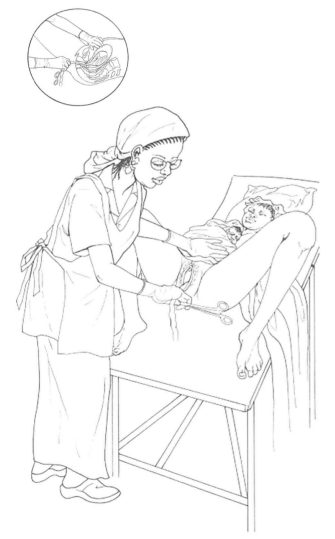

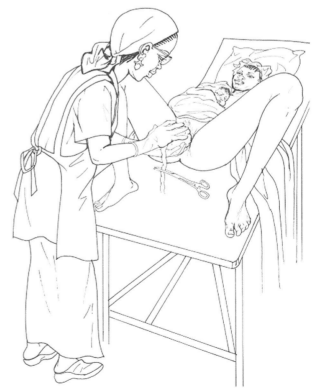

Figure 6   Perform controlled cord traction with counter traction. From POPPHI. Managing the third stage of labor in peripheral health care settings: a guide to train auxillary midwives. Seattle, WA: PATH, with permission

Figure 7   Only release support of the uterus when the placenta is visible at the vulva. From POPPHI. Managing the third stage of labor in peripheral health care settings: a guide to train auxillary midwives. Seattle, WA: PATH, with permission

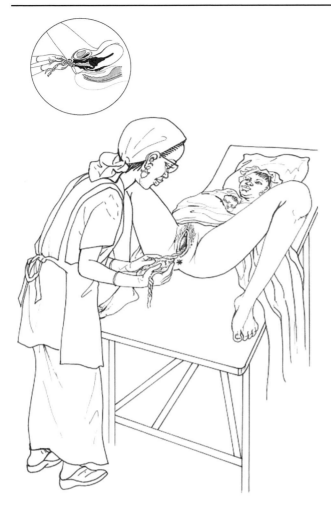

Figure 8 Hold and gently turn the placenta as it is delivered. From POPPHI. Managing the third stage of labor in peripheral health care settings: a guide to train auxillary midwives. Seattle, WA: PATH, with permission

(7) Examine the genitalia and repair lacerations/ episiotomy if necessary.

(8) Evaluate blood loss.

(9) Explain all examination findings to the woman and, if she desires, her family.

GLOBAL RECOMMENDATIONS BASED ON CLINICAL EVIDENCE

In 2003, a global push was made to promote AMTSL. This initiative was part of the world's effort to achieve Millennium Development Goal 5, which calls for a 75% reduction in the maternal mortality ratio between 1990 and 2015. At that time, there were three clear 'categories' of practitioners:

(1) Practitioners in the UK and Commonwealth countries and much of Europe who were aware of the evidence supporting the use of AMTSL and practiced it routinely;

(2) Practitioners in Latin America, the United States, Franco-phone Africa and other non-Commonwealth countries who were either

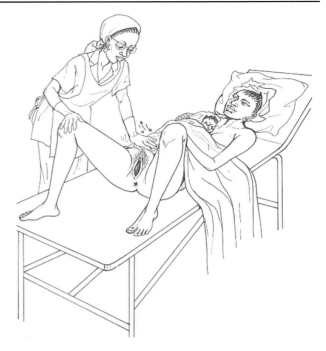

Figure 9 Massage the uterus until it is firm. From POPPHI. Managing the third stage of labor in peripheral health care settings: a guide to train auxillary midwives. Seattle, WA: PATH, with permission

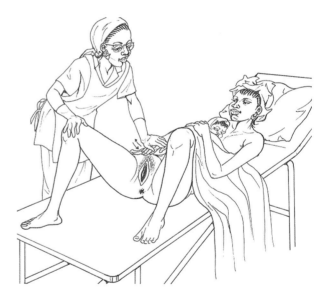

Figure 10 Instruct the woman how to massage her own uterus. From POPPHI. Managing the third stage of labor in peripheral health care settings: a guide to train auxillary midwives. Seattle, WA: PATH, with permission

unaware of AMTSL or if aware, unconvinced or against the its application;

(3) Practitioners in countries where AMTSL was part of routine care during childbirth, who were either not applying AMTSL or applying it incorrectly, because they were not trained in its correct application or because they lacked the necessary supplies, medications and consumables.

In an effort to reach political leaders, opinion leaders and decision-makers, FIGO, ICM and WHO

120

developed two important policy documents: (1) 2003 Joint statement by FIGO and ICM on the *Management of the Third Stage of Labor to Prevent Postpartum Haemorrhage*[17] and (2) *WHO Recommendations for the Prevention of Postpartum Haemorrhage*[5].

Joint Statement by FIGO and ICM on *Management of the Third Stage of Labor to Prevent Postpartum Hemorrhage*

The 2003 Joint Statement was a pivotal document that provided a platform upon which to build a global effort to save women from dying of PPH[17]. Signed in Chile by the leaders of both organizations, it was later ratified by the respective leadership councils and members, and has served as a seminal document for joint efforts and collaboration with WHO and others.

The two premier professional organizations responsible for leadership in maternity care pledged to work through their national membership organizations to promote the practice of AMTSL and ensure that obstetricians, other physicians, midwives and those caring for women during childbirth offered women this evidence-based practice. FIGO and ICM, in collaboration with partners, became leaders in an effort to share data on the efficacy and effectiveness of this intervention and increase the uptake by countries.

During the process of developing the Joint Statement, data were presented on the importance of delayed cord clamping for the newborn. Recognizing that the definition used in the Bristol and Hinchingbrooke trials included immediate cord clamping, FIGO and ICM experts determined that 'immediate cord clamping' was unlikely to be a key component of AMTSL, and its removal would have little impact on the incidence or severity of PPH. Immediate cord clamping was removed from the definition of AMTSL in the 2006 joint statement[18].

The importance of surveillance of a woman in the immediate postpartum period was highlighted and immediate massage of the fundus of the uterus after delivery of the placenta until the uterus was contracted was included in the definition as well as palpation for a contracted uterus every 15 minutes for 2 hours.

WHO guidance

WHO staff drafted questions on the various interventions used or suggested for prevention of atonic PPH and shared them for review by an international panel of experts. WHO commissioned an external organization to review and grade the evidence to answer the questions using the GRADE methodology. When completed, WHO held a Technical Consultation in Geneva in 2006 to review the evidence provided by the GRADE process and to discuss the various issues related to the prevention of PPH. Based on the data, the experts developed recommendations. Key recommendations from the report are listed below[5]. For a complete report on the WHO PPH Technical Consultation, visit http://whqlibdoc.who.int/hq/2007/WHO_MPS_07.06_eng.pdf.

The WHO technical consultation made five key recommendations to prevent PPH:

(1) AMTSL should be offered by skilled attendants to all women (strong recommendation, moderate quality evidence).

(2) Recommendations for choice of uterotonic drug in the context of AMTSL:

   (a) If all injectable uterotonic drugs are available, skilled attendants should offer oxytocin to all women for prevention of PPH in preference to ergometrine/methylergometrine (strong recommendation, low quality evidence).

   (b) If oxytocin is not available, skilled attendants should offer ergometrine/methylergometrine or the fixed drug combination of oxytocin and ergometrine to women without hypertension or heart disease for prevention of PPH (strong recommendation, low quality evidence).

   (c) Skilled attendants should offer oxytocin for prevention of PPH in preference to oral misoprostol (600 μg) (strong recommendation, high quality evidence).

   (d) Skilled attendants should not offer sublingual misoprostol, rectal misoprostol, or carboprost/sulprostone for prevention of PPH in preference to oxytocin (strong recommendation, very low quality evidence).

(3) In the absence of AMTSL, a uterotonic drug (oxytocin or misoprostol) should be offered by a health worker trained in its use for prevention of PPH (strong recommendation, moderate quality evidence).

(4) Because of the benefits to the baby, the cord should not be clamped earlier than necessary for applying cord traction in AMTSL (weak recommendation, low quality evidence).

   (a) For the sake of clarity, it is estimated that this will normally take around 3 minutes.

   (b) Early clamping may be required if the baby is asphyxiated and requires immediate resuscitation.

(5) Given the current evidence, the panel recommends no change in the practice of CCT as one of the components of AMTSL (strong recommendation, low quality evidence). However, further research was recommended.

THE PREVENTION OF POSTPARTUM HEMORRHAGE INITIATIVE (POPPHI): A GLOBAL EFFORT TO TACKLE THE BIGGEST MATERNAL KILLER

In August 2004, the US Agency for International Development developed and funded the Prevention of Postpartum Hemorrhage Initiative (POPPHI). It was a 5 year project focused on the reduction of PPH, the single most important cause of maternal deaths worldwide. Partners in the effort were the Program for Appropriate Technology in Health (PATH), Research Triangle International (RTI), FIGO, ICM and EngenderHealth.

POPPHI started with one simple but immensely challenging mandate: to catalyze the expansion of AMTSL practices worldwide as a key step to reducing maternal mortality by preventing PPH. As evidence emerged about the effectiveness of misoprostol to prevent PPH, POPPHI participated in global discussions about and evaluation of the research on this promising intervention. In addition to its work to expand the use of AMTSL, POPPHI began prioritizing (supporting) community-based strategies for preventing PPH, particularly as data demonstrated the effectiveness of misoprostol, and the Uniject™ device prefilled with oxytocin became commercially available.

One of POPPHI's first activities was to conduct national surveys in ten diverse developing countries. The survey helped to advance understanding of current AMTSL practices, and to provide Ministries of Health (MOHs) and their international partners with the descriptive information necessary to assess AMTSL practices and to identify major barriers to and enabling factors for its use (http://pphprevention.org/Surveytools.php). The research used nationally representative samples of observed facility-based deliveries. The survey results showed that correct use of AMTSL was low: only 0.5–32% of observed deliveries (Figure 11). These findings suggest that as many as 1.4 million women per year who gave birth vaginally did not receive AMTSL.

As part of the development of the survey tools, POPPHI identified the determinants to the use of AMTSL and requirements for introduction and expansion/scale-up of the use of AMTSL in a country (Figure 12).

After identifying the determinants to use, POPPHI and its partners identified key activities and approaches that proved to be highly effective in increasing the uptake of AMTSL. The approaches used by POPPHI included:

- Partnering with global leaders of maternal health

- Partnering with MOH and in-country professional organizations

- Strengthening policy

- Conducting pilot and demonstration projects and programs

- Strengthening provider practice through innovations and standardized trainings

- Expanding monitoring and evaluation systems to include PPH and AMTSL

- Strengthening and updating uterotonic drug storage and logistics systems

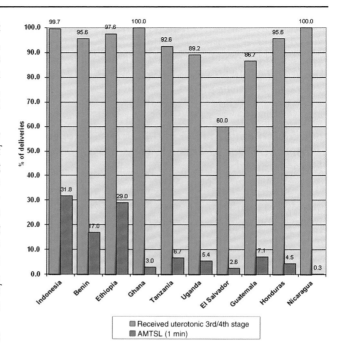

Figure 11 Percentage of observed deliveries in which uterotonic drugs were given during the third/fourth stages of labor and AMTSL was used correctly (including uterotonic administration within 1 minute). From POPPHI. Managing the third stage of labor in peripheral health care settings: a guide to train auxillary midwives. Seattle, WA: PATH, with permission

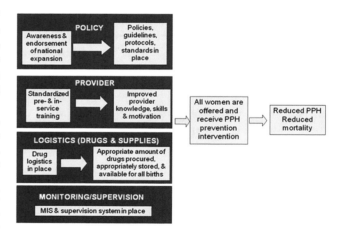

Figure 12 Determinants of uptake and use of PPH prevention interventions. MIS, management information system. From POPPHI. Managing the third stage of labor in peripheral health care settings: a guide to train auxillary midwives. Seattle, WA: PATH, with permission

- Providing small grants to national professional associations to promote PPH prevention initiatives

- Supporting expansion or scale-up of AMTSL in multiple countries.

The POPPHI project also developed tools and resources to strengthen providers' skill in the practice. These included AMTSL learning materials, a toolkit for providers, on-site and individual learning package, website, CD-ROM, fact sheets, job aids, posters and more. The website (www.pphprevention.org)

remains active and contains all of these documents and many more.

POPPHI created a consistent message on AMTSL using the strong evidence base for its use, demonstrated that AMTSL could have a large impact on maternal mortality, and provided clear examples for how countries could implement programs to prevent PPH. Overall, POPPHI and its various partners had a 'footprint' in more than 40 countries by conducting activities, collaborating with various groups or providing virtual or on the ground support to the various organizations working to save lives through prevention of PPH.

It is likely that POPPHI's most significant work was in the area of policy and advocacy where it continued the momentum and catalyzed additional work by WHO, FIGO, ICM, USAID, other research institutions, such as the US National Institute for Health, and others. Country governments and national professional associations were key partners, and many of the efforts and activities of POPPHI continue through government programs.

Although POPPHI was successfully terminated in 2010, FIGO has made a 10 year commitment to pursue the decrease in mortality and severe morbidity from PPH and with these efforts and many others, the efforts to save women from dying of PPH continues.

COUNTRY EXAMPLES

Benin

The Benin Government made a commitment to scale up AMTSL throughout the country after the practice was introduced in 2002 and 2003. POPPHI's AMTSL survey conducted in 2007 found that while 84% of women in Benin gave birth in a facility where providers had received training in AMTSL and 62% of health districts had a PPH/AMTSL initiative, only 18% of women in the sample received AMTSL that was practiced according to standard. Results of the survey catalyzed several key activities:

- In 2008, a national task force developed a set of recommendations and a national action plan for improving AMTSL practice. Some of these recommendations included:

  - Development of a national-level post for a person responsible for promoting and monitoring AMTSL use

  - AMTSL is now integrated into the national safe motherhood plan

  - AMTSL is integrated into pre-service education programs for nurses, midwives and physicians as well as other in-service training programs, such as those for emergency obstetric and newborn care

  - To improve monitoring, evaluation and tracking of AMTSL coverage rates, the three elements of AMTSL were integrated into the partograph,

    and AMTSL was integrated into the delivery register

- In 2008, survey results and recommendations made by the national task force were disseminated regionally. Each district subsequently developed action plans to improve AMTSL practice and improve quantification and storage of oxytocin

- In 2008, national protocols related to PPH prevention and management were reviewed and updated to include evidence-based practices

- In 2009, national protocols were developed for quantification, transport and storage of uterotonic drugs

- In 2009, the Beninese midwifery association and the Beninese and Togolese Society for Obstetrics and Gynecology ratified revised protocols and signed a joint statement on the prevention of PPH and rational use of uterotonic drugs

- In 2009, Benin's Minister of Health made a commitment to increasing the number of midwives hired by the government to ensure that all women giving birth in facilities would be assisted by a skilled birth attendant and receive AMTSL.

Mali

Mali developed a national commitment to scaling up AMTSL for all providers attending births in health care facilities since the practice was introduced in 2002 and 2003. The PPH prevention initiative was launched in 2007 and national and regional plans for preventing PPH were developed. Since then, the government has implemented the following activities that are part of the national and regional plans:

- A national task force with members from the National Department of Health and international partners was established to develop a plan for scaling up AMTSL and monitoring progress. Achievements include:

  - Procurement of oxytocin in the Uniject® device was included in the national plan for AMTSL scale-up

  - The three elements of AMTSL were integrated into the partograph

  - AMTSL was integrated into pre-service education programs for nurses, midwives and physicians and in other in-service training programs, such as emergency obstetric and newborn care

  - AMTSL is tracked in districts and regions targeted by USAID

- In 2006, an operational research study in three districts (Gao, Koulikoro and Sikasso) on the feasibility and safety of training auxiliary midwives (*matrones*) to use AMTSL. On April 2, 2009, Mali's Minister of Health authorized *matrones* to provide AMTSL and use oxytocin when practicing AMTSL

- In 2008, PPH was featured as the theme for the National Midwifery Day. At this event, a joint statement on the prevention of PPH and rational use of uterotonic drugs was signed by the Malian Midwifery Association (the Association des Sages-Femmes du Mali, or ASFM) and the Malian Society for Obstetrics and Gynecology

- In 2009, the National Order of Midwives published a bulletin on PPH prevention and rational use of uterotonic drugs.

CONCLUSIONS: CURRENT GUIDANCE FOR CLINICIANS

AMTSL is a highly effective intervention that decreases the incidence of PPH from uterine atony by approximately 60%, decreases the cost of maternity care as shown in studies in Guatemala and Zambia, and decreases the use of additional uterotonic drugs or other more invasive interventions to manage PPH. It also decreases the length of the third stage of labor – which is important in very busy labor and delivery wards or in short-staffed facilities. All skilled birth attendants – obstetricians/gynecologists, midwives and other practitioners – should therefore become competent to practice AMTSL through their pre-service education or simple in-service training programs.

While the proportion of deliveries attended by skilled health personnel rose from 58% in 1990 to 68% in 2008, it has remained low in the WHO African Region and the WHO South-East Asia Region where only around 50% of deliveries were attended by skilled health personnel[19], meaning a large percentage of women are not being cared for by a skilled birth attendant during the third stage of labor. In these situations, two strategies should be promoted: (1) fewer skilled birth attendants should be trained to actively manage the third stage of labor without CCT and (2) community health workers and pregnant women should be trained in the use of misoprostol to prevent PPH. These strategies will increase the number of women having uterotonic coverage through simplified AMTSL and have great potential to save additional women's lives and markedly decrease maternal mortality and serious morbidity associated with PPH.

New research identifies the uterotonic as the key component of AMTSL's effectiveness. If not already a focus of program managers' and clinicians' activities, the importance of procuring sufficient quality medication is highlighted. Adequate training on proper storage and management of the medication is also necessary. It is critical to ensure that the system can complete appropriate quantification exercises, procure from manufacturers using current good manufacturing practices (cGMP), distribute in a timely fashion to all facilities and eliminate stock-outs. All facilities providing childbirth services must keep quality uterotonic drugs on hand at all times and use them consistently, as per protocol.

The Millennium Development Goal (MDG) 5 is to achieve a 75% reduction in maternal mortality between 1990 and 2015. Despite global efforts to reduce mortality, WHO reports that the global maternal mortality ratio (i.e. the number of maternal deaths per 100,000 live births) declined by only 2.3% per year between 1990 and 2008[20]. This is far from the annual decline of 5.5% required to achieve MDG 5. Achieving MDG 5 will continue to be an overwhelming challenge and an elusive goal if we cannot address the biggest killer in childbirth, PPH. Implementation of strategies to prevent PPH at all points of care where women are giving birth will significantly contribute to reductions in maternal morbidity and mortality.

References

1. McCormick ML, Sanghvi HCG, Kinzie B, McIntosh N. Preventing postpartum hemorrhage in low-resource settings. Int J Gynecol Obstet 2002;77:267–75
2. Everett F, Magann EF, Evans S, et al. the length of the third stage of labor and the risk of postpartum hemorrhage. Obstet Gynecol 2005;105:290–3
3. Prendiville WJ, Harding JE, Elbourne DR, Stirrat GM. The Bristol third stage trial: active versus physiological management of the third stage of labor. BMJ 1988;297:1295–300
4. Rogers J, Wood J, McCandlish R, Ayers S, Truesdale A, Elbourne D. Active versus expectant management of the third stage of labor: the Hinchingbrooke randomized controlled trial. Lancet 1998;351:693–9
5. World Health Organization (WHO) Department of Making Pregnancy Safer. WHO Recommendations for the Prevention of Postpartum Haemorrhage. Geneva, Switzerland: World Health Organization, 2007 Available at: www.who.int/making_pregnancy_safer/publications/WHORecommendationsforPPHaemorrhage.pdf
6. Hogerzeil HV, Walker GJ. Instability of (methyl)ergometrine in tropical climates: An overview. Eur J Obstet Gynecol Reprod Biol 1996;69:25–29
7. Gulmezoglu AM, Villar J, Ngoc NN, et al. WHO Collaborative Group to Evaluate Misoprostol in the Management of the Third Stage of Labor. WHO multicentre randomised trial of misoprostol in the management of the third stage of labor. Lancet 2001;358:689–95
8. Derman RJ, Kodkany BS, Goudar SS, et al. Oral misoprostol in preventing postpartum haemorrhage in resource-poor communities: a randomised controlled trial. Lancet 2006;368:1248–53
9. Mobeen N, Durocher J, Zuberi N, et al. Administration of misoprostol by trained traditional birth attendants to prevent postpartum haemorrhage in homebirths in Pakistan: a randomised placebo-controlled trial. BJOG 2011;118:353–61
10. Høj L, Cardoso P, Nielsen BB, Hvidman L, Nielsen J, Aaby P. Effect of sublingual misoprostol on severe postpartum haemorrhage in a primary health centre in Guinea-Bissau: randomised double blind clinical trial. BMJ 2005;331:723–7
11. Abalos E. Effect of timing of umbilical cord clamping of term infants on maternal and neonatal outcomes: RHL commentary (last revised: 2 March 2009). The WHO Reproductive Health Library. Geneva: World Health Organization. 2009 http://apps.who.int/rhl/pregnancy_childbirth/childbirth/3rd_stage/cd004074_abalose_com/en/index.html
12. Yao AC, Moinian M, Lind J. Distribution of blood between infant and placenta after birth. Lancet 1969;7626:871–3
13. Van Rheenen PJ, Brabin BJ. A practical approach to timing cord clamping in resource poor settings. BMJ 2006;333:954–8

14. World Health Organization (WHO) Department of Making Pregnancy Safer. MPS Technical Update: Prevention of Post-partum Haemorrhage by Active Management of the Third Stage of Labor. Geneva, Switzerland: WHO, October 2007. http://www.who.int/making_pregnancy_safer/publications/PPH_TechUpdate2.pdf

15. Cotter A, Ness A, Tolosa J. Prophylactic oxytocin for the third stage of labor (Review). Cochrane Database Syst Rev 2001;(12):Issue 4

16. Gulmezoglu AM, Lumbiganon P, Landoulsi S, et al. Active management of the third stage of labor without controlled cord traction: a randomized non-inferiority controlled trial. Lancet 2012;379:1721–7

17. International Confederation of Midwives International Federation of Gynaecology and Obstetrics. Joint statement management of the third stage of labour to prevent post-partum haemorrhage. The Hague: ICM; London: FIGO, 2003

18. International Confederation of Midwives (ICM), International Federation of Gynaecology and Obstetrics (FIGO). Prevention and Treatment of Post-partum Haemorrhage: New Advances for Low Resource Settings Joint Statement. The Hague: ICM; London: FIGO, 2006

19. World Health Organization. World Health Statistics 2011. http://www.who.int/gho/publications/world_health_statistics/EN_WHS2011_Part1.pdf

20. World Health Organization. Maternal mortality Fact sheet N°348. November 2010. http://www.who.int/mediacentre/factsheets/fs348/en/index.html

Addendum A: Comparison of physiologic (expectant) and active management of the third stage of labor (AMTSL)

	Physiologic (expectant) management	Active management*
Uterotonic	Uterotonic is not given before the placenta delivered	Uterotonic is given within 1 minute of the baby's birth (after ruling out the presence of a second baby)
Cord clamping	The cord is neither clamped nor cut early	Clamp and cut the cord following strict hygienic techniques after cord pulsations have ceased or approximately 2–3 minutes after birth of the baby, whichever comes first
Signs of placental separation	Wait for signs of separation: Gush of blood Lengthening of cord Uterus becomes rounder and smaller as the placenta descends	Do not wait for signs of placental separation. Instead: Palpate the uterus for a contraction Wait for the uterus to contract Apply CCT with counter traction
Delivery of the placenta	Placenta delivered by gravity assisted by maternal effort	Placenta delivered by CCT while supporting and stabilizing the uterus by applying counter traction
Uterine massage	Massage the uterus after the placenta is delivered	Massage the uterus *after* the placenta is delivered
Advantages	Does not interfere with normal labor process Does not require special drugs/supplies May be appropriate when immediate care is needed for the baby (such as resuscitation) and no trained assistant is available May not require a birth attendant with injection skills	Decreases length of third stage Decrease likelihood of prolonged third stage Decreases average blood loss Decreases the number of PPH cases Decreases need for blood transfusion
Disadvantages	Length of third stage is longer compared to AMTSL Blood loss is greater compared to AMTSL Increased risk of PPH	Requires uterotonic and items needed for injection/injection safety Requires a birth attendant with experience and skills giving injections and using CCT

*This definition differs from the original research protocol in the Bristol and Hinchingbrooke trials because the original protocols included immediate cord clamping and did not include massage of the uterus. In the Hinchingbrooke trial, midwives used either CCT or maternal effort to deliver the placenta.
CCT, controlled cord traction; PPH, postpartum hemorrhage

Section 3

Demographic Considerations

16

Definitions and Classifications

A. Coker and R. Oliver

INTRODUCTION

Conventionally, the term 'postpartum hemorrhage' (PPH) is applied to pregnancies beyond 20 weeks' gestation. Although bleeding at an earlier gestation may have a similar etiology, these are usually referred to as spontaneous miscarriages.

Despite numerous advances in medical and surgical treatment over the past 50 years, no significant changes have been made in the definitions or classification of PPH[1]. The World Health Organization (WHO) definition was proposed in 1990 and is widely used: 'any blood loss from the genital tract during delivery above 500 ml'[2] and updated in 2003 to include the first 24 hours after delivery[3].

The average blood loss during a normal vaginal delivery is widely described as 500 ml; however, approximately 5% of women lose more than 1000 ml during a vaginal birth[4–7]. On the other hand, cesarean deliveries are associated with an average estimated blood loss of 1000 ml[8]. Under these circumstances, a considerable degree of overlap exists in the acceptable range of blood loss for vaginal and cesarean deliveries. It is interesting to note that these definitions may be subject to further revision in the future when accurate studies of measured blood loss become available.

PURPOSE OF CLASSIFICATION

Classification of PPH is desirable for the following reasons. First, due to the rapidity of disease progression there is an overriding clinical need to determine the most suitable line of management. Although the urgency of intervention depends on the rate of decline or deterioration, the rate of decline or deterioration may also influence the urgency of intervention.

The second reason for classification is to assess the prognosis. This may help to determine the immediate, medium- and long-term clinical outcome. Therefore, a prognostic classification will guide the degree of aggressiveness of the intervention, especially as management may involve more than one clinical specialty. It will also help to decide on the optimal site for subsequent care, e.g. high dependency unit (HDU) or intensive care unit (ITU), if such exist in the hospital.

The third reason is to allow effective communication based on standardization of the estimate of the degree of hemorrhage, thus standardizing differing management options. The initial assessment is usually made by the staff available on site, and these are often relatively junior medical, midwifery, or nursing personnel. They in turn have to assess the severity of bleeding and summon help or assistance as required. Thus, a standardized easily applicable working classification facilitates effective communication and obviates interobserver variation.

CLASSIFICATIONS IN USE

Conventional temporal classification

Traditionally the classification of PPH has been based on the timing of the onset of bleeding in relation to the delivery. Hemorrhage within the first 24 hours of vaginal delivery is termed either early or primary PPH, whereas bleeding occurring afterwards, but within 12 weeks of delivery, is termed late or secondary PPH[9]. Secondary PPH is less common than primary PPH, affecting 1–3% of all deliveries. In both cases, the true blood loss is often underestimated due to the difficulty with visual quantitation[10,11].

Classification based on quantification of blood loss

Amount of blood lost

Blood loss at delivery is estimated using various methods. These range from the less modern methods of counting blood soaked pieces of cloth or 'kangas' used by traditional birth attendants in rural settings to more modern techniques such as using a calibrated drape that is placed under the buttocks (see Chapters 9 and 11) or calculating the blood loss by subtraction after weighing all swabs using sensitive weighing scales[12].

Change in hematocrit

The American College of Obstetrics and Gynecology advocates the definitions of PPH of either a 10% change in hematocrit between the antenatal and postpartum period, or a need for erythrocyte transfusion[13].

Rapidity of blood loss

In attempts to overcome these inconsistencies, PPH has also been classified based on the rapidity of blood loss. *Severe hemorrhage has been classified as blood loss of more than 150 ml/min (within 20 min causing a loss of more than 50% of blood volume) or a sudden blood loss of more than 1500–2000 ml* (uterine atony; loss of 25–35% of blood volume)[14].

Volume deficit

A form of standardized classification described by Benedetti considers four classes of hemorrhage[15]. The class of hemorrhage reflects the volume deficit, and this is not necessarily the same as the volume of blood loss (Table 1).

Class 1

The average 60 kg pregnant woman has a blood volume of 6000 ml at 30 weeks' gestation. A volume loss of less than 900 ml in such a woman will rarely lead to any symptoms and signs of volume deficit and will not require any acute treatment. This has been described as class 1.

Class 2

A blood loss of 1200–1500 ml will manifest clinical signs, such as a rise in pulse and respiratory rate. There may also be recordable blood pressure changes, but not the classic cold, clammy extremities.

Class 3

Class 3 denotes patients where the blood loss is sufficient to cause overt hypotension. The blood loss is usually around 1800–2100 ml, and is accompanied by signs of tachycardia (120–160 bpm), cold clammy extremities and tachypnea.

Class 4

Class 4 is commonly described as massive obstetric hemorrhage. When the volume loss exceeds 40%, profound shock ensues, and the blood pressure and pulse are not easily recordable. Immediate and urgent volume therapy is necessary, as a fatal outcome secondary to circulatory collapse and cardiac arrest is not far away unless resuscitation is immediate and aggressive.

Classification based on causative factors

The causes of PPH can also form a basis of classification.

Causes of primary PPH

Primary PPH is traditionally considered as a disorder of one or more of the four processes: uterine atony, retained clots or placental debris, genital lesions or trauma, and disorders of coagulation. The oft quoted acronym (aide memoire) for these conditions is the 'four Ts': tone, tissue, trauma and thrombin. Uterine atony alone accounts for 75–90% of PPH (Table 2).

Table 1 Classification of hemorrhage[15]

Hemorrhage class	Acute blood loss (ml)	Percentage lost
1	900	15
2	1200–1500	20–25
3	1800–2100	30–35
4	2400	≥40

Table 2 Classification of postpartum hemorrhage (PPH) according to causative factors. Adapted from Wac *et al.*, *The Female Patient* 2005;30:19

Causes of primary PPH

Tonus (uterine atony)
Uterine overdistention: multiparity, polyhydramnios, macrosomia
Uterine relaxants: nifedipine, magnesium, beta-mimetics, indomethacin, nitric oxide donors
Rapid or prolonged labor
Oxytoxics to induce labor
Chorioamnionitis
Halogenated anesthetics
Fibroid uterus

Tissue
Impediment to uterine contraction/retraction: multiple fibroids, retained placenta
Placental abnormality: placenta accreta, succenturiate lobe
Prior uterine surgery: myomectomy, classical or lower segment cesarean section
Obstructed labor
Prolonged third stage of labor
Excessive traction on the cord

Trauma
Vulvovaginal injury
Episiotomy/tears
Macrosomia
Precipitous delivery

Thrombin (coagulopathy)
Acquired during pregnancy: thrombocytopenia of HELLP syndrome, DIC, eclampsia, intrauterine fetal death, septicemia, placenta abruptio, amniotic fluid embolism, pregnancy-induced hypertension, sepsis
Hereditary: Von Willebrand's disease
Anticoagulant therapy: valve replacement, patients on absolute bed rest

Causes of secondary PPH
Uterine infection
Retained placental fragments
Abnormal involution of placental site

HELLP, hemolysis, elevated liver enzymes, low platelets; DIC, disseminated intravascular coagulation

Classification based on clinical signs and symptoms

Any bleeding that results in or could result in hemodynamic instability, if untreated, is considered as PPH (Table 3).

PITFALLS OF CURRENT CLASSIFICATIONS

Although the WHO definition is widely used, no single definition of PPH is used worldwide. This creates problems in translation and uniformity of treatment and results in obstacles to providing management programs with the best possible outcomes. The International Statistical Classification of Diseases and Related Health Problems, Tenth Revision, Australian Modification (ICD-10-AM) describes PPH as a blood loss of 500 ml or more for a vaginal delivery and 750 ml or more in association with cesarean delivery[16]. In the United States and Canada, on the other hand, a blood loss of 500 ml for a vaginal delivery and 1000 ml for a cesarean birth are often used[17].

The drawbacks of a classification system based solely on quantity of blood loss or decline in hematocrit include the fact that this is a retrospective assessment and may not represent the current clinical situation. Moreover, such a classification is of limited use to a clinician faced with active and continuous bleeding. For example, the change in hematocrit depends on the timing of the test and the amount of fluid resuscitation given[18]. It could also be affected by extraneous factors such as prepartum hemoconcentration, which may exist in conditions such as pre-eclampsia.

Significant underestimation impairs the diagnosis of PPH when it is made by a clinical estimate of blood loss. The WHO definition of 500 ml is increasingly becoming irrelevant as most healthy mothers in the developed world can cope with a blood loss of more than 500 ml without any hemodynamic compromise. Visually assessed bleeding is more likely than not inaccurate, and studies have shown underestimation of measured blood loss by an average of 100–150 ml[19,20]. This has been reiterated in the systematic review by Carroli *et al.* which found the prevalence of PPH to be 10.55% in studies that measured postpartum blood loss[19], compared with 7.23% in studies where blood loss was estimated visually[21]. In the clinical realm, many authorities state that underestimation generally is by a factor of two.

Classifications based on the need for blood transfusion alone are also of limited value as the practice of blood transfusion varies widely according to local circumstances and attitudes to transfusion on the part of patients as well as physicians. The clinical application of such a classification may, in addition, be limited because of inherent individual differences in response to blood loss. Hemodynamic compensation depends on the initial hemoglobin levels prior to onset of bleeding, and this varies among healthy individuals. For these reasons, reliance on a classification solely based on the amount of blood loss and without consideration of clinical signs and symptoms may lead to inconsistency of management.

NEED FOR A CLINICAL AND PROGNOSTIC CLASSIFICATION

Universally, guidelines on the management of PPH have reiterated the importance of accurate estimation of blood loss and the clinical condition of the hemorrhaging patient. This proposition was further emphasized in the 1988–1990 Confidential Enquiries into Maternal Deaths in the United Kingdom (CEMD)[22] and reiterated in the 1991–1993 report as a list of six bullet points, the first being 'accurate estimation of blood loss'[23].

In 2009, the International Postpartum Hemorrhage Collaborative Group recommended that it was fundamental that the definitions of PPH should be unified

and further research should investigate how existing definitions are applied in practice to the coding of data[24]. The ideal classification of PPH should take into consideration both the volume loss and the clinical consequences of such loss. The recorded parameters should be easily measurable and reproducible. This will help in providing an accurate and consistent assessment of loss, which can readily be communicated and incorporated into most labor ward protocols.

PROPOSED CLASSIFICATION

The 500 ml limit as defined by WHO[2] should be considered as an alert line; the action line is then reached when vital functions of the woman are endangered. In healthy women this usually occurs after the blood loss has exceeded 1000 ml, but as *blood loss is notoriously underestimated it may be dangerous not to institute simple therapeutic measures as described in this volume (bimanual massage, uterotonic agents, inspection of the lower genital tract) and be ready to institute more aggressive actions should it be necessary (see below).*

We propose a classification (Table 4) wherein the volume loss is assessed in conjunction with clinical signs and symptoms. We propose this classification is mainly useful in fully equipped hospitals and obstetric units, and it is not being proposed for full

Table 3 Symptoms related to blood loss with postpartum hemorrhage. Adapted from Bonnar J. *Baillieres Best Pract Res Clin Obstet Gynaecol* 2000;14:1

Blood loss		Blood pressure	
ml	%	(mmHg)	*Signs and symptoms*
500–1000	10–15	Normal	Palpitations, dizziness, tachycardia
1000–1500	15–25	Slightly low	Weakness, sweating, tachycardia
1500–2000	25–35	70–80	Restlessness, pallor, oliguria.
2000–3000	35–45	50–70	Collapse, air hunger, anuria

Table 4 Proposed classification. Adapted from Benedetti T. Obstetric haemorrhage. In: Gabbe SG, Niebyl JR, Simpson JL, eds. *A Pocket Companion to Obstetrics*, 4th edn. New York: Churchill Livingstone, 2002[5]

Hemorrhage class	Estimated blood loss (ml)	Blood volume loss (%)	Clinical signs and symptoms
0 (normal loss)	<500	<10	None
	ALERT LINE		
1*	500–1000	15	Minimal
	ACTION LINE		
2†	1200–1500	20–25	↓Urine output ↑Pulse rate ↑Respiratory rate Postural hypotension Narrow pulse pressure
3‡	1800–2100	30–35	Hypotension Tachycardia Cold clammy Tachypnea
4§	>2400	>40	Profound shock

*Need observation ± replacement therapy; †Replacement therapy and uterotonics; ‡Urgent active management; §Critical active management (50% mortality if not managed actively)

implementation in areas which are resource poor. In such areas, the action line should be moved forward in time and minimal therapy instituted earlier.

Our adaptation of a previously described classification[15] will fulfill most of these criteria. This guideline adopts a practical approach whereby a perceived loss of 500–1000 ml (in the absence of clinical signs of shock) prompts basic measures of monitoring and readiness for resuscitation (alert line), whereas a perceived loss of more than 1000 ml or a smaller loss associated with clinical signs of shock (hypotension, tachycardia, tachypnea, oliguria or delayed peripheral capillary filling) prompts a full protocol of measures to resuscitate, monitor and arrest bleeding.

References

1. El-Refaey H, Rodeck C. Post partum haemorrhage: definitions, medical and surgical management. A time for change. Br Med Bull 2003;67:205–17
2. WHO. The Prevention and Management of Postpartum Haemorrhage. Report of a Technical Working Group. Geneva 3–6 July 1989. Unpublished document. WHO/MCH/90.7.Geneva:World Health Organization,1990
3. WHO. Managing Complications in Pregnancy and Childbirth: A guide for midwives and doctors. Department of Reproductive Health and Research. Geneva: World Health Organization, 2003
4. Pritchard JA, Baldwin, RM Dickey JC, Wiggins KM. Blood volume changes in pregnancy and the puerperium. Am J Obstet Gynecol 1962;84:1271
5. Newton M. Postpartum hemorrhage. Am J Obstet Gynecol 1966;94:711–7
6. De Leeuw NKM, Lowenstein L, Tucker EC, Dayal S. Correlation of red cell loss at delivery with changes in red cell mass. Am J Obstet Gynecol 1968;100:1092–101
7. Letsky E. The haematological system. In: Hytten F, Chamberlain G, eds. Clinical Physiology in Obstetrics, 2nd edn. Oxford, UK: Blackwell, 1991
8. Baskett TF. Complications of the third stage of labour. In: Essential Management of Obstetrical Emergencies, 3rd edn. Bristol, UK: Clinical Press, 1999:196–201
9. Alexander J, Thomas P, Sanghera J. Treatments for secondary postpartum haemorrhage. Cochrane Database Syst Rev 2002;(1):CD002867
10. Ghares EE, Albert SN, Dodek SM . Intrapartum blood loss measured with Cr 51-tagged erythrocytes. Obstet Gynecol 1962;19:455–62
11. Newton M, Mosey LM, Egli GE, Gifford WB, Hull CT. Blood loss during and immediately after delivery. Obstet Gynecol 1961;17:9–18
12. Prata N, Mbaruku G, Campbell M. Using the Kanga to measure post partum blood loss. Int J Gynaecol Obstet 2005;89:49–50
13. American College of Gynecologists and Obstetricians. Quality Assurance in Obstetrics and Gynecology. Washington DC: American College of Obstetricians and Gynecologists, 1989
14. Sobieszczyk S, Breborowicz GH. Management recommendations for postpartum hemorrhage. Arch Perinatal Med 2004;10:1–4
15. Benedetti T. Obstetric haemorrhage. In: Gabbe SG, Niebyl JR, Simpson JL, eds. A pocket Companion to Obstetrics, 4th edn. New York: Churchill Livingstone, 2002
16. National Centre for Classification in Health. Australian Coding Standards. The International Statistical Classification of Diseases and Related Health Problems, Tenth Revision, Australian Modification (ICD-10-AM). Sydney, Australia: National Centre for Classification in Health, 2002
17. American College of Obstetricians and Gynecologists. ACOG Practice Bulletin: Clinical Management Guidelines for Obstetrician-Gynecologists Number 76, October 2006: postpartum hemorrhage. Obstet Gynecol 2006;108:1039–47
18. Cunningham FG, Gant NF, Leveno KJ, et al. Conduct of normal labor and delivery. In: Cunningham FG, Williams JW, eds. Williams Obstetrics, 21st edn. New York, NY: McGraw-Hill, 2001:320–5
19. Patel A, Goudar SS, Geller SE, et al. Drape estimation vs. visual assessment for estimating postpartum hemorrhage. Int J Gynaecol Obstet 2006;93:220–4
20. Prasertcharoensuk W, Swadpanich U, Lumbiganon P. Accuracy of the blood loss estimation in the third stage of labor. Int J Gynecol Obstet 2000;71:69–70
21. Carroli G, Cuesta C, Abalos E, Gulmezoglu AM. Epidemiology of postpartum hemorrhage: a systematic review. Best Pract Res Clin Obstet Gynaecol 2008;22:999–1012
22. Hibbard B, Milner D . Report on Confidential Enquiries into Maternal Deaths in the United Kingdom. 1988–1990. London: HMSO, 1994
23. Anonymous Report on Confidential Enquiries into Maternal Deaths in the United Kingdom. 1991–1993. London: HMSO, 1996
24. Knight M, Callaghan WM, Berg C, et al. BMC Pregnancy Childbirth. Trends in postpartum hemorrhage in high resource countries: a review and recommendations from the International Postpartum Hemorrhage Collaborative Group. Oxford, UK: National Perinatal Epidemiology Unit, University of Oxford, 2009;9:55

17

Definitions, Vital Statistics and Risk Factors: an Overview

M. J. Cameron

INTRODUCTION

A recent systematic review suggests that the prevalence of postpartum hemorrhage (PPH) (blood loss of 500 ml or more) and severe PPH (defined by authors as blood loss of 1000 ml or more) is 1.85% and 6%, respectively, of all deliveries, albeit with significant regional variations[1]. This chapter describes the incidence of primary PPH, the difficulties in reporting epidemiological data on primary PPH and the etiology and precipitating factors for primary PPH. Because of its broad scope, this discussion invariably includes several points mentioned in greater detail elsewhere. Regardless, these statistics should provide additional insights as many derive from secondary analyses.

DEFINING POSTPARTUM HEMORRHAGE

The traditional definition of primary PPH used in most textbooks of obstetrics is a visually estimated blood loss of 500 ml or more within the first 24 h after delivery[2]. In contrast, secondary PPH generally is defined as 'excessive bleeding' from the genital tract after 24 h and up to 6 weeks postdelivery (see Chapter 16). As such, this latter definition only contains quantification of the time period rather than the extent of blood loss. However, according to older and commonly quoted data, measured blood loss during a vaginal delivery averages 500 ml, whereas during a cesarean section the average is 1000 ml[3]. Given this reality, the 'classic' definition of primary PPH is a reflection of the almost universal tendency to underestimate delivery blood loss (see below and Chapters 9 and 11).

Because a loss of 500 ml at delivery for most women in the developed world does not result in significant morbidity, one might argue that the classic definition of primary PPH is clinically inappropriate and should be revised to identify a group of women who manifest symptoms or become 'ill' and thus are at real risk of morbidity after the hemorrhage. If the classic definition were to be changed, definitions of any event leading to severe obstetric morbidity could then be based on 'pathophysiology', 'management' or a combination of both parameters[4]. The problem with using a management-based definition of hemorrhage, such as number of units of blood transfused, is that it can only be used retrospectively and is of no value to the clinician attempting to treat this condition. Further, such a definition is likely to be highly influenced by local practitioner/hospital beliefs about when to transfuse as well as the local facilities available for transfusion. Consequently, it may be better to think of the term 'significant obstetric hemorrhage', using a definition of loss of more than 1000 ml or more than 1500 ml, rather than define primary PPH as more than 500 ml blood loss[5].

In the average non-pregnant adult, circulating blood represents a total of 7% of body weight, or approximately 5 liters. Loss of 30–40% of the circulating volume (1500–2000 ml) results in tachycardia, tachypnea, a measurable fall in systolic blood pressure and alterations in mental state[6]. Therefore, the concept of defining a 'significant primary PPH' as one resulting in a blood loss of 1500 ml or more is meritorious as this reflects the point when physiological compensatory mechanisms begin to fail. Whether this concept will find universal acceptance remains to be seen, however. Even if it does, its implementation would depend on the accuracy of the estimation, a circumstance which is more often than not lacking in clinical practice.

DIFFICULTIES OF COMPARING STUDIES

Two key factors must be considered when comparing published studies of primary PPH: first, the method used to determine blood loss, and, second, the method of managing the third stage of labor. In addition, confounding represents a potential problem in case–control studies that examine risk factors for primary PPH.

Determining blood loss: estimating versus measuring

Accurate measurement of blood loss at delivery is possible but must be planned for in advance (see also Chapter 11). The most obvious is collection of blood into receptacles and direct measurement. This can be combined with a gravimetric procedure which depends upon converting the increase in weight of sponges and linen into milliliters of blood on a ml/g basis. Gulmezoglu and Hofmeyr proposed a method for directly measuring blood loss objectively which does not interfere with routine care[7]. They suggest 'after delivery of the baby, the amniotic fluid is allowed to drain away and amniotic fluid-soaked bed linen is covered with a dry disposable 'linen saver'. A low-profile, wedge-shaped plastic 'fracture bedpan' is slipped under the woman's buttocks for blood collection, with blood and clots decanted into a measuring cylinder. Weighing of blood-soaked swabs and linen savers occurs, with the known dry weight subtracted and calculated volume added to that from the bedpan.' They particularly recommend this method for all future trials of interventions to reduce primary PPH. Strand and colleagues suggested a novel method with a combination of a plastic sheet and a bucket below a cholera bed on which the woman rested during postpartum observation[8]. As interesting as these methods are, they are cumbersome, time-consuming and may not be widely available. In contrast, the BRASSS-V collection drape and the instructions for its use as described in Chapter 11 is cheap, can be produced locally and has been enthusiastically accepted in a variety of circumstances. As with any direct measurement of blood loss, however, contamination with amniotic fluid and urine is not uncommon.

Laboratory-based methods for measuring blood loss include photometric techniques, whereby sanitary protection is collected and blood pigment converted to acid or alkaline hematin and the concentration then compared in a colorimeter with the patient's own venous blood[9]. Alternatively, volumetric methods involve labelling the woman's plasma or erythrocytes with dyes or radioactive substances and then calculating the reduction in blood volume. Unfortunately, both techniques require expertise, are time-consuming and expensive to perform compared to simple measurement of blood loss.

Visual estimation has long been considered to be unreliable. Duthie and colleagues compared visual estimation and measured blood loss using the alkaline-hematin method during normal delivery in 37 primigravid and 25 multigravid women. These investigators found that, for both groups, the mean estimated blood loss (261 ml and 220 ml, respectively) was significantly lower than the mean measured blood loss (401 ml and 319 ml, respectively)[10]. This observation is consistent with studies of simulated scenarios that suggest trained and experienced midwives and doctors underestimate blood loss at delivery by 30–50%[11]. Importantly, estimates are particularly unreliable for very small and very large amounts of blood[12] (see Chapter 9).

Reported rates of PPH also differ widely depending on the method of measuring blood loss. Older studies that directly measured blood loss reported rates of primary PPH (>500 ml) of between 22% and 29%[13,14] compared to rates of 5–8% with visual estimation. More recently, Prasertcharoensuk and colleagues compared visual estimation with direct measurement in 228 women who had a spontaneous vaginal delivery[15]. The incidences of PPH more than 500 ml and more than 1000 ml were 5.7% and 0.44%, respectively, by visual estimation, whereas direct measurements showed incidences of 27.63% and 3.51%, respectively. These differences are five and seven times higher, respectively. The authors concluded that visual estimation underestimated the incidence of PPH by 89%. Razvi and colleagues conducted a similar prospective study and showed a similar degree of underestimation[16].

Conduct of third stage of labor

Active management of the third stage (AMTSL) involves early clamping of the umbilical cord before pulsations have stopped, controlled cord traction using the Brandt–Andrews technique and the use of prophylactic uterotonics, usually with the delivery of the fetal anterior shoulder (see also Chapter 14). In contrast, expectant or 'physiological' third stage involves late clamping of the cord after pulsations have stopped, waiting for spontaneous separation of the placenta from the uterine wall and avoidance of synthetic uterotonics. Nipple stimulation has been used to promote the release of endogenous oxytocin and reduce the length and amount of bleeding in the third stage of labor[17], but is not part of active or expectant management. A meta-analysis of five randomized, controlled trials (involving over 6000 women) indicates that active management results in a reduction in maternal blood loss at delivery and a reduction in the risks of PPH, defined as an estimated blood loss of more than 500 ml (relative risk (RR) 0.38, 95% confidence interval (CI) 0.32–0.46), and severe PPH, defined as an estimated blood loss of 1000 ml or more (RR 0.33, 95% CI 0.21–0.51) as well as prolonged third stage[18].

Clearly, the reported incidence of PPH in any population is influenced by the conduct of the third stage. As active management is less widely practiced in some areas of the developing world, this must be considered when making international comparisons of PPH rates.

CONFOUNDING FACTORS IN EPIDEMIOLOGICAL STUDIES

Confounding is a potential problem in epidemiologic studies exploring risk. A confounder is associated with the risk factor and causally related to the outcome. Thus, a researcher may attempt to relate an exposure to an outcome, but actually measures the effect of a third factor, the confounding variable[19]. As an example, parity, particularly grand multiparity, is generally considered a risk factor for primary PPH. However, grand multiparas tend to be older and therefore have higher rates of age-related medical diseases, such as diabetes mellitus, which could be the 'true' risk factors for PPH.

Methods used to control confounders include:

(1) Restriction – in the example cited in the preceding paragraph, women with diabetes mellitus could be excluded. However, restriction limits the external validity of the findings and reduces the sample size.

(2) Matching – here, if diabetes mellitus is deemed a confounder, then for every woman recruited with diabetes mellitus who has a PPH, she is matched to a control with diabetes mellitus who did not have PPH.

(3) Stratification – can be thought of as *post hoc* restriction performed at the analysis phase.

Multivariate analysis is a statistical tool for determining the relative contributions of different causes to a single event or outcome[20]. Epidemiological studies that use multivariate methods are more likely to eliminate confounders. For readers who require further information about the problems of epidemiological studies, please refer to Grimes and Schultz[21] and Mamdani and colleagues[22].

INCIDENCE OF PRIMARY POSTPARTUM HEMORRHAGE

Denominator data

Studies that attempt to quantify the incidence and impact of PPH need a denominator value over a time period to calculate rates. Common denominators used to calculate maternal mortality and morbidity rates[23] are illustrated in Table 1.

Developed countries, including the UK, have the advantage of accurate denominator data, including both livebirths and stillbirths. Consequently, the UK Confidential Enquiries into Maternal Deaths have used maternities for denominator data, because this enables establishment of a more detailed picture of maternal death rates. However, for many countries, particularly in the developing world, no process of stillbirth (or even livebirth) registration exists.

Table 1 Denominators used in calculating maternal mortality and morbidity

Denominator	Definition	Advantages and disadvantages
Livebirths	Number of pregnancies that result in a livebirth at any gestational age	Easier to collect than maternities
Maternities	Number of pregnancies that result in a livebirth at any gestational age or stillbirths occurring at or after 24 weeks of completed gestation and required to be notified by law	Includes the majority of women at risk from death from obstetric causes but requires infrastructure for notification of stillbirths
Women aged 15–44 years	Number of women of reproductive age in a given population	Lacks rigor of confining rate to women who were pregnant, but enables comparison with other causes of death

Denominator data are, therefore, likely to be based on livebirths, rather than maternities. Indeed, in some countries even livebirth data collection may not be reliable. As a result, it is often extremely difficult to compare maternal mortality and morbidity from different geographic areas.

Maternal mortality

One method of attempting to quantify the magnitude of PPH is to determine its contribution to maternal deaths around the world, and in a particular country over time. Trends over time within one country are an important audit tool in examining the care of women with PPH, as can be seen from the UK Confidential Enquiries into Maternal Deaths. However, differences between countries often reflect differences in health care provision, general economic prosperity and geographic and climactic conditions that affect access to obstetric care.

Global picture

WHO estimates that obstetric hemorrhage complicates 10.5% of all livebirths in the world, with an estimated 13,795,000 women experiencing this complication in 2000[23]. Around 132,000 maternal deaths are directly attributable to hemorrhage, comprising 28% of all direct deaths. In comparison, the following numbers relate to other conditions: 79,000 deaths from sepsis, 63,000 deaths from pre-eclampsia/ eclampsia, 69,000 from abortion and 42,000 from obstructed labor.

United Kingdom

A triennial report on Confidential Enquiries into Maternal Death has been published since 1985, with reports for England and Wales commencing in 1952 (see Chapter 20). Direct deaths are reported that result from obstetric complications of the pregnant state (pregnancy, labor and puerperium up to 42 days), from interventions, omissions, incorrect treatment or from a chain of events resulting from any of the above. Obstetric hemorrhage comprising placental abruption, placenta previa and PPH is one example of direct deaths[24]. In the 2006–2008 triennium, there were 107 direct maternal deaths. Nine (8%) of these were attributed to obstetric hemorrhage with five (4.7%) principally attributed to PPH. Since the UK-wide triennium report began in 1985, 106 deaths from obstetric hemorrhage have been recorded, of which half (55 women) were caused by PPH, resulting in a death rate for PPH of 3.1 per million maternities. Calculated death rates for PPH for each triennium are shown in Table 2 as is a decline during the most recent three reports.

At first glance there appears to be a marked increase in PPH in the 2000–2002 triennial report compared to the one that immediately preceded it. However, two patients who died had no contact at all with health services and another two refused blood products that

Table 2 Maternal mortality from PPH in UK (extrapolated from CMACE[25])

Triennium	Postpartum hemorrhage (n)	Total maternities (n)	Rate per million maternities
1985–87	6	2,268,766	2.6
1988–90	11	2,360,309	4.6
1991–93	8	2,315,204	3.4
1994–96	5	2,197,640	2.2
1997–99	1	2,123,614	0.4
2000–02	10	1,997,472	5.0
2003–05	9	2,114,004	4.3
2006–08	5	2,291,493	2.2

would probably have saved their lives. Excluding these four deaths results in a rate per million maternities comparable to the reports published between 1985 and 1996. Of the eight women who sought care in the 2000–2002 cohort and ultimately died from PPH, elements of substandard care were present in seven (88%) including:

(1) Organizational problems – including inappropriate booking at hospitals with inadequate blood transfusion and intensive care facilities;

(2) Poor quality of resuscitation – including inadequate transfusion of blood and blood products;

(3) Equipment failure, e.g. malfunctioning of specimen transport system;

(4) Inadequate staffing of recovery areas;

(5) Failure to recognize or treat antenatal medical conditions, e.g. inherited bleeding disorders;

(6) Failure of senior staff to attend;

(7) Concerns about the quality of surgical treatment given. The recognition of these diverse elements provides a blue-print to health care authorities to institute remedial action (see Chapter 40).

The 2003–2005 report recommended the use of Maternity Obstetric Early Warning Scoring (MEOWS) charts to help recognize the deteriorating patient. In the 2006–2008 report, there is a non-statistical reduction in death from major obstetric hemorrhage making it the 6th most common cause of direct maternal deaths[25]. Where suboptimal care was identified, the report concludes there were issues with 'lack of early senior multidisciplinary involvement, lack of close postoperative monitoring and the failure to act on symptoms and signs that a woman is seriously unwell, including readings from MEOWS charts; such factors remain important contributors to maternal death from hemorrhage.'

United States of America

The Center for Disease Control (CDC) conducted a pregnancy-related mortality survey in the USA between 1991 and 1999[26]. Hemorrhage in pregnancy was responsible for 17% of maternal deaths, although this figure includes hemorrhage from first-trimester pregnancy complications. Of the 2519 maternal deaths that were associated with livebirth and the 275 maternal deaths associated with stillbirth, 2.7% and 21.1%, respectively, were considered to be a direct result of obstetric hemorrhage. Unfortunately, no separate data were provided about PPH. Comparison with the 1987–1990 data shows a reduction in the percentage of maternal deaths from pregnancy-related hemorrhage from 28.7% to 17%[27]. The trend may no longer be present at the time of this writing.

France

A confidential enquiry into maternal deaths in five of the 22 administrative areas of France found that five deaths from 39 obstetric causes were due to PPH[28], implicating PPH in 13% of the obstetric deaths. No denominator data were collected, and therefore it is not possible to estimate rates.

Africa

Bouvier-Colle and colleagues performed a population-based survey of pregnant women from seven West African areas from 1994 to 1996[29]. Overall, 55 women died from direct or indirect obstetric causes among 17,694 livebirths. Hemorrhage accounted for 17 deaths (31%), with delivery hemorrhage (third stage) and postdelivery hemorrhage (retention of placenta) accounting for six and four deaths, respectively. This equates to a maternal mortality rate of 565 per 1,000,000 livebirths, a rate approximately 200-fold higher compared to the UK.

Another study in South Africa, involving one tertiary center, reported a maternal mortality rate of 1710 per 1,000,000 livebirths during the period 1986–1992, with 25% of deaths attributed to obstetric hemorrhage[30]. Within this setting, hemorrhage was the leading cause of death.

Maternal morbidity

Because maternal death in the developed world is a rare event, clinicians have attempted to quantify significant morbidity, which is often labelled as a maternal adverse event or a near miss (see Chapter 60). Studies have generally included massive obstetric hemorrhage as one indicator of severe maternal morbidity. As with mortality, comparisons between studies are often difficult because of variations in definition of 'massive obstetric hemorrhage'. Both antenatal and intrapartum bleeding are sometimes included within the definition of 'obstetric hemorrhage'.

Scotland

The Scottish Programme for Clinical Effectiveness in Reproductive Health (SPCERH) conducted a prospective investigation into 14 severe maternal morbidity categories for all maternity units in Scotland in 2003[4]. Within this audit, major obstetric hemorrhage was defined as estimated blood loss of 2500 ml or more, or transfusion of 5 units or more of blood or the need for fresh frozen plasma or cryoprecipitate. Of the 375 events, 176 (46%) were reported to be related to obstetric hemorrhage. Because some patients experienced more than one morbid event, major obstetric hemorrhage occurred in 65% of 'near-miss patients' (176/270). Using a denominator of 50,157 livebirths, the authors calculated a rate of major obstetric hemorrhage of 3.5/1000 births (CI 3.0–4.1). Of the 176 cases notified to the investigators, full disclosure of data was obtained in 152 cases; 70% of the cases were due to primary PPH, 26% to intrapartum hemorrhage and 17% to antepartum hemorrhage with some women falling into more than one category.

England

In the South East Thames region, 19 maternity units participated in a 1-year study between 1997 and 1998 to determine the incidence of severe obstetric morbidity[31]. Severe obstetric hemorrhage was defined as estimated blood loss of 1500 ml or more or a peripartum fall in hemoglobin concentration of 40 g/l or more or the need for an acute transfusion of 4 or more units of blood. A total of 588 cases of severe obstetric morbidity were observed among 48,856 women delivered over the year, giving an incidence of 12/1000 deliveries. Hemorrhage was the leading cause of obstetric morbidity at 6.7 (CI 6.0–7.5) occurrences per 1000 deliveries, representing nearly two-thirds of cases. However, this study did not include thromboembolic disease, which is the leading cause of direct maternal deaths in the UK.

United States and Canada

One large US study demonstrated that PPH has increased 26% (from 2.3% to 2.9%) between 1994 and 2006, with the increase mainly attributed to an increase in uterine atony[32]. Wen and colleagues in Canada conducted a retrospective cohort study of severe maternal morbidity involving 2,548,824 women who gave birth in over a 10-year period from 1991, using information on hospital discharges compiled by the Canadian Institute for Health Information[33]. Their criteria for severe maternal morbidity included PPH requiring hysterectomy or transfusion. Their overall rate of all severe maternal morbidity was 4.38 per 1000 deliveries. Overall rates for severe PPH in the 10-year time frame are illustrated in Table 3 along with time analysis for rates at the beginning and end of the study.

Within this study, rates for PPH requiring transfusion halved (RR 0.5, CI 0.44–0.55), but hysterectomy rates for PPH almost doubled (RR 1.76, CI 1.48–2.08). Because the definition of PPH was based on management rather than pathophysiology, it is difficult to tease out whether the temporal change reflects a true reduction in the incidence of PPH or simply a change in clinical management.

Australia

Roberts and colleagues demonstrated an increase in maternal morbidity outcome indicator from 11.5 per 1000 to 13.8 per 1000 in women delivering in New South Wales between 1999 and 2004, with this increase being attributed to PPH[34].

Africa

Filippi and colleagues conducted prospective and retrospective data extraction on near-miss obstetric events in nine referral hospitals in three countries (Benin, Cote d'Ivoire and Morocco)[35]. Obstetric hemorrhage was defined as hemorrhage leading to clinical shock, emergency hysterectomy and blood transfusion. The incidence of near-miss cases varied widely between hospitals. Most of the women were already in a critical condition on arrival, with two-thirds being referred from another facility. The study identified a total of 507 cases of late pregnancy obstetric hemorrhage (i.e. previa, abruption and other non-classified hemorrhage and PPH) from 33,478 deliveries, representing a near-miss late obstetric hemorrhage rate of 15.1/1000 deliveries. In total there were 266 cases of PPH, representing a near-miss PPH rate of 7.9/1000 deliveries.

Prual and colleagues examined severe maternal morbidity from direct obstetric causes in West Africa between 1994 and 1996[36]. A severe obstetric event was defined as 'prepartum', 'peripartum' or 'PPH leading to blood transfusion, or hospitalization for more than 4 days or to hysterectomy'. A total of 1307 severe maternal morbidity events were identified, with obstetric hemorrhage representing the largest group involving 601 cases, 342 of which were PPH. The near miss obstetric hemorrhage rate was 30.5 (CI 28.1–33.0)/1000 live births and the near-miss PPH rate was 17.4 (CI 15.6–19.3)/1000 live births.

The Pretoria region of South Africa has used the same definition of 'near miss' for over 5 years, allowing comparison of temporal changes[37]. Rates per 1000 births for near misses plus maternal deaths over 5 years

Table 3 Postpartum hemorrhage (PPH) rates in Canada 1991–2000. Adapted from Wen[33]

	Number of cases (1991–2000)	Rate per 1000 deliveries (95% CI)	Rate per 1000 deliveries (1991–1993)	Rate per 1000 deliveries (1998–2000)	Relative risk (95% CI)*
PPH requiring transfusion	2317	0.91 (0.87–0.95)	1.27	0.63	0.5 (0.44–0.55)
PPH requiring hysterectomy	892	0.35 (0.33–0.37)	0.26	0.46	1.76 (1.48–2.08)

*The 1991–1993 period was the reference period

from severe PPH are shown in Table 4. These rates are not dissimilar to those in Canada or the UK.

ETIOLOGY AND PRECIPITATING FACTORS

Causes of primary postpartum hemorrhage

In recent years, individual authors and academic groups have used the four Ts pneumonic to provide a simplistic categorization of the causes of PPH. This is shown in Table 5[38].

Uterine atony

Uterine atony, the most common cause of PPH, is reported in 70% of cases[38]. It can occur after normal vaginal delivery, instrumental vaginal delivery and abdominal delivery. A large cohort study found an incidence of uterine atony after primary cesarean section of 1416/23,390 (6%)[39]. Multiple linear regression analysis demonstrates the following factors as being independently associated with risk of uterine atony: multiple gestation (odds ratio (OR) 2.40, 95% CI 1.95–2.93), Hispanic race (OR 2.21, 95% CI 1.90–2.57), induced or augmented labor for more than 18 h (OR 2.23, 95% CI 1.92–2.60), infant birth weight more than 4500 g (OR 2.05, 95% CI 1.53–2.69) and clinically diagnosed chorioamnionitis (OR 1.80, 95% CI 1.55–2.09).

Surprisingly, it is more difficult to find comparable studies of risk factors for uterine atony in women achieving vaginal delivery. A single center, case–control study from Pakistan reporting on women who had either assisted or non-assisted vaginal delivery found only two factors had a strong association with uterine atony: gestational diabetes mellitus (OR 7.6, 95% CI 6.9–9.0) and prolonged second stage of labor in multiparas (OR 4.0, 95% CI 3.1–5.0)[40]. They found no association with high parity, age, pre-eclampsia, augmentation of labor, antenatal anemia and a history of poor maternal or perinatal outcomes.

Trauma

Trauma is reported as the primary cause of PPH in 20% of cases[38] (see also Chapter 23). Genital tract trauma at delivery is associated with an odds ratio of

1.7 (95% CI 1.4–2.1) for PPH (measured blood loss more than 1000 ml)[41]. Similar results were found in a Dutch study with a reported OR of 1.82 (CI 1.01–3.28) for PPH (≥1000 ml) with perineal trauma of first degree tears or more[42]. Trauma to the broad ligament, uterine rupture, cervical and vaginal tears and perineal tears are all associated with increased blood loss at normal vaginal delivery.

Inversion of the uterus is a rare cause of PPH (see Chapter 23). The incidence of inversion varies from 1 in 1584 deliveries in Pakistan[43] to around 1 in 25,000 deliveries in the USA, UK and Norway[44]. Blood loss at delivery with a uterine inversion is usually at least 1000 ml[45], with 65% of uterine inversions being complicated by PPH and 47.5% requiring blood transfusion in a large series of 40 cases[46].

Tissue

Retained placenta accounts for approximately 10% of all cases of PPH[38]. Effective uterine contraction to aid hemostasis requires complete expulsion of the placenta. Most retained placentas can be removed manually, but rarely the conditions of placenta percreta, increta and accreta may be responsible for placental retention (see Chapters 28 and 59). Retained placenta occurs after 0.5–3% of deliveries[47]. Several case–control and cohort studies show that retained placenta is associated with increased blood loss and increased need for blood transfusion. Stones and colleagues reported that retained placenta had a RR of 5.15 (99% CI 3.36–7.87) for blood loss of 1000 ml or more within the first 24 h of delivery[48]. Bais and colleagues found an incidence of 1.8% for retained placenta in Holland[42]. Using multiple regression, these authors determined that retained placenta was associated with an OR of 7.83 (95% CI 3.78–16.22) and 11.73 (95% CI 5.67–24.1) for PPH of 500 ml or more and PPH of 1000 ml or more, respectively. In addition, retained placenta was found to have an OR of 21.7 (95% CI 8.9–53.2) for red cell transfusion in this Dutch cohort.

Tandberg and colleagues reported an incidence of retained placenta of 0.6% in a large Norwegian cohort of 24,750 deliveries and showed that hemoglobin fell by a mean of 3.4 g/dl in the retained placental group compared to no fall in the controls[49]. In addition, blood transfusion was required in 10% of the retained placental group but only 0.5% of the control group. A similar incidence of retained placenta was found in a Saudi Arabian case–control study which demonstrated increased blood loss in women with a retained placenta (mean 437 ml) compared with controls (mean 263 ml)[50]. A large study from Aberdeen of over 36,000 women reported PPH in 21.3% of women with retained placenta compared to 3.5% in vaginal deliveries without retained placenta[51]. Both studies confirmed that women with a history of retained placenta have an increased risk of recurrence in subsequent pregnancies[50,51]. In the study by Adelusi and colleagues, 6.1% of the patients with retained placenta had a prior history of retained placenta, compared

Table 4 Rates per 1000 births for near misses plus maternal deaths from severe postpartum hemorrhage in Pretoria. Adapted from Pattinson et al.[37]

	1997–99	2000	2001	2002
Rate/1000 births	0.96	1.37	2.38	2.28

Table 5 The four Ts of PPH (from ALSO[38])

Tone – uterine atony
Trauma – of any part of the genital tract, inverted uterus
Tissue – retained placenta, invasive placenta
Thrombin – coagulopathy

to none in their control group of normal vaginal deliveries[50].

Placental accreta is a rare and serious complication, occurring in about 0.001–0.05% of all deliveries[52,53] (see also Chapters 29 and 30). Makhseed and colleagues found an increasing risk for accreta with increasing numbers of cesarean sections OR 4.11 (95% CI 0.83–19.34) after one previous cesarean section and an OR of 30.25 (95% CI 9.9–92.4) after two previous cesarean sections, compared with no previous cesarean section. Kastner and colleagues found that placenta accreta was implicated in 49% of their 48 cases of emergency hysterectomy[54]. Zaki and co-workers found an incidence of 0.05% of placenta accreta in a population of 23,000 women[53]. They found that rates of PPH and emergency hysterectomy were higher in the accreta group compared to the placenta previa group undergoing cesarean section. PPH occurred in 91.7% of the accreta group compared to 18.4% of the previa group (OR 48.9, 95% CI 5.93–403)[27], whereas 50% of accreta cases required emergency hysterectomy compared to 2% in the previa group (OR 48, 95% CI 7.93–290)[52]. Within the accreta group, 75% of patients had a previous history of cesarean section, compared to 27.5% in the previa group (OR 7.9, 95% CI 1.98–31)[38].

Thrombin

Disorders of the clotting cascade and platelet dysfunction are the cause of PPH in 1% of cases[38]. Known associations with coagulation failure include placental abruption, pre-eclampsia, septicemia and intrauterine sepsis, retained dead fetus, amniotic fluid embolus, incompatible blood transfusion, abortion with hypertonic saline and existing coagulation abnormalities[5,55,56] (see Chapter 25).

ANTENATAL RISK FACTORS FOR PRIMARY POSTPARTUM HEMORRHAGE

Age

Increasing maternal age appears to be an independent risk factor for PPH. In Japan, Ohkuchi and colleagues studied 10,053 consecutive women who delivered a singleton infant[57]. Excessive blood loss (≥90th centile) was defined separately for vaginal and cesarean deliveries (615 ml and 1531 ml, respectively). On multivariate analysis, age of 35 years or older was an independent risk factor for PPH in vaginal deliveries (OR 1.5, 95% CI 1.2–1.9) and cesarean deliveries (OR 1.8, 95% CI 1.2–2.7). In Nigeria, Tsu reported that advanced maternal age (≥35 years) was associated with an adjusted RR of 3.0 (95% CI 1.3–7.3) for PPH (defined as visual estimation of ≥600 ml)[58]. Ijaiya and co-workers in Nigeria found that the risk of PPH in women over 35 years was two-fold higher compared to women less than 25 years, although no consideration of confounding was made in this study[59]. Rates of obstetric hysterectomy have also been reported

to increase with age; Okogbenin and colleagues in Nigeria reported an increase from 0.1% at 20 years to 0.7% at 40 years or older[60]. However, others have found no relationship between delaying childbirth and PPH[61].

Ethnicity

Several studies have examined whether ethnicity is a factor for PPH. Magann and co-workers, using a definition of PPH as measured blood loss of more than 1000 ml and/or need for transfusion[41], found Asian race to be a risk factor (OR 1.8, 95% CI 1.4–2.2)). Other studies have observed similar findings in Asians[62] (OR 1.73, 95% CI 1.20–2.49) and the Hispanic races (OR 1.66, 95% CI 1.02–2.69)[62] and for low postnatal hematocrit value of less than 26%, (OR 3.99, 95% CI 0.59–9.26)[63].

Body mass index

Women who are obese have higher rates of intrapartum and postpartum complications. Usha and colleagues performed a population-based observational study of 60,167 deliveries in South Glamorgan, UK; women with a body mass index (BMI) more than 30 had an OR of 1.5 (95% CI 1.2–1.8) for blood loss more than 500 ml, compared to women with a BMI of 20–30[64]. Stones and colleagues reported a RR for major obstetric hemorrhage of 1.64 (95% CI 1.24–2.17) when the BMI was over 27[48].

Parity

Although grand multiparity has traditionally been considered a risk factor for PPH, Stones and colleagues and Selo-Ojeme did not demonstrate any relation between grand multiparity and major obstetric hemorrhage[48,65]. This observation was confirmed in a large Australian study which used multivariate regression analysis and found no association between grand multiparity (five or more previous births) and PPH (>500 ml)[66]. Tsu reported an association with low parity (0–1 previous birth) with an adjusted RR without intrapartum factors of 1.7 (95% CI 1.1–2.7) and an adjusted RR with intrapartum factors of 1.5 (95% CI 0.95–2.5) but not with grand multiparity (defined as five or more births)[58]. Ohkuchi also found primiparity to be associated with excessive blood loss at vaginal delivery (OR 1.6, 95% CI 1.4–1.9)[57]. Studies from Pakistan[67] and Nigeria[59] reported an association between grand multiparity and PPH, but failed to account for other confounding factors such as maternal age.

Other medical conditions

Several medical conditions are associated with PPH. Women with type 2 diabetes mellitus have an increased incidence of PPH of more than 500 ml (34%) compared to the non-diabetic population

(6%)[68,69]. Epilepsy is also associated with PPH with odds ratio of 1.2 (95% CI 1.1–1.4)[70] . A large Norwegian cohort study demonstrated an association between PPH (both mild >500 ml and severe >1500 ml) and pre-eclampsia[71]. Connective tissue disorders such as Marfans and Ehlers-Danlos syndrome have also been associated with PPH[69,72]. Blood loss at delivery is also increased with inherited coagulopathies[56]. The most common inherited hemorrhagic disorder is von Willebrand's disease, with a reported prevalence of between 1 and 3%. Most patients (70%) have type 1 disease characterized by low plasma levels of factor VIII, von Willebrand factor antigen and von Willebrand factor activity. Less common inherited bleeding disorders include carriage of hemophilia A (factor VIII deficiency) or hemophilia B (factor IX deficiency) and factor XI deficiency. In their review, Economaides and colleagues suggest that the risks of primary PPH in patients with von Willebrand's disease, factor XI deficiency and carriers of hemophilia are 22%, 16%, and 18.5%, respectively, compared with 5% in the general obstetric population[56]. James also reviewed the numerous case series and the more limited case–control studies of women with bleeding disorders and came to similar conclusions[73] (see Chapter 25).

Prolonged pregnancy

A large Danish cohort study compared a post-term group (gestational age ≥42 weeks or more) of 77,956 singleton deliveries and a term group of 34,140 singleton spontaneous deliveries[74]. The adjusted odds ratio for PPH was 1.37 (95% CI 1.28–1.46), suggesting an association between prolonged pregnancy and PPH. A large American study of 119,254 women reported increased incidence of PPH at 41 weeks of gestation with OR 1.21 (95% CI 1.1–1.32)[75].

Fetal macrosomia

Fetal macrosomia is associated with PPH. Jolly and colleagues examined 350,311 completed singleton pregnancies in London[76]. Linear regression analysis suggested that a birth weight of more than 4 kg was better at predicting maternal morbidity than birth weight of more than the 90th centile. PPH was increased in women with fetal macrosomia (OR 2.01, 95% CI 1.93–2.10). In a large cohort of 146,526 mother–infant pairs in California, Stotland and co-workers also demonstrated an adjusted OR for PPH of 1.69 (95% CI 1.58–1.82) in infants of 4000–4499 g compared to 2.15 (95% CI 1.86–2.48) and 2.03 (95% CI 1.33–3.09) with weights of 4500–4999 g and 5000 g or more, respectively[77]. In Nigeria, a case–control study of 351 infants weighing more than 4 kg with 6563 term infant controls found an incidence of PPH of 8.3% and 2.1%, respectively[78]. Bais and colleagues, in their Dutch study, also demonstrated an increase in risk for PPH (≥500 ml) and severe PPH (≥1000 ml)

with infants with weights of 4 kg or more (OR 2.11, 95% CI 1.62–2.76 and 2.55, 95% CI 1.5–4.18)[42].

Multiple pregnancies

Twins and higher-order pregnancies are at increased risk for PPH. Walker and co-workers conducted a retrospective cohort study involving 165,188 singleton pregnancies and 44,674 multiple pregnancies in Canada[79]. Multiple pregnancies were associated with an increased risk for PPH (RR 1.88, 95% CI 1.81–1.95), hysterectomy (RR 2.29, 95% CI 1.66–3.16) and blood transfusion (RR 1.67, 95% CI 1.13–2.46). Several additional studies estimated the RR of PPH associated with multiple pregnancies to be between 3.0 and 4.5[48,62,80]. Bais and colleagues, in a Dutch population-based cohort study of 3464 women, used multiple regression analysis and found that the OR for PPH of 500 ml or more for multiple pregnancy was 2.6 (95% CI 1.06–6.39)[42]. Albrecht and co-workers conducted a retrospective review of 57 triplet deliveries and found an incidence of 12.3% for PPH requiring transfusion[81], and a case series of 71 quadruplet pregnancies conducted by Collins and colleagues estimated that the frequency of PPH and transfusion to be 21% (95% CI 11–31%) and 13% 95% CI 5–21%), respectively[82]. Magann and colleagues demonstrated an OR for PPH of 2.2 (95% CI 1.5–3.2) in multiple pregnancies[41], and Stones and colleagues showed a relative risk of 4.46 (95% CI 3.01–6.61) for obstetric hemorrhage with multiple pregnancies[48].

Fibroids

The suggestion that leiomyomas can cause PPH is mainly based on case reports[83], but one cohort study of 10,000 women in Japan found that women with leiomyomas had an OR of 1.9 (95% CI 1.2–3.1) and 3.6 (95% CI 2.0–6.3) for excessive blood loss at vaginal and cesarean delivery, respectively[57].

Antepartum hemorrhage

Antepartum hemorrhage is associated with a risk of PPH with an OR of 1.8 (95% CI 1.3–2.3)[41]. Stones and co-workers found a RR for major obstetric hemorrhage (>1000 ml) of 12.6 (95% CI 7.61–20.9), 13.1 (95% CI 7.47–23) and 11.3 (95% CI 3.36–38.1) for proven abruption, previa with bleeding, and previa with no bleeding, respectively[48]. Ohkuchi and colleagues, in their 10,000 women, demonstrated that a low-lying placenta was associated with odds ratios of 4.4 (95% CI 2.2–8.6) and 3.3 (95% CI 1.4–7.9) for excess blood loss at the time of vaginal and cesarean delivery, respectively[57]. This study also reported that placenta previa was associated with an OR of 6.3 (95% CI 4.0–9.9) for excessive blood loss at cesarean delivery.

Previous history of PPH

Magann and colleagues found previous PPH to be associated with an increased risk for subsequent PPH (OR 2.2, 95% CI 1.7–2.9)[41]. Similar findings have been reported by Ford and colleagues[84].

Previous cesarean delivery

A Japanese study demonstrated an odds ratio of 3.1 (95% CI 2.1–4.4) for excessive blood loss at vaginal delivery in women with a previous cesarean section[57].

INTRAPARTUM RISK FACTORS FOR PRIMARY POSTPARTUM HEMORRHAGE

Induction of labor

Meta-analysis of trials of induction of labor at or beyond term indicates that induction does not increase cesarean section or operative vaginal delivery rates[85]. However, this meta-analysis did not examine blood loss at delivery. Epidemiological studies suggest a link between induction of labor and PPH. Brinsden and colleagues reviewed 3674 normal deliveries and found that the incidence of PPH was increased after induction of labor[86]; among primipara, the incidence was nearly twice that of spontaneous labor, even when only normal deliveries were considered. The study of Magann and colleagues suggested an OR of 1.5 (95% CI 1.2–1.7) for PPH after induction of labor[41] and Bais and co-workers found an OR of 1.74 (95% CI 1.06–2.87) for severe PPH of more than 1000 ml after induction of labor[42].

Tylleskar and colleagues performed a prospective, randomized, controlled trial of term induction of labor with amniotomy plus oxytocin versus waiting for spontaneous labor in 84 women and found no difference in the amount of bleeding at the third stage[87]. A Cochrane review[88] of amniotomy versus vaginal prostaglandin for induction of labor reported no difference in PPH rates. Another Cochrane[89] review of amniotomy plus intravenous oxytocin included only one placebo-controlled trial, but no data on PPH were reported. This review compared amniotomy plus intravenous oxytocin against vaginal prostaglandin (two trials, 160 women) and found a higher rate of PPH in the amniotomy/oxytocin group (13.8% vs. 2.5%, respectively, RR 5.5, 95% CI 1.26–24.07)[89].

A review of intravenous oxytocin alone for cervical ripening[90] found no difference in PPH rates compared to the placebo/expectant management group (three trials, 2611 women; RR 1.24, 95% CI 0.85–1.81) or vaginal prostaglandin (PG) E2 (four trials, 2792 women; RR 1.02, 95% CI 0.75–1.4). Use of mechanical methods to induce labor[91] was not associated with any difference in PPH rates when compared to placebo (one study, 240 women, RR 0.46, 95% CI 0.09–2.31), vaginal PGE2 (one study, 60 women, RR 3.0, 95% CI 0.33–27.24), intracervical PGE2 (three studies, 3339 women, RR 0.91, 95% CI 0.40–2.11), misoprostol (one study, 248 women, RR 2.34, 95% CI 0.46–11.85) or to oxytocinon alone (one study, 60 patients, RR 1.0, 95% CI 0.22–4.56).

Meta-analysis[92] of trials of membrane sweeping for induction of labor found a reduction in PPH compared to no intervention (three trials, 278 women, RR 0.31, 95% CI 0.11–0.89). A review of oral misoprostol for induction of labor[93] did not include any trial that compared this agent with placebo. However, one trial reported in this review, involving 692 women and using PGE2 in the control arm, found no difference in PPH rate (RR 0.98, 95% CI 0.73–1.31). Other reviews of induction of labor methods have reported no difference in PPH rates between vaginal misoprostol when compared to placebo (two trials, 107 women, RR 0.91, 95% CI 0.13–6.37)[94], vaginal prostaglandins (five trials, 1002 women, RR 0.88, 95% CI 0.63–1.22), intracervical prostaglandins (two trials, 172 women, RR 1.62, 95% CI 0.22–12.19), or with oxytocin (two trials, 245 women, RR 0.51, 95% CI 0.16–1.66). Finally, a review of vaginal PGE2 for induction of labor suggested an increased risk of PPH compared to placebo[95] (eight studies, 3437 women, RR 1.44, 95% CI 1.01–2.05).

Duration of labor

First stage

Compared with the second stage of labor, limited evidence is available regarding the influence of the duration of the first stage of labor on PPH[96]. Magann and colleagues defined a prolonged first stage of labor as a latent phase of more than 20 h in nulliparous and more than 14 h in multiparous and/or an active phase of less than 1.2 cm per hour in nulliparous and less than 1.4 cm in multiparous patients[41]. These investigators found an OR of 1.6 for prolonged first stage of labor, but the 95% CI ranged from 1 to 1.6.

Second stage

Several large studies have explored the relationship between the length of the second stage and adverse maternal and neonatal outcomes. Cohen analysed obstetric data from 4403 nulliparas and found an increase in PPH rate after more than 3 h in the second stage[97]. He attributed this to the increased need for mid-forceps delivery. A large retrospective study involving 25,069 women in spontaneous labor at term with a cephalic presentation found that second-stage duration had a significant independent association with the risk of PPH[98]. A more recent retrospective cohort study of 15,759 nulliparous term, cephalic singleton births in San Francisco divided the second stage of labor into 1-h intervals[99]. PPH was defined as estimated blood loss of more than 500 ml after vaginal delivery or more than 1000 ml after cesarean delivery. The frequency of PPH increased from 7.1% when the second stage lasted 0–1 h to 30.9% when it lasted more than 4 h. The risk for PPH with a second stage of more than 3 h remained statistically significant when controlled for confounders (including operative vaginal delivery, episiotomy, birth weight and fetal position) (OR 1.48, 95% CI 1.24–1.78). Myles and colleagues examined 6791 cephalic singleton births and found that the incidence of PPH was 2.3% in women experiencing a second stage less than 2 h compared to 6.2% in women with a longer second stage[100]. Janni and co-workers compared 952 women with a singleton cephalic pregnancy after 34 weeks' gestation with a 'normal' second stage to 248 women with a second stage more than 2 h[101]. The median difference between intrapartum and postpartum hemoglobin levels was lower in the normal group (−0.79 g/dl) compared to the prolonged second-stage group (−1.84 g/dl). Multivariate regression confirmed duration of the second stage as an independent predictor of PPH (RR 2.3, 95% CI 1.6–3.3). Magann and colleagues also found an OR of 1.6 (95% CI 1.1–2.1) for prolonged second stage[41]. Recently, a French group has published data on the duration of passive and active phases of the second stage of labor in low risk nulliparous women finding that severe PPH (≥1000 ml blood loss) was increased with active second stage exceeding 40 minutes (adjusted OR 3.5, 95% CI 1–12.3) and exceeding 50 minutes (adjusted OR 10.6; 95% CI 2.8–40.3) but a prolonged passive second stage was not associated with increased risk for severe PPH[102].

Third stage

Strong evidence indicates that, despite the use of active management, prolongation of the third stage of labor increases the risk for PPH. Combs and colleagues studied 12,979 singleton, vaginal deliveries and found that the median duration of the third stage was 6 min (interquartile range 4–10 min)[103]. The incidence of PPH and blood transfusion remaining constant until the third stage reached 30 min (3.3% of deliveries). Thereafter, it increased progressively, reaching a plateau at 75 min[103]. Dombrowski and colleagues studied the third stage in 45,852 singleton deliveries of 20 weeks' gestation or more[104]. PPH was defined as an estimated blood loss of 500 ml or more. At all gestational ages, the frequency of PPH increased with increasing duration of the third stage, reaching the peak at 40 min. Magann and colleagues performed a prospective observational study of 6588 vaginal deliveries[105]. PPH was defined as a blood loss of more than 1000 ml or hemodynamic instability requiring blood transfusion. PPH risk was significant (and increased in a dose-related fashion with time) at 10 min (OR 2.1, 95% CI 1.6–2.6), 20 min (OR 4.3, 95% CI 3.3–5.5) and at 30 min (OR 6.2, 95% CI 4.6–8.2). Using receiver operating characteristic (ROC) curves, the best predictor for PPH was a third stage of 18 min or more[105]. Similarly, a Dutch population-based cohort study of 3464 nulliparous women suggested that a third stage of 30 min or more was associated with a blood loss of 500 ml or more (OR 2.61, 95% CI 1.83–3.72) and 1000 ml or more (OR 4.90, 95% CI 2.89–8.32)[42]. Blood loss was determined by a combination of measurement and visual estimation.

Analgesia

A retrospective case–control study involving 1056 and 6261 women with and without epidural analgesia, respectively, found that use of epidural analgesia was associated with intrapartum hemorrhage of 500 ml or more[106]. Magann and colleagues also found an OR of 1.3 for PPH with epidural analgesia, but the 95% CI extended from 1 to 1.637[105]. However, if cesarean delivery is required, regional analgesia is superior to general anesthesia in reducing blood loss, according to evidence from one randomized, controlled trial involving 341 women[107].

Delivery method

The UK NICE guideline on cesarean section examined maternal morbidity in a comparison of planned cesarean section with planned vaginal birth from available randomized, controlled trials on an intention-to-treat basis[108]. For maternal obstetric hemorrhage (defined as blood loss >1000 ml), an absolute risk of 0.5% for planned cesarean section and 0.7% for vaginal birth (RR 0.8, 95% CI 0.4–4.4) was reported, suggesting there is no difference in risk. Magann and colleagues examined the incidence and risk factors for PPH in 1844 elective cesarean sections and 2933 non-elective cesarean sections[109]. Two criteria were used to define PPH: measured blood loss more than 1000 ml and/or need for blood transfusion and measured blood loss more than 1500 ml and/or need for blood transfusion. Six per cent of all cesarean deliveries were complicated by a blood loss more than 1000 ml. The PPH rates for elective cesarean section (blood loss >1000 ml – 4.84%, blood loss >1500 ml – 1.9%) were lower than for non-elective cesarean delivery (6.75% and 3.04%, respectively). During the 4-year period of this study, there were 13,868 vaginal deliveries with a PPH rate of 5.15% (blood loss >1000 ml) and 2.4% (blood loss >1500 ml)[109]. No data on operative vaginal delivery rate were reported. Although the PPH rate was higher in women undergoing non-elective cesarean delivery than after vaginal delivery, the difference in rate for elective cesarean delivery was not statistically different. Using linear regression, risk factors for PPH at elective cesarean delivery were leiomyomas, placenta previa, preterm birth and general anesthesia. For non-elective cesarean delivery, risk factors were blood disorders, retained placenta, antepartum transfusion, antepartum/intrapartum hemorrhage, placenta previa, general anesthesia and macrosomia.

Combs and colleagues performed a case–control study involving 3052 cesarean deliveries[110]. They reported a PPH incidence (based on fall in hematocrit and/or need for blood transfusion) of 6.4% for cesarean delivery, similar to Magann and colleagues. However, Combs and colleagues did not differentiate elective from non-elective deliveries.

This group also examined 9598 vaginal deliveries and found an overall incidence of PPH of 3.9%[62]. Using linear regression, they reported an adjusted OR of 1.66 (95% CI 1.06–2.60) for forceps or vacuum extraction use, suggesting that operative vaginal delivery is associated with PPH. In addition, the use of sequential instruments (forceps after unsuccessful vacuum extraction) to achieve vaginal delivery is a further risk factor (OR 1.9, 95% CI 1.1–3.2)[41] or relative risk of 1.6 (95% CI, 1.3–2.0)[111] for PPH.

Episiotomy

A Cochrane review argues for restrictive use of episiotomy because this policy is associated with fewer complications[112]. Surprisingly, this meta-analysis does not address the question of PPH incidence with episiotomy. Iatrogenic trauma by the indiscriminate use of a mid-line or mediolateral episiotomy is associated with increased blood loss and PPH in most studies, with blood loss increases of between 300 and 600 ml compared with no episiotomy[113,114]. Stones and colleagues reported a relative risk of 2.06 (95% CI 1.36–3.11) for PPH when episiotomy occurred[48]. Bais and co-workers reported similar results with an OR of 2.18 (95% CI 1.68–2.81)[42] and Combs and colleagues reported that a mediolateral episiotomy is associated with an odds ratio of 4.67 (95% CI 2.59–8.43) for PPH[62]. However, one recent randomized, controlled trial of the use of episiotomy when perineal tears appear imminent suggested no difference in PPH rates[115].

Chorioamnionitis

Several studies report an increased risk for PPH in the presence of chorioamnionitis, with ORs ranging from 1.3 (95% CI 1.1–1.7) at vaginal birth[41] to 2.69 (95% CI 1.44–5.03) at cesarean section[110].

CONCLUSIONS

PPH remains an extremely important cause of maternal mortality and morbidity throughout the world. Sadly, substandard care continues to contribute to mortality and morbidity from PPH, regardless of the country in which death takes place. Major obstetric hemorrhage complicates around 10% of live births and is responsible for 28% of direct deaths, globally. Marked differences exist between countries; in the UK there are two deaths per million maternities, whereas the figure is 200 times higher in parts of Africa. Severe obstetric hemorrhage is increasingly used as a measure of quality of health care in women. In the UK, severe obstetric hemorrhage occurs in three to seven cases per 1000 livebirths, with PPH implicated in 70% of cases. In contrast, rates as high as 30.5 per 1000 livebirths are reported in parts of Africa, with PPH rates of 17.4 per 1000.

References

1. Carroli G , Cuesta C, Abalos E, Gulmezoglu AM. Epidemiology of postpartum haemorrhage : a systematic review. Best Practice Res Clin Obstet Gynaecol 2008;22:999–1012
2. Park EH, Sachs BP. Postpartum hemorrhage and other problems of the third stage. In James DK, Steer PJ, Weiner CP, Gonik B, eds. High Risk Pregnancy: Management Options. London: WB Saunders, 1999:1231–46
3. Pritchard JA, Baldwin RM, Dickey JC, et al. Red blood cell loss and changes in apparent blood volume during and following vaginal delivery, caesarean section and caesarean section plus total hysterectomy. Am J Obstet Gynecol 1962; 84:1271
4. Brace V, Penney GC. Scottish Confidential Audit of Severe Maternal Morbidity: First Annual Report 2003. 22, 5–31. Aberdeen: Scottish Programme for Clinical Effectiveness in Reproductive Health, 2005
5. Griffiths D, Howell C. Massive obstetric haemorrhage. In Johanson R, Cox C, Grady K, Howell C, eds. Managing Obstetric Emergencies and Trauma (MOET) course manual. London: RCOG Press, 2003:151–62
6. Grady K, Cox C. Shock. In: Johanson R, Cox C, Grady K, Howell C, eds. Managing Obstetric Emergencies and Trauma. London: RCOG Press, 2003:81–90
7. Gulmezoglu AM, Hofmeyr GJ. Prevention and treatment of postpartum haemorrhage. In: MacLean AB, Neilson J, eds. Maternal Morbidity and Mortality. London: RCOG Press, 2002:241–51
8. Strand RT, da Silva F, Bergstrom S. Use of cholera beds in the delivery room: a simple and appropriate method for direct measurement of postpartum bleeding. Trop Doctor 2003;33:215–16
9. Chua S, Ho LM, Vanaja K, Nordstrom L, Roy AC, Arulkumaran S. Validation of a laboratory method of measuring postpartum blood loss. Gynecol Obstet Invest 1998;46:31–3
10. Duthie SJ, Ven D, Yung GL, Guang DZ, Chan SY, Ma HK. Discrepancy between laboratory determination and visual estimation of blood loss during normal delivery. Eur J Obstet Gynecol Reprod Biol 1991;38:119–24
11. Glover P. Blood loss at delivery: how accurate is your estimation? Aust J Midwifery 2003;16:21–4
12. Higgins PG. Measuring nurses' accuracy of estimating blood loss. J Adv Nursing 1982;7:157–62
13. Newton M, Mosey LM, Egli GE, Gifford WB, Hull CT. Blood loss during and immediately after delivery. Obstet Gynecol 1961;17:9–18
14. Hill JA, Fadel HE, Nelson MC, Nelson RM, Nelson GH. Blood loss at vaginal delivery. South Med J 1986;79:188–92
15. Prasertcharoensuk W, Swadpanich U, Lumbiganon P. Accuracy of the blood loss estimation in the third stage of labor. Int J Gynaecol Obstet 2000;71:69–70
16. Razvi K, Chua S, Arulkumaran S, Ratnam SS. A comparison between visual estimation and laboratory determination of blood loss during the third stage of labour. Aust N Z J Obstet Gynaecol 1996;36:152–4
17. Irons DW, Sriskandabalan P, Bullough CH. A simple alternative to parenteral oxytocics for the third stage of labor. Int J Gynaecol Obstet 1994;46:15–8
18. Prendiville WJ, Elbourne D, McDonald S. Active versus expectant management in the third stage of labour. Cochrane Database Syst Rev 2000;(2):CD000007
19. Grimes DA, Schulz KF. Bias and causal associations in observational research. Lancet 2002;359:248–52
20. Katz MH. Multivariable analysis: A practical guide for clinicians. Cambridge: Cambridge University Press, 1999
21. Grimes DA, Schulz KF. Clinical research in obstetrics and gynecology: a Baedeker for busy clinicians. Obstet Gynecol Survey 2002;57:S35–S53
22. Mamdani M, Sykora K, Li P, et al. Reader's guide to critical appraisal of cohort studies. 2. Assessing potential for confounding. BMJ 2005;330:960–2

23. Anonymous. Introduction. In: Lewis G, ed. Why Mothers Die 2000–2002. London: RCOG, 2004:1–24
24. Hall M. Haemorrhage. In Lewis G, ed. Why Mothers Die 2000–2002. London: RCOG Press, 2004:86–93
25. Norman J. Chapter 4 : Haemorrhage. In: Saving Mothers' Lives: Reviewing maternal deaths to make motherhood safer: 2006–2008. BJOG 2011;118 (Suppl 1)
26. Chang J, Elam-Evans LD, Berg CJ, et al. Pregnancy-related mortality surveillance, United States, 1991–1999. CDC. http//www.cdc.gov/mmwr/preview/mmwrhtml/ss5202a1. htm 52(SS02), 1–8. 2003
27. Berg CJ, Atrash HK, Koonin LM, Tucker M. Pregnancy-related mortality in the United States, 1987–1990. Obstet Gynecol 1996;88:161–7
28. Bouvier-Colle MH, Varnoux N, Breart G. Maternal deaths and substandard care: the results of a confidential survey in France. Medical Experts Committee. Eur J Obstet Gynecol Reproduct Biol 1995;58:3–7
29. Bouvier-Colle MH, Ouedraogo C, Dumont A, et al. Maternal mortality in West Africa. Rates, causes and substandard care from a prospective survey. Acta Obstet Gynecol Scand 2001;80:113–9
30. Spies CA, Bam RH, Cronje HS, Schoon MG, Wiid M, Niemand I. Maternal deaths in Bloemfontein, South Africa, 1986–1992. South Afri Med J 1995;85:753–5
31. Waterstone M, Bewley S, Wolfe C. Incidence and predictors of severe obstetric morbidity: case–control study. BMJ 2001;322:1089–93
32. Callaghan Wm , Kuklina EV, Berg CJ. Trends in postpartum hemorrhage: United States, 1994–2006. Am J Obstet Gynecol 2010;202:353 e1–6
33. Wen SW, Huang L, Liston R, et al. Severe maternal morbidity in Canada, 1991–2001. Can Med Assoc J 2005;173: 759–64
34. Roberts CL, Ford JB, Algert CS, Bell JC, Simpson JM, Morris JM. Trends in adverse maternal outcomes during childbirth: a population-based study of severe maternal morbidity. BMC Pregnancy Childbirth 2009;25:7
35. Filippi V, Ronsmans C, Gohou V, et al. Maternity wards or emergency obstetric rooms? Incidence of near-miss events in African hospitals. Acta Obstet Gynecol Scand 2005;84: 11–6
36. Prual A, Bouvier-Colle MH, de Bernis L, Breart G. Severe maternal morbidity from direct obstetric causes in West Africa: incidence and case fatality rates. Bull WHO 2000;78: 593–602
37. Pattinson RC, Hall M. Near misses: a useful adjunct to maternal death enquiries. Br Med Bull 2003;67:231–43
38. Anderson J, Etches D, Smith D. Postpartum haemorrhage. In: Damos JR, Eisinger SH, eds. Advanced Life Support in Obstetrics (ALSO) provider course manual. Kansas: American Academy of Family Physicians, 2000:1–15
39. Rouse DJ, Leindecker S, Landon M, et al. The MFMU Cesarean Registry: uterine atony after primary cesarean delivery. Am J Obstet Gynecol 2005;193:1056–60
40. Feerasta SH, Motiei A, Motiwala S, Zuberi NF. Uterine atony at a tertiary care hospital in Pakistan: a risk factor analysis. J Pak Med Assoc 2000;50:132–6
41. Magann EF, Evans S, Hutchinson M, Collins R, Howard BC, Morrison JC. Postpartum hemorrhage after vaginal birth: an analysis of risk factors. S Med J 2005;98:419–22
42. Bais JM, Eskes M, Pel M, Bonsel GJ, Bleker OP. Postpartum haemorrhage in nulliparous women: incidence and risk factors in low and high risk women. A Dutch population-based cohort study on standard (> or = 500 ml) and severe (> or = 1000 ml) postpartum haemorrhage.Eur J Obstet Gynecol Reprod Biol 2004;115:166–72
43. Hussain M, Jabeen T, Liaquat N, Noorani K, Bhutta SZ. Acute puerperal uterine inversion. J Coll Phys Surg–Pakistan 2004;14:215–7
44. Milenkovic M, Kahn J. Inversion of the uterus: a serious complication at childbirth. Acta Obstet Gynecol Scand 2005;84:95–6
45. Beringer RM, Patteril M. Puerperal uterine inversion and shock. Br J Anaesthes 2004;92:439–41
46. Baskett TF. Acute uterine inversion: a review of 40 cases. J Obstet Gynaecol Can 2002;24:953–6
47. Weeks AD, Mirembe FM. The retained placenta – new insights into an old problem. Eur J Obstet Gynecol Reprod Biol 2002;102:109–10
48. Stones RW, Paterson CM, Saunders NJ. Risk factors for major obstetric haemorrhage. Eur J Obstet Gynecol Reprod Biol 1993;48:15–8
49. Tandberg A, Albrechtsen S, Iversen OE. Manual removal of the placenta. Incidence and clinical significance. Acta Obstet Gynecol Scand 1999;78:33–6
50. Adelusi B, Soltan MH, Chowdhury N, Kangave D. Risk of retained placenta: multivariate approach. Acta Obstet Gynecol Scand 1997;76:414–8
51. Hall MH, Halliwell R, Carr-Hill R. Concomitant and repeated happenings of complications of the third stage of labour. Br J Obstet Gynaecol 1985;92:732–8
52. Makhseed M, el-Tomi N, Moussa M. A retrospective analysis of pathological placental implantation – site and penetration. Int J Gynaecol Obstet 1994;47:127–34
53. Zaki ZM, Bahar AM, Ali ME, Albar HA, Gerais MA. Risk factors and morbidity in patients with placenta previa accreta compared to placenta previa non-accreta. Acta Obstet Gynecol Scand 1998;77:391–4
54. Kastner ES, Figueroa R, Garry D, Maulik D. Emergency peripartum hysterectomy: experience at a community teaching hospital. Obstet Gynecol 2002;99:971–5
55. Walker ID, Walker JJ, Colvin BT, Letsky EA, Rivers R, Stevens R. Investigation and management of haemorrhagic disorders in pregnancy. Haemostasis and Thrombosis Task Force. J Clin Pathol 1994;47:100–8
56. Economides DL, Kadir RA, Lee CA. Inherited bleeding disorders in obstetrics and gynaecology. Br J Obstet Gynaecol 1999;106:5–13
57. Ohkuchi A, Onagawa T, Usui R, et al. Effect of maternal age on blood loss during parturition: a retrospective multivariate analysis of 10,053 cases. J Perinat Med. 2003;31: 209–15
58. Tsu VD. Postpartum haemorrhage in Zimbabwe:a risk factor analysis. Br J Obstet Gynaecol 1993;100:327–33
59. Ijaiya MA, Aboyeji AP, Abubakar D. Analysis of 348 consecutive cases of primary postpartum haemorrhage at a tertiary hospital in Nigeria. J Obstet Gynaecol 2003;23: 374–7
60. Okogbenin SA, Gharoro EP, Otoide VO, Okonta PI. Obstetric hysterectomy: fifteen years' experience in a Nigerian tertiary centre. J Obstet Gynaecol 2003;23:356–9
61. Roberts CL, Algert CS, March LM. Delayed childbearing – are there any risks? Med J Aust 1994;160:539–44
62. Combs CA, Murphy EL, Laros RK Jr. Factors associated with postpartum hemorrhage with vaginal birth. Obstet Gynecol 1991;77:69–76
63. Petersen LA, Lindner DS, Kleiber CM, Zimmerman MB, Hinton AT, Yankowitz J. Factors that predict low hematocrit levels in the postpartum patient after vaginal delivery. Am J Obstet Gynecol 2002;186:737–44
64. Usha KT, Hemmadi S, Bethel J, Evans J. Outcome of pregnancy in a woman with an increased body mass index. Br J Obstet Gynaecol 2005;112:768–72
65. Selo-Ojeme DO, Okonofua FE. Risk factors for primary postpartum haemorrhage. A case control study. Arch Gynecol Obstet 1997;259: 179–87
66. Humphrey MD. Is grand multiparity an independent predictor of pregnancy risk? A retrospective observational study. Med J Aust 2003;179:294–6
67. Munim S, Rahbar MH, Rizvi M, Mushtaq N. The effect of grandmultiparity on pregnancy related complications: the Aga Khan University experience. J Pak Med Assoc 2000;50: 54–8
68. Dunne F, Brydon P, Smith K, Gee H. Pregnancy in women with Type 2 diabetes: 12 years outcome data 1990–2002.

Diabet Med 2003;20:734–8 65. Dunne F. Type 2 diabetes and pregnancy. Semin Fetal Neonat Med 2005;10:333–9

69. Rahman J, Rahman FZ, Rahman W, al-Suleiman SA, Rahman MS. Obstetric and gynecologic complications in women with Marfan syndrome. J Reprod Med 2003;48: 723–8

70. Borthen I, Eide M, Daltveit A, Gilhus N. Delivery outcome of women with epilepsy: a population-based cohort study. BJOG 2010;117:1537–43

71. Eskild A, Vatten LJ. Abnormal bleeding associated with preeclampsia: a population study of 315,085 pregnancies. Acta Obstet Gynecol Scand 2009;88:154–8

72. Lind J, Wallenburg HC. Pregnancy and the Ehlers-Danlos syndrome: a retrospective study in a Dutch population. Acta Obstet Gynecol Scand 2002;81:293–300

73. James AH. More than menorrhagia: a review of the obstetric and gynaecological manifestations of bleeding disorders. Haemophilia 2005;11:295–307

74. Olesen AW, Westergaard JG, Olsen J. Perinatal and maternal complications related to postterm delivery: a national register-based study, 1978–1993. Am J Obstet Gynecol 2003;189:222–7

75. Caughey AB, Stotland NE, Washington EW, Escobar GJ. Maternal and obstetric complications of pregnancy are associated with increasing gestational age at term. Am J Obstet Gynecol 2007;196:155.e1–6

76. Jolly MC, Sebire NJ, Harris JP, Regan L, Robinson S. Risk factors for macrosomia and its clinical consequences: a study of 350,311 pregnancies. Eur J Obstet Gynecol Reprod Biol 2003;111:9–14

77. Stotland NE, Caughey AB, Breed EM, Escobar GJ. Risk factors and obstetric complications associated with macrosomia. Int J Gynaecol Obstet 2004;87:220–6

78. Fakeye O. The incidence, sociobiological factors and obstetric complications associated with large infants at Ilorin, Nigeria. Int J Gynaecol Obstet 1988;27:343–7

79. Walker MC, Murphy KE, Pan S, Yang Q, Wen SW. Adverse maternal outcomes in multifetal pregnancies. Br J Obstet Gynaecol 2004;111:1294–6

80. Klapholz H. Blood transfusion in contemporary obstetric practice. Obstet Gynecol 1990;75:940–3

81. Albrecht JL, Tomich PG. The maternal and neonatal outcome of triplet gestations. Am J Obstet Gynecol 1996;174: 1551–6

82. Collins MS, Bleyl JA. Seventy-one quadruplet pregnancies: management and outcome. Am J Obstet Gynecol 1990;162: 1384–91

83. Akrivis C, Varras M, Bellou A, Kitsiou E, Stefanaki S, Antoniou N. Primary postpartum haemorrhage due to a large submucosal nonpedunculated uterine leiomyoma: a case report and review of the literature. Clin Exp Obstet Gynecol 2003;30:156–8

84. Ford JB, Roberts CL, Bell JC, Algert CS, Morris JM Postpartum haemorrhage occurrence and recurrence: a population-based study. Med J Aust 2007;187:391–3

85. Crowley P. Interventions for preventing or improving the outcome of delivery at or beyond term (Review). Cochrane Database Syst Rev 2000;(4):CD000170

86. Brinsden PR, Clark AD. Postpartum haemorrhage after induced and spontaneous labour. Br Med J 1978;2:855–6

87. Tylleskar J, Finnstrom O, Leijon I, Hedenskog S, Ryden G. Spontaneous labor and elective induction – a prospective randomized study. I. Effects on mother and fetus. Acta Obstet Gynecol Scand 1979;58:513–8

88. Bricker L, Luckas M. Amniotomy alone for induction of labour. (Review). Cochrane Database Syst Rev 2000;(4): CD002862

89. Howarth GR, Botha DJ. Amniotomy plus intravenous oxytocin for induction of labour. (Review). Cochrane Database Syst Rev 2001;(3):CD003250

90. Kelly AJ, Tan B. Intravenous oxytocin alone for cervical ripening and induction of labour. (Review). Cochrane Database Syst Rev 2001;(3):CD003246

91. Boulvain M, Kelly A, Lohse C, Stan C, Irion O. Mechanical methods for induction of labour. (Review). Cochrane Database Syst Rev 2001;(4):CD001233

92. Boulvain M, Stan C, Irion O. Membrane sweeping for induction of labour. [update of Cochrane Database Syst Rev 2001;(2):CD000451; PMID: 11405964]. (Review). Cochrane Database Syst Rev 2001;(2):CD000451

93. Alfirevic Z. Oral misoprostol for induction of labour. [update of Cochrane Database Syst Rev 2000;(4): CD001338; PMID: 11034716]. (Review). Cochrane Database Syst Rev 2001;(2):CD001338

94. Hofmeyr GJ, Gulmezoglu AM. Vaginal misoprostol for cervical ripening and induction of labour.[update of Cochrane Database Syst Rev 2001;(3):CD000941; PMID: 11686970]. (Review). Cochrane Database Syst Rev 2003; (1):CD000941

95. Kelly AJ, Kavanagh J, Thomas J. Vaginal prostaglandin (PGE2 and PGF2a) for induction of labour at term.[update of Cochrane Database Syst Rev. 2001;(2):CD003101; PMID: 11406078]. (Review). Cochrane Database Syst Rev 2001;(2):CD003101

96. Mahon TR, Chazotte C, Cohen WR. Short labor: characteristics and outcome. Obstet Gynecol 1994;84:47–51

97. Cohen WR. Influence of the duration of second stage labor on perinatal outcome and puerperal morbidity. Obstet Gynecol 1977;49:266–9

98. Saunders NS, Paterson CM, Wadsworth J. Neonatal and maternal morbidity in relation to the length of the second stage of labour. Br J Obstet Gynaecol 1992;99:381–5

99. Cheng YW, Hopkins LM, Caughey AB. How long is too long: Does a prolonged second stage of labor in nulliparous women affect maternal and neonatal outcomes? Am J Obstet Gynecol 2004;191:933–8

100. Myles TD, Santolaya J. Maternal and neonatal outcomes in patients with a prolonged second stage of labor. Obstet Gynecol 2003;102:52–8

101. Janni W, Schiessl B, Peschers U, et al. The prognostic impact of a prolonged second stage of labor on maternal and fetal outcome. Acta Obstet Gynecol Scand 2002;81:214–21

102. Le Ray C, Fraser W, Rozenberg P, et al. Duration of passive and active phases of the second stage of labour and risk of severe postpartum haemorrhage in low-risk nulliparous women. Eur J Obstet Gynecol Reprod Biol 2011;158: 167–72

103. Combs CA, Laros RK Jr. Prolonged third stage of labor: morbidity and risk factors. Obstet Gynecol 1991;77:863–7

104. Dombrowski MP, Bottoms SF, Saleh AA, Hurd WW, Romero R. Third stage of labor: analysis of duration and clinical practice. Am J Obstet Gynecol 1995;172:1279–84

105. Magann EF, Evans S, Chauhan SP, Lanneau G, Fisk AD, Morrison JC. The length of the third stage of labor and the risk of postpartum hemorrhage. Obstet Gynecol 2005;105: 290–3

106. Ploeckinger B, Ulm MR, Chalubinski K, Gruber W. Epidural anaesthesia in labour: influence on surgical delivery rates, intrapartum fever and blood loss. Gynecol Obstet Invest 1995;39:24–7

107. Lertakyamanee J, Chinachoti T, Tritrakarn T, Muangkasem J, Somboonnanonda A, Kolatat T. Comparison of general and regional anesthesia for cesarean section: success rate, blood loss and satisfaction from a randomized trial. J Med Assoc Thailand 1999;82:672–80

108. Anonymous. Women – centred care. In National Collaborating Centre for Women's and Children's Health, ed. Caesarean Section. London: RCOG Press, 2004:20–5

109. Magann EF, Evans S, Hutchinson M, Collins R, Lanneau G, Morrison JC. Postpartum hemorrhage after cesarean delivery: an analysis of risk factors. S Med J 2005;98:681–5

110. Combs CA, Murphy EL, Laros RK Jr. Factors associated with hemorrhage in cesarean deliveries. Obstet Gynecol 1991;77:77–82

111. Gardella C, Taylor M, Benedetti T, Hitti J, Critchlow C. The effect of sequential use of vacuum and forceps for

assisted vaginal delivery on neonatal and maternal outcomes. Am J Obstet Gynecol 2001;185:896–902

112. Carroli G, Belizan J. Episiotomy for vaginal birth. (Review). Cochrane Database of Systematic Reviews 2000;(2): CD000081

113. Myers–Helfgott MG, Helfgott AW. Routine use of episiotomy in modern obstetrics. Should it be performed?. Obstet Gynecol Clin North Am 1999;26:305–25

114. House MJ, Cario G, Jones MH. Episiotomy and the perineum: A random controlled trial. J Obstet Gynaecol 1986;7: 107–10

115. Dannecker C, Hillemanns P, Strauss A, Hasbargen U, Hepp H, Anthuber C. Episiotomy and perineal tears presumed to be imminent: randomized controlled trial. Acta Obstet Gynecol Scand 2004;83:364–8

18

Maternal Morbidity and Near Misses: Determining the Real Numbers

M. E. Campbell and J. Barrett

INTRODUCTION

Maternal morbidity, and in particular severe acute maternal morbidity (SAMM), is important in that it reflects a threat to maternal life. In many jurisdictions, maternal mortality is so low that studying maternal deaths alone provides an exceedingly narrow scope of information. With a fuller understanding of maternal morbidity and mortality, however, trends can be observed and gaps in care indentified, such that these parameters can be improved. Improving the health of mothers is a global priority, as reflected in the United Nations Millennium Development Goals[1].

To date, collection of maternal morbidity and mortality data has been hindered by variations in terminology and approach. First, several terms have been used to describe a significant threat to maternal life: severe maternal morbidity, SAMM and maternal near miss. Second, no standard approach exists for identifying a case where a maternal life was in jeopardy. To this end, World Health Organization (WHO) has sought to standardize terminology and case identification[2].

Research underway in Canada uses the new standardized terminology and case identification system proposed by WHO. Using this approach at the hospital level, and ultimately synthesizing these results with existing national database research, can provide much more comprehensive data on maternal near misses.

UNDERSTANDING WHO STANDARD TERMINOLOGY: MATERNAL NEAR MISS

As noted by Say *et al.*, three differing definitions of near miss or SAMM are found in the literature:

(1) A severe life-threatening obstetric complication necessitating an urgent medical intervention in order to prevent likely death of the mother;

(2) Any pregnant or recently delivered woman in whom immediate survival is threatened and who survives by chance or due to hospital care;

(3) A very ill woman who would have died had it not been that luck and good care was on her side[2].

Following a review of the literature and consultation with an international group of experts, the WHO Working Group on Maternal Mortality and Morbidity Classifications came up with a standard definition to describe severe threats to maternal life.

In the deliberations, the term 'near miss' was thought to best capture the intended meaning when considering a severe threat to maternal life[2]. This term has traditionally been used by the airline industry to describe a close call, or accident that was possible, but avoided[3]. In the medical field, it has been used similarly to refer to a situation that had the potential to cause harm, illness or injury, but did not[3].

In the context of maternal health, however, the near miss term historically has been used to refer to a condition where a woman experienced a severe complication, nearly died, but survived. Considering the term 'maternal near miss' best reflects the concept of 'nearly dying but surviving', the WHO Working Group recommended the use of this term instead of SAMM[2].

Next, a standard definition was proposed which would capture the meaning of the three differing definitions used in the literature. Furthermore, this definition is aligned with the International Statistical Classification of Diseases and Related Health Problems (ICD) 10th version[2].

A *maternal near miss* case[2] is therefore defined as: '*A woman who nearly died but survived a complication that occurred during pregnancy, childbirth or within 42 days of termination of pregnancy.*'

UNDERSTANDING WHO STANDARD APPROACH TO MATERNAL NEAR MISS CASE IDENTIFICATION

As identified by Say *et al.*[2], three main approaches facilitate maternal near miss case identification. First, *disease-specific criteria* use particular diseases, each with specific end-points that signify severe maternal morbidity. An example is pre-eclampsia, where the occurrence of specific negative sequelae (convulsions, hepatic involvement) signals a maternal near miss. Second, using *intervention-based criteria*, admission to an intensive care unit (ICU), for example, indicates a near miss. Third, *organ dysfunction criteria* can be applied, whereby certain markers, such as failure to form clots or the need for a massive transfusion, represent a maternal near miss.

The WHO Working Group suggests that the organ dysfunction-based approach is 'the most promising frame for establishing a standard set of criteria'[2]. Although this approach would ideally rely on a minimum standard of critical care, including laboratory investigations, clinical criteria alone could be used to identify severe organ dysfunction in resource limited settings. Furthermore, the organ dysfunction-based approach is more comprehensive and more readily applied to a range of settings compared with disease-specific criteria, where there has been wide variation in outcomes used to identify maternal near miss, and when considering the likely exclusion of cases due to variable access to care when management-based criteria are used[2,4]. Table 1 describes advantages and disadvantages of each approach.

Organ system dysfunction-based approach

Specific criteria have been proposed to identify a near miss using the organ dysfunction-based approach.

These include clinical criteria, laboratory marker and management-based proxies. Figure 1 outlines these criteria, delineated by organ system.

Means to collect maternal near miss data: the Canadian approach

Canadian stakeholders recently convened to improve maternal morbidity and mortality surveillance nationwide. Canada has unique barriers to efficient maternal health surveillance, including a large geographic area and division into multiple provinces and territories, each of which is separately responsible for health care delivery.

Multiple stakeholders are currently engaged in research or policy work to improve maternal health surveillance in Canada (not inclusive):

(1) The Public Health Agency of Canada (PHAC), which houses the Canadian Perinatal Surveillance System (CPSS) – the CPSS monitors, analyses and reports on the health of pregnant women, mothers and infants in Canada[9];

Table 1 Advantages and disadvantages of three approaches for use as a quality of care tool to identify maternal near miss cases. Reproduced from Say et al.[2], with permission

	Advantages	Disadvantages
Clinical criteria related to a specific disease entity	Straight forward to interpret Data can be obtained retrospectively from case notes and registers The quality of care of a particular disease can be assessed Complication rates for a particular disease can be calculated	Common direct causes of maternal mortality may be omitted* The criteria used to define morbidity often have too low a threshold of morbidity to be called maternal near miss Retrospectively collected information might be problematic due to poor documentation and hence bias† Difficult to use for ongoing audits for all morbidities‡
Intervention-based criteria	Simple to identify the cases usually on the basis of retrospective analysis of a register in the hospital Could be useful to identify the potential maternal near miss cases	Allows the identification of only a fraction of all severe morbidity cases, because of variation in accessibility of the intervention, eligibility criteria for an intervention, or in the case of ICU, what constitutes intensive care Biased by resources available**
Organ system dysfunction-based criteria	Mimics the confidential enquires into maternal death systems, thus the same system could be used to complement maternal death enquires. It might allow calculation of more stable summary measures of morbidity/mortality†† Allows for identification of critically ill women thereby establishing the pattern of diseases causing morbidity and their relative importance Allows for the identification of new and emerging disease priorities, and studying health system's response Keeps focus on severe diseases that should not cause death with appropriate care, such as severe PPH‡‡ Many hospitals have a severe adverse events committee and these can be a source of identifying cases Variation in defining identification criteria can be avoided particularly for similar settings, allowing the establishment of reliable summary estimates for maternal near miss	Dependent on existence of a minimum level of care including functioning laboratories and basic critical care monitoring Retrospective identification of cases might be difficult because of the inability to identify cases from registers

*In Waterstone et al.[5] pulmonary embolus was omitted because of the difficulty of diagnosing pulmonary emboli accurately when they are not fatal. Early pregnancy complications such as ectopic pregnancies and abortions are also often omitted
†Potentially the cases with the worst care would have the poorest notes
‡This system is useful to audit the care of a specific disease entity, but is not suitable for ongoing audits. The ability to examine the quality of care of a specific disease entity has been well illustrated by Bouvier et al.[6]
**A condition that is life threatening in a country where no appropriate response can be given may not be classified as a maternal near miss and interventions such as cesarean section may often be performed on women who are not suffering from severe morbidity
††As is currently being undertaken in Scotland[7]. The difference being the definition of the end point. Maternal death is easy to define, however, severe morbidity is more difficult, hence the need for objective criteria
‡‡It is not a common cause of death in high-income countries but is the most frequent cause of maternal near miss[7,8]

Box: Maternal life-threatening conditions			
Dysfunctional system	**Clinical criteria**	**Laboratory markers**	**Management based proxies**
Cardiovascular	( ) Shock ( ) Cardiac arrest	( ) Severe hypoperfusion (lactate>5 mmol/L or >45mg/dL) ( ) Severe Acidosis (pH<7.1)	( ) Use of continuous vasoactive drugs ( ) Cardio-pulmonary resuscitation
Respiratory	( ) Acute cyanosis ( ) Gasping ( ) Severe tachypnea (Respiratory rate >40 bpm) ( ) Severe bradypnea (Respiratory rate <6 bpm)	( ) Severe hypoxemia (Oxygen saturation < 90% for ≥ 60 minutes or PaO2/FiO2<200)	( ) Intubation and ventilation not related to anaesthesia
Renal	( ) Oliguria non responsive to fluids or diuretics	( ) Severe acute azotemia (Creatinine ≥300μmol/l or ≥3.5 mg/dL)	( ) Dialysis for acute renal failure
Haematologic/ Coagulation	( ) Failure to form clots	( ) Severe acute thrombocytopenia (<50,000 platelets/ml)	( ) Massive transfusion of blood / red cells (≥ 5 units)
Hepatic	( ) Jaundice in the presence of preeclampsia	( ) Severe acute hyperbilirubinemia (Bilirubin>100 μmol/l or >6.0 mg/dL)	
Neurologic	( ) Prolonged unconsciousness (lasting >12h) ( ) Stroke ( ) Uncontrollable fit / status epilepticus ( ) Global paralysis		
Alternative severity proxy			( ) Hysterectomy following infection or haemorrhage

Figure 1 WHO near miss identification and classification tool. Adapted for Say *et al.*[2], with permission

(2) The Society of Obstetricians and Gynecologists of Canada (SOGC), a professional organization for gynecologists, obstetricians, family physicians, nurses, midwives and allied health professionals in Canada[10];

(3) Statistics Canada, a government agency that produces statistical information[11];

(4) The Canadian Institute for Health Information (CIHI), an independent, not-for-profit corporation that provides essential information on Canada's health system and the health of Canadians[12];

(5) The Canadian Maternal Morbidity Working Group, a group of researchers affiliated with various Canadian universities engaged in maternal morbidity and mortality research.

These stakeholders engage via national meetings and committees. Recent activities include a Joint SOGC–CPSS Committee on Maternal Mortality and Severe Morbidity aiming to make recommendations to improve national surveillance of maternal mortality and severe morbidity in Canada (written communication from Joint SOGC–CPSS Committee on Maternal Mortality and Severe Morbidity co-chair Kimberly Elmslie, PHAC, Ottawa, 2011 Feb 24). In addition, the Canadian Maternal Morbidity Working Group met with SOGC, Statistics Canada and CIHI representatives in late 2009 to discuss and create a consensus document on solutions for 'enhanced and consistent national surveillance of maternal mortality and severe maternal morbidity in Canada'[13].

To date, the primary research on maternal morbidity and mortality in Canada that looks at these entities broadly uses available databases[14–16]. Although database research is important in that it is simple, cost-effective and timely[16], it does have specific limitations which prevent a complete and comprehensive understanding of maternal near misses.

The Canadian Maternal Morbidity Working Group's consensus document outlined current deficiencies with maternal mortality and near miss surveillance in Canada. First, administrative databases in Canada, such as Canadian Institute for Health Information Discharge Abstract Database, Statistics Canada's Canadian Vital Statistics System, and provincial administrative and perinatal databases, do provide information on maternal mortality and maternal near miss, but without a systematic mechanism to compile these data nationally[13,14]. Furthermore, certain provinces may be excluded because of lack of participation in or alignment with existing databases[14,16]. Moreover, database research is subject to coding errors[13,15], and may not provide complete information regarding the relationship between various disease entities and conditions that threaten maternal life[15]. For example, a recent publication using data from the Discharge Abstract Database of CIHI identified temporal trends of increasing rates of severe PPH as well as acute renal failure and assisted ventilation. Based on information available from this particular database, it is not clear whether these trends were related or represented distinct pathological processes (Figure 2)[15].

Hospital-based maternal near miss research

Hospital-based research provides a more in-depth perspective on the relationship between certain disease entities and also can provide insight into the means by which social determinants of health factor into emerging trends. Although hospitals generally review cases of severe morbidity and mortality, these data are rarely available outside the respective institution, severely limiting national and international synthesis of data[13,14]. A standard approach to hospital-based data collection would allow for hospital to hospital comparisons as well as pooling of data to compare, for example, tertiary (i.e. high risk) centers with others.

Such a process would also identify trends based on patient features (i.e. obesity), hospital facilities (i.e. presence of ICU) or geographic considerations (i.e. distance to nearest hospital).

Hospital-based case identification is additionally advantageous in that any practitioner can use this approach, as it is simple and does not require detailed statistical knowledge. Furthermore, with the emergence of standardized case identification criteria from the WHO Working Group on Maternal Mortality and Morbidity Classifications, data can be pooled and compared across jurisdictions.

In accordance with the Canadian Maternal Morbidity Working Group's recommendations, efforts are currently underway to pilot an approach to maternal near miss research using the criteria proposed by the WHO Working Group. This approach is outlined in Figure 3.

Near miss cases will be defined using an organ-system dysfunction-based approach as outlined, and described in detail in the WHO near miss identification and classification tool in Figure 1.

All obstetric patients (more than 20 weeks pregnant) cared for at the piloting Canadian hospitals and meeting WHO near miss identification and classification tool criteria will be included as cases. No

specific exclusion criteria are operational. The protocol will be circulated to all staff obstetricians and posted in the relevant clinical areas. If a patient fulfills any criteria listed in the WHO tool, the most responsible physician will be asked to report the case to the research team.

As a method of cross-reference, in order to ensure that no cases are overlooked, the research team will liaise with the blood bank and intensive care unit at their respective hospitals.

A time period of 1 year was chosen for this study to account for seasonal trends (i.e. illness related to flu), and because it is expected that there will be relatively few cases. One year of data collection should allow for an adequate initial pool of cases in order to:

(1) Assess the incidence of near misses at the piloting hospitals;

(2) Understand the major causes of maternal near miss at the piloting hospitals;

(3) Develop trial software designed to compile maternal near miss cases;

(4) Provide feedback to the Canadian Maternal Morbidity Working Group in advance of broader data collection nationally.

Being an exploratory pilot study, the goals are not to perform statistical analysis or derive specific conclusions, but rather to obtain an initial overview of the problem on which further research can be based.

Collected data will be stripped of identifying material, although age and health information relevant to the study will be maintained. Data will be entered into a software program, and will include details such as gravidity, parity, whether antenatal care was received, current pregnancy outcome, route of delivery, whether anesthesia was required, details regarding the primary obstetric problem (including pre-existing conditions like obesity and hypertension), details related to the near miss markers (using the organ system dysfunction-based approach) and details regarding the care received. Names of care providers involved in the case will NOT be included.

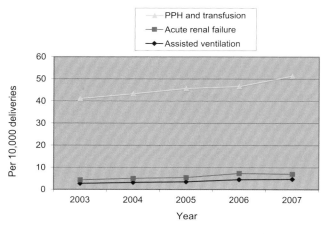

Figure 2 Near miss trends. Adapted from Liu et al.[11]

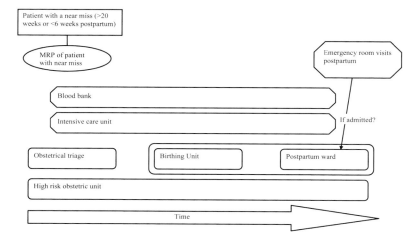

Figure 3 Hospital-based case identification flow chart. MRP, most responsible person

Upon completion of data collection, the data will be analysed and summarized according to recurring themes. These themes may be related to the primary obstetric problem (including predisposing conditions), details related to management (i.e. whether the patient underwent cesarean section) or any other commonality apparent on reviewing the data.

Ethical considerations in hospital-based maternal near miss research

Current estimates of the incidence of maternal near miss cases in Canada range from 4.62/1000 deliveries[14] to 13.8/1000 deliveries[16]. Thus, a large hospital with 3000 deliveries per year would expect anywhere from 13 to 42 cases. This is a relatively small number. When specific scenarios are considered, for example, the number of women requiring hysterectomy following infection or hemorrhage, the numbers will be even smaller when considered for only one institution. This may create a dilemma in that patient confidentiality must be maintained; however, there is great interest in understanding the circumstances surrounding particular cases. Thus, when data are published for an individual institution, there may be limitations in the number of details that can be included to ensure patient confidentiality. This barrier can be overcome when multiple institutions pool data.

Although the pilot studies in Canada will be subject to this barrier, once the hospital-based maternal near miss research is expanded more broadly, a wealth of data is expected that will surely compensate for this early limitation.

CONCLUSION

The development of a standardized definition and classification system by WHO is a critical tool in advancing maternal near miss research both in Canada and internationally. This tool will allow for cross-jurisdictional comparisons in maternal near miss research, and will ultimately advance understanding of current threats to maternal health.

Hospital-based maternal near miss research will supplement and fill gaps in existing database research currently conducted in Canada. With a more complete and comprehensive understanding of threats to maternal health, interventions can be designed to improve the health of mothers, in line with the United Nations Millennium Development Goals.

PRACTICE POINTS

- A complete and comprehensive understanding of threats to maternal health is required in order to improve the health of mothers

- Various approaches to maternal near miss research complement each other and provide a better understanding of emerging trends, interactions among different pathological processes, and interactions between pathology and social determinants of health

- Standardized terminology and classification systems to identify maternal near miss cases allow for cross-jurisdictional pooling and comparing of data, and ultimately a deeper understanding of threats to maternal health.

References

1. United Nations. Millennium Development Goals – Goal 5: Improve Maternal Health. 2011. http://www.un.org/millenniumgoals/maternal.shtml
2. Say L, Souza JP, Pattison RC. Maternal near miss – towards a standard tool for monitoring quality of maternal health care. Best Pract Res Clin Obstet Gynaecol 2009;23:287–96
3. Nashef SA. What is a near miss? Lancet 2003;361:180–1
4. Say L, Pattinson R, Gulmezoglu AM. WHO systematic review of maternal morbidity and mortality: the prevalence of severe acute maternal morbidity (near miss). Reprod Health 2004;1:3
5. Waterstone M, Bewley S, Wolfe C. Incidence and predictors of severe obstetric morbidity: case-control study. BMJ 2001; 322:1089–94
6. Bouvier-Colle M-H, Salanave B, Ancel PY. Obstetric patients in intensive care units and maternal mortality. RegionalTeams for the Survey. Eur J Obstet Gynecol Reprod Biol 1996;65:121–5
7. Brace V, Penney G, Hall M. Quantifying severe maternal morbidity: a Scottish population study. Br J Obstet Gynaecol 2004;111:481–4
8. Hall MH. Near misses and severe maternal morbidity. Why mothers die 1997–1999: The confidential enquiries into maternal deaths in the United Kingdom. London: RCOG Press: Department of Health, Welsh Office, Scottish Home and Health Department, Department of Health and Social Sciences, Northern Ireland, 2001:323–5
9. The Public Health Agency of Canada. Overview of the Canadian Perinatal Surveillance System. 2004. http://www.phac-aspc.gc.ca/rhs-ssg/overview-apercu-eng.php
10. The Society of Obstetricians and Gynaecologists of Canada. About SOGC. 2009. http://www.sogc.org/about/index_e.asp
11. Statistics Canada. About us. 2010. http://www.statcan.gc.ca/about-apercu/about-apropos-eng.htm
12. Canadian Institute for Health Information. Vision and Mandate. 2010. http://www.cihi.ca/CIHI-ext-portal/internet/EN/SubTheme/about+cihi/vision+and+mandate/cihi010703
13. Allen VM, Campbell M, Carson G, et al. Maternal mortality and severe morbidity surveillance in Canada. J Obstet Gynaecol Can 2010;32:1140–6
14. Maternal Health Study Group of the Canadian Perinatal Surveillance System. Special report on maternal mortality and severe morbidity in Canada. Enhanced surveillance: the path to prevention. Ottawa: Health Canada; 2004. http://www.phac-aspc.gc.ca/rhs-ssg/srmm-rsmm/index-eng.php
15. Liu S, Joseph KS, Bartholomew S, et al; Maternal Health Study Group of the Canadian Perinatal Surveillance System. http://www.ncbi.nlm.nih.gov/pubmed/21050517 Temporal trends and regional variations in severe maternal morbidity in Canada, 2003 to 2007. J Obstet Gynaecol Can 2010;32: 847–55
16. Joseph KS, Liu S, Rouleau J, et al; Maternal Health Study Group of the Canadian Perinatal Surveillance System. http://www.ncbi.nlm.nih.gov/pubmed/21050516 Severe maternal morbidity in Canada, 2003 to 2007: surveillance using routine hospitalization data and ICD-10CA codes. J Obstet Gynaecol Can 2010;32:837–46

19

Problems in Determining Accurate Rates of Postpartum Hemorrhage

J. C. Bello-Munoz and L. Cabero-Roura

INTRODUCTION

Postpartum hemorrhage (PPH) plays a major role in maternal mortality. It represents a risk that attends every delivery, and is an impending danger to every childbearing woman in the world. The chance of dying is not the same for everyone[1], as a number of factors may lead to a severe, life-threatening condition and to an adverse outcome. These conditions are not the same in every region of the world, but tend to worsen as do economic conditions. For many years, PPH was considered a public health issue, primarily in low resource countries. In recent years, however, often because of an improvement in the quality of patients' clinical records, industrialized countries have witnessed what appears to be a slow but steady increase in the incidence of PPH, particularly due to post-partum uterine atony (PPUA)[2]. PPUA is the most common cause of PPH[3]. However, all sources do not share the same definition or accept the same criteria of what is PPH; the very definition of PPH is not uniform in all jurisdictions; and the same may be said for the method of measuring the amount of blood loss. Remarkable differences also exist regarding what is accepted as immediate, early, or late PPH. Therefore, it is difficult to quantify and even to analyse to what extent it is true that this pathology is increasing[4]. Possible causes of the variations cited here remain unclear, and no single cause has yet been identified as being responsible. However, as described later in this chapter, many different elements may be involved[5].

Notwithstanding these limitations, some indirect indicators point towards similar trends during recent years, for example, the number of transfusions administered within the first 12 hours postdelivery or the number of transfused blood derivatives (erythrocyte concentrates, platelets, etc.)[6]. In addition, population-based studies from Canada, Ireland, Australia, France, Norway, USA and other countries have demonstrated an increase in the incidence of PPH during the past decade[7–13]. It is true that during this same period a number of changes in obstetric practice as well as maternal demographic characteristics may have contributed to an increased risk of PPH; these include an increase in the rate of cesarean delivery[14], a larger proportion of multiple births[15], and more pregnant women of advanced maternal age[16,17]. However, there is insufficient evidence to support the proposition that these changes alone can be responsible for this increase. Furthermore, some well designed studies fail to find these reputed causative factors, but find other possible risk factors[1,18].

To date, there are surprisingly few population-based studies on PPH, particularly longitudinal studies. Most studies investigating risk factors for this condition have been small[11], case-controlled[13] or hospital-based[13,15–17] in design. These studies vary regarding the classification of PPH in terms of amount of blood loss, actual measurement of hemorrhage and the accompanying markers of hemodynamic compromise. Moreover, very few have considered the covariates in multivariate analysis[2,5]. Despite the wide variation in design and results, the coinciding trends towards an increase is striking when the results are plotted (Figure 1).

Recently, several collaborative studies have searched for the relationship between specific risk factors and the increased incidence of PPH. Unfortunately most of the data are heterogeneous and reliable comparison of collected data remains a difficult task. In 2009, the International Collaborative Group, which included representatives from Australia, Belgium, Canada, France, UK and USA, presented the results of pooled data from studies carried out in their respective countries[4]. Some of the issues raised at that meeting are summarized here.

Australia

Some of the sources employed by the International Collaborative Group were national registers, for example, in Australia, the data came from the Admitted Patient Data Collection (APDC), which carries the registers of every hospital discharge record in New South Wales (NSW)[19]. Diagnoses and procedures are coded according to the International Statistical Classification of Diseases and Related Health Problems, Australian Modification (ICD-9 to July 1998 and ICD-10 subsequently) and the affiliated Australian Classification of Health Interventions. PPH is defined as a hemorrhage of 500 ml or more following vaginal

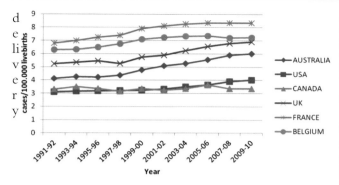

Figure 1 Maternal death attributable to PPH in developed countries. Data adapted from Knight *et al.* 2009[4], with permission

or 750 ml or more following a cesarean delivery resulting in a recorded clinical diagnosis of PPH and identified during the birth hospitalization from the hospital data. Data for Victoria were derived from the perinatal data collection form. The ICD-10AM definition of PPH was also used.

In the case of the Australian registers, in at least two regions, NSW and Victoria, a continuous increase in PPH was registered between 1991 and 2006 despite a stepped change between 1998/1999 which might be related to a change in definition of PPH from 600 to 500 ml)[20]. *In NSW*, Cameron *et al.*[21] assessed trends and outcomes of PPH in a population-based descriptive study of 52,151 women who had PPH either at the time of delivery or requiring a re-admission to hospital for this condition in the years between 1994 and 2002. The outcome measures included maternal death, hysterectomy, admission to intensive care unit (ICU), transfusion and major maternal morbidity, including procedures to reduce blood supply to the uterus, acute renal failure and postpartum coagulation defects. The author found that, during that period, both the number and adjusted (for under-reporting) rate of PPH during the birth admission increased from 8.3% to 10.7% of deliveries. The rate of PPH adjusted for maternal age and mode of delivery was similar to the unadjusted rate. There was a six-fold increase in the rate of transfusions among women who hemorrhaged from 1.9% to 11.7%. At the same time, the hospital re-admissions for PPH declined from 1.2% of deliveries to 0.9%. These changes were statistically significant, although no significant changes occurred in the rates of hysterectomies, procedures to reduce blood supply to the uterus, admissions to ICU, acute renal failure or coagulation defects.

Canada

In Canada, information was based on all hospital deliveries as documented in the Discharge Abstract Database of the Canadian Institute for Health Information from 1991 to 2005[7,8,22]. All medical diagnoses were coded according to the ICD, whereas specific procedures were coded using the Canadian

Classification of Diagnostic, Therapeutic and Surgical Procedures (CCP) and the Canadian Classification of Interventions (CCI). PPH was coded if blood loss after childbirth exceeded 500 ml after a vaginal delivery, 1000 ml after a cesarean delivery or when the physician made a notation of PPH in the medical chart.

The Canadian authors used code the ICD-9, registering PPH and, lately, ICD-10 codes for PPH due to retained placenta (third stage hemorrhage), uterine atony (immediate PPH, within the first 24 hours following delivery of placenta), delayed and secondary PPH (after the first 24 hours following delivery) and PPH due to coagulation defects, respectively. It is important to emphasize that those women whose deliveries were complicated by PPH and who additionally had an abdominal hysterectomy were identified using the relevant CCP and CCI codes. Blood transfusions were identified using a specific code introduced in the database in 1994 (blood transfusion rates were unavailable before that year).

France

The information from France came through the published PPH data by Dupont *et al.*[23]. According to these data, PPH occurred in 1144 of 21,350 deliveries, an overall incidence of $5.4 \pm 0.3\%$. Among these, 316 cases were coded as severe. Diagnosis was clinical in 82.5% of severe cases and 77.5% of non-severe cases; the remainder were detected by postpartum laboratory tests. Uterotonic agents were given prophylactically to 46.7% of the 896 patients following vaginal delivery. In cases in which PPH was due to uterine atony, 83.1% of women underwent examination of the uterine cavity and 96.3% received oxytocin, which proved to be therapeutic. Sulprostone was administered to 39.5% cases of persistent PPH. Regarding cesarean delivery, a uterotonic was given prophylactically to 85.4% of the 247 patients delivered. Oxytocin was therapeutic in 94.8% of cases of uterine atony. Sulprostone was administered in 84.4% of cases of persistent PPH. However, the median delay for second-line pharmacological treatment was significantly shortened (from 80 min, range 35–130, in 2002 to 32.5 min, range 20–75 in 2005). An increase was observed in the use of surgery for PPH (0.06% versus 0.12% of deliveries; $p = 0.03$) and in blood transfusions (0.18% versus 0.33%; $p = 0.01$). Nonetheless, the prevalence of major PPH did not change (0.80% versus 0.86% of deliveries; $p = 0.62$)[24].

United Kingdom

In the UK, the information from Scottish sources was obtained from the Scottish Confidential Audit of Severe Maternal Morbidity[25]. UK data on PPH, including data from England, Scotland, Wales and Northern Ireland were obtained from the UK Obstetric Surveillance System (UKOSS) survey of hemorrhage-associated peripartum hysterectomy and severe obstetric hemorrhage in UK between 2003 and

2007[26]. In their registers, 318 women underwent peripartum hysterectomy. The most commonly reported causes of hemorrhage were uterine atony (53%) and morbidly adherent placenta (39%). Women were not universally managed with uterotonic therapies. Fifty women were unsuccessfully managed with B-Lynch or other brace suture prior to hysterectomy, 28 with activated factor VII and nine with arterial embolization. Twenty-one per cent of women suffered damage to other structures, 20% required a further operation and 19% were reported to have additional severe morbidity. Bladder damage was more likely in women with placenta accreta than in women with uterine atony. There were no significant differences in outcomes between women undergoing total or subtotal hysterectomy. Two women died resulting in a case fatality rate of 0.6% (95% CI 0–1.5%). Regarding changes in incidence, a mild increase in the numbers of PPH was documented during the study period, particularly when evaluating the past 6 years.

Belgium

In Belgium, data came from the hospital discharge data for the Flanders region, and to determine the proportion of women receiving a blood transfusion within 24 h of birth as a proxy for PPH[12,27]. A population-based study reported an increase in the risk of severe PPH associated with induction of labor (OR 1.71)[12]. However, further analysis of data on peripartum hysterectomy to control PPH in the region did not show an association with induction of labor even after adjustment for previous cesarean delivery. According to authors' findings, labor induction and other changes in obstetric practice could lead to an increased duration of labor, in both first and second stage, which might contribute to the already documented increase in the frequency of PPH.

United States

In the US data used by the International Collaborative Group were obtained from the Nationwide Inpatient Sample (NIS) for 1994–2006 (partially summarized in Figure 1)[28–30]. The NIS is a large public-use administrative dataset that includes approximately 20% of all of the discharges from non-Federal, acute-care hospitals in the US. The database is maintained by the Agency for Healthcare Research and Quality as part of the Healthcare Utilization Project. The database contains up to 15 diagnosis fields and 15 procedure fields; diagnoses and procedures are coded at the hospital at the time of discharge using the ICD-9-CM[15]. Patients were subsequently stratified based on the presumed etiology of their PPH according to the categories defined in the ICD-9 classification: 666.0 for PPH from retained placenta (including placenta accreta), 666.1 for PPH from uterine atony, 666.2 for delayed and secondary PPH (after the first 24 hours after delivery), and 666.3 for PPH caused by coagulation defects.

Patients who received transfusion of blood products or who underwent a peripartum hysterectomy were also identified using the ICD-9 codes. Deliveries in which maternal age was not recorded were excluded from analysis.

In summary, findings indicated that, during the period 1996–2004, the percentage of deliveries with a diagnostic code of PPH increased by 26% (from 2.3 to 2.9% of all deliveries). This change in incidence was mainly due to uterine atony. It is worth mentioning that the highest rate of uterine atony occurred among women whose labor was induced and who delivered vaginally. This was followed by women whose induction ended in cesarean delivery and women who had vaginal births without induction of labor. Women, who had cesarean deliveries and did not have induced labor, consistently had the lowest rates of PPH caused by atony.

According to this particular register, women who had vaginal deliveries were at increased risk for PPH. However, the data from the past 2 years show that, the incidence of PPH is similar for all groups (spontaneous, induced, failed induction and scheduled cesarean section). Thus, the percentage change in uterine atony was dramatically greater for cesarean deliveries compared with vaginal deliveries.

COLLABORATIVE GROUP OBSERVATIONS

The International Collaborative Group, observed an increasing trend in coded PPH between 1991 and 2006 in Canada, NSW (Australia) and the USA. The observed increase in coded PPH was limited solely to immediate/atonic PPH, rather than late PPH, which is a noteworthy finding[4].

Severity of PPH was also documented in some areas, with increasing transfusion rates at childbirth in the USA and Australia, but not in Canada or Flanders[5,15,16,20]. The rate of hysterectomy for peripartum hemorrhage remained stable between 1997–1998 and 2005–2006 in the UK[12,17], although in Canada rates of hysterectomy for atonic PPH increased from 24.0 per 100,000 deliveries in 1991 to 41.7 per 100,000 deliveries in 2004 (a 73% increase, 95% CI 27–137)[31]. On the other hand, maternal mortality from hemorrhage appeared to be relatively static (Australia between 1994–1996 and 2003–2005[18,19], France between 1997–1999 and 2000–2002[10], UK between 1985–1987 and 2003–2005[20], US between 1998 and 2004)[9], although the rate of Sheehan's syndrome increased in Canada from 3.7 per million deliveries in 1991–1993 to 12.6 in 2002–2004 (241% increase, 95% CI 8% decrease to 1,158% increase $p = 0.10$; p value or increasing annual linear trend = 0.008)[32]. Unfortunately, similar data were not available from other countries. In Canada no evidence of an increase in maternal mortality from PPH and/or in blood transfusion for PPH was seen.

In all populations examined, maternal age at childbirth was increasing[12,16,33–35], cesarean delivery was becoming more common[14,17,36], and multiple pregnancy rates were also increasing[15,37,38]. The proportion of induced labors increased over a similar time period as the observed increase in PPH[7,16,27,39]

The International Collaborative Group also investigated possible associations between environmental contaminants, toxins or environmental toxins, alternative/complementary medicine, antidepressants and PPH but failed to identify environmental factors that may have been responsible for these recent increases[23].

RELATED ISSUES

Variations in definition

It is unfortunate that no single definition of PPH is accepted. In some countries definitions are 500 ml for a vaginal delivery and 1000 ml for a cesarean section. In contrast, a blood loss of 500 ml for a vaginal delivery and 750 ml for a cesarean delivery is used in Australia[20], and in others the 500 ml blood loss is used to define PPH irrespective of the mode of delivery; further research is required to investigate how definitions are applied in practice to the coding of data. Regardless of the specific definitions used, routine visual estimates of blood loss are frequently inaccurate[30,31] (see Chapters 9 and 11), and recent analyses using calculated blood losses demonstrate that many and perhaps most women lose sufficient blood at delivery to meet the diagnostic criteria for PPH[31,32].

Alternatively, PPH has been defined as a 10% or more drop in hematocrit[1]. The use of blood transfusions and procedures to control bleeding have both been used as markers of the severity of PPH and to identify women with severe pregnancy morbidity[2,3,6,25,40]. How these definitions are used, their inherent inaccuracies, and the translation of definitions to administrative ICD coding may complicate the interpretation of trend data. In Australia, Scotland and the USA, for example, increases in the reported rates of severe complications of childbirth have been almost entirely due to increases in the use of blood transfusions and/or severe obstetric hemorrhage[10,41–45]. In these countries, it appears that not only are PPH rates increasing, but so is the hemorrhage severity. In contrast, Canadian rates of severe maternal morbidity remained stable between 1991 and 2000 in the context of comparatively low and stable rates of transfusion[4,7,15]. Such international differences may reflect differing attitudes among obstetricians about blood transfusions[16,37,46].

It has been suggested that restriction of a definition of PPH to 500 ml or 750 ml of blood loss is somewhat arbitrary and does not take into account other markers of hemodynamic compromise and the wide variation in maternal blood volume that can be lost without risking the patient's life[24]. As noted previously in this chapter and in many other chapters in this volume, the visual estimation of blood loss almost invariably results in underestimation[47,48] (Chapter 9). Thus, while assessing severity of PPH was attempted in every

cited study by including transfused cases only, different authors were unable to model risk factors due to the relatively few well documented cases of transfusion in the early years of the different surveys and the considerably broad variation in transfusion numbers over the periods the studies were carried out. Similarly, coexistence of coding indicating a hysterectomy had been used as a marker for severity, but here again too few studies attempting a multivariate analysis were found.

It is important to keep in mind that a diagnosis of PPH must be reported in the medical record by a clinician, obstetrician or midwife for a case to be coded as such by medical coders. Clinicians might be unwilling to record a diagnosis of PPH unless there are accompanying signs of compromise.

Regarding the issue of potential differences in the recording of PPH, the ICD-9 has a universal code for this diagnosis. Also, a single code is available for all types of retained, trapped and adherent placenta with hemorrhage. Considering that the necessity of separating codes for adherent placenta might be useful, given the increases in the frequency of cesarean delivery, such a code was added to the ICD-10. The Australian local modification introduced in 2002 (adding a code for morbidly adherent placenta, including placenta accreta, increta and percreta), enabled subsequent study on this population[34]. One of the suggestions made by the International Collaborative Group was that future revisions of the ICD should include separate codes for atonic PPH and PPH immediately following childbirth due to other causes. Also, additional codes are required for placenta accreta/percreta/increta. This recommendation is supported by the fact that currently collected data do not allow adequate categorization of PPH according to severity; this deficiency inhibits the ability to determine outcomes for women with differing degrees of blood loss.

Despite the quite well described pathways for solution, for example by recording actual estimated blood loss using a simple blood collector bag[48], the different strategies to manage the third stage of labor, and the different guidelines pointing to the timing and route of prophylactic oxytocic administration, as well as surgical procedures and therapies undertaken to control PPH as fully described in the other chapters of this volume[6–8,13,17,23,29,44], the fact remains that PPH and uterine atony both are slightly and steadily increasing in their respective incidences.

Additional factors

[Editor's note: The factors described below are also mentioned in greater or lesser detail in other chapters of this volume L.G.K.]

A number of factors appear to be acting in concert to influence the increased incidence of PPH in developed countries. In the populations cited above, *maternal age* at childbirth has been increasing significantly[6,16,49], and although, the vast majority of studies failed to demonstrate a clear impact of aging on PPH rates[5,6,39], increasing maternal age has been consistently described to be a substantial risk factor in all registers of obstetric hysterectomy for PPH[5,12,40].

At the same time, in the UK, Australia and in the vast majority of the European countries, births of *immigrant women* are increasing[22,23,41–45], and the rates of severe maternal morbidity, although not specifically PPH, are higher in women from *ethnic minority groups* albeit not consistently[22,50–54]. Also, the rising rates of *obesity* demonstrated in many countries[55–61] may also impact on the incidence of PPH; an increased body mass index (BMI) is a reported risk factor for hemorrhage[62–70].

Cesarean delivery is not only more frequent globally, but also results in a higher blood loss when compared to normal delivery[1,7,42]. Of interest, validation of data on PPH from NSW showed that there is significant under-recording of blood loss after cesarean delivery (60% of cesarean deliveries with recorded blood loss versus 96% of vaginal births)[19]. Additionally, post-cesarean transfusion for low hematocrit or post-cesarean section laparotomy for evacuation of hematoma are not captured as a part of the PPH code[14], which may explain the lack of increase in risk of PPH in women undergoing cesarean section in this population. Other studies have shown that the antecedent of a previous delivery by cesarean section is associated with increased risk of abnormal placentation, hemorrhage and peripartum hysterectomy[34,26,71,72]. In Canada, where PPH following cesarean delivery by definition requires a blood loss over 1000 ml, cesarean delivery was shown to have a protective effect on atonic PPH (adjusted odds ratio 0.52)[73].

Strikingly, the planned cesarean section seems to play a role in protection against PPH, and this has not been an isolated finding[74–81]. While, modeling yielded similar results to models including all singleton deliveries and also tended to confirm the major contribution of vaginal/instrumental deliveries to PPH[14,71,78, 80,82,83]; it remains possible, however, that there is a considerable underestimation of blood loss at cesarean delivery and consequent under-enumeration of cesarean deliveries with PPH[84]. Another possible explanation for the deceiving and apparently protective effect of cesarean section is that postsurgical patients may be under closer observation and are more likely to have early diagnosis of hemorrhage with earlier interventions than patients who deliver vaginally[71].

Another potential factor is the practice of *labor induction*, which is currently performed more often[13,23,25,28] than in the past. In some areas, this practice was associated with significantly increased odds for PPH[85]. In addition, after adjustment for mode of delivery, maternal age, birth weight and public/private admission status, the use of oxytocin infusion for augmentation also independently increased the odds for PPH (adjusted (a)OR 1.19)[35]. A population-based Norwegian study also reported an increase in the risk of severe PPH associated with induction of labor (aOR 1.71)[86]. Despite this,

secondary analysis of data on peripartum hysterectomy to control PPH in the UK did not show an association with induction of labor even after adjustment for previous cesarean delivery[66].

Labor induction and other changes in obstetric practice may lead to an increased duration of labor, in both first and second stage, which may contribute to an increase in the frequency of PPH. An increasing duration of labor over time has been demonstrated in Victoria (Australia) as well as in Nova Scotia (Canada)[20,36,37,85,87]. The Nova Scotia study found an increase in the risk of PPH related to an increasing duration of the second stage of labor[88]. A role for increased labor duration in PPH is also supported by the above mentioned UK study of hemorrhage-associated peripartum hysterectomy, which showed an independent association between peripartum hysterectomy and labor of 12 hours or greater duration. After adjusting for the effects of age, parity, previous cesarean section delivery, other uterine surgery and multiple pregnancy, the aOR remained at 3.04 (95% CI 1.52–6.08)[11]. This finding is also supported by data on atonic PPH in Canada, which show an increased risk after a prolonged first stage, prolonged second stage and prolonged labor (without specifying a definition)[84,89–91].

Multiple pregnancy rates are also increasing[10,15,17,38]; possible contributory factors include assisted reproductive techniques and, again, an aging population of women giving birth[90]. Multiple pregnancy has been associated with an increased risk of PPH and associated complications in a number of studies[5,12,57,58], and the observed rise in the rate of multiple pregnancy may logically contribute to increasing PPH incidence. However, although there was a significant increase in multiple pregnancies in NSW between 1994 and 2002 (1.4–1.7% of all pregnancies), there was no significant change in the proportion of PPH among multiple pregnancies. The PPH rate among multiple pregnancies varied from 2.5% in 1994 to 3.1% in 1996 and 2002 (with an average rate of 2.9%), representing an increase of 183 pregnancies, which in the overall context of PPH risk could be considered as inconsequential[85].

A secondary analysis of Canadian PPH data showed that multiple pregnancy, even after adjustment for cesarean delivery, labor induction, maternal characteristics and obstetric practices, failed to explain the increase in PPH rates, although it did explain some of the increase in hysterectomy for PPH[22].

Finally, it is quite possible that the rise in PPH rates may be associated with risk factors not included in the different models cited previously, including *chorioamnionitis*[92], *pyrexia* in labor[28,93,94], *overweight* leading to peripartum obesity[55,62,95], duration of the *third stage* of labor[86], *previous PPH*[37] and *placenta accreta*[72], although some studies have included *retained placenta* as a separate risk factor[96–99]. The role it plays in PPH could not be investigated in the vast majority of publications, due to retained placenta being included in the definition of PPH in the ICD-9 coding[8,9].

Other potential risk factors that could have a possible role include, the increased use of oxytocin in the management of *first stage of delivery*[24,27,100,101], and increased rates of coagulation disorders in the puerperium when using *dinoprostone* for cervical ripening, although this risk seems to be low[101]. However, when all these facts act together, even if only slightly, they can account for a change which has impacted on the overall risk of PPH.

Furthermore, changes in the management of the third stage of labor may have affected rates of PPH. There is clear evidence that *active management of the third stage* of labor reduces PPH when compared to physiological or expectant management. It also substantially, decreases bleeding and transfusion requirements as well as postpartum hysterectomies[7,46,86,99,100,102,103]. Active management involves drug administration, early umbilical cord clamping and controlled cord traction, whereas expectant management involves waiting for signs of separation and allowing the placenta to deliver spontaneously or aided by gravity or nipple stimulation.

Over the period of these studies (1994–2002) and across the world, it is likely that variations in third stage management occurred. A Cochrane systematic review was not published until 2000 and state and national policies/recommendations regarding third stage management not introduced until 2002–2003. A more recent report indicates there has been considerable variation in active or expectant management, midwifery practices such as fundal massage and in the choice and dose of prophylactic drug used (i.e. ergometrine–oxytocin or oxytocin)[30]. Oxytocin is now more commonly used than ergometrine–oxytocin, having fewer maternal side-effects; however, it has been shown to be slightly less effective in reducing the risk of PPH of 500–1000 ml[12]. Misoprostol has been shown to play a role in controlling PPUA with higher success rates than oxytocin[7,93,104,105]. Competing interests of mothers and babies have also complicated third stage management with delayed cord clamping recommended for preterm babies. Completed studies on management or length of the third stage of labor were not available at the time of this review[35,91,106,107].

Matters of controversy

Studies findings are not always consistent with the commonly held belief that increasing rates of PPH are due to changes in maternal characteristics and obstetric procedures. In particular, increased PPH rates were not consistently explained by increases in maternal age, cesarean section, multiple pregnancy, induction/augmentation of labor or epidural use.

It is also noteworthy that, the 'classic' risk factors for PPH reflected in the recent literature corroborate those found in older series: *large babies*[108,109], *placental abnormalities*[72], *induction*[30] and *instrumental delivery*[38,110], which were the strongest predictors of PPH after adjustment for other factors[8,28,111,112]. Yet, those risk factors are claimed to be under control in the developed world.

So, if the increase in PPH rates is not related to increases in the proportion of cesarean deliveries, or trends in other risk factors, what is it due to? One possible explanation may be changes in reporting or ascertainment. Changes in reporting, such as the change from ICD-9 to ICD-10 in 1998 (which did not alter PPH coding), and the introduction of a statewide policy for management and reporting of PPH in 2002 do not coincide with observed increases in the PPH rate, which occurred primarily between 1994 and 1999. It is possible that hospitals may have been directed by state health authorities or their own administrators to vary their coding practice from the national/state standard for local reasons, thus introducing inconsistent practices between hospitals[20,23,26,41,102], although there is no reason to assume this is widespread or would have resulted in a false increase in reported cases.

Accounting for changes in risk factors

As we noted earlier in this chapter, attempts to explain the increase in PPH rates by taking into account changes in the observed risk factors for PPH over time cannot convincingly explain the rise in these rates. Ford *et al.* investigated risk factors for any PPH among singleton deliveries in Australia over the period 1994–2002[85], while Joseph *et al.* investigated risk factors for atonic PPH among deliveries in Canada over the period 1991–2004[8]. Using different methods, the two studies took into account maternal age, parity, year of birth, country of birth, onset of labor, mode of delivery, epidural analgesia, abnormal labor (precipitate labor, incoordinate contractions, etc.), prolonged or obstructed labor, hypertensive disorders, placental abnormalities (placenta or vasa previa), placental abruption, gestational age, birth weight, perineal trauma, cervical laceration, previous cesarean, multiple pregnancy, polyhydramnios and amniotic cavity infection. Both studies concluded that although the frequency of many risk and protective factors for PPH changed during the studies period, controlling for these factors did not seem to alter temporal trends, suggesting factors other than those considered were responsible for the rising PPH rates.

The authors postulated that other factors such as a more liberal approach to duration of labor, which allows women to labor for longer (information which was not collected with sufficient detail in any of the series), increases in obesity (not recorded in all hospital records) or changes in the management of third stage of labor (not always recorded in hospital data) may play a part in rising PPH rates. Other possible risk factors merit further investigation and should include the effect of induction of labor − taking into account agents used − or the infinitely more complex interactions of risk factors such as the interplay between body mass index, oxytocin agents or misoprostol during third stage management and subsequent blood loss[7,97,104,113,114].

Better and comparable data, particularly in areas where ascertainment is available from multiple datasets, will help to resolve some of the limitations of previous studies that rely on hospital discharge data which may under-ascertain the above-mentioned risk factors[115], lack information on sociodemographic factors[45,50,116–119], and not accurately capture antenatal history[120].

CONCLUSION AND KEY RECOMMENDATIONS

The incidence of PPH seems to be rising in the industrialized countries. In spite of multiple possible confounding factors, this appears as a real and concerning problem. An important number of risk factors could be considered as directly involved; however, none accounts substantially for the situation. The most likely scenario is a gathering of all these factors, which leads to this increase as the final outcome.

References

1. Rath WH. Postpartum hemorrhage—update on problems of definitions and diagnosis. Acta Obstet Gynecol Scand 2011;90:421–8
2. Deneux-Tharaux C, Dupont C, Colin C, et al. Multifaceted intervention to decrease the rate of severe postpartum haemorrhage: the PITHAGORE6 cluster-randomised controlled trial. BJOG 2010;117:1278–87
3. Lutomski J, Byrne B, Devane D, Greene R. Increasing trends in atonic postpartum haemorrhage in Ireland: an 11-year population-based cohort study. BJOG 2012;119:306–14
4. Knight M, Callaghan WM, Berg C, et al. Trends in postpartum hemorrhage in high resource countries: a review and recommendations from the International Postpartum Hemorrhage Collaborative Group. BMC Pregnancy Childbirth 2009;9:55
5. Gissler M, Alexander S, MacFarlane A, et al. Stillbirths and infant deaths among migrants in industrialized countries. Acta Obstet Gynecol Scand 2009;88:134–48
6. Burtelow M, Riley E, Druzin M, Fontaine M, Viele M, Goodnough LT. How we treat: management of life-threatening primary postpartum hemorrhage with a standardized massive transfusion protocol. Transfusion 2007;47:1564–72
7. Leduc D, Senikas V, Lalonde AB, et al. Active management of the third stage of labour: prevention and treatment of postpartum hemorrhage. J Obstet Gynaecol Can 2009;31:980–93
8. Kramer MS, Dahhou M, Vallerand D, Liston R, Joseph KS. Risk factors for postpartum hemorrhage: can we explain the recent temporal increase? J Obstet Gynaecol Can 2011;33:810–9
9. Callaghan WM, Kuklina EV, Berg CJ. Trends in postpartum hemorrhage: United States, 1994–2006. Am J Obstet Gynecol 2010;202:353.e1–6
10. Kayem G, Kurinczuk J, Lewis G, Golightly S, Brocklehurst P, Knight M. Risk factors for progression from severe maternal morbidity to death: a national cohort study. PLoS ONE 2011;6:e29077
11. Hinshaw K, Simpson S, Cummings S, Hildreth A, Thornton J. A randomised controlled trial of early versus delayed oxytocin augmentation to treat primary dysfunctional labour in nulliparous women. BJOG 2008;115:1289–1295; discussion 1295–1296
12. Cammu H, Martens G, Van Maele G, Amy J-J. The higher the educational level of the first-time mother, the lower the fetal and post-neonatal but not the neonatal mortality in Belgium (Flanders). Eur J Obstet Gynecol Reprod Biol 2010;148:13–6
13. Wong TY. Emergency peripartum hysterectomy: a 10-year review in a tertiary obstetric hospital. N Z Med J 2011;124:34–9.
14. Chang C-C, Wang I-T, Chen Y-H, Lin H-C. Anesthetic management as a risk factor for postpartum hemorrhage after cesarean deliveries. Am J Obstet Gynecol 2011;205:462.e1–7
15. Walker MC, Murphy KE, Pan S, Yang Q, Wen SW. Adverse maternal outcomes in multifetal pregnancies. BJOG 2004;111:1294–6
16. Montan S. Increased risk in the elderly parturient. Curr Opin Obstet Gynecol 2007;19:110–2
17. Attilakos G, Psaroudakis D, Ash J, et al. Carbetocin versus oxytocin for the prevention of postpartum haemorrhage following caesarean section: the results of a double-blind randomised trial. BJOG 2010;117:929–36
18. Ford JB, Algert CS, Kok C, Choy MA, Roberts CL. Hospital data reporting on postpartum hemorrhage: under-estimates recurrence and over-estimates the contribution of uterine atony. Matern Child Health J [Internet]. 2011; http://www.ncbi.nlm.nih.gov/pubmed/22109815
19. Roberts CL, Ford JB, Algert CS, Bell JC, Simpson JM, Morris JM. Trends in adverse maternal outcomes during childbirth: a population-based study of severe maternal morbidity. BMC Pregnancy Childbirth 2009;9:7
20. Ford JB, Roberts CL, Simpson JM, Vaughan J, Cameron CA. Increased postpartum hemorrhage rates in Australia. Int J Gynaecol Obstet 2007;98:237–43
21. Cameron CA, Roberts CL, Olive EC, Ford JB, Fischer WE. Trends in postpartum haemorrhage. Aust N Z J Public Health 2006;30:151–6
22. Fuller-Thomson E, Rotermann M, Ray JG. Elevated risk factors for adverse pregnancy outcomes among Filipina-Canadian women. J Obstet Gynaecol Can 2010;32:113–9
23. Dupont C, Deneux-Tharaux C, Touzet S, et al. Clinical audit: a useful tool for reducing severe postpartum haemorrhages? Int J Qual Health Care 2011;23:583–9
24. Audureau E, Deneux-Tharaux C, Lefèvre P, et al. Practices for prevention, diagnosis and management of postpartum haemorrhage: impact of a regional multifaceted intervention. BJOG 2009;116:1325–33
25. Peacock L, Clark V. Cell Salvage in obstetrics: a review of data from the 2007 Scottish Confidential Audit of Severe Maternal Morbidity. Int J Obstet Anesth 2011;20:196–8
26. Knight M. Peripartum hysterectomy in the UK: management and outcomes of the associated haemorrhage. BJOG 2007;114:1380–7
27. Belghiti J, Kayem G, Dupont C, Rudigoz R-C, Bouvier-Colle M-H, Deneux-Tharaux C. Oxytocin during labour and risk of severe postpartum haemorrhage: a population-based, cohort-nested case-control study. BMJ Open 2011;1:e000514
28. Mousa HA, Alfirevic Z. Treatment for primary postpartum haemorrhage. In: The Cochrane Collaboration, Mousa HA, eds. Cochrane Database of Systematic Reviews [Internet]. Chichester, UK: John Wiley & Sons, Ltd; 2007 http://doi.wiley.com/10.1002/14651858.CD003249.pub2
29. Chu SY, Kim SY, Bish CL. Prepregnancy obesity prevalence in the United States, 2004–2005. Matern Child Health J 2009;13:614–20
30. Caughey AB, Sundaram V, Kaimal AJ, et al. Maternal and neonatal outcomes of elective induction of labor. Evid Rep Technol Assess 2009;(176):1–257
31. Knight M, Kurinczuk JJ, Spark P, Brocklehurst P. Extreme obesity in pregnancy in the United Kingdom. Obstet Gynecol 2010;115:989–97
32. East CE, Leader LR, Sheehan P, Henshall NE, Colditz PB. Intrapartum fetal scalp lactate sampling for fetal assessment

in the presence of a non-reassuring fetal heart rate trace. Cochrane Database Syst Rev 2010;3:CD006174

33. Clark SL. Strategies for reducing maternal mortality. Semin. Perinatol 2012;36:42–7

34. Benson MD, Cheema N, Kaufman MW, Goldschmidt RA, Beaumont JL. Uterine intravascular fetal material and coagulopathy at peripartum hysterectomy. Gynecol Obstet Invest 2012;73:158–61

35. Clark SL, Hankins GDV. Preventing maternal death: 10 clinical diamonds. Obstet Gynecol 2012;119:360–4

36. Dupont C, Touzet S, Colin C, et al. Incidence and management of postpartum haemorrhage following the dissemination of guidelines in a network of 16 maternity units in France. Int J Obstet Anesth 2009;18:320–7

37. Ossola MW, Somigliana E, Mauro M, Acaia B, Benaglia L, Fedele L. Risk factors for emergency postpartum hysterectomy: the neglected role of previous surgically induced abortions. Acta Obstet Gynecol Scand 2011;90:1450–3

38. Zeeman GG. Obstetric critical care: a blueprint for improved outcomes. Crit Care Med 2006;34(9 Suppl): S208–14

39. Khaskheli M, Baloch S, Baloch AS. Obstetrical trauma to the genital tract following vaginal delivery. J Coll Physicians Surg Pak 2012;22:95–7

40. Markova V, Sørensen JL, Holm C, Nørgaard A, Langhoff-Roos J. Evaluation of multi-professional obstetric skills training for postpartum hemorrhage. Acta Obstet Gynecol Scand 2012;91:346–52

41. Saucedo M, Deneux-Tharaux C, Bouvier-Colle M-H. Understanding regional differences in maternal mortality: a national case-control study in France. BJOG 2011 [Epub ahead of print]

42. Kozuki N, Lee AC, Katz J. Moderate to severe, but not mild, maternal anemia is associated with increased risk of small-for-gestational-age outcomes. J Nutrit 2012;142: 358–62

43. De M, Biswas S, Ganguly RP, et al. Impact of increased rate of caesarean section on perinatal outcome: sociolegal evaluation. J Indian Med Assoc 2011;109:312–4

44. Belghiti J, Kayem G, Dupont C, Rudigoz R-C, Bouvier-Colle M-H, Deneux-Tharaux C. Oxytocin during labour and risk of severe postpartum haemorrhage: a population-based, cohort-nested case-control study. BMJ Open 2011;1: e000514

45. Kayem G, Kurinczuk J, Lewis G, Golightly S, Brocklehurst P, Knight M. Risk factors for progression from severe maternal morbidity to death: a national cohort study. PLoS ONE 2011;6:e29077

46. Su CW. Postpartum hemorrhage. Prim Care 2012;39: 167–87

47. Amat L, Sabrià J, Martínez E, Rodríguez NL, Querol S, Lailla JM. Cord blood collection for banking and the risk of maternal hemorrhage. Acta Obstet Gynecol Scand 2011;90: 1043–5

48. Zhang W-H, Deneux-Tharaux C, Brocklehurst P, Juszczak E, Joslin M, Alexander S. Effect of a collector bag for measurement of postpartum blood loss after vaginal delivery: cluster randomised trial in 13 European countries. BMJ 2010;340:c293

49. Holm C, Langhoff-Roos J, Petersen K, Norgaard A, Diness B. Severe postpartum haemorrhage and mode of delivery: a retrospective cohort study. BJOG 2012;119:1018

50. Haelterman E, Qvist R, Barlow P, Alexander S. Social deprivation and poor access to care as risk factors for severe pre-eclampsia. Eur J Obstet Gynecol Reprod Biol 2003; 111:25–32

51. Ramos GA, Caughey AB. The interrelationship between ethnicity and obesity on obstetric outcomes. Am J Obstet Gynecol 2005;193:1089–93

52. Taveras EM, Gillman MW, Kleinman K, Rich-Edwards JW, Rifas-Shiman SL. Racial/ethnic differences in early-life risk factors for childhood obesity. Pediatrics 2010;125: 686–95

53. Stacey T, Thompson JMD, Mitchell EA, Ekeroma AJ, Zuccollo JM, McCowan LME. Relationship between obesity, ethnicity and risk of late stillbirth: a case control study. BMC Pregnancy Childbirth 2011;11:3

54. Maternal, pregnancy, and birth characteristics of Asians and Native Hawaiians/Pacific Islanders—King County, Washington, 2003–2008. MMWR Morb Mortal Wkly Rep 2011;60:211–3

55. Tsoi E, Shaikh H, Robinson S, Teoh TG. Obesity in pregnancy: a major healthcare issue. Postgrad Med J 2010;86: 617–23

56. Beyerlein A, Lack N, von Kries R. Within-population average ranges compared with Institute of Medicine recommendations for gestational weight gain. Obstet Gynecol 2010; 116:1111–8

57. Gould Rothberg BE, Magriples U, Kershaw TS, Rising SS, Ickovics JR. Gestational weight gain and subsequent postpartum weight loss among young, low-income, ethnic minority women. Am J. Obstet Gynecol 2011;204:52.e1–11

58. Heslehurst N, Simpson H, Ells LJ, et al. The impact of maternal BMI status on pregnancy outcomes with immediate short-term obstetric resource implications: a meta-analysis. Obes Rev 2008;9:635–83

59. Shaikh H, Robinson S, Teoh TG. Management of maternal obesity prior to and during pregnancy. Semin Fetal Neonatal Med 2010;15:77–82

60. Magriples U, Kershaw TS, Rising SS, Westdahl C, Ickovics JR. The effects of obesity and weight gain in young women on obstetric outcomes. Am J Perinatol 2009;26:365–71

61. Galtier-Dereure F, Boegner C, Bringer J. Obesity and pregnancy: complications and cost. Am J Clin Nutr 2000;71(5 Suppl):1242S–8S

62. Nohr EA, Vaeth M, Baker JL, Sørensen TIA, Olsen J, Rasmussen KM. Pregnancy outcomes related to gestational weight gain in women defined by their body mass index, parity, height, and smoking status. Am J Clin Nutr 2009;90: 1288–94

63. Narchi H, Skinner A. Overweight and obesity in pregnancy do not adversely affect neonatal outcomes: new evidence. J Obstet Gynaecol 2010;30:679–86

64. McDonald SD, Han Z, Mulla S, Beyene J. Overweight and obesity in mothers and risk of preterm birth and low birth weight infants: systematic review and meta-analyses. BMJ 2010;341:c3428

65. Liu X, Du J, Wang G, Chen Z, Wang W, Xi Q. Effect of pre-pregnancy body mass index on adverse pregnancy outcome in north of China. Arch Gynecol Obstet 2011;283: 65–70

66. Mantakas A, Farrell T. The influence of increasing BMI in nulliparous women on pregnancy outcome. Eur J Obstet Gynecol Reprod Biol 2010;153:43–6

67. Usha Kiran TS, Hemmadi S, Bethel J, Evans J. Outcome of pregnancy in a woman with an increased body mass index. BJOG 2005;112:768–72

68. Jarvie E, Ramsay JE. Obstetric management of obesity in pregnancy. Semin Fetal Neonatal Med 2010;15:83–8

69. Higgins CA, Martin W, Anderson L, et al. Maternal obesity and its relationship with spontaneous and oxytocin-induced contractility of human myometrium in vitro. Reprod Sci 2010;17:177–85

70. Arrowsmith S, Wray S, Quenby S. Maternal obesity and labour complications following induction of labour in prolonged pregnancy. BJOG 2011;118:578–88

71. Skupski DW, Lowenwirt IP, Weinbaum FI, Brodsky D, Danek M, Eglinton GS. Improving hospital systems for the care of women with major obstetric hemorrhage. Obstet Gynecol 2006;107:977–83

72. Tikkanen M, Paavonen J, Loukovaara M, Stefanovic V. Antenatal diagnosis of placenta accreta leads to reduced blood loss. Acta Obstet Gynecol Scand 2011;90:1140–6

73. Ogueh O, Morin L, Usher RH, Benjamin A. Obstetric implications of low-lying placentas diagnosed in the second trimester. Int J Gynaecol Obstet 2003;83:11–7

74. Singh S, McGlennan A, England A, Simons R. A validation study of the CEMACH recommended modified early obstetric warning system (MEOWS). Anaesthesia 2012;67: 12–8

75. Ogueh O, Morin L, Usher RH, Benjamin A. Obstetric implications of low-lying placentas diagnosed in the second trimester. Int J Gynaecol Obstet 2003;83:11–7

76. Selo-Ojeme D, Rogers C, Mohanty A, Zaidi N, Villar R, Shangaris P. Is induced labour in the nullipara associated with more maternal and perinatal morbidity? Arch Gynecol Obstet 2011;284:337–41

77. Fox R, Evans K. Severe antepartum haemorrhage following membrane sweep. J Obstet Gynaecol 2005;25:211

78. Tussing AD, Wojtowycz MA. The effect of physician characteristics on clinical behavior: cesarean section in New York State. Soc Sci Med 1993;37:1251–60

79. Robson MS, Scudamore IW, Walsh SM. Using the medical audit cycle to reduce cesarean section rates. Am J Obstet Gynecol 1996;174:199–205

80. Goyert GL, Bottoms SF, Treadwell MC, Nehra PC. The physician factor in cesarean birth rates. N Engl. Med 1989; 320:706–9

81. Irion O, Hirsbrunner Almagbaly P, Morabia A. Planned vaginal delivery versus elective caesarean section: a study of 705 singleton term breech presentations. Br J Obstet Gynaecol 1998;105:710–7

82. Barnsley JM, Vayda E, Lomas J, et al. Cesarean section in Ontario: practice patterns and responses to hypothetical cases. Can J Surg 1990;33:128–32

83. Lilford RJ, van Coeverden de Groot HA, Moore PJ, Bingham P. The relative risks of caesarean section (intrapartum and elective) and vaginal delivery: a detailed analysis to exclude the effects of medical disorders and other acute pre-existing physiological disturbances. Br J Obstet Gynaecol 1990;97:883–92

84. Zhang W-H, Deneux-Tharaux C, Brocklehurst P, et al. Effect of a collector bag for measurement of postpartum blood loss after vaginal delivery: cluster randomised trial in 13 European countries. BMJ 2010;340:c293

85. Ford JB, Roberts CL, Simpson JM, Vaughan J, Cameron CA. Increased postpartum hemorrhage rates in Australia. Int J Gynaecol Obstet 2007;98:237–43

86. Winter C, Macfarlane A, Deneux-Tharaux C, et al. Variations in policies for management of the third stage of labour and the immediate management of postpartum haemorrhage in Europe. BJOG 2007;114:845–54

87. Leung NYW, Lau ACW, Chan KKC, Yan WW. Clinical characteristics and outcomes of obstetric patients admitted to the Intensive Care Unit: a 10-year retrospective review. Hong Kong Med J 2010;16:18–25

88. Allen VM, Baskett TF, O'Connell CM, McKeen D, Allen AC. Maternal and perinatal outcomes with increasing duration of the second stage of labor. Obstet Gynecol 2009;113: 1248–58

89. Oxman AD, Fretheim A, Lavis JN, Lewin S. SUPPORT Tools for evidence-informed health Policymaking (STP) 12: Finding and using research evidence about resource use and costs. Health Research Policy Syst 2009;7(Suppl 1):S12

90. Wang Y, Tanbo T, Åbyholm T, Henriksen T. The impact of advanced maternal age and parity on obstetric and perinatal outcomes in singleton gestations. Arch Gynecol Obstet 2010;284:31–7

91. Lalonde A, Daviss BA, Acosta A, Herschderfer K. Postpartum hemorrhage today: ICM/FIGO initiative 2004–2006. Int J Gynaecol Obstet 2006;94:243–53

92. Papanna R, Mann LK, Johnson A, Sangi-Haghpeykar H, Moise KJ. Chorioamnion separation as a risk for preterm premature rupture of membranes after laser therapy for twin-twin transfusion syndrome. Obstet Gynecol 2010;115: 771–6

93. Durocher J, Bynum J, León W, Barrera G, Winikoff B. High fever following postpartum administration of sublingual misoprostol. BJOG 2010;117:845–52

94. Gülmezoglu AM, Forna F, Villar J, Hofmeyr GJ. Prostaglandins for preventing postpartum haemorrhage. In: The Cochrane Collaboration, Gülmezoglu AM, ed. Cochrane Database of Systematic Reviews [Internet]. Chichester, UK: John Wiley & Sons, Ltd; 2007 http://doi.wiley.com/10.1002/14651858.CD000494.pub3

95. Sirimi N, Goulis DG. Obesity in pregnancy. Hormones (Athens) 2010;9:299–306

96. Weeks AD. The retained placenta. Best Pract Res Clin Obstet Gynaecol 2008;22:1103–17

97. van Beekhuizen HJ, Pembe AB, Fauteck H, Lotgering FK. Treatment of retained placenta with misoprostol: a randomised controlled trial in a low-resource setting (Tanzania). BMC Pregnancy Childbirth 2009;9:48

98. Tandberg A, Albrechtsen S, Iversen OE. Manual removal of the placenta, Incidence and clinical significance. Acta Obstet Gynecol Scand 1999;78:33–6

99. Dombrowski MP, Bottoms SF, Saleh AAA, Hurd WW, Romero R. Third stage of labor: Analysis of duration and clinical practice. Am J Obstet Gynecol 1995;172:1279–84

100. Ozalp E, Tanir HM, Sener T. Dinoprostone vaginal insert versus intravenous oxytocin to reduce postpartum blood loss following vaginal or cesarean delivery. Clin Exp Obstet Gynecol 2010;37:53–5

101. De Abajo FJ, Meseguer CM, Antiñolo G, et al. Labor induction with dinoprostone or oxytocine and postpartum disseminated intravascular coagulation: a hospital-based case-control study. Am J Obstet Gynecol 2004;191: 1637–43

102. Begley CM, Gyte GM, Devane D, McGuire W, Weeks A. Active versus expectant management for women in the third stage of labour. Cochrane Database Syst Rev 2011;11: CD007412

103. Dixon L, Tracy SK, Guilliland K, Fletcher L, Hendry C, Pairman S. Outcomes of physiological and active third stage labour care amongst women in New Zealand. Midwifery 2011 [Epub ahead of print]

104. Fawole AO, Sotiloye OS, Hunyinbo KI, et al. A double-blind, randomized, placebo-controlled trial of misoprostol and routine uterotonics for the prevention of postpartum hemorrhage. Int J Gynaecol Obstet 2011;112:107–11

105. Elati A, Weeks AD. The use of misoprostol in obstetrics and gynaecology. BJOG 2009;116(Suppl 1):61–9

106. Esler MD, Douglas MJ. Planning for hemorrhage. Steps an anesthesiologist can take to limit and treat hemorrhage in the obstetric patient. Anesthesiol Clin North Am 2003;21: 127–144

107. Shakur H, Elbourne D, Gulmezoglu M, et al. The WOMAN Trial (World Maternal Antifibrinolytic Trial): Tranexamic acid for the treatment of postpartum haemorrhage: an international randomised, double blind placebo controlled trial. Trials 2010;11:40

108. Narchi H, Skinner A. Infants of diabetic mothers with abnormal fetal growth missed by standard growth charts. J Obstet Gynaecol. 2009;29:609–13

109. Ben-Haroush A, Hadar E, Chen R, Hod M, Yogev Y. Maternal obesity is a major risk factor for large-for-gestational-infants in pregnancies complicated by gestational diabetes. Arch Gynecol Obstet 2009;279:539–43

110. Keriakos R, Chaudhuri S. Operative interventions in the management of major postpartum haemorrhage. J Obstet Gynaecol 2012;32:14–25

111. Vergani P, Locatelli A, Ratti M, et al. Predictors of adverse perinatal outcome in twins delivered at <37 weeks. J Matern Fetal Neonatal Med 2004;16:343–7

112. Bricker L, Peden H, Tomlinson AJ, et al. Titrated low-dose vaginal and/or oral misoprostol to induce labour for prelabour membrane rupture: a randomised trial. BJOG 2008;115:1503–11

113. Umar NI, Abdul MA, Jido TA, Tukur J, Dattijo LM. Disseminated intravascular coagulation following induction of labour with misoprostol: a case report. Niger J Med 2008; 17:156–8

114. Lokugamage AU, Refaey HE, Rodeck CH. Misoprostol and pregnancy: ever-increasing indications of effective usage. Curr Opin Obstet Gynecol 2003;15:513–8

115. Cedergren MI. Non-elective caesarean delivery due to ineffective uterine contractility or due to obstructed labour in relation to maternal body mass index. Eur J Obstet Gynecol Reprod Biol 2009;145:163–6

116. Souza JP, Cecatti JG, Faundes A, et al. Maternal near miss and maternal death in the World Health Organization's 2005 global survey on maternal and perinatal health. Bull World Health Organ 2010;88:113–9

117. Dempsey JC, Ashiny Z, Qiu C-F, Miller RS, Sorensen TK, Williams MA. Maternal pre-pregnancy overweight status and obesity as risk factors for cesarean delivery. J Matern Fetal Neonatal Med 2005;17:179–85

118. Galtier F, Raingeard I, Renard E, Boulot P, Bringer J. Optimizing the outcome of pregnancy in obese women: from pregestational to long-term management. Diabetes Metab 2008;34:19–25

119. Smith DM, Whitworth M, Sibley C, et al. The design of a community lifestyle programme to improve the physical and psychological well-being of pregnant women with a BMI of 30 kg/m2 or more. BMC Public Health 2010;10:284

120. Dodd JM, Grivell RM, Crowther CA, Robinson JS. Antenatal interventions for overweight or obese pregnant women: a systematic review of randomised trials. BJOG 2010;117:1316–26

20

Maternal Deaths from Major Obstetric Hemorrhage in the UK: Changing Evidence from the Confidential Enquiries (1985–2011)

D. Fleming, R. Gangopadhyay, M. Karoshi and S. Arulkumaran

INTRODUCTION

Tragically, despite the UK having one of the best maternity services in the world, women still die of a variety of causes related to childbirth. To understand better these causes and prevent their recurrence, the UK developed a process of reporting maternal mortality in the middle of the 19th century. It was not until 1952, however, that these Confidential Enquiries into Maternal Deaths began to assess formally the principal causes of maternal deaths, identify avoidable factors and recommend improvements in clinical care and service provision[1]. This continuing effort has been recognized as the world's finest medical audit and its presence has not only reshaped maternity services across UK, but also has a broad international influence.

Since 1985–1987, a single report published triennially has incorporated all maternal deaths in England, Wales, Scotland and Northern Ireland. As of 2003, the reports have been titled 'Saving Mothers' Lives'; previously, they were known as 'Why Mothers Die'.

The Confidential Enquiry into Maternal and Child Health (CEMACH) was established in April 2003, replacing the combined CEMD (Confidential Enquiries into Maternal Deaths) and CESDI (Confidential Enquiry into Stillbirths and Deaths in Infancy). The editorial efforts were incorporated into the Centre for Maternal and Child Enquiries (CMACE), a free standing charity in its own right since July 2009, and the triennial report in 2011 was published under the auspices of CMACE[2].

Of the important causes of maternal death in the UK, major obstetric hemorrhage (MOH) remained the third leading direct cause of maternal death between 1985 and 2005 except in 2000–2002 when it ranked second[3–9]. In the 2006–2008 report, it ranked as sixth[10].

Although encouraging, this decline is not statistically significant, and there is no place for complacency. It is unfortunate that even with a reduction in maternal deaths from MOH, the majority still result from substandard care (Figure 1). Occasionally, however, deaths are deemed unavoidable despite excellent care, as some cases have unusual presentations which delay clinical diagnosis and treatment[10].

This chapter follows the trends in maternal death contributed by MOH as described in the Confidential Enquiry reports over the past 23 years (since 1985). Table 1 summarizes the absolute numbers of maternal deaths from different causes of MOH. The evolutions of the different major causes of maternal deaths are outlined below.

PLACENTAL ABRUPTION

Substandard management of complications

Women died due to complications secondary to abruption such as disseminated intravascular coagulopathy (DIC) and end organ failures (renal, hepatic and respiratory including acute respiratory distress syndrome (ARDS)) when these complications were managed inadequately.

In earlier reports, substandard care due to fluid overload resulted in pulmonary edema, highlighting inadequacies in critical care in obstetrics, especially that not involving the anesthetists. However, since 2000–2002 maternal deaths secondary to inadequate supportive care have reduced significantly, although isolated deaths have occurred where abruption

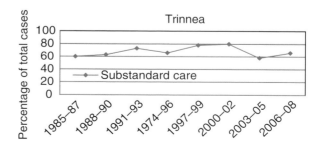

Figure 1 Trends in substandard care

Table 1 Direct deaths by type of obstetric hemorrhage and mortality rate UK: 1985–2008

Triennium	Causes of maternal deaths from MOH					
	Placental abruption	Placenta previa	PPH	Genital tract trauma	Total	Rate (per 100,000 maternities)
1985–1987	4	0	6	6	16	0.71
1988–1990	6	5	11	3	25	1.06
1991–1993	3	4	8	4	19	0.82
1994–1996	4	3	5	5	17	0.77
1997–1999	3	3	1	2	9	0.42
2000–2002	3	4	10	1	18	0.90
2003–2005	2	3	9	3	17	0.80
2006–2008	2	2	5	0	9	0.39

MOH, major obstetric hemorrhage

was complicated with amniotic fluid embolism (2000–2002).

Substandard care occurred in one case (1991–1993) after cesarean section for abruption when the patient developed bowel perforation secondary to active ulcerative colitis that was managed inappropriately by not involving surgeons at an early stage[5].

Complex clinical scenarios

Challenging cases included management of intra-uterine fetal death in women with previous uterine scars where differentiation between scar dehiscence and abruption delayed onset of appropriate treatment.

Other contributory factors

In the 1997–1999 report, a maternal death was considered unavoidable in a case of placental abruption where contributory factors (domestic violence and pulmonary hypertension) were present[6]. Such occurrences are rare and no further fatal outcomes of a similar nature have been reported to date.

PLACENTA PREVIA

Lack of consultant involvement

In late 1980s and early 1990s, a common cause of the provision of substandard care was the undertaking of a cesarean section for placenta previa by inexperienced obstetric registrars and, in a few instances, by inexperienced anesthetists. These conditions were accompanied by poor postoperative care and monitoring which led to delays in detecting intraperitoneal hemorrhage. Since 2000–2002, however, consultant (anesthetist and obstetrician) involvement in the management of placenta previa, especially in elective case therapy, has improved[8].

Inadequate diagnosis of placenta previa/accreta

The 1991–1993 report highlighted that less than optimal quality ultrasound scans could miss detection of low-lying placenta, especially in cases where the pelvic

anatomy was distorted. This led to many unexpected findings of placenta previa/accreta during emergency cesarean sections which were followed by MOH and maternal mortality[5].

Thereafter, subsequent recommendations emphasized the importance of confirming placental location in all cases, especially in women with previous uterine scars (cesarean section, myomectomy, uterine surgery). Later reports showed significant improvement in assessing placental location and in the diagnosis of morbidly adherent placenta.

Management of morbidly adherent placenta

The problem of placenta previa/accreta appears to be increasing, perhaps reflecting the increasing number of operative births. One key recommendation is to ensure that all women with previous cesarean sections undergo placental localization with ultrasound. Additional investigations are warranted using trans-abdominal and transvaginal probes and magnetic resonance imaging (MRI) if persisting anterior placenta previa is found. Although this is a standard practice in most UK units, it is not followed universally[9]. Despite excellent preoperative planning and management in placenta accreta/percreta, women still die from MOH and surgical complications as optimum management is still not uniform and often patients receive operations that may not be optimal for the site of the placental invasion (see Chapters by Palacios at the beginning of the book).

Failure to admit women with placenta previa at term

The 1994–1996 report[6] highlighted the importance of admitting women with placenta previa at term, especially in the presence of vaginal bleeding. Lessons were learnt and there were no further maternal deaths from this factor.

POSTPARTUM HEMORRHAGE

Deaths from PPH continue to outnumber those from antepartum hemorrhage.

Cesarean section (intra- and postoperative)

Lack of surgical competency

Inadequate primary hemostasis during cesarean section, followed by massive postoperative intraperitoneal hemorrhage, has been a constant and important cause of maternal mortality in most reports.

Inexperience of the trainees was highlighted since the 1994–1996 reports, whereby inexperienced trainees performed complex cesarean sections without adequate supervision leading to catastrophic complications in the immediate postoperative period. Although this may have been due to the introduction of a new training structure for the junior obstetric trainees, the involvement of more senior and experienced consultant obstetricians has been repeatedly emphasized in subsequent reports[5–7]. This has been followed by improvements in consultant involvement in recent reports[8–10], especially in elective cases.

Control of hemorrhage and resuscitation

Failure to seek consultant help early and delay in decision-making for radical surgery (such as hysterectomy) was crucial in many maternal deaths throughout the reports. The 1997–1999 report first mentioned conservative surgical techniques such as B-Lynch sutures and internal iliac artery ligations.

Some obstetric consultants may not have the necessary surgical skills such as cesarean hysterectomy. In these cases, early involvement of experienced gynecology consultants has been strongly recommended.

Lack of clinical leadership and poor communication between multidisciplinary teams also has been highlighted, especially since the 1997–1999 report, as contributing to the substandard care in emergency situations[7].

Failure to diagnose intraperitoneal hemorrhage in the postoperative period

This had been an important contributor to delay in resuscitation leading to maternal death. Inexperience of trainees again was highlighted as the most important cause of intraperitoneal hemorrhage in recent reports. Although the need for regular 'fire drills' has been highlighted in reports since 1991–1993[5], it was the 2003–2005 report that first recommended the modified obstetric early warning system (MEOWS) chart and regular training on maternal collapse. The recommendation was followed by significant improvement in postoperative care, as evident in the latest report. The MEOWS charts are now standard in many UK units[9].

Improper case selection

Routine booking of women with a high risk of bleeding during delivery/cesarean section was frequently reported till the late 1990s. Maternal deaths as a result of MOH, not surprisingly after cesarean section in cases complicated by severe thrombocytopenia, for example, occurred after booking in small district general hospitals without the facilities of a blood bank and intensive care units[3–5].

Instrumental delivery

Genital tract trauma following instrumental delivery leading to maternal death is rare but has been reported on occasion. Substandard care included lack of continuous vigilance by senior obstetricians, including the delegation to a senior house officer (SHO) of the repair of an extensive vaginal tear in a hypotensive patient (1998–2000).

In another instance, a broad ligament hematoma occurred after a difficult instrumental delivery by an SHO, and the woman later died of ARDS (1985–1987). Finally, an intractable atonic PPH followed an instrumental delivery but was unrelated to the procedure (1994–1996).

Spontaneous vaginal delivery

MOH secondary to atonic PPH following spontaneous vaginal delivery has declined since the 1997–1999 report[5]. Previously important contributory factors for atonic PPH were failure of diagnosis of clotting disorders (1985–1987), retained placenta (1988–1990), associated amniotic fluid embolism (AFE) and severe pre-eclamptic toxemia (PET) (1991–1993). Substandard care included delayed transfer to intensive therapy unit (ITU) for adequate supportive care after initial resuscitation.

Uterine rupture

There has been a significant decline in maternal deaths following uterine rupture since the 2003–2005 report. The main causes for uterine ruptures were prescribing high doses of prostaglandin for induction of labor in multiparous women and Syntocinon® augmentation in vaginal birth after cesarean section (VBAC)[9].

Coagulation disorders

Coagulation disorders often complicate MOH. A common cause of substandard care was failure of early diagnosis and treatment of DIC. In earlier reports (1985–1987), the occurrence of DIC was as high as 70% in the cases of maternal death due to MOH. Subsequent reports, however, have shown a decline in coagulation failure (less than 50% in 1988–1990 and approximately 27% in 1991–1993). No specific data have been presented on coagulation failure in association with MOH in subsequent reports. However, the incidence of DIC is still thought to be high, and recent reports repeatedly emphasize the need for early involvement of consultant hematologists in MOH to prevent and treat DIC[3–10].

Inaccurate estimation of blood loss

This remains a recurring contributory factor for maternal deaths due to MOH in all triennial reports. Reports since 1993–1995 have emphasized the awareness of health care professionals of the rapidly fatal consequences of MOH. Underestimation of blood loss leads to improper assessment of patients, delayed resuscitation and development of the coagulopathy, leading to maternal death.

In response to this recurring theme, the 2006–2008 report advocated the use of early warning scoring systems. These are used in other clinical areas, but need to be modified to account for the differences in maternal physiology in pregnancy. It is hoped that they will help in the more timely recognition, treatment and referral of women who have or are developing a critical response to illness. Such systems should not only be used in delivery suite settings, but also in all other clinical areas where pregnant women are managed (e.g. early pregnancy units, emergency departments and critical care).

The vital role of the anesthetic team has been highlighted in almost all reports. During resuscitation, the anesthetists have a major role in monitoring fluid, blood and blood product replacement. Management includes early use of invasive monitoring such as arterial and central venous pressure lines (specifically mentioned since the 1997–1999 report)[5].

Antenatal care

Correction of anemia

The importance of correcting anemia prior to delivery has been recommended since the 1985–1987 report. Despite this, correcting anemia in women with a high risk of hemorrhage still requires attention.

Early booking

Organizational failures with early booking have been highlighted since the 2000–2002 report. The 2003–2005 report specifically raised concerns regarding the adverse effects of late booking for women of ethnic minorities and women who do not speak English.

Women refusing antenatal care

This has contributed to maternal death in almost all triennial reports. These women mainly conceal their pregnancy due to a fear of the child being taken away after birth. Maternal deaths are considered almost unavoidable in such cases, especially if obstetric complications go undetected throughout antenatal period.

Women refusing blood products

In almost all triennial reports, women have died as a result of their religious beliefs and their refusal of blood products. It is inappropriate to influence these women's religious beliefs, but it is important that they are recognized and suitable plans put into place. The 1991–1993 CEMACH report added guidelines for 'The treatment of obstetric haemorrhage in women who refuse blood transfusion'. This was re-issued in 2000–2002 as 'Guidelines for the management and treatment of obstetric haemorrhage in women who decline blood transfusion'. Despite the presence of such guidelines, two deaths occurred in 2003–2005 in women refusing blood products. Specific recommendations included ensuring that guidelines are available to and discussed with all maternity staff. The roles of consultant obstetricians and anesthetic care are paramount in planning antenatal care and delivering these

women. Red blood cell salvage was recognized as a very effective intervention. These women ideally should be delivered in units which are familiar with this practice if they consent to the intervention.

Encouraging improvement in care

Place of care

High risk women need to be cared for in units with on-site blood bank and intensive care facilities. There has been significant improvement with proper case selection in low risk units.

Input from experienced operators

In early reports, it was not uncommon for inexperienced house officers or junior registrars to be managing complicated cases with indirect supervision. This delayed early active intervention with subsequent maternal deaths. With time this has been recognized and addressed, with calls for increased consultant presence on the labor ward. As junior training hours decrease, it is possible that consultants of the future may not have the full range of competencies. Accordingly, it is important to note that the attending clinician should have the appropriate experience as well as seniority.

Newer interventions

The triennial reports have emphasized the safety and effectiveness of the newer techniques such as B-Lynch sutures, intrauterine balloons and interventional radiology[8].

Recommendations

Early recognition of serious illness and effective, multidisciplinary, team working are key to avoiding potentially avoidable maternal deaths. Highlights of the important recommendations in the last eight reports are summarized in Figure 2.

Maternal morbidity

Since the 2003–2005 report, there has been mention on occasions of severe maternal morbidity following peripartum hysterectomy. The UK Obstetric Surveillance System (UKOSS) data on peripartum hysterectomy 2005–2006 revealed that the most common cause of hemorrhage was uterine atony (53%)[11].

Can maternal deaths secondary to MOH be entirely eliminated?

Based on the principles of modern medicine, in an ideal world, no mother should die of MOH. However, the reality may be far from this naive assumption. As noted above, there have been other causes of maternal deaths apart from substandard clinical care. The examples include women refusing blood products

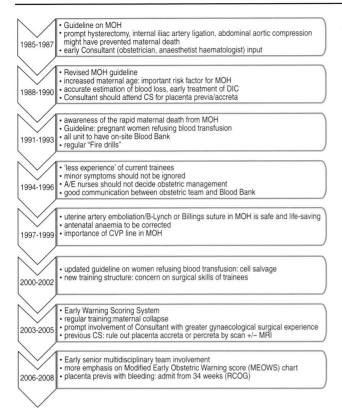

| 1985-1987 | • Guideline on MOH
• prompt hysterectomy, internal iliac artery ligation, abdominal aortic compression might have prevented maternal death
• early Consultant (obstetrician, anaesthetist haematologist) input |

| 1988-1990 | • Revised MOH guideline
• increased maternal age: important risk factor for MOH
• accurate estimation of blood loss, early treatment of DIC
• Consultant should attend CS for placenta previa/accreta |

| 1991-1993 | • awareness of the rapid maternal death from MOH
• Guideline: pregnant women refusing blood transfusion
• all unit to have on-site Blood Bank
• regular "Fire drills" |

| 1994-1996 | • 'less experience' of current trainees
• minor symptoms should not be ignored
• A/E nurses should not decide obstetric management
• good communication between obstetric team and Blood Bank |

| 1997-1999 | • uterine artery emboliation/B-Lynch or Billings suture in MOH is safe and life-saving
• antenatal anaemia to be corrected
• importance of CVP line in MOH |

| 2000-2002 | • updated guideline on women refusing blood transfusion: cell salvage
• new training structure: concern on surgical skills of trainees |

| 2003-2005 | • Early Warning Scoring System
• regular training:maternal collapse
• prompt involvement of Consultant with greater gynaecological surgical experience
• previous CS: rule out placenta accreta or percreta by scan +/– MRI |

| 2006-2008 | • Early senior multidisciplinary team involvement
• more emphasis on Modified Early Obstetric Warning score (MEOWS) chart
• placenta previs with bleeding: admit from 34 weeks (RCOG) |

Figure 2 Summary of recommendations from the Confidential Enquiry reports 1985-2008. A/E, accident and emergency; CS, cesarean section; CVP, central venous pressure; DIC, disseminated intravascular coagulopathy; MOH, major obstetric hemorrhage; RCOG, Royal College of Obstetricians and Gynaecologists. Adapted from CEMACH[3–9]

and concealed pregnancy, where regardless of excellent care, maternal deaths were deemed unavoidable. Therefore, all health care professionals involved in care of pregnant women should aim towards elimination of substandard care. This may not prevent all maternal deaths but will certainly reduce them significantly.

Actions by professional bodies

To ensure a robust system of preventing maternal morbidity and mortality, the following standards have been laid out by relevant professional bodies (UK).

Royal College of Obstetricians and Gynaecologists (RCOG)[12]

Intervention radiology RCOG has strongly recommended the availability of interventional radiology to prevent and treat MOH. This technique is effective to prevent and treat MOH and reduce transfusion, hysterectomy, maternal morbidity and mortality. It can be used either to embolize bleeding vessels in acute hemorrhage or prophylactically to occlude (with a special balloon) internal iliac or uterine arteries in suspected placenta accreta.

Maternity dash board This is a tool to benchmark activity and monitor performance against the standards for the maternity unit on a monthly basis. It essentially follows the principles of a car dashboard, so that appropriate action can be taken before the car breaks down. The following are monitored as an integral part of the dash board: clinical activity, workforce, clinical outcomes and risk incidents/complaints or patient satisfaction surveys.

Consultant involvement It is quite clear that early consultant involvement is crucial to prevent maternal mortality in MOH. Apart from 24 hour consultant cover in the delivery suite, RCOG has also recommended that in the following situations, the consultant should attend in person, irrespective of the level of the trainee:

(1) Maternal collapse (such as massive abruption, septic shock);

(2) Cesarean section for major placenta previa;

(3) PPH of more than 1.5 liters where:

(a) The hemorrhage is continuing and a MOH;

(b) The protocol has been instigated;

(4) Return to theater – laparotomy;

(5) When requested.

Improving communication Poor communication can lead to fatal consequences. It has been suggested that one-to-one handover should follow the SBAR (situation background assessment recommendation) tool. SHARING (staff, high risk, awaiting theatre, recovery ward, inductions, NICU, gynecology) is a structured form of written handover that takes place at the beginning and end of each shift (between in-coming and out-going on-call teams).

In most UK maternity units, there is an established system of emergency call to get the relevant staff (such as obstetric, anesthetist and hematology on-call teams and porters) in case of a MOH. In such a situation, this is usually by calling the hospital switchboard with the number '2222' and asking for relevant codes (in different units, it is variously called 'MOH call', 'code red' or 'code blue' call).

Guidelines Guidelines have been developed on 'Prevention and management of PPH' and 'Blood transfusion in Obstetrics' to standardize the management of MOH in all maternity units in UK. Figure 3 summarizes the RCOG recommended algorithm in the management of MOH described in the 'Prevention and management of PPH'.

National Patient Safety Agency (NPSA)[14]

The placenta previa after cesarean section (PPCS) care bundle All women undergoing cesarean section at high risk of placenta accreta should be managed in

MOH

Call for help

To call senior midwife/obstetrician and anesthetist

To alert hematologist, blood transfusion laboratory, consultant obstetrician on-call

Resuscitation

Assess: Airway (A), Breathing (B), Circulation (C)

Oxygen mast (15 liters), Fluid balance (2 liters Hartmann's 1.5 liters colloid)

Blood transfusion (O RhD negative or group-specific blood), Blood products (FFP, PLT, cyroprecipitate, factor VIIa); to keep patient warm

Investigations: 14-g cannulae (x2) and send bloods (FBC, coagulation, U&Es, LFTs), Crossmatch (4 units, FFP, PLT, cryoprecipitate), Hb bedside testing.

Monitoring: ECG, oximeter, Foley catheter, to consider central and arterial lines, to commence record chart, weigh all swabs and estimate blood loss

Medical management

Bimanual uterine compression, Empty bladder, Oxytocin 5 iu x 2, Erogmetrine 500 micrograms, Oxytocin infusion (40 u in 500 ml)

Carboprost 250 micrograms IM every 15 minutes up to 8 times, Carboprost (intramyometrial) 0.5 mg, Misoprostol 1000 micrograms rectally

Transfer to theater

Examination Under Anesthesia (EUA), to check and correct any coagulation abnormality

To consider: Balloon tamponade (intrauterine), Brace suture, Interventional radiology

Surgery

Bilateral uterine artery ligation/Bilateral internal iliac ligation

Hysterectomy (second consultant)

Consider: transfer to High Dependency/Intensive care Unit

Figure 3 Algorithm to manage PPH/major obstetric hemorrhage[13]. FFP, fresh frozen plasma; PLT, platelets; FBC, full blood count; U&Es, urea and electrolytes; HB, hemoglobin; LFTs, liver function tests; ECG, electrocardiogram

line with this care bundle. The important considerations of the bundle include:

(1) Consultant obstetrician and anesthetist directly supervising the delivery;

(2) Blood and blood products available on site;

(3) Patient's consent for possible interventions (hysterectomy, cell salvage, interventional radiology and leaving placenta *in situ*);

(4) Multidisciplinary involvement in preoperative planning;

(5) Local availability of level 2 critical care bed.

SUMMARY

MOH remains an important direct cause of maternal death in the UK. The triennial reports have indicated areas of substandard care and directions for further research and audits. Improvement of care in women with MOH is taking place. For example, blood bank facilities have been made available on site, experienced operators are more readily accessible, and skills and drills have been introduced to facilitate team work and communication.

Even so, the obstetric care team continues to face challenges as not all areas of substandard care have been addressed. Adequate resuscitation in MOH is often 'too little and too late'. The tendency to underestimate the effect of massive blood loss can continue because women in pregnancy can compensate for a period of time and then decompensate very rapidly. It is hoped that early warning scoring systems may address this issue. As the work force becomes more specialized with fewer training hours, appropriately experienced operators must be available to carry out complex surgical procedures. A multidisciplinary approach should be pursued in all aspects of care, anticipating, managing and caring for women at risk of and experiencing PPH.

References

1. Weindling A. The Confidential Enquiry into Maternal and Child Health (CEMACH). Arch Dis Child 2003;88:1034–7
2. Yentis SM. From CEMD to CEMACH to CMACE to...? Where now for the Confidential Enquiries into Maternal Deaths? Anaesthesia 2011;66:859–60
3. CEMD. Report on Confidential Enquiries into Maternal Deaths in the United Kingdom 1985–87. Chapter 3. Antepartum and Postpartum Haemorrhage. London: HMSO, 1991:73–87
4. CEMD. Report on Confidential Enquiries into Maternal Deaths in the United Kingdom 1988–90. Chapter 3. Antepartum and Postpartum Haemorrhage. London: HMSO, 1994
5. CEMD. Report on Confidential Enquiries into Maternal Deaths in the United Kingdom 1991–93. Chapter 3.

Antepartum and Postpartum Haemorrhage. London: HMSO, 1996

6. CEMD. Report on Confidential Enquiries into Maternal Deaths in the United Kingdom 1994–96. Chapter 4. Antepartum and Postpartum Haemorrhage. London: HMSO, 1998

7. CEMACH. Why Mothers Die 1997–1999. Chapter 4. Haemorrhage. London: RCOG, 2001

8. CEMACH. Why Mothers Die 2000–2002. Chapter 4. Haemorrhage. London: RCOG, 2004

9. CEMACH. Saving Mothers Lives: reviewing maternal deaths to make motherhood safer (2003 – 2005). Chapter 4. Haemorrhage. London: RCOG, 2007

10. Cantwell R, Clutton-Brock T, Cooper G, et al. The Eighth Report on Confidential Enquiries into Maternal Deaths in the United Kingdom. BJOG 2011;118(Suppl 1):1–203

11. Knight M, Kurinczuk JJ, Spark P, Brocklenhurst P on behalf of UKOSS. United Kingdom Obstetric Surveillance System (UKOSS) Annual Report 2007. Oxford: National Perinatal Epidemiology, 2007

12. RCOG. Guidelines. http://www.rcog.org.uk/guidelines

13. RCOG. Postpartum Hemorrhage Prevention and Management. Green Top Guideline 52. London, UK: RCOG

14. NHS. Placenta Praevia afer Caesarean Section Care Bundle. 2010. http://www.nrls.npsa.nhs.uk/resources/?EntryId45= 66359

21

Declining Mortality Rate from Postpartum Hemorrhage in Japan and Factors Influencing the Changes, 1950–2009

Y. Imaizumi, T. Ikeda and L. G. Keith

INTRODUCTION

Although WHO[1] continues to list postpartum hemorrhage (PPH) as a major cause of maternal mortality, especially in the developing world, Japan, as an important member of the group of developed nations, has had small numbers of deaths from PPH in recent years. This chapter describes a 60-year trend of mortality from PPH using data from vital statistics[2]. It also outlines factors influencing PPH death rates.

MATERIALS AND METHODS

The International Classification of Diseases (ICD) for 1950–1967 assigned PPH with the codes 672 (ICD-6 and ICD-7)[3,4], 652–653 (ICD-8)[5] for 1968–1978, 666 (ICD-9)[6] for 1979–1994, and O72 (ICD-10)[7] for 1995–2009. ICD for 1909–1922 assigned puerperal hemorrhage with the codes 135 (ICD-2)[8], and 144 (ICD-3 and ICD-4)[9,10] for 1923–1943. In computing the PPH death rate, the number of PPH deaths was divided by the numbers of births (live and fetal births).

RESULTS

Yearly change of the PPH death rate

Table 1 shows the number of PPH deaths and the death rate during the period from 1950 to 2009. The PPH death rate was 23.0 per 100,000 births in 1954 and rapidly decreased to 2.1 in 1987, only to further decrease to 1.0 in 2009. Table 1 also shows the ratio of maternal deaths due to PPH. For the past 18 years, these ratios have fluctuated annually owing to the small numbers involved.

Figure 1 depicts the PPH death rate and maternal mortality from 1950 to 2009. The maternal death rate was 166.7 per 100,000 births in 1954, but rapidly declined to 15.1 in 1985 and gradually decreased further to 4.8 in 2009. Figure 1 also shows the 3-year average of maternal deaths due to PPH. The proportion of PPH deaths as a percentage of all maternal deaths was 11.8% in 1950, increased to 23.0% in 1985, declined again to 9.2 in 1996, and, finally, increased

thereafter to 20.5 in 2009. Despite these constant reductions in maternal death rates and the rate of deaths from PPH, the percentage of maternal deaths due to PPH varied from 9% to 23% during the entire period.

Table 1 Death rate due to postpartum hemorrhage (PPH), number of PPH deaths, ratio of the PPH deaths to maternal deaths and mean age at death during 1950–2009

Year	No. of deaths	Death rate (per 100,000)	Ratio* (%)	Mean age at death†	Year	No. of deaths	Death rate (per 100,000)	Ratio* (%)	Mean age at death†
1950	448	17.5	10.9	32.0	1980	61	3.7	18.9	32.1
1951	472	20.0	12.8	32.0	1981	68	4.2	23.1	32.0
1952	410	18.6	12.0	32.0	1982	46	2.9	16.5	32.3
1953	423	20.5	12.5	31.6	1983	45	2.8	19.2	32.6
1954	450	23.0	13.8	31.2	1984	53	3.4	23.2	33.3
1955	406	21.2	13.1	30.9	1985	55	3.7	24.3	33.2
1956	374	20.3	13.2	30.6	1986	40	2.8	21.4	32.7
1957	370	21.2	13.8	30.5	1987	29	2.1	17.9	33.0
1958	338	18.4	13.2	30.4	1988	18	1.3	14.2	32.2
1959	338	18.7	14.2	30.2	1989	17	1.3	12.6	33.9
1960	278	15.6	13.3	30.2	1990	13	1.0	12.4	33.3
1961	284	16.1	14.8	30.1	1991	18	1.4	16.4	33.8
1962	246	13.7	13.6	30.2	1992	21	1.7	19.0	32.8
1963	219	11.9	12.9	30.3	1993	9	0.7	9.9	33.4
1964	241	12.8	14.2	30.1	1994	13	1.0	17.2	32.4
1965	240	12.1	15.0	30.1	1995	4	0.3	4.7	33.0
1966	158	10.5	12.5	29.9	1996	10	0.8	13.8	33.5
1967	234	11.0	16.8	29.9	1997	7	0.6	9.0	33.6
1968	215	10.7	16.9	30.2	1998	12	1.0	14.0	34.1
1969	182	9.0	16.6	30.2	1999	9	0.7	12.5	32.8
1970	152	7.3	15.1	30.7	2000	11	0.9	14.2	33.7
1971	144	6.8	15.9	30.6	2001	7	0.6	9.2	31.7
1972	140	6.5	16.9	30.2	2002	14	1.2	16.6	32.7
1973	117	5.3	14.6	30.1	2003	17	1.5	24.4	33.3
1974	113	5.3	16.1	30.3	2004	10	0.9	20.3	33.5
1975	71	3.5	13.0	30.7	2005	6	0.5	9.6	33.5
1976	65	3.4	13.7	31.3	2006	7	0.6	13.0	34.1
1977	73	3.9	18.0	31.3	2007	9	0.8	25.9	34.4
1978	60	3.3	15.9	31.7	2008	6	0.5	15.3	34.6
1979	68	3.9	18.1	31.9	2009	11	1.0	20.9	33.4

*PPH deaths to number of maternal deaths; †3-year moving average at death

169

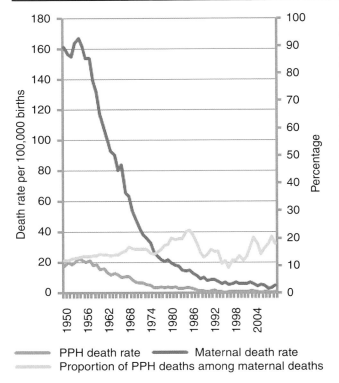

PPH death rate — Maternal death rate
Proportion of PPH deaths among maternal deaths

Figure 1 Death rate due to postpartum hemorrhage (PPH), maternal mortality and percentage of maternal deaths due to PPH, 1950–2009

Death rate by maternal age

Table 2 shows the PPH death rate according to maternal age for three consecutive periods of two decades each, beginning in 1950–1969 and ending with 1990–2009. In the first 20-year period, the PPH death rate was lowest (9.4–9.8 per 100,000 births) when the mother was under 25 years of age, increasing to 63.1 at 40–44 years and slightly decreasing thereafter (60.9). In the middle period, the overall death rate decreased to 25% compared with the earlier period, while the death rate by maternal age shows a similar pattern to

the first 20-year period. More recently, in the past 20 years, the overall death rate decreased to 25% compared with the middle period. The death rate was 0.2 per 100,000 births in mothers under 20 years of age, but not unexpectedly increased with maternal age up to 45 years and over (7.9). Comparing the PPH death rates of the first and the most recent 20-year periods, the greatest declining rate was noted among mothers under 20 years of age (1/45), and this decreased with maternal age up to 45 years and over (1/8). Accordingly, the vast improvement of the PPH mortality was observed remarkably in the younger maternal years.

Table 1 demonstrates that the 3-year moving average of maternal age at death remained nearly constant (29.9–34.6 years) for 60 years. Table 2 shows averages of maternal age at death from PPH and live birth for the three time periods. Average ages at death are 30.8 years for 1950–1969, 31.4 years for 1970–1989, and 33.5 years for 1990–2009. The corresponding average maternal age at live birth is 27.8, 28.0 and 29.7 years, respectively. The differences between average ages at birth and at the time of death are 3–3.8 years, a very narrow range that has not changed in 40 years.

Geographical variations

Table 3 shows the PPH death rates according to prefectures during the periods from 1950–1979 and 1980–2009. The highest PPH death rate (per 100,000 births) occurred in Shimane Prefecture for both periods (18.9 and 4.0, respectively), whereas the lowest was noted in Okinawa Prefecture for both periods (3.2 and 0.4); these values were 6 and 10 times higher, respectively, in Shimane Prefecture compared with Okinawa Prefecture. In 1951 and 1953, the number of deaths from PPH was compared in urban and rural areas. The PPH death rate was 17.2 (139 deaths in 1951 and 140 in 1953) in urban areas and 22.1 (333 in 1951 and 283 in 1953) in rural areas. The difference between the death rates in the urban and in rural areas is significant at the 5% level (odds ratio 1.28 and 95%

Table 2 Postpartum hemorrhage (PPH) death rate according to maternal age, mean maternal age at death due to PPH and mean maternal age at live birth from 1950–1969 to 1990–2009

Maternal age	1950–1969			1970–1989			1990–2009			Ratio of death rates for the oldest and the recent period
	Number of deaths	Death rate*	%	Number of deaths	Death rate*	%	Number of deaths	Death rate*	%	
Under 20	68	9.8	1.1	15	3.1	1.0	1	0.2	0.5	44.5
20–24	988	9.4	15.6	141	1.8	9.9	10	0.3	4.7	32.6
25–29	2009	12.2	31.8	464	2.7	32.4	43	0.5	20.1	25.6
30–34	1690	21.6	26.7	435	5.7	30.4	75	1.0	35.0	22.8
35–39	1104	40.4	17.5	292	17.3	20.4	61	2.3	28.5	17.9
40–44	434	63.1	6.9	78	32.5	5.5	23	6.2	10.7	10.1
Over 45	29	60.9	0.5	5	30.4	0.3	1	7.9	0.5	7.7
Total	6322	16.2	100	1430	4.1	100	214	0.9	100	18.2
Mean maternal age										
at death due to PPH		30.8			31.4			33.5		
at live birth		27.8			28.0			29.7		

*per 100,000 births

Table 3 Death rates for postpartum hemorrhage, 1950–2009

Prefecture	1950–1979			1980–2009		
	Number	Rate*	Ratio†	Number	Rate*	Ratio†
Hokkaido	411	12.7	13.8	28	1.6	21.7
Aomori	146	15.1	13.0	6	1.3	10.9
Iwate	157	17.4	14.2	3	0.7	5.8
Miyagi	118	10.6	13.1	18	2.4	24.3
Akita	117	15.5	13.4	6	1.8	18.2
Yamagata	77	10.7	12.2	6	1.6	18.2
Fukushima	192	15.2	15.6	15	2.2	22.7
Ibaraki	204	15.7	15.1	17	1.9	18.5
Tochigi	124	13.0	12.5	17	2.7	25.4
Gunma	156	16.1	16.2	7	1.1	14.9
Saitama	254	11.8	13.7	37	1.8	15.7
Chiba	208	11.4	14.3	35	2.0	20.8
Tokyo	506	8.8	12.3	62	1.8	18.7
Kanagawa	256	9.2	13.5	52	2.0	20.1
Niigata	162	11.6	13.2	6	0.8	11.3
Toyama	60	10.6	12.2	3	0.9	13.6
Ishikawa	62	10.8	13.3	4	1.1	14.3
Fukui	61	14.1	14.2	2	0.8	12.5
Yamanashi	77	17.4	16.8	5	1.9	17.9
Nagano	144	13.5	15.4	17	2.5	23.0
Gifu	88	8.8	9.4	13	2.0	19.7
Shizuoka	173	9.7	11.8	15	1.3	13.0
Aichi	255	8.6	12.0	25	1.1	12.2
Mie	112	13.2	14.8	11	2.0	25.0
Shiga	68	13.5	13.1	7	1.6	18.9
Kyoto	133	11.7	13.0	8	1.0	9.6
Osaka	429	10.7	12.8	55	2.0	19.4
Hyogo	332	13.3	14.2	25	1.5	15.9
Nara	74	15.1	14.2	8	1.9	22.9
Wakayama	76	13.6	12.5	7	2.2	25.9
Tottori	60	17.9	18.6	3	1.6	21.4
Shimane	86	18.9	15.6	9	4.0	30.0
Okayama	143	15.5	16.9	8	1.3	19.1
Hiroshima	204	15.4	17.2	11	1.2	20.4
Yamaguchi	109	12.5	12.0	9	2.0	19.6
Tokushima	89	19.3	16.3	4	1.7	16.7
Kagawa	62	12.5	12.8	5	1.6	25.0
Ehime	123	14.4	15.9	5	1.1	12.2
Kochi	80	18.5	16.4	4	1.7	14.8
Fukuoka	276	11.4	12.4	21	1.3	15.9
Saga	81	14.7	12.3	4	1.4	13.8
Nagasaki	167	15.0	14.2	12	2.3	19.1
Kumamoto	180	16.9	15.3	7	1.2	17.5
Oita	119	16.9	14.3	5	1.3	12.5
Miyazaki	116	16.1	14.2	5	1.3	14.3
Kagoshima	191	17.2	13.2	11	1.9	12.6
Okinawa	5	3.2	11.9	2	0.4	4.3
Total	7325	12.4	13.7	646	1.7	17.6

*Death rate per 100,000 births; †percentage of PPH deaths to maternal deaths

Table 4 Death rates (per 100,000 births) from postpartum hemorrhage (PPH) and maternal deaths (MD) and ratio of the PPH in each district, 1950–1979 and 1980–2009

District	1950–1979					1980–2009				
	Number		Death rate		PPH/MD (%)	Number		Death rate		PPH/MD (%)
	PPH	MD	PPH	MD		PPH	MD	PPH	MD	
Hokkaido	411	2983	12.7	92.0	13.8	28	129	1.6	7.6	21.7
Tohoku	807	5858	14.1	102.3	15.6	54	313	1.8	10.2	17.3
Kanto	1708	12,643	10.9	80.3	13.5	227	1191	1.9	10.0	19.1
Chubu	1194	9282	10.8	83.8	14.8	101	651	1.4	8.9	15.5
Kinki	1112	8364	12.1	91.0	12.5	110	622	1.7	9.6	17.7
Chugoku	602	3814	15.4	97.5	12.0	40	186	1.7	7.8	21.5
Shikoku	354	2294	15.7	101.9	16.4	18	112	1.5	9.0	16.1
Kyushu	1130	8337	14.7	108.4	13.2	65	426	1.5	9.8	15.3
Okinawa	5*	42*	3.2*	26.7*	11.9*	2	47	0.4	8.5	4.3

*1973–1979

1950–1979 and 1980–2009 in Table 4. The PPH death rate was the lowest in the Okinawa District (3.2 for the earlier period and 0.4 for the later period), and death rates in other districts ranged between 10.8 and 15.7 in 1950–1979 and 1.4 and 1.9 in 1980–2009. Therefore, with exception of the Okinawa District, the rate was similar among the other eight districts. However, the highest maternal death rate was seen in Kyushu District (108.4) in the period 1950–1979 and in Tohoku District (10.2) in the period 1980–2009, whereas the corresponding lowest values were seen in Okinawa District (26.7) and in Hokkaido District (7.6), respectively. The highest value was 1.2–1.3 times higher than the lowest for both periods. The variations of maternal death rates in the other nine districts were small.

Behind maternal deaths from PPH

Nakabayashi *et al.*[11] performed a nationwide study of critical obstetric cases in 2004 by sending an inquiry questionnaire to 834 departments of obstetric and gynecology and 164 emergency departments in Japan. A total of 335 departments responded, which covered 124,595 cases or 11.2% of all the deliveries in Japan. PPH was present in 934 cases (749 cases per 100,000 live births). Transfusion was carried out in 868 cases (696 cases per 100,000 live births) and hysterectomy or arterial embolization was performed in 134 cases (108 cases per 100,000 live births). Four maternal deaths were reported in the 934 PPH cases, which corresponds to a mortality rate of 0.4% or 3 per 100,000 live births. This mortality rate due to PPH was significantly lower than the death rate from maternal cerebrovascular disease (mainly cerebral hemorrhage, 38.9%), pulmonary embolization (33.3%) and sepsis and severe infective disease (7.1%) in Japan at the same time. It is important to note, however, that almost 7460 cases of PPH deaths were prevented each year by the management and effort of medical staff including obstetricians. (There are almost one million

confidence interval 1.11–1.48 between urban and rural areas).

The ratio of PPH deaths to maternal deaths was 13.7% for Japan overall in the period 1950–1979 where the highest ratio was 18.6% in Tottori Prefecture and the lowest (9.4%) in Gifu Prefecture (Table 3). Corresponding values in the period 1980–2009 were 17.6% for the whole of Japan, 30.0% in Shimane Prefecture and 4.3% in Okinawa Prefecture.

The PPH and maternal death rates and the ratio of PPH are recomputed in each district in the period for

life births per year in Japan, the number of PPH cases occurring per year is 749×10 (one million/100,000) = 7490. With three deaths due to PPH per 100,000 live births per year, 30 PPH deaths occur per year. Therefore, death is assumed to have been prevented in $7490 - 30 = 7460$ cases.)

Prevention of maternal death due to PPH: current projects

In 2010, the Japan Society of Obstetrics and Gynecology published 'Guidelines for management of critical bleeding in obstetrics' in conjunction with the other related academic societies[12]. In the guidelines, the severity of the patient's hemorrhage is stratified into three levels or 'codes', according to vital signs and reactivity to treatment: III bleeding but stable, II requiring vasopressor, and I threatening to cardiac arrest.

Furthermore, and of equal importance, a new nationwide survey of maternal death was commenced in 2010. To emulate work from the Center for Maternal and Child Enquiries (CMACE) in the UK, all maternal deaths should be reported, evaluated and examined for preventive strategy. The maternal deaths are reported to the Society of Obstetrics and Gynecology, which anonymizes the cases, so that they can be evaluated by experts. From January to December in 2010, a total of 39 cases of maternal deaths were investigated for cause. Of these, seven (23%) deaths were as a result of PPH and 12 (31%) from amniotic fluid embolism. PPH cases comprised two examples of uterine rupture, two of uterine inversion, one of cervical laceration, one placental abruption and three listed as miscellaneous.

Amniotic fluid embolism

Amniotic fluid embolism is a fatal obstetric condition characterized by hypotension, respiratory distress with cyanosis, disseminated intravascular coagulopathy (DIC) and neurological manifestations such as seizures. As a cause of maternal death, it is usually categorized as pulmonary embolism with thrombotic pulmonary embolism in the ICD-9 and 10. However, a Japanese study recently revealed that almost half of amniotic fluid embolism cases also manifested PPH[13]. We surveyed autopsy cases of maternal deaths from 1989 to 2004 in Japan. Out of 193 cases, amniotic fluid embolism was the leading cause (28% of all maternal deaths). Out of 42 cases of pathological amniotic fluid embolism, 21 (50%) cases were clinically diagnosed. The other 21 cases were diagnosed as DIC or shock after delivery.

Because of the lack of diagnostic techniques to differentiate amniotic fluid embolism-related PPH from all PPH, the present categorization of PPH for maternal death should be re-evaluated.

Death rate from puerperal hemorrhage before World War II

Data on vital statistics in Japan have been available since 1899, except for the period 1944–1946 due to World War II. Before World War II, the number of PPH deaths was not obtained, but data on deaths from puerperal hemorrhage were obtained during the period from 1909 to 1943. The cause of deaths for PPH and puerperal hemorrhage are not the same. The latter include PPH and other hemorrhage.

Table 5 shows the number of deaths from the puerperal hemorrhage, the puerperal hemorrhage death rate, and the ratio of the puerperal hemorrhage (the percentage of maternal deaths due to puerperal hemorrhage) during the period from 1909 to 1943. The puerperal hemorrhage death rate was 46.6 in 1909 and gradually increased to 63.2 in 1940 and decreased to 53.1 in 1943. The ratio of the puerperal hemorrhage was 13.5% in 1909 and increased to 27.4% in 1943. Table 5 also shows the maternal mortality rate from 1899 to 1943. The maternal mortality rate decreased from 409.8 in 1899 to 193.6 in 1943.

Table 6 shows the number of puerperal hemorrhage deaths, the death rate and ratio of PPH to maternal deaths during the periods 1909–1922 and 1933–1942 in each prefecture. For the earlier period, the highest puerperal hemorrhage death rate was 75.0 in Okinawa Prefecture and the lowest was 30.2 in Miyagi Prefecture. For the later period, the corresponding rates were 76.2 in Nara Prefecture and 37.5 in Aichi Prefecture. Therefore, the highest rates were 2.5 times higher than the lowest death rate in

Table 5 Puerperal hemorrhage (PH) and maternal death (MD) rates for 1899–1943

Year	No. of deaths PH	No. of deaths MD	Death rate (per 100,000) PH	Death rate (per 100,000) MD	Year	No. of deaths PH	No. of deaths MD	Death rate (per 100,000) PH	Death rate (per 100,000) MD
1899	–	6240	–	409.8	1922	1116	6565	53.1	312.4
1900	–	6200	–	397.8	1923	1114	6897	51.2	316.8
1901	–	6671	–	402.6	1924	1154	6273	54.3	295.3
1902	–	6556	–	392.9	1925	1268	6309	57.4	285.4
1903	–	6071	–	369.3	1926	1179	5721	52.9	256.7
1904	–	5742	–	361.7	1927	1207	5765	55.4	264.7
1905	–	6185	–	387.8	1928	1213	5997	53.8	265.8
1906	–	6237	–	403.9	1929	1234	5867	56.2	267.4
1907	–	6728	–	379.4	1930	1250	5681	56.7	257.9
1908	–	7091	–	388.4	1931	1254	5667	56.5	255.4
1909	864	6399	46.6	344.9	1932	1318	5530	57.2	240.2
1910	843	6228	45.1	333.0	1933	1347	5763	60.3	257.8
1911	812	6192	42.7	325.4	1934	1307	5709	60.6	264.7
1912	706	5770	37.4	306.1	1935	1322	5698	57.3	247.1
1913	778	5900	40.8	309.7	1936	1241	5384	56.1	243.3
1914	782	6418	40.0	328.4	1937	1268	5444	55.3	237.5
1915	824	6452	42.5	332.5	1938	1186	4877	58.5	240.5
1916	871	6337	44.8	325.8	1939	1206	4818	60.3	240.9
1917	870	6368	44.6	326.1	1940	1402	5070	63.2	228.6
1918	1056	6812	54.6	352.1	1941	1370	4929	57.5	207.0
1919	910	5910	47.6	309.2	1942	1192	4586	51.2	196.9
1920	1100	7158	51.2	329.9	1943	1245	4542	53.1	193.6
1921	1092	7181	51.3	337.3					

Table 6 Death rates of puerperal hemorrhage (PH), and ratio of PH to maternal deaths, 1909–1942

Prefecture	1909–1922		1933–1942		Ratio of PH to maternal deaths	
	No. of PH	Death rate	No. of PH	Death rate	1909–1922	1933–1942
Hokkaido	615	57.0	692	62.2	17.27	27.2
Aomori	150	24.5	168	42.5	10.4	19.8
Iwate	223	50.3	206	49.9	11.7	18.3
Miyagi	149	30.2	286	63.5	11.2	32.1
Akita	231	47.1	295	73.0	11.8	25.0
Yamagata	208	41.5	248	62.6	15.0	32.8
Fukushima	308	47.5	338	60.3	15.9	31.7
Ibaraki	238	36.1	300	56.4	11.5	28.0
Tochigi	268	50.4	261	63.5	16.0	30.1
Gunma	305	58.7	315	73.3	19.1	33.3
Saitama	322	46.7	319	60.3	15.3	27.5
Chiba	265	40.5	307	60.9	12.2	25.2
Tokyo	866	65.2	1271	67.0	15.3	26.1
Kanagawa	278	51.1	433	71.6	15.4	28.8
Niigata	468	50.0	422	60.6	15.1	30.0
Toyama	168	41.9	125	45.1	11.5	20.9
Ishikawa	166	42.9	127	53.0	11.7	19.9
Fukui	115	36.7	91	44.9	12.5	20.5
Yamanashi	174	61.4	155	72.0	16.4	28.7
Nagano	365	52.7	380	71.5	15.3	32.4
Gifu	191	35.3	206	49.7	11.3	23.1
Shizuoka	322	42.4	345	52.7	13.9	26.0
Aichi	359	36.8	352	37.5	14.0	21.0
Mie	200	39.2	197	53.1	13.9	24.5
Shiga	164	52.4	117	57.1	17.9	25.5
Kyoto	333	63.7	242	54.3	14.2	21.0
Osaka	560	60.0	803	69.6	13.0	22.6
Hyogo	524	54.7	433	51.0	15.2	20.8
Nara	133	47.7	135	76.2	13.6	24.7
Wakayama	162	47.4	138	57.3	13.0	22.4
Tottori	84	42.2	85	58.7	13.2	23.9
Shimane	179	58.2	126	55.0	13.2	21.1
Okayama	262	51.1	189	49.6	12.4	20.3
Hiroshima	361	50.9	224	42.4	15.4	20.8
Yamaguchi	248	60.3	213	61.8	13.4	19.7
Tokushima	224	66.5	118	48.5	19.1	22.4
Kagawa	175	48.6	95	40.7	16.7	19.8
Ehime	224	45.5	188	49.5	13.4	25.1
Kochi	117	40.4	121	60.3	12.1	24.8
Fukuoka	437	52.1	495	56.8	13.6	21.9
Saga	166	52.0	112	49.8	15.3	22.7
Nagasaki	277	61.9	239	56.2	17.3	24.1
Kumamoto	249	49.2	230	54.1	11.9	22.9
Oita	184	48.7	186	59.0	12.8	21.7
Miyazaki	156	58.6	162	57.3	14.8	24.1
Kagoshima	322	55.6	277	53.3	13.5	22.7
Okinawa	129	75.0	69	43.0	9.5	12.5
Total	12,624	49.9	12,836	57.9	14.1	24.6

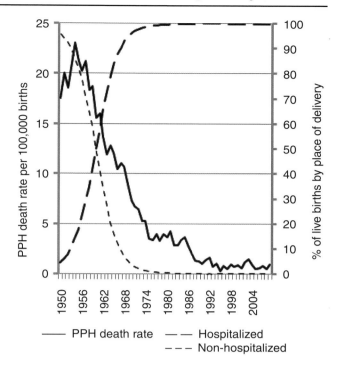

Figure 2 Relationship between PPH death rate and percentage of live births by place of delivery, 1950–2009

DISCUSSION – WHY DID POSTPARTUM HEMORRHAGE DECREASE IN JAPAN?

Our results indicate that of the common risk factors for PPH (prolonged third stage of labor, pre-eclampsia, mediolateral episiotomy, previous PPH, maternal age, twin pregnancy, arrest of descent, soft-tissue lacerations, Asian ethnicity, augmented labor, forceps or vacuum delivery, Hispanic ethnicity, midline episiotomy and nulliparity)[14,15], maternal age (over 35 years) plays an important role. A prior Japanese study by Ohkuchi et al.[16] had indicated that age was a risk factor among Japanese parturients, but this study was hospital based, much shorter in duration and could not, by definition, consider moving averages at age of death. Figure 2 shows the relationship between the PPH death rate and the percentage of live births by place of delivery: institutional (hospital, clinic or maternity home) and non-institutional (home and others) from 1950 to 2009. The percentage of non-institutional deliveries was 95% in 1950, and decreased to 50% in 1960 and, finally, drastically decreased to 1% in 1975. However, the percentage of institutional deliveries was only 5% in 1950, but rapidly increased to 50% by 1960, 90% by 1967, and then became 99% in 1974 and nearly 100% for the period 1980–2009. The relationship between the PPH death rate and the percentage of non-hospitalized deliveries is strongly correlated (correlation coefficient 0.92). According to Nagaya et al.[17], during 1991–1992, 197 maternal deaths occurred within a hospital and 22 outside a medical facility; 11 deaths were without available records. The percentage of maternal deaths due to PPH was 55% (12/22) outside medical facilities, but there was no information about deaths due to PPH in the hospital. According to

1909–1922 and 2 times higher in 1933–1942. The ratio of puerperal hemorrhage deaths to maternal deaths was 14.1% for Japan overall in the period 1909–1922, where the highest ratio was 19.1% in Tokushima Prefecture and the lowest was 9.5% in Okinawa Prefecture. The corresponding values were 24.6% for Japan overall, 33.3% in Gunma Prefecture and 12.5% in Okinawa Prefecture, in the period 1933–1942.

the Japanese vital statistics[2], the percentage of maternal deaths due to PPH was 17.6% (39/221) for the period 1991–1992. Even assuming that there were no PPH deaths in the 11 maternal deaths without records, the percentage due to PPH is 13.7% (27/197) in hospital, which is an overestimated value. However, it is of great importance to Asian countries that deaths due to PPH will decline as a higher percentage of institutional deliveries becomes the norm.

The traditional definition of PPH is a blood loss of more than 500 ml, but this definition is now considered questionable, as it is based on a study published in 1964 which was uncontrolled and underpowered. More recently, Kubo[18] undertook a hospital-based study on blood loss of PPH in Japan. They retrospectively analysed 253,607 cases for the blood loss at delivery in the years from 2001 to 2005. Their definitions of usual blood loss of PPH by means of 90% of distribution as normal were 800 ml or more in singleton vaginal births, 1500 ml or more for singleton of cesarean birth, 1600 ml or more for multiple birth delivered vaginally, and 2300 ml or more for multiple births delivered by cesarean. Given these values, it is entirely reasonable to suggest that the definition of PPH be modified in such a manner as to include fetal multiplicity and delivery route. Of interest, the American College of Obstetrician and Gynecologists mentioned in its practice bulletin that PPH was defined as blood loss in excess of 500 ml following a vaginal birth or a loss of greater than 1000 ml following cesarean birth[19]. If more articles such as those by Kubo[18] and Nakabayashi[11] continue to appear, it would be reasonable for practitioners to call upon their respective national colleges to rethink their positions.

Nagaya et al.[17] investigated 220 cases of maternal deaths in 1993 and 1994 in Japan. PPH with antepartum hemorrhage was the leading cause of maternal death, accounting for 40% of all deaths. These authors compared the results with the corresponding results in the UK, and attributed the higher rate of PPH in maternal deaths to the thinly distributed number of hospitals for labor and delivery. In other words, there were more hospitals but fewer numbers of doctors to conduct deliveries in Japan compared with in the UK. These authors thought that the scarcity of staff could have caused delay for patients to be transferred to a tertiary center or to be managed intensively with transfusion. Although this article was not published until 2000, the data obviously were made available to the proper authorities, because the Japanese government took the initiative in 1998 to establish comprehensive maternal hospitals to centralize medical staff and materials for high risk pregnancy and delivery such as PPH.

References

1. World Health Organization. WHO recommendations on the prevention of postpartum hemorrhage: A summary of the results from a WHO technical consultation. Geneva, Switzerland: World Health Organization, 2006
2. Japan, Ministry of Health and Welfare. Vital Statistics, 1950–2009, Health and Welfare Statistics and Information Department, Ministry of Health and Welfare, Tokyo, 1952–2010. Japan: Ministry of Health and Welfare [in Japanese]
3. World Health Organization. International Classification of Diseases, 6th Revision. Geneva, Switzerland: World: World Health Organization, 1950
4. World Health Organization. International Classification of Diseases, Seventh Revision. Geneva, Switzerland: World Health Organization, 1957
5. World Health Organization. International Classification of Diseases, 8th Revision. Geneva, Switzerland: World Health Organization, 1968
6. World Health Organization. International Classification of Diseases, Ninth Revision. Geneva, Switzerland: World Health Organization, 1977
7. World Health Organization. International Classification of Diseases, 10th Revision. Geneva, Switzerland: World Health Organization, 1993
8. The International Statistical Institute. International List of Causes of Death, 2nd Revision. Paris, France: International Statistical Institute, 1909
9. The International Statistical Institute. International List of Causes of Death, 3rd Revision. Paris, France: International Statistical Institute, 1920
10. The International Statistical Institute. International List of Causes of Death, 4th Revision. Paris, France: International Statistical Institute, 1929
11. Nakabayashi M, Asakura H, Kubo T, Kobayashi T, Saito S, Sato S. Committee report of maternal death and critical obstetrical cases. Nippon Sanka Fujinka Gakkai Zasshi 2007;59:1222–4 [in Japanese]
12. Irita K, Inada E. Guidelines for management of critical bleeding in obstetrics. Masui 2011;60:14–2213
13. Kanayama N, Inori J, Ishibashi-Ueda H, et al. Maternal death analysis from the Japanese autopsy registry for recent 16 years: significance of amniotic fluid embolism. J Obstet Gynecol Res 2011;37:58–63
14. Combs CA, Murphy EL, Laros RK Jr. Factors associated with postpartum hemorrhage with vaginal birth. Obstet Gynecol 1991;77:73
15. Cameron MJ, Robson SC. Vital statistics: an overview. In: B-Lynch C, Keith LG, Lalonde A, Karoshi M, eds. A Textbook of Postpartum Hemorrhage. London: Sapiens Publishing, 2006:17–34
16. Ohkuchi A, Onagawa T, Usui R, et al. Effect of maternal age on blood loss during parturition: a retrospective multivariate analysis of 10,053 cases. J Perinat Med 2003;31:209–15
17. Nagaya K, Fetters MD, Ishikawa M, et al. Cause of maternal mortality in Japan. JAMA 2000;283:2661–7
18. Kubo T. Clinical conference 2, Management of obstetrical abnormal hemorrhage: A new concept for abnormal blood loss at delivery. Nippon Sanka Fujinka Gakkai Zasshi 2010;62:121–5 [in Japanese]
19. American College of Obstetricians and Gynecologists. Practice bulletin 76: Postpartum Hemorrhage. Obstet Gynecol 2006;108:1039–47

Section 4

Causation

22

Hemodynamic Changes in the Uterus and its Blood Vessels in Pregnancy*†

F. Burbank

INTRODUCTION

Postpartum hemorrhage (PPH) most commonly originates from disrupted blood vessels of the uterus, a unique circulation supplied by two arterial systems and drained by two venous plexes. At term, the uterus receives one-tenth of the output of the heart.

During pregnancy fetal tissue invades the uterus and transforms a few hundred tiny arterioles into large, trumpet-shaped arteries that supply the placenta. At delivery, these huge arteries are torn apart, spilling blood into the uterine cavity.

All women do not die from hemorrhage during delivery because the potential for blood clotting and the accumulation of fibrinolytic substances build up in the mother's circulation during pregnancy. At the onset of true labor, clotting starts in the uterine circulation to prevent blood loss. A few hours following delivery, fibrinolysis ensues to ensure that blood flow resumes to the uterus.

It is the balance between blood clotting and fibrinolysis that determines the outcome of PPH.

Vascular imaging studies are performed using film-based or digital angiography, ultrasound with or without Doppler encoding, contrast medium-enhanced computed tomography (CT), and unenhanced and contrast medium-enhanced magnetic resonance imaging (MRI). At one extreme, an ultrasound examination could be restricted to visualization of the right uterine artery, in cross-section, at the level of uterine isthmus. At the other extreme, a dynamic arteriogram recorded on multiple 14 × 14 inch cut-films or on a 14 inch image intensifier, could display all the blood vessels in the pelvis on a sequence of images beginning with arterial filling and ending with venous drainage. A contrast medium-enhanced, spiral CT can study all major arteries in the chest, abdomen and pelvis during a single injection of contrast medium within one breath-hold! Finally, imaging studies can examine blood flow during the whole cardiac cycle, providing information from systole through diastole, and they can characterize the entire vascular tree, from arteries to capillaries and veins. Vascular imaging is the foundation of modern vascular surgery, cardiac surgery, interventional cardiology and interventional radiology. Anatomic, surgical and imaging studies each have a place in developing a coherent understanding of the vasculature of the uterus.

UTERINE BLOOD VESSELS BEFORE PREGNANCY – ARTERIES OF THE UTERUS

Arteries that touch or are within the uterus – extrinsic arteries of the uterus

Uterine arteries

Blood reaches the uterus primarily from the right and left uterine arteries, secondarily from small right and left communicating arteries that connect ipsilateral ovarian and ascending uterine arteries, and to a minor extent from tiny, unnamed, randomly distributed arteries that reach the uterus through the broad ligament (Figure 1)[1–14]. Uterine arteries are of medium

*Excerpted from selected chapters in: Burbank F. Fibroids, Menstruation, Childbirth, and Evolution: The Fascinating Story of Uterine Blood Vessels. Tucson, AZ: Wheatmark, 2009; ISBN: 978–1–60494–170–8.

†Editor's comments: The first edition of this Textbook was directed towards treatment modalities. In this second edition, the editors have made great effort to expand the thrust beyond traditional and non-traditional therapeutic measures. This chapter is an effort to make the complexity of the vascular supply of the uterus more easily understandable. It supplements much of the material presented in the chapters by Professor Palacios-Jaraquemada and his colleagues which clearly points out the differences between the therapeutic measures required when PPH is from the upper uterine segment (S1) as opposed to the lower uterine segment (S2). Moreover, the language selected by Dr Burbank is simple and straightforward. In other words, this chapter deals with anatomy but it is not written in anatomical jargon.

This chapter is a synopsis of material presented in the full chapter available at www.glowm.com in *The Global Library of Women's Medicine* by Dr Fred Burbank, a radiologist residing in California USA. The editors are grateful to Dr Burbank for presenting readers with a easily understandable impression of what every obstetrician/gynecologyst deals with everyday but certainly cannot always be expected to have at his/her fingertips when PPH arises. L.G.K.

size. As a point of reference, the common iliac artery – which is a large artery – is approximately 13 mm in diameter[15].

Ultrasound measurements of uterine artery diameters have been published and, in general, these diameters are smaller than angiographically measured diameters. Because angiographic measurements of arterial sizes have to be corrected for magnification, the process is imprecise, and ultrasound size measurements are probably more accurate. Each method visualizes only the internal lumen of an artery or vein. Average diameter of the left uterine artery in one series which examined 27 non-pregnant women was 1.6 mm[16]. Palmer *et al.* reported the average diameter of the right and left uterine arteries to be 1.4 mm in 12 non-pregnant women[17]. Taken together, these ultrasound and angiographic studies place the range of normal, non-pregnant uterine artery diameters somewhere between 1.5 and 5 mm, considerably smaller than the internal iliac artery, approximately the size range of the coronary arteries. As is shown later, the uterine arteries increase in diameter during pregnancy.

Each uterine artery arises from the ipsilateral internal iliac artery or from one of its major branches or divisions (Figure 1)[7,18]. Variation exists in the division of the internal iliac artery into branches[19].

During angiography, the uterine arteries are definitively identified by their unique shape and by their insertion into the uterus, not by their origin from the internal iliac artery origin (Figure 1). The proximal third of each uterine artery descends inferiorly, in a relatively straight line. In their mid and distal thirds, however, the uterine arteries undulate in a tortuous pattern that angiographically looks like loops. They are not loops; rather they are undulations.

The undulations in the uterine arteries are not acquired features. They are redundant arterial length which is present in both fetuses and nulliparous women[20]. As is shown later, the uterine arteries grow rapidly in diameter in response to increasing blood flow during pregnancy, but do not appear to have the capacity to grow rapidly in length. The undulations seem to be reserve arterial length that is used when the uterus expands into the abdominal cavity during pregnancy.

A triangular space described by Beliaeva as the 'cavity of the broad ligament' is present at the base of the broad ligament (Figure 2)[14]. Within this cavity the uterine arteries join the lateral borders of the uterus at the level of the isthmus. The junction of the uterine arteries with the isthmus is almost always within 15 mm of the lateral vaginal fornices[21]. When the cervix is viewed as a clock face from the perspective of a vaginal examination, the right uterine artery joins the uterus at approximately 9:00 o'clock; the left, at approximately 3:00 o'clock. Very little variation in this clock pattern exists[21].

Ovarian arteries

The ovarian arteries originate in the abdomen where the ovaries and their arterial supply form during the embryologic period (see Figure 1). During intrauterine development the ovaries migrate from the abdomen to the pelvis and drag their blood supply along with them. The ovarian arteries most commonly arise directly from the abdominal aorta but can originate as branches of the right or left renal arteries, from lumbar, adrenal, or iliac arteries, and can be duplicated[7,19,22–24]. In the lower abdomen and pelvis the ovarian arteries undulate in a pattern similar to the tortuosity seen in the uterine arteries[8,25]. Like the uterine arteries, tortuosity in the ovarian arteries appears to provide redundant arterial length that is

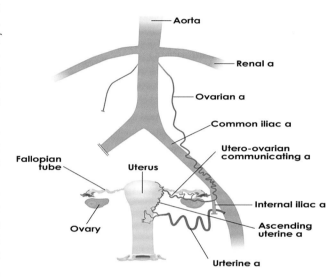

Figure 1 Diagram showing the extrinsic arteries of the left side of the uterus, including the aorta and renal and ovarian arteries arising from the abdominal aorta, the uterine artery arising from the internal ialiac artery, and the utero-ovarian communicating artery. Symmetrical arteries are present on th right but are not shown

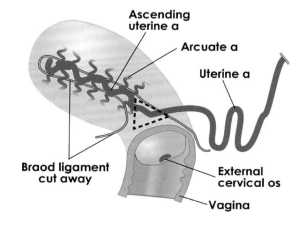

Figure 2 Drawing of the uterus as seen from the left lateral perspective with the broad ligament and vagina partially cut away to show the cavity of the broad ligament which is shown as a dashed line triangle. The left uterine artery reaches the uterus within this triangle at the 3:00 o'clock position of the cervix, approximately at the level of the internal cervical os. Note: Like coronary arteries, the ascending uterine arteries are surface vessels. The arcuate arteries are not; they cannot be seen from outside of the uterus. They traverse the uterus within the vascular layer of the myometrium

called upon during rapid enlargement of the uterus in pregnancy.

Utero-ovarian communicating arteries

Blood flow within the communicating arteries is tidal. Flow can pass from the uterine circulation to the ovarian circulation or from the ovarian circulation to the uterine depending on resistance differences between the two systems. In most women, the utero-ovarian communicating arteries are smaller in diameter than the uterine arteries or the ovarian arteries[26,27].

The communicating arteries are small enough to be difficult to visualize on routine angiography.

In general, each communicating artery is much smaller than its corresponding uterine artery. Consequently, each ovarian artery can only *potentially* supply the full blood flow needs of the uterus. To fully supply the uterus, the communicating arteries and their ipsilateral parent ovarian arteries must first experience increased blood flow. Once increased blood flow occurs, the ovarian and communicating arteries grow in diameter. When their diameters are equal to the diameter of the uterine arteries, they can supply the full metabolic needs of the uterus.

Broad ligament arteries

Broad ligament arteries are tiny vessels that arise from the main uterine arteries along their paths within the broad ligament[14]. They connect the main uterine arteries with the ascending uterine artery, and other branches, at random locations.

Arteries that touch or are within the uterus – intrinsic arteries of the uterus

Anatomy

Just prior to contact with the uterus, the uterine arteries give rise to branches that run along the right and left lateral borders of the cervix and vaginal dome. These arteries are referred to as either the 'descending' uterine arteries or 'vaginal' branches of the uterine arteries. The descending uterine arteries supply the isthmus, cervix and upper vagina[28,29]. After joining the uterus, the uterine arteries ascend along the right and left lateral margins of the body of the uterus and are referred to as the right and left 'ascending' uterine arteries (Figures 1 and 2). As they ascend, the uterine arteries undulate and give rise to a dozen or more arteries that course between the outer and middle thirds of the myometrium[30]. This zone is referred to as the 'vascular zone' or in older literature as the 'stratum vasculare'. Because of their semicircular course, these arteries are referred to as 'arcuate' arteries (Figure 3)[31]. Arcuate arteries arise from the ascending uterine arteries in a haphazard manner with thicker branches compensating for thinner ones. Direct and continuous anastomotic connections are present between right and left arcuate arteries which connect anteriorly and posteriorly near the uterine sagittal midline forming

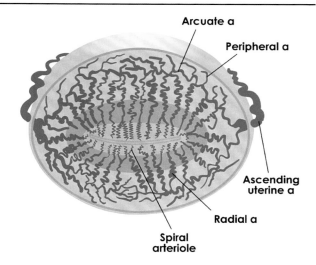

Figure 3 Drawing of transverse section through the body of the uterus showing the intrinsic arteries of the uterus: the ascending uterine, arcuate, peripheral and radial arteries and the spiral arterioles. Ascending uterine arteries are shown in perspective. This arterial pattern is repeated throughout the body of the uterus. Mucus on the surface of the endometrium is depicted as the innermost zone; the endometrium next; the junctional zone next; the myometrium next; and finally the serosa. Adapted from Sampson[31]

an arterial grid throughout the uterus[32]. The arcuate arteries give rise to peripheral arteries that course towards the serosal surface of the uterus and radial arteries that course toward the endometrial cavity.

Like the ovarian, uterine and ascending uterine arteries, the radial arteries undulate along their path. Again, the undulation is most likely present to provide reserve arterial length during the rapid volume growth of the uterus during pregnancy. They terminate at the endometrial–junctional zone border by giving off multiple branches that enter and supply the endometrium. Longer, tortuous branches are described as 'spiral arterioles'. They are termed 'spiral' for their corkscrew or spiral appearance and are classified as arterioles since most cannot be seen by the naked eye. Shorter, straight arterioles also arise from the terminal radial arteries. These supply the basal layer of the endometrium, that portion that does not slough during menstruation. Compared with the density of arteries in the myometrium, endometrial arterioles are sparse[30].

Vascular embryology

All of the intrinsic arteries of the uterus are formed prior to birth.

Arteries that do not touch the uterus – collateral uterine arterial pathways

Although the uterine arteries originate from the internal iliac artery, the proximal occlusion of an internal iliac artery does not stop blood flow in the ipsilateral uterine arteries to the uterus. A network of collateral arteries supplies blood to the uterine arteries when the internal iliac arteries are occluded. Collateral flow reaches the uterus from multiple branches of the aorta (inferior mesenteric artery, lumbar and vertebral arteries, and middle sacral), from multiple branches of the external iliac artery (deep iliac circumflex and inferior epigastric artery) and from femoral artery branches (medial femoral circumflex and lateral femoral circumflex)[5,33–35]. When bilateral internal iliac artery occlusion was performed *proximal* to the posterior division of the internal iliac artery, reversed collateral flow from the iliolumbar and lateral sacral arteries filled the anterior divisions of the internal iliac arteries and re-established antegrade blood flow in each uterine artery. When bilateral internal iliac occlusion was performed *distal* to the posterior division, reverse flow in the middle hemorrhoidal artery reconstituted antegrade flow in each uterine artery. Under these two conditions, antegrade flow in each uterine artery persisted, but flow was not normal. Pulse pressure was dampened, resembling pressure variations in a venous system instead of an arterial system. Bilateral occlusion of the internal iliac arteries changes the character of perfusion to the uterus; it does not stop antegrade perfusion of the uterus through the uterine arteries. Following bilateral iliac artery occlusion during cesarean delivery, Chitrit *et al.* noted no change in Doppler flow velocity waveforms in the uterine arteries[36].

If the right and left uterine arteries are occluded, the uterus does not die. This is a unique organ response. For example, if the right and left coronary or renal arteries were occluded, the heart or kidneys, respectively, would die. The uterus does not die because the ovarian and broad ligament arteries can supply sufficient blood to the uterus to keep it alive while they increase in diameter and eventually provide the full needs of the uterus. If an ascending uterine artery were occluded, blood flow from the contralateral ascending uterine artery could supply the uterus[37]. If the right anterior arcuate arteries were be occluded, the left anterior arcuate arteries could supply the right-sided territory, and so on. As a result of these redundant extrinsic and intrinsic uterine arterial connections, the vasculature of the uterus functions like a big-city electric power grid. Short of hysterectomy, long-term power outage in the uterus is nearly impossible.

UTERINE BLOOD VESSELS DURING PREGNANCY – EMBRYO AND FETUS NOURISHMENT BY PLACENTA

The mature placenta

The discoid, hemochorial placenta is an organ in which maternal blood comes into direct contact with fetal trophoblast cells that cover placental villi. Maternal and fetal circulatory systems come into very, very close contact, separated only by a lining of trophoblasts. However, they are separate, and the separation of the maternal and fetal circulation has been known since 1786[38]. The maternal side of the mature placental circulation is shown in Figure 4. Blood is delivered to the intravillous space by uteroplacental

arteries which spray oxygenated blood over fetal villi. Blood returns to the maternal circulation from the placenta by way of uteroplacental veins.

The mature placenta – growth and 'migration' later in pregnancy

Until the end of the fourth month of pregnancy, the normal placenta grows in both thickness and circumference. After this period there is no appreciable increase in placental thickness but the placenta continues to grow circumferentially until near the end of pregnancy.

The absolute position of the placenta on the surface of the uterus is fixed at the time of implantation. Over time, the placenta grows centrifugally. At the same time as the placenta grows in mass, the uterus expands in volume due to fetal and amniotic fluid growth and by myometrial growth. The growth is *pari passu* with that portion of the wall of the uterus to which the placenta is attached (Figure 5)[39]. A placenta cannot pick up and move like a crab or a spider. It is firmly connected to the underlying myometrium and has large arterial and venous connections that cannot move. However, differential growth of the placenta and the uterine cavity does occur over time resulting in an apparent shift or 'migration' of placental location. Most commonly, the apparent shift is away from the internal cervical os[40–42].

At 18 weeks, 45.1% of placentas were posterior and 42.1% anterior. By 34 weeks, slight variations in placental location were seen with more apparent 'migration' for placentas attached to the posterior wall than the anterior. All of the posterior low lying placentas and all but 3.4% of the anterior low lying placentas 'migrated' away from the cervical os.

When the placenta does remain within or very near to the internal cervical os, placenta previa is present.

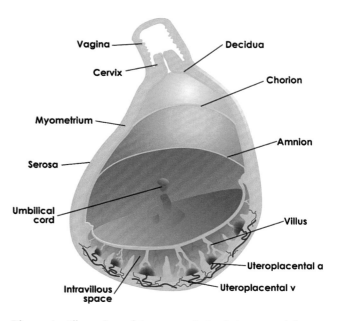

Figure 4 Illustration of the maternal circulation to and from a mature placenta. Fetal circulation in not shown

Placenta previa is variously described as 'total' if the internal os is covered by the placenta, 'partial' if the os is only partially covered, and 'marginal' if the edge of the placenta is at the edge of the os. Because the cervix dilates during labor, bleeding from separation of the placenta from the uterine wall can occur. The risk of placenta previa increases with maternal age and parity[44]. Preterm detachment of the normally implanted placenta, commonly termed 'abruptio placenta', is attributed variously to abnormal myometrial arteries at the placental base, abnormal uterine contractions, or is considered idiopathic[45–49].

The mature placenta – term placental size in relation to uterine surface area

At term the average placenta is 185 mm in diameter, 23 mm in thickness, 497 mm^3 in volume and weighs 508 g[39]. The term placenta is in contact with approximately 20% of the surface area of the uterus (Figure 6). Average placental base surface area is 252 cm^2 which corresponds to a diameter of 18 cm[39,50–53]. This area is referred to as the 'placental footprint' which is the area where hemostasis must occur if the mother is to survive placental separation.

UTERINE BLOOD VESSELS DURING PREGNANCY – HEMODYNAMIC CHANGES DURING PREGNANCY

Parallel blood flow circuits in the uterus

Of all the thousands of spiral arterioles in the uterus, however, only 200 spiral arterioles are transformed into uteroplacental arteries. To feed decidua and myometrium throughout the uterus, spiral and straight arterioles remain arterioles, with their high vascular resistance. As a result, two classes of arteries exist in the uterus. A small number of spiral arterioles and radial arteries are transformed into uteroplacental arteries, and a much larger number of arterioles are not transformed.

Placental and non-placental circulations are parallel sub-systems within the uterus. In parallel blood flow, some blood flow is distributed to one limb of the sub-systems and some to the other. Blood does not flow first through one sub-system and then another as in the serial sub-system.

Uterine artery resistance drops dramatically between weeks 8 and 16, decreasing little thereafter. Over an entire pregnancy, uterine artery resistance in a pregnant woman drops to approximately half the level of that in a non-pregnant woman by 24 weeks.

Uterine artery diameter increases during pregnancy

As vascular resistance in the arterioles of the uterus drops, blood flow increases, and the diameter of the uterine arteries increases during pregnancy. Average uterine artery diameter increases from 3 mm at the beginning of pregnancy to 7 mm at term.

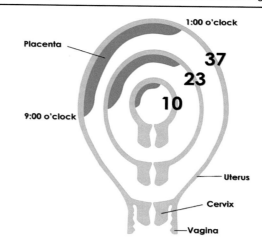

Figure 5 An illustration in the coronal plane showing placental attached to the uterus from 9:00 o'clock to 1:00 o'clock at 10 weeks, 23 weeks and 37 weeks of gestation. Adapted from a published figure in reference 43

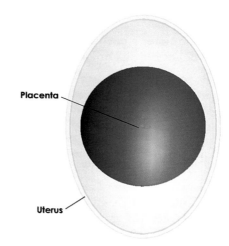

Figure 6 Illustration showing the area of contact between a term uterus and a term placenta based on a circular placenta and a prolate ellipse uterus. In this illustration the anterior wall of the uterus is cut away and the placenta is attached to the posterior wall of the uterus. The placental is in contact with 20% of the wall of the internal surface of the uterus

Uterine artery blood flow

At term

Wide variations in uterine artery blood flow values at term pregnancy have been published. Uterine artery blood flow near term is considered to be approximately 800 ml/min[54]. This places a boundary for bilateral uterine artery blood flow change during pregnancy: 100 ml/min before pregnancy to 800 ml/ min near term. Blood flow during pregnancy must fall between these two extremes.

Throughout pregnancy, blood flow increases week by week. The rate of change, however, is not constant and the overall shape of the blood flow curve during pregnancy is the typical 'S' shaped curve seen throughout biology. Twenty weeks' gestation, or mid-pregnancy, appears to be the inflection point of the curve. Before 20 weeks, the increase in uterine blood flow accelerates; after that, it decelerates.

Uterine artery blood flow increases secondary to increases in both uterine artery diameter and uterine artery red blood cell velocity (Figure 7).

Ovarian vein diameter – increase during pregnancy

The ovarian and uterine veins grow sufficiently in diameter during pregnancy to accommodate the large increase in blood flow to the uterus. No published uterine vein diameter measurements exist taken during pregnancy.

If one uses the surgical estimate of 9 mm for the non-pregnant ovarian vascular pedicle diameter and compares that with 3.9 mm by CT measurement of the ovarian vein alone, then proportionately at 38.9 weeks the ovarian vein, alone, would be 18.4 mm in diameter, a growth in diameter of 372%.

Ovarian vein diameter – decrease following pregnancy (smaller but still enlarged)

After delivery, when blood flow to the uterus returns to normal, the uterine and ovarian veins decrease in diameter. However, they do not return to their nulliparous diameters.

Arteries and veins in the pregnant woman

Taken together the anatomical changes of the arteries and veins of the uterus and ovary during mid-pregnancy are shown in Figure 8. See Figure 9 for a comparison with a non-pregnant woman. The ovarian and uterine veins have grown in diameter but growth is much more pronounced in the ovarian veins which empty into the inferior vena cava below the insertions

of the renal veins. The ovarian and uterine arteries have grown, too, but the growth of the uterine arteries has outstripped growth of the ovarian arteries. The tortuosity of the uterine and ovarian arteries has been extended as they were stretched with enlargement of the uterus. Though quite rare, spontaneous rupture of enlarged uterine or ovarian veins and uterine arteries has been reported[54,55].

UTERINE BLOOD VESSELS DURING PREGNANCY – LABOR AND DELIVERY

Mechanics of placental separation

After delivery of a baby, the uterus continues to contract. During these postpartum contractions, the

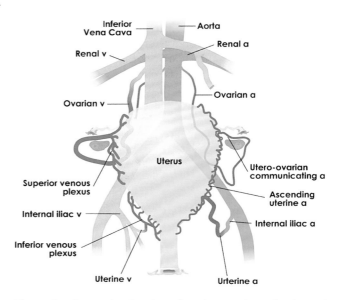

Figure 8 Composite drawing of uterine arteries and veins and their systematic origins and insertions, respectively, at 24 weeks of gestation

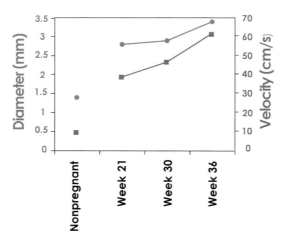

Figure 7 Graph of uterine artery diameter and red blood cell velocity in women not pregnant and at 21, 30 and 36 weeks of gestation. Uterine artery diameter is displayed as circles; velocity, as squares. Adapted from published tabular data[17]. The most rapid increases in diameter and red blood cell velocity occur between the time a woman gets pregnant and 21 weeks pregnancy

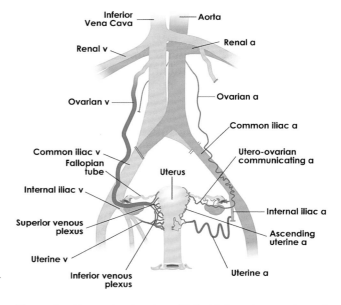

Figure 9 Composite drawing of left-sided uterine arteries and right-sided uterine veins showing their systematic origins and insertions in a non-pregnant woman

myometrium of the placental footprint becomes smaller and smaller, while the placenta, itself, being a solid structure, remains fixed in shape. The drop in the myometrial contact area of the placental footprint without change in the shape of the placental causes shear stress between the placenta and the uterus. The shear stresses at the junction between the placental base and the placental footprint tear the placenta away from the uterus, creating 200 torn and ragged uteroplacental arteries and veins!

Goto[56] defined three types of placental separation. In type I separation (53.0%), as a whole, the placenta smoothly slides off the wall of the uterus. In type II (35.5%), a portion of the placenta and fetal membranes adhere to the uterine wall preventing smooth separation. In type III (11.5%), a retroplacental hematoma forms between the uterine wall and the placenta during separation.

PRACTICE POINTS

- The uterus is a highly vascular organ with two arterial and two venous systems intertwined

- During pregnancy clotting and fibrinolytic factors in the blood build up in concentration in mother's blood. Throughout pregnancy both systems are active. However, the clotting system is a little more active than the fibrinolytic system. This imbalance during pregnancy has consequences for maternal health

- To stop hemorrhage following delivery, during true labor clotting commences within the uterine circulation

- Two hours following delivery, fibrinolysis commences in the uterus to restore blood flow.

References

1. Lipshutz B. A composite study of the hypogastric artery and its branches. Ann Surg 1918;67:584–608
2. Borell U, Fernstrom I. The adnexal branches of the uterine artery. An arteriographic study in human subjects. Acta Radiol 1953;40:561–82
3. Fernstrom I. Arteriography of the uterine artery. Acta Radiol 1955;S122:3–128
4. Radberg C, Wickbom I. Pelvic angiography and pneumo-peritoneum in the diagnosis of gynecologic lesions. Acta Radiol Diagn (Stockh) 1967;6:133–44
5. Merland JJ, Chiras J. Arteriography of the pelvis. Diagnostic and therapeutic procedures. Berlin, Heidelberg, New York: Springer-Verlag, 1981
6. Pron GE, Common AA, Sniderman KW, Bell SD, Simons ME, Vanderburgh LC. Radiological embolization of uterine arteries for symptomatic fibroids: preliminary findings of a Canadian multicenter trial [Abstract]. Minim Invasive Ther AlliedTechnol 1998;7(Suppl 1):26
7. Pelage JP, De Dref O, Soyer P, et al. Arterial anatomy of the female genital tract: Variations and relevance to transcatheter embolization of the uterus [Pictorial Essay]. AJR 1999;172: 989–94
8. Borell U. [Arteriography of uterine and adnexal vessels]. Geburtshilfe Frauenheilkd 1955;15:497–513
9. Nikolic B, Spies JB, Abbara S, Goodwin SC. Ovarian artery supply of uterine fibroids as a cause of treatment failure after uterine artery embolization: A case report. J Vasc Interv Radiol 1999;10:1167–70
10. Binkert CA, Andrews RT, Kaufman JA. Utility of non-selective abdominal aortography in demonstrating ovarian artery collaterals in patients undergoing uterine artery embolization for fibroids. J Vasc Interv Radiol 2001;12:841–5
11. Razavi MK, Wolanske KA, Hwang GL, Sze DY, Kee ST, Dake MD. Angiographic classification of ovarian artery-to-uterine artery anastomoses: initial observations in uterine fibroid embolization. Radiology 2002;224:707–12
12. Pelage JP, Walker WJ, Le Dref O. Re: utility of nonselective abdominal aortography in demonstrating ovarian artery collaterals in patients undergoing uterine artery embolization for fibroids. J Vasc Interv Radiol 2002;13:656
13. Worthington-Kirsch RL, Andrews RT, Siskin GP, et al. Uterine fibroid embolization: Technical aspects. Tech Vasc Interv Radiol 2002;5:17–34
14. Beliaeva YA. [Age-related properties of the arteries of the large ligament]. Arkhiv Anatomii 1965;48:98–107
15. Zamudio S, Palmer SK, Droma T, et al. Effect of altitude on uterine artery blood flow during normal pregnancy. J Appl Physiol 1995;79:7–14
16. Thaler I, Manor D, Itskovitz J, et al. Changes in uterine blood flow during human pregnancy. Am J Obstet Gynecol 1990; 162:121–5
17. Palmer SK, Zamudio S, Coffin C, Parker S, Stamm E, Moore LG. Quantitative estimation of human uterine artery blood flow and pelvic blood flow redistribution in pregnancy. Obstet Gynecol 1992;80:1000–6
18. Gomez-Jorge J, Keyoung A, Levy EB, Spies JB. Uterine artery anatomy relevant to uterine leiomyomata embolization. Cardiovasc Intervent Radiol 2003;26:522–7
19. Lippert H, Pabst R. Arterial variations in man. Munich: Bergmann, 1985
20. Holmgren B. Some observations on the blood vessels of the uterus under normal conditions and in myoma. Acta Obstet Gynecol Scand 1938;18:192–213
21. Cooper JM, Dickner SK. A Doppler-guided transvaginal approach leading to uterine artery occlusion may be a less invasive means to control uterine perfusion [Abstract]. J Am Assoc Gynecol Laparosc 2002;9:S12
22. Frates RE. Selective angiography of the ovarian artery. Radiology 1969;92:1014–9
23. Shlansky-Goldberg R. Uterine artery embolization: Historical and anatomic considerations. Semin Intervent Radiol 2000;17:223–36
24. Pelage JP, Cazejust J, Pluot E, et al. Uterine fibroid vascularization and clinical relevance to uterine fibroid embolization. Radiographics 2005;25 (Suppl 1):S99–117
25. Borell U, Fernstrom I. The ovarian artery: an arteriographic study in human subjects. Acta Radiol 1954;42:253–65
26. Kozik W. [Arterial vasculature of ovaries in women of various ages in light of anatomic, radiologic and microangiographic examinations]. Ann Acad Med Stetin 2000;46:25–34
27. Kozik W, Czerwinski F, Pilarczyk K, Partyka C. [Arteries of the hilum and parenchymal part of the ovary in reproductive age in microangiographic studies]. Ginekol Pol 2002;73: 1173–8
28. Ide P, Bonte J. [Arterial supply of the uterine isthmus and cervix]. Bull Soc Roy Belg Gynec Obstet 1964;34: 365–73
29. Palacios Jaraquemada JM, Monaco RG, Barbosa NE, Ferle L, Iriarte H, Conesa HA. Lower uterine blood supply: Extra-uterine anastomotic system and its application in surgical devascularization techniques. Acta Obstet Gynecol Scand 2007;86:228–34
30. Farrer-Brown G, Beilby JO, Tarbit MH. The blood supply of the uterus. 1. Arterial vasculature. J Obstet Gynaecol Br Commonw 1970;77:673–81
31. Sampson JA. The blood supply of uterine myomata. Surg Gynecol Obstet 1912;14:215–34

32. Lindenbaum E, Brandes JM, Itskovitz J. Ipsi- and contralateral anastomosis of the uterine arteries. Acta Anat 1978;102: 157–61

33. Chait A, Moltz A, Nelson JH Jr. The collateral arterial circulation in the pelvis. An angiographic study. Am J Roentgenol Radium Ther Nucl Med 1968;102:392–400

34. Mattingly RF, Thompson JD. Te Linde's Operative Gynecology, 6th edn. Philadelphia: J. B. Lippincott Company, 1985

35. Nasu K, Fujimoto H, Yamamoto S, Naitou H, Maekawa I, Yasuda S, Itou H. [Collaterals after flow alternation in pelvic arteries: precondition for pelvic reservoir therapy]. Nippon Igaku Hoshasen Gakkai Zasshi 1998;58:204–11

36. Chitrit Y, Guillaumin D, Caubel P, Herrero R. Absence of flow velocity waveform changes in uterine arteries after bilateral internal iliac artery ligation. Am J Obstet Gynecol 2000;182:727–28

37. Lindenbaum E, Brandes JM, Itskovitz J. Ipsi- and contralateral anastomosis of the uterine arteries. Acta Anat 1978;102: 157–61

38. Hunter J. On the structure of the placenta. In: Hunter J (Editor). Observations on certain parts of the animal economy. London: No. 13, Castle-Street, Leichester-Square, 1786:127–40

39. Boyd JD, Hamilton WJ. The Human Placenta. Cambridge, England: W. Heffer & Sons Ltd, 1970

40. King DL. Placental migration demonstrated by ultrasonography. A hypothesis of dynamic placentation. Radiology 1973;109:167–70

41. McClure N, Dornal JC. Early identification of placenta praevia. Br J Obstet Gynaecol 1990;97:959–61

42. Taipale P, Hiilesmaa V, Ylostalo P. Transvaginal ultrasonography at 18–23 weeks in predicting placenta previa at delivery. Ultrasound Obstet Gynecol 1998;12:422–5

43. Hamilton WJ, Boyd JD, Mossman HW. Human embryology. Baltimore: Williams & Wilkins Company, 1962

44. Ananth CV, Wilcox AJ, Savitz DA, Bowes WA Jr, Luther ER. Effect of maternal age and parity on the risk of uteroplacental bleeding disorders in pregnancy. Obstet Gynecol 1996;88:511–6

45. Alvarez H, Caldeyro R. [Contractility and premature separation of placenta]. An Fac Med Montevideo 1950;35:682–95

46. Minh HN, Smadja A, Orcel L. [Intimate mechanism of premature separation of the normally inserted placenta]. J Gynecol Obstet Biol Reprod (Paris) 1977;6:301–10

47. Amoa AB, Augerea L, Klufio CA. Antepartum haemorrhage at the Port Moresby General Hospital: a retrospective study of 130 consecutive cases. P N G Med J 1992;35:17–22

48. Pumarino R. [Premature seperation of placenta and uterine apoplexia]. Bol Hosp Vina Del Mar 1951;7:30–4

49. Dommisse J, Tiltman AJ. Placental bed biopsies in placental abruption. Br J Obstet Gynaecol 1992;99:651–4

50. Bekova KS. [The relationship between the weight of the fetus, the weight and surface area of the placenta and the structure of the veins of the fetal surface of the placenta]. Vopr Okhr Materin Det 1972;17:20–2

51. Woods DL, Malan AF, de V Heese H, van Schalkwyk DJ. Placental size at birth. S Afr Med J 1978;54:778–9

52. Mapfurira MJ, Msamati BC, Banadda BM. Correlations between weights of newborn babies, placental parameters and gestational age. Cent Afr J Med 1992;38:414–20

53. Blickstein I, Ron A. Can placental surface area and neonatal weight be predicted from placental surface measurements? Preliminary observations on normal-term pregnancies. Gynecol Obstet Invest 1995;40:253–6

54. Maguire P. Sponaneous rupture of utero-ovarian vessels during pregnancy. J Okla Med Ass 1962;55:123–4

55. Steinberg LH, Goodfellow C, Rankin L. Spontaneous rupture of the uterine artery in pregnancy. Br J Obstet Gynaecol 1993;100:184

56. Goto M. [A survey of placental separation by real-time B-mode scanning]. Nippon Sanka Fujinka Gakkai Zasshi 1984;36:1171–9

23

Obstetric Trauma

D. G. Evans and C. B-Lynch

ACUTE UTERINE INVERSION

Acute uterine inversion, defined as when the uterus is turned inside out, is a rare but serious complication of the third stage of labor. The estimated incidence is approximately 1 in 20–25 000 deliveries[1–3]. As the estimate of a later report was <1 : 2000[4], the true incidence is unclear because some of the milder forms correct themselves spontaneously and are thus not recognized or reported.

Classification

Uterine inversion may be complete or incomplete, depending on whether the fundus has passed through the cervix[5]. When the uterine inversion occurs within the first 24 h post-delivery, it is classified as acute. Inversion occurring after the first 24 h and up to 4 weeks postpartum is classified as sub-acute, and the rare chronic inversion occurs after the 4th week postpartum.

Etiology

The expulsion of the placenta was probably intended by Nature to occur as a result of gravitational forces, with the mother in the same squatting position that is often adopted for defecation. When the third stage is conducted in the dorsal position, however, help may be necessary for placental expulsion. Accordingly, the inappropriate management of the third stage of labor is often implicated in the etiology of acute uterine inversion. Indeed, Crede's method of placental delivery with uncontrolled cord traction, referred to in most textbooks of midwifery and older textbooks of obstetrics, may indeed increase the risk of acute uterine inversion. The firmly contracted uterus is used as a piston to push the placenta out, in the same manner that a piston is used to push fluid out of the barrel of a syringe. Pressure is applied with the palm of the hand in the axis of the pelvic inlet, in a downward and backward direction with the aim of forcing the placenta out through the lower genital tract. Unfortunately, application of Crede's maneuver when the uterus is not contracted may well facilitate acute inversion. On the other hand, the Brandt Andrews maneuver, also mentioned in standard textbooks of midwifery and obstetrics, a modification of Aristotle's method of delivering the placenta by cord traction, recommends applying tension, but not traction, to the umbilical cord with one hand, whilst the other hand is placed on the abdomen gently moving the uterus upwards and backwards. Today, controlled cord traction is standard practice for the third stage of labor.

Other etiological factors include forcibly attempting to expel the placenta by using fundal pressure when the uterus is atonic, and traction on the umbilical cord in a fundally placed placenta when the uterus is relaxed. It may also be brought about by a local atony, more particularly of the fundal placental site together with active contractions of the rest of the uterus. Other etiological factors include macrosomia, polyhydramnios, multiple pregnancy, primiparity and oxytocin administration[5]. In other instances, however, the inversion occurs spontaneously from sudden increased abdominal pressure as a result of coughing, sneezing or straining.

Chronic inversion may result from an acute inversion left unrecognized or from a sub-mucous fibroid which has prolapsed through the cervix. A placental polyp resulting from a retained cotyledon of the placenta may present in the same fashion.

Diagnosis

Symptoms are acute and pronounced. Generally, the mother is aware of something coming down and this is usually quickly followed by unanticipated profound shock. The uterus may appear at the introitus outside the vagina and the fundus is no longer palpable abdominally. In partial inversion, the fundus of the uterus may be indented and may or may not pass through the cervical os. In such instances, it is neither palpable abdominally nor visible at the vulva. Vaginal examination detects the inverted body of the uterus, and, above and encircling it, the ring of the cervix. In all instances, pain may be severe due to stretching of the infundibulo-pelvic ligaments and other viscera.

Shock is the outstanding sign, and may in part be neurogenic due to stretching of the viscera and in part due to hemorrhage and hypovolemia. The degree of shock is proportional to blood loss and hemorrhage is variable, depending on whether any attempt has been made to remove the placenta. Some bleeding will always be present unless the placenta is completely adherent to the uterine wall. It is important to recognize that severe hemorrhage will accompany any attempt at removing the placenta before the uterus is replaced[5,6]. This eventuality is a special risk if the birth has been attended by a traditional birth attendant (TBA) in parts of the underdeveloped world.

Management

Acute uterine inversion is a true obstetric emergency[6], and clearly one which may lead to severe postpartum hemorrhage. If present and available, a supportive team should be summoned to the delivery suite for resuscitation and protocol management. Uterotonics, if started, are to be stopped and manual replacement attempted under adequate and appropriate anesthesia followed by delivery of the placenta assisted by restart of oxytocin[7].

Elevation of the foot of the delivery table or bed may relieve the tension on the viscera and reduce the pain and shock. Immediate resuscitation with intravenous fluids is indicated via large-gauge venous access. Adequate analgesia must be instituted prior to attempting replacement, and the bladder should be catheterized. Antibiotic prophylaxis is advisable.

Any delay increases the difficulty in replacing the uterus, and the first health-care professional present should make the initial attempt at replacement. This will be aided if regional anesthetic is already in place[8]. The placenta should be left *in situ* and no attempt made to remove it. The portion of the uterus that came down last should go back first, that is, the lower segment initially and the fundus later. The hand is lubricated with hibitane cream (or other suitable antiseptic if available) and placed inside the vagina. With gentle maneuvers of the fingers around the cervical rim and simultaneous upward pressure with the palm of the hand, the uterus is gradually replaced. The employment of force is dangerous, as the thinned-out lower segment may be torn or otherwise traumatized. The vaginal vault may already have been torn in some cases. The degree of shock does not diminish until the uterus is replaced. In the majority of instances, replacement of the uterus is successful using this conservative method[9]. If replacement is successful, the placenta should be manually removed with the aid of ergometrine or an oxytocic infusion. In underdeveloped countries or in a home setting, boiled water brought to a bearable temperature can be used to soak clean towels or cloths to assist in pushing and packing the vagina. This may facilitate replacement attempts and control further blood loss. Bimanual massage of the fundus may improve contraction.

If replacement is unsuccessful, measures to relax the cervical retraction ring should be the next line of therapy. Beta mimetics or amyl nitrite inhalation can often relax the retraction ring sufficiently to allow uterine replacement[9]. A similar effect is seen with the administration of halothane anesthesia, but, unfortunately, use of this agent in sufficient doses can result in the unwanted and life-threatening complications of uterine atony, hypotension and severe hemorrhage.

Halothane is no longer used for these and other reasons. A 2 g intravenous bolus of magnesium sulfate can be used in the hypotensive patient (0.25 mg of intravenous terbutaline in the stable patient) to relax the cervical contraction ring[10]. Intravenous nitroglycerine can be tried although it is not commonly used.

Further attempts at replacement of the uterus should take place under general anesthesia in an operating theater equipped and ready to perform a laparotomy. Before resorting to a laparotomy, however, the tried and tested O'Sullivan hydrostatic technique[11] should be attempted. Here, the patient is first resuscitated to restore vital signs including adequate blood volume and pressure. The obstetric team and anesthetist are summoned.

Adequate analgesia is essential before:

(1) Attempt at repositioning without the use of uterine relaxant;

(2) If response is not imminent or sustained, an anesthetist should provide uterine relaxation to facilitate repositioning and the administration of uterotonics;

(3) General anesthesia is preferable, administered by an obstetric anesthetist. Digital repositioning should be maintained to support and establish good uterine muscle tone;

(4) 1–2 liters of saline at body temperature should be infused into the vagina through rubber tubes placed in the posterior fornix, whilst obliterating the introitus with the obstetrician's hand. As the vaginal walls distend, the fundus of the uterus rises and the inversion is usually promptly corrected. Once this is achieved, fluid is allowed to slowly escape from the vagina whilst the placement of the uterine fundus is achieved and maintained.

When O'Sullivan first described this technique, he used a douche-can and wide rubber tubing to deliver the solution. More recently, a silastic vacuum cup has been used to instil the sterile solution into the vagina[12]. Until replacement is effected, however, towels soaked in warm hypertonic saline solution and draped over the inverted uterus may reduce the edema which will inevitably occur and which further impedes replacement of the uterus. In extremely difficult cases, replacement may require mid-line laparotomy, with the patient cleansed and draped in the Lloyd Davis (frog-legged) position with a head-down (Trendelenberg) tilt. The patient is catheterized with an indwelling catheter and broad-spectrum antibiotics are administered. With the bowels packed upward and away from the uterus, the obstetric surgeon places his hands in front and back of the lower segment with the finger tips between and below the level of the inverted fundus. With progressive pressure on the fingertips of both hands which flip up simultaneously, the internal dimple is replaced progressively by the rising uterine fundus (Figure 1a–e)[13]. Uterine perfusion returns with re-establishment of uterine pulse pressure.

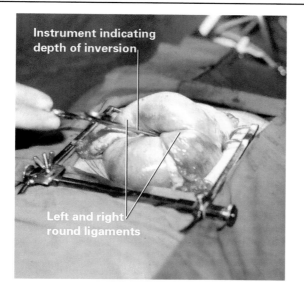

Figure 1a Acute uterine inversion

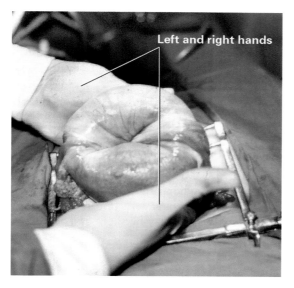

Figure 1b Acute uterine inversion. Finger tips placed below fundus of uterus to facilitate reduction

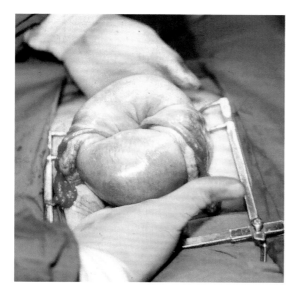

Figure 1c Acute uterine inversion. Progressive reduction with some ischemia

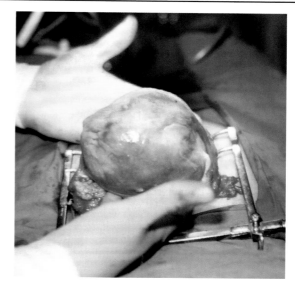

Figure 1d Acute uterine inversion. Return of vascularity

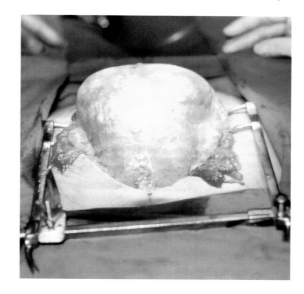

Figure 1e Acute uterine inversion. Complete reduction and revascularization with normal clinical features. (B-Lynch technique of non-instrumental reduction of acute uterine inversion at laparotomy. ©Copyright '05)

If this technique fails, then the mid-line abdominal incision can be extended upwards if necessary. The inverted uterus resembles a funnel; it is best to exteriorize the uterus. Instrumental upward traction is applied to the round ligaments bilaterally using Allis or ring forceps, while the assistant exerts upward pressure on the inverted parts from the vagina below. This maneuver is the Huntington technique[14,15].

Failure at this stage warrants employing the Haultain technique whereby an incision is made vertically in the posterior cervix via the abdominal route, following the dimple as a guide to relieve the constriction at this level. The assistant exerts upward pressure from the vagina to effect reduction and replacement[16].

On return of the uterus to its normal position, the placenta should be removed manually from the vagina, and uterine contraction maintained abdominally by bi-manual stimulation. Ergometrine, oxytocic intra-venous infusion, or mesoprostyl can be administered. The posterior uterine incision, if used, is then repaired in layers, and the abdomen closed in the usual fashion. The patient should be monitored in the intensive care or the high-dependency unit for 24 h.

A sub-acute inversion is managed in a similar manner but may resolve spontaneously as the uterus involutes[4].

In chronic inversion, the uterus involutes in its inverted position and remains in the vagina as a soft swelling, which bleeds readily to touch and shows areas of superficial ulceration. Prolonged inversion may result in conversion of the columnar epithelium of the uterine wall into a stratified squamous epithelium. Replacement of a chronic inversion can prove extremely difficult, due partly to the inevitable edema present and the friable nature of the tissues. The techniques adopted for replacing the acutely inverted uterus are no longer helpful in this chronic situation. Bed rest, elevation of the foot of the bed, antibiotic prophylaxis, and vaginal cleansing with hibitane packs may be helpful to reduce the edema and treat any infections, but it may eventually be necessary to perform a hysterectomy. If the chronic inversion is due to the presence of a fibroid or a placental polyp, initial removal of the polyp by ligating and cutting the pedicle as near to the base as possible may facilitate replacement of the inverted uterus.

RUPTURED UTERUS

Uterine rupture is a serious obstetric complication with high morbidity and mortality. In developed countries, the increasing number of cesarean sections performed for minor degrees of disproportion, fetal distress or pre-eclampsia in primiparae is of considerable importance in calculating the long-term risks associated with cesarean section, particularly in terms of the incidence and risk of uterine rupture. Both the short- and long-term risks are accentuated in resource-poor countries.

Uterine rupture may be complete when the tear extends into the peritoneal cavity, or incomplete when the serosa remains intact. The rupture may be spontaneous, traumatic or the result of scar dehiscence and may occur either during pregnancy, early in labor or following a prolonged labor[17].

In developed countries, the most common cause of uterine rupture is dehiscence of a previous lower segment transverse cesarean section scar. Rupture of a classical scar is eight times more common than that of a previous lower segment incision, and is far more apt to occur before rather than during labor. Previous rupture of a scar confers a 10–20-fold increase in risk of a subsequent rupture[18,19].

Rupture of the uterus is generally sudden, accompanied by severe abdominal pain and followed by vascular collapse. In many cases, however, asymptomatic dehiscence takes place during a vaginal delivery after a previous cesarean section, when the dehiscence is

gradual and retraction of the uterus arrests hemorrhage from the wound. Because of this possibility, it is always necessary to exclude silent dehiscence by manual exploration of the uterus after delivery of the fetus when a scar is present on the uterus.

A major factor in spontaneous uterine rupture is obstructed labor, especially in the developing world when women routinely delivery without the benefit of the presence of trained health-care providers. Rupture may be due to maternal or fetal causes (generally macrosomia). Examples of maternal causes are cephalopelvic disproportion from pelvic contraction due to developmental, constitutional or nutritional causes, abnormal presentation such as shoulder presentation, breech or brow, persistent mentoposterior face presentation, transverse lie, fetal abnormality, hydrocephalus, fetal tumor, fetal ascites, conjoined twins, maternal tumors, intrinsic cervical lesions, extrinsic fibroids or tumor, locked twins, and rarely uterine misalignment such as incarcerated retroverted uterus, and pathological uterine anteversion. Additionally, grand multiparity, the use of uterotonic drugs to induce or augment labor, placenta percreta, and intra-uterine manipulation have all been implicated as causes of uterine rupture[19,20].

The most common predisposing cause of rupture during pregnancy is a weak scar following a previous cesarean section[20]. Rarely, rupture can occur following unrecognized injury to the uterus at a previous difficult delivery. It may present with sudden severe abdominal pains and collapse, or the symptoms may present gradually, when rupture is based on scar dehiscence. If the onset is gradual, diagnosis may be difficult as the abdominal pain may be slight and accompanied only by alterations in the fetal heart tracing, maternal tachycardia and minimal vaginal bleeding. This triad is then followed by patient collapse, cessation of fetal movement and easy palpation of the fetal parts if the fetus has been expelled completely into the peritoneal cavity. If the patient is in a hospital and the catastrophe recognized at its onset, the outcome should be the safe delivery of the baby and repair of the uterus. If the patient is not in a hospital, on the other hand, the catastrophe is just that, a catastrophe of a dead child and its mother.

Uterine rupture during labor is also most commonly due to dehiscence of a previous cesarean scar with pain over the scar, followed by sudden severe abdominal pain and collapse. In grand multiparae with a friable inelastic uterine wall, rupture may occur in early labor even where there has been no previous scar or difficult delivery, although this eventuality is not nearly as common as rupture in the previously scarred uterus. Here, however, diagnosis may be difficult initially as the presentation may be confused with a small accidental hemorrhage and therefore missed.

Rupture after a prolonged labor is commonly due to obstructed labor, with marked thinning of the lower segment and increased retraction of the upper segment resulting in the formation of a retraction or Bandl's ring. The tear begins in the lower uterine segment, may extend up to the fundus or down into the vagina, or proceed laterally into the broad ligament. If the tear is posterior, it may go through the posterior vaginal fornix into the Pouch of Douglas (colporrhexis)[20]. If the rupture is in the lower anterior segment, the bladder is stripped from its attachment to the lower segment. The peritoneum remains intact and so the rupture is characterized as incomplete. A multiparous patient in obstructed labor will continue to have tetanic contractions until the uterus ruptures, whilst a primiparous patient will usually go out of labor. Classical clinical signs of a rupture in a multiparous patient can be dramatic; abdominal pain is constant, the contractions become virtually continuous initially with only short intervals between them and later no interval between contractile forces, with the formation of a Bandl's ring followed by rupture and collapse. The contractions then usually stop[20–22], the fetus is expelled into the peritoneal cavity, the fetal parts are easily palpable and the uterus adopts an altered shape.

Rarely, the uterus may rupture during early to midpregnancy or during labor in patients who have had a previous cornual ectopic pregnancy. Here also, the rupture is dramatic, is located over the repair site of the ectopic and is characterized as a fundal blow-out. Sudden severe abdominal pain is experienced over the fundus of the uterus followed by collapse.

Rupture of a previously unscarred uterus is usually a catastrophic event resulting in death of the infant, extensive damage to the uterus and a very high risk of maternal death from blood loss. The damage to the uterus may be so extensive that repair is impossible and a hysterectomy is required. In developed countries, the incidence of ruptured uterus in an unscarred uterus is approximately 1 : 10 000 deliveries[22]; in the underdeveloped countries, the data are unknown. The incidence of rupture of a uterus with a previous cesarean section scar is 1%[22,23]. A trial of labor following a previous cesarean section increases the risk of perinatal death and rupture of the uterus compared to elective repeat cesarean section. In one large Canadian study, a trial of labor following a previous cesarean section was associated with an increased risk of rupture (by 0.56%) but fewer maternal deaths than in an elective section (1.6 vs. 5.6 per 100 000)[19].

In less developed countries, the incidence of uterine rupture varies from 1.4% to 25%, with 25% in Ethiopian women with obstructed labor[23]. Uterine rupture accounted for 9.3% of maternal mortality in one study from India and 6.2% in a study from South Africa[24].

A laparotomy is indicated when rupture of the uterus is suspected. The patient is anesthetized, cleansed, draped and the bladder catheterized with an indwelling catheter. A mid-line lower abdominal incision should be used as this may be extended cephalad if necessary. The fetus should be delivered expeditiously and the uterus delivered from the abdominal incision to assist in controlling the bleeding and assessing the situation while resuscitative measures are

undertaken. In the series of over 1300 world-wide reported successful applications of the B-Lynch (Brace) suture, 25 cases were applied for persistent uterine atony after repair of a uterine rupture. In these cases, successful bleeding control and hemostasis were achieved (CBL world-wide communication www.CBLynch. com)[25].

Hysterectomy may be necessary and should have been consented, if at all possible. It is not necessary to remove the ovaries merely because this is easier in a crisis. As with a cesarean hysterectomy performed in late labor, the cervix is no longer a discrete and circumscribed solid structure, easily delineated and permitting accurate placement of vaginal clamps. In the acute situation, hemostasis and avoidance of further dissection are of paramount importance, and the removal of the distal cervix is not critical. The most difficult surgical situation occurs when the rupture is extraperitoneal into the broad ligament, with a massive hematoma distorting the anatomy and obscuring the bleeding points. Here, it may be necessary to pack the space, the end of the pack being brought out through a gap in the uterine repair[20]. A balloon catheter with light traction may be used for enhanced tamponade with or without the application of the B-Lynch (Brace) suture application[26].

Other conservative surgery may be appropriate on occasions, for example, when simple repair of the tear may be preferable to hysterectomy. With an anterior rupture, the bladder may be involved; the appearance of hematuria is almost pathognomonic. Repair is undertaken and the bladder catheterized for 2 weeks. A posterior fornix rupture (colporrhexis) is relatively easy to repair. Incomplete rupture is not usually apparent until delivery has been achieved. It will commonly declare itself by intrapartum or postpartum hemorrhage. It should always be excluded by manual exploration after delivery of the fetus. Both bladder tears and colporrhexis may be missed if not anticipated. If this is the case, bleeding may continue, to the surgeon's dismay.

BLUNT ABDOMINAL TRAUMA

The three main causes of serious blunt abdominal trauma in pregnancy are motor vehicle accidents, falls and domestic or intimate partner physical abuse. In the developed world, the most common cause of blunt abdominal trauma is motor vehicle accidents[27,28]. In the less developed countries, the incidence of domestic physical abuse or intimate partner physical abuse can be as high as 13.5%[29]. Developed countries are not immune from this problem, however, and a large review of the prevalence of abuse during pregnancy in the United States documented that between 0.9% and 20.1% of pregnant women were abused by their partners. This figure covers all forms of abuse, emotional, physical and sexual[30].

Direct abdominal trauma by punching or kicking the abdomen increases the risk of adverse outcome of the pregnancy. Adverse outcomes are more common with direct physical assaults than with motor vehicle accidents[29,30]. Partner abuse also tends to be a repetitive event, increasing the risk to the fetus[31]. In some countries, partner abuse and violence against women is accepted as a cultural norm, thus reducing the numbers of reported cases. Even in the Chinese community in Hong Kong and despite western socialization, it is not uncommon for women to submit to their husbands and endure humiliation for the sake of keeping their family together. Providing help for these pregnant women is challenging[32].

Motor vehicle accidents account for 60–75% of cases of blunt trauma. Most injuries are minor, but, in the United States, between 1300 and 3900 women each year suffer a fetal loss as a result of a motor vehicle accident[27,28]. Despite the majority of the injuries being minor, the fetus is always at risk and careful assessment must be carried out in all cases of blunt abdominal trauma resulting from motor vehicle accidents. Assessments must be frequent and repeated with special attention to conditions commonly seen after such trauma. These include abruptio placentae, preterm labor, uterine rupture, fetomaternal hemorrhage, direct fetal injury and fetal demise[33].

The pattern of injury following automobile accidents depends on the type of seat belt restraints. An unbelted driver or passenger is usually ejected from the vehicle or sustains injuries when they hit the interior of the car. The injuries are mainly to the face, head, chest, abdomen and pelvis. With shoulder and abdominal restraints, rib, sternum and clavicular fractures are common, whereas in the lap-only belted, lumbar spine and hollow viscus injuries are more frequent. Sharp objects in the pockets of the clothing on the person can cause additional trauma; a fountain pen may perforate the lungs or heart. Even bulky outdoor overclothing represents a hazard. With thick clothing, there is a short distance between the body of the person and the restraint. On impact, the weight of the body causes acceleration forwards. The speed of contact between the person and the restraint can compound the damage sustained to the body.

During the first trimester, the uterus is well protected within the pelvis and sustains very little damage from blunt trauma. With advancing pregnancy, however, the uterus becomes an abdominal organ and therefore more susceptible to trauma. The blood supply to the pelvis is markedly increased the more advanced the pregnancy, giving rise to retroperitoneal hemorrhage which can be life-threatening. Bowel injuries are less common, as the bowel occupies the upper abdominal space later in pregnancy, is a more movable entity and is not in the direct line of the trauma.

Assessing the extent of trauma can be difficult, as clinical signs initially may be sparse. Patients should be assessed frequently to detect deterioration in their condition. The presence of bony injuries should raise suspicion of intraperitoneal hemorrhage: rib fractures are associated with liver and spleen injuries and pelvic fractures with retroperitoneal hemorrhage and injury to the genitourinary system.

Difficulty is often encountered in detecting a small amount of bleeding into the peritoneal cavity. As blood may be non-irritant, ultrasound examination may be equivocal, and CT scanning exposes the fetus to a large radioactive dose. The decision to proceed to a laparotomy may therefore be entirely based on clinical judgement.

The most common cause of fetal death in non-fatal accidents is abruptio placentae. In minor injuries, the incidence is between 1 and 5%, in contrast to major trauma where the incidence may be as high as 30%. At the time of impact, the intrauterine pressure may be as high as ten times the pressure reached at the height of a labor contraction. Blunt trauma causes the uterus to compress and then expand and the placenta shears away from the uterine wall. The degree of separation may bear no relationship to the degree of trauma; abruption may occur with very little evidence of injury to the mother. It usually, but not always, follows soon after the trauma.

Vaginal bleeding, abdominal pain, increased uterine tone, uterine tenderness, high frequency contractions, and abnormal fetal cardiotocography are the classical clinical signs of a placental abruption. In a posteriorly inserted placenta, severe backache and vaginal bleeding may be significant symptoms. The bleeding may be revealed or concealed within the uterus. If concealed, in severe cases, the uterus becomes woody hard as described by Couvelaire, blood having been extravasated into the muscular wall of the uterus. Fetal parts are impossible to feel and the patient's condition rapidly deteriorates due to hypovolemia and pain.

The management of abruptio placentae depends on the severity of the abruption, the nature of the general injuries sustained, the condition of the fetus and the duration of the pregnancy. The trauma surgeon and the obstetrician should work together in managing the patient. Establishing wide-bore intravenous access is essential. The hematologist should also be involved. A complete thrombophilia screen should be requested and cross-matched blood organized, together with fresh frozen plasma.

A preterm uncompromised fetus should be observed by continuous cardiotocography for a minimum of 6–12 h or by a Pinard stethoscope in less developed communities and, if the gestation is under 34 weeks, the mother should be given corticosteroids to mimimize the adverse effect of prematurity on lung maturation. If the fetus is previable and compromised, vaginal delivery is the safest for the mother.

In a term pregnancy with abruptio and an uncompromised fetus, vaginal delivery is an option. However, cesarean section is advised if the fetus is compromised. If the fetus, on the other hand, has died, induction of labor and vaginal delivery are appropriate and safe for the mother.

Preterm labor following blunt abdominal trauma may be precipitated by extravasation of blood into the myometrium stimulating uterine contraction. Prostaglandin release may stimulate uterine activity. Preterm labor requiring tocolysis occurs in 10–30% of cases of blunt abdominal trauma, but less than 1% deliver before 34 weeks. Tocolytics should be used guardedly, lest they mask the sign of abruption. Contractions following blunt abdominal trauma abate without treatment in 90% of cases. All tocolytics have side-effects which the obstetrician should be familiar with: beta mimetics induce tachycardia and may mask the early signs of abruption; non-steroidal anti-inflammatory agents affect platelet and renal function; and calcium channel blockers cause hypertension. The fetal heart rate and the uterine contractions should be continuously monitored[34].

Uterine rupture is a rare (1%) occurrence in blunt abdominal trauma; when it does occur, it is usually in association with a fractured pelvis. The site of rupture is commonly the fundus of the uterus or the site of a previous uterine scar. Fetal mortality in such cases is 100%, and maternal mortality 10%[35-38]. Diagnosis may be difficult with vague abdominal pain, uterine tenderness, but with easily palpable fetal parts, and a poor trace or absence of a fetal heart on cardiotocography. Fetal demise and maternal shock are more dramatic presentations.

If suspected, exploratory laparotomy in the presence of the trauma surgeon is indicated. Uterine repair should be undertaken only if the patient is hemodynamically stable. If not, hysterectomy should be performed. However, the risk of a rupture in a subsequent pregnancy is high, and the patient and her family should be advised this at an appropriate time.

Fetal injury occurs very infrequently following blunt abdominal trauma. Fracture of the long bones or the skull is the most common injury and occurs in approximately 1% of cases. If the fetus is distressed, immediate delivery is called for. In the preterm non-compromised fetus, delivery may be delayed, but serial monitoring is advised[39,40].

Fetomaternal hemorrhage occurs in up to 30% of cases of blunt abdominal trauma, especially if the placenta is situated anteriorly. Most fetuses will have a normal outcome, although anemia, supraventricular tachycardia and fetal demise can occur depending on the extent of the fetomaternal hemorrhage[41,42]. Victims of blunt abdominal trauma should be screened for Rhesus factor, and all Rhesus-negative mothers given Anti-D immunoglobulin to prevent sensitization. Sensitization can occur as early as the 5th week of pregnancy. A Kleihauer–Betke test is essential to assess the magnitude of the fetomaternal hemorrhage and adjust the dose of Anti-D immunoglobulin accordingly.

In all cases of blunt abdominal injuries, fetal assessment is of paramount importance. Cardiotocography is the most sensitive method of immediate fetal surveillance. Ultrasonography is only accurate in predicting 40% of cases of abruption. Uterine activity is the most sensitive indicator for predicting abruption following blunt abdominal trauma. Frequent contractions have an adverse effect on fetal outcome.

As a guideline, patients who have sustained blunt abdominal trauma, but have no abdominal tenderness, no vaginal bleeding and no contractions should be monitored 2-hourly for 6–12 hours. Patients with abdominal tenderness, vaginal bleeding and contractions should be monitored continuously[43,44].

References

1. Spain AW. Acute inversion of the uterus. J Obstet Gynaecol Br Empire 1946;53:219
2. Das P. Inversion of the uterus. J Obstet Gynaecol Br Empire 1940;47:525–48
3. Fahmy M. Acute inversion of the uterus. Int J Surg 1977; 62:100
4. Watson P, Besch N, Bowes WA. Management of acute and subacute puerperal inversion of the uterus. Obstet Gynecol 1980;55:12
5. Brar HS, Greenspoon JS, Platt LD, Paul RH. Acute puerperal uterine inversion. J Reprod Med 1989;34:173–7
6. Wendel PJ, Cox SM. Emergent obstetric management of uterine inversion. Obstet Gynecol Clin N Am 1995;22: 261–74
7. Abouleish E, Ali V, Joumaa B, et al. Anaesthetic management of acute puerperal uterine inversion. Br J Anaesth 1995;75: 486–7
8. Catanzarite VA, Moffitt KD, Baker ML, et al. New approach to the management of acute puerperal uterine inversion. Obstet Gynecol 1986; 68(Suppl):7–10
9. Clark SL. Use of ritodrine in uterine inversion. Am J Obstet Gynecol 1984;151:705
10. Grossman RA. Magnesium sulphate for uterine inversion. J Reprod Med 1981;26:261–2
11. O'Sullivan JV. Acute inversion of the uterus. Br Med J 1945; ii:282–3
12. Ogueh O, Ayida G. Acute uterine inversion: a new technique of hydrostatic replacement. Br J Obstet Gynaecol 1997; 104,951–2
13. B-Lynch C. Non instrumental atraumatic stepwise reduction of acute uterine inversion. In press
14. Huntington JL. Acute inversion of the uterus. Boston Med Surg J 1921;184:376–80
15. Huntington JL, Irving PC, Kellogg PS. Abdominal reposition in acute inversion of the puerperal uterus. Am J Obstet Gynecol 1928;15:34–40
16. Haultain FWN. The treatment of chronic uterine inversion by abdominal hysterotomy with a successful case. Br Med J 1901;ii:974
17. Schrinsky DC, Benson RC. Rupture of the pregnant uterus: a review. Obstet Gynaecol Surv 1978;33:217–32
18. Ritchie EH. Pregnancy after rupture of the pregnant uterus. J Obstet Gynaecol Br Commonwealth 1971;78:642–8
19. Aguero O, Kizer S. Obstetric prognosis of the repair of uterine rupture. Surg Gynaecol Obstet 1968;127:528–30
20. Hudson CN. Obstructed labour and its sequelae. In Lawson JB, Harrison KA, Bergstrom S, eds. Maternity Care in Developing Countries. London: RCOG Press, 2001
21. Wen SW, Rusen ID, Walker M, et al. Comparison of maternal mortality and morbidity between trial of labor and elective Caesarean among women with previous caesarean delivery. Am J Obstet Gynecol 2004;19:1263–9
22. Miller DA, Goodwin TM, Cherman RB, Oaul RH. Intrapartum rupture of the unscarred uterus. Obstet Gynecol 1997;89:671–3
23. Gaym A. Obstructed labour in a district hospital. Ethiop Med J 2002;40:11
24. Rajaram P, Agarwal A, Swain S. Determinants of maternal mortality: a hospital based study from South India. Ind J Matern Child Health 1995;6:7–10
25. B-Lynch C. Persistent uterine atony after successful repair of ruptured uterus treated by Brace suture, world-wide reports and personal communication. www.cblynch.com

26. Danso D, Reginald P. Intrauterine balloon catheter with B-Lynch suture. Br J Obstet Gynaecol 2002;109:963

27. Esposito TJ, Gens DR, Smith IG, Scorpio R, Buchman T. Trauma during pregnancy. A review of 79 cases. Arch Surg 1991;126:1073–8

28. Hoff WS, D'Amelio LF, Tinkoff GH, et al. Maternal predictors of fetal demise in trauma during pregnancy. Surg Gynecol Obstet 1991;172:175–80

29. Valladares E, Pena R, Oersson LA, Hogberg U. Violence against pregnant women: prevalence and characteristics. A population-based study in Nicaragua. Br J Obstet Gynaecol 2005;112:1234–48

30. Gazmararian JA, Lazorick S, Spitz AM, Ballard TJ, Saltzman LE, Marks JS. Prevalence of violence against women: a review of the literature. JAMA 1996;275:1915–20

31. Godwin TM, Breen MT. Pregnancy outcome and feto-maternal hemorrhage after non catastrophic trauma. Am J Obstet Gynecol 1990;162:665–71

32. Tiwari A, Leung WC, Leung TW, Humphreys J, Parker B, Ho PC. A randomised controlled trial of empowerment training for Chinese abused pregnant women in Hong Kong. Br J Obstet Gynaecol 2005;112:1249–56

33. Connolly A, Katz VL, Bash KL, McMahon MJ, Hansen WF. Trauma and pregnancy. Am J Perinatol 1997;14:331–6

34. Elliott M. Vehicular accidents and pregnancy. Aust NZ J Obstet Gynaecol 1966;6:279–86

35. Williams JK, McClain L, Rosemurgy AS, Colorado NM. Evaluation of blunt abdominal trauma in the third trimester of pregnancy: maternal, and fetal considerations. Obstet Gynecol 1990;75:33–7

36. American College of Obstetricians and Gynecologists. Trauma during pregnancy. ACOG Technical Bulletin No. 161, November 1991, Washington DC

37. Mighty H. Trauma in pregnancy. Crit Care Clin 1994;10:623–34

38. Dahmus MA, Sibai BN. Blunt abdominal trauma. Are there any predictive factors for abruptio placentae or maternal-fetal distress. Am J Obstet Gynecol 1993;169:1054–9

39. Lavin JP, PolSky SS. Abdominal trauma during pregnancy. Clin Perinatol 1983;10:423–38

40. Goodwin TM, Breen MT. Pregnancy outcome and feto-maternal hemorrhage after non-catastrophic trauma. Am J Obstet Gynecol 1990;162:665–71

41. Pearlman MD, Tintinalli JE, Lorenz RP. A prospective controlled study of outcome after trauma during pregnancy. Am J Obstet Gynecol 1990;162:1502–10

42. Rose PG, Strohm PL, Zuspan FP. Fetomaternal hemorrhage following trauma. Am J Obstet Gynecol 1985;153:844–7

43. Pearlman MD, Phillips ME. Safety belt use during pregnancy. Obstet Gynecol 1996;88:1026–9

44. Pearlman MD, Tintinalli JE, Lorenz RP. Blunt trauma during pregnancy. N Engl J Med 1991;323:1609–13

24

Bleeding from the Lower Genital Tract

A. Duncan and C. von Widekind

INTRODUCTION

In the first comprehensive English Language textbook on the subject, William Smellie, in his 1752 *Treatise on the Theory and Practise of Midwifery*[1], correctly identifies the atonic uterus as a major cause of postpartum hemorrhage with his statement 'This dangerous efflux is occasioned by every thing that hinders the emptied uterus from contracting'. Although he refers to vaginal packing with *Tow or linen rags* (dipped in astringents such as oxycrate, red tart wine, alum or Sacchar-saturni), he does not specifically refer to bleeding from the lower genital tract. Because this omission was repeated in subsequent years by many standard textbooks and reviews of postpartum hemorrhage, it is not surprising that the present evidence base is poor, and a 2005 MESH search in PubMed of the National Library USA combining the terms 'Postpartum hemorrhage' AND 'Lacerations' OR 'Rupture' NOT 'Uterine rupture' came up with only 28 publications.

Maternal deaths specifically from lower genital tract bleeding as the cause of postpartum hemorrhage are rare in the developed world. The 2000–2002 United Kingdom Confidential Enquiries[2] reported only one death from this cause. World-wide, no accurate figures exist, but it is likely that the numbers are significant, particularly where there is significant co-morbidity and a poorly resourced maternity infrastructure[3].

CLASSIFICATION

Possible sources of bleeding from the lower genital tract include:

(1) Cervical tears;

(2) Vaginal tears (above and below the levator ani muscle, see Figure 1);

(3) Vulva and perineal tears;

(4) Episiotomies.

With the exception of cervical tears without vaginal extension, all of the above can lead to paravaginal hematomas, which in turn can be divided into those above and below the levator ani muscle (Figure 1). Infralevator hematomas include those of the vulva, perineum, paravaginal space and ischiorectal fossa. Supralevator bleeding

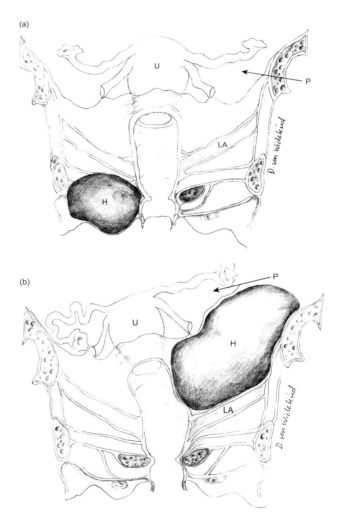

Figure 1 Paravaginal hematomas. (a) The hematoma lies beneath the levator ani muscle; (b) the hematoma lies above the levator ani and is spreading upwards into the broad ligament. H, hematoma; LA, levator ani, U, uterus; P, pelvic peritoneal reflection

is more dangerous, as it is more difficult to identify and control the source of bleeding, and blood loss into the retroperitoneal space can be massive.

INCIDENCE

In the UK, postpartum hemorrhage of more than 500 ml occurs in between 5 and 17% of all deliveries and postpartum hemorrhage of more than 1000 ml in 1.3% of deliveries.

Cervical tears

Minor cervical tears are common and are likely to remain undetected. However, bleeding which occurs despite a well-contracted uterus and which does not appear to be arising from the vagina or perineum is an indication for examining the cervix. Numerous cases have been described of women dying from hemorrhage due to a cervical tear, following operative vaginal delivery.

Postpartum hematoma

Because there is no agreed definition, there is no consensus as to the incidence. After spontaneous delivery, up to 50% of parturients develop a minor self-limiting infralevator/vulva hematoma[5]. In contrast, the formation of a significant postpartum hematoma is an uncommon but serious complication after delivery, with the reported incidence of around 1 in 500–700 deliveries[6]. Major pelvic (supralevator) hematomas are rare, with widely varying reported incidence of between 1 in 500 and 1 in 20 000[7].

Episiotomy

An episiotomy can bleed heavily, and, although there are no data on the incidence of hemorrhage from this cause alone, observational studies suggest that the relative risk of postpartum hemorrhage is increased four to five times if an episiotomy is performed[8].

RISK FACTORS

The major causes of postpartum hemorrhage are uterine atony, retained placental fragments, morbid adherence of the placenta and lower genital tract lacerations. Data from the North West Thames District of the UK (Table 1) reviewed the obstetric factors associated with a blood loss of more than 1000 ml and apportioned a relative risk to each factor[4]. Of these, assisted delivery (forceps or vacuum extraction), prolonged labor, maternal obesity (and associated large baby) and episiotomy were most relevant to the risks of lower genital tract hemorrhage. It is worth noting that episiotomy, with a relative risk of 5, carried the same weight as a cause of postpartum hemorrhage as did multiple pregnancy and retained placenta. Rotational forceps are a particular risk factor for spiral vaginal tears[9].

Coagulation disorders, if present, are likely to significantly increase the risk of lower genital tract hemorrhage and hematoma and therefore should always be corrected where possible. If vaginal lacerations require repair in this situation, the threshold for the use of a vaginal pack should be low.

Table 1 Risk factors for postpartum hemorrhage and approximate increase in risk[4]

Antenatal	Relative risk	Intrapartum	Relative risk
Placenta previa	13	Emergency cesarean section	9
Obesity	2	Assisted delivery	2
		Prolonged labor (> 12 h)	2
		Placental abruption	13
		Multiple pregnancy	5
		Retained placenta	5
		Elective cesarean section	4
		Mediolateral episiotomy	5
		Pyrexia in labor	2

PREVENTION

The three main areas in which risk can be reduced all require a proactive approach:

(1) Antenatal co-morbidities such as anemia and diabetes should be treated so that women entering labor are as healthy as possible.

(2) A consistent proactive approach is required in both the first and second stages of labor. Active monitoring (partogram) and early intervention are essential where progress is inadequate or cephalic-pelvic disproportion is diagnosed. Coagulation defects (including iatrogenic defects due to anti-coagulation) should be corrected where possible (see Chapter 25).

(3) Postpartum, the early identification of excessive blood loss and a proactive approach to resuscitation/fluid replacement as well as identification of the source of bleeding and stopping it, are vital.

Because operative delivery and episiotomy are both significant risk factors for postpartum hemorrhage from the lower genital tract, efforts to reduce the incidence of both are likely to reduce the risk of hemorrhage. Where operative vaginal delivery is required, however, then a proper technique as described in standard textbooks[10] will reduce the risk of vaginal and cervical tears.

DIAGNOSIS

Careful and well-documented observation after delivery is imperative as the seriousness of concealed or persistent low-grade blood loss can be underestimated.

Bleeding, especially after instrumental vaginal delivery, that occurs despite a well-contracted uterus and that does not appear to be arising from the lower vagina or perineum is an indication for examination of the upper vagina and cervix. The characteristic feature of bleeding from upper vaginal and cervical tears is a steady loss of fresh red blood.

Exclusion of upper vaginal and cervical tears requires examination in the lithotomy position with good relaxation, good light and proper assistance[7]. A tagged vaginal tampon to absorb blood loss from the uterine cavity and the use of flat-bladed vaginal retractors will assist in visualizing the vaginal walls.

The cervix should always be examined where there is continuing bleeding despite a well-contracted uterus and also after use of all rotational forceps, which are associated with a significant increase in the risk of upper vaginal and cervical tears[11]. The method for doing this is to grasp the anterior lip with one ring forceps and to place a second ring forceps at the 2-o'clock position, followed by progressively 'leap-frogging' the forceps ahead of one another until the entire circumference has been inspected.

TREATMENT

Hemorrhage from the lower genital tract should always be suspected when there is ongoing bleeding despite a well-contracted uterus. Generally, high vaginal or cervical tears require repair under regional anesthesia in theater.

The Scottish Obstetrics Guidelines and Audit Project (SOGAP) group provides detailed guidelines on the management of postpartum hemorrhage[12]. A summary of the ORDER protocol as described by Bonnar[13] is shown in Figure 2, with additional boxes relating to hemorrhage from the lower genital tract.

Perineal tear repair

The technique has been well described elsewhere[14]. The principles include ensuring that the first suture is inserted above the apex of the tear or episiotomy incision, use of a continuous polyglactin/polyglycolic acid suture on a taper-cut needle, obliteration of dead spaces and taking care that sutures are not inserted too tightly. If dead spaces cannot be closed securely, then a vaginal pack should be inserted.

Vaginal tear repair

The technique for repair of superficial vaginal tears is similar to that of perineal repair, as described above. Use an absorbable, continuous interlocking stitch, which must start and finish beyond the apices of the laceration, and should where possible reach the full depth of the tear in order to reduce the risk of subsequent hematoma formation.

For deeper tears, an attempt should be made to identify the bleeding vessel and ligate it. If there is any significant dead space or if the vagina is too friable to accept suturing, then packing is indicated (see below), because access to deeper tears is usually difficult in an inadequately anesthetized patient. Thus, repair of such lacerations should be done in theater with adequate anesthesia.

Lacerations high in the vaginal vault and those extending up from the cervix may involve the uterus or be the cause of broad ligament or retroperitoneal hematomas. The proximity of the ureters to the lateral vaginal fornices, and the base of the bladder to the anterior fornix, must be kept in mind when any extensive repair is undertaken in these areas. Poorly placed stitches can lead to genitourinary fistulas. Vaginal packing for at least 24 h is always wise under these conditions.

Vaginal packing using gauze is the most common method to achieve vaginal tamponade. As with uterine packing, the technique of vaginal packing involves ribbon gauze inserted uniformly side-to-side, front-to-back and top-to-bottom. Vaginal packing using thrombin-soaked packs, as described for uterine packing, can also be considered[15], especially where closure of all lacerations has not been possible.

Because of the risk that the raw vaginal surface will bleed on removal of the pack, povidone iodine-soaked double lengths of 4.5 × 48 inch packs can be inserted inside sterile plastic drapes (this has been well described for the management of uterine hemorrhage, but the principle is the same for vaginal packing) to allow for easy removal[16]. Generally, packs are left in place for 24–36 h before removal[17]. A urinary Foley catheter and broad-spectrum antibiotic cover should be given where packs are used. Balloon tamponade using Rüsch catheters[18] or Blakemore-Sengstaken[19] tubes, as described for treatment of uterine bleeding (see Chapters 46–48), can also be used.

Pinborg and colleagues[20] described the successful use of the blood pressure cuff in two patients to control intractable vaginal bleeding following evacuation of vaginal hematoma that developed after spontaneous vaginal delivery. A blood pressure cuff was inserted into a sterile glove, which in turn was inserted into the vagina and the pressure then gradually increased to 120 mmHg, 10 mmHg above the systolic pressure, to stop the bleeding. Eight hours later, the pressure of the cuff was reduced by 10 mmHg/h and the cuff then taken out after 32 h. Both patients made an uneventful recovery.

Cervical tear

Any cervical tear extending above the internal os warrants laparotomy. Small, non-bleeding lacerations of the cervix do not need to be sutured. Any bleeding cervical tear, and certainly any tear longer than 2 cm, however, should be sutured by using an absorbable suture on a tapered (rather than a cutting) needle. A suitable method for suturing is shown in Figure 3.

Both edges of the most caudal part of the laceration are grasped with a ring forceps and then sutured with an interrupted or figure-of-eight stitch. This is then held with a hemostat to bring down into view the next part of the tear, which is sutured in the same way, and so on until the apex is secured. The laceration should be observed for a few minutes after suturing, to ensure adequate hemostasis. The ring forceps can be replaced and left on for some time if oozing persists.

Cervical and vaginal vault lacerations that continue to ooze despite treatment as detailed above or those that are associated with hematomas may be amenable to selective arterial embolization (see below).

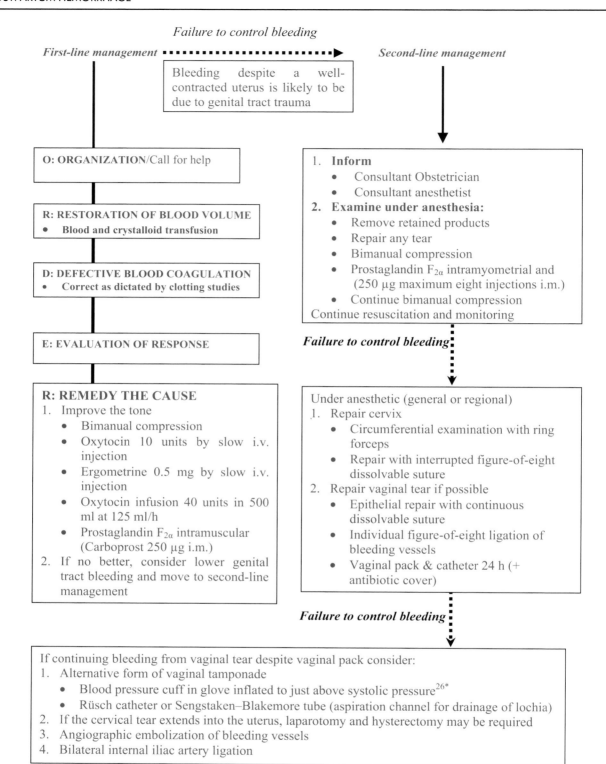

Failure to control bleeding

First-line management ■■■■■■■■■■■■■■■■■■■■■■■■■▶ *Second-line management*

Bleeding despite a well-contracted uterus is likely to be due to genital tract trauma

O: ORGANIZATION/Call for help

R: RESTORATION OF BLOOD VOLUME
- **Blood and crystalloid transfusion**

D: DEFECTIVE BLOOD COAGULATION
- **Correct as dictated by clotting studies**

E: EVALUATION OF RESPONSE

R: REMEDY THE CAUSE
1. Improve the tone
   - Bimanual compression
   - Oxytocin 10 units by slow i.v. injection
   - Ergometrine 0.5 mg by slow i.v. injection
   - Oxytocin infusion 40 units in 500 ml at 125 ml/h
   - Prostaglandin $F_{2\alpha}$ intramuscular (Carboprost 250 µg i.m.)
2. If no better, consider lower genital tract bleeding and move to second-line management

1. **Inform**
   - Consultant Obstetrician
   - Consultant anesthetist
2. **Examine under anesthesia:**
   - Remove retained products
   - Repair any tear
   - Bimanual compression
   - Prostaglandin $F_{2\alpha}$ intramyometrial and (250 µg maximum eight injections i.m.)
   - Continue bimanual compression
   Continue resuscitation and monitoring

Failure to control bleeding

Under anesthetic (general or regional)
1. Repair cervix
   - Circumferential examination with ring forceps
   - Repair with interrupted figure-of-eight dissolvable suture
2. Repair vaginal tear if possible
   - Epithelial repair with continuous dissolvable suture
   - Individual figure-of-eight ligation of bleeding vessels
   - Vaginal pack & catheter 24 h (+ antibiotic cover)

Failure to control bleeding

If continuing bleeding from vaginal tear despite vaginal pack consider:
1. Alternative form of vaginal tamponade
   - Blood pressure cuff in glove inflated to just above systolic pressure[26*]
   - Rüsch catheter or Sengstaken–Blakemore tube (aspiration channel for drainage of lochia)
2. If the cervical tear extends into the uterus, laparotomy and hysterectomy may be required
3. Angiographic embolization of bleeding vessels
4. Bilateral internal iliac artery ligation

Figure 2 Management of major postpartum hemorrhage (blood loss >1000 ml or clinical shock) (see reference 13)

Hematoma management

The literature on the management of paragenital hematomas is limited and no randomized studies of the efficacy of various treatments exist[21].

Infralevator hematomas

As always, initial management consists of resuscitation measures and analgesia followed by a period of observation. For hematomas that are less than 5 cm and not expanding, conservative treatment with ice packs, pressure dressing and analgesia is recommended[22]. The visible skin margin of the hematomas should be marked to help establish whether it is expanding. For hematomas that are expanding or more than 5 cm in size, surgical intervention is recommended. Where possible, the surgical incision should be made via the vagina to minimize visible scarring.

(a)

(b)

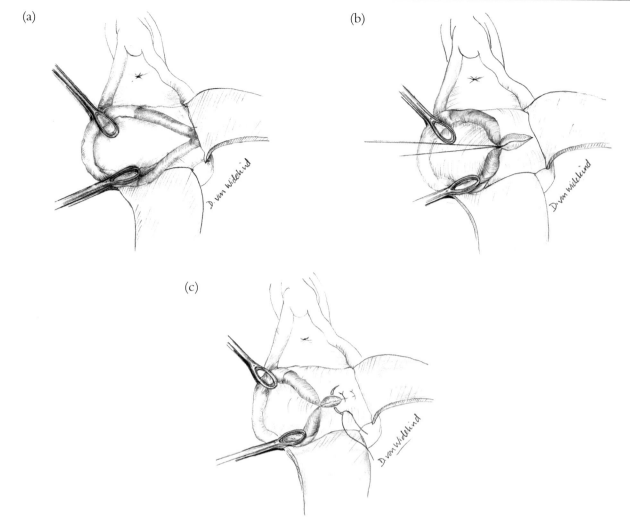

(c)

Figure 3   (a)–(c) Suturing cervical tear

Distinct bleeding points should be under-run with figure-of-eight dissolvable sutures. The presence of any residual bleeding or a hematoma cavity is an indication for insertion of a drain, a vaginal pack and a Foley catheter, all of which should be left in place for at least 24 h. Usually, however, no distinct bleeding point can be seen, in which case a drain and pack should be inserted[10].

Supralevator hematomas

Approximately 50% of broad ligament hematomas present early with symptoms of lower abdominal pain, hemorrhage and in severe cases, shock. The other 50% present after 24 h. Broad ligament and retroperitoneal hematomas are initially managed expectantly if the patient is stable and the lesions are not expanding[23]. Ultrasound, CT scanning and MRI may all be used to assess the size and progress of these hematomas. Close observation, intravenous fluid resuscitation, blood transfusion, vaginal packing or balloon/blood pressure cuff tamponade and antibiotics are commenced as appropriate, but, if it is not possible to maintain a stable hemodynamic state, then active

intervention is indicated, with options including the following:

(1) *Laparotomy ± total abdominal hysterectomy*   This is indicated where there is any possibility that a supralevator/broad ligament hematoma is due to a ruptured uterus or where a cervical tear appears to have extended up into the uterus. At laparotomy, if there is continuing bleeding from the upper vagina, then the anterior division of the internal iliac artery should be ligated in continuity, which will reduce the pulse pressure to the distal internal iliac artery branches (that supply the uterus and vagina) by 85% and the blood flow by about 50%[24] (see Chapters 52 and 55). A further vaginal pack should be inserted.

(2) *Selective arterial embolization*   Where there is continuing expansion of a supralevator hematoma without extension into the cervix or uterus, selective arterial embolization is seen as the treatment of choice[25] over internal iliac artery ligation, which in itself has an uncertain chance of success[26] and involves imposing a laparotomy on an already unstable patient. The blood supply to the upper

vagina is from a rich anastomotic network of vessels, arising mainly from branches of the anterior trunk of the internal iliac artery (vaginal, uterine, middle rectal arteries) and the internal pudendal artery, which is the most inferior branch of the posterior trunk of the internal iliac artery. The technique of selective arterial embolization investigates these vessels by preliminary transfemoral arteriography, followed by embolization using Gelfoam (gelatin) pledglets. Pelage and colleagues[25] reported a series of 35 patients who underwent this procedure for unanticipated postpartum hemorrhage. Bleeding was controlled in all but one, who required hysterectomy 5 days later for re-bleeding. All women who had successful embolization resumed menstruation. The procedure, however, is not without risk and deaths have been reported due to sepsis and multiple organ failure[27].

SUMMARY

In summary, bleeding from the lower genital tract should always be considered as a possible cause of primary postpartum hemorrhage where there is continuing bleeding despite a well-contracted uterus. Primary repair of vaginal or cervical tears with full-thickness sutures using a dissolving suture on a taper-cut needle, followed by insertion of a vaginal pack and catheter for at least 24 h will stem most bleeding. Urgent resort to laparotomy is necessary if there is a cervical tear extending beyond the internal cervical os up into the uterus, or if bleeding fails to settle despite an attempt at vaginal tamponade. Internal iliac artery ligation or selective arterial embolization should be considered where there is continuing expansion of a supralevator hematoma or upper vaginal bleeding despite the above measures. As always, regular assessments, clear documentation, a proactive approach and early intervention are vital to obtain a good outcome.

References

1. Smellie W. A Treatise on the Theory and Practice of Midwifery, 1792
2. Millward-Sadler H. Why Mothers Die 2000–2002. The Confidential Enquiries into Maternal Deaths in the United Kingdom. London: Royal College of Obstetricians and Gynaecologists, 2004:227
3. Etuk S, Asuqo E. Effects of community and health facility interventions on postpartum haemorrhage. Int J Gynaecol Obstet 2000;70:381–3
4. Stones R, Paxton C, Saunders N. Risk factors for major obstetric haemorrhage. Eur J Obstet Gynecol Reprod Biol 1993;48:15–18
5. Drife J. Management of primary postpartum haemorrhage. Br J Obstet Gynaecol 1997;104:275–7
6. Hankins G, Zahn C. Puerperal haematomas and lower genital tract lacerations. In Hankins G, et al., eds. Operative Obstetrics. Connecticut: Appleton & Lange, 1995:57–72
7. Cheung TH, Chang A. Puerperal haematomas. Asia-Oceania J Obstet Gynaecol 1991;17:119–23
8. Combs C, Murphy E, Laros R. Factors associated with postpartum hemorrhage with vaginal birth. Obstet Gynecol 1991;77:69–76
9. Stones R, Paterson C, Saunders N. Risk factors for major obstetric haemorrhage. Eur J Obstet Gynecol Reprod Biol 1993; 48:15–18
10. James D, Steer P, Weiner C, et al. High-risk Pregnancy Management Options, 2nd edn. London: WB Saunders, 1999:1187–204
11. Healy D, Quinn M, Pepperell R. Rotational delivery of the fetus: Kielland's forceps and two other methods compared. Br J Obstet Gynaecol 1982;89:501–6
12. Management of Postpartum haemorrhage – A Clinical Practice Guideline for Professionals involved in Maternity Care in Scotland. Aberdeen: Scottish Programme for Clinical Effectiveness in Reproductive Health, 1998
13. Bonnar J. Massive obstetric hemorrhage. Baillieres Best Pract Res Clin Obstet Gynaecol 2000;14:1–18
14. Johanson R. Continuous vs. interrupted sutures for perineal repair. In Keirse M, Renfrew M, Neilson J, Crowther C, eds. Pregnancy and Childbirth Module. The Cochrane Pregnancy and Childbirth Database. London: BMJ Publishing Group, 1994
15. Bobrowski R, Jones T. A thrombogenic uterine pack for postpartum hemorrhage. Obstet Gynecol 1995;85:836–7
16. Wax J, Channell J, Vandersloot J. Packing of the lower uterine segment: new approach to an old technique? Int J Gynaecol Obstet 1993;43:197–8
17. Maier R. Control of postpartum haemorrhage with uterine packing. Am J Obstet Gynecol 1993;169:317
18. Johanson R, Kumar M, Obhrai M, et al. Management of massive postpartum haemorrhage: use of a hydrostatic balloon catheter to avoid laparotomy. Br J Obstet Gynaecol 2001;108:420–2
19. Katesmark M, Brown R, Raju K. Successful use of a Sengstaken-Blakemore tube to control massive postpartum haemorrhage. Br J Obstet Gynaecol 1994;101:259–60
20. Pinborg A, Bodker B, Hogdall C. Postpartum haematoma and vaginal packing with a blood pressure cuff. Acta Obstet Gynecol Scand 2000;79:887–9
21. Ridgway LE. Puerperal emergency. Vaginal and vulvar haematomas. Obstet Gynecol Clin North Am 1995;22:275–83
22. Zahn C, Yeomans E. Postpartum haemorrhage: placenta accrete, uterine inversion and puerperal haematomas. Clin Obstet Gynaecol 1990;33:422
23. Lingam K, Hood V, Carty M. Angiographic embolisation in the management of pelvic haemorrhage. Br J Obstet Gynaecol 2000;107:1176–8
24. Burchell R. Physiology of internal iliac artery ligation. J Obstet Gynaecol Br Commonwealth 1968;75:642–51
25. Pelage J, Le Dref O, Jacob D, et al. Selective arterial embolisation of the uterine arteries in the management of intractable postpartum haemorrhage. Acta Obstet Gynecol Scand 1999;78:698–703
26. Evans S, McShane P. The efficacy of internal iliac artery ligation in obstetric haemorrhage. Surg Gynecol Obstet 1985;160:250–3
27. Ledee N, Ville Y, Musset D, et al. Management in intractable obstetric haemorrhage: an audit study on 61 cases. Eur J Obstet Gynecol Reprod Biol 2001;94:189–96

25

Acquired and Congenital Hemostatic Disorders in Pregnancy and the Puerperium

R. V. Ganchev and C. A. Ludlam

During normal pregnancy, a series of progressive changes in hemostasis occur that are overall procoagulant and help prevent excessive bleeding at the time of delivery. The concentrations of coagulation factors VII, VIII, X and von Willebrand factor (vWF) rise significantly (Table 1) and are accompanied by a pronounced increase in fibrinogen levels (up to two-fold from non-pregnant levels). Factor V and factor IX levels remain unchanged or increase only slightly. Factor XIII levels tend to decrease in late pregnancy after an initial increase in early pregnancy. Markers of coagulation activation such as prothrombin fragments (PF1+2), thrombin–antithrombin complexes (TAT) and D-dimer are increased, while a decrease in physiological anticoagulants is manifested by a significant reduction in protein S activity and acquired activated protein C (APC) resistance. Fibrinolysis is inhibited not only by the rise in endothelium-derived plasminogen activator inhibitor-1 (PAI-1), but also by placenta-derived PAI-2. Microparticles derived from maternal endothelial cells and platelets, and from placental trophoblasts, may contribute to the procoagulant effect[1]. Although concentrations of soluble tissue factor (TF) remain constant during normal pregnancy[2], monocyte TF activity and expression are lower when compared with those in non-pregnant women, possibly acting to counterbalance the procoagulant changes[3,4]. Local hemostasis at the placental

trophoblast level is characterized by increased TF expression and low expression of tissue factor pathway inhibitor (TFPI)[1]. Approximately 4 weeks post-delivery, the hemostatic system returns to that of the non-pregnant state[5].

Although the overall balance shifts towards hypercoagulability, occasionally medical conditions coincident with pregnancy and complications of pregnancy itself put excessive demands on maternal physiology and may result in a bleeding tendency. This chapter describes acquired and congenital hemostatic disorders that may lead to hemorrhagic complications in the obstetric patient. Though many of these conditions are rare and the average health care provider may see few if any during a long career, their recitation here is appropriate as some are associated with a tendency for the parturient to have postpartum hemorrhage (PPH).

ACQUIRED DISORDERS OF HEMOSTASIS

Thrombocytopenia

Thrombocytopenia is the most common hemostatic abnormality and may complicate up to 10% of all pregnancies. The normal platelet count ranges from $150–400 \times 10^9/l$, and thrombocytopenia is defined as a count of less than $150 \times 10^9/l$. The platelet count may decline by approximately 10% during normal pregnancy[6]. Spontaneous bleeding is unusual unless the count has fallen to below $30 \times 10^9/l$, but surgical bleeding or PPH may occur as a consequence of a platelet count of less than $50 \times 10^9/l$. Thrombocytopenia in pregnancy may result from a variety of causes (Table 2). The timing of onset of these disorders during pregnancy and their clinical manifestations often overlap, making the identification of individual causes of thrombocytopenia sometimes problematic.

It is important to consider spurious thrombocytopenia as a possible cause of decreased platelet count before embarking on extensive investigations or treatment. This is a laboratory artifact due to platelet aggregation *in vitro* caused by EDTA-induced antibodies against platelet GPIIb/IIIa receptors[7] and can be diagnosed by visual inspection of the blood film, when platelet changes are readily visible.

Table 1 Coagulation system changes in normal pregnancy

	Increased	*Decreased*	*No change*
Systemic changes			
Procoagulant factors	I, V, VII, VIII, IX, X	XIII	V, IX, PC, AT
Anticoagulant factors	Soluble TM	PS	
Adhesive proteins	vWF		
Fibrinolytic proteins	PAI-1, PAI-2	t-PA	Soluble TF
Tissue factor (TF)		Monocyte TF	
Microparticles (MP)	MP		
Local placental changes	TF	TFPI	

TM, thrombomodulin; PS, protein S; PC, protein C; AT, antithrombin; vWF, von Willebrand factor; PAI, plasminogen activator inhibitor; t-PA, tissue plasminogen activator; TFPI, tissue factor pathway inhibitor. Modified from Brenner B. Haemostatic changes in pregnancy. *Thromb Res* 2004;114:409–14

Table 2 Causes of pregnancy-associated thrombocytopenia

Pregnancy-specific	Not pregnancy-specific
Gestational (incidental) thrombocytopenia	Idiopathic thrombocytopenic purpura (ITP)
Pre-eclampsia	Thrombotic thrombocytopenic purpura (TTP)
HELLP syndrome (hemolysis, elevated liver enzymes and low platelets)	Hemolytic uremic syndrome (HUS)
	Systemic lupus erythematosus
	Viral infection (HIV, CMV, EBV)
	Antiphospholipid antibodies
Acute fatty liver of pregnancy (AFLP)	Consumptive coagulopathy
	Drug-induced thrombocytopenia
	Type 2B von Willebrand disease
	Congenital

CMV, cytomegalovirus; EBV, Epstein-Barr virus
From McCrae KR. Thrombocytopenia in pregnancy: differential diagnosis, pathogenesis and management. *Blood Rev* 2003;17:7–14

Gestational thrombocytopenia

Gestational, or incidental, thrombocytopenia (GT) is the most common cause of thrombocytopenia in pregnancy, affecting 5% of all pregnant women and accounting for more than 75% of cases of pregnancy-associated thrombocytopenia. It presents as a mild to moderate thrombocytopenia ($100–150 \times 10^9$/l), which is detected incidentally often for the first time during the third trimester of pregnancy. The platelet count returns to normal within 7 days of delivery. GT is the physiologic thrombocytopenia that accompanies normal pregnancy and is thought to be due to hemodilution and/or accelerated platelet clearance[8,9]. It is an entirely benign condition and is not associated with maternal hemorrhage or fetal or neonatal thrombocytopenia. It is, however, necessary to monitor the platelet count during pregnancy and, if it falls below 100×10^9/l, the diagnosis must be reviewed. Rare cases, subsequently confirmed as GT, have had counts as low as 50×10^9/l[10]. Epidural anesthesia is considered safe if the maternal platelet count is greater than 80×10^9/l. Delivery should proceed according to obstetric indications. Traumatic delivery, use of fetal scalp electrodes and fetal scalp blood sampling should be avoided. If it is difficult to distinguish between GT and idiopathic thrombocytopenic purpura (ITP), a cord platelet count should be obtained.

Idiopathic thrombocytopenic purpura

ITP accounts for one to five cases of thrombocytopenia per 10,000 pregnancies[11] and 5% of cases of pregnancy-associated thrombocytopenia[8]. It is the most common cause of significant thrombocytopenia in the first trimester. Concepts surrounding the mechanisms of thrombocytopenia in ITP have shifted from the traditional view of increased platelet destruction mediated by autoantibodies to more complex mechanisms in which both impaired platelet production and T-cell mediated effects play a role[12,13]. The most common presentation is the finding of an asymptomatic thrombocytopenia on a routine blood count, when the distinction from GT may be difficult. Patients occasionally present for the first time with severe thrombocytopenia in pregnancy, and women with previously diagnosed ITP often experience an exacerbation in pregnancy[14]. Symptomatic patients present with minor bruises or petechiae, bleeding from mucosal surfaces, or rarely fatal intracranial bleeding.

As in the non-pregnant patient, ITP is a diagnosis of exclusion with thrombocytopenia and normal or increased megakaryocytes in the bone marrow in the absence of other causes. There is no confirmatory laboratory test, and documentation of a low platelet count outside pregnancy is invaluable. Practically, however, in the absence of a platelet count prior to pregnancy, significant thrombocytopenia ($<100 \times 10^9$/l) in the first trimester, with a declining platelet count as gestation progresses, is most consistent with ITP. In contrast, mild thrombocytopenia developing in the second or third trimester and not associated with hypertension or proteinuria most likely represents GT[15]. Bone marrow examination is unnecessary unless there is suspicion of leukemia, lymphoma or malignant infiltration.

The decision to treat a pregnant woman with ITP is based on assessment of the risk of significant maternal hemorrhage. The count usually falls as pregnancy progresses, with a nadir in the third trimester[14], and active treatment may have to be instituted to ensure a safe platelet count at the time of delivery. The incidence of antepartum hemorrhage is not increased in maternal ITP, but there is a small increased risk of PPH complications, not from the placental bed but from surgical incisions such as episiotomies and from soft-tissue lacerations[16].

Asymptomatic patients with platelet counts $>20 \times 10^9$/l do not require treatment until delivery is imminent but should be carefully monitored. Platelet counts of $>50 \times 10^9$/l are regarded as safe for normal vaginal delivery, and those $>80 \times 10^9$/l are safe for cesarean section, spinal or epidural anesthesia[17].

The major treatment options for maternal ITP are corticosteroids or intravenous immunoglobulin (IVIg). There is no evidence, however, that either of these treatment modalities administered to the mother affects the platelet count in the fetus or neonate. If the duration of treatment is likely to be short, i.e. starting in the third trimester, corticosteroids are an effective option. An initial dose of 1 mg/kg prednisolone (based on pre-pregnancy weight) is recommended[14,17], which can be subsequently tapered. In addition to their toxicities in non-pregnant individuals, such as osteoporosis and weight gain, corticosteroids increase the incidence of pregnancy-induced hypertension and gestational diabetes, and may promote premature rupture of the fetal membranes.

Concerns about potential adverse maternal effects of steroids have led some to use IVIg as a first-line therapy in pregnancy[15,18]. Others reserve this treatment for patients in whom steroid therapy is likely to be prolonged or in whom an unacceptably high maintenance dose is required (>7.5 mg prednisolone daily). The conventional dose of IVIg is 0.4 g/kg/day for

5 days, although 1 g/kg/day for 2 days has been used successfully and may be more convenient[14]. A persistent and predictable response is obtained in 80% of the cases. The response to therapy usually occurs within 24 h (more rapid than with steroids) and is maintained for 2–3 weeks. After an initial response, repeat single infusions can be used to prevent hemorrhagic symptoms and ensure an adequate platelet count for delivery.

Therapeutic options for those women with severely symptomatic ITP refractory to oral steroids or IVIg include high-dose intravenous methylprednisolone (1.0 g), perhaps combined with IVIg, or azathioprine[17], but these should only be considered after careful assessment of the potential risks. Splenectomy is now rarely performed in pregnancy. It remains an option if all other attempts to increase the platelet count fail and is best performed in the second trimester. Approximately two-thirds of patients have a useful response to splenectomy. Prophylaxis against infections with organisms such as pneumococci, *Haemophilus influenzae* and *Neisseria meningitidis* is necessary. When splenectomy is performed during pregnancy, penicillin V prophylaxis should be given in the prenatal period, and vaccination against these organisms should be performed postnatally. Anecdotal reports exist of successful use of anti-D[19] and of the anti-CD20 monoclonal antibody rituximab in pregnancy[20]; however, until further studies are available, use of these agents in pregnancy should be restricted to refractory cases in which alternatives are unsuitable or have failed.

The offspring of mothers with ITP may also develop thrombocytopenia, as a result of the transplacental passage of maternal antiplatelet IgG[8,15]. The incidence of severe neonatal thrombocytopenia ($<50 \times 10^9$/l) has been reported between 9 and 15%, with intracranial hemorrhage occurring in 0–1.5% of infants[21]. Due to the inability of maternal clinical characteristics to predict neonatal thrombocytopenia, antenatal (cordocentesis) and perinatal (fetal scalp blood sampling) procedures for determination of fetal platelet count have been considered in the past. Cordocentesis carries a mortality of 1–2%, however, whereas scalp blood sampling is associated with artifactually low results and risk of significant hemorrhage. For these reasons, both procedures are now largely abandoned in the management of ITP in pregnancy. The most reliable predictor of fetal thrombocytopenia is a history of thrombocytopenia at delivery in a prior sibling[22].

In view of the very low risk of serious neonatal hemorrhage, it is now agreed that the mode of delivery in ITP should be determined by purely obstetric indications[14,17]. If the maternal platelet count remains low at the time of delivery, despite optimal antenatal management, platelet transfusion may be required to treat maternal bleeding. Fetal scalp electrodes, fetal blood samples, ventouse delivery and rotational forceps should be avoided. Mothers with thrombocytopenia are unlikely to bleed from the uterine cavity after the third stage of labor, provided that there are no retained products of conception. However, bleeding may occur from surgical wounds, episiotomies or perineal tears. Non-steroidal anti-inflammatory drugs should be avoided for postpartum analgesia. ITP should not exclude women from consideration for peripartum thrombosis prophylaxis. Prophylactic doses of low-molecular weight heparin (LMWH) are generally safe if the platelet count is greater than 50×10^9/l. Following delivery, a cord blood platelet count should be determined in all cases. Intramuscular injections, such as vitamin K, should be avoided until platelet count is known. Since the neonatal platelet count may decline for 4–5 days after delivery[14], daily monitoring is indicated. Infants should be closely observed and treatment is rarely required. In those with clinical hemorrhage or platelet count $<20 \times 10^9$/l, treatment with IVIg produces a rapid response. Life-threatening hemorrhage should be managed with platelet transfusion combined with IVIg[14].

Secondary autoimmune thrombocytopenia

Antiphospholipid syndrome

The diagnosis of primary antiphospholipid syndrome requires the coexistence of clinical manifestations (either vascular thrombosis or recurrent miscarriages) with laboratory evidence of reproducible antiphospholipid antibodies (either lupus anticoagulant or anticardiolipin antibody)[23]. Primary antiphospholipid syndrome is associated with autoimmune thrombocytopenia in 20–40% of cases[24]. Thrombocytopenia is rarely severe and usually does not require treatment. If treatment is necessary, management options during pregnancy are similar to those for primary ITP. However, primary antiphospholipid syndrome is associated with recurrent spontaneous abortions before 10 weeks of gestation, and women with the condition are at risk of intrauterine fetal growth restriction or death, pre-eclampsia and maternal thrombosis[23,25].

A combination of low-dose aspirin and prophylactic heparin is helpful in preventing recurrent spontaneous abortions in antiphospholipid syndrome[26]. Antenatal and postnatal thrombosis prophylaxis is indicated in women with antiphospholipid syndrome and a history of thrombosis[27]. Moderate thrombocytopenia should not alter decisions about antiplatelet or antithrombotic therapy in antiphospholipid syndrome[24].

Systemic lupus erythematosus

Immune platelet destruction may occur in systemic lupus erythematosus (SLE) because of antiplatelet antibodies or immune complexes, but thrombocytopenia is seldom severe; less than 5% of cases have a platelet count $<30 \times 10^9$/l during the course of the disease[16]. Thrombocytopenia is often the first presenting feature and may precede any other manifestations of the condition by months or years. The management of isolated thrombocytopenia associated with SLE in pregnancy is governed by the principles outlined for ITP. Women with SLE are also at risk for pre-eclampsia which may be complicated by thrombocytopenia.

HIV-associated thrombocytopenia

HIV-related thrombocytopenia can be caused by increased platelet destruction by antiplatelet antibodies or immune complexes, commonly during early-onset HIV. In advanced disease, drugs and infection may lead to marrow dysfunction that results in thrombocytopenia. In one series of HIV-positive women, approximately 3% were thrombocytopenic and, in most cases, thrombocytopenia was believed to be directly related to HIV infection[28]. Slightly fewer than half of the thrombocytopenic women had a platelet count $<50 \times 10^9/l$, and 20% had hemorrhagic complications[28].

Treatment with antiretroviral therapy tends to improve the defective thrombopoiesis and increase the platelet count in HIV-positive patients, but some antiretroviral drugs may also cause thrombocytopenia. When immune destruction is believed to be a significant component of thrombocytopenia, IVIg may be required to treat hemorrhagic symptoms or to increase the platelet count before delivery in thrombocytopenic HIV-positive women[28]. Corticosteroids are also effective but may be associated with increased risk of further immunosuppression and infection. Thrombotic thrombocytopenic purpura is found more frequently in HIV-infected patients and should be treated accordingly. Cesarean delivery reduces the risk of transmission of HIV from mother to fetus.

Drug-induced thrombocytopenia

Drug-induced thrombocytopenia may be caused by immune- or non-immune-mediated platelet destruction or suppression of platelet production. Both are uncommon in pregnancy, but drug-induced causes should be considered and excluded. Drugs which are commonly associated with thrombocytopenia are shown in Table 3.

Heparin-induced thrombocytopenia A unique form of drug-induced thrombocytopenia is heparin-induced thrombocytopenia. It occurs in 1–5% of patients receiving unfractionated heparin but is considerably less common in patients treated with LMWH. Heparin-induced thrombocytopenia (HIT) is caused by an antibody directed against the heparin–platelet factor 4 complex, which can induce platelet activation and aggregation *in vivo*. Unlike other thrombocytopenias, HIT is complicated by arterial and/or venous thrombosis which may be life-threatening. Laboratory tests are available to confirm the diagnosis. HIT has been reported in pregnancy[29,30], although it may be less common in pregnant than in non-pregnant individuals[31]. Fetal thrombocytopenia does not occur because heparin does not cross the placenta. Heparin should be withdrawn immediately on clinical suspicion of HIT. If ongoing anticoagulation is

Table 3 Drugs causing thrombocytopenia

Immune mediated
Acetaminophen
Aminosalicylic acid
Amiodarone
Amphotericin B
Cimetidine
Diclofenac
Gold/gold salts
Levamisole
Methyldopa
Quinine and quinidine
Ranitidine
Sulfasalazine
Vancomycin
Unique antibody-mediated process
Heparin
Suppression of platelet production
Anagrelide
Valproic acid
Suppression of all hematopoietic cells
Chemotherapeutic agents

Adapted from George JN, Raskob GE, Shah SR, *et al*. Drug-induced thrombocytopenia: a systematic review of published case reports. *Ann Intern Med* 1998;129:886–90

urgently required, the heparinoid danaparoid may be used in most patients. Danaparoid has been used successfully to treat HIT in pregnancy[30]. Hirudin is an alternative in non-pregnant patients, but experience is limited in pregnancy and its use is not recommended unless there is no suitable alternative[32]. Fondaparinux, a parenteral synthetic pentasaccharide which inhibits factor Xa indirectly, is not licensed for use in HIT but there are reports of its successful use in the management of HIT in pregnant women[33,34]. Platelet transfusion should be avoided in patients with HIT. Routine monitoring of the platelet counts in pregnant women on prophylactic LMWH is no longer required because of the very low incidence of HIT in this situation[35,36], but regular monitoring is still required in pregnant women receiving unfractionated heparin (UFH)[35,36]. British Committee for Standards in Haematology guidelines advise that the platelet count should be monitored in women receiving treatment doses of LMWH[35]; however, the Royal College of Obstetricians and Gynaecologists venous thromboembolism guidelines recommend that monitoring is not necessary unless a woman has received UFH[36].

Thrombocytopenia with microangiopathy

Several syndromes are associated with thrombocytopenia as a result of platelet activation, red cell fragmentation and a variable degree of hemolysis (microangiopathic hemolytic anemia, MAHA). Some syndromes are unique to obstetric practice. The differential diagnosis is particularly pertinent for obstetricians and is important because management options differ. The differential diagnosis is summarized in Table 4.

Table 4 Differentiation of pregnancy-associated microangiopathies

Diagnosis	TTP	HUS	HELLP	Pre-eclampsia	AFLP
Time of onset	2nd trimester	Postpartum	3rd trimester	3rd trimester	3rd trimester
Hemolysis	+++	++	++	+	+
Thrombocytopenia	+++	++	++	++	+/±
Coagulopathy	—	—	±	±	+++
Liver disease	±	±	+++	±	+++
Renal disease	±	+++	+	+	±
Hypertension	Rare	±	±	+++	±
CNS disease	+++	±	±	±	+
Effect of delivery on disease	None	None	Recovery	Recovery	Recovery
Management	Early plasma exchange	Supportive ± plasma exchange	Supportive consider plasma exchange if persists	Supportive plasma exchange rarely required	Supportive

TTP, thrombotic thrombocytopenic purpura; HUS, hemolytic uremic syndrome; HELLP, hemolysis, elevated liver enzymes, and low platelets; AFLP, acute fatty liver of pregnancy
Adapted from Horn EH. Thrombocytopenia and bleeding disorders. In: James DK, Steer PJ, Weiner CP, Gonik B, eds. *High-Risk Pregnancy: Management Options*, 3rd edn. Elsevier, 2006:901–24

Pre-eclampsia and HELLP syndrome

Pre-eclampsia affects approximately 6% of all pregnancies, most often those of primigravidas less than 20 or more than 30 years of age[8]. The criteria for the diagnosis include hypertension and proteinuria >300 mg/24 h developing after 20 weeks of gestation[6]. Although the clinical manifestations of pre-eclampsia generally do not become evident until the third trimester, the lesions underlying this disorder occur early in pregnancy and involve deficient remodeling of the maternal uterine vasculature by placental trophoblast cells[37,38]. Thrombocytopenia develops in approximately 50% of patients, with the severity usually proportional to the severity of the pre-eclampsia. Occasionally, the onset of thrombocytopenia precedes other manifestations of pre-eclampsia[8]. Current understanding of the pathogenesis of thrombocytopenia in pre-eclampsia is that it is due to excessive platelet activation, adhesion of platelets to damaged or activated endothelium, and/or clearance of IgG-coated platelets by the reticuloendothelial system[8].

Activation of the coagulation cascade occurs in most patients with pre-eclampsia; however, screening coagulation tests such as activated partial thromboplastin time (APTT), prothrombin time (PT) and fibrinogen are usually normal. Regardless, more sensitive markers of hemostatic activity such as D-dimer and TAT complexes are often elevated. In severe pre-eclampsia, the activation of coagulation results in consumption of clotting factors and therefore prolongation of the clotting test times and a fall in plasma fibrinogen.

The HELLP (hemolysis, elevated liver enzymes and low platelets) syndrome is often considered to be a variant of pre-eclampsia and is the most common cause of severe liver disease in pregnant women[39]. Criteria for the diagnosis of the HELLP syndrome include microangiopathic hemolytic anemia, aspartate aminotransferase (AST) more than 70 U/l and thrombocytopenia, with a platelet count less than $100 \times 10^9/l$[40]. Patients may present with severe epigastric and right upper quadrant pain, which need not be accompanied by hypertension and proteinuria.

Exacerbation of HELLP syndrome may occur postpartum, and there is a recurrence risk of approximately 3% in subsequent pregnancies. The syndrome occasionally presents postpartum, usually within 48 h, but rarely as late as 6 days after delivery. Despite their similarities, HELLP is associated with significantly greater maternal and fetal morbidity and mortality than pre-eclampsia *per se*[8].

Management of the pre-eclampsia/HELLP syndrome is supportive and should be focused on stabilizing the patient medically prior to early delivery of the fetus. Platelet transfusions may be needed if bleeding occurs or if thrombocytopenia is severe and cesarean delivery is planned, though the survival time of transfused platelets in patients with pre-eclampsia is diminished[6]. Regional analgesia is an option if the maternal platelet count is greater than $80 \times 10^9/l$ and the results of the coagulation screening tests are normal. If required, the consumptive coagulopathy resulting from pre-eclampsia should be treated with fresh frozen plasma (FFP). Consumptive coagulopathy severe enough to result in depletion of fibrinogen is uncommon in these disorders, but, if severe hypofibrinogenemia is present, plasma fibrinogen levels can be raised with cryoprecipitate or fibrinogen concentrate. In most cases, the clinical manifestations of pre-eclampsia resolve within several days after delivery, although the platelet count may decline for additional 24–48 h[41]. If severe thrombocytopenia, hemolysis or organ dysfunction persists after delivery, plasma exchange may be considered[42], but the diagnosis should also be reviewed.

Thrombotic thrombocytopenic purpura and hemolytic uremic syndrome

Thrombotic thrombocytopenic purpura (TTP) and hemolytic uremic syndrome (HUS) share the central features of microangiopathic hemolytic anemia and thrombocytopenia. Though neither disease occurs exclusively during pregnancy, the incidence of both is increased in this setting, and up to 10% of all cases of TTP occur in pregnant patients[6]. TTP is defined by a pentad of symptoms that include MAHA, thrombocytopenia, neurological abnormalities, fever and renal dysfunction, although the complete pentad is present at the time of diagnosis in less than 40% of patients[41]. The clinical manifestations of HUS are similar. Neurological abnormalities are a particular feature of patients with TTP; renal dysfunction is more severe in patients with HUS. Congenital or acquired deficiency of a specific von Willebrand factor-cleaving protease, ADAMTS 13, and the consequent increased level of high-molecular weight multimers of vWF play a central role in the pathogenesis of TTP. Interestingly, levels of ADAMTS 13 decrease during normal pregnancy, perhaps accounting, at least in part, for the predisposition to development of thrombotic microangiopathy in this setting[43].

TTP and HUS may be difficult to discern from one another, as well as from other pregnancy-associated microangiopathies such as pre-eclampsia or the HELLP syndrome. The extent of microangiopathic hemolysis is generally more severe in TTP or HUS than in pre-eclampsia or HELLP, and the former disorders are not associated with hypertension. The time of onset of these disorders is also helpful in differentiating between them. TTP usually presents in the second trimester, HUS in the postpartum period, and pre-eclampsia and the HELLP syndrome almost exclusively in the third trimester[8,41,44]. Plasma antithrombin levels are normal in TTP and HUS and reduced in pre-eclampsia and HELLP[41]. Another feature distinguishing these disorders is their response to delivery. Whereas pre-eclampsia and the HELLP syndrome usually improve following delivery, the courses of TTP and HUS do not. Hence, pregnancy termination should not be considered therapeutic in patients with TTP or HUS[45]. However, TTP responds equally well to plasma exchange in pregnant and non-pregnant patients with more than 75% of patients achieving remission[6]. Plasma exchange should be instituted as soon as possible after the diagnosis of TTP and should be continued daily until at least 48 h after complete remission is obtained. Repeated plasma exchange cycles are usually maintained until delivery. There is a rationale for use of immunosuppressive therapy in those patients with inhibitors of ADAMTS 13. The use of low dose aspirin has been advocated when the platelet count increases to more than 50×10^9/l. Platelet transfusion is contraindicated and may lead to rapid worsening of the condition. Management of HUS is supportive and includes renal dialysis and red cell transfusion. Plasma exchange has no proven benefit in the treatment of HUS.

The placental ischemia and increased incidence of premature delivery that complicate pregnancies in patients with TTP and HUS may lead to poor fetal outcomes, but these are markedly improved by good management of the conditions.

Acute fatty liver of pregnancy

Acute fatty liver of pregnancy (AFLP) affects one of every 5000–10,000 pregnancies and is most common in primagravidas during the third trimester[46]. The cause of the condition is unknown in the majority of instances, but some patients may have a long-chain 3-hydroxy-acyl CoA dehydrogenase (LCHAD) deficiency[47].

Patients present with overt signs of hepatic damage and may have hemorrhagic manifestations, perhaps the result of decreased synthesis of clotting factors and consumptive coagulopathy. Evidence for consumptive coagulopathy is provided by thrombocytopenia, prolonged APTT and PT, and by decrease in fibrinogen and antithrombin levels.

AFLP is most aptly viewed as part of the pregnancy-associated microangiopathies; up to 50% of patients with AFLP may also meet criteria for pre-eclampsia. The extent of microangiopathic hemolysis and thrombocytopenia is generally mild compared with that observed in HELLP, TTP, or HUS[48].

Delivery is the most important aspect of management, as it starts the reversal of the pathological process. Coagulation defects are managed supportively with FFP, cryoprecipitate or fibrinogen concentrate and platelet concentrates. In these patients, normalization of hemostatic abnormalities may not occur for up to 10 days after delivery. Fetal mortality in this disorder approaches 15%, though maternal mortality occurs in less than 5% of cases[46].

CONSUMPTIVE COAGULOPATHY

Disseminated intravascular coagulation (DIC) is an acquired clinicopathologic syndrome, characterized by activation of the coagulation system, and resulting in widespread intravascular deposition of fibrin-rich thrombi. Consumption of clotting factors usually leads to a bleeding diathesis, although a small percentage of affected individuals may go on to develop widespread thrombosis with peripheral organ ischemia. *Some degree of consumptive coagulopathy accompanies most forms of obstetric hemorrhage; however, the greater risk of coagulopathy usually arises from consumption of clotting factors and platelets as a result of massive obstetric hemorrhage. The combination of massive hemorrhage and coagulation failure is recognized as one of the most serious complications in pregnancy.*

Obstetric consumptive coagulopathy is usually acute in onset (except as an uncommon late complication of retained dead fetus) and can be caused by a variety of disease processes. It is triggered by several mechanisms including release of TF into the circulation, endothelial damage to small vessels and production of procoagulant phospholipids in response to intravascular hemolysis[49] (Table 5). Blood loss itself with transfusion and volume replacement may also trigger consumptive coagulopathy. When obstetric complications are associated with coagulation failure, several mechanisms may interact. These triggers lead to the generation of thrombin, cause defects in inhibitors of coagulation and suppress fibrinolysis. Thrombin promotes platelet activation and aggregates formation, which occlude the microvasculature and

Table 5 Mechanism of consumptive coagulopathy in pregnancy

Injury to vascular endothelium
Pre-eclampsia
Hypovolemic shock
Septicemic shock

Release of tissue factor (TF)
Placental abruption
Amniotic fluid embolism
Retained dead fetus
Placenta accreta
Acute fatty liver

Production of procoagulant
Fetomaternal hemorrhage
Phospholipids
Incompatible blood transfusion
Septicemia
Intravascular hemolysis

From Anthony J. Major obstetric hemorrhage and disseminated intravascular coagulation. In: James DK, Steer PJ, Weiner CP, Gonik B, eds. *High-Risk Pregnancy: Management Options*, 3rd edn. Elsevier, 2006:1606–23

result in thrombocytopenia. Thrombin becomes bound to antithrombin (AT) and thrombomodulin, and these proteins are soon consumed. Following binding to thrombomodulin, thrombin activates the anticoagulant protein C, which also becomes depleted, predisposing to microvascular thrombosis. In consumptive coagulopathy secondary to sepsis, increased levels of C4b-binding protein result in the binding of more free protein S, and therefore render it unavailable to be a cofactor of the anticoagulant protein C. PAI-1 is increased out of proportion to the level of tissue plasminogen activator (tPA), resulting in depressed fibrinolysis. Fibrin is formed, but its removal is impaired, leading to thrombosis of small and middle-size vessels. The passage of erythrocytes through partially occluded vessels leads to red cell fragmentation and microangiopathic hemolytic anemia.

Placental abruption is the most common cause of obstetric consumptive coagulopathy (60% of cases; 5% of all abruptions), but the syndrome is uncommon unless the abruption is severe enough to cause fetal death. Initially, increased intrauterine pressure forces TF-rich decidual fragments into the maternal circulation. However, in severe abruption, hypovolemic shock, large volume transfusion and high levels of fibrin degradation products (FDPs) that act as anticoagulants themselves exacerbate the situation. Retained dead fetus may cause chronic consumptive coagulopathy by release of TF from the dead fetus into the maternal circulation, but generally only if the fetus is at least of 20 weeks' size and the period of death is more than 4 weeks. Amniotic fluid embolism occurs during labor, cesarean section or within a short time of delivery. Amniotic fluid is rich in TF and may enter uterine veins when there has been a tear in the uterine wall. The condition may lead to maternal death as a result of severe pulmonary hypertension following embolization of the pulmonary vessels by fetal squames. If the mother survives this acute event, there may be an

anaphylactoid reaction to the presence of the fetal tissues in the maternal circulation associated with cardiovascular collapse, pulmonary edema and the development of consumptive coagulopathy.

Sepsis causes consumptive coagulopathy via the release of proinflammatory cytokines such as tumor necrosis factor α (TNFα), interleukin 1 (IL-1) and IL-6, which may trigger TF expression by monocytes and endothelial cells[50]. Severe pre-eclampsia with intense vasospasm and resulting ischemia causes endothelial injury and expression of TF.

Acute consumptive coagulopathy in pregnancy presents almost invariably with bleeding – either as a genital tract bleeding from the placental site or bleeding from the wound after cesarean section. There may be excessive bleeding from venepuncture sites.

Laboratory investigations are essential to establish the diagnosis of consumptive coagulopathy. The characteristic changes are a low or falling platelet count and a prolongation of the APTT and PT. Fibrinogen level falls with the progression of the coagulopathy; the normal range in late pregnancy is 4–6 g/l which is significantly higher than the non-pregnant range, 2–4 g/l; coagulation fails at levels of less than 1 g/l. FDPs are increased, reflecting the excessive deposition of fibrin and enhanced fibrinolysis. The D-dimer is the most commonly used parameter to assess FDP levels, as it is specific for fibrin breakdown. Normal D-dimer levels are below 200 ng/ml, but often exceed 2000 ng/ml in cases of consumptive coagulopathy. The blood film may show evidence of microangiopathic hemolysis with fragmentation of red cells.

The basic principles in treatment of consumptive coagulopathy are removal of the precipitating cause if possible, correction of aggravating factors, and replacement of missing coagulation factors and platelets. Any etiological condition should be promptly treated; delivery of the fetus is often required. Correction of aggravating factors such as shock and hypoxia is important. This includes red cell transfusion if necessary and oxygen administration. Intravenous antibiotics should be given if sepsis is suspected. Replacement of clotting factors is most effectively performed with FFP at a dose of 15–20 ml/kg. If there is severe hypofibrinogenemia, cryoprecipitate or virally inactivated fibrinogen concentrate may be required; two cryoprecipitate pools (10 donor units) or 3–5 g of fibrinogen concentrate are expected to raise plasma fibrinogen by approximately 1 g/l. Platelets should be maintained above 50×10^9/l in the presence of active bleeding by the administration of blood group-compatible platelets. Heparin use often leads to excessive bleeding and therefore does not usually have a role in obstetric consumptive coagulopathy except in cases of a retained dead fetus. Similarly, antifibrinolytic drugs (tranexamic acid, aprotinin) are not helpful and are usually contraindicated because they inhibit the removal of deposited fibrin by fibrinolysis.

The D-dimer, platelet count and fibrinogen level are clinically useful tests in monitoring replacement therapy if the patient is bleeding. The aim should be to achieve a platelet count above $50 \times 10^9/l$, a fibrinogen level of more than 1.0 g/l and significant shortening of the APTT and PT to approach their normal values.

Although recombinant activated factor VII (rFVIIa) is not licensed for use in pregnancy, it has been used in obstetric patients with consumptive coagulopathy and severe bleeding not responsive to other treatment options[51,52]. Consumptive coagulopathy is not a contraindication to the use of rFVIIa if massive bleeding is occurring. However, caution should be used in patients with major consumptive coagulopathy because there are occasional reports of thrombosis and consumptive coagulopathy after the use of rFVIIa[53].

Recombinant activated protein C (raPC) has been successfully used in sepsis-related obstetric consumptive coagulopathy at a dose of $24 \mu g/kg/h$ in a 96 h infusion[54,55]. Caution is needed in patients with severe thrombocytopenia ($<30 \times 10^9/l$) because of the increased incidence of intracerebral hemorrhage associated with its use; monitoring platelet count and platelet transfusion as necessary are important considerations. In addition to acting as an anticoagulant, raPC has direct anti-inflammatory and anti-apoptotic properties[56]. This may explain in part why the other endogenous anticoagulants (antithrombin and TFPI) used in severe sepsis have not shown such good efficacy.

FACTOR VIII INHIBITORS

Acquired hemophilia is due to the development of an autoantibody to factor VIII (FVIII). The estimated incidence is approximately 1 per 1,000,000 per annum. Most cases occur in healthy individuals without discernible risk factors, but the condition is associated with autoimmune disorders such as rheumatoid arthritis and SLE, inflammatory bowel disease, multiple sclerosis and malignancies. In up to 11% of cases, the associated factor is a recent or ongoing pregnancy[57].

Acquired hemophilia may occur in relation to any pregnancy, but the risk appears to be greatest after the first delivery. Onset is usually at term or within 3 months postpartum, but may only become evident 12 months postdelivery[58]. Clinical manifestations do not necessarily correlate with inhibitor levels and can range from spontaneous bruising to life-threatening hemorrhage. FVIII inhibitors may cross the placenta and persist in the neonate for up to 3 months, but neonatal complications are rare[58]. Spontaneous resolution occurs in almost 100% of women first diagnosed in the postpartum period after 30 months[57].

Basic coagulation studies in acquired hemophilia demonstrate a prolonged APPT with a normal PT and thrombin time (TT). If plasma from the patient is mixed with normal plasma, the APPT remains prolonged due to the inhibitor antibody neutralizing the FVIII in the normal plasma. FVIII inhibitors must be differentiated from a lupus inhibitor by specific tests because the clinical implications are profoundly different. Quantification of FVIII inhibitor is by the Bethesda assay, and checking this level may help in determining the choice of therapy and monitoring the progress of the patient.

Treatment is aimed at control of bleeding and accelerating the elimination of inhibitors. Hematological measures to minimize blood loss aim to compensate for the loss of FVIII. Choice of product to attempt to normalize hemostasis depends on various considerations, including the severity of bleeding, availability of clotting factor concentrates, inhibitor level and cross-reactivity of inhibitor to porcine FVIII. Human FVIII may be effective if the titer of inhibitor is low, i.e. less than 10 Bethesda units. At higher levels, use of porcine FVIII which may not cross-react with the inhibitor, and rFVIIa or prothrombin complex concentrate (PCC) become necessary[59].

Inhibiting the production of the inhibitor is the second management aim. Prednisolone at a dose of 1 mg/kg is associated with a loss of inhibitor in 50% of patients with acquired hemophilia[59]. Other immunosuppressives should be considered if there is no response to steroids. Addition of cyclophosphamide (2–3 mg/kg) should be considered at 3 weeks if there is no decline in the inhibitor titer, or earlier if there is continued bleeding. Other methods to reduce inhibitor levels include azathioprine or infusion of IVIg; plasma exchange is rarely effective. Rituximab has been used in the management of postpartum acquired hemophilia[60].

ANTICOAGULANT THERAPY DURING PREGNANCY AND THE PERIPARTUM PERIOD

Anticoagulant therapy is indicated during pregnancy for the prevention and treatment of venous thromboembolism (VTE), for the prevention and treatment of systemic embolism in patients with mechanical heart valve prostheses and, in combination with aspirin, for the prevention of recurrent pregnancy loss in women with antiphospholipid syndrome (APS) or other thrombophilias.

The anticoagulants currently available for the prevention and treatment of VTE and arterial thromboembolism include UFH, LMWH, vitamin K antagonists and direct thrombin and factor Xa inhibitors. Among these, heparins and warfarin are the principal drugs. The novel oral anticoagulants, direct inhibitors of thrombin and factor Xa, are promising but their role is not established and there are no data on their use in pregnancy.

Heparins are the anticoagulant of choice during pregnancy for situations in which their efficacy is established. Neither UFH nor LMWH cross the placenta[61]. Heparins are not associated with any known teratogenic risk, and the fetus is not anticoagulated as a result of maternal heparin use. LMWHs have potential advantages over UFH during pregnancy because they have a longer plasma half-life and a more predictable dose-response than UFH, with the potential for once-daily administration. In addition, LMWHs are associated with a lower risk of HIT and osteoporosis than UFH.

Coumarin derivatives such as warfarin cross the placenta and have the potential to cause teratogenicity as well as to anticoagulate the fetus predisposing to bleeding *in utero*. It is probable that oral anticoagulants are safe during the first 6 weeks of gestation, but there is an approximately 5% risk of developmental abnormalities of fetal cartilage and bone if they are taken between 6 and 12 weeks' gestation[62]. The risk of warfarin embryopathy is dose dependent, with an increased risk when the daily warfarin dose exceeds 5 mg[63]. Fetal intracranial bleeds *in utero* are a well-established complication after exposure to these drugs during any trimester. In general, coumarins should not be used for the prevention or treatment of VTE in pregnancy, but they remain the anticoagulants of choice for the management of pregnant women with mechanical heart valve prostheses.

Fondaparinux is used for prophylaxis and treatment of VTE and treatment of acute coronary syndrome (ACS). It is not licensed for use in pregnancy, but there are reports of its successful use in the management of VTE in pregnant women[33].

LMWHs are currently widely used for the prevention and treatment of gestational VTE. In our institution, women on prophylactic doses of LMWH are advised to have the dose of the LMWH tailed off at the end of pregnancy and omit their dose if labor is suspected. Women on a therapeutic dose of LMWH are admitted in advance of planned induction to be converted to the therapeutic dose of intravenous UFH. They should omit LMWH on the day of admission and should be started on UFH, aiming for an APTT ratio of 1.5–2.0. UFH should be reduced to 500 IU/h when contractions start, aiming for an APTT ratio of less than 1.5 and should be stopped at the second stage of labor or earlier if a cesarean section may be required. In the latter case, protamine sulfate may be needed for reversal of UFH if the APTT ratio remains above 1.5. Postpartum, the heparin infusion can be restarted 4 h postdelivery at 500 IU/h, providing there is no bleeding. Patients are restarted on a therapeutic dose of LMWH 2–3 days after delivery. Warfarin can be started 4–5 days postpartum, and LMWH should be continued until an international normalized ratio (INR) of 2.0 or greater is reached on two consecutive days. Breastfeeding is safe on UFH, LMWH and warfarin.

Epidural anesthesia is generally safe in women following discontinuation of UFH, providing their coagulation screen is normal and their platelet count is more than 80×10^9/l. It remains unclear what period of time should elapse between the last dose of LMWH and insertion or removal of an epidural or spinal catheter, or how long the time interval should be until the next dose. The guidelines of the Royal College of Obstetricians and Gynaecologists suggest that, in women on treatment dose of LMWH, 24 hours should elapse after the last dose of the LMWH before insertion of an epidural catheter or spinal catheter, the cannula not to be removed within 12 hours of the most recent injection, and no further dose of LMWH should be given for at least 4 hours after its removal[36]. For women on prophylactic doses of LMWH, regional anesthetic techniques should not be used until 12 hours have elapsed since the last injection. As above, the cannula should not be removed within 12 hours of the most recent injection, and no further dose of LMWH should be given for at least 4 hours after its removal.

Women with mechanical heart valve prostheses require anticoagulation throughout pregnancy. They have a high thrombotic risk with older type of mechanical prostheses (e.g. Starr-Edwards or Bjork-Shiley), a prosthesis in the mitral position, multiple prosthetic valves, atrial fibrillation and a history of previous thrombotic event.

On the other hand, women with newer less thrombogenic bileaflet valves, particularly if they are in the aortic position (and providing they are in sinus rhythm and have normal left ventricular function), may be regarded as being at lower thromboembolic risk.

There is controversy surrounding the optimal choice of anticoagulation in pregnant women with mechanical heart valve prostheses. Both LMWH and UFH have been associated with an increased incidence of valve thrombosis compared with warfarin[64].

Despite the fetal consequences associated with oral anticoagulation, the European Society of Cardiology recommends warfarin as the anticoagulant of choice for pregnant women with mechanical heart valve prostheses[65]. UFH may be considered during the first trimester; warfarin is then used with a switch to UFH at 36 weeks to decrease the risk of fetal bleeding complications at delivery.

The American College of Chest Physicians recommends one of three anticoagulant regimens consisting of UFH, LMWH, or warfarin with UFH or LMWH during the first trimester and at the end of pregnancy, in women with mechanical heart valves[61]. The lack of well designed trials does not allow identification of one approach as clearly superior to others.

Decisions about the most appropriate anticoagulant regimen during pregnancy for women with mechanical heart valve prostheses must be made on an individual patient basis after careful counseling, and should be based as much as possible on the relative risks of the various thromboprophylaxis regimens and whether the patient is perceived to be at high or low thromboembolic risk.

On the basis of the report that the risk of fetal complications with warfarin appears to be dose-related, providing their daily warfarin requirement does not exceed 5 mg[63], some women may feel reassured about the relatively low risk to their fetus if they use warfarin throughout pregnancy, or with substitution of UFH or LMWH from 6 to 12 weeks' gestation. However, women whose daily warfarin requirement exceeds 5 mg, particularly if they are classified into the lower thromboembolic risk group, may wish to minimize the risk of fetal complication and may be prepared to rely on adjusted doses of LMWH. The peak anti-Xa level 4 hours postinjection should be between 1.0 and 1.2 U/ml[61].

CONGENITAL DISORDERS OF HEMOSTASIS

Congenital platelet disorders

Bernard–Soulier syndrome is a rare autosomal recessive platelet disorder due to a variety of mutations in membrane glycoproteins Ib, IX and V. Patients usually present early in life with spontaneous bruising, epistaxis or bleeding after minor trauma; menorrhagia is a common presentation. Laboratory findings include thrombocytopenia, large platelets, prolonged bleeding time and poor platelet aggregation *in vitro* to ristocetin.

In a review of 30 pregnancies in 18 women with Bernard–Soulier syndrome, primary PPH was reported in 10 pregnancies (33%) and secondary PPH in 12 pregnancies (40%)[66]. Options for management of bleeding in Bernard–Soulier syndrome in pregnancy include tranexamic acid, desmopressin (DDAVP), rFVIIa and platelet transfusion. It is preferable to avoid platelet transfusion if at all possible because of its associated risk of alloantibody formation; maternal alloantibodies can cross the placenta and cause fetal or neonatal alloimmune thrombocytopenia. In the above review, alloimmune thrombocytopenia was reported in six neonates, with one intrauterine death and one neonatal death. The use of rFVIIa combined with tranexamic acid is recommended for uncomplicated vaginal delivery. However, HLA-matched platelet infusion with tranexamic acid is recommended as a first line treatment for cesarean sections or if bleeding occurs during vaginal delivery.

Regional analgesia is contraindicated because of the risk of spinal/epidural hematoma. The safest mode of delivery for the fetus and the mother is controversial. In most of the reported cases, cesarean section was the preferred mode of delivery. PPH has been reported in patients delivered vaginally and by cesarean section. However, the risk of bleeding to the fetus is only in association with alloimmune thrombocytopenia. If this diagnosis is excluded, cesarean section should be reserved for obstetric indications. When vaginal delivery is contemplated, prolonged labor especially during the second stage and instrumental deliveries should be avoided.

Glanzmann's thrombasthenia is due to a spectrum of mutations in platelet membrane GP IIb/IIIa, resulting in failure to bind fibrinogen. It is characterized by excessive menstrual blood loss, bleeding from mucous membranes, and major hemorrhage following trauma or surgery. The platelet count is normal, but clot retraction is greatly impaired and agents such as adenosine diphosphate (ADP), epinephrine and collagen fail to induce platelet aggregation. In a review of 31 detailed case reports of 40 pregnancies in 35 women with Glanzmann's thrombasthenia, antenatal bleeding was described in 50% of pregnancies but was usually mild and occurred at mucocutaneous sites[67]. Primary PPH was reported in 34% of the pregnancies and secondary PPH in 24%. PPH was frequently severe and occurred up to 20 days after delivery. There was a wide variation in approach to prevention and treatment of PPH, but most women received platelet transfusion, sometimes with additional rFVIIa and antifibrinolytics. Maternal alloimmunization against platelets was reported in 73% of pregnancies and was associated with four neonatal deaths[67]. Regional anesthesia is contraindicated in Glanzmann's thrombasthenia. Elective cesarean section was performed in 31% of the reported pregnancies, but there was no discernible relationship between this mode of delivery and the frequency of maternal or fetal bleeding. Many centers would now consider elective cesarean section in mothers with Glanzmann's thrombasthenia for obstetric indications or in situations of high fetal bleeding risk such as maternal alloimmunization.

The May-Hegglin anomaly is a rare autosomal dominant condition with thrombocytopenia and giant platelets. Platelet count varies between 40 and $80 \times 10^9/l$, but platelet function appears normal. Excess hemorrhage is uncommon, but patients may need a platelet transfusion to achieve hemostasis at delivery[68].

von Willebrand disease

von Willebrand disease (vWD) is the most common of the inherited bleeding disorders, reportedly found in approximately 1% of the general population without ethnic variations. It is caused by a reduced plasma concentration of structurally normal von Willebrand factor (vWF) or the presence of a structurally abnormal molecule with reduced activity. vWF is the carrier protein in plasma for FVIII, and it also acts as a bridge between platelets and subendothelial collagen fibers.

vWF is synthesized in endothelial cells as a polypeptide of 2813 amino acids, which undergoes initial dimerization and then multimerization up to a multimer with a molecular weight of 20,000 kDa. High-molecular weight (HMW) multimers are functionally more effective in promoting platelet adhesion and aggregation. The vWF protein is stored in Weibel–Palade bodies in the endothelial cells from where it is released into the plasma. vWF is also synthesized in megakaryocytes, stored in the platelet α-granules and, on activation, secreted by the platelet release reaction. This allows accumulation of vWF at the site of vascular injury where it can promote further platelet adhesion and thus hemostasis. The mature vWF protein possesses a number of specific binding sites, which represent its different activities (Figure 1). Circulating HMW multimers are cleaved by a protease, known as ADAMTS 13, which is lacking in patients with the rare congenital thrombotic thrombocytopenic purpura.

vWD is subclassified into seven categories (Table 6), which correspond to distinct pathophysiological

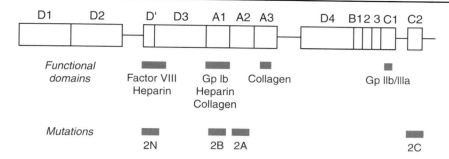

Figure 1 The von Willebrand factor. The protein consists of a series of domains with different binding sites for factor VIII, heparin, collagen and platelet glycoprotein (Gp) Ib and IIb/IIIa. The sites of gene mutations giving rise to different subtypes of VWD are marked. From Green D, Ludlam CA. VWD in bleeding disorders. *Health Press* 2004:63–9

mechanisms and are important in determining therapy. Of all the categories, about approximately 70–80% of patients have type 1 disease.

The condition commonly presents as a mild to moderate bleeding disorder, typically with easy bruising or bleeding from mucosal surfaces. The most frequent problem found in the non-pregnant female is menorrhagia, which may be quite severe. Patients with mild abnormalities may be asymptomatic, with the diagnosis made only after significant hemostatic challenges such as operations and trauma.

Laboratory tests in patients with vWD reveal a prolonged bleeding time and may show a prolonged APTT. More definitive diagnostic tests depend on the finding of reduced vWF activity measured by ristocetin cofactor activity (vWF:RCo) and collagen-binding assay (vWF:CB), accompanied by variable reductions in vWF antigen (vWF:Ag) and FVIII. Several further tests that aid in classification include analysis of ristocetin-induced platelet aggregation (RIPA), vWF multimer and assay of FVIII binding to vWF[69]. Mild thrombocytopenia may occur in patients with vWD type 2B.

The diagnosis may not be straightforward, as one or more of the activities of FVIII and vWF may be borderline and even normal. It is often necessary to repeat the estimations on at least three occasions. Stress, physical exercise, recent surgery and pregnancy all increase plasma vWF and FVIII levels, and diagnosis may be difficult in these circumstances[70]. When investigating patients with borderline results, it should be taken into account that FVIII and vWF levels are 15–20% lower in individuals with blood group O compared to individuals with blood group A[70]. Molecular genetic analysis may be useful as an aid to diagnosis in type 2 or 3 vWD. Knowledge of the mutation may also aid genetic counseling and allow the option of prenatal diagnosis to be offered to women at risk of having a child with severe type 3 vWD.

The aim of therapy for vWD is to correct impaired primary hemostasis and impaired coagulation. Treatment choice depends on the severity and the type of disease, and on the clinical setting. Treatment options usually include DDAVP and vWF-containing blood products[71].

Table 6 Classification of von Willebrand disease (vWD)

Type 1	Partial quantitative deficiency of apparently normal vWF
Type 2	Qualitative deficiency of vWF
Type 2A	Qualitative variants with decreased HMW multimers
Type 2B	Qualitative variants with increased affinity for platelet GP Ib
Type 2M	Qualitative variants with normal HMW multimers appearance
Type 2N	Qualitative variants with markedly decreased affinity for factor VIII
Type 3	Virtually complete deficiency of vWF

vWF, von Willebrand factor; HMW, high-molecular weight
Adapted from Sadler JE. *Thromb Haemost* 1994;71:520–5

DDAVP, a synthetic vasopressin analogue, releases vWF from endothelial stores; it also increases plasma FVIII level. It is usually given by slow intravenous infusion of 0.3 µg/kg over 20 min, which can be repeated every 4–6 h on two or three occasions. The drug can also be given subcutaneously or as a nasal spray. Side-effects include hypotension, facial flushing, fluid retention for up to 24 h and consequent hyponatremia. DDAVP can safely be used during pregnancy and after delivery[72,73]. It is effective in many situations in type 1 vWD in which a 3–5-fold increase in the plasma vWF and FVIII levels could be seen. It is of no therapeutic benefit in type 3 vWD because of the very low basal levels of vWF and FVIII. The response in type 2s is less predictable. DDAVP is contraindicated in patients with type 2B because it may exacerbate the co-existing thrombocytopenia. Patients should have a test of DDAVP (if possible when not pregnant) to see if it increases the vWF/ FVIII level sufficiently to prevent or stop hemorrhage.

Plasma-derived vWF containing concentrates are necessary in patients who do not respond adequately to DDAVP or in whom it is contraindicated. The loading dose is 40–60 IU/kg, and this can be followed by repeat doses every 12–24 h to maintain vWF activity (vWF:RCoF) more than 50%. All currently available concentrates are derived from plasma. As at least one viral inactivation step is included in their manufacture, they are unlikely to transmit hepatitis or HIV, but there is still a risk of parvovirus infection.

von Willebrand disease and pregnancy

von Willebrand disease is the most common congenital hemostatic disorder in pregnancy. In a normal pregnancy, both FVIII and vWF levels progressively increase (Figure 2)[74]. vWF starts to rise as early as the 6th week and by the third trimester may have increased 3–4-fold. FVIII and vWF levels also increase in most women with vWD, which may explain the frequent improvement in minor bleeding manifestations during pregnancy. The hemostatic response to pregnancy depends on both the type and severity of disease. Most women with type 1 vWD have an increase in FVIII and vWF levels into the normal non-pregnant range, which may mask the diagnosis during pregnancy. However, levels may remain low in severe cases. FVIII and vWF antigen levels often increase in pregnant women with type 2 vWD with minimal or no increase in vWF activity levels. In type 2B vWD, the increase in the abnormal vWF can cause progressive and severe thrombocytopenia, but intervention is not usually required. Most women with type 3 vWD have no improvement in FVIII or vWF levels during pregnancy[75]. After delivery, FVIII and vWF in normal women fall slowly to baseline levels over a period of 4–6 weeks. As the individual hemostatic response to pregnancy is variable, vWF and FVIII levels should be checked at booking, 28 weeks', 34 weeks' gestation and prior to invasive procedures[73]. vWF and FVIII levels may fall rapidly after delivery and should be checked a few days postpartum.

Antepartum hemorrhage is uncommon in women with vWD, but may occur after spontaneous miscarriage or elective termination, occasionally as the initial presentation of vWD. The risk of bleeding in patients with vWD is usually greatest postpartum; PPH may be the first presentation of vWD. One series showed an 18.5% incidence of primary PPH and a 20% incidence of secondary PPH[76]. The risk is greater in women with type 2 and 3 disease and those whose FVIII and vWD levels are less than 50%. vWD may also exacerbate bleeding due to other obstetric causes, such as uterine atony or a trauma to the birth canal. Other pregnancy-associated reasons for bleeding in women with vWD include extensive bruising and hematomas at intramuscular injection, episiotomy and surgical wound sites.

For patients whose vWD profile has normalized in pregnancy, no specific hemostatic support is required. For patients whose vWF activity (vWF:RCo) has not normalized, hemostatic supportive therapy is necessary to cover vaginal delivery or cesarean section. Treatment is indicated to raise FVIII level and vWF activity above 50%[76]. Patients with type 1 vWD may receive DDAVP if they are responsive and there are no current contraindications; patients with type 2 and 3 vWD will usually require vWF concentrate.

Ventouse delivery, fetal blood sampling and fetal scalp electrodes should be avoided if the fetus is at risk for type 2 or 3 vWD or more severe forms of type 1 vWD. Because of the high incidence of secondary PPH in patients with vWD, efforts should be made to ensure that the placenta is complete upon expulsion or removal. Careful and prompt repair of episiotomy wounds or perineal tears is advisable.

Decisions about regional analgesia should be individualized[77]. In type 1 vWD when FVIII and vWF activity have spontaneously corrected, epidural anesthesia is likely to be safe. Alternatives should be used for patients with type 2 or 3 vWD and in type 1 vWD where vWF activity has remained low, as bleeding in such cases does not always correlate with laboratory parameters after corrective treatment.

After delivery, all patients should be closely observed for PPH and uncorrected hemostatic defects treated. In responsive patients, DDAVP is the treatment of choice to prevent and treat mild to moderate postpartum bleeding. FVIII level and vWF activity should be maintained at greater than 50% for 3 days following vaginal delivery and for 5–7 days following cesarean section.

It is difficult and unnecessary to diagnose type 1 or type 2 vWD in the neonate. If type 3 vWD is suspected, a cord blood sample should be sent for assay of FVIII and vWF activity. Intramuscular injections should be avoided for both mother and newborn.

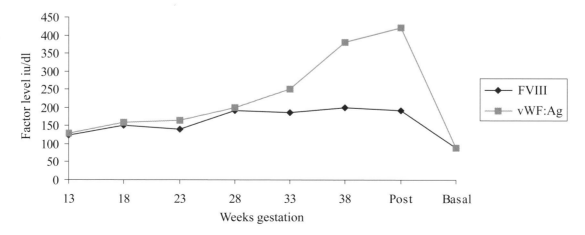

Figure 2 Levels of factor VIII and vWF in normal pregnancy. From Giangrande PL. Management of pregnancy in carriers of haemophilia. *Haemophilia* 1998;4:779–84

HEMOPHILIAS

Hemophilias A and B are the most common severe congenital bleeding disorders associated with reduced or absent coagulation FVIII and FIX, respectively. Hemophilia A affects approximately one in 5000 live male births and hemophilia B affects approximately one in 30,000 live male births. The genes for both conditions are located on the X-chromosome; they are therefore sex-linked disorders that almost exclusively affect males. Clinically, the hemophilias cause a spectrum of bleeding manifestations varying from easy bruising to spontaneous deep muscle and joint hemorrhages and intracranial bleeding. Hemophilias can only be distinguished by measuring plasma levels of the specific clotting factors. The clinical severity is directly related to plasma concentrations of FVIII/FIX. Individuals with levels of below 1% of normal have severe hemophilia and the most frequent bleeds. Females in families with a history of hemophilia may be obligate, potential or sporadic carriers, depending on the details of the pedigree[78]. An obligate carrier is a woman, whose father has hemophilia, or a woman who has family history of hemophilia and who has given birth to a hemophilic son, or a woman who has more than one child with hemophilia. A potential carrier of hemophilia is a woman who has a maternal relative with the disorder. A woman with one affected child and no family history is likely to be a sporadic carrier[78]. Female carriers of hemophilia are expected to have clotting factor levels around 50% of normal as they have only one affected chromosome. However, a wide range of values (5–219%)[79] has been reported as a result of random inactivation of the X-chromosomes (lyonization). If the FVIII/IX level is less than 50%, abnormal bleeding may occur after trauma or surgery.

There are two main risks for a female carrier of hemophilia in pregnancy. First, women with a low FVIII/IX level may be at risk of bleeding after delivery or during invasive procedures in the first trimester. Second, there is a 50% chance of each son inheriting hemophilia and 50% of her daughters being carriers.

As discussed earlier, the levels of FVIII tend to increase during normal pregnancy (Figure 2). The increase is particularly marked during the third trimester, when levels of FVIII may rise to double the normal baseline value. Similarly, the vast majority of carriers of hemophilia A will have increased their FVIII production to within the normal range by late gestation; factor replacement therapy is thus only rarely required during delivery in carriers of hemophilia A. The risk of bleeding in carriers of hemophilia A is greatest in the postpartum period because FVIII levels may decrease rapidly after delivery. By contrast, the level of FIX does not increase significantly during pregnancy, and thus a woman with a low initial baseline FIX is more likely to require replacement to control bleeding complications during delivery.

All women who are obligate or potential carriers of hemophilia should be offered genetic testing and counseling. In particular, they should have their carrier status determined to allow for the optimal management of their pregnancies. Genetic testing should be offered when the individual is able to understand the issues concerned (usually at age of 13–15 years) and after having given informed consent[80]. In many individuals in the UK with hemophilia A and B, the causative mutation has been identified. If the mutation within the family is known, it is straightforward to screen the potential carrier. If, on the other hand, the mutation is not known, then linkage analysis using informative genetic polymorphisms may be possible. If neither of these approaches is suitable, then direct mutation detection may be possible by sequencing the FVIII/FIX gene.

Coagulation studies should also be carried out to identify carriers with low FVIII/FIX levels. Phenotypic data may be helpful in assessing the statistical risk of carriership if molecular diagnosis is not possible. However, normal levels of FVIII/FIX do not exclude carrier status[80]. Women who have low levels of FVIII may have a useful hemostatic response to DDAVP. To establish whether this response is occurring, a trial of DDAVP can be attempted, with measurement of the response in FVIII levels over the next 24 h.

Once carrier status has been established, women should be offered pre-pregnancy counseling to provide them with the information necessary to make informed reproductive choices. Preimplantation diagnosis is potentially useful for carriers of hemophilia who, after counseling, do not wish to contemplate bringing up a hemophilic child, but would not consider termination of an affected fetus. Following *in vitro* fertilization (IVF) treatment, it is possible to remove a single embryonic cell at the 8–16-cell stage and carry out genetic diagnosis. Female or unaffected male embryos can then be transferred into the uterus. In the UK, each such test requires a license from the Human Fertilisation and Embryology Authority.

If prenatal diagnosis is requested and a suitable molecular marker exists, testing is usually carried out by chorionic villus sampling (CVS) at 11–12 weeks; DNA extracted from fetal cells is analyzed. The principal advantage of this procedure is that it may be applied during the first trimester, so that, if termination of the pregnancy is required, this is easier to accomplish. The main adverse event related to CVS is miscarriage, which is estimated at about 1–2%. Cells as a source of DNA can also be obtained from amniotic fluid (amniocentesis) after 15 weeks' gestation; here, the miscarriage rate is about 0.5–1%. Fetal blood sampling by cordocentesis is now rarely carried out because of the inherent hazards associated with this procedure. The use of prenatal diagnosis is decreasing in developed countries; as hemophilia care improves, more couples are willing to contemplate bringing up a child with hemophilia[74].

Fetal sex should be determined in all pregnancies in which the fetus is at risk of hemophilia. Non-invasive determination of fetal gender is now possible in the first trimester by ultrasound and/or analysis of free fetal DNA in maternal blood and has been shown to be a reliable method of avoiding invasive prenatal diagnostic tests in pregnancies[81]. Women may not wish to know the sex of the infant as they would not consider termination of pregnancy. However, this information is important for the appropriate management of labor and delivery.

Factor VIII/IX levels in female carriers of hemophilia should be monitored regularly in pregnancy. UK guidelines recommend measurement of coagulation factor levels at booking, at 28 weeks and at 34 weeks[73]. It is particularly important to measure coagulation factor levels toward the end of the third trimester (34–36 weeks) to plan management of delivery[74]. If maternal FVIII/FIX levels remain low at 34–36 weeks in hemophilia carriers, treatment is necessary for delivery[74]. FVIII/FIX plasma levels should be maintained at greater than 50% for all modes of delivery[73]. Epidural anesthesia may be used if coagulation defects have been corrected and the relevant factor level is above 50% or has been raised to more than 50%[73]. Recombinant FVIII/FIX or DDAVP (for carriers of hemophilia A only) should be used. Plasma-derived factor concentrate products, including those subjected to dual inactivation processes, have the potential to transmit non-lipid coated viruses, e.g. parvovirus, and should be avoided if possible. Recombinant FVIII/FIX concentrates avoid the risk of potential viral transmission. Infection of the fetus with parvovirus may result in hydrops fetalis and fetal death.

The optimal mode of delivery for a fetus at risk of hemophilia remains the subject of debate due to continuing uncertainty regarding the risk of intracranial (ICH) and extracranial hemorrhage (ECH). In a recently published population based study, infants of maternal carriers of hemophilia were more often delivered by cesarean section[82]. In the same survey, 17 cases of intracranial hemorrhage were reported, two of which were associated with assisted delivery, while 14 followed spontaneous vaginal delivery and one followed emergency cesarean delivery. In cases of vaginal delivery, ventouse delivery is absolutely contraindicated because of the risk of major cephalohematoma and intracranial bleeding. Mid-cavity rotational forceps delivery should be avoided, but simple lift-out forceps delivery is allowed. Fetal scalp sampling and scalp electrodes should not be used if the fetus may have hemophilia.

Most bleeding problems in carriers of hemophilia occur postpartum. In a series of 65 live births in 53 carriers of hemophilia the incidence of primary and secondary PPH was reported at 19% and 2%, respectively, compared with 5% and 0.7%, respectively, in the general population[81]. Replacement therapy should be given immediately after delivery to mothers with an uncorrected hemostatic defect. Treatment options at this stage are the same as those during labor and delivery. Supportive therapy to maintain hemostasis should be continued for at least 3 days after vaginal delivery and for at least 5 days after cesarean section[73].

Cord blood should be obtained for FVIII/FIX assay[83]. In the infant, intramuscular injections should be avoided until hemophilia has been excluded. Both ICH and ECH are observed in newborn infants with hemophilia and the incidence of ICH in neonates with severe hemophilia is estimated to be 1–4%[83]. Routine cranial ultrasound scan may be a useful screening investigation, but cannot be relied upon to detect all cases of early ICH. In neonates with non-specific symptoms which could represent ICH, or in neonates with a documented ECH, computed tomography (CT) or MRI scanning should be considered even in the presence of an apparently normal cranial ultrasound scan. Where there is a strong clinical suspicion of ICH or other bleeding, factor concentrate should be given immediately and not withheld pending definitive imaging studies.

RARE COAGULATION DISORDERS

Inherited abnormalities of fibrinogen

Inherited abnormalities of fibrinogen consist of quantitative (afibrinogenemia and hypofibrinogenemia) and qualitative deficiencies (dysfibrinogenemia). Afibrinogenemia refers to a total absence of fibrinogen, while hypofibrinogenemia is a milder form of the disorder with a decreased level of both antigenic and functional (Clauss) fibrinogen. These conditions can also coexist as hypodysfibrinogenemia. In normal pregnancy fibrinogen levels may increase to up to two-fold from non-pregnant levels, whereas the hemostatic abnormality in women with fibrinogen deficiency/dysfunction is expected to continue throughout pregnancy. Afibrinogenemia is an autosomal recessive disorder in contrast to hypofibrinogenemia which can be inherited as either a dominant or a recessive trait. Both are associated with recurrent miscarriages as well as placental abruption and PPH[84].

In women with afibrinogenemia, regular replacement therapy throughout pregnancy to keep fibrinogen levels above 1 g/l is recommended and should be commenced as soon as possible in pregnancy to prevent early fetal loss[85]. Replacement therapy may be required in women with hypofibrinogenemia depending on the fibrinogen level and the bleeding tendency. Options for replacement therapy include plasma-derived fibrinogen concentrate and cryoprecipitate. Cryoprecipitate is a good source of fibrinogen but should not usually be used, as it is not virally inactivated. Fibrinogen concentrate is heat treated and the preferred option. Fibrinogen clearance increases as the pregnancy progresses and the amount of the infused fibrinogen will need to increase with advancing gestation. Thrombotic events have also been reported in patients with inherited afibrinogenemia[84]; hence, the risk of bleeding and thrombosis should be considered and balanced during pregnancy.

For labor and delivery, in women with afibrinogenemia, replacement therapy to maintain a minimum fibrinogen level of 1.5 g/l has been suggested for the prevention of placental abruption and PPH[85]. For women with hypofibrinogenemia, intrapartum replacement is required if the fibrinogen level is below

1.5 g/l and/or if the woman has a significant bleeding history[84].

Afibrinogenemia and hypofibrinogenemia are associated with a high risk of PPH. In a literature review of congenital hypofibrinogenemia, PPH was found to be the most common obstetric complication occurring in 45% (14/31 deliveries) among 10 patients[86]. Paradoxically thrombotic events during puerperium have also been reported in afibrinogenemia and hypofibrinogenemia[84]. The postpartum management of these patients should take into account any personal and family history of bleeding and thrombosis. Standard measures such as compression stockings, adequate hydration and early mobilization are recommended.

Dysfibrinogenemia is inherited as an autosomal dominant trait and the diagnosis is made by demonstrating a low functional fibrinogen with a normal antigenic fibrinogen. This condition has an unpredictable clinical phenotype; as such, the management of pregnant women with dysfibrinogenemia needs to be individualized, taking into account the fibrinogen level and personal and family history of bleeding and thrombosis. In asymptomatic women no specific treatment is required during pregnancy. Women with a personal or family history of thrombosis should be offered antenatal thromboprophylaxis with LMWH; fibrinogen replacement is given only if bleeding occurs. Conversely, replacement therapy should be considered in women with a personal or family bleeding phenotype, and concomitant thromboprophylaxis with LMWH should also be considered as fibrinogen may precipitate venous thrombosis[87].

Women with dysfibrinogenemia are also at risk of both postpartum thrombosis and hemorrhage; therefore, their intrapartum and postpartum management should be individualized. In asymptomatic women or those with a mild bleeding phenotype, no specific treatment other than close observation is required. Vaginal delivery can be managed conservatively with treatment given to raise fibrinogen level to more than 1 g/l above baseline if bleeding occurs. However, if the bleeding tendency is significant or if the woman is undergoing cesarean section, prophylactic treatment is recommended to raise the fibrinogen level to more than 1 g/l baseline and to maintain it above 0.5 g/l until wound healing has occurred[87]. Standard measures for venous thrombosis should be followed in all women with dysfibrinogenemia. Postpartum thromboprophylaxis with LMWH is recommended for those with personal or family history of thrombosis or following cesarean section as such surgery is usually performed under replacement cover[87].

As dysfibrinogenemia is usually transmitted as an autosomal dominant trait, it is important to regard the neonate as potentially affected and avoid invasive monitoring procedures and instrumental deliveries.

Factor VII deficiency

Congenital FVII deficiency is the most common of the rare inherited coagulation disorders with an estimated prevalence of 1 in 500,000. It is inherited in an autosomal recessive manner and its frequency is significantly increased in countries where consanguineous marriages are common. FVII levels are usually less than 10% in homozygotes and around 50% in heterozygotes. Although there is a poor correlation between FVII levels and bleeding risk, hemorrhages occur in patients with factor VII levels below 10%[84]. Individuals with a moderate FVII deficiency often bleed from the mucous membranes, and epistaxis, bleeding gums and menorrhagia are common. In severe FVII deficiency (FVII level <2%), bleeding into the central nervous system very early in life leads to a high morbidity and mortality. Congenital FVII deficiency is usually suspected when an isolated prolongation of the PT is found in a patient without liver disease, and a normal APTT and fibrinogen level.

A significant rise in FVII level is seen during pregnancy in non-deficient women. This has also been observed in women with mild/moderate forms of FVII deficiency (heterozygotes)[88] but not in women with severe deficiency[89]. In women with mild/moderate deficiency, FVII level may normalize at term; therefore, replacement therapy may not be required for labor and delivery. However, this decision should be individualized and should take into account the mother's bleeding history, FVII level in the third trimester and the mode of delivery. Women with FVII level of less than 10–20% at term or significant bleeding history are more likely to be at risk of PPH and require prophylactic treatment[89].

Recombinant activated FVII (rFVIIa) has been approved in the European Union for use in congenital FVII deficiency[90]. In places where this product is not available, FFP, PCC or plasma-derived FVII concentrate may be used. Recombinant FVIIa is given in boluses of 20 µg/kg; higher doses may be associated with thrombosis.

Factor V deficiency

Hereditary FV deficiency is a very rare autosomal recessive condition. The prevalence of the homozygous state is approximately 1 in 1,000,000. Parental consanguinity is often present. In homozygote individuals, FV levels range from less than 1% to 10% and in heterozygotes FV level is around 50%[87]. FV deficiency is associated with prolongation of both the PT and the APTT, but a normal TT and is confirmed by performing a FV assay. Homozygous deficiency is associated with a moderately severe bleeding disorder in the form of easy bruising and mucous membrane bleeding, but patients may also develop hemarthroses and muscle hematomas. Pregnancy and delivery are not usually accompanied by any bleeding complications in women with FV levels of around 50%. Women with FV deficiency especially those with low FV levels appear to be at increased risk of PPH. In women with partial (heterozygous) deficiency and no history of bleeding, labor and delivery could be managed expectantly[87]. However, in women with severe (homozygous) deficiency substitution therapy with FFP (as no FV concentrate is available) is recommended to raise FV level above 15–25%[84]. Further doses may be necessary to maintain these levels during and after delivery. If cesarean section is performed, it is recommended that FV levels are maintained above this level until wound healing is established[87].

Combined factor V and VIII deficiency

Combined FV and FVIII deficiency is a rare autosomal recessive disorder which usually arises as a consequence of consanguinity. It is caused by mutations in one of two different genes, LMAN1 and MCFD2, which encode proteins that form a complex involved in the transport of FV and FVIII from the endoplasmic reticulum to the Golgi apparatus. Although mild bleeding symptoms such as easy bruising and epistaxis are not uncommon in affected individuals, circulating levels of FV and FVIII are usually sufficient to prevent more severe spontaneous bleeding episodes. The combined deficiency disorder is associated with a prolongation of both the PT and the APTT, with the APTT prolongation disproportionate to that of the PT. Factor assays reveal levels of between 5 and 20% for both FV and FVIII[91]. There are no published data on the management of pregnant women with this combined deficiency. As FV levels in pregnancy do not change significantly and FVIII levels rise throughout the pregnancy, any possible bleeding, especially during labor and delivery, is likely to be dependent on the FV level. However, both levels should be monitored with FV levels kept above 15–20% and FVIII levels above 50% during delivery or for any invasive procedures[87].

Factor X deficiency

Congenital FX deficiency is an autosomal recessive disorder. The prevalence of the severe (homozygous) form is 1 in 1,000,000 in the general population and is much higher in countries where consanguineous marriages are more common. The prevalence of heterozygous FX deficiency is about 1:500, but individuals are usually clinically asymptomatic. Severe FX deficiency (FX level <1%) is associated with a significant risk of intracranial hemorrhage in the first weeks of life and umbilical stump bleeding. The most frequent symptom is epistaxis, which is seen with all severities of deficiency. Menorrhagia occurs in half of the women. Severe arthropathy may occur as a result of recurrent joint bleeds. Mild deficiency is defined by FX levels of 6–10%; these individuals are often diagnosed incidentally, but may experience easy bruising or menorrhagia. The diagnosis of FX deficiency is suspected following the finding of a prolonged APTT and PT and is confirmed by measuring plasma FX levels.

Fourteen pregnancies in nine women with isolated FX deficiency have been reported in the literature[92]. The complications described include spontaneous abortions, placental abruptions, premature births and PPH. FX levels increase during pregnancy and antenatal replacement therapy is not usually needed. However, women with severe FX deficiency and a history of adverse outcome in pregnancy may benefit from aggressive replacement therapy[87]. FX is present in PCCs. FFP may be an alternative when PCCs are not available. As the half-life of FX is 24–40 h, a single daily infusion is usually adequate. FX levels of 10–20% are generally sufficient for hemostasis[87] and are required at the time of delivery. FX levels should be monitored as caution is required because of the prothrombotic properties of these concentrates.

Combined deficiencies of the vitamin K-dependent factors II, VII, IX and X

Congenital combined deficiency of factors II, VII, IX and X is an autosomal recessive bleeding disorder. It is caused by deficiency of enzymes associated with vitamin K metabolism (e.g. γ-glutamyl carboxylase) as a result of homozygous genetic mutations. Mucocutaneous and postoperative related bleeding have been reported. Severe cases may present with intracranial hemorrhage or umbilical cord bleeding in infancy. Some individuals have associated skeletal abnormalities (probably related to abnormalities in bone vitamin K-dependent proteins such as osteocalcin). Severe bleeding is usually associated with activities of the vitamin K-dependent factors of less than 5%. Affected individuals show prolongation of the APTT and PT associated with variable reductions in the specific activities of factors II, VII, IX and X.

The clinical picture and response to vitamin K is variable, some responding to low-dose oral vitamin K, but others are non-responsive even to high-dose intravenous replacement. In those individuals who are non-responsive to vitamin K, PCCs are the product of choice.

There is a single report of a pregnancy progressing to term in an individual with severe congenital vitamin K-dependent clotting factor deficiency managed with oral vitamin K 15 mg daily throughout pregnancy. Bleeding from an episiotomy wound in this case required fresh frozen plasma[93].

Factor XI deficiency

FXI deficiency is an autosomally inherited condition, which is particularly common in Ashkenazi Jews in whom heterozygote frequency is 8%. Overall, the prevalence of severe deficiency is approximately 1 in 1,000,000, but partial deficiency is much more common. The deficiency is classified as severe if the FXI level is less than 15% (homozygotes) and as partial at 15–70% (heterozygotes); the lower limit of the normal range is 70%. It is associated with a variable bleeding tendency, and bleeding can occur in heterozygous as well as homozygous individuals. Spontaneous bleeding is extremely rare, even in those with undetectable FXI levels. Bleeding is provoked by injury or surgery, particularly in areas of high fibrinolytic activity (e.g. genitourinary tract). Menorrhagia is common, and women with FXI deficiency may be diagnosed as a consequence of this. The bleeding tendency can be inconsistent with an individual and the family, and could not clearly be related to the factor levels. This unpredictable nature of FXI deficiency makes management for pregnancy and delivery difficult. The APTT is usually prolonged and diagnosis is confirmed by finding a low FXI level.

As FXI level does not increase during pregnancy, many women will continue to have a subnormal factor level at term, and thus be at risk of excessive bleeding during delivery. Women with FXI deficiency are also at increased risk of both primary and secondary PPH. In a case series of 11 women with FXI deficiency, the incidence of primary and secondary PPH was 16% and 24%, respectively[76].

Due to the unpredictable bleeding tendency in FXI deficiency, the decision for prophylaxis during labor and delivery needs to be individualized and must take into consideration FXI level, personal/family bleeding history and the mode of delivery. In women with partial FXI deficiency and no bleeding history but previous hemostatic challenge, treatment is not usually required during vaginal delivery. In women with partial deficiency and significant bleeding history or no previous hemostatic challenges, tranexamic acid is often used for 3 days, with the first dose being administered during labor. Tranexamic acid is also used to manage prolonged mild intermittent secondary PPH which is a common presentation of FXI-deficient patients[94]. FXI concentrate is needed for severely deficient women to cover vaginal delivery and also for cesarean section. The aim is to maintain the FXI level between 50% and 70% during labor and for 3–4 days after vaginal delivery and 7 days after cesarean section. FXI concentrate is potentially thrombogenic; the single dose should not exceed 30 IU/kg with the aim of raising FXI level to no greater than 70%[94]. Concurrent use of tranexamic acid or other antifibrinolytic drugs with FXI concentrate should be avoided. FFP can be used, but in patients with severe deficiency, it is difficult to produce a sufficient rise (to more than 30%) without the risk of fluid overload[87]. Recombinant FVIIa has been used successfully to manage adult patients with FXI deficiency undergoing surgery, although it is not licensed for this indication[87].

Factor XIII deficiency

Congenital FXIII (fibrin stabilizing factor) deficiency is an autosomal recessive disorder. FXIII circulates in plasma as a tetramer composed of two A-subunits and two B-subunits. There are three types of FXIII deficiency: type I is a combined deficiency of both subunits A and B, type II is a deficiency of subunit A and type III is a deficiency of subunit B[84].

The condition is characterized by features of delayed and impaired wound healing with bleeding occurring 24–36 h after surgery or trauma. Umbilical bleeding in the first few weeks of life is very suggestive of the disorder. Soft tissue bleeds are more common than hemarthroses, which usually only occur after trauma. Spontaneous intracranial bleeds are a characteristic feature. The severity of the bleeding state varies markedly between individuals with apparently similar FXIII plasma levels. The routine tests (APTT and PT) are normal and the FXIII level has to be specifically requested of the laboratory.

Women with types I and III usually conceive and deliver normally, whereas the majority of women with type II deficiency miscarry without appropriate replacement therapy started preconception. Regular therapy to maintain the FXIII level at more than 3%[87] and if possible more than 10%[95] is recommended to prevent bleeding and pregnancy loss in women with type II deficiency. A FXIII level of more than 20%, and if possible, more than 30% during labor/delivery has been suggested to minimize the risk of bleeding complications[95]. FXIII concentrate, either plasma-derived or recombinant, is the treatment of choice and is superior to FFP and cryoprecipitate. FXIII has a half-life of 7–10 days and therefore only needs to be given at 4–6-weekly intervals.

The incidence of PPH in women with FXIII deficiency is not known. Successful pregnancy in women with FXIII subunit A deficiency is generally only achieved with replacement therapy throughout pregnancy and at delivery[95] and as the administered FXIII concentrate has a long circulating half-life most of these cases are not complicated by PPH. Women with types I and III FXIII deficiency usually conceive and deliver normally without replacement therapy, but PPH and postpartum prophylaxis should be considered in these cases.

References

1. Brenner B. Haemostatic changes in pregnancy. Thromb Res 2004;114:409–14
2. Bellart J, Gilabert R, Miralles RM, et al. Endothelial cell markers and fibrinopeptide A to D-dimer ratio as a measure of coagulation and fibrinolysis balance in normal pregnancy. Gynecol Obstet Invest 1998;46:17–21
3. Øian P, Omsjø I, Maltau JM, Østerud B. Reduced thromboplastin activity in blood monocytes and reduced sensitiviaty to stimuli in vitro of blood monocytes from pregnant women. Br J Haematol 1985;59:133–7
4. Holmes VA, Wallace JMW, Gilmore WS, et al. Tissue factor expression on monocyte subpopulations during normal pregnancy. Thromb Haemost 2002;87:953–8
5. Holmes VA, Wallace JM. Haemostasis in normal pregnancy: a balancing act? Biochem Soc Trans 2005;33:428–32
6. McCrae KR. Thrombocytopenia in pregnancy: differential diagnosis, pathogenesis and management. Blood Rev 2003; 17:7–14
7. Casonato A, Bertomoro A, Pontara E, et al. EDTA dependent pseudothrombocytopenia caused by antibodies against the cytoadhesive receptor of platelet gpIIB-IIIA. J Clin Pathol 1994;47:625–30
8. McCrae KR, Samuels P, Schreiber AD. Pregnancy-associated thrombocytopenia: pathogenesis and management. Blood 1992;80:2697–714
9. Shehata N, Burrows RF, Kelton JG. Gestational thrombocytopenia. Clin Obstet Gynecol 1999;42:327–34
10. Guidelines for the investigation and management of idiopathic thrombocytopenic purpura in adults, children and in pregnancy. Br J Haematol 2003;120:574–96

11. Kessler I, Lancet M, Borenstein R, et al. The obstetrical management of patients with immunologic thrombocytopenic purpura. Int J Gynaecol Obstet 1982;20:23–8

12. Olsson B, Andersson PO, Jernas M, et al. T-cell-mediated cytotoxicity toward platelets in chronic idiopathic thrombocytopenic purpura. Nat Med 2003;9:1123–24

13. Chang M, Nakagawa PA, Williams SA, et al. Immune thrombocytopenic purpura (ITP) plasma and purified ITP monoclonal autoantibodies inhibit megakaryocytopoiesis in vitro. Blood 2003;102:887–95

14. Burrows RF, Kelton JG. Thrombocytopenia during pregnancy. In Greer IA, Turpie AG, Forbes CD, eds. Haemostasis and Thrombosis in Obstetrics and Gynaecology. London: Chapman & Hall, 1992

15. Gill KK, Kelton JG. Management of idiopathic thrombocytopenic purpura in pregnancy. Sem Hematol 2000;37:275–83

16. Letsky EA. In de Swiet, ed. Coagulation Defects in Medical Disorders in Obstetric Practice, 4th edn. Oxford: Blackwell Science, 2002:61–96

17. Letsky EA, Greaves M. Guidelines on the investigation and management of thrombocytopenia in pregnancy and neonatal alloimmune thrombocytopenia Maternal and Neonatal Haemostasis Working Party of the Haemostasis and Thrombosis Task Force of the British Society for Haematology. Br J Haematol 1996;95:21–6

18. Crowther MA, Burrows RF, Ginsberg J, Kelton JG. Thrombocytopenia in pregnancy: diagnosis, pathogenesis and management. Blood Rev 1996;10:8–16

19. Cromwell C, Tarantino M, Aledort LM. Safety of anti-D during pregnancy. Am J Hematol 2009;84:261–2

20. Gall B, Yee A, Berry B, Birchman D, et al. Rituximab for management of refractory pregnancy-associated immune thrombocytopenic purpura. J Obstet Gynaecol Can 2010;32:1167–71

21. Bussel JB, Druzin ML, Cines DB, Samuels P. Thrombocytopenia in pregnancy. Lancet 1991; 337: 251

22. Godelieve C, Christiaens ML, Nieuwenhuis HK, Bussel JB. Comparison of platelet counts in first and second newborns of mothers with immune thrombocytopenic purpura. Obstet Gynecol 1997;90:546–52

23. Miyakis S, Lockshin MD, Atsumi T, et al. International consensus statement on an update of the classification criteria for definite antiphospholipid syndrome (APS). J Thromb Haemost 2006;4:295–306

24. Galli M, Finazzi G, Barbui T. Thrombocytopenia in the antiphospholipid syndrome: pathophysiology, clinical relevance and treatment. Ann Med Intern 1996;147:24–7

25. Harris EN. A reassessment of the antiphospholipid syndrome. J Rheumatol 1990;17:733–5

26. Rai R, Cohen H, Dave M, Regan L. Randomised controlled trial of aspirin and aspirin plus heparin in pregnant women with recurrent miscarriage associated with phospholipid antibodies (or antiphospholipid antibodies). BMJ 1997;314:253–7

27. Royal College of Obstetricians and Gynaecologists: Guidelines. Reducing the risk of thrombosis and embolism during pregnancy and the puerperium. Guidelines No 37a. London: RCOG, 2009

28. Mandelbrot L, Schlienger I, Bongain A, et al. Thrombocytopenia in pregnant women infected with human immunodeficiency virus: maternal and neonatal outcome. Am J Obstet Gynecol 1994;171:252–7

29. Van Besien K, Hoffman R, Golichowski A. Pregnancy associated with lupus anticoagulant and heparin induced thrombocytopenia: management with a low molecular weight heparinoid. Thromb Res 1991;62:23–9

30. Greinacher A, Eckhardt T, Mussmann J, Mueller-Eckhardt C. Pregnancy complicated by heparin associated thrombocytopenia: management by a prospectively in vitro selected heparinoid (Org 10172). Thromb Res 1993;71:123–6

31. Fausett MB, Vogtlander M, Lee RM, et al. Heparin-induced thrombocytopenia is rare in pregnancy. Am J Obstet Gynecol 2001;185:148–52

32. Huhle G, Geberth M, Hoffmann U, et al. Management of heparin-associated thrombocytopenia in pregnancy with subcutaneous r-hirudin. Gynecol Obstet Invest 2000;49:67–9

33. Schindewolf M, Daemgen-von-Brevern G, Mani H, Lindhoff-Last E. Alternative anticoagulation with fondaparinux in pregnant patients with heparin intolerance. J Thromb Haemost 2007; 5 Supplement 2:P-W-590

34. Ciurzyński M, Jankowski K, Pietrzak B, et al. Use of fondaparinux in a pregnant woman with pulmonary embolism and heparin-induced thrombocytopenia. Med Sci Monit 2011;17:56–9

35. Baglin T, Barrowcliffe TW, Cohen A, et al. Guidelines on the use and monitoring of heparin. Br J Haematol 2006;133:19–34

36. Royal College of Obstetricians and Gynaecologists: Guidelines. The acute management of thrombosis and embolism during pregnancy and the puerperium Guidelines No 37b. London: RCOG, 2007

37. Khong TY, De Wolf F, Robertson WB, Brosens I. Inadequate maternal vascular response to placentation in pregnancies complicated by preeclampsia and by small for gestational age infants. Am J Obstet Gynecol 1987;157:360–3

38. Goldman-Wohl D, Yagel S. Regulation of trophoblast invasion: from normal implantation to preeclampsia. Mol Cell Endocrinol 2002;187:233–8

39. Tank PD, Nadanwar YS, Mayadeo NM. Outcome of pregnancy with severe liver disease. Int J Gynaecol Obstet 2002;76:27–31

40. Sibai BM. The HELLP syndrome (hemolysis, elevated liver enzymes, and low platelets): much ado about nothing? Am J Obstet Gynecol 1990;162:311–16

41. McCrae KR, Cines DB. Thrombotic microangiopathy during pregnancy. Sem Hematol1997;34:148–58

42. Martin JN, Files JC, Blake PG, et al. Plasma exchange for preeclampsia: Postpartum use for persistently severe preeclampsia-eclampsia with HELLP syndrome. Am J Obstet Gynecol 1990;162:126–37

43. Mannucci PM, Canciani T, Forza I, et al. Changes in health and disease of the metalloprotease that cleaves von Willebrand Factor. Blood 2001;98:2730–5

44. Lain KY, Roberts JM. Contemporary concepts of the pathogenesis and management of pre-eclampsia. JAMA 2002;287:3183–6

45. Esplin MS, Branch DW. Diagnosis and management of thrombotic microangiopathies during pregnancy. Clin Obstet Gynecol 1999;42:360–8

46. Bacq Y. Acute fatty liver of pregnancy. Sem Perinatol 1998;22:134–40

47. Tyni T, Ekholm E, Pihko H. Pregnancy complications are frequent in long-chain 3-hydroxyacyl-coenzyme A dehydrogenase deficiency. Am J Obstet Gynecol 1998;178:603–8

48. Vigil-De Gracia P. Acute fatty liver and HELLP syndrome: two distinct pregnancy disorders. Int J Gynaecol Obstet 2001;73:215–21

49. Anthony J. Major obstetric hemorrhage and disseminated intravascular coagulation. In James DK, Steer PJ, Weiner CP, Gonik B, eds. High Risk Pregnancy: Management Options, 3rd edn. Amsterdam: Elsevier, 2006:1606–23

50. Levi M. Current understanding of disseminated intravascular coagulation. Br J Haematol 2004;124:567–76

51. Moscardo F, Perez F, de la Rubia J, et al. Successful treatment of severe intra-abdominal bleeding associated with disseminated intravascular coagulation using recombinant activated factor VII. Br J Haematol 2001;114:174–6

52. Zupancic S, Sokolic V, Viskovic T, et al. Successful use of recombinant factor VIIa for massive bleeding after caesarean section due to HELLP syndrome. Acta Haematol 2002;108:162–3

53. Ludlam CA. The evidence behind inhibitor treatment with recombinant factor VIIa. Patophysiol Haemost Thromb 2002;32(Suppl 1):13–18

54. Maclean A, Almeida Z, Lopez P. Complications of acute fatty liver of pregnancy treated with activated protein C. Arch Gynecol Obstet 2005;273:119–21

55. Mikaszewska-Sokolewicz M, Mayzner-Zawadzka E. Use of recombinant human activated protein C in treatment of severe sepsis in a pregnant patient with fully symptomatic ovarian hyperstimulation syndrome. Med Sci Monit 2005;11: 27–32

56. Toh CH, Dennis M. Disseminated intravascular coagulation: old disease, new hope. BMJ 2003;327:974–7

57. Kashyap R, Choudhry VP, Mahapatra M, et al. Postpartum acquired haemophilia: clinical recognition and management. Haemophilia 2001;7:327–30

58. Porteous AO, Appleton DS, Hoveyda F, Lees CC. Acquired haemophilia and postpartum haemorrhage treated with internal pudendal embolisation. Br J Obstet Gynaecol 2005;112: 678–9

59. Boggio LN, Green D. Acquired hemophilia. Rev Clin Exp Hematol 2001;5:389–404

60. Dedeken L, St-Louis J, Demers C, et al. Postpartum acquired haemophilia: a single centre experience with rituximab. Haemophilia 2009;15:1166–8

61. Bates SM, Greer IA, Pabinger I, et al. Venous thromboembolism, thrombophilia, antithrombotic therapy and pregnancy. ACCP Evidence-Based Clinical Practice Guidelines (8th Edition). Chest 2008;133;844S–6S

62. Ginsberg JS, Hirsh J, Turner C, et al. Risks to the fetus of anticoagulant therapy during pregnancy. Thromb Haemost 1989;61:197–203

63. Vitale N, De Feo M, De Santo LS, et al. Dose-dependent fetal complications of warfarin in pregnant women with mechanical heart valves. J Am Coll Cardiol 1999;33:1637–41

64. Chan WS, Anand S, Ginsberg JS. Anticoagulation of pregnant women with mechanical heart valves: a systematic review of the literature. Arch Intern Med 2000;160:191–6

65. Vahanian A, Baumgartner H, Bax J, et al. Guidelines on the management of valvular heart disease: The task Force on the Management of Valvular Heart Disease of the European Society of Cardiology. Eur Heart J 2007; 28:230–68

66. Peitsidis P, Datta T, Pafilis I, et al. Bernard Soulier syndrome in pregnancy: a systematic review. Haemophilia 2010;16: 584–91

67. Siddiq S, Clark A and Mumford A. A systematic review of the management and outcomes of pregnancy in Glanzmann thrombasthenia. Haemophilia 2011;[Epub ahead of print]

68. Pajor A, Nemes L, Demeter J. May Hegglin anomaly and pregnancy. Eur J Obstet Gynecol Reprod Biol 1999;85: 229–31

69. Favaloro EJ. Laboratory assessment as a critical component of the appropriate diagnosis and sub-classification of von Willebrand's disease. Blood Rev 1999;13:185–204

70. Laffan M, Brown SA, Collins PW, et al. The diagnosis of von Willebrand disease: a guideline from the UKHCDO. Haemophilia 2004;10:199–217

71. Pasi KJ, Collins PW, Keeling DM, et al. Management of von Willebrand disease: a guideline from the UKHCDO. Haemophilia 2004;10:218–31

72. Mannucci PM. How I treat patients with von Willebrand disease. Blood 2001;97:1915–19

73. Lee CA, Chi C, Pavord SR, et al. The obstetric and gynaecological management of women with inherited bleeding disorders – review with guidelines produced by a taskforce of UKHCDO. Haemophilia 2006;12:301–36

74. Giangrande PL. Management of pregnancy in carriers of haemophilia. Haemophilia 1998;4:779–84

75. Kujovich JL. Von Willebrand disease and pregnancy. J Thromb Haemost 2005;3:246–53

76. Kadir RA, Lee CA, Sabin CA, et al. Pregnancy in women with von Willebrand's disease or factor XI deficiency. Br J Obstet Gynaecol 1998; 105;314–21

77. Stedeford JC, Pittman JA. Von Willebrand's disease and neuroaxial anaesthesia. Anaesthesia 2000;55:1228–9

78. Miller R. Counselling about diagnosis and inheritance of genetic bleeding disorders: haemophilia A and B. Haemophilia 1999;5:77–83

79. Plug I, Mauser-Bunschoten EP, Brocker-Vriends AHJ, et al. Bleeding in carriers of haemophilia. Blood 2006;108:52–6

80. Ludlam CA, Pasi KJ, Bolton-Maggs P, et al. A framework for genetic service provision for haemophilia and other inherited bleeding disorders. Haemophilia 2005;11:145–63

81. Chi C, Lee CA, Shiltagh N, et al. Pregnancy in carriers of haemophilia, Haemophilia 2008;14:56–64

82. Kulkarni R, Soucie JM, Lusher J, et al. Sites of initial bleeding episodes, mode of delivery and age of diagnosis in babies with haemophilia diagnosed before the age of 2 years: a report from The Centers for Disease Control and Prevention's (CDC) Universal Data Collection (UDC) project. Haemophilia 2009;15:1281–90

83. Chalmers E, Williams M, Brennand J, et al. The management of haemophilia in the fetus and neonate. A UKHCDO guideline approved by the BCSH, www.bcshguidelines.com

84. Kadir R, Chi C, Bolton-Maggs P. Pregnancy and rare bleeding disorders. Haemophilia 2009;15:990–1005

85. Kobayashi T, Kanayama N, Tokunaga N, et al. Prenatal and peripartum management of congenital afibrinogenemia. Br J Haematol 2000;109:364–6

86. Goodwin TM. Congenital hypofibrinogenemia in pregnancy. Obstet Gynecol Surv 1989;44:157–61

87. Bolton-Maggs PH, Perry DJ, Chalmers EA, et al. The rare coagulation disorders – review with guidelines for management from the UKHCDO. Haemophilia 2004;10: 593–628

88. Kulkarni AA, Lee CA, Kadir RA. Pregnancy in women with congenital factor VII deficiency. Haemophilia 2006;12: 413–6

89. Eskandari N, Feldman N, Greenspoon JS. Factor VII deficiency in pregnancy treated with recombinant factor VIIa. Obstet Gynecol 2002;99:935–7

90. Mariani G, Konkle BA, Ingerslev J. Congenital factor VII deficiency: therapy with recombinant activated factor VII – a critical appraisal. Haemophilia 2006;12:19–27

91. Mannucci PM, Duga S, Peyvandi F. Recessively inherited coagulation disorders. Blood 2004;104:1243–52

92. Girolami A, Randi ML, Ruzzon E, et al. Pregnancy and oral contraceptives in congenital bleeding disorders of the vitamin K-dependent coagulation factors. Acta Haematol 2006;115: 58–63

93. McMahon MJ, James AH. Combined deficiency of factors II, VII, IX, and X (Borgschulte– Grigsby deficiency) in pregnancy. Obstet Gynecol 2001;97:808–9

94. Kadir RA, Economides DL, Lee CA. Factor XI deficiency in women. Am J Hematol 1999;60:48–54

95. Asahina T, Kobayashi T, Takeuchi K, et al. Congenital blood coagulation factor XIII deficiency and successful deliveries: a review of the literature. Obstet Gynecol Surv 2007;62: 255–60

26

Vascular Malformations as a Cause of Postpartum Hemorrhage

K. Hayes

INTRODUCTION

Uterine vascular malformations (UVM) leading to postpartum hemorrhage (PPH) are rare. The world-wide literature consists of case reports and small case series, and while the true incidence is unknown, it is likely to represent a very small proportion of causes of PPH. UVM can be congenital but are more commonly acquired when they tend to present with secondary PPH, although in rare instances they present with primary or even tertiary bleeding[1]. As a general rule, primary PPH occurring temporally close to delivery most likely is a result of a pre-existing arterio-venous malformation (AVM), whereas secondary or tertiary PPH is more likely due to an acquired pseudoaneurysm.

Secondary PPH occurs in up to 0.5–1.5% of pregnancies[2] and the vast majority of women who present with secondary or tertiary PPH will have endometritis with or without retained products of conception (RPOC). Their management usually consists of broad spectrum antibiotics and, if necessary, an evacuation of RPOC. The vast majority of these women stop bleeding thereafter. Because some women receive multiple courses of antibiotics and evacuation procedures without evidence of infection or RPOC, clinicians finally start to consider vascular malformations rather than persevering with repeated ineffective treatments.

VASCULAR MALFORMATIONS

Vascular malformations may be congenital or acquired and consist of true AVMs, arteriovenous fistulae and pseudoaneurysms.

Congenital arteriovenous malformations

Congenital AVMs are abnormal arteriovenous connections that can occur anywhere in the body. These are rare as primary uterine lesions and no true estimate of their incidence is possible. The majority are usually found in the head and neck, and a 10 year review in a tertiary referral vascular center found only one uterine case out of 145 AVMs[3]. They result from abnormal development of primitive vessels that form connections between pelvic arteries and veins in the uterus[4].

They are characterized by several feeding and draining vessels with an interconnecting nidus with turbulent flow[5]. When they occur in the uterus they have the potential to cause obstetric and/or gynecological bleeding. The majority of significant bleeds occur as a result of either iatrogenic intervention (uterine instrumentation) or placental implantation involving the AVM[6].

AVMs are so rare that they are only likely to contribute truly to less than 1% of PPH. Moreover, the diagnosis is usually only made in a hysterectomy specimen or by interventional radiology on the basis of an arteriogram when bleeding is intractable and the patient remains stable enough for possible embolization.

Due to their rarity, the diagnosis of an AVM is usually retrospective if it is made at all. From the clinical point of view, the PPH is managed as any other PPH. Not surprisingly, however, many conservative measures fail to work, as it is likely that the abnormal vascular compartment of the AVM has been opened.

Acquired vascular malformations

Acquired vascular malformations invariably result from iatrogenic or traumatic injury to the uterine artery vascular bed[7]. This is particularly so when significant intractable secondary PPH occurs and where uterine artery pseudoaneurysm needs to be considered. A recent review of case reports and series of pseudoaneurysms[1] found 16 cases of which 10 had recently undergone cesarean section, three uterine evacuation procedures, and three had had normal spontaneous vaginal deliveries (of these, two had had previous gynecological surgery).

A pseudoaneurysm is characterized by a complete lack of vascular layers (intima, media and adventitia) surrounding the blood collection which communicates with the parent artery through the injury. The boundary of the 'aneurysm' is in fact the surrounding connective tissue. In terms of etiology, cesarean section at advanced dilatation with uterine angle extension is the commonest antecedent event, where direct trauma and suturing around the uterine artery bed cause abnormal vascular connections. Failure to completely secure the bleeding vessels at the apex of an angular tear leads to leakage into the surrounding tissues. Recent curettage, particularly if difficult or if the placental tissue was very adherent, also can cause direct vascular trauma. When these abnormalities present after an uncomplicated vaginal delivery, it is proposed that the myometrial vascular bed is disrupted by the mechanics of delivery or, in fact, more likely the malformation pre-existed and only presented after delivery.

Due to the abnormal vascular connections, the normal controls over hemostasis fail, and increases in blood pressure due to activity lead to rupture of the fragile structure with blood draining from the lesion into the uterine cavity. This often happens spontaneously with no obvious provocation but may be exacerbated by repeated uterine evacuation. Bleeding may be intermittent, and it is proposed that the boundaries of the pseudoaneurysm act intermittently as a valve[1].

If the lesion is deeper into the myometrium and does not connect with the cavity, then a pelvic hematoma will ensue or rarely lead to an intraperitoneal hemorrhage. This is especially dangerous, as bleeding is covert and patients may delay seeking medical help.

CLINICAL PRESENTATION

When should a clinician suspect this rare phenomenon? The following characteristics are most indicative of a pseudoaneurysm as the underlying cause of a PPH:

(1) There is usually secondary heavy vaginal bleeding.

(2) There are repeated episodes of bleeding requiring medical attention with secondary or tertiary PPH.

(3) Many women will even have received one or more blood transfusions.

(4) Bleeding is usually painless.

(5) There is usually a history of recent emergency cesarean section (typically at advanced dilatation) or uterine curettage.

(6) There is a failure to respond to medical treatment or uterine evacuation.

(7) There is no evidence of an alternative cause such as infection or RPOC on transvaginal sonography.

The recent review of 16 cases of pseudoaneurysm outlined above, reported in 15 centers, were diagnosed at a mean of 18 days postpartum with a range from 3 hours to 76 days postdelivery[1]. In this clinical situation when faced with recurrent disproportionately heavy bleeding that has failed to respond to 'routine management' with no apparent underlying cause, the need for senior input and a search for a vascular malformation should be apparent.

DIAGNOSIS

Diagnosis is likely only if sufficient clinical suspicion exists, as the pseudoaneurysm may be small and easy to miss[1]. Although angiography is considered the gold standard diagnostic test for vascular abnormalities, good quality transvaginal sonography with Doppler is generally the initial key to diagnosis. Transvaginal sonography will be diagnostic for most cases, and Abu Ghazza *et al.*[1] showed that transvaginal sonography alone was diagnostic in 12 of the aforementioned 16 cases of pseudoaneurysm. The use of transvaginal sonography not only makes the diagnosis, but also lateralizes the lesion so that management can be directed more selectively. The following characteristics establish the diagnosis of pseudoaneurysm on transvaginal sonography:

- A discrete mass usually in the right or left paracervical region (see Figures 1 and 2)

- Doppler flow within the mass showing a 'to and fro' mixed pattern in diastole and systole (see Figures 3 and 4)

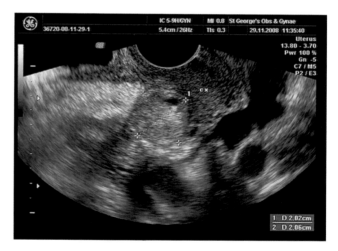

Figure 1 An inhomogenous mass in the left paracervical region on transvaginal sonography in longitudinal section

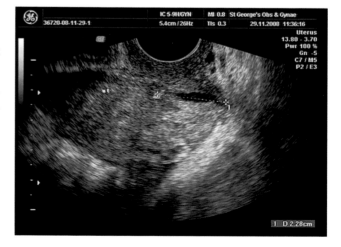

Figure 2 The same mass in transverse section demonstrating vascular caliber

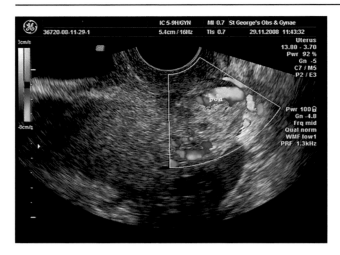

Figure 3 The same mass in Figure 2 with Doppler demonstrating mixed 'to' flow in systole

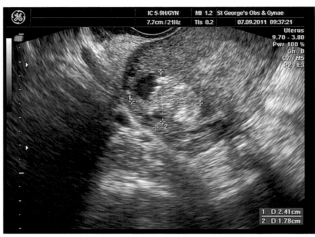

Figure 5 A mass is seen in the right upper myometrial region in transverse section

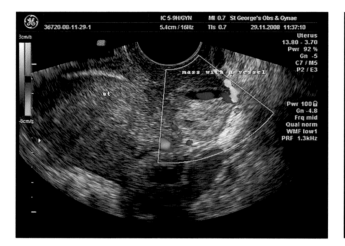

Figure 4 The same mass in Figure 2 with Doppler demonstrating 'fro' flow in diastole

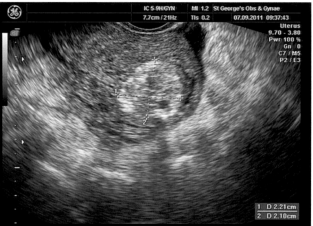

Figure 6 The same mass seen in longitudinal section

- Doppler flow within the mass showing turbulent mixed flow
- No evidence of products of conception in the uterine cavity.

In this clinical situation differential diagnosis of a mass includes an incidental fibroid, hematoma, or an abscess. The characteristic vascular appearance with the 'to and fro' sign first described by Abu-Yousef et al. in 1988[8] is only seen in a pseudoaneurysm and differentiates a pseudoaneurysm from the other diagnoses. It is important to image the whole myometrium and paracervical regions, as the pseudoaneurysm may also be found in both of these sites[9,10]. The other characteristic sonographic pattern is high flow with low resistance on Doppler examination[11,12]. The same is true if congenital AVM is suspected, as by definition they invariably lie within the myometrium. Figures 5–8 are transvaginal sonography images of a congenital AVM that was diagnosed in the author's unit after primary major PPH that fortunately diminished spontaneously.

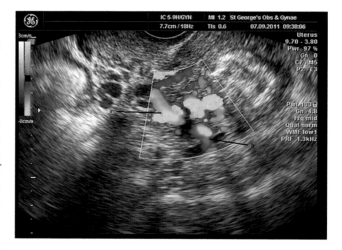

Figure 7 A congenital AVM demonstrating a feeding artery (arrow a) and draining vein (arrow b)

Computed tomography (CT) and magnetic resonance imaging (MRI) angiography are increasingly used in the diagnosis of pseudoaneurysm[13], and MRI in particular seems to be at least as good as transvaginal

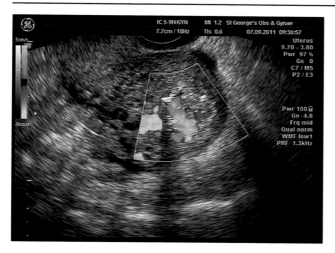

Figure 8 The same AVM as shown in Figure 7 showing a different pattern of flow during a single examination

sonography, though not necessarily any better in terms of sensitivity[4]. Due to the extra cost and sparse availability of these latter diagnostic modalities, MRI is only likely to be helpful where there is doubt over the diagnosis on transvaginal sonography and where invasive angiography may be avoided, where transvaginal sonography is negative but clinical suspicion is high or when the diagnosis has not been considered specifically and MRI picks it up as an 'incidental finding'.

Because of the high pick up rates associated with transvaginal sonography and other imaging techniques, angiography will generally be used as a confirmatory test for definitive management with the added advantage of mapping the vascular tree including any collateral supply to the malformation. Endovascular treatment can obviously be performed at the same time.

MANAGEMENT

By the time the diagnosis is considered, the patient will already have received antibiotics and will often have had at least one evacuation of retained products of conception (ERPC). Inevitably this fails to resolve the problem and bleeding either continues or resumes after an initial period of quiescence; bleeding is usually heavy and hemodynamic support including blood transfusion is common. In this situation the following need to be considered:

- Seek senior obstetric help

- Continue hemodynamic support if required

- Do not instrument the uterus further unless there is convincing evidence of RPOC on ultrasound

- If pseudoaneurysm is considered, then expert transvaginal ultrasound examining the paracervical regions, adnexae along the uterine artery, the myometrium in its entirety and the broad ligaments has a high pick up rate

- In theory, uterine balloon tamponade may be effective with a known pre-existing congenital AVM or pseudoaneurysm if pressure is applied to the discrete area that is bleeding. This will only be temporary to stabilize the patient before definitive treatment

- Once diagnosed, discuss the case with interventional radiology – an arteriogram will confirm the transvaginal sonography findings

- Selective uterine artery embolization is usually simple to perform at this time and its efficacy can be seen immediately with a postembolization angiogram

- In the presence of continued uterine bleeding despite selective embolization, then bilateral uterine artery embolization or internal iliac anterior division embolization may be possible, particularly if the arteriogram demonstrates any collateral supply from other pelvic vessels

- Postprocedural care should be routine as long as there is no significant bleeding from the uterus and/or femoral puncture sites

- De-briefing regarding future pregnancies is important – fertility should be essentially unchanged and there are no major obstetric issues regarding future antenatal care or delivery

- Ultimately hysterectomy is the treatment of last resort if uterine bleeding is intractable despite the above measures or hemodynamic instability makes interventional radiology inappropriate.

Embolization of the pelvic vascular system is not only a well established treatment for PPH in general (see Chapter 49), but also has been shown to be particularly useful in the context of a demonstrable discrete vascular malformation. The advantages of this procedure are that it is minimally invasive and can be performed under local anesthesia, it preserves the uterus and if the site of hemorrhage can be accurately identified, selective embolization can be performed with minimal disruption of the normal vascular supply to the uterus[1]. The source of hemorrhage may be identified as either an abnormality of the parent artery such as a pseudoaneurysm or by contrast extravasation. If such a source is not readily identified, however, empirical embolization of the uterine arteries or anterior divisions of the internal iliac arteries bilaterally can still be performed. In addition angiography may identify alternative, unsuspected sources of hemorrhage which can similarly be embolized. The literature describes a high degree of success in managing vascular malformations with embolization, though it is impossible to quote a success rate, as intrinsic bias exists when failed cases leading to hysterectomy are likely to be either not reported or at best under-reported. Figures 9 and 10 demonstrate angiographically confirmed pseudoaneurysms in two different patients, and Figures 11 and 12 show the contrast extravasation into the uterine cavity in the latter patient followed by its cessation after selective embolization.

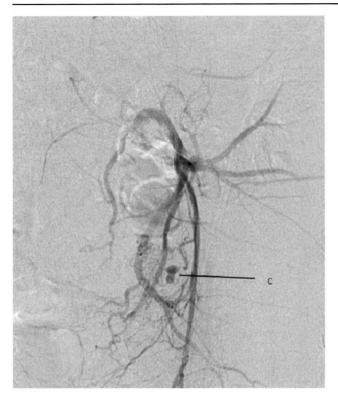

Figure 9 Angiographic 'proof' of a pseudoaneurysm of the right uterine supply diagnosed on transvaginal sonography – arrow c

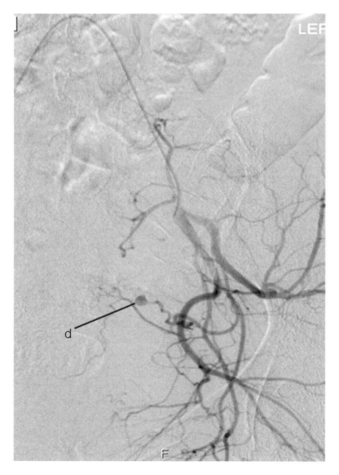

Figure 10 A second left pseudoaneurysm confirmed on angiography – arrow d

Embolization is performed with percutaneous catheterization of the femoral artery; the type of material used for embolization depends on the findings. Typically a temporary agent, gelatine sponge, is used for general PPH to reduce perfusion pressure, stop hemorrhage and allow eventual re-canalization. However, if a discrete vascular malformation such as pseudoaneursym can be identified and a catheter introduced into it, particulate emboli, of which there are a variety, are usually used.

Clearly, the more proximal and non-selective the embolization, the greater the risk of compromise to the pelvic vascular supply subsequently. Pregnancies following embolization are reported including a series for known AVMs[14], but the long-term reproductive sequelae are not yet defined, and the procedure itself carries potential documented morbidity including infection, neurological damage and bladder necrosis[15,16]. These short- and long-term risks need to be weighed against the risk of PPH on an individual basis and discussed with the patient and her partner including honesty about the uncertainties of the current worldwide data.

A recent case report describes successful direct injection of embolization particles into a known lesion at laparotomy following failed endovascular embolizaton[17], though this is a one-off case.

Ultimately hysterectomy is considered the only treatment if uterine bleeding is intractable despite the above measures or hemodynamic instability makes interventional radiology unsafe. It is clearly surgically important to get below the level of the origin of the pseudoaneurysm (usually the uterine artery) and tie off its supply or bleeding will inevitably continue.

In the rare cases where a known congenital AVM exists, PPH may be anticipated in a subsequent pregnancy or if there is the need for gynecological intervention. Unfortunately there is a paucity of evidence to guide whether expectant management or pre-pregnancy embolization is the most appropriate means to reduce the risk of future PPH. The likelihood of PPH is impossible to predict, but pragmatically if there is a normal obstetric history compared with a history of significant PPH this fact is likely to influence individual management. Elective embolization after a delivery can be considered to prevent future bleeding risk, but again the pros and cons should be discussed on an individual basis.

PREVENTION OF VASCULAR MALFORMATIONS

Clearly congenital malformations cannot be prevented, but pseudoaneurysm is nearly always due to iatrogenic causes. The vast majority of women with this problem have had obstetric or gynecological surgery as the underlying cause, many operations being emergency lower segment cesarean section at advanced dilatation but occasionally after curettage or open gynecological surgery.

Failure to secure angular tears of the uterus involving the uterine artery or one of its branches leads to

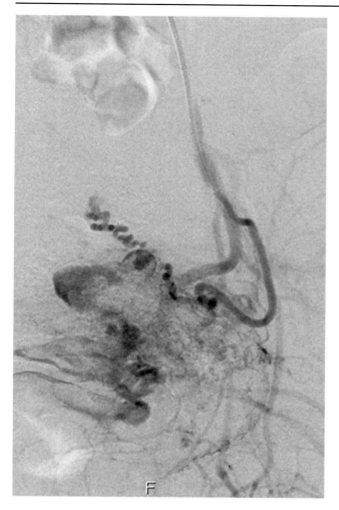

Figure 11 Contrast extravazation into the uterine cavity demonstrated in the pseudoaneurysm in Figure 10

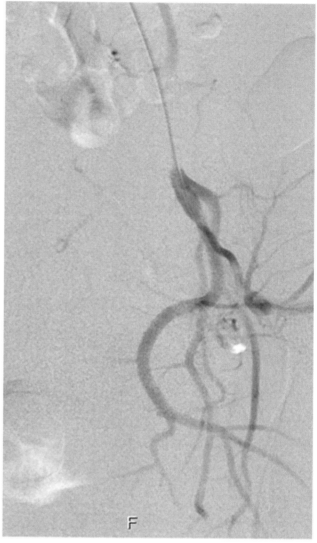

Figure 12 The same patient's angiogram demonstrating occlusion of the pseudoaneurysm after selective uterine artery embolization

pseudoaneurysm formation. All those who work in obstetric units understand that emergency lower segment cesarean section at full dilatation can lead to a difficult delivery, usually from occipital malposition and/or deflexion of the fetal head. Greater diligence when delivering the fetal head at advanced dilatation to try and prevent angular tears is very important; in the event that they occur, however, repairing them and ensuring the uterine vessels are completely secured should reduce the risk of pseudoaneurysm formation. Also, correcting any dextro-rotation of the uterus before incision will also reduce the risk of inadvertent uterine artery injury. Lesions seem to occur slightly more often on the left side, but are reported on both sides of the uterus.

CONCLUSION

Arteriovenous malformations are a rare phenomenon, and no clinician or center will deal with large numbers. They are undoubtedly more common than we realize, but many are likely to be clinically irrelevant, contributing only a very small proportion of the pathology causing PPH. When they do occur, however, they tend to cause a disproportionate amount of

bleeding. Little or nothing can be done about congenital AVMs, as they cannot be predicted. Regardless, they need serious consideration when acute primary PPH is intractable; these patients usually end up with embolization or hysterectomy as they respond poorly to conservative treatment.

Acquired pseudoaneurysms nearly always occur following lower segment cesarean section in advanced labor and more rarely after gynecological surgery. Although prevention is in theory possible, it is more important to have a high index of suspicion when there is sudden and major secondary PPH with little evidence of RPOC, a poor response to initial therapy and following a lower segment cesarean section in the late stages of labor.

Good quality transvaginal ultrasound with Doppler studies will diagnose most lesions, which can be confirmed on arteriography. Further uterine instrumentation should be avoided as this will exacerbate the problem; selective uterine artery embolization is a highly effective treatment with few side-effects. If recognized in a timely fashion, the need for peripartum hysterectomy can usually be avoided with preservation of a woman's future fertility.

PRACTICE POINTS

- Arteriovenous malformations are a rare but important cause of PPH, usually secondary

- AVMs are usually associated with a history of emergency lower segment cesarean section in the late stages of labor

- AVMs are characterized by heavy bleeding with no other apparent cause that fails to respond to conservative and medical treatment

- High quality transvaginal ultrasound is an excellent diagnostic tool if clinical suspicion is sufficiently high

- Uterine artery embolization is the highly effective treatment of choice.

References

1. Abu-Ghazza O, Hayes K, Chandraharan E, Belli AM. Vascular malformations in relation to obstetrics and gynaecology: diagnosis and treatment. The Obstetrician Gynaecologist 2010;12:87–93

2. Uchil D. Complications of the puerperium. In: Arulkumaran S, et al. eds. The Management of Labour, 2nd edn. Andhra Pradesh, India: Orient Longman, 2005

3. Kim JY, Kim DI, Do YS, et al. Surgical treatment for congenital arteriovenous malformation: 10 years' experience. Eur J Vasc Endovasc Surg 2006;32:101–6

4. Cura M, Martinez N, Cura A, Dalsaso TJ, Elmerhi F. Arteriovenous malformations of the uterus. Acta Radiol 2009;50:823–9

5. Tanaka R, Miyasaka Y, Fujii K, Kan S, Yagashita S. Vascular structure of arteriovenous malformations. J Clin Neurosci 2000;7:24–8

6. Grivell RM, Reid KM, Mellor A. *Uterine* arteriovenous malformations: a review of the current literature. Obstet Gynecol Surv 2005;60:761–7

7. Kwon JH, Kim GS. Obstetric iatrogenic arterial injuries of the uterus: diagnosis with US and treatment with transcatheter arterial embolization. Radiographics 2002;22:35–46

8. Abu-Yousef M, Wiese J, Shamma A. The "to and fro" sign: duplex Doppler evidence of femoral artery pseudoaneurysm. AJR Am J Roentgenol 1988;150:632

9. Eason D, Tank R. Avoidable morbidity in a patient with pseudoaneurysm of the uterine artery after Caesarean section. J Clin Ultrasound 2006;34:407–11

10. Ho S. A case of uterine pseudoaneurysm. Singapore Med J 2002;43:202–4

11. Kelly SM, Belli AM, Campbell S. Arteriovenous malformation of the uterus associated with secondary postpartum hemorrhage. Ultrasound Obstet Gynecol 2003;21:602–5

12. Müngen E, Yergök YZ, Ertekin AA, Ergür AR, Uçmakli E, Aytaçlar S. Color Doppler sonographic features of uterine arteriovenous malformations: report of two cases. Ultrasound Obstet Gynecol 1997;10:215–9

13. Grivell RM, Reid KM, Mellor A. Uterine arteriovenous malformations: a review of the current literature. Obstet Gynecol Surv 2005;60:761–7

14. Delotte J, Chevallier P, Benoit B, Castillon JM, Bongain A. Pregnancy after embolization therapy for uterine arteriovenous malformation. Fertil Steril 2006;85:228

15. Hare WSC, Holland CJ. Paresis following internal iliac artery embolization. Radiology 1983;146:47–51

16. Sibour PR. Bladder necrosis secondary to pelvic artery embolization: case report and literature review. J Urol 1994; 151:422

17. Przybojewski SJ, Sadler DJ. Novel image-guided management of a uterine arteriovenous malformation. Cardiovasc Intervent Radiol 2011;34(Suppl 2):S161–6

Section 5

Placental Abnormalities

27

Placental Abnormalities

C. E. M. Aiken, M. K. Mehasseb and J. C. Konje

INTRODUCTION

In the UK, hemorrhage was the major factor in more than 150 maternal deaths between 1985 and 1996[1], and remains one of the main causes of admission of pregnant women to intensive care units[2–4]. In countries with limited resources, the toll from obstetric hemorrhage is greater[5,6] and a significant number of the deaths from hemorrhage are associated with substandard care and/or inadequate obstetric facilities[1,7].

Placental abnormalities are a major contributor to obstetric hemorrhage. Placental abruption and placenta previa are associated with odds ratios for postpartum hemorrhage (PPH) of 13 (99% CI 7.6–12.1) and 12 (99% CI 7.2–23), respectively, representing the highest of any major risk factors identified by the Royal College of Obstetricians and Gynaecologists (RCOG)[8]. Placental abnormalities including morbidly adherent placentas (accreta, increta, percreta) are rare conditions, but increasing in incidence and associated with high risk of catastrophic hemorrhage. In one series, placental abnormalities accounted for 36% of pregnancy-related deaths due to hemorrhage[9].

PLACENTAL ABRUPTION

The Latin term 'abruptio placentae' means 'rending asunder of the placenta', a valid clinical characteristic of most cases implying a sudden accident. The bleeding associated with abruption follows premature separation of a normally sited placenta once fetal viability has been attained. The initial event begins with bleeding into the decidua basalis, usually from the spiral arteries. The exact mechanism of abruption is unclear in many cases, but incomplete trophoblastic invasion, chronic inflammation and subclinical trauma all have been suggested as playing a role[10]. The condition is an increasingly important cause of maternal hemorrhage, with overall incidence increasing from 0.6% to 0.8% worldwide over the past decade[11]. This change may be as a result at least in part to the increase in cesarean section rate in developed countries. According to one large retrospective cohort study from the US, a previous cesarean section confers a 40% increased risk in a subsequent pregnancy[12]. According to the Confidential Enquiry into Maternal Deaths (2011)[13], between 2006 and 2008 two maternal deaths in the UK were ascribed to placental abruption, although in developing countries the overall maternal mortality rate is probably much higher[14].

Incidence and risk factors

Placental abruption occurs in approximately 1 in 200 pregnancies (0.5%)[15], although higher incidences have been reported[16]. The incidence is much higher (4.5%) when placentas are examined routinely, suggesting that small episodes are more common than those diagnosed clinically[17]. Placental abruptions are characteristically revealed (apparent, with external bleeding) or concealed (no external bleeding is present); the former occurs in 65–80% of cases (Figure 1). Concealed abruptions are clinically more dangerous as they often are associated with more severe complications. Risk factors for placental abruption are shown in Table 1.

Domestic violence, maternal stress and depression represent independent risk factors for placental abruption and subsequent hemorrhage[23,24]. These specific aspects of social history should help the process of making care decisions and should not be overlooked in routine antenatal care.

Diagnosis

Unlike placenta previa where ultrasound is the mainstay of diagnosis, diagnosis is usually on clinical grounds in cases of placental abruption (Table 2). The specificity and sensitivity of correlating the clinical and histological diagnoses of placental abruption have been reported as 30% and 100%, respectively[26]. In certain cases, however, ultrasonography may be helpful, for example when a large retroplacental hematoma is present, although this is uncommon even in severe cases. Symptoms and signs will be diagnostic in moderate to severe cases. In the mild forms, however, the diagnosis may not become obvious until after delivery when a retroplacental clot is identified. In clinical practice, a retroplacental clot is identified at later histological examination in 77% of clinically diagnosed cases of placental abruption[26].

Classically, placental abruption presents with vaginal bleeding, abdominal pain, uterine contractions and abdominal tenderness (Table 2). Vaginal bleeding, however, is present in no more than 70–80% of

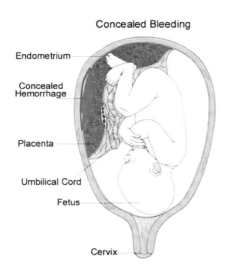

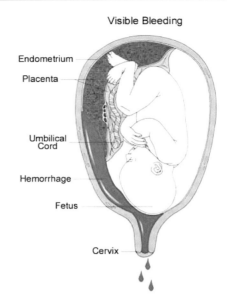

Figure 1 Concealed and revealed (visible) placental abruption

Table 1 Risk factors associated with placental abruption[18–22]

Risk factor	Relative risk
Increased age and parity	1.3–1.5
Pre-eclampsia	2.1–4.0
Chronic hypertension	1.8–3.0
Preterm rupture of membranes	2.4–4.9
Multifetal gestation	2.1
Hydramnios	2.0
Cigarette smoking	1.4–1.9
Thrombophilias	3–7
Cocaine use	NA
Prior abruption	10–25
Uterine leiomyomas	NA
Trauma	NA
Early vaginal bleeding	1.6–3.1
Autoimmune thyroid disorders	1.51–2.7

NA, Not available

Table 2 Clinical picture of placental abruption[25]

Symptom/sign	Frequency (%)
Vaginal bleeding	78
Uterine tenderness or back pain	66
Fetal distress	60
Preterm labor	22
High-frequency contractions	17
Hypertonus	17
Dead fetus	15

Table 3 Grading of placental abruption[29]

Grade	Description
0	Asymptomatic abruption with a small retroplacental clot (<150 ml)
1	Vaginal bleeding (150–500 ml); uterine tetany and tenderness may be present; no signs of maternal shock or fetal distress
2	Vaginal bleeding; no signs of maternal shock; signs of fetal distress present
3	Vaginal bleeding; marked uterine tetany yielding a board-like consistency on palpation; persistent abdominal pain, with maternal shock and fetal demise; coagulopathy may be evident in 30% of cases

cases[27]. If it occurs after the 36th week of gestation (50% of cases), it is characteristically dark and non-clotting, especially in severe cases. Because labor most commonly precipitates placental separation[28], nearly 50% of patients with placental abruption are in established labor. In cases where labor has also commenced, uterine contractions may be difficult to distinguish from the abdominal pain of abruption. Where this distinction is possible, the contractions are characteristically very frequent often with a rate of more than five in 10 minutes[25].

Sher and Statland[29] divided placental abruption into four grades of severity upon which management can be based. These are shown in Table 3. The absence of abdominal pain does not exclude placental abruption, especially where the placenta is located posteriorly. This is evidenced by the so called 'unsuspected or silent abruption' referred to by Notelovitz *et al.*[30] and the higher histological incidence of placental abruption found by Fox[17]. The presence of pain is probably indicative of extravasation of blood into the myometrium. In severe cases (grade 3) (Table 3) the pain is sharp, severe and sudden in onset. Some patients may, in addition, present with nausea, anxiety, thirst, restlessness and a feeling of faintness, whereas others characteristically complain of absent or reduced fetal movements.

When blood loss has been significant, some patients will present with signs of shock, tachycardia being more important than hypotension in this context. The presence of hypertension, on the other hand, may mask true hypovolemia, whereas an increasing abdominal girth or a rising fundal height heightens suspicion of significant concealed hemorrhage. Typically, the uterus is 'woody hard' in severe cases and the fetus is difficult, if not impossible, to palpate. In such instances, a continuous fetal heart rate monitor or real-time ultrasonography is essential to identify the fetal heart beat. The fetus may be 'distressed' and display heart rate abnormalities (grade 1–2) or may be dead (grade 3)[31]. In severe cases complicated by disseminated intravascular coagulation (DIC; often late presentations), clotting is absent in the vaginal blood loss, which is dark colored. The incidence of coagulopathy is variable but significant (35–38%)[32,33], occurring mainly in the severe forms.

A vaginal examination reveals blood clots in the vagina, although serous fluid from a retroplacental clot may be confused with liquor. The cervix may be dilating, as 50% of cases are in labor and if the membranes are ruptured, blood stained liquor is commonly seen. Ultrasound scan can exclude coincident placenta previa, which is present in 10% of cases. When the retroplacental clot is large, it appears on ultrasonography as hyperechogenic or isoechogenic compared to the placenta. On occasion, such findings are misinterpreted as a thick placenta[34]. In contrast, a resolving retroplacental clot, often found earlier in the pregnancy and of a self-limited nature, appears hyperechogenic within 1 week and sonolucent within 2 weeks. Though the accuracy of ultrasound as a diagnostic tool is less than ideal, it is useful in monitoring those cases managed conservatively. The size of the hematoma, its location, changes over time and fetal growth are all parameters routinely monitored by ultrasound scan. A Kleihauer-Betke test has previously been used to help in the diagnosis but is of limited value in guiding management[35,36].

Management

Management depends on the severity of the abruption, the state of the fetus and the gestational age of the pregnancy. Management can be divided into general and specific measures.

General management is similar to that for any patient presenting with bleeding. The specific measures include immediate delivery, expectant management and management of complications.

Immediate delivery

Immediate delivery depends on the severity of abruption and whether the fetus is alive or dead.

When the fetus is alive (80% of cases), the decision on how best to achieve delivery is not easy. It is compounded by the fact that the outlook for the fetus is poor, not only in terms of immediate survival, but also because studies have shown that as many as 15.4% of live born infants do not survive[37]. Accepting these facts, delivering by cesarean section when the fetus is alive has been shown in non-randomized controlled trials to have a better outcome than vaginal delivery which would necessitate a delay and further extension of the retroplacental hematoma 52% versus 16%[38] and 20% versus 15%[31], respectively. Indecision and unnecessary delays in performing immediate abdominal delivery are responsible for most poor results associated with cesarean section for abruption in the last quarter of pregnancy[28]. Indecision is particular

reprehensible in all cases where the fetus is alive, especially if there is evidence of fetal distress. The presence of DIC adds considerable risk to the mother whose morbidity and mortality could be increased by surgery, but DIC is considered by most authorities to be rare with a living fetus[14]. Once the decision is made to deliver and the fetus is alive, the degree of abruption and the state of the fetus must be taken into consideration. When the abruption is severe, cesarean section must be performed promptly once initial maternal resuscitative measures have been undertaken, as most post-admission fetal deaths occur if more than 2 hours have elapsed after admission.

In contrast, when the abruption is mild to moderate (i.e. grade 1 or 2), the mode of delivery should be determined by the condition of the baby, its presentation and the state of the cervix. In the presence of abnormal fetal heart rate patterns, immediate operative abdominal delivery is the option of choice. However, if the decision is to deliver vaginally, continuous fetal monitoring must be available to enable early identification of abnormal fetal heart rate patterns. Golditch and Boyce[39], Lunan[40] and Okonufua and Olatubosun[38] have all shown that the perinatal mortality is higher with vaginal delivery in the absence of electronic fetal monitoring. Although there is a place for prostaglandins in cervical ripening in women with mild abruption, the danger of inducing tetanic contractions must always be borne in mind. Where amniotomy is feasible, this often (but by no means always) hastens delivery; when it is not possible, Syntocinon® can be used while maintaining vigilance for hyperstimulation.

Where the fetus is dead (20% of cases), placental detachment is usually greater than 50%, and approximately 30% of patients manifest coagulopathy. Vaginal delivery should be the goal after maternal resuscitation, recognizing that the average blood loss is often more than 2500 ml. Under such circumstances, at least 4 units of blood should be cross-matched and transfusion commenced with packed red blood cells regardless of the initial vital signs, as the initial hematocrit or hemoglobin levels may be normal due to hemoconcentration. Once resuscitation has been established, subsequent hypotension and tachycardia are likely to supervene.

Unless there is an obstetric contraindication to vaginal delivery or hemorrhage is so brisk that it cannot be safely managed with vigorous blood transfusion, every attempt should be made to deliver such patients vaginally without jeopardizing maternal health. Once resuscitation has been initiated, fetal membranes should be ruptured (amniotomy) to hasten the onset of labor. Rupture of the membranes may provide the additional benefit of reducing the thromboplastins entering the maternal circulation through a reduction in intrauterine pressure, but this remains to be proven[14]. Amniotomy is effective in most cases, but augmentation with Syntocinon may be needed if no rhythmic uterine contractions are superimposed on the background uterine hypertonus. The rigidity of the uterus or the presence of a high intrauterine pressure should not deter the use of Syntocinon. The benefits of achieving a vaginal delivery override the risks of using Syntocinon, but careful monitoring is essential because uterine rupture may follow vigorous stimulation and the pain from the abruption may be confused with that of the rupture. There is no evidence that the use of Syntocinon is associated with enhanced passage of thromboplastin into the maternal circulation thereby either initiating or enhancing maternal consumptive coagulopathy[41]. Maternal outcome is mainly dependent on the diligence with fluid and blood replacement rather than on the interval to delivery[42]. Where the cervix is unfavorable and maternal health is not in danger, prostaglandins may be used to induce delivery.

Expectant management

This is recommended when neither the fetus nor the mother are at risk. Unfortunately, the lack of signs of fetal compromise on monitoring does not guarantee absence of deterioration in the fetal condition. In general, however, pregnancy is prolonged with expectant management in the hope of improving fetal maturity and therefore survival.

Such an approach is ideal for pregnancies that are less than 37 completed weeks of gestation; however, as neonatal survival is virtually guaranteed at more than 34–35 weeks' gestation, there is no place in persisting with such an approach for pregnancies more than 34 weeks where fetal monitoring cannot reliably predict outcome. Expectant management is recommended for patients whose vaginal bleeding is slight, abdominal pain is mild and usually localized, and who are cardiovascularly stable. Once a decision has been made on conservative management, the fetal condition must be monitored closely as it may change very rapidly.

Expectant management can take place in the community or in the hospital; no evidence suggests that admission is associated with a better outcome. However, when patient education as well as access to hospital is poor, admission may provide a safer option. Unfortunately, it is perhaps in such communities that admission may be rejected because it is expensive or causes significant family disruptions.

During expectant management, fetal growth should be monitored by regular ultrasound scan, as fetal growth restriction is common. The timing of delivery depends on further vaginal bleeding, fetal condition, gestational age and available neonatal care facilities. If bleeding episodes are recurrent, induction at 37–38 weeks is advisable provided there is no fetal compromise. Where the initial episode is small and self-limiting and there are no acute features (e.g. abnormal cardiotocography or a biophysical profile score <6) or chronic fetal compromise (growth restriction, oligohydramnios or abnormal umbilical artery Doppler recording) available evidence does not support induction of labor. Despite this lack of evidence, it is common practice to advocate induction of labor at term using the speculative argument that some undetected

damage might have occurred to the integrity and function of the placenta and, in the face of such uncertainty, delivery at term confers more advantages.

In a small proportion of cases, mild abruption may coexist with labor. Whether abruption provoked labor, or vice versa, is difficult to establish. The use of tocolytics in such patients is controversial, as their use in the presence of placental abruption is regarded by many as contraindicated, since they may worsen this process[43]. Sholl[44], however, stated that a trial of tocolytics in the presence of mild placental abruption and labor may successfully prolong pregnancy without jeopardizing the mother and fetus. One retrospective case series reported on 131 cases of placental abruption where tocolysis had been administered to 73% of patients with no additional increase in maternal or fetal morbidity or mortality[45]. At present, there is insufficient evidence to truly guide expectant management of placental abruption; decisions regarding treatment should be made on a case by case basis.

Management of complications of placental abruption

Complications of placental abruption include:

(1) *Maternal shock* This may be disproportionate to the revealed blood loss. The type and nature of the resuscitation should therefore be determined by the clinical state of the patient. In most cases of shock, DIC requires exclusion, as its presence requires additional measures to replace coagulation factors.

(2) *DIC* Treatment is aimed at volume replacement and correction of coagulation factor deficits and is best accomplished in consultation with a hematologist. Monitoring of renal function is essential, as acute tubular necrosis is a recognized complication. Heparin has no role in the modern management of consumptive coagulopathy. The presence of coagulopathy *per se* is not an indication for cesarean delivery but rather a strong contraindication. Also, the presence of an unfavorable cervix is not an indication for cesarean delivery, unless the condition of the mother necessitates prompt delivery. Abdominal and uterine incisions can bleed excessively when coagulation defects persist.

(3) *Ischemic necrosis of the distal organs (e.g. kidneys and brain)* This requires adequate fluid replacement and vigilance for the integrity of such organs (see Chapter on classification of near misses by Barrett).

(4) *PPH (secondary to DIC or Couvelaire uterus)* Treatment is with uterotonic drugs and other methods of managing PPH.

(5) *Isoimmunization* The administration of anti-D needs to be within 72 hours of delivery, but the quantity administered should be determined by a Kleihauers–Betke test.

PLACENTA PREVIA

Placenta previa is defined as a partial or completely sited placenta in the lower uterine segment after fetal viability (20 weeks in developed countries and 24–28 in developing countries). Four grades of placenta previa are recognized (Figure 2):

- *Grade I* Placenta in the lower segment but its edge does not reach the internal os

- *Grade II* Lower placental edge reaches the os but does not cover it

- *Grade III* Placenta covers the os and is asymmetrical

- *Grade IV* Placenta symmetrically covers the os.

Although this is the most commonly used classification/grading system in textbooks, it is important to recognize others that reflect the ultrasound definition of the placental site. The RCOG classifies placenta previa in clinical terms as major or minor. When the placenta lies over the internal os, it is considered a major previa; in contrast, it is considered a minor placenta previa when the placenta lies within the lower segment, but does not cover the os.

Incidence and risk factors

The overall incidence is variable but approximates to 1 in 300 deliveries (0.3%)[15,46]. Risk factors include:

(1) *Maternal age* Placenta previa is more common with advanced maternal age, but this may be a reflection of increased parity rather than age. In general, the doubling in incidence from 0.3% to 0.7% over a 10-year period is attributed to a shift to an older obstetric population[47].

(2) *Parity* Women of higher parity have a higher incidence[48].

(3) *Multifetal gestation* This is thought to be secondary to an increase in the surface area occupied by the placental mass[49].

(4) *Prior cesarean section delivery* The incidence increases with the number of previous cesarean deliveries[50,51]. A single cesarean section increases the risk by 0.65%, two by 1.5%, three by 2.2% and four or more by 10%. In addition, a previous cesarean section in association with placenta previa increases the risk of cesarean hysterectomy almost 4-fold[47].

(5) *Smoking* Doubles the risk of placenta previa[49,52]. This may be attributed to placental hypertrophy secondary to carbon monoxide hypoxemia[52].

(6) *Fetal anomalies* Patients with placenta previa have 12 times the usual risk of having a recurrent previa in subsequent pregnancies. For unclear reasons, fetal anomalies are increased with placenta previa even after controlling for maternal age[46]. It is also uncertain whether an association with intrauterine fetal growth restriction is present[53,54].

Diagnosis

Diagnosis is made either by clinical presentation or by imaging.

Clinical presentation

The most characteristic feature of placenta previa is painless vaginal bleeding, commonly recurrent and unprovoked and typically not appearing until after the end of the second trimester. The first episode is usually self-limiting and is rarely so profuse as to prove fatal. However, the earlier in pregnancy the first presentation of bleeding occurs, the more likely is the subsequent need for early intervention. 'Fetal distress' is unusual unless the hemorrhage is severe enough to cause maternal shock.

Abdominal palpation is not diagnostic but where the presenting part is free (unengaged) in late pregnancy or the lie is abnormal/unstable, placenta previa should be suspected. Sometimes, especially with minor degrees of placenta previa, bleeding might not appear until the onset of labor. This may mimic abruption clinically. In women who present with bleeding in the latter half of pregnancy, the possibility of placenta previa should always be considered, but the diagnosis can seldom be made solely on clinical grounds. Nonetheless, such presentations may provoke reimaging to check the placental site.

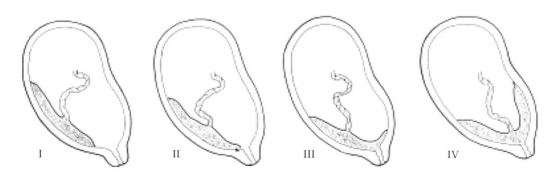

Figure 2 Grades of placenta previa. I, Encroaching on the lower segment; II, reaching the internal os; III, asymmetrically covering the internal os; IV, symmetrically covering the internal os

There is no role for digital examination in the diagnosis of placenta previa unless in the operating theater as part of a double set-up with adequate preparation for proceeding to cesarean section. Fortunately, this is now an uncommon (and costly) practice, especially where imaging (see below) should be easily available and reliable.

Imaging

The most commonly used method for placental localization in modern obstetrics is ultrasound scan (Figure 3). Because it is safe, accurate and non-invasive, it is the method of choice for making the diagnosis, although the gestational age at which the diagnosis is made significantly influences its accuracy. The earlier the scan is performed, the more likely is the placenta found in the lower pole of the uterus. Consequently, it is not recommended that ultrasound be carried out at 20–22 weeks for the purpose of placental localization alone, but that the position should be noted during the routine anomaly scan if it is carried out at this time.

About 28% of placentas in women scanned transabdominally before 24 weeks are 'low', but by 24 weeks this figure drops to 18%; only 3% are low lying by term[55]. Conversely, a false negative scan for a low placenta is found in as many as 7% of cases at 20 weeks[56]. Such results are commoner when the placenta is posterior, the bladder is over filled, the fetal head obscures the placental margin or the operator fails to scan the lateral uterine wall[57]. A low-lying placenta is more common in early pregnancy, because the lower segment does not exist. This apparent 'placental migration' is due to enlargement of the upper segment and formation of the lower segment, with many apparently low-lying placentas being found to be above the lower segment. Comeau et al.[58] and Ruparelia and Chapman[59] have shown that the more advanced is the pregnancy, the more accurate is a scan diagnosis of placenta previa.

Transvaginal ultrasound is not only more accurate in diagnosing placenta previa but also is more precise in defining the relationship of the lower edge of the placenta to the internal os. The safety of transvaginal scanning in the context of managing low-lying placentas has been shown in multiple observational trials, and the use of such scanning allowed reclassification of a considerable number of suspected low-lying placentas[60]. When the distance between the lower edge of the placenta and the internal cervical os is actually measured, the persistence of a low-lying placenta is higher at a later gestation. Taipale et al.[61], for example, observed that if a placenta overlapped the internal os by at least 25 mm at 18–23 weeks, the positive predictive value for previa at the time of delivery was 40%, with a sensitivity of 80%. In a similar type of study, Becker et al.[62] found that when the lower edge overlapped the os by at least 25 mm at 20–23 weeks, a vaginal delivery was not possible at all at term (i.e. it had a 100% positive predictive value).

Although the practice of localizing the placenta at the time of the routine anomaly scan at 19–21 weeks will continue, its limitations should be recognized and, wherever possible, transvaginal ultrasound scans should be offered to improve the accuracy of localization as well as to measure the distance from the os to the placental edge in order to help define the degree of 'low-lying'. Dashe et al.[63] observed that persistence of placental previa diagnosed at 20–23 weeks occurred in 34% of cases at delivery, while 73% of those with a low placenta, but not covering the os present at 32–35 weeks persisted at delivery. In view of this observation, the latest consensus guidance from the Royal College of Obstetrician and Gynaecologists[8] suggests that in a woman with minor previa who has an unscarred uterus diagnosed transvaginally at 20–24 weeks and who is asymptomatic, further imaging may safely be left until 36 weeks. This policy aims to avoid the financial and psychological cost to the patient and medical staff of repeated imaging late in pregnancy. The situation is altered, however, for women in whom the transvaginal ultrasound at 20–24 weeks has shown a placenta that covers the internal os. In these patients, the likelihood of a placenta previa diagnosed at 32 weeks persisting until term is 90%[62]. Accordingly, these women should have repeated scanning in order to allow appropriate planning for delivery. Repeated scanning should also occur earlier in patients who have had a previous cesarean section (in whom the risk of a low-lying placenta persisting until term has been estimated at approximately 50%).

The third major criterion that must be met in order to allow rescanning to be delayed safely until 36 weeks is that there should be no episodes of bleeding. Women with a low-lying placenta who are experiencing small self-limiting episodes of bleeding should be managed on a case-by-case basis, in the absence of any high quality evidence to guide clinical practice. Transperineal sonography has been used by some investigators[64], allowing visualization of the internal os in all cases and carryng a positive predictive value of 90% and a negative predictive value of 100% for placenta previa.

Magnetic resonance imaging (MRI) also has been used to visualize placental abnormalities including

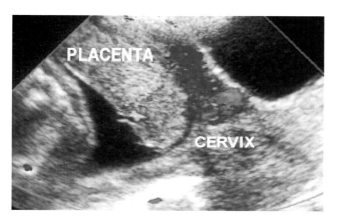

Figure 3 Transabdominal ultrasound scan with superimposed color Doppler signal showing an anterior placenta previa

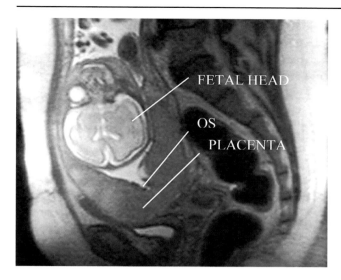

Figure 4 MRI of a grade IV placenta previa (completely covering the internal os)

placenta previa (Figure 4). This has the advantage of being objective and reproducible, thus minimizing operator error. However, due to its cost and logistic limitations, it is unlikely that it will replace ultrasonography for routine evaluation[65,66].

Management

Asymptomatic patients (where the diagnosis is made on ultrasound scan) are managed expectantly, often in a similar way to those with mild symptoms that are non-threatening to either the mother or fetus.

Those with symptoms can be divided into four categories depending on maternal condition, severity of hemorrhage, gestational age and the neonatal facilities available in the unit. These categories are:

(1) Pregnancy <37 weeks' gestation and with no threat to the mother;

(2) Pregnancy >37 weeks with no threat to the mother;

(3) Severe life-threatening and continuing hemorrhage;

(4) Hemorrhage associated with uterine contractions.

The management of the third and fourth categories is immediate delivery by cesarean section. Where there is non-life threatening hemorrhage after 37 weeks' gestation, a planned delivery is advisable. This decision must, however, be made with the recognition that such a hemorrhage could very rapidly become life threatening. For category 1, the best approach is expectant management, although this must not be at the detriment of maternal life.

Expectant management

Perinatal mortality in placenta previa is directly related to gestational age at delivery[67–70]. Macafee[68] and Johnson *et al.*[70] introduced expectant management of

placenta previa with the aim of achieving maximum fetal maturity possible, while minimizing the risks to both mother and fetus, the overall objective being to reduce perinatal mortality while at the same time reducing maternal mortality. This concept was based on the assumption that most episodes of bleeding are usually small, self-limited and are not fatal to the fetus or mother in the absence of provoking trauma (e.g. intercourse, vaginal examination) or labor, and that a relatively high proportion of cases, particularly those presenting early with lesser degrees of previa, may resolve to permit vaginal delivery.

Recent work shows that the incidence of resolving placenta previa, in the absence of a previously scarred uterus, is higher than previously described. Improvements in perinatal mortality attributed mainly to prolongation of pregnancy following expectant management have been recorded[44,71]. In those who are to be managed expectantly on an inpatient basis, the RCOG[8] recommends that thromboprophylaxis be instituted in the form of good hydration and compression hosiery, but that anticoagulation may be considered on an individual basis in high risk patients.

Although most experts advocate immediate delivery in the presence of severe hemorrhage (heavy vaginal bleeding producing maternal hypovolemia), heavy bleeding is not, however, considered a contraindication to expectant management[72]. An aggressive approach involving admission and repeated transfusions improves perinatal morbidity and mortality, especially when the bleeding occurs very early in pregnancy. In one study, where approximately 20% of the women lost over 500 ml of blood, half were successfully managed expectantly with a mean gain in gestation of 16.8 days[73]. Crenshaw *et al.*[69], on the other hand, managed only 43–46% of patients successfully with an aggressive expectant approach, whereas Cotton *et al.*[67], also with an aggressive approach, successfully managed 66% of women expectantly.

During expectant management, preterm labor remains a problem. Brenner *et al.*[74] found that 40% of women with placenta previa developed prelabor rupture of membranes, went into spontaneous labor or developed other problems that resulted in delivery before 37 weeks' gestation. Inhibiting contractions in those with preterm labor would seem logical, but some authors regard antepartum hemorrhage as a contraindication to the use of tocolytics[42]. In the presence of vaginal bleeding and uterine contractions, placental abruption, widely regarded as a contraindication to tocolysis, cannot be excluded. In addition, placental abruption is said to coexist with placenta previa in 10% of cases, and tocolytics cause maternal tachycardia and palpitations, two important features that could be confused with hypovolemia. Sampson *et al.*[75] advocate the use of tocolytics in cases of placenta previa and uterine contractions occurring after 21 weeks and demonstrated a reduction in perinatal mortality from 126 to 41 per 1000. The largest available trial shows at least no excess morbidity or mortality from tocolysis used in tertiary centers in the third trimester[44].

High perinatal mortality is directly related to the total amount of blood lost before delivery; thus light blood loss is not associated with significantly high perinatal mortality. Liberal use of blood transfusion reportedly nullifies this effect[67]. Although in theory there is no limit to the number of blood transfusions a patient can have, praticality and patient wishes, along with cost considerations, dictate otherwise. To optimize oxygen supply to the fetus and protect the mother against anticipated future blood loss, transfusion therapy should maintain a hemoglobin of at least 10 g/dl or a hematocrit of 30%.

Despite the use of expectant management, 20% of women with placenta previa are delivered earlier than 32 weeks, accounting for 73% of perinatal deaths[67]. These deaths remain a major problem. Neonatal mortality and morbidity are reduced by maternal corticosteroid administration.

Although Macafee[68] in his regimen proposes that the patient remains as an inpatient in a fully equipped and fully staffed maternity hospital from the time of initial diagnosis to delivery, a policy of permitting some women to return home has been advocated as part of expectant management, but this remains controversial[76]. Cotton et al.[67] reported no difference in the perinatal and maternal mortality rates in those sent home and those managed in hospitals, whereas D'Angelo and Irwin[77] suggested that keeping the mother in hospital until delivery was justified on the grounds that neonatal mortality and morbidity, and cost of later treatment were reduced. Kaunitz et al.[78] in a review of 355 maternities managed at home, however, reported one intrapartum death from placenta previa. In a review of 15,930 deliveries in Edinburgh, Love and Wallace[72] concluded that while clinical outcomes were highly variable and cannot be predicted from antenatal events, the majority of cases with or without bleeding irrespective of the degree of previa could be managed on an outpatient basis.

Interpretation of this evidence has led to a recommendation by the RCOG that major placenta previa should be managed on a inpatient basis from 34 weeks completed gestation onwards[63]. However, continuous hospitalization is costly and is associated with psychological morbidity among the women and their families. In developing countries, inpatient care may be unavailable and/or unaffordable. However, the advantages of such a program include easy access to resuscitation and prompt delivery as well as ensuring bed rest (which anecdotally has been thought to decrease the occurrence of hemorrhage) and limitation of activities. Evidence demonstrating a benefit from hospitalization at 34 weeks is lacking, with only one small randomized control trial available to guide decision making[79]. With improvement in transportation facilities and ambulance services in developed countries, highly motivated women who clearly understand the necessity of restriction of activity, have the constant presence of a companion and are within, for example, 15–30 min of the hospital perhaps may be monitored at home during the third trimester. This dictum will only apply to cases of grade I–III placenta previa or asymptomatic grade IV placental previa. The most recent RCOG Green-top guidelines[8] advocate that home management is most appropriate within a research context. In all cases of expectant management, regardless of location, local hematology services should be involved in the planning stages and rapid availability of blood products ensured.

Method of delivery

A diagnosis of placenta previa often precedes delivery by cesarean section, but this outcome is not inevitable, especially where the previa is a minor degree. For minor degrees of placenta previa (grade I or II anterior) and an engaged fetal head, pregnancy may continue beyond 37–38 weeks with anticipated vaginal delivery. In such patients, amniotomy followed by Syntocinon can be considered.

On the other hand, patients with a major placenta previa (grade II posterior, grade III–IV), should be delivered by elective or emergency cesarean section. The former is ideal since emergency delivery has a negative effect on perinatal mortality and morbidity, independent of gestational age. Perhaps it is related to the necessity of performing the operation in the absence of a fully prepared staff, a common occurrence during night, weekend and holiday shifts. Of interest, Cotton et al.[67] found that 27.7% of babies born as emergencies had anemia compared to 2.9% delivered electively. Perhaps this difference is also related to staffing differences or the hope that things will clear up by the morning, but this opinion is speculative.

Cesarean section for placenta previa poses several problems. It should ideally never be performed by an inexperienced obstetrician. The RCOG recommends that such operations are performed by consultants. Although general was preferred to regional anesthesia in the past, it is now acceptable practice to use the latter especially as Frederiksen et al.[80] demonstrated not only its safety but also a reduction in intrapartum blood loss compared to that with general anesthesia.

Procedure

The anesthetic requirements for a cesarean section in the context of placenta previa are a matter of debate, and often depend on the experience of the anesthetist and the available resources. Indeed, an increasing number of anesthetists either offer or strongly suggest that regional anesthesia is preferable for these patients[65,66]. A large retrospective study of operative deliveries for placenta previa, with outcomes stratified by type of anesthetic, demonstrated that the requirements for transfusion were higher in the general compared with the regional anesthesia groups[81]. This may be because epidurals, by lowering blood pressure, critically reduce uterine and placenta perfusion. Where the patient's condition is stable and there is no active bleeding, epidural or spinal anesthesia should not be regarded as contraindicated provided an experienced anesthetist is available. It is no longer considered acceptable for the same physician to administer the anesthetic, position the patient, and subsequently perform the operation as was so often the case only a few decades ago.

The uterine incision should be a transverse lower segment incision (if possible), provided there is a lower segment. Where the lower segment is non-existent or is very vascular, some obstetricians advocate a classical or a De Lee's incision. Scott[82], however, believes that such incisions are rarely justified because of their consequences and long-term disadvantages. When difficulties are encountered with transverse lower segment incisions, these may be converted to inverted T, J or U shaped incisions.

Where the placenta is anterior, two approaches are available after incising the uterus, going through the placenta or defining its edge and going through the membranes above or below the placenta. The former approach requires speed and may result in significant fetal blood loss[83]. The latter approach, however, may be associated with undue delay in the delivery of the fetus, more troublesome bleeding from a partially separated placenta and therefore fetal blood loss and anoxia. Myerscough[83] advises against cutting or tearing through the placenta because of the inevitable fetal blood loss that will occur as fetal vessels are torn. Because the lower segment is less muscular, contraction and retraction which result in the occlusion of the sinuses of the placental bed is inadequate, and intraoperative hemorrhage is therefore not uncommon[84]. Where hemostasis is difficult to achieve, bleeding sinuses could be oversewn with atraumatic sutures[82]. If this is unsuccessful, packing the uterus is possible, but the major disadvantage of this technique is that by leaving the pack *in situ* during closure of the uterus the bleeding may continue but remain concealed for some time as the pack is soaking through. The use of balloons with a tamponading effect on the bleeding placenta bed or intramyometrial injection of prostaglandin $F_{2\alpha}$ has been shown to be useful in such cases[83] (see Section 8 for information on balloons). Bleeding can also be stabilized with use of the B-Lynch brace suture (see Chapter 51). Where facilities are available, uterine artery embolization has been used with excellent results (see Chapter 49). The difficulty with this is planning to ensure that the facilities and the interventional radiologist are available in the interventional radiology suite when needed. When the bleeding remains uncontrollable, ligation of the internal iliac artery or even hysterectomy may be necessary as the last resort (see Chapter 55).

PLACENTA ACCRETA, INCRETA AND PERCRETA

This is a group of pathologically invasive placentations of varying severity. Such morbid adherence occurs when the implantation site is lacking a sufficient decidua. Consequently, the physiological cleavage plane through the decidual spongy layer is missing. This leads to one or more cotyledons being firmly anchored to the decidua basalis and to or through the myometrium (see also Chapter 28–30).

The term placenta accreta is used to describe any placental implantation that is adherent firmly to the uterine wall. Placental villi are anchored to the myometrium due to defective decidualization. If villi invade the myometrium, the condition is called placenta increta. If the invasion goes as deep as reaching the serosal surface, this is called placenta percreta.

Although uncommon, such placental aberrations are associated with a significantly higher maternal morbidity and sometimes mortality, primarily due to the risk of torrential hemorrhage, uterine perforation, infection and the associated surgical difficulties and complications[85].

Incidence

Morbidly adherent placentation occurs in about 1 in 2500 term (0.04%) pregnancies. A marked increase in incidence has been noted over the past 50 years, probably secondary to rising cesarean section delivery rates, with the risk of accreta increasing dramatically with the number of previous sections[86].

Risk factors include implantation over the lower uterine segment overlying a previous surgical scar or excessive uterine curettage resulting in Asherman's syndrome. Placenta previa is identified in 30% of cases, and 25% of the women would have had a previous cesarean delivery. Nearly a quarter have previously undergone curettage and another quarter are grand multigravida (six or more)[87].

Diagnosis

Recent advances in ultrasound technology enhance diagnosis in patients at high risk – i.e. those with a low-lying placenta on early ultrasound scan, or who have had at least one previous cesarean section – as well as among those not considered to be at risk. When ultrasound is used in combination with MRI, the diagnosis of accreta/percreta can be made with reasonable accuracy with regard to the existence and extent of placental invasion[88–90]. In patients without previous uterine surgery, however, the diagnosis may not be made until after delivery. Some patients may present with vague features which include a raised maternal serum α-fetoprotein[91] and bleeding before delivery, although this is usually a consequence of placenta previa. Uterine rupture may occur antenatally due to myometrial invasion by chorionic villi at the site of a cesarean section scar[92].

Using ultrasound color Doppler flow mapping improves the diagnostic sensitivity. The two most sensitive criteria are: (1) a distance less than 1 mm between the uterine serosal bladder interface and the retroplacental vessels; and (2) the presence of large intraplacental lakes[93]. Preliminary work suggests that the application of three-dimensional color power Doppler ultrasound complements other techniques for antenatal imaging. The additional benefit of MRI scanning in cases where insufficient anatomical information is obtained from Doppler scanning is a matter of debate, but in the absence of harm demonstrated by this screening modality, many authorities recommend the additional use of MRI imaging. At least one study demonstrated that depth of placental invasion may be more accurately determined from MRI[89]. The main MRI features of placenta accreta include uterine bulging, heterogeneous signal intensity within the placenta, and dark intraplacental bands on T2-weighted imaging[88].

Management

In most cases, problems arise after delivery of the baby. Most of the complications of morbid adherence are related to the problems of delivery or failure to deliver the placenta as anticipated. Management must therefore aim to minimize these complications.

Hemorrhage is the most common complication and this is associated with attempts to detach the placenta from the uterus. Delay in recourse to hysterectomy in attempts to conserve future reproductive potential is a major factor in maternal mortality and morbidity from placenta accreta. Clinicians are understandably reluctant to perform a peripartum hysterectomy until other options have been considered and exhausted, but this should not delay the life-saving intervention of arresting bleeding. A decision to perform a peripartum hysterectomy should ideally be made by two obstetric consultants. In cases where the placental anomaly is identified predelivery, this must be taken into account in the planning stages, and the woman counseled appropriately. Recent research has focused on the value of embolization of the internal iliac or uterine vessels in units where interventional radiology is readily available[63]. Radiological interventions are unlikely to be helpful in the emergency situation of unanticipated hemorrhage, but in cases where the management has been planned prenatally, the value of prophylactic catheterization of the vessels has been studied. Current evidence of benefit is equivocal, and pending further evaluation, the optimal management is to avoid catheterization as a prophylactic measure. Sometimes, the percreta type might even invade the bladder base, further complicating the surgical procedure required and making the control of hemorrhage very difficult. It is agreed by most authorities that delivery in placenta accreta is optimal at 36–37 weeks, with corticosteroid therapy to the mother for fetal lung maturity.

In cases of extensive placenta accreta (involving most of the placental surface), bleeding might be very limited until attempts at manual removal are made. At times, traction on the cord may lead to uterine inversion. Manual removal is usually not successful as the plane of cleavage between the uterus and the placenta cannot be developed. The safest treatment is usually hysterectomy.

Attempts at uterine conservation include piecemeal removal of as much placental tissue as possible

followed by packing of the uterine cavity, but this approach has been reported to carry an unacceptably high mortality rate of 25%[87]. Another option to conserve the uterus is to leave the entire placenta in situ if there is no bleeding. For women wishing to preserve their fertility, where the placenta has not separated, a review of reported cases revealed that among women whose placentas were left in situ, hysterectomy was avoided in 80%[94]. This is now thought to be the optimal strategy when the placenta is not separated[95]. In cases where the placenta partially separates despite morbidly adherent sections, adherent parts should be left in situ to minimize the risk of severe bleeding. Hysterectomy or alternative removal strategies can then be attempted electively at a later date. Kayem describes a case where spontaneous resorption of the placenta occurred over 6 months following uterine artery embolization[96]. Another group described a similar approach, but their patient was treated by methotrexate. The placenta spontaneously delivered after 4 weeks[97,98]. Chapters 28–30 provide further discussion on this topic as does Chapter 31 on one-step conservative therapy.

RARE TYPES OF PLACENTAL ABNORMALITIES: SHAPE

Some anatomical variations in placental shape can lead to serious PPH. These include bipartite placentas, succenturiate lobes and placenta membranacea.

Bipartite placenta

This occurs when the placenta is occasionally separated into two lobes, and the division is incomplete with vessels of fetal origin extending from one lobe to the other before ending in the umbilical cord. Its incidence is about 1 in 350 deliveries[99].

Succenturiate lobe

In this abnormality, one or more small accessory lobes develop in the membranes at a distance from the main placenta. The succenturiate lobe is usually linked to the main placenta by vascular connections of fetal origin. The process can be considered a small version of the lobate placenta. The accessory lobe may be retained in the uterus after delivery, causing serious hemorrhage. Its incidence has been reported to be as high as 5%[100].

Placenta membranacea

This type of placenta develops as a thin membrane-like structure with the whole of the fetal membranes covering the functioning villi. The diagnosis can be made with ultrasound scan. This abnormality can lead to serious hemorrhage as an association with placenta previa or accreta. One variation is the 'ring-shaped' or 'horse-shoe' placenta where the process is not involving the whole placenta, but only a central part. This might occur in about 1 in 6000 deliveries[100].

References

1. Bonnar J. Massive obstetric hemorrhage. Baillieres Best Pract Res Clin Obstet Gynaecol 2000;14:1–18
2. Gilbert TT, Smulian JC, Martin AA. Obstetric admissioin to the intensive care unit: Outcomes and severity of illness. Obstet Gynecol 2003;102:897
3. Hazelgrove JF, Price C, Pappachan VJ, Smith GB. Multicenter study of obstetric admission to 14 intensive care units in southern England. Crit Care Med 2001;29:770
4. Zeeman GG, Wendel GD Jr, Cunningham FG. A blueprint for obstetric critical care. Am J Obstet Gynecol 2003;188:532
5. Jegosathy R. Sudden maternal deaths in Malaysia: a case report. J Obstet Gynaecol Res 2002;28:186
6. Rahman MH, Akhter HH, Khan Chowdhury ME, Yusuf HR, Rochat RW. Obstetric deaths in Bangladesh. Int J Gynaecol Obstet 2002;77:161
7. Nagaya K, Fetters MD, Ishikawa M, et al. Causes of maternal mortality in Japan. JAMA 2000;283:2661
8. RCOG Green-top Guideline no 27, January 2011. Placental praevia, placental accreta and vasa praevia. London: RCOG, 2011
9. Chichakli LO, Atrash HK, MacKay AP, Musani AS, Berg CJ. Pregnancy-related mortality in the United States due to hemorrhage: 1979–1992. Obstet Gynecol 1999;94:721
10. Ananth CV, Oyelese Y, Prasad V, Getahun D, Smulian JC. Evidence of placental abruption as a chronic process: associations with vaginal bleeding early in pregnancy and placental lesions. Eur J Obstet Gynecol Reprod Biol 2006;128:15–21
11. Pariente G, Wiznitzer A, Sergienko R, Mazor M, Holcberg G, Sheiner E. Placental abruption: critical analysis of risk factors and perinatal outcomes. J Matern Fetal Neonatal Med 2011;24:698–702
12. Yang Q, Wen SW, Oppenheimer L et al. Association of cesarean delivery for first birth with placenta praevia and placental abruption in second pregnancy. BJOG 2007;114:609–13
13. Royal College of Obstetricians and Gynaecologists. Confidential Enquiries into Maternal Deaths: Saving Mothers' Lives. London, UK: RCOG, 2011
14. Hall DR. Abruptio placentae and disseminated intravascular coagulopathy. Semin Perinatol 2009;33:189–95
15. Martin JA, Hamilton BE, Sutton PD, et al. Births: Final data for 2001. I:n National Vital Statistics report 2002. Hyattsville, MD: National Centre for Health Statistics, 2002
16. Rasmussen S, Irgens LM, Bergsjo P, Dalaker K. The occurrence of placental abruption in Norway 1967–1991. Acta Obstet Gynecol Scand 1996;75:222–8
17. Fox H. Pathology of the placenta. London, UK: Saunders, 1978
18. Kramer MS, Usher RH, Pollack R, Boyd M, Usher S. Etiologic determinants of abruptio placentae. Obstet Gynecol 1997;89:221–6
19. Kupferminc MJ. Thrombophilia and pregnancy. Curr Pharm Des 2005;11:735–48
20. Ananth CV, Oyelese Y, Yeo L, Pradhan A, Vintzileos AM. Placental abruption in the United States, 1979 through 2001: temporal trends and potential determinants. Am J Obstet Gynecol 2005;192:191–8
21. Ananth, C.V., et al., Placental abruption and adverse perinatal outcomes. JAMA 1999;282:1646–51
22. Eskes TK. Clotting disorders and placental abruption: homocysteine—a new risk factor. Eur J Obstet Gynecol Reprod Biol 2001;95:206–12
23. de Paz NC, Sanchez SE, Huaman LE, et al. Risk of placental abruption in relation to maternal depressive, anxiety and stress symptoms. J Affect Disord 2011;130:280–4
24. Leone JM, Lane SD, Koumans EH, et al. Effects of intimate partner violence on pregnancy trauma and placental abruption. J Womens Health (Larchmt) 2010;19:1501–9
25. Hurd WW, Miodovnik M, Hertzberg V, Lavin JP. Selective management of abruptio placentae: A prospective study. Obstet Gynecol 1983;61:467
26. Elsasser DA, Ananth CV, Prasad V, Vintzileos AM; New Jersey-Placental Abruption Study Investigators. Diagnosis of placental abruption: relationship between clinical and histopathological findings. Eur J Obstet Gynecol Reprod Biol 2010;148:125–30
27. Knuppel AR, Drukker JE. Bleeding in late pregnancy: Antepartum bleeding. In: Hayashi RH, Castillo MS, eds. High risk Pregnancy: A Team Approach. Philadelphia: Saunders, 1986
28. Hibbard B.M. Bleeding in late pregnancy. In: Hibbard BM, ed. Principles of Obstetrics. London: Butterworths, 1988
29. Sher G, Statland BE. Abruptio placentae with coagulopathy: a rational basis for management. Clin Obstet Gynecol 1985;28:15–23
30. Notelovitz M, Bottoms SF, Dase DF, Leichter PJ. Painless abruptio placentae. Obstet Gynecol 1979;53:270–2
31. Page EW, King EB, Merrill JA. Abruptio placentae; dangers of delay in delivery. Obstet Gynecol 1954;3:385–93
32. Pritchard JA, Brekken AL. Clinical and laboratory studies on severe abruptio placentae. Am J Obstet Gynecol 1967;97:681–700
33. Green-Thompson RW. Antepartum hemorrhage. Clin Obstet Gynaecol 1982;9:479–515
34. Nyberg DA, Cyr DR, Mack LA, Wilson DA, Shuman WP. Sonographic spectrum of placental abruption. AJR Am J Roentgenol 1987;148:161–4
35. Emery CL, Morway LF, Chung-Park M, et al. The Kleihauer-Betke test. Clinical utility, indication, and correlation in patients with placental abruption and cocaine use. Arch Pathol Lab Med 1995;119:1032–7
36. Cahill, A.G., et al., Minor trauma in pregnancy—is the evaluation unwarranted? Am J Obstet Gynecol 2008;198:208 e1–5.
37. Abdella TN, Sibai BM, Hays JM Jr, Anderson GD. Relationship of hypertensive disease to abruptio placentae. Obstet Gynecol 1984;63:365–70
38. Okonofua FE, Olatubosun OA. Cesarean versus vaginal delivery in abruptio placentae associatedwith live fetuses. Int J Gynaecol Obstet 1985;23:471–4
39. Golditch IA, Boyce NE. Management of abruptio placentae. JAMA 1970;212:288–93
40. Lunan CB. The management of abruptio placentae. J Obstet Gynaecol Br Commonw 1973;80:120–4
41. Clark S, Cotton, DB, Gonik, B, et al. Central hemodynamic alterations in amniotic fluid embolism. Am J Obstet Gynecol 1995;158:1124
42. Brame RG, Harbert GM Jr, McGaughey HS Jr, Thornton WN Jr. Maternal risk in abruption. Obstet Gynecol 1968;31:224–7
43. Besinger RE, Niebyl JR. The safety and efficacy of tocolytic agents for the treatment of preterm labour. Obstet Gynecol Surv 1990;45:415–40
44. Sholl JS. Abruptio placentae: Clinical management in nonacute cases. Am J Obstet Gynecol 1987;156:40
45. Towers CV, Pircon RA, Heppard M. Is tocolysis safe in the management of third-trimester bleeding? Am J Obstet Gynecol 1999;180:1572–8
46. Crane JM, van den Hof MC, Dodds L, Armson BA, Liston R. Neonatal outcomes in placenta previa. Obstet Gynecol 1999;93:541
47. Frederiksen MC, Glassenberg R, Stika CS. Placenta previa: A 22-yEar analysis. Am J Obstet Gynecol 1999;180:1432
48. Babinszki A, Kerenyi T, Torok O, Grazi V, Lapinski RH, Berkowitz RL. Perinatal outcome in grand and great-grand multiparity: effects of parity on obstetric risk factors. Am J Obstet Gynecol 1999;181:669–74
49. Ananth CV, Smulian JC, Vintzileos AM. The effect of placenta previa on neonatal mortality: a population-based study in the United States, 1989 through 1997. Am J Obstet Gynecol 2003;188:1299–304

50. Gesteland K, Oshiro B, Henry E, et al. Rates of placenta previa and placental abruption in women delivered only vaginally or only by cesarean section. J Soc Gynecol Investig 2004;11:208A

51. Gilliam M, Rosenberg D, Davis F. The likelihood of placenta previa with greater number of cesarean deliveries and higher parity. Obstet Gynecol 2002;93:973

52. Williams MA, Mittendorf R, Lieberman E, et al. Cigarette smoking during pregnancy in relation to placenta previa. Am J Obstet Gynecol 1991;165:28–32

53. Brar HS, Platt LD, DeVore GR, Horenstein J. Fetal umbilical velocimetry for the surveillance of pregnancies complicated by placenta previa. J Reprod Med 1988;33:741–4

54. Ananth CV, Demissie K, Smulian JC, Vintzileos AM. Relationship among placenta previa, fetal growth restriction, and preterm delivery: a population-based study. Obstet Gynecol 2001;98:299–306

55. Chapman MG, Furness ET, Jones WR, Sheat JH.. Significance of the location of placenta site in early pregnancy. BJOG 1989;86:846–8

56. McLure N, Dornan JC. Early identification of placenta previa. BJOG 1990;97:959–61

57. Laing FC. Placenta previa: avoiding false-negative diagnoses. J Clin Ultrasound 1981;9:109–13

58. Comeau J, Shaw L, Marcell CC, Lavery JP. Early placenta previa and delivery outcome. Obstet Gynecol 1983;61:577–80

59. Ruparelia BA, Chapman MG. Early low-lying placentae—ultrasonic assessment, progress and outcome. Eur J Obstet Gynecol Reprod Biol 1985;20:209–13

60. Smith RS, Lauria MR, Comstock CH, et al. Transvaginal ultrasonography for all placentas that appear to be low-lying or over the internal cervical os. Ultrasound Obstet Gynecol 1997;9:22–4

61. Taipale P, Hiilesmaa V, Ylostalo P. Transvaginal ultrasonography at 18–23 weeks in predicting placenta previa at delivery. Ultrasound Obstet Gynecol 1998;12:422–5

62. Becker RH, Vonk R, Mende BC, Ragosch V, Entezami M. The relevance of placental location at 20–23 gestational weeks for prediction of placenta previa at delivery: evaluation of 8650 cases. Ultrasound Obstet Gynecol 2001;17:496–501

63. Dashe JS, McIntire DD, Ramus RM, Santos-Ramos R, Twickler DM. Persistence of placenta previa according to gestational age at ultrasound detection. Obstet Gynecol, 2002;99:692–7

64. Hertzberg BS, Bowie JD, Carroll BA, Kliewer MA, Weber TM. Diagnosis of placenta previa during the third trimester: role of transperineal sonography. AJR Am J Roentgenol 1992;159:83–7

65. Powell MC, Buckley J, Price H, Worthington BS, Symonds EM. Magnetic resonance imaging and placenta previa. Am J Obstet Gynecol 1986;154:565–9

66. Fraser R, Watson R. Bleeding during the latter half of pregnancy. In: Chalmers I, ed. Effective Care in Pregnancy and Childbirth. London: Oxford University Press, 1989

67. Cotton DB, Read JA, Paul RH, Quilligan EJ. The conservative aggressive management of placenta previa. Am J Obstet Gynecol 1980;137:687–95

68. Macafee CH, Millar WG, Harley G. Maternal and foetal mortality in placenta praevia. J Obstet Gynaecol Br Emp, 1962;69:203–12

69. Crenshaw C Jr, Jones DE, Parker RT. Placenta previa: a survey of twenty years experience with improved perinatal survival by expectant therapy and cesarean delivery. Obstet Gynecol Surv 1973;28:461–70

70. Johnson HW, Williamson JC, Greeley AV. The conservative management of some varieties of placenta praevia. Am J Obstet Gynecol 1945;49:398–406

71. Besinger RE, Moniak CW, Paskiewicz LS, Fisher SG, Tomich PG. The effect of tocolytic use in the management of symptomatic placenta previa. Am J Obstet Gynecol 1995;172:1770–5; discussion 1775–8

72. Love CD, Wallace EM. Pregnancies complicated by placenta praevia: what is appropriate management? Br J Obstet Gynaecol 1996;103:864–7

73. Ananth CV, Smulian JC, Vintzileos AM. The association of placenta previa with history of cesarean delivery and abortion: a metaanalysis. Am J Obstet Gynecol 1997;177:1071–8

74. Brenner WE, Edelman DA, Hendricks CH. Characteristics of patients with placenta previa and results of "expectant management". Am J Obstet Gynecol 1978;132:180–91

75. Sampson MB, Lastres O, Tomasi AM, Thomason JL, Work BA Jr. Tocolysis with terbutaline sulfate in patients with placenta complicated by premature labor. J Reprod Med 1984;29:248–50

76. Silver R, Depp R, Sabbagha RE, Dooley SL, Socol ML, Tamura RK. Placenta previa: aggressive expectant management. Am J Obstet Gynecol 1984;150:15–22

77. D'Angelo LJ, Irwin LF. Conservative management of placenta previa: a cost-benefit analysis. Am J Obstet Gynecol 1984;149:320–6

78. Kaunitz AM, Spence C, Danielson TS, Rochat RW, Grimes DA. Perinatal and maternal mortality in a eligious group avoiding obstetric care. Am J Obstet Gynecol, 1984;150:826–31

79. Wing DA, Paul RH, Millar LK. Management of the symptomatic placenta previa: a randomized, controlled trial of inpatient versus outpatient expectant management. Am J Obstet Gynecol 1996;175:806–11

80. Frederiksen MC, Glassenberg R, Stika CS. Placenta previa: A 22-year analysis. Am J Obstet Gynecol 1999;180:1432

81. Parekh N, Husaini SW, Russell IF. Cesarean section for placenta praevia: a retrospective study of anaesthetic management. Br J Anaesth 2000;84:725–30

82. Scott JS, Antepartum hemorrhage. In: Whitefield CR, ed. Dewhurst's Textbook of Obstetrics and Gynaecology for Postgraduates. Blackwell: Oxford: Blackwell, 1986

83. Myerscough PR. Munro Kerr's operative obstetrics, 10th edn. London: Bailliere Tindall, 1982

84. Williamson HC, Greeley AV. Management of placenta praevia: 12 year study. Am J Obstet Gynecol 1945;50:987–91

85. Zelop CM, Harlow BL, Frigoletto FD Jr, Safon LE, Saltzman DH. Emergency peripartum hysterectomy. Am J Obstet Gynecol 1993;168:1443–8

86. Comstock CH. Antenatal diagnosis of placenta accreta: a review. Ultrasound Obstet Gynecol 2005;26:89–96

87. Fox H. Placenta accreta, 1945–1969. Obstet Gynecol Surv 1972;27:475

88. Lax A, Prince MR, Mennitt KW, Schwebach JR, Budorick NE. The value of specific MRI features in the evaluation of suspected placental invasion. Magn Reson Imaging 2007;25:87–93

89. Masselli G, Brunelli R, Casciani E, et al., Magnetic resonance imaging in the evaluation of placental adhesive disorders: correlation with color Doppler ultrasound. Eur Radiol 2008;18:1292–9

90. Palacios Jaraquemada JM, Bruno CH. Magnetic resonance imaging in 300 cases of placenta accreta: surgical correlation of new findings. Acta Obstet Gynecol Scand 2005;84:716–24

91. Hung TH, Shau WY, Hsieh CC, Chiu TH, Hsu JJ, Hsieh TT. Risk factors for placenta accreta. Obstet Gynecol 1999;93:545–50

92. Liang HS, Jeng CJ, Sheen TC, Lee FK, Yang YC, Tzeng CR. First-trimester uterine rupture from a placenta percreta. A case report. J Reprod Med 2003;48:474–8

93. Twickler DM, Lucas MJ, Balis AB et al., Color flow mapping for myometrial invasion in women with a prior cesarean delivery. J Matern Fetal Med 2000;9:330–5

94. Timmermans S, van Hof AC, Duvekot JJ. Conservative management of abnormally invasive placentation. Obstet Gynecol Surv 2007;62:529–39

95. Eller AG, Porter TF, Soisson P, Silver RM. Optimal management strategies for placenta accreta. BJOG 2009;116:648–54

96. Kayem G, Davy C, Goffinet F, Thomas C, Clément D, Cabrol D. Conservative versus extirpative management in cases of placenta accreta. Obstet Gynecol 2004;104:531–6

97. Henrich W, Fuchs I, Ehrenstein T, et al., Antenatal diagnosis of placenta percreta with planned in situ retention and methotrexate therapy in a woman infected with HIV. Ultrasound Obstet Gynecol 2002;20:90–3

98. Nijman RG, Mantingh A, Aarnoudse JG. Persistent retained placenta percreta: methotrexate treatment and Doppler flow characteristics. BJOG 2002;109:587–8

99. Fox H. Pathology of the placenta. Clin Obstet Gynaecol 1986;13:501–19

100. Benirschke K, Kaufman P. Pathology of the human placenta, 4th edn. New York: Springer-Verlag, 2000

28

Management of Placenta Accreta

G. Kayem, L. Sentilhes, G. Grangé, T. Schmitz, V. Tsatsaris, D. Cabrol and F. Goffinet

INTRODUCTION

The occurrence of placenta accreta is linked to abnormal invasion at the placental implantation site due to a defect within the decidua basalis[1]. The term *increta* is used in the case of invasion of the myometrium, while *percreta* refers to invasion of the serosa or even adjacent organs, most frequently the bladder. Nonetheless, the term *accreta* is frequently used more generally to cover all three definitions.

Placenta accreta is often diagnosed after the baby's birth, when the placenta fails to deliver. Trying to force this delivery can result in severe postpartum hemorrhage (PPH), emergency hysterectomy and even death. Abnormalities of placental insertion are responsible for 35–38% of peripartum hysterectomies in recent population-based studies[2,3]. Other potential complications include multiple organ failure, in cases of severe hemorrhage, as well as damage to adjacent organs, such as the bladder. This is particularly true for placenta percreta, for which peri- and postoperative morbidity is high; a maternal mortality rate of 7% has been reported[4]. Finally, and more rarely, case reports of percreta describe spontaneous uterine rupture in the second or third trimester of pregnancy, combined with massive hemoperitoneum[5–7].

Management of placenta accreta involves two principal difficulties: first, its identification, which is aided by risk factor assessment and complementary examinations, and second, its management which strives to reduce maternal complications as much as possible.

INCIDENCE AND RISK FACTORS OF PLACENTA ACCRETA

The incidence of placenta accreta is rising, apparently in correlation with cesarean rates, and has multiplied by 10 in 50 years. Miller *et al.* reported that among 155,670 deliveries between 1985 and 1994, placenta accreta complicated 1/2510 births[8]. In a more recent study, covering 1982–2002, Wu *et al.* found a still higher incidence in their facility: 1 per 533 pregnancies[9]. It is important to note, however, that because of recruitment bias in these two tertiary reference centers, the incidence rates calculated from their data are not representative of the real incidence in the general population.

The principal risk factors for placenta accreta are placenta previa or a history of cesarean delivery. Other reported risk factors are maternal age greater than 35 years, multiparity, a history of uterine surgery with an endometrial breach and curettage. Miller *et al.* showed that placenta accreta occurred in 55 of 590 (9.3%) women with placenta previa compared to seven of 155,080 (1/22,154) without placenta previa (relative risk (RR) 20.7, 95% confidence interval (95% CI) 9.4–45.2)[8]. Moreover, among women with placenta previa, placenta accreta was diagnosed in 36 of 124 (29%) women for whom placental implantation overlaid a cesarean scar and in four of 62 (6.5%) women for whom it did not (RR 4.5, 95% CI 1.7–12.1). Among women with placenta previa, age greater than 35 years and a history of cesarean delivery were also independent risk factors of placenta accreta. Finally, among women with placenta previa, the risk of placenta accreta ranged from less than 2% for those younger than 35 years with no previous cesarean to 39% for those with two or more previous cesarean sections.

PRENATAL SCREENING FOR PLACENTA ACCRETA

Comprehensive management of placenta accreta must involve multidisciplinary care, if at all possible planned in advance, including obstetricians, anesthetists and radiologists experienced in interventional radiology. Moreover, in cases of placenta percreta, potential damage to adjacent organs may require the participation of urologists or general surgeons. Prenatal screening for placenta accreta is therefore essential for scheduling the delivery and reducing maternal risk. Diagnosis is generally suspected by ultrasound and magnetic resonance imaging (MRI) in women with risk factors.

Numerous studies have assessed the performance of ultrasound for predicting placenta accreta. The classically described ultrasound criteria are the absence of a hypoechoic zone or clear space between the placenta and the myometrium (Figure 1), interruptions of the echogenic area at the interface of the serosa and the bladder, a pseudotumoral appearance of the placenta in/around the uterine serosa, and the presence of

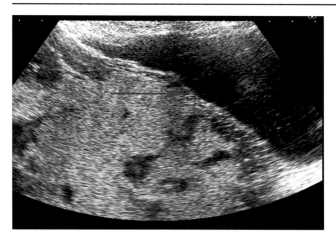

Figure 1 A classic ultrasound characteristic predicting placenta accreta is absence of clear space between the placenta and the myometrium

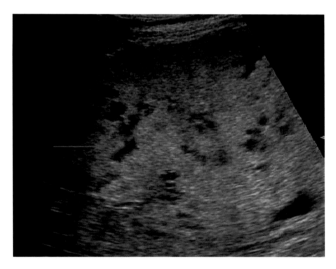

Figure 2 Intraplacental lacunae (grade 3) giving placenta a 'moth-eaten' appearance

intraplacental lacunae in the accreta zone, which give the placenta a 'swiss cheese' or 'moth-eaten' appearance (Figure 2). Guy *et al.* reported that the use of these criteria had a positive predictive value (PPV) of 62% for placenta accreta[10]. Similarly, Finberg and Williams obtained a PPV of 78% and a negative predictive value (NPV) of 93% with the use of ultrasound[11]. Ultrasound signs can appear quite early. Comstock *et al.* showed that at 15–20 weeks, the presence of intraplacental lacunae was the best predictive marker of placenta accreta, with a sensitivity of 79% and a PPV of 92%[12]. The absence of a retroplacental hypoechoic clear space, although considered to be a good predictive sign of placenta accreta, had a sensitivity of only 57% with 48% false positives. After 20 weeks, the sensitivity of these diagnostic criteria increased, reaching 93% for the lacunae and 80% for the absence of the retroplacental clear space. Finally, an ultrasound appearance of a convex or 'tented' bladder was associated with placenta accreta, even in the absence of increta or percreta implantation. It was not specific for bladder invasion[12].

Yang *et al.* studied the predictive value of placental lacunae for maternal morbidity in 51 patients with placenta previa and a history of cesarean delivery[13]. These authors classified the intraplacental lacunae according to a score based on Finberg's criteria[11]: the absence of lacuna was classified as grade zero, one to three small lacunae as grade 1, four to six large, irregular lacunae as grade 2, and numerous lacuna including some that were large and irregular as grade 3. Grade 1 lacunae had the best predictive value, with a sensitivity of 86%, a specificity of 78%, PPV of 76% and NPV of 88%. No hysterectomy was performed in women without lacunae.

Three-dimensional power ultrasound, with Doppler energy data acquisition, has also been tested in a prospective study including 170 women with placenta previa, 39 of whom also had accreta[14]. Both two- and three-dimensional Doppler criteria were analysed. The three-dimensional criteria were: (1) confluent vessels at the junction between the bladder and uterine serosa; (2) hypervascularization on lateral view; and (3) inseparable cotyledonal and intervillous circulations, with a chaotic appearance. These three-dimensional power Doppler signs had excellent diagnostic value, with a sensitivity of 100% and a specificity of 85% when at least one of the three was present. The best sign was that of vascular confluence at the basal plate, which had a sensitivity of 97% and a specificity of 92%. The diagnostic value of both standard two-dimensional gray scale and Doppler color signs in this study was of a lesser magnitude. In particular, the presence of placental lacunae had a sensitivity of 54% and a specificity of 85%.

Finally, MRI is useful for this diagnosis[15,16], especially for a posterior placenta[17]. Among the diagnostic criteria proposed are abnormal bulging of the lower segment, heterogeneity of signal intensity in T2-weighted (T2) imaging, and dark intraplacental bands, also in T2 imaging[18]. The most interesting study, because it came closest to daily clinical practice, is that reported by Warshak *et al.*[19]. All the women who had a history of uterine scar (or myomectomy) and either placenta previa or a low-lying placenta had an initial Doppler ultrasound. If placenta accreta was suspected (uterine scar and placental implantation near the scar), MRI was performed with gadolinium injection. Placentation was then considered abnormal if manual removal of the placenta was difficult (due to its adhesion to the myometrium) and it resulted in PPH (clinical diagnosis), or if the pathology examination found villi but no decidual cells in the myometrium (pathology diagnosis). Of the 453 patients studied, 9% had placenta accreta. MRI allowed a diagnosis of placenta accreta to be ruled out in 14 of the 16 Doppler ultrasound false-positive results. Performing MRI when ultrasound findings suggest placenta accreta thus seems useful for improving the performance of Doppler ultrasound. Gadolinium appears to improve the specificity of MRI in marking the border between the placenta and the myometrium more clearly. The safety of gadolinium has not been demonstrated in the fetus, but its use is authorized by the European Society of Urogenital Radiology when required and without any specific follow-up.

MANAGEMENT OF PLACENTA ACCRETA SUSPECTED BEFORE DELIVERY

A consensus approach to placenta accreta is to leave it *in situ*[20,21], as trying to detach it can induce a massive hemorrhage[22]. Two types of management are possible: a cesarean hysterectomy or conservative treatment, consisting in leaving the placenta in the uterine cavity without hysterectomy. In both instances, however, the difficulty is that there is no diagnostic technique that provides a PPV of 100% for the diagnosis of placenta accreta.

CESAREAN HYSTERECTOMY

For women who do not desire further children, a hysterectomy following the cesarean is appropriate if the risk factors and imaging strongly indicate the diagnosis. In this case, the placenta is left in place after removal of the newborn by a hysterotomy incision, preferably at a distance from the placental bed. A prudent attempt at placental delivery includes the injection of 5 IU of oxytocin and moderate cord traction to confirm the diagnosis; this strategy seems reasonable in view of the possibility of false-positive images, although it does include the risk of inducing bleeding. If this effort fails, an experienced team performs a hysterectomy. During this procedure, which must be planned, blood loss is assessed and units of packed red blood cells and ideally fresh frozen plasma are available should a hemorrhage or disseminated intravascular coagulation develop (see Chapter 5). Some teams recommend the use of a 'cell saver' to compensate for blood loss[22] (see Chapter 70).

The American College of Obstetrics and Gynecology (ACOG) currently recommends a cesarean hysterectomy without attempting manual removal of the placenta when prenatal suspicion of placenta accreta is strong[23]. Very few series have assessed maternal morbidity after cesarean hysterectomy. In a series of 76 such procedures for placenta accreta, Eller *et al.* found the following outcomes: transfusion (≥4 units of packed red blood cells) 42%, ureteral injuries 7%, cystotomy 29% and infectious complications 33%[24]. Another single-center study of cesarean hysterectomies due to placenta accreta in one California hospital[25] reported a similar morbidity rate in a comparison of 62 cesarean hysterectomies diagnosed prenatally with 37 cases discovered per partum. These authors showed that the risk of hemorrhage was lower when the diagnosis preceded the cesarean, but 52% of the patients with predelivery diagnoses had placenta accreta; among those without prenatal diagnoses, the rate of bladder injury was 23% and that of ureteral injury 8%.

Among the strategies proposed for planned cesarean hysterectomies is intraoperative embolization as soon as the fetus is removed or the preoperative placement of intravascular balloons that can be inflated during the surgery. Uterine artery embolization performed after fetal extraction and before hysterectomy has also been proposed. In a series of 26 women who had a preventive arterial embolization before the hysterectomy, Angtsmann *et al.* observed significant reductions in blood loss, percentage of patients receiving transfusions and number of units of packed red blood cells transfused[26]. Placement of intravascular balloons has also been studied. A series of 11 women found encouraging results with reduced bleeding[27], while others reported no significant benefits from this procedure[28,29]. In a retrospective study, Bodner *et al.* examined[29] consecutive patients treated for placenta accreta, divided into two groups: those with ($n = 6$) and without temporary balloon occlusion ($n = 22$)[29]. In this study, temporary occlusion or embolization before hysterectomy failed to reduce the risk of hemorrhage. Similarly, Shrivastava *et al.* found no beneficial results for 69 women managed for placenta accreta by cesarean hysterectomy[28]. Nonetheless, this type of study is difficult to perform, especially because of inclusion bias, which can result in including the most serious cases in the group with balloon treatment. For this reason, and because the possibility of controlling hemorrhage by the endovascular pathway during surgery is so seductive for the physician, this technique is still under evaluation, but should generally be reserved for the most complex cases (see Chapter 49).

MANAGEMENT OF PLACENTA ACCRETA WITHOUT HYSTERECTOMY

Hysterectomy results in permanent sterility, something often not at all desired by the younger parturient, especially if her family is not complete. Moreover, in the context of placenta accreta/percreta, hysterectomy can be accompanied by high morbidity and be life-threatening. To try to minimize these complications, particularly when the patient expresses a desire for more children, a conservative alternative to extirpative treatment or cesarean hysterectomy has been offered in some institutions[20,30].

Conservative treatment that leaves the placenta in the uterine cavity

The management strategies are outlined below and shown in the algorithm of Figure 3.

When placenta accreta is strongly suspected before delivery, based on risk factors and imaging studies that support this diagnosis, management should include the following:

(1) The exact position of the placenta is determined by preoperative ultrasound. Cesarean delivery is scheduled.

(2) The operation begins with a midline cutaneous incision, enlarged above the umbilicus if necessary.

(3) The uterine approach uses a midline incision at a distance from the placental bed. After removal of the child, the obstetrician carefully attempts to remove the placenta; failure to do so confirms the diagnosis. In this case, the cord is cut at the site of insertion and the uterine cavity is closed (Figure 4).

(4) Postoperative antibiotic therapy (amoxicillin and clavulanic acid) is usually administered prophylactically for 10 days to minimize the risk of infection.

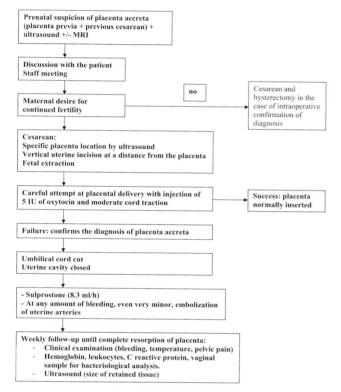

Figure 3 Algorithm for proposed management strategy of prenatal diagnosis of placenta accreta

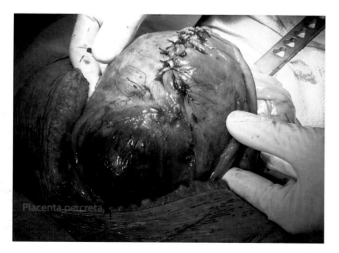

Figure 4 Conservative management at the end of intervention. The baby has been delivered by a fundal hysterotomy and the uterus has been closed. The placenta has been left in place and is still visible through the lower segment of the uterus

If the diagnosis is not suspected until the third stage of labor:

(1) Manual uterine examination is gentle and unforced.

(2) The adherent placenta is left in place partially or completely, especially if the patient's hemodynamic status is stable and there are no clinical or laboratory signs of infections.

(3) Subsequent follow-up requires weekly visits until complete resorption of the placenta. The visits include a clinical examination, pelvic ultrasound and laboratory tests for infection (vaginal sample and C reactive protein).

One study from our group compared an extirpative strategy with conservative treatment performed consecutively during two different periods[31,32]. Conservative treatment was associated with a reduced risk of hemorrhage and a lower hysterectomy rate than extirpative management, but with a higher risk of maternal infection (Table 1).

Case reports also describe similar conservative management and underline in particular the risk of complications from hemorrhage and infection[33]. Two French series have described women with placenta accreta managed conservatively. Bretelle *et al.* used conservative management for 26 women, but had a final hysterectomy rate of 19%[34]. Sentilhes *et al.* report morbidity in 167 cases of placenta accreta treated conservatively at 40 university hospital centers throughout France (Table 2). Severe maternal morbidity occurred in 6% of these cases and the final hysterectomy rate was 22%. One maternal death occurred in a woman with aplastic anemia, nephrotoxicity and septic shock (peritonitis) 3 months after a methotrexate injection in the umbilical cord. After a median delay of 13.5 weeks (4–60 weeks), an empty uterus was obtained spontaneously in 75% of the women, while hysteroscopic resection or curettage was required to obtain an empty

Table 1 Comparison of maternal morbidity between extirpative management and conservative management. From Kayem *et al.*[32], with permission

	Extirpative management (n = 13)	Conservative management (n = 38)	p-Value
Hysterectomies, n (%)	11 (84.6)	10 (26.3)	<0.001
Transfusion	12 (92.3)	25 (65.8)	0.13
Patients (n (%))			
Packed red blood cells, ml (mean ± SD)	3230 ± 2170	1081 ± 1357	<0.001
Fresh frozen plasma, ml (mean ± SD)	2238 ± 1415	197 ± 632	<0.001
Disseminated intravascular coagulation	5 (38.5)	1 (2.6)	0.003
Transfer to ICU, n (%)	7 (53.8)	11 (28.9)	0.19
Time spent in ICU, days (mean ± SD)	2.42 ± 2.6	2.27 ± 0.9	0.85
Postpartum endometritis, n (%)	0	7 (18.4)	0.22

ICU, intensive care unit

Table 2 Maternal morbidity after conservative treatment for placenta accreta. Data shown as *n* (%), mean ± standard deviation or median (interquartiles). Some patients had several types of maternal morbidity. From Sentilhes *et al.*[21], with permission

Immediate maternal morbidity	Placenta accreta (n = 167)
Emergency hysterectomy	18 (10.8%)
Postpartum antibiotic treatment >5 days	54 (32.3%)
Patients receiving transfusions	70 (41.9%)
Units of packed red cells or fresh frozen plasma >5	25 (15.0%)
Transfer to intensive care	43 (25.7%)
Time spent in intensive care (days)	2.36 ± 1.93
Acute pulmonary edema	1 (0.6%)
Acute kidney failure	1 (0.6%)
Lesion of adjacent organ	1 (0.6%)
Septic shock	1 (0.6%)
Sepsis	7 (4.2%)
Infection	47 (28.1%)
Endometritis	15 (9.0%)
Infection of uterine wall	8 (4.7%)
Peritonitis	2 (1.2%)
Pyelonephritis	2 (1.2%)
Vesicouterine fistula	1 (0.6%)
Uterine necrosis	2 (1.2%)
Isolated postpartum fever >38.5°C for 24 hours	17 (10.2%)
Thromboembolic complications	3 (1.8%)
Secondary third-stage hemorrhage stopped after	18 (10.8%)
Uterotonics	2/18 (11.1%)
Manual uterine examination	2/18 (11.1%)
Hysteroscopy and curettage	2/18 (11.1%)
Embolization	4/18 (22.2%)
Delayed hysterectomy	8/18 (50.0%)
Delayed hysterectomy	18 (44.8%)
Mean time since birth	22 (9–45)
Indication for delayed hysterectomy	
Secondary third-stage hemorrhage	8/18 (44.4%)
Sepsis	2/18 (11.1%)
Secondary third-stage hemorrhage and sepsis	3/18 (16.7%)
Vesicouterine fistula	1/18 (5.6%)
Uterine necrosis and sepsis	2/18 (11.1%)
Arteriovenous malformation	1/18 (5.6%)
Maternal request	1/18 (5.6%)
Death	1 (0.6%)
Uterine preservation	131 (78.4%)
Severe maternal morbidity	10 (6.0%)

uterus in 25% of the cases, with a median delay of 20 weeks (2–45 weeks)[21]. Finally and most importantly, the fertility and obstetric outcome of patients treated conservatively for placenta accreta were not impaired, although the risk of placenta accreta in the next pregnancy appears high (30%)[35].

Conservative treatment with resection of the placental bed

Palacios-Jaraquemada *et al.* have proposed a different approach to conservative treatment[36], suggesting resection of the entire placental bed after detaching and pushing the bladder in a caudad direction. Hemorrhage was prevented by suturing the uterine arteries. After resection of the placenta and adjoining uterine wall, the uterine edges are brought together and sutured with U stitches. Uterine compression sutures,

somewhat more penetrating than B-Lynch sutures, are used to control possible bleeding[37,38]. Finally, a resorbable vicryl mesh (polyglycolic acid) is placed above the uterine scar and coated with a non-adhesive cellulose layer. This series included 68 cases of placenta percreta resulting in 18 hysterectomies. The complications observed included two ureteral injuries as well as complications due to both hemorrhage and infection.

A somewhat different case of resection of the placenta and lower segment was also published by our group. It involved placenta percreta of a cervicoisthmic pregnancy for which more standard conservative treatment was impossible[39]. The woman had a subsequent pregnancy without postpartum complications.

Adjuvant treatment with conservative management

Methotrexate, uterine artery embolization and sulprostone are the three adjuvant treatments described for attempting to manage placenta accreta conservatively[40–44].

The impact of methotrexate on placental resorption has not been fully assessed. Overall, placental resorption in the reported cases has been variable, ranging from expulsion of the placenta on the 7th day to progressive resorption over a period of 6 months[40–42,44]. No comparative series have studied methotrexate use for this purpose. Moreover, the slow rate of placental cell renewal at term, compared with at the beginning of pregnancy, suggests that methotrexate might be far less effective than in ectopic pregnancies. For these reasons, no convincing evidence favors the use of methotrexate. Finally, the only maternal death in the study of Sentilhes *et al.* was due in part to aplastic anemia associated with administration of methotrexate[21].

Similarly, few studies report placental outcome after uterine artery embolization[45,46]. The objective is to prevent a secondary hemorrhage, to reduce the risk of blood loss and to accelerate the disappearance of the placenta by necrosis. Nonetheless, arterial embolization is not an innocuous procedure, and complications have been described, in particular, cases of uterine necrosis, ischemia of the lumbar plexus, hemoperitoneum due to dissection of an epigastric artery and ischemia of the lower limbs due to embolism[3,21,47–50].

MANAGEMENT OF PLACENTA ACCRETA DIAGNOSED AFTER DELIVERY

In numerous cases, the diagnosis of accreta is made only in the third stage of labor. This can occur during delivery, when the placenta is not delivered, and no plane of cleavage can be found between the uterus and the placenta. If this attempt was careful, without force or insistence, and the patient's hemodynamic status is stable, conservative treatment can be attempted. In other cases, the situation requires management of a severe PPH, except that the uterotonics used alone are less effective than in the case, for example, of uterine atony.

Accordingly, uterine artery embolization or ligation of the hypogastric arteries can be used[51,52]. Other techniques that have been described include an emergency uterine ligation for hemostasis[52,53], placement of an intrauterine balloon to ensure hemostatic compression, argon laser coagulation or even aortic compression[54–56]. Numerous techniques for uterine compression by B-Lynch or similar sutures, including Haymann's modification, have been suggested but have not been specifically evaluated for this indication[53,57–63].

Finally, the failure of these measures or an initial massive hemorrhage requires an emergency hysterectomy. Any delay increases the risk of maternal complications which are discussed more fully in other chapters of this book.

CONCLUSION

The standard guidelines for placenta accreta are to avoid forcing placental delivery and to perform a hysterectomy. A more conservative approach that leaves the placenta in place can nonetheless be proposed in specific cases where the woman wants to preserve her ability to have children. This strategy must nonetheless be used carefully and in an appropriately equipped facility because of the possible risk of severe maternal morbidity associated with it.

References

1. Khong TY, Robertson WB. Placenta creta and placenta praevia creta. Placenta 1987;8:399–409
2. Knight M. Peripartum hysterectomy in the UK: management and outcomes of the associated haemorrhage. BJOG 2007; 114:1380–7
3. Zwart JJ, Richters JM, Ory F, de Vries JI, Bloemenkamp KW, van Roosmalen J. Uterine rupture in The Netherlands: a nationwide population-based cohort study. BJOG 2009; 116:1069–78, discussion 78–80
4. O'Brien JM, Barton JR, Donaldson ES. The management of placenta percreta: conservative and operative strategies. Am J Obstet Gynecol 1996;175:1632–8
5. Baruah S, Gangopadhyay P, Labib MM. Spontaneous rupture of unscarred uterus at early mid-trimester due to placenta percreta. J Obstet Gynaecol 2004;24:705
6. Hlibczuk V. Spontaneous uterine rupture as an unusual cause of abdominal pain in the early second trimester of pregnancy. J Emergency Med 2004;27:143–5
7. Topuz S. Spontaneous uterine rupture at an unusual site due to placenta percreta in a 21-week twin pregnancy with previous cesarean section. Clin Exp Obstet Gynecol 2004;31: 239–41
8. Miller DA, Chollet JA, Goodwin TM. Clinical risk factors for placenta previa-placenta accreta. Am J Obstet Gynecol 1997; 177:210–4
9. Wu S, Kocherginsky M, Hibbard JU. Abnormal placentation: twenty-year analysis. Am J Obstet Gynecol 2005;192: 1458–61
10. Guy GP, Peisner DB, Timor-Tritsch IE. Ultrasonographic evaluation of uteroplacental blood flow patterns of abnormally located and adherent placentas. Am J Obstet Gynecol 1990;163:723–7
11. Finberg HJ, Williams JW. Placenta accreta: prospective sonographic diagnosis in patients with placenta previa and prior cesarean section. J Ultrasound Med 1992;11:333–43
12. Comstock CH, Love JJ Jr., Bronsteen RA, et al. Sonographic detection of placenta accreta in the second and third trimesters of pregnancy. Am J Obstet Gynecol 2004;190:1135–40
13. Yang JI, Lim YK, Kim HS, Chang KH, Lee JP, Ryu HS. Sonographic findings of placental lacunae and the prediction of adherent placenta in women with placenta previa totalis and prior Cesarean section. Ultrasound Obstet Gynecol 2006; 28:178–82
14. Shih JC, Palacios Jaraquemada JM, Su YN, et al. Role of three-dimensional power Doppler in the antenatal diagnosis of placenta accreta: comparison with gray-scale and color Doppler techniques. Ultrasound Obstet Gynecol 2009;33: 193–203
15. Maldjian C, Adam R, Pelosi M, Pelosi M. MRI appearance of cervical incompetence in a pregnant patient. Magn Reson Imaging 1999;17:1399–402
16. Tanaka YO. [MRI of the female pelvis: useful information for daily practice]. Nippon Igaku Hoshasen Gakkai Zasshi 2002;62:471–8
17. Levine D, Hulka CA, Ludmir J, Li W, Edelman RR. Placenta accreta: evaluation with color Doppler US, power Doppler US, and MR imaging. Radiology 1997;205:773–6
18. Lax A, Prince MR, Mennitt KW, Schwebach JR, Budorick NE. The value of specific MRI features in the evaluation of suspected placental invasion. Magn Reson Imaging 2007;25: 87–93
19. Warshak CR, Eskander R, Hull AD, et al. Accuracy of ultrasonography and magnetic resonance imaging in the diagnosis of placenta accreta. Obstet Gynecol 2006;108:573–81
20. Kayem G, Grange G, Goffinet F. [Management of placenta accreta]. Gynecol Obstet Fertil 2007;35:186–92
21. Sentilhes L, Ambroselli C, Kayem G, et al. Maternal outcome after conservative treatment of placenta accreta. Obstet Gynecol 2010;115:526–34
22. Goncalves LF, Chaiworapongsa T, Romero R. Intrauterine infection and prematurity. Ment Retard Dev Disabil Res Rev 2002;8:3–13
23. Ramsey PS, Tamura T, Goldenberg RL, et al. The preterm prediction study: elevated cervical ferritin levels at 22 to 24 weeks of gestation are associated with spontaneous preterm delivery in asymptomatic women. Am J Obstet Gynecol 2002;186:458–63
24. Eller A, Porter T, Soisson P, Silver R. Optimal management strategies for placenta accreta. BJOG 2009;116:648–54
25. Warshak CR, Ramos GA, Eskander R, et al. Effect of predelivery diagnosis in 99 consecutive cases of placenta accreta. Obstet Gynecol 2010;115:65–9
26. Angstmann T, Gard G, Harrington T, Ward E, Thomson A, Giles W. Surgical management of placenta accreta: a cohort series and suggested approach. Am J Obstet Gynecol 2010; 202:38 e1–9
27. Tan CH, Tay KH, Sheah K, et al. Perioperative endovascular internal iliac artery occlusion balloon placement in management of placenta accreta. AJR Am J Roentgenol 2007;189: 1158–63
28. Shrivastava V, Nageotte M, Major C, Haydon M, Wing D. Case-control comparison of cesarean hysterectomy with and without prophylactic placement of intravascular balloon catheters for placenta accreta. Am J Obstet Gynecol 2007;197: 402e1–5
29. Bodner LJ, Nosher JL, Gribbin C, Siegel RL, Beale S, Scorza W. Balloon-assisted occlusion of the internal iliac arteries in patients with placenta accreta/percreta. Cardiovasc Intervent Radiol 2006;29:354–61
30. Kayem G, Pannier E, Goffinet F, Grange G, Cabrol D. Fertility after conservative treatment of placenta accreta. Fertil Steril 2002;78:637–8
31. Kayem G, Davy C, Goffinet F, Thomas C, Clement D, Cabrol D. Conservative versus extirpative management in cases of placenta accreta. Obstet Gynecol 2004;104:531–6
32. Kayem G, Anselem O, Schmitz T, et al. [Conservative versus radical management in cases of placenta accreta: a historical study]. J Gynecol Obstet Biol Reprod 2007;36:680–7

33. Timmermans S, van Hof AC, Duvekot JJ. Conservative management of abnormally invasive placentation. Obstet Gynecol Surv 2007;62:529–39

34. Bretelle F, Courbiere B, Mazouni C, et al. Management of placenta accreta: morbidity and outcome. Eur J Obstet Gynecol Reprod Biol 2007;133:34–9

35. Sentilhes L, Kayem G, Ambroselli C, et al. Fertility and pregnancy outcomes following conservative treatment for placenta accreta. Hum Reprod 2010;25:2803–10

36. Palacios-Jaraquemada JM, Pesaresi M, Nassif JC, Hermosid S. Anterior placenta percreta: surgical approach, hemostasis and uterine repair. Acta Obstet Gynecol Scand 2004;83:738–44

37. Allahdin S, Aird C, Danielian P. B-Lynch sutures for major primary postpartum haemorrhage at caesarean section. J Obstet Gynaecol 2006;26:639–42

38. Cho JH, Jun HS, Lee CN. Hemostatic suturing technique for uterine bleeding during cesarean delivery. Obstet Gynecol 2000;96:129–31

39. Kayem G, Deis S, Estrade S, Haddad B. Conservative management of a near-term cervico-isthmic pregnancy, followed by a successful subsequent pregnancy: a case report. Fertil Steril 2008;89:1826e13–5

40. Arulkumaran S, Ng CS, Ingemarsson I, Ratnam SS. Medical treatment of placenta accreta with methotrexate. Acta Obstet Gynecol Scand 1986;65:285–6

41. Buckshee K, Dadhwal V. Medical management of placenta accreta. Int J Gynaecol Obstet 1997;59:47–8

42. Gupta D, Sinha R. Management of placenta accreta with oral methotrexate. Int J Gynaecol Obstet 1998;60:171–3

43. Jaffe R, DuBeshter B, Sherer DM, Thompson EA, Woods JR Jr. Failure of methotrexate treatment for term placenta percreta. Am J Obstet Gynecol 1994;171:558–9

44. Mussalli GM, Shah J, Berck DJ, Elimian A, Tejani N, Manning FA. Placenta accreta and methotrexate therapy: three case reports. J Perinatol 2000;20:331–4

45. Lemercier E, Genevois A, Descargue G, Clavier E, Benozio M. [MRI evaluation of placenta accreta treated by embolization. Apropos of a case. Review of the literature]. J Radiol 1999;80:383–7

46. Sentilhes L, Gromez A, Marpeau L. Fertility after pelvic arterial embolization, stepwise uterine devascularization, hypogastric artery ligation, and B-Lynch suture to control postpartum hemorrhage. Int J Gynaecol Obstet 2009;108:249

47. Touboul C, Badiou W, Saada J, et al. Efficacy of selective arterial embolisation for the treatment of life-threatening post-partum haemorrhage in a large population. PLoS ONE. 2008;3:e3819

48. Chauleur C, Fanget C, Tourne G, Levy R, Larchez C, Seffert P. Serious primary post-partum hemorrhage, arterial embolization and future fertility: a retrospective study of 46 cases. Hum Reprod 2008;23:1553–9

49. Kirby JM, Kachura JR, Rajan DK, et al. Arterial embolization for primary postpartum hemorrhage. J Vasc Interv Radiol 2009;20:1036–45

50. Maassen MS, Lambers MD, Tutein Nolthenius RP, van der Valk PH, Elgersma OE. Complications and failure of uterine artery embolisation for intractable postpartum haemorrhage. BJOG 2009;116:55–61

51. Kayem G, Sentilhes L, Deneux-Tharaux C. Management of placenta accreta. BJOG 2009;116:1536–7; author reply 7–8

52. Sentilhes L, Kayem G, Descamps P. Factors associated with peripartum hysterectomy. Obstet Gynecol 2009;114:927

53. Sentilhes L, Gromez A, Razzouk K, Resch B, Verspyck E, Marpeau L. B-Lynch suture for massive persistent postpartum hemorrhage following stepwise uterine devascularization. Acta Obstet Gynecol Scand 2008;87:1020–6

54. Komulainen MH, Vayrynen MA, Kauko ML, Saarikoski S. Two cases of placenta accreta managed conservatively. Eur J Obstet Gynecol Reprod Biol 1995;62:135–7

55. Scarantino SE, Reilly JG, Moretti ML, Pillari VT. Argon beam coagulation in the management of placenta accreta. Obstet Gynecol 1999;94:825–7

56. Johanson R, Kumar M, Obhrai M, Young P. Management of massive postpartum haemorrhage: use of a hydrostatic balloon catheter to avoid laparotomy. BJOG 2001;108:420–2

57. Price N, Whitelaw N, B-Lynch C. Application of the B-Lynch brace suture with associated intrauterine balloon catheter for massive haemorrhage due to placenta accreta following a second-trimester miscarriage. J Obstet Gynaecol 2006;26:267–8

58. Hayman RG, Arulkumaran S, Steer PJ. Uterine compression sutures: surgical management of postpartum hemorrhage. Obstet Gynecol 2002;99:502–6

59. Bhal K, Bhal N, Mulik V, Shankar L. The uterine compression suture—a valuable approach to control major haemorrhage at lower segment caesarean section. J Obstet Gynaecol 2005;25:10–4

60. Hwu YM, Chen CP, Chen HS, Su TH. Parallel vertical compression sutures: a technique to control bleeding from placenta praevia or accreta during caesarean section. BJOG 2005;112:1420–3

61. Wu HH, Yeh GP. Uterine cavity synechiae after hemostatic square suturing technique. Obstet Gynecol 2005;105:1176–8

62. Ochoa M, Allaire AD, Stitely ML. Pyometria after hemostatic square suture technique. Obstet Gynecol 2002;99:506–9

63. Cho JY, Kim SJ, Cha KY, Kay CW, Kim MI, Cha KS. Interrupted circular suture: bleeding control during cesarean delivery in placenta previa accreta. Obstet Gynecol 1991;78:876–9

29

The Management of Placenta Accreta at Queen's Hospital, Romford, UK

M. O. Thompson, C. Otigbah, A. Kelkar, A. Coker, A. Pankhania and S. Kapoor

GENERAL COMMENTS

Introduction

Placenta accreta, increta and percreta are all forms of morbidly adherent placenta (MAP) with abnormally invasive placentation. Histologically defined by trophoblastic invasion of the myometrium in the absence of intervening decidua, superficial myometrial invasion is classed as accreta, deeper myometrial invasion as increta, and invasion through the serosa or into adjacent pelvic organs as percreta[1]. The condition was of such rarity 60 years ago that many experienced practicing obstetricians had never encountered a case, and the associated maternal mortality rate was extremely high (37–67% of cases managed)[2]. Although associated maternal mortality is now significantly lower (7–10% of cases)[3,4], it remains a much dreaded obstetric complication primarily because of the risk to the mother. Although awareness of the condition and its attendant risks is increasing, no consensus exists regarding the best management strategies to maximize outcomes. This paucity of information hampers service planning and decisions on optimal management strategies and presents difficulties in conducting meaningful research, particularly comparative studies (see Chapter 1).

Clinical significance

Women with placenta accreta or any of its variants are at high risk of life-threatening massive obstetric hemorrhage, bladder or ureteric injury, uterine perforation and rupture, peripartum hysterectomy and maternal death[1]. The prevalence is apparently on the increase globally due to the increasing cesarean delivery rates and advancing maternal age[5]. Reported prevalence in the 1930s was less than 1 in 30,000 deliveries, increasing to 1 in 2510 deliveries in the 1980s and up to 1 in 540 deliveries as reported in some centers by 2006[5,6].

Local significance

The Maternity Unit at Queen's Hospital, Romford, is the high-risk section of one of the largest acute hospital trusts in the UK, with an average annual delivery rate of 10,000 births. The Trust serves a population of 750,000 from a wide range of social and ethnic groups. Active screening for MAP commenced after a maternal death from a morbidly adherent placenta in 2006. In the subsequent 4-year period, a positive antenatal diagnosis was made in 17 of the 39,120 pregnancies. There was one false positive diagnosis, giving an annual prevalence of 1:2445 deliveries for MAP. This chapter reviews the medical literature on MAP and draws on the experience provided by these cases.

Diagnosis

Traditionally, a diagnosis of MAP was made either clinically following difficult or failed attempts at manual placental removal of a MAP or histopathologically following peripartum hysterectomy or autopsy (Figure 1). In our unit, as is the case in many centers worldwide, antenatal diagnosis is now increasingly made using a combination of ultrasound and magnetic resonance imaging (MRI).

Diagnosis of a MAP in the first trimester is exceedingly rare. It is usually encountered acutely following unexpectedly severe uterine bleeding during pregnancy[7], termination or evacuation of retained

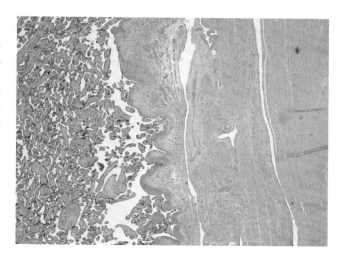

Figure 1 Histological slide showing placenta accreta

products of conception. Some cases present with heavy genital tract bleeding a few weeks or months after the evacuation of a spontaneous, missed or incomplete miscarriage and the diagnosis of a retained placenta accreta, increta or percreta is made only after histological examination following surgery[8–10].

Currently, most cases are detected in the second trimester, although the diagnosis may remain inconclusive until the later stages of pregnancy if or when there are no symptoms of vaginal bleeding to prompt earlier investigation. When vaginal bleeding occurs early on in the first and second trimesters, however, near-catastrophic blood loss is the usual result in most cases. As a consequence, there have been calls to commence ultrasound screening for MAP early, as part of the 11–14 week nuchal translucency screening scan[11,12]. Indeed, close scrutiny of the uterine wall, umbilical cord insertion and placentation at the 11–14 week ultrasound screening may be helpful in establishing a diagnosis of MAP at such early gestations.

Risk factors

The commonest etiologic factors seen with MAP are a previous endomyometrial injury in conjunction with a low lying placenta[13]. Women with placenta previa and a previous cesarean delivery are now well established as being at greatest risk for MAP[14]. Screening for MAP is therefore possible by combining the previous obstetric history with a thorough ultrasound examination of the placenta. In women who are found to have placenta previa on ultrasound, the association with previous cesarean section delivery is strong, and the risk of MAP increases from 24% with one previous cesarean to 67% with three or more previous cesareans[15]. Other important associated factors include a short birth interval following a cesarean delivery[16,17], increasing parity and advancing maternal age above 35 years[1].

Biochemical markers

Biochemical detection is not established for MAP. However, elevated maternal serum levels of α fetoprotein (AFP) and serum free β human chorionic gonadotropin (β hCG) have been reported with MAP in the absence of fetal abnormality[18–20]. The rationale is probably similar to other conditions where a breach or leak occurs at fetoplacental–maternal interfaces, although the elevation in AFP is postulated to be more likely related to coexisting placenta previa[21]. An elevated level of creatine kinase, possibly secondary to an endomyometrial breach or increased breakdown, is also reported as a possible marker[20,22]. More sophisticated laboratory tests, including the possibility of antenatal diagnosis from fetal cells in maternal blood are being studied[23].

Ultrasound imaging

Grayscale ultrasound is the mainstay of antenatal diagnosis with a high sensitivity and specificity. Multiple ultrasound diagnostic signs are usually seen in cases later confirmed to have MAP, and, although there is no single pathognomonic feature, most have a strong association. The greater the number of characteristic ultrasound features seen, the more likely is the diagnosis[24], and there may be an increase in the number and clarity of diagnostic ultrasound parameters as gestation increases. Although the superiority and accuracy of one route over another is often debated, the transabdominal and transvaginal routes are often complementary.

Our personal observations suggest that the more severe and extensive the morbid adherence, the easier the antenatal ultrasound diagnosis. Ultrasound appearances, however, do not always accurately predict the clinical severity of bleeding, as perforation and torrential bleeding remain possible, occurring even with small or focal lesions. Ultrasound imaging has a good negative predictive value for the diagnosis of MAP ranging between 92 and 98%, a fact which is invaluable in any good screening program[25,26].

Characteristic findings for MAP on grayscale ultrasound include:

(1) The presence of lacunae;

(2) Loss of the normal hypoechogenic retroplacental myometrial zone;

(3) Irregularity of the retroplacental sonolucent zone;

(4) Thinning, especially less than 1 mm, or disruption of the uterine serosa–bladder interface;

(5) The presence of focal exophytic masses;

(6) Lacunar flow within the placenta[25,27] (Figure 2).

Color Doppler ultrasound

The use of color Doppler can improve the accuracy of diagnosis of MAP by providing a more detailed assessment of the depth of trophoblastic invasion into the myometrium or serosa, especially in an anterior placenta[28–30]. The sensitivity and specificity of color

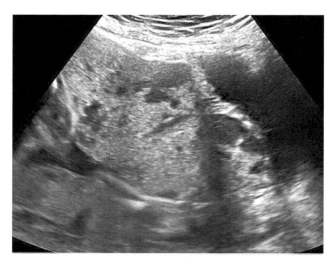

Figure 2 Grayscale image showing presence of lacunae

Doppler in diagnosing placenta previa accreta range between 82.4 and 100% and 92 and 96.8%, respectively[31]. A finding of color Doppler flow within lacunae further increases diagnostic sensitivity to 100%, with an associated 83% positive predictive value for morbid placental adherence[28].

Characteristic findings on color Doppler ultrasound include:

(1) A diffuse lacunar flow pattern with high-velocity pulsatile venous-type flow (peak systolic velocity more than 15 cm/s) spread throughout the placenta, myometrium and cervix;

(2) A central lacunar flow pattern with turbulent flow distributed regionally or focally in the parenchyma;

(3) Bladder–uterine serosal interphase hypervascularity;

(4) Markedly dilated vessels over the peripheral subplacental zone;

(5) An absence of subplacental vascular signals in the areas lacking the peripheral subplacental hypoechoic zone;

(6) Abnormal vascular channels linking the placenta to the bladder[31] (Figure 3).

Three-dimensional ultrasound

It is unclear whether three-dimensional ultrasonography adds any benefit to diagnostic accuracy for MAP[29]. However, viewing planes can be more easily manipulated to enhance views of the vascular framework of the placenta and adjacent tissues, thus improving detection of bladder and parametrial extension. Four-dimensional ultrasound, on the other hand, permits instantaneous multiplanar reconstructions in real time. This gives an added ability to display and rotate reconstructed images from any desired angle, and from any of the three planes: sagittal, coronal, or axial (Figure 4).

Three-dimensional color power Doppler ultrasound

The role of three-dimensional color power Doppler is better established. Color power Doppler ultrasound is reportedly the most sensitive and specific single criterion (sensitivity 97% and specificity 92%), with the highest positive predictive value currently reported for diagnosis[24,32] (Figure 5). *This is the single most reliable diagnostic modality* and it increases diagnostic confidence in determining the exact site, depth and extent of invasion. Characteristic findings on three-dimensional color power Doppler ultrasound include:

(1) Numerous dilated and coherent vessels involving the serosa–bladder interface on a basal view;

(2) Increased intraplacental hypervascularity;

(3) Inseparable cotyledonal and intervillous circulations;

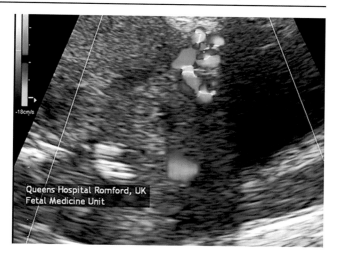

Figure 3   Color Doppler image of placenta increta

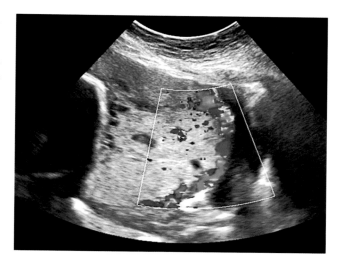

Figure 4   Three-dimensional color Doppler image showing placenta percreta

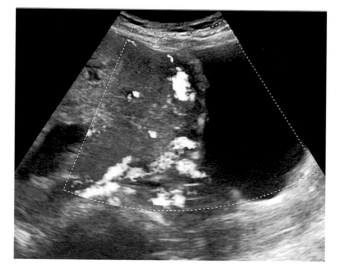

Figure 5   Color power Doppler image of placenta increta

(4) Tortuous vascularity with chaotic branching;

(5) Detour vessels on the lateral view[24,32] (Figure 6).

Magnetic resonance imaging

MRI is an imaging modality that does not require the use of ionizing radiation, provides excellent tissue definition and additionally allows multiplanar imaging. MRI is increasingly useful in planning surgery, particularly in the evaluation of posteriorly sited placentas, in obese women and in pregnancies complicated by a reduced amniotic fluid volume, although claustrophobia in some women may limit its use[33–36]. The additional use of an image enhancing contrast material such as gadolinium is controversial because of the maternal and fetal risks, but this has been used in circumstances where the benefits of an accurate diagnosis appear to far outweigh potential complications. MRI is a valuable diagnostic tool for MAPs with a good negative predictive ability. *Characteristic MRI findings include lower uterine segment thinning, protrusions from the uterine wall, heterogeneous signal intensity within the placenta and dark intraplacental bands on T2-weighted imaging[33–37]* (Figure 7).

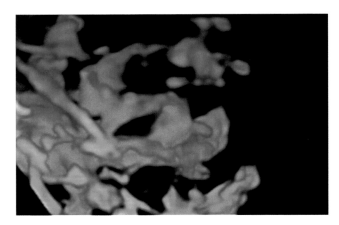

Figure 6 Three-dimensional power color Doppler image of placenta increta

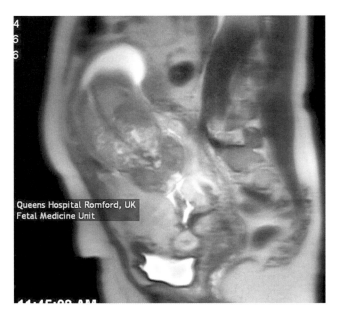

Figure 7 MRI scan showing placenta increta

Screening for morbidly adherent placentas

The role of screening for MAP has yet to be established, even though a more widespread use of this modality would offer clear advantages. In our unit, screening commenced in 2006, using the antenatal booking history and ultrasound as the starting points for our search. Any woman with a history of previous uterine surgery receives a thorough placental assessment at the 20 week second trimester ultrasound scan by a sonographer. A check is made for the diagnostic pointers described above and, if any positive findings are present, the woman is referred to the fetal medicine unit for a consultant's assessment. Where required, an MRI scan is performed at 32 weeks' gestation to help confirm or reject the diagnosis. A diagnosis made in the third trimester is usually conclusive, and adequate preparations for a safe delivery can begin.

Management of morbidly adherent placentas

The most important aspects of management are:

(1) The early identification of women at high risk of MAP;

(2) Intensive multidisciplinary care;

(3) Care and delivery in an appropriately equipped unit.

The care of women diagnosed at any stage of pregnancy with MAP should be conducted by obstetricians working as part of a multidisciplinary team. In our unit two senior obstetricians specialized in fetomaternal medicine supervise the care of women with a diagnosis of MAP. This ensures that routine pregnancy assessments and care are not ignored as a result of the overriding concerns about the risks of placental bleeding. In the 5-year period since screening commenced and our multidisciplinary care team was constituted, we have now encountered 23 cases exhibiting the entire spectrum of MAP across the gestational range.

Planned management in antenatally diagnosed cases

After the antenatal diagnosis of MAP, a multidisciplinary team is assembled. Ideally the team should include specialist obstetricians, anesthetists, urologists, interventional radiologists, hematologists, neonatologists, blood transfusion specialists, operating department practitioners, portering staff and theater nurses and assistants trained to assist in performance of cesarean hysterectomy and laparotomy, along with a full complement of gynecological, vascular surgery and urology instruments. In reality, this list needs to be modified to comply with local needs, requirements and resources.

At Queen's Hospital, Romford, because of the level of risk involved, emergency contact telephone numbers for the delivery suite and senior specialist obstetric team are provided to the woman and her family with 24-hour availability of at least one senior member of the obstetric team. Details of her diagnosis; the grade and extent of morbid adherence; possible risks and complications to mother and baby; mode, details and risks of planned conservative or extirpative management; the likely need for transfusion with blood products; cystoscopy; ureteric stenting; arterial embolization in the interventional radiology theater suite; selective arterial ligation; planned abdominal incision, type of cesarean section planned; and type of hysterectomy planned are all documented in the hospital antenatal hand-held records. An agreed, signed birth plan with all these details boldly marked on the risk assessment page is also attached to the woman's hand-held hospital notes for contingency reasons.

Counseling

Counseling the woman and her family is crucial and is undertaken primarily by obstetric members of the team who are the point of first contact. The gravity of this condition often dictates prolonged and detailed discussions with multiple family members present in order to ensure a clear understanding. We, therefore hold our discussion sessions in the Fetal Medicine Unit (FMU) counseling room separately, and apart from the routine antenatal clinic sessions for this purpose. After the initial counseling sessions, a definitive management plan is agreed in consultation with the woman and her family by the 32nd week of pregnancy when the diagnosis would have been confirmed by the ultrasound and MRI examinations.

Counseling includes advice to refrain from sexual intercourse until after delivery, to ensure that the woman is not left unattended or on her own at home, and to arrange ambulance transfer to hospital immediately if vaginal bleeding occurs. Advice is also given to report any genital tract discharge, hematuria, abdominal pain or uterine contractions to hospital immediately via the delivery suite emergency telephone hotline. Ambulance services can then be contacted by our midwifery staff or directly via a telephone call from the woman to arrange hospital transfer.

It must be ascertained that the woman lives within easy commuting distance of the hospital and that there have been no prior episodes of vaginal bleeding or other complications before agreeing to outpatient care following the diagnosis. The plans for operative delivery, possible need for blood transfusion, uterine preservation and hysterectomy are discussed in detail with the woman and her relatives before the third trimester and any concerns regarding these are thoroughly discussed. All the discussions are carefully recorded in the hospital notes. Women who live more than 10 miles from the hospital are either managed as inpatients or referred to their local hospital with all their results to date and a copy of the plan of care and delivery.

Consent

Consent for surgical treatment options should be obtained early, soon after the diagnosis, because of the risk of urgent radical operative intervention before the end of the second trimester or emergency preterm delivery. The consent form we use details the planned conservative or extirpative management, associated risks and complications, need for transfusion with blood products, preoperative cystoscopy, ureteric stenting, arterial embolization in the interventional radiology theater suite, selective arterial ligation, planned abdominal incision, type of cesarean section planned, and type of hysterectomy planned with extirpative management. This is individualized, with these details entered manually on the routine National Health Service operation consent form.

Coordination

Antenatal care and multidisciplinary team coordination is handled by the FMU consultant obstetricians, a designated senior midwife and blood transfusion specialist practitioners who all liaise closely with each other and inform and update other team members regularly. Close monitoring for any other incidental pregnancy associated complications continues under the care of the specialist obstetricians. Serial ultrasound scans to assess fetal growth and maternal assessments are arranged at 24, 28 and 32 weeks of gestation. The anesthetic and neonatology team members are involved once viability has been attained.

Gestational age at delivery

This is decided upon on an individual basis depending on the risk to the mother including severe maternal genital tract bleeding, any associated medical or obstetric conditions, fetal status and available facilities for neonatal intensive care. Timing of delivery is discussed at 32 weeks with the multidisciplinary team. In the absence of significant antenatal complications, delivery is usually aimed for 37 weeks' gestation. Early transfer to an appropriate unit should be arranged if appropriate local facilities for neonatal care are deemed suboptimal.

Multidisciplinary team involvement and planning

Preoperative review

A multidisciplinary team review is held at 32 weeks where clinical status of both mother and baby, all imaging, hematology and other test results are discussed, and the plan for delivery is reassessed with any new findings. A diagnosis of parametrial invasion is particularly important in planning surgery[37]. This is assessed antenatally using three-dimensional color Doppler ultrasound and MRI at 32 weeks to enable planning of the surgical technique at the multidisciplinary team meeting with the team's interventional radiologists, urologists and obstetricians.

The final multidisciplinary review takes place in the week before delivery, usually between 34 and 36 weeks. An evaluation of the items listed in Figure 8 is

Checklist for 32-week multidisciplinary team meeting	Details
1. Operation consent forms	
2. Planned anesthesia	
3. Choice of abdominal incision	
4. Planned uterine preservation	
5. Planned placental retention	
6. Anticipated parametrial or paravesical dissection	
7. Anticipated interventional radiology procedures	
8. Anticipated blood transfusion requirements	
9. Any concurrent medical or obstetric complications?	

Figure 8 Morbidly adherent placenta (MAP) multidisciplinary team management checklist

performed and each item is crossed off the checklist once dealt with. At this stage decisions are taken regarding the team members required to attend the delivery, the sterile packs required, which operating theater is to be used and the theater staff who will attend. In order to allow ample time and preparation for the delivery and after care the number of cases booked for other elective surgery in the delivery suite theaters on that morning is curtailed.

Pre-delivery specialist anesthetic reviews are also arranged to decide on the anesthetic plan in consultation with the woman in time for discussion at this meeting along with the neonatology review.

The hematology team members are closely involved in antenatal care; any pre-existing anemia is corrected where possible prior to delivery, and all women who decline blood products are identified to explore means of boosting their hemoglobin levels, avoid excessive blood loss and identify what blood products, if any, they would accept under emergency life-threatening conditions (Chapter 72). This is particularly important because even minimal blood loss in an anemic or undernourished woman could have more profound consequences[38].

This activity is especially valuable in developing countries where access to blood transfusion facilities may be quite a distance away, thereby necessitating early referral and transfer to an appropriate center for hospital-based care until delivery.

Women with a previous cesarean delivery and placenta previa or antenatally suspected morbid placental adherence should be delivered in units where at least a level 2 critical care bed is available. For women who decline blood products, transfer to delivery units where cell salvage and interventional radiology are available is recommended[39]. Women living in developing countries or in areas where no surgical or blood transfusion services are available should be transferred early to secondary or tertiary units where these exist[38,40].

MANAGEMENT OPTIONS

The definitive treatment strategy for MAP is either conservative or extirpative, with the surgical removal of the placenta, uterus or both. Overall, the planned management depends on the degree of placental invasion and the woman's desire to retain her reproductive capacity.

Conservative management

Conservative management is defined by uterine preservation and retention of fertility. Various conservative management methods are described, but, in general, the practice is either to undertake manual placental removal immediately after the delivery of the baby or to proceed with planned placental retention, awaiting either spontaneous expulsion or resorption. In some case reports, manual placental removal has been undertaken after a delayed interval to permit regression of the vascular supply. In other reported cases, immediate placental morcellation, curettage or removal piecemeal followed by the insertion of a uterine pack, uterine tamponade device, balloon catheter or the application of uterine hemostatic or compression sutures have been successful[2,41–47].

Other semiconservative interventions, improvized on the spur-of-the-moment in critical emergency situations to avoid further bleeding complications or more drastic surgery are reported. These include oversewing of the placental bed, or suturing flaps of cervix or surgical mesh to cover defects[41,48].

In cases presenting acutely in the first or second trimester, simple excision and repair of defects caused by the implantation, curettage or removal followed by insertion of a tamponade balloon[49], hysterotomy and evacuation of products or, rarely, wedge resection and repair of myometrium have been reported[48,50].

Those presenting acutely in the third trimester are more often seen during the third stage of labor, after the delivery of the infant. The commonest presentation is of a retained placenta with the finding of an absent cleavage plane for its safe removal. *Conservative management under these circumstances involves leaving the entire placenta in situ for removal later or awaiting spontaneous complete resorption.*

The woman is carefully counseled about the findings and her risks, and closely followed up weekly for at least 6 weeks with regular clinical and ultrasound examinations, monitoring her white cell count and differential along with inflammatory markers such as C-reactive protein to assess for signs of infection. A broad-spectrum prophylactic antibiotic such as amoxicillin and clavulanic acid is given for 10 days.

Complications have been reported with the conservative management of MAP. These include immediate to late postpartum vaginal bleeding up to 3 months after delivery which could result in disseminated intravascular coagulation (DIC), infectious morbidity, fever secondary to tissue necrosis, prolonged retention of products of conception and placental polyps. Rarely, vesicouterine fistulas or urethral strictures may occur from placental necrosis secondary to placenta percreta[44,46]. There is no respite until the placenta is completely reabsorbed or expelled and at the 6 week follow-up visit the histopathology findings should be reviewed.

In acutely presenting cases postpartum where there is continued or heavy bleeding, radiological embolization or selective surgical arterial ligation of the internal iliac and uterine arteries should be arranged immediately. In some instances, the placenta is then expelled shortly afterwards, within 48 hours to 6 weeks, although it may take up to 6 months and sometimes over a year for the placenta to be entirely reabsorbed[46]. If bleeding does not cease, despite uterotonic administration and arterial occlusion, uterine balloon tamponade, or uterine compression sutures should be tried[49,50].

True MAPs do not undergo complete spontaneous separation from the uterine wall in the third stage, leading to significant attendant risks of secondary hemorrhage, infection and the need for a hysterectomy at a later time. An awareness of these risks has motivated the introduction of interventions to attempt to hasten placental involution. These include reducing blood supply to the uterus through transcatheter arterial embolization, selective surgical arterial ligation or stepwise devascularization[50–54]. Attempts to expedite resorption by inducing placental necrosis using cytotoxic therapy, especially methotrexate, are also well reported in the literature[55–58].

Methotrexate efficacy is not well substantiated, and no standard mode of administration, treatment dosages or protocols exist. Moreover, reports of failed conservative management associated with its use exist[56,57], as do reports of maternal mortality associated with low dose administration for ectopic gestations or with intraumbilical cord injections[59,60]. Because successful conservative management without the use of methotrexate is now reported[46], it may be advisable to refrain from its use as an adjunct. In our unit adjunctive methotrexate in the treatment of MAP was discontinued following catastrophic complications associated with a maternal death secondary to fulminant sepsis and tissue necrosis.

Radiological transcatheter pelvic arterial embolization, on the other hand, is reportedly more effective with conservative management[62], although its prophylactic value is still debated and repeat embolizations may have to be performed[63]. There are no known randomized controlled trials of the use of arterial embolization in the management of MAPs. A review conducted for the World Health Organization in 2009 concluded that although there may be resource issues, it should be considered a recommended intervention for the control of obstetric hemorrhage where readily available[38].

The various adjunctive measures described above are used to prevent, reduce or treat the massive obstetric hemorrhage associated with placental retention or removal, and each is discussed fully in the pertinent chapters. *In the context of MAPs, the usual primary cause of dangerous vaginal bleeding is attempted manual removal which at any stage is fraught with danger and should be strongly resisted[64,65].*

Extirpative management

Extirpative management could be conducted as either an emergency or electively, and is characterized by removal of the placenta and the uterus[64]. Although surgery can be performed immediately, it may need to be deferred depending on the type of presentation and clinical status, to undertake planned placental retention with or without an adjunctive modality, followed by an interval hysterectomy.

Emergency management in acutely presenting cases

Management of MAP presenting acutely in the first and second trimesters is individualized according to the mode of presentation, maternal condition and severity. Definitive management includes hemodynamic stabilization with immediate fluid and blood replacement, followed by diagnostic imaging in the form of an emergency ultrasound, computed tomography (CT) or MRI scan when the woman is hemodynamically stable. Based on the results of the scan, the presence or absence of hemoperitoneum and the woman's clinical condition, an operative procedure is planned. As the risk is very high in those presenting at earlier gestational ages, consent for surgery should always include permission for a hysterectomy.

In cases presenting in the third trimester, the placenta should also be left undisturbed while preparations are quickly made for surgery. The intraoperative findings dictate the mode of treatment. A hysterectomy is the treatment of choice in most severe cases, while selective radiological arterial embolization or other hemostatic methods may be useful in facilitating surgery and arresting hemorrhage. In desperate cases, aortic compression may be required to control uterine bleeding and can be done safely for up to 4 hours until it is controlled or help becomes available[65].

A primary decision required with extirpative management is whether to perform an immediate or interval hysterectomy. It also has to be decided whether a total or subtotal (supracervical) hysterectomy is more appropriate. A subtotal hysterectomy is more expedient particularly in moribund cases, but a total hysterectomy with removal of the cervix is advocated by some surgeons because of concerns about delayed hemorrhage from the hypervascularized vault especially in cases of placenta previa accreta.

In practice, the decision is often best taken intraoperatively based on the patient's physical condition, the degree of distortion of the pelvic anatomy by placental infiltration or scarring from previous surgery and the severity of bleeding. Surgical skill and experience significantly influence the decisions because of the distorted anatomy that often accompanies morbid placental adherence, and situations may arise where a subtotal operation is preferred because of the woman's clinical status, or limited operator experience. Interested readers should consult Chapter 31.

Elective management in antenatally diagnosed cases

Since commencing our screening program, the vast majority of cases presenting in our unit are now diagnosed prior to the late second trimester and are delivered electively in the daytime when proper arrangements for major operative interventions can be made. This helps to prevent major complications such as those described above.

Immediate preoperative preparation

The equipment and supplies checklist (Figure 9) is reviewed the day prior to surgery, and the blood transfusion specialist practitioner checks hematology and blood bank supplies. On the morning of surgery, the woman is admitted from home after an overnight fast or is transferred from the antenatal ward if already admitted, and the consent forms and theater checklist are reviewed once again.

The color Doppler and MRI findings accurately predict the need for preoperative ureteric stenting[37], a fact which has been our experience during the past 5 years. If required, intravascular balloon embolization catheters are inserted in the interventional radiology theater suite, before the woman is transferred to the delivery suite operating theater with the catheters ready in place. The preoperative checklist is then reviewed.

Preoperative placental site mapping is performed with a review of the ultrasound and MRI scans by the urologist, interventional radiologist and obstetricians to identify areas of potential difficulty with dissection, areas of particular hypervascularity and, very importantly, specific areas of parametrial, inferolateral pelvic or bladder extension. An ultrasound scan can be performed intraoperatively to map the placental coverage area using a sterile probe cover. At Queen's, we usually mark the placental outlines on the abdominal skin prior to skin preparation and draping, using a surigcal skin marker fiber-tip pen.

Intraoperative management

Cystoscopy

A preoperative cystoscopy is performed in all our cases with placenta previa or suspected bladder invasion. Complete penetration or excrescences through the bladder mucosa are rare, but venous congestion and areas of hypervascularity are commonly visible in cases with placenta increta–percreta (Figure 10).

Ureteric stenting

The place of ureteric stenting in the management of the MAP remains in question[68]. The potential benefits include earlier intraoperative diagnosis of ureteric injury and more rapid and easier identification of injured ureters even in the presence of profuse bleeding[68]. However, some surgeons argue that the process

Checklist for operative equipment and supplies	Details
1. Cell salvage machine	
2. Central arterial line	
3. High pressure suction pumps	
4. Wide bore intravenous access x 2	
5. High volume intravascular infusion pumps	
6. 4 units of crossmatched packed red blood cells (2 units in the delivery suite fridge for immediate use)	
7. Clotting factors and fresh frozen plasma	
8. Body warmers and warming blankets, Bair-Hugger® and space blankets	
9. Intraoperative calf-compression devices – Flowtron® boots	
10. Instruments for cystoscopy, ureteric stenting, bowel and bladder resection and a vascular surgery set	

Figure 9 Morbidly adherent placenta (MAP) preoperative checklist: equipment and supplies

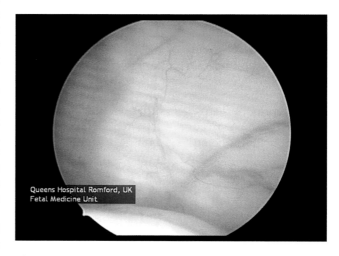

Figure 10 Cystoscopic image showing dilated venous channels with a placenta increta

of stenting abolishes the elasticity of the ureters and makes them more liable to injury than when normal recoil and peristaltic activity is present[69]. In addition, stenting could possibly kink or displace (and thereby relocate) the ureters, increasing their risk of damage during surgery[69].

Perhaps of greater relevance to the more invasive grades of MAP, it has been argued that even if ureteric stenting does not prevent ureteric injuries, it does not permit such injury to go unrecognized at surgery. This is important, because non-recognition of ureteric injury leads to serious complications. That being said, ureteric stenting is not without risk of complications itself[67–69], including urinary tract infection, reflex anuria secondary to ureterovesical junction edema, renocortical vasoconstriction following catheter stimulation, and even the rare ureterovenous fistula[70]. In a recent study, it was determined that although ureteric stenting did not seem to lead to a reduction in ureteric injury, its use was associated with a reduction in early postoperative morbidity[71].

Direct visualization of the ureters during surgery is the only proven preventive measure against injury[73]. Prophylactic ureteric stenting does not eliminate ureteric injuries and can therefore not replace direct visualization of the ureters and meticulous surgical technique to avoid complications[72–74].

In summary, although ureteric stenting cannot eliminate ureteric injuries, it may be advisable where an increased risk of injury is present[69]. The greatest blood loss occurs during dissection of the bladder from the lower uterine segment, and the presence of ureteric stents allows more rapid, continuous localization of the ureters, a process that may reduce operative time and blood loss as well as the likelihood of ureteric injury[73].

In our unit, we insert ureteric catheters in cases with bladder base involvement, posteroinferior bladder wall infiltration or parametrial extension because of the likelihood that more extensive dissection would be required, thereby increasing the risk of ureteric damage (Figure 11).

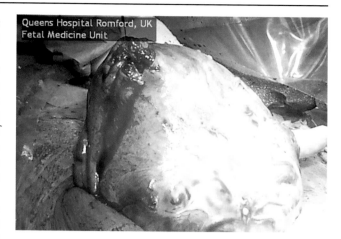

Figure 11   Intraoperative image showing placenta increta

Operative delivery of the infant

The fetal presentation and position are checked preoperatively by ultrasound in anticipation of any manipulations that may be required to effect delivery. A classical cesarean or transfundal uterine incision[75] is made away from the upper placental margin that has been marked preoperatively, to effect delivery of the infant without impinging on the placenta (an image of fundal delivery is found in Chapter 1). The umbilical cord is then ligated, transected and trimmed close to its placental insertion. Where antenatal ultrasound and MRI scans have shown morbid adherence and there is intraoperative evidence of the same, no attempt is made at placental removal. *Forceful or delayed attempts at placental removal are not to be made because of the risk of severe life-threatening hemorrhage,* therefore uterotonics are given at this stage, and the uterine incision is closed.

Selective arterial embolization (Figure 12) or surgical ligation is then performed to reduce the uteroplacental blood supply. In most of our cases, we clamp both internal iliac arteries temporarily until the hysterectomy is completed, only surgically ligating these where there is or has been significant bleeding. In cases with moderate bladder involvement, we perform a wide anterior uterine wall dissection next, reflecting the bladder to expose the lower segment and cervix, and the hysterectomy then follows. The bipolar diathermy forceps and hemostatic clips such as the titanium ligaclips (Ethicon Inc, Sommerville NJ, USA), instruments not routinely used in gynecological surgery, are useful in this endeavor. In other, more severe cases, a bladder wedge resection or partial cystectomy may be required. Complete vault closure or re-peritonealization of the vault is not advisable in such cases, because leaving the cuff open permits any postoperative bleeding to become apparent. In other circumstances, faced with brisk ongoing hemorrhage, it is a good idea to perform a subtotal hysterectomy first to arrest the bleeding, as both the uterine and ovarian arteries are usually ligated with the first pedicles taken[65].

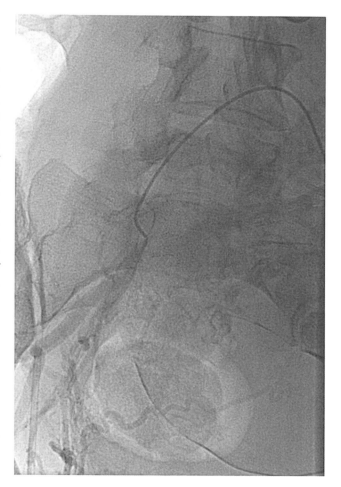

Figure 12   Selective endovascular arterial embolization

An alternative one-step, conservative surgical method has also been proposed as treatment for placenta percreta[45]. The report emanates from a unit with vastly experienced surgeons who have extensive experience with this method which involves extensive dissection and the use of surgical mesh. Although it may hold a place in the management of the more severely invasive placenta percreta, it may not be as appropriate in treating lesser degrees of the condition, particularly in the hands of surgeons who are unfamiliar with the extensive dissection techniques required for its completion[45].

In our experience, during the immediate postnatal period a substantial degree of the florid vascularization and engorgement subsides; therefore, in cases with severe bladder or extensive parametrial invasion, we retain the placenta and an interval hysterectomy is arranged. Where vascular clamps or embolization catheters have been applied, these are removed after the hysterectomy is complete and hemostasis is ensured.

Tissue reconstruction is commenced once this has been achieved. The suture lines created between the bladder and posterior vaginal wall are then covered with an interpositional peritoneal or omental flap if the latter is easily accessible. A U-shaped flap of peritoneum covering the bladder dome is inverted and tacked down onto the vaginal suture line to provide support as previously described by a member of our team[77]. A wide bore Robinson's or corrugated Yates drain is left behind, with mass closure of the abdomen using loop nylon sutures followed by skin closure with sutures or staples.

Various means are available for measuring operative and immediate postpartum blood loss to ensure that blood replacement is adequate[38]. At Queen's, all surgical swabs and sponges are weighed to quantify the blood loss at surgery. We commence blood replacement intraoperatively with the use of the cell salvage machine as guided by the estimation, the patient's vital signs and central venous pressure monitoring.

Postpartum management

After surgery in elective cases, the woman is transferred to either the delivery suite or the obstetric high dependency unit for close postoperative monitoring, further stabilization and care. In the acutely ill or where maternal condition has deteriorated during surgery, transfer to the intensive care unit is arranged for close monitoring, blood and fluid replacement, and correction of any acidosis, hypothermia, or coagulopathy.

Because postpartum hemorrhage is the commonest complication of morbid placental adherence, close observation of blood loss, abdominal drains and intensive monitoring of fluid input and output is crucial. Central venous pressure line monitoring helps reduce the well known underestimation of blood loss at surgery. Stable vital signs and a good hourly urine output are favorable prognostic signs.

Postoperative thromboprophylaxis

There is an increased risk of venous thromboembolism because of the prolonged operating time, heavy blood loss, the extensive pelvic dissection and tissue manipulation, and reduced mobility postoperatively. Prophylactic heparin should therefore be given[39]. We use pneumatic limb compression devices (Flowtron® boots) intraoperatively and administer prophylactic low molecular weight heparins postoperatively for 6 weeks.

SUMMARY AND CONCLUSIONS

We have discussed the contemporary diagnosis and management of MAPs against the background of the 5-year experience in our obstetric unit. Traditionally, management of MAP centered around hysterectomy[71], but recently the emphasis has changed to favor other, minimally invasive and fertility preserving options[41–46,52,79]. Although conservative management strategies carry a significant risk of maternal morbidity and mortality, they remain viable options that can be safely exercised.

Proper management should be based on accurate early diagnosis with appropriate perioperative multidisciplinary planning to anticipate and avoid massive obstetric hemorrhage at delivery. Previously novel treatment options and appliances such as the Bakri tamponade balloon and radiological transcatheter arterial embolization have rapidly acquired key management roles in the management of MAP.

Women at risk should be delivered at centers with appropriate expertise and resources for managing this condition. The evidence base for the management of MAPs is not always clear, leaving room for debate over some of the strategies recommended. Further clinical evidence and reports are needed to guide appropriate service planning, provide accurate information to support the counseling of women about the associated risks, and develop management guidelines to enhance patient safety.

ACKNOWLEDGMENTS

We would like to acknowledge the tremendous contributions of all those involved in the multidisciplinary management of MAP at our institution without whom none of this would have been possible. This includes all the sonographers, blood transfusion specialist practitioners, members of the midwifery teams, delivery suite, operating theater staff, the interventional radiology team and staff from the hospital portering service.

References

1. Oyelese Y, Smulian JC. Placenta previa, placenta accreta, and vasa previa. Obstet Gynecol 2006;107:927–41
2. McKeogh RP, D'Errico E. placenta accreta: clinical manifestations and conservative management. N Engl J Med 1951;245:159–65
3. Kayem G, Davy C, Goffinet F, Thomas C, Clement D, Cabrol D. Conservative versus extirpative management in cases of placenta accreta. Obstet Gynecol 2004;104:531–6
4. Sonin A. Nonoperative treatment of placenta percreta: value of MR imaging. AJR 2001;177:1301–3
5. Wu S, Kocherginsky M, Hibbard JU. Abnormal placentation: twenty-year analysis. Am J Obstet Gynecol 2005;192:1458–61
6. Silver RM, Landon MB, Rouse DJ, et al. Maternal morbidity associated with multiple repeat cesarean deliveries. Obstet Gynecol 2006;107:1226–32

7. Shih JC, Cheng WF, Shyu MK, Lee CN, Hsieh FJ. Power Doppler evidence of placenta accreta appearing in the first trimester. Ultrasound Obstet Gynecol 2002;19:623–5

8. Amoh Y, Watanabe Y, Saga T, et al. Retained placenta accreta: MRI and pathologic correlation. J Comput Assist Tomogr 1995;19:827–9

9. Davis JD, Cruz A. Persistent placenta increta: a complication of conservative management of presumed placenta accreta. Obstet Gynecol 1996;88:653–4

10. Avva R, Shah HR, Angtuaco TL. Retained placenta increta following missed miscarriage. US Case of the day. Radiographics 1999;19:1089–92

11. Fisher SJ, Zhou Y, Huang L, Winn VD. When is seeing believing? The use of color Doppler ultrasound to diagnose placenta accreta in the first trimester of pregnancy. Ultrasound Obstet Gynecol 2002;19:540–2

12. Stirnemann J, Forner S, Bernard J, Ville Y. Screening for placenta accreta by ultrasound in the first trimester. Ultrasound Obstet Gynecol 2010;36:139–40

13. Beuker JM, Erwich JJHM, Khong TY. Is endomyometrial injury during termination of pregnancy or curettage following miscarriage the precursor to placenta accreta? J Clin Pathol 2005;58:273–5

14. Esakoff TF, Sparks TN, Kaimal AJ, et al. Diagnosis and morbidity of placenta accreta. Ultrasound Obstet Gynecol 2011;37:324–7

15. Clark SL, Koonings PP, Phelan JP. Placenta previa/accreta and prior Cesarean section. Obstet Gynecol 1985;66:89–92

16. Wax JR, Seiler A, Horowitz S, Ingardia CJ. Interpregnancy interval as a risk factor for placenta accreta. Conn Med 2000; 64:659–61

17. Shipp TD, Zelop CM, Repke JT, Cohen A, Lieberman E. Interdelivery interval and risk of symptomatic uterine rupture. Obstet Gynecol 2001;97:175–7

18. Zelop C, Nadel A, Frigoletto FD Jr, Pauker S, MacMillan M, Benacerraf BR. Placenta accreta/percreta/ increta: a cause of elevated maternal serum alphafetoprotein. Obstet Gynecol 1992;80:693–4

19. Kupferminc MJ, Tamura RK, Wigton TR, et al. Placenta accreta is associated with elevated maternal serum alphafetoprotein. Obstet Gynecol 1993;82:266–9

20. Hung TH, Shau WY, Hsieh CC, Chiu TH, Tsu JJ, TC Hsieh. Risk factors for placenta accreta. Obstet Gynecol 1999;93:545–50

21. Butler EI, Dashe JS, Ramus RM. Association between maternal serum alpha-fetoprotein and adverse outcomes in pregnancies with placenta praevia. Obstet Gynecol 2001;97:35–8

22. Ophir E. Tendler R, Odeh M, et al. Creatine kinase as a biochemical marker in diagnosis of placenta increta and percreta. Am J Obstet Gynecol 1999;180:1039–40

23. Miura S, Yamasaki K, Yoshida A, et al. Increased level of cell-free placenta mRNA in a subgroup of placenta previa that needs hysterectomy. Prenat Diagn 2008;28:805–9

24. Shih JC, Palacios Jaraquemada JM, Su YN, et al. Role of three-dimensional power Doppler in the antenatal diagnosis of placenta accreta: comparison with gray-scale and color Doppler techniques. Ultrasound Obstet Gynecol 2009;33: 193–203

25. Dwyer BK, Belogolovkin V, Tran L, Rao A, Carroll I, Barth R, Chitkara U. Prenatal diagnosis of placenta accreta: sonography or magnetic resonance imaging? J Ultrasound Med 2008;27:1275–81

26. Warshak CR, Eskander R, Hull AD, et al. Accuracy of ultrasonography and magnetic resonance imaging in the diagnosis of placenta accreta. Obstet Gynecol 2006;108:573–81

27. Comstock CH. Antenatal diagnosis of placenta accreta: a review. Ultrasound Obstet Gynecol 2005;26:89–96

28. Lerner JP, Deane S, Timor-Tritsch IE. Characterization of placenta accreta using transvaginal sonography and color Doppler imaging. Ultrasound Obstet Gynecol 1995;5: 198–201

29. Levine D, Hulka CA, Ludmir J, Li W, Edelman RR. Placenta accreta: evaluation with color Doppler ultrasound, power Doppler ultrasound and MR imaging. Radiology 1997;205:773–6

30. Twickler DM, Lucas MJ, Balis AB, et al. Color flow mapping for myometrial invasion in women with a prior Cesarean delivery. J Matern Fetal Med 2000;9:330–5

31. Chou MM, Ho ES, Lee YH. Prenatal diagnosis of placenta previa accreta by transabdominal color Doppler ultrasound. Ultrasound Obstet Gynecol 2000;15:28–35

32. Chou MM, Tseng JJ, Ho ESC, Hwang JI. Three-dimensional color power Doppler imaging in the assessment of uteroplacental neovascularization in placenta previa increta-percreta. Am J Obstet Gynecol 2001;185:1257–60

33. Kirkinen P, Helin-Martikainen HL, Vanninen R, Partanen K. Placenta accreta: Imaging by gray-scale and contrast-enhanced color Doppler sonography and magnetic resonance imaging. J Clin Ultrasound 1998;26:90–4

34. Lam G, Kuller J, McMahon M. Use of magnetic resonance imaging and ultrasound in the antenatal diagnosis of placenta accreta. J Soc Gynecol Invest 2002;9:37–40

35. Taipale P, Orden MR, Berg M, Manninen H, Alafuzof I. Prenatal diagnosis of placenta accreta and percreta with ultrasonography, color Doppler, and magnetic resonance imaging. Obstet Gynecol 2004;104:537–40

36. Laifer-Narin S. Utility of MRI in the evaluation of abnormal placentation. Ultrasound Obstet Gynecol 2007;30: 456–546

37. Palacios Jaraquemada JM, Bruno CH. Magnetic resonance imaging in 300 cases of placenta accreta: surgical correlation of new findings. Acta Obstet Gynecol Scand 2005;84:716–24

38. World Health Organization. WHO Guidelines for the Management of Postpartum Haemorrhage and Retained Placenta. Geneva, Switzerland: WHO Press, 2009:21–3

39. Royal College of Obstetricians and Gynaecologists. Placenta praevia, placenta praevia accreta and vasa praevia: diagnosis and management. Clinical guideline no 27. London: RCOG Press, 2011

40. Snelgrove JW. Postpartum haemorrhage in the developing world; a review of clinical management strategies. McGill J Med 2009;12:61–6

41. Cox SM, Carpenter RJ, Cotton DB. Placenta percreta: ultrasound diagnosis and conservative surgical management. Obstet Gynecol 1988;71:454–6

42. O'Brien JM, Barton JR, Donaldson ES. The management of placenta percreta: conservative and operative strategies. Am J Obstet Gynecol 1996;175:1632–8

43. Panoskaltsis TA, Ascarelli A, de Souza N, et al. Placenta increta: evaluation of radiological investigations and therapeutic options of conservative management. Br J Obstet Gynaecol 2000;107:802–6

44. Kayem G, Davy C, Goffinet F, Thomas C, Clement D, Cabrol D. Conservative versus extirpative management in cases of placenta accreta. Obstet Gynecol 2004;104:531–6

45. Palacios Jaraquemada J, Pesaresi M, Nassif JC, Hermosid S. Anterior placenta percreta: surgical approach, hemostasis and uterine repair. Acta Obstet Gynecol Scand 2004;83:738–44

46. Timmermans S, van Hof AC, Duvekot JJ. Conservative management of abnormally invasive placentation. Obstet Gynecol Surv 2007;62:529–39

47. Frenzel D, Condous GS, Papageorghiou AT, McWhinney NA. The use of the 'tamponade test' to stop massive obstetric haemorrhage in placenta accreta. BJOG 2005;112:676–7

48. Schnorr JA, Singer JS, Udoff EJ, Taylor PT. Late uterine wedge resection of placenta increta. Obstet Gynecol 1999;94: 823–5

49. Bakri YN. Uterine tamponade-drain for hemorrhage secondary to placenta previa-accreta. Int J Gynaecol Obstet 1992;37: 302–3

50. Morken NH, Henriksen H. Placenta percreta – two cases and review of the literature. Eur J Obstet Gynecol Reprod Biol 2001;100:112–5

51. Alanis M, Hurst BS, Marshburn PB, Matthews ML. Conservative management of placenta increta with selective arterial embolization preserves future fertility and results in a

favourable outcome in subsequent pregnancies. Fertil Steril 2006; 86:1513–7

52. Sentilhes L, Ambroselli C, Kayem G, et al. Maternal outcome after conservative treatment of placenta accreta. Obstet Gynecol 2010;115:526–34

53. Joshi V, Otiv S, Majumder R, Nikam Y, Shrivastava M. Internal iliac artery ligation for arresting postpartum-haemorrhage. BJOG 2007;114:356–61

54. AbdRabbo SA. Step wise uterine devascularization: a novel technique for management of uncontrollable postpartum hemorrhage with preservation of the uterus. Am J Obstet Gynecol 1994;171:694–700

55. Arulkumaran S, Ng CS, Ingemarsson I, Ratnam SS. Medical treatment of placenta accreta with methotrexate. Acta Obstet Gynecol Scand 1986;65:285–6

56. Jaffe R, DuBester B, Sherer DM, Thompson EA, Woods JR. Failure of methotrexate treatment for term placenta previa. Am J Obstet Gynecol 1994;171:558–9

57. Butt K, Gagnon A, Delisle MF. Case report; failure of methotrexate and internal iliac balloon catheterization to manage placenta percreta. Obstet Gynecol 2002;99:981–2

58. Chauleur C, Fanget C, Tourne G, Levy R, Larchez C, Seffert P. Serious primary post-partum hemorrhage, arterial embolization and future fertility: A retrospective study of 46 cases. Hum Reprod 2008;23:1553–9

59. Kelly H, Harvey D, Moll S. A cautionary tale: fatal outcome of methotrexate therapy given for management of ectopic pregnancy. Obstet Gynecol 2006;107:439–41

60. Teal SB. A cautionary tale: fatal outcome of methotrexate therapy given for management of ectopic pregnancy. Obstet Gynecol 2006;107:1420–1

61. Sentilhes L, Gromez A, Clavier E, Resch B, Verspyck E, Marpeau L. Predictors of failed pelvic arterial embolization for severe postpartum hemorrhage. Obstet Gynecol 2009; 113:992–9

62. Deux JF, Bazot M, Le Blanche AF, et al. Is selective embolization of uterine arteries a safe alternative to hysterectomy in patients with postpartum haemorrhage? AJR 2001; 177:145–9

63. Teo SB, Kanagalingam D, Tan HK, Tan LK. Massive postpartum haemorrhage after uterus-conserving surgery in placenta percreta: the danger of the partial placenta percreta. BJOG 2008;115:789–92

64. Palacios-Jaraquemada JM. Diagnosis and management of placenta accreta. Best Pract Res Clin Obstet Gynaecol 2008; 22:1133–48

65. Steer PJ. The surgical approach to postpartum haemorrhage. Obstet Gynaecologist 2009;11:231–8

66. ACOG Committee Opinion. Placenta accreta. Number 266, January 2002. American College of Obstetricians and Gynecologists. Int J Gynaecol Obstet 2002;77:77–8

67. Kyzer S, Gordon PH. The prophylactic use of ureteral catheters during colorectal operations. Am Surg 1994;60:212–6

68. Shingleton HM: Repairing injuries to the urinary tract: update on general surgery. Contemp Obstet Gynecol 1984; 23:76–90

69. Bothwell WN, Bleicher RJ, Dent TL. Prophylactic ureteral catheterization in surgery. Dis Colon Rectum 1994;37: 330–4

70. Bhargava A, Yusuf R. Ureterovenous fistula: an unusual complication of ureteric catheterisation. Br J Urol Int 1987; 60:373–4

71. Eller AG, Porter TF, Poisson P, Silver RM. optimal management strategies for placenta accreta. BJOG 2009;116:648–54

72. Grainger DA, Soderstrom RM, Schiff SF, Glickman MG, DeCherney AH, Diamond MP. Ureteral injuries at laparoscopy: insights into diagnosis, management, and prevention. Obstet Gynecol 1990;75:839–43

73. Kuno K, Menzin A, Kauder HH, Sison C, Gal D. Prophylactic ureteral catheterization in gynecologic surgery. Urology 1998;52:1004–8

74. Chou MT, Wang CJ, Lien RC. Prophylactic ureteral catheterization in gynecologic surgery: a 12-year randomized trial in a community hospital. Int Urogynecol J 2009;20: 689–93

75. Ogawa M, Sato A, Yasuda K, Shimnizu D, Hosoya N, Tanaka T. Cesarean section by transfundal approach for placenta previa percreta attached to anterior uterine wall in a woman with a previous repeat cesarean section: case report. Acta Obstet Gynecol Scand 2004;83:115–6

76. Morgan M, Atalla R. Mifepristone and misoprostol for the management of placenta accreta – a new alternative approach. BJOG 2009;116:1002–3

77. Punekar SV, Prem AR, Kelkar AR, Ridhorkar VR. Repair of complex vesicovaginal interposition : a different design fistulas using peritoneal flap. Indian J Urol 1997;13:24–8

30

Mifepristone and Misoprostol for the Management of Placenta Accreta: an Alternative Approach

R. K. Atalla

INTRODUCTION

The incidence of morbidly adherent placentas has increased ten-fold in the past 50 years, currently occurring at a frequency of 1 per 1000–2500 deliveries[1,2]. It is contributing to a large proportion of postpartum hemorrhages (PPH) and has led to some maternal mortalities and several surgical interventions.

Current management of morbidly adherent placentas – accreta, increta and especially percreta – reportedly result in a maternal mortality rate of up to 7%, and extensive morbidity due to massive hemorrhage, blood transfusions, infection, ureteral damage and fistula formation[3–5]. In developing countries, adherent placenta contributed to 13% of maternal deaths[6].

Traditionally there was a tendency to ensure complete removal of the placental tissue after the delivery to avoid the risk of PPH. This led to a high risk of intervention that sometimes was associated with higher morbidity. In reality, management of adherent placenta should be altered according to the cause of failed delivery of placenta and whether it is associated with PPH.

Several options have been developed over recent years for the management of placenta accreta with limited success rates[7–16]. Recently, the combination of mifepristone/misoprostol was introduced for the treatment of placenta accreta. Both drugs were used over several years for the management of termination of pregnancy with a high success rate to reach complete expulsion of products of conception.

MIFEPRISTONE

Mifepristone is a synthetic steroid compound that is a progesterone antagonist. It also has an anti-implantation effect in early gestation. It causes decidual necrosis which leads to placental detachment. It also increases uterine contractility, softens the cervix and encourages cervical dilatation as well as sensitizes the myometrium to respond to natural or externally administered prostaglandin. It was used successfully in the termination of pregnancy in the first and second trimester, and has been gradually introduced for the induction of labor in the third trimester. Its side-effects are minimal including nausea, vomiting, diarrhea, dizziness, fatigue and fever. Pelvic inflammatory disease (PID) is a very rare but serious complication[17]. Mifepristone's success rate in achieving a complete miscarriage varies around 88% and is sometimes associated with excessive bleeding and incomplete termination of pregnancy requiring further intervention.

MISOPROSTOL

Prostaglandin E1 analogue 'misoprostol' was developed to promote healing of gastric and duodenal ulcers. It soon became apparent that it stimulates uterine contractions[18]. Misoprostol, binds to myometrial cells to cause strong myometrial contractions leading to expulsion of tissue. It also causes cervical ripening with softening and dilatation of the cervix. It has been used successfully to treat uterine atony and hemorrhage in the third stage of labor. As it does not need to be stored refrigerated, it replaced oxytocin for the management of third stage of labor in developing countries and remote areas (see Chapter 15), it was then introduced for the management of PPH in developed countries[19,20] (see Chapter 32). When given in the postpartum period, it is known to cause only minimal side-effects, such as mild shivering and pyrexia. It has been used for induction of labor and induction of abortion[18,20–22].

Misoprostol can be administered orally, sublingually, vaginally or rectally[21]. Oral and sublingual misoprostol are faster and more practical than rectal administration[23,24]. Vaginal and oral misoprostol are of similar efficacy; however, vaginal application has been found to have lower gastrointestinal side-effects, while the oral route was preferred by women[25,26].

Misoprostol alone has been used for the management of adherent placenta with a limited success rate, although it is effective with the added benefit of decreased blood loss.

THE USE OF MIFEPRISTONE/MISOPROSTOL IN THE MANAGEMENT OF PLACENTA ACCRETA AND COMPARISON WITH OTHER TREATMENTS

It was expected that the combination of both drugs would significantly potentiate the success rate for the treatment of placenta accreta in parallel to the increase in the success rate of complete miscarriage from 88% to 96% when mifepristone was used as a pre-treatment to misoprostol[27–31]. Maximum effect of this regimen is achieved when misoprostol is administered 36–48 h after mifepristone. The choice of doses and best regimen has been debated as has the route of administration. The manufacturer recommends a dose of 600 mg of mifepristone prior to prostaglandin administration[32]. However, evidence from a randomized trial indicates that a dose of 200 mg has similar efficacy when compared with 400 mg or 600 mg[33].

When the above regimen is followed 36–48 h later, by a maximum of five doses of misoprostol 400 μg administered at 3 hourly intervals, vaginally or orally, completed abortions were achieved in 94.6% of pregnancies between 9 and 13 weeks and in nearly 91% of mid-trimester medical abortion[34,35].

The insight to use mifepristone and misoprostol in the management of placenta accreta followed on from the high success rate of this regimen to induce a complete abortion. The dose of the medications in such a specific indication has not been established due to the small number of cases treated. However, the safety of this combination has been established in several studies examining termination of pregnancy[36]. Due to the minimally reported possible side-effects, the choice of such a regimen will establish its place rapidly as a safer alternative for the management of placenta accreta[37]. The use of the mifepristone and misoprostol regimen in the management of placenta accreta has been reported in the literature in only two cases both of which resulted in expulsion of the placenta. In both instances manual removal of placenta was attempted and failed to remove any part of the placenta and a postpartum magnetic resonance imaging (MRI) and ultrasound scan established the diagnosis of placenta accreta. However, the timing and dosage of the medication varied between the two.

An attempt to avoid the complications of expectant management and close monitoring led to the first use of mifepristone/misoprostol combination for expulsion of the placenta 15 weeks after delivery. This combination was chosen instead of methotrexate due to the limited success rate and high risk of complications in the latter.

When compared with methotrexate, the mifepristone/misoprostol combination was preferred, as methotrexate has limited success in the treatment of placenta accreta with spontaneous loss of placental tissues occurring in 26% of cases. Furthermore, case reports have shown that intramuscular methotrexate may not have shortened the duration of management treatment from delivery till resorption of placenta. In all 13% of women had complications such as delayed

hemorrhage, infection as well as added possible side-effects of vomiting, alopecia and bone marrow suppression, renal or hepatic impairment; and fatality has been reported[38,39]. Furthermore, in one case the human chorionic gonadotropin levels returned to normal, but the placenta was still attached; this raised more doubt about the success of methotrexate.

In the second case report, the expectant management also had to be abandoned within a few days of the delivery. The patient was developing severe infection and a rapid delivery of the placenta was needed. A dose of mifepristone 600 mg was given and 40 hours later, the placenta was expelled with minimal bleeding prior to the start of the misoprostol regimen[37].

As the mother showed severe signs of infection, surgical options – mainly hysterectomy or more recently myometrial resection – were the only other alternatives[40]. Again medical treatment with the combination of mifepristone/misoprostol compares favorably as a result of the high risk of complications with surgical options and the desire of the mother to preserve her fertility. Only 68 patients with anterior placenta accreta were included in a trial of myometrial resection and uterine repair, and in 18 patients hysterectomies had to be performed[40]. Furthermore, there were a large number of serious reported complications including pelvic hemorrhage, coagulopathies, uterine infection, low ureteral ligations, iatrogenic foreign bodies and collection[40]. Future fertility has only been recorded in 20% of those who had their uterus conserved.

The incidence of peripartum hysterectomy is approximately 1 in 2000 deliveries[41]. Emergency hysterectomy should be reserved only for the treatment of placenta accreta if associated with uncontrollable bleeding due to the associated high maternal morbidity and mortality from hemorrhage, blood transfusion, disseminated intravascular coagulopathy, infection and potential injury to the adjacent lower urinary tract[42–44].

THE POSSIBLE ROLE OF THE MIFEPRISTONE/ MISOPROSTOL REGIMEN IN THE MANAGEMENT OF PLACENTA ACCRETA

Following these successful experiences in our unit, further patients of different gestations were treated with the combination of mifepristone/ misoprostol within a few hours of delivery after failed attempts at manual removal of placenta. In our practice, we offer ultrasound evaluation after delivery which is usually beneficial in assessing placental separation, possibly avoiding intervention especially if the mother has not had any regional analgesia. An attempt at manual removal of the placenta is made if the placenta is adherent; however, the obstetrician should be aware of the other management options available and try to avoid aggressive piece meal removal of the placenta especially if no separation plane can be identified. The regimen of mifepristone 600 mg followed by 200 μg of misoprostol orally at 3 hourly intervals to a maximum of five doses has been used to expel placenta accreta after confirmation of the diagnosis by MRI.

The treatment has been successful in all conditions; however, in one patient vaginal bleeding followed 1 week after completion of treatment and expulsion of the placenta. The bleeding led to hospital admission but did not necessitate any medical intervention. Such a treatment regimen has to be weighed against alternative treatment options.

Advantages of mifepristone/misoprostol regimen

Nearly all maternity units are familiar with the mifepristone/misoprostol combination. The patients do not need any special monitoring as the side-effects of the drugs are minimal and uncommon; however, most units will administer the mifepristone under medical supervision and ask the patient to remain in the unit for 1 hour. Mifepristone should be avoided if the patient suffers from severe asthma, chronic adrenal failure renal or hepatic impairment or acute porphyria, and caution should be used if she suffers from mild asthma, hemorrhagic disorders or is on anticoagulant therapy, or has risk factors for cardiovascular disease or adrenal suppression.

The cost of such a regimen is minimal compared with any alternative. The completed course will be less than £100 and the cost of 1 day of hospital admission if the misoprostol is administered as an inpatient – though this is not essential.

Mifepristone/misoprostol combination has been used successfully to shorten the duration of the conservative management of placenta accreta; therefore, it can be introduced at any time after the delivery, although administration soon after delivery is encouraged. More importantly, mifepristone/misoprostol combination has been shown not to affect future fertility and hence to be superior to surgical options.

The success rate of mifepristone/misoprostol management protocol compares favorably with all surgical interventions which should be avoided and only offered to the patient if there is severe bleeding or when other methods have been exhausted[45].

CONCLUSION

Placenta accreta is difficult to diagnose antenatally by imaging techniques and the diagnosis is usually established after delivery at the time of the manual removal of the retained placenta[46–51]. In hospitals lacking emergency access to an intervention radiologist or vascular surgeon, forcible traumatic removal of placenta accreta could initiate severe hemorrhage and should be avoided. Placenta accreta does not usually cause severe bleeding unless disturbed and partly removed manually. It is essential for the obstetrician to be aware of all management options for such a potential dangerous condition. With the established safety of the new mifepristone/misoprostol combination regimen and growing evidence of its potential efficacy in managing

placenta accreta, this combination should have a role in sparing invasive procedures for the management of placenta accreta associated with severe PPH. This new regimen could be used soon after delivery or in association with conservative management. Furthermore, the treatment is cost-effective, easy to use and may be life-saving in many low-resource settings. A large study is needed to establish the overall success rate as well as possible future fertility rate. Meanwhile, obstetricians should be encouraged to report their experience with the use of the combination.

References

1. Miller DA, Chollet JA, Goodwin TM. Clinical risk factors for placenta previa-placenta accreta. Am J Obstet Gynecol 1997; 177:210–14

2. Committee on Obstetric Practice. American College of Obstetricians and Gynecologists Committee Opinion. Placenta accreta. Number 266, January 2002. Int J Gynaecol Obstet 2002;77:77–8

3. O'Brien JM, Barton JR, Donaldson ES. The management of placenta percreta: conservative and operative strategies. Am J Obstet Gynecol 1996;175:1632–8

4. Dombrowski MP, Bottoms SF, Saleh AA, Hurd WW, Romero R. Third stage of labor: Analysis of duration and clinical practice. Am J Obstet Gynecol 1995;172:1279–84

5. Tandberg A, Albrechtsen S, Iversen OE. Manual removal of the placenta. Incidence and clinical significance. Acta Obstet Gynecol Scand 1999;78:33–6

6. MacLeod J, Rhode R. Retrospective follow-up of maternal deaths and their associated risk factors in a rural district of Tanzania. Trop Med Int Health 1998;3:130–7

7. van Beekhuizen HJ, de Groot AN, De Boo T, Burger D, Jansen N, Lotgering FK. Sulprostone reduces the need for the manual removal of the placenta in patients with retained placenta: a randomized controlled trial. Am J Obstet Gynecol 2006;194:446–50

8. Carroli G, Bergel E. Umbilical vein injection for management of retained placenta. Cochrane Database Syst Rev 2001; (4):CD001337

9. Chan AS, Ananthanarayan C, Rolbin SH. Department of Anaesthesia, Mount Sinai Hospital, University of Toronto, Ontario. Alternating nitroglycerin and syntocinon to facilitate uterine exploration and removal of an adherent placenta. Can J Anaesth 1995;42:335–7

10. Clement D, Kayem G, Cabrol D. Conservative treatment of placenta percreta: a safe alternative. Eur J Obstet Gynecol Reprod Biol 2004;114:108–9

11. Greenberg JA, Miner JD. Uterine artery embolization and hysteroscopic resection to treat retained placenta accreta: A case report. J Minim Invasive Gynecol 2006;13:342–4

12. Jung HN, Shin SW, Choi SJ, et al. Uterine artery embolization for emergent management of postpartum hemorrhage associated with placenta accreta. Acta Radiol 2011;52:638–42

13. Tong SYP, Tay KH, Kwek YCK. Conservative management of placenta accreta: review of three cases. Singapore Med J 2008;49:156

14. Khan GQ, John IS, Wani S, Dohety T, Sibai BM. Controlled cord traction versus minimal intervention techniques in delivery of the placenta: a randomized controlled trial. Am J Obstet Gynecol 1997;177:770–4

15. Rogers MSYP, Wong S. Avoiding manual removal of the placenta: evaluation of intra-umbilical injection of uterotonics using the Pipingas technique for management of adherent placenta. Acta Obstet Gynaecol 2007;86:48–56

16. Sherer DM, Gorelick C, Zigalo A, Sclafani S, Zinn HL, Abulafia O. Placenta previa percreta managed conservatively with methotrexate and multiple bilateral uterine artery embolizations. Ultrasound Obstet Gynecol 2007;30:227–30

17. Lawton BA, Rose SB, Shepherd J. Atypical presentation of serious pelvic inflammatory disease following mifepristone-induced abortion. Contraception 2006;73:431–2

18. Misoprostol in Obstetrics and Gynaecology. http://www.misoprostol.org/

19. Hofmeyr GJ, Walraven G, Gülmezoglu AM, Maholwana B, Alfirevic Z, Villar J. Misoprostol to treat postpartum haemorrhage: a systematic review. BJOG 2005;112:547–53

20. Walley RL, Wilson JB, Crane JMG, Matthews K, Sawyer E, Hutchens D. A double-blind placebo controlled randomised trial of misoprostol and oxytocin in the management of the third stage of labour. BJOG 2000;107:1111–5

21. Weeks A, Faundes A. Misoprostol in obstetrics and gynecology. Int J Gynaecol Obstet. 2007;99:S156–9

22. Surbeck DV, Fehr PM, Hosli I, Holzgreve W. Oral misoprostol for the third stage of labor: a randomized placebo-controlled trial. Am J Obstet Gynecol 1999;94:255–8

23. van Stralen G, Roosmalen van JJM. Regarding Rogers MS, Yuen PM, Wong S. Avoiding manual removal of placenta: evaluation of intra-umbilical injection of uterotonics using the Pipingas technique for management of adherent placenta. Acta Obstet Gynecol 2007;86:48–54 [Letter]. Acta Obstet Gynaecol 2007;86:764

24. Tang OS, Schweer H, Seybert HW, Lee SWH, Ho PC. Pharmacokinetics of different routes of administration of misoprostol. Hum Reprod 2002;17:332–6

25. Gemzell-Danielsson K, Bygdeman M, Aronsson A. Studies on uterine contractility following mifepristone and various routes of misoprostol. Contraception 2006;74:31–5

26. Ngai SW, Tang OS, Ho PC. Randomized comparison of vaginal (200 micrograms every 3 h) and oral (400 micrograms every 3 h) misoprostol when combined with mifepristone in termination of second trimester pregnancy. Hum Reprod 2000;15:2205–8

27. Jain JK, Dutton C, Harwood B, Meckstroth KR, Mishell DR Jr. A prospective randomized, double-blinded, placebo-controlled trial comparing mifepristone and vaginal misoprostol alone for elective termination of pregnancy. Hum Reprod 2002;17:1477–82

28. Rose B, Shand C, Simmons A. Mifepristone- and Misoprostol-induced mid-trimester termination of pregnancy: a review of 272 cases. Aust N Z J Obstet Gynaecol 2006;46:479–85

29. Rodger MW, Baird DT. Pretreatment with mifepristone (RU 486) reduces interval between prostaglandin administration and expulsion in second trimester abortion. Br J Obstet Gynaecol 1990;97:41–5

30. Cameron IT, Baird DT. The use of 16, 16-dimethyl-trans delta2 prostaglandin E1 methyl ester (gemeprost) vaginal pessaries for the termination of pregnancy in the early second trimester. A comparison with extra amniotic prostaglandin E2 Br J Obstet Gynaecol 1984;91:1136–40

31. Urquhart DR, Templeton AA. Mifepristone (RU486) for cervical priming prior to surgically induced abortion in the late first trimester. Contraception 1990;42:191–9

32. Electronic Medicines Compendium. Mifegyne. 2001 http://emc.medicines.org.uk/emc/assets/c/html/DisplayDoc.asp

33. World Health Organization Task Force on Post-ovulatory Methods of Fertility Regulation. Termination of pregnancy with reduced doses of mifepristone. BMJ 1993;307:532–7

34. Ashok PW, Kidd A, Flett GMM, Fitzmaurice A, Graham W, Templeton A. A randomized comparison of medical abortion and surgical vacuum aspiration at 10–13 weeks of gestation. Hum Reprod 2002;17:92–8

35. Webster D, Penney GC, Templeton A. A comparison of 600 and 200 mg mifepristone prior to second trimester abortion with the prostaglandin misoprostol. Br J Obstet Gynaecol 1996;103:706–9

36. Peyron R, Aubeny E, Targosz V, et al. Early termination of pregnancy with mifepristone (RU 486) and the orally active prostaglandin misoprostol. N Engl J Med 1993;38:1509–13

37. Morgan M, Atalla R. Mifepristone and misoprostol for the management of placenta accreta – a new alternative approach. BJOG 2009;116:1002–3

38. Mussalli GM, Shah J, Berck DJ, et al. Placenta accreta and methotrexate therapy: three case reports. J Perinatol 2000;20:331–4

39. Tong SYP, Tay KH, Kwek YCK. Conservative management of placenta accreta: review of three cases. Singapore Med J 2008;49:156

40. Palacios-Jaraquemada JM, Pesaresi M, Nassif JC, Hermosid S. Anterior placenta percreta: surgica l approach, hemostasis and uterine repair. Acta Obstet Gynecol Scand 2004;83:738–44

41. Baskett TF, O'Connell CM. Severe obstetric maternal morbidity: a 15-year population-based study. J Obstet Gynaecol 2005;25:7–9

42. Ozumba BC, Mbagwu SC. Emergency obstetric hysterectomy in Eastern Nigeria. Int Surg 1991;76:109–11

43. Bakshi S, Meyer BA. Indications for and out- comes of emergency peripartum hysterectomy. A five-year review. J Reprod Med 2000;45:733–7

44. Engelsen IB, Albrechsten S, Iverson OE. Peri- partum hysterectomy – incidence and maternal morbidity. Acta Obstet Gynecol Scand 2001;80:409–12

45. Morgan M, Atalla R. Conservative therapy in placenta accreta: unexpected problems after drug-induced uterine contractions. BJOG 2009;116:1821–2

46. Kerr de Mendonca, L. Sonographic diagnosis of placenta accreta. Presentation of six cases. J Ultrasound Med 1988;7:211–5

47. Hoffman-Tretin JC, Koenigsberg M, Rabin A, Anyaegbunam A. Placenta accreta. Additional sonographic observations. J Ultrasound Med 1992;11:29–34

48. Finberg HJ, Williams JW. Placenta accreta: Prospective sonographic diagnosis in patients with placenta previa and prior Cesarean section. J Ultrasound Med 1992;11:333–43

49. Comstock CH. Antenatal diagnosis of placenta accreta: a review. Ultrasound Obstet Gynecol 2005;26:89–96

50. Chou MM, Ho ES, Lee YH. Prenatal diagnosis of placenta previa accreta by transabdominal color Doppler ultrasound. Ultrasound Obstet Gynecol 2000;15:28–35

51. Lam G, Kuller J, McMahon M. Use of magnetic resonance imaging and ultrasound in the antenatal diagnosis of placenta accreta. J Soc Gynecol Invest 2002;9:37–40

31

One-Step Conservative Surgery for Abnormal Invasive Placenta (Placenta Accreta–Increta–Percreta)

J. M. Palacios-Jaraquemada

INTRODUCTION

Fifty years ago, placenta accreta was an obstetric rarity. Today, however, placenta accreta and its variations represent one of the principal causes of maternal morbidity and mortality. That this is the case is often attributed to the increased number of cesarean deliveries, but close examination of the numbers involved suggests that other factors may also be in operation.

The potential for the compromise of neighboring organs, as well as the development of neovascularization, implies specific technical difficulties associated with the treatment of placenta accreta, all of which directly relate to morbidity and mortality secondary to hemorrhage. Placenta accreta, characterized by the abnormal adherence of the placenta to the myometrium, may present different degrees of invasion, which are categorized as placenta accreta, increta and percreta. Since these terms are all based on histological examination, their proper use should be postoperative as well as retrospective. From a clinical perspective, the different degrees of invasion are more appropriately termed placenta accreta or abnormal invasive placenta.

The most common location of placenta accreta is the anterior lower uterine wall, especially when associated with a prior cesarean scar[1-3]. This association implies difficulties from a technical surgical point of view including adherence to bladder, development of neovascularization, destruction of myometrial tissue and access to the pelvic subperitoneal spaces. The uteroplacental tissues of placenta accreta are noticeably fragile and tend to bleed excessively. Absence of surgical planes for dissection makes it difficult or nearly impossible to apply the usual hemostatic procedures if an accurate tissue dissection between invaded tissues cannot be made.

Understanding the behavior and development of placenta accreta is essential in order to plan an appropriate surgical approach. Various vascular occlusive mechanisms have been used to reduce the tendency for bleeding[4-6], but they have not always been effective and, in some cases, have been deficient. Issues such as these have led to the need for a detailed study of each aspect related to the treatment of placenta accreta. One of the most important is to understand how both the pelvic anastomotic system and the collateral uterine vascular anastomoses work (see Chapters 1 and 22).

Predicting the surgical difficulty, as well as understanding the specific invaded areas, is essential in order to know which vascular pedicles are involved in a given case. A combination of vascular control, fascial dissection and identification of specific pelvic elements (ureter or specific vessels) makes it possible to prevent injuries and to avoid complications. Once a primary diagnosis has been arrived at, the next priority is to know how and where the placenta invades the adjacent tissues.

Designing a one-time surgery implies solving all the problems caused by placenta accreta at one operation. This involves vascular disconnection of the invaded organs (uterus, placenta and bladder), correct compartment exposure of the pelvic organs (necessary for the hemostatic procedures), total resection of the invaded myometrium and, finally, uterine and vesical reconstruction[7].

One-step conservative surgery for abnormal placentation (OSCS) was first implemented in 1990 and, 20 years later, has been applied in more than 450 patients. This series includes the most diverse types and degrees of placental invasion, operated upon electively as well as in emergency circumstances. To date, 106 consecutive postrepair pregnancies have been reported; of these, only two cases of partial recurrence were noted. This number represents the lowest relapse rate reported for conservative treatments in abnormal invasive placenta.

PLACENTAL INVASION

For years, the absence of Nitabuch's layer was considered the main phenomenon that led to abnormal placental invasion. However, numerous cases have been reported where absence of Nitabuch's layer coexisted with normal placentation. This observation suggests that the absence of this membrane might be a secondary process, rather than the primary cause of abnormal adherence[8]. In mammals, damage to the uterine collagen modifies decidualization; as such, it is logical to propose that a deformed collagen scar (repeated cesarean, postsurgical damage, radiation, etc.) may have a similar effect in the human being.

Placental invasion represents a highly complex phenomenon associated with numerous biochemical interactions. A series of myometrial mediators promote a physiological limit to trophoblastic invasion. In cases of extreme myometrial thinning (e.g. previous cesarean scar), the placenta might not find this physiological limitation and thus invade the myometrium excessively[9]. The absence of adequate vascular support would induce the secretion of vascular growth factors, the purpose of which would be to ensure sufficient placental flow to the fetus. This phenomenon would promote the opening and hypertrophy of microscopic anastomotic collaterals between the uteroplacental tissue, the bladder and the vagina. The vascular growth factors allow the newly formed vessels to grow rapidly and with a high flow. These characteristics are ideal to maintain an optimal placental blood supply; on the other hand, they also represent a surgical nightmare.

Fortunately, not all placental invasions have characteristic newly formed vessels. This is because the mechanism through which the placenta reaches the serosa is different. For placental advancement to occur through the myometrium there must be a prior tissue lesion. That is to say that placental advancement is a physical fact secondary to rupture of the myometrium. If, on the other hand, this fact depended on an invasive characteristic of the placenta, we would be able to see a similar percentage of invasions on all sides of the uterus, a phenomenon which has not been observed to date. All the evidence seems to indicate that if placental implantation is adequately supplied with blood, the placenta only advances through the myometrial defect. In contrast, if the placenta does not obtain an adequate vascular supply, the intense release of vascular growth factors promotes the thickening of the vascular microanastomoses (newly formed vessels, also called neovascularization).

SURGICAL ANATOMY

Morphological classification

Although three types of adherent placenta are found throughout the obstetrics literature (accreta, increta and percreta), this classification is retrospective, histopathological in nature and of uncertain use in surgical practice. Moreover, efforts to find the corresponding diagnostic images of this histological classification have been elusive. Finally, not even pathologists consider the histological examination of placenta accreta as a diagnostic gold standard[10,11]. This apparent contradiction is supported by the fact that, in one specimen, all types and degrees of invasion may coexist. Therefore,

histological diagnosis only provides a report of the site from which the sample was taken, and this area may or may not be representative of the remainder of the invaded area. Unfortunately, however, histological classification is relative to the degree of surgical difficulty; therefore, it is not always necessary to persist with presurgical studies. For example, countless cases describe simple surgery for placenta percreta, and extremely difficult surgery with bleeding for localized placenta accreta. In contrast, classification according to invasion areas bears a close correlation with the possibility of bleeding and surgical complexity; both features correspond to the origin of the blood supply and to the difficulty in pelvic dissection. The classification based on invaded areas makes it possible to know and plan how and on which vessels to perform vascular control[12,13].

From a surgical morphological point of view, three main types of anterior placental adherences may be distinguished[14]. In type 1 the anterior segment is noticeably thinner and the placenta reaches the serous surface, no newly formed placental–vesical or vesicouterine vessels are identified, and there is a lax dividing plane between the posterior bladder wall and the anterior surface of the uterine segment (Figure 1). In type 2 both the lower uterine segment and the posterior wall of the bladder are noticeably thinner, there is no lax plane between both organs and a fibrous scar connects them, and no newly formed placental–vesical or vesicouterine vessels are observed (Figure 2). Type 3 is characterized by a thinner uterine segment, vesical wall of variable thickness, presence of placental–vesical and vesicouterine neovascular circulation and vesicouterine plane with or without fibrous adherence (Figure 3).

This morphological, diagnostic and intrasurgical division establishes the type of approach advisable for each type. Type 1 usually constitutes the typical case labelled diagnostic false positive. In this type, both ultrasound and placental magnetic resonance imaging (pMRI) show dehiscence with placental advancement which reaches the serosa; therefore, and from an

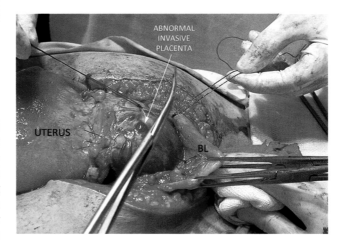

Figure 1 Superior view of anterior placental invasion. The placenta reaches to the uterine serosa, but there is a lax dissectible tissue between posterior bladder wall and the placenta. BL, bladder

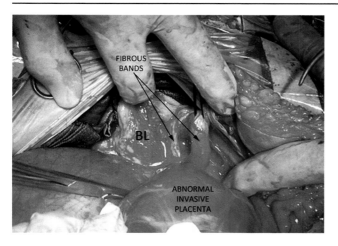

Figure 2 Superior view of anterior placental invasion. Notice the dense fibrous bands between the posterior bladder wall and the placenta. BL, bladder

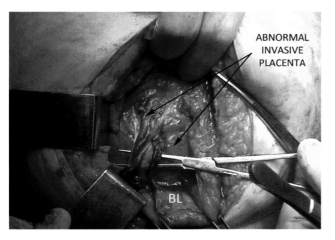

Figure 3 Superior view of anterior placental invasion. Newly formed vessels are present between posterior bladder wall and the abnormal placental invasion (black arrows) is evident. BL, bladder

exclusively diagnostic point of view, these are cases of placenta percreta. However, once the newborn is delivered, placental detachment can be performed without difficulty. There is no bleeding, and on direct examination no remains of adherent placenta are observed. A more detailed examination – which includes dissection of the retrovesical plane – would show a circular area of dehiscence hardly detectable if it is not explored specifically.

Type 2 provides an apparent sensation of safety when the vesicouterine pouch is opened; the dissection plane is narrow though manageable. While dissection progresses, small and persistent hemorrhagic foci occur which are difficult to control. The dissection plane continues to be identifiable until the surgeon unexpectedly sees the vesical mucosa or the Foley catheter. Access inside the bladder is almost imperceptible because dissection is performed on a fibrosed plane that connects the posterior vesical wall with the uterine scar. If, during dissection, the anterior side of the placental invasion is injured, a severe high-pressure hemorrhage ensues, aggravated by the fetal

content. Attempts to achieve hemostasis or suture of the placental invaded area (extremely thinning) usually aggravate the blood loss due to uterine tissue rupture, making it essential to evacuate the uterus in order to control the hemorrhage.

In type 3 the neovascular component must be ligated and divided between double ligatures so as to access the vesicouterine space; the ligature maneuver must always leave the main segment of the ligated vessel on the uterine side, because if the ligature is cut or released, the vessel which was cut off may easily be clamped with a hemostatic clamp. If this happens over the vesical sector, it is convenient to perform a vascular suture with polyglactin 000, which will include the vesical muscular tunic, to provide the mechanical support when suture is adjusted.

For the cases of fibrosis of the vesicouterine plane, it is advisable to open the anterior side of the parametrium and to dissect medially the cervicovesical space. This plane is only rarely invaded; however, if this occurs, it may be dissected through stepwise vascular ligatures and vascular section. Once inside this space, both fingers can be introduced laterally (Pelosi's maneuver) through the vesicocervical plane. After this, dissection and ligature can be performed on all the newly formed vessels towards the cephalic sector[15].

Induced neovascularization

Neovascularization is one of the main surgical problems in abnormal invasive placenta. These vessels are usually of high caliber and flow, and even though they may initially appear to have an anarchical pattern, they do not. From an embryological point of view, the vascular growth to the pelvis is formed by magma of interanastomosed vessels. Once organ differentiation has been established, many vessels develop whereas others regress until they become invisible. However, when the appropriate conditions are present (vascular growth factors), these vessels can develop and establish anatomical connections not described in normal conditions.

In cases of anterior placenta accreta, newly formed vessels can be observed between the uterine, vesical and vaginal arteries. Preoperative identification of the abnormal placental invasion enables planning of the approach and the technical tactics necessary to perform the specific vascular control of the pedicles involved.

Anatomy of newly formed vessels

It is usual to associate placenta accreta with newly formed vessels that communicate with the placenta, uterus, bladder and neighboring tissues. Newly formed vessels are generally of a large axial diameter, and they make adequate vascular exchange with the placenta possible. Once abnormal placentation has been established, the proliferation of angiogenic growth factors enables the development of high-volume newly formed vessels with fragile and less developed medial muscular layers. Although these latter vessels initially appear to have an anarchic pattern, this specific arterial and venous vascular group has an organized distribution[14] at three anastomotic levels: (1) vesicouterine system (VUS), (2) placental–vesical system (PVS) and (3) colpouterine system (CUS). The VUS habitually involves vessels that connect the uterine artery with the posterior-superior bladder wall and also with the contralateral uterine artery. These are superficial vessels, and can be observed through the vesicouterine fold running transversally. The presence of direct anastomoses of considerable size between the uterine arteries and the bladder must be considered during embolization, because this communication can be a direct means to perform an undesired occlusion in the vesical parenchyma (Figure 4).

The PVS is probably the best known, as it establishes a connection between the placental vasculature and the vesicular muscular layer, and is perpendicular to the vesicouterine plane. Anastomoses between the bladder and placenta (PVS) could be observed as thin interconnected net (Figure 5) as well as easily identifiable thick cords (Figure 6). The PVS can send and receive vessels from the entire surface of the posterior bladder wall, and therefore make connections with branches of the upper and lower vesical arteries, although it frequently does so with the upper vesical pedicle.

Finally, the CUS is the anatomically most hidden (obscure) system, though probably it is the most important physiologically. The CUS is located in the thickness of the anterior bladder wall and is parallel to its long axis; thus, it can only be identified through deep dissection of the retrovesical space. Nevertheless, on occasions CUS may not be visible at first sight, because its macroscopic visualization depends on the degree of anastomotic vascular development, which may vary from imperceptible cords to the replacement of the vaginal muscular tunic for a noticeably developed vascular plexus. The CUS connects the lower, middle and upper vaginal pedicles to the caudal branches of the uterine artery, as well as the anastomotic intrauterine arcade, and is anatomically located between its muscular fibers.

From a merely vascular point of view, the vesicouterine and placental–vesical anastomotic pedicles are likely to be controlled by endovascular occlusion of the uterine arteries (via transanastomotic flow). However, hemostasis of the colpouterine pedicle can be very difficult or nearly impossible, since it would represent a high-flow anastomotic arcade between the vaginal and uterine pedicles. Endovascular access to CUS is improved by catheterization of the internal pudendal artery, which is a branch of the posterior division of the iliac internal artery. On the other hand, CUS hemostasis can be performed in a simple, efficient and safe manner through square compression sutures, as described by Cho et al.[16]. This method stops bleeding from specific areas regardless of vessel origin.

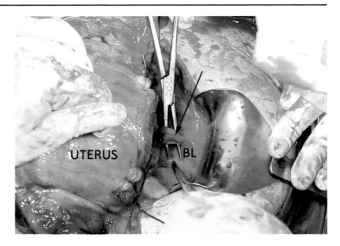

Figure 4 Superior view of lower uterus after reconstructive surgery for abnormal invasive placenta. Black arrow shows a direct anastomosis between transmedial interuterine anastomosis and the bladder

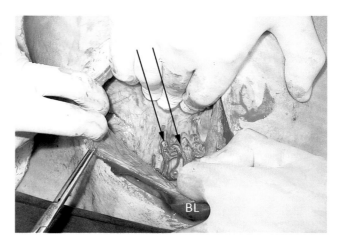

Figure 5 Superior viewing of anterior placental invasion. Black arrows show a group of thin newly formed vessels between the posterior bladder wall and the placenta. BL, bladder

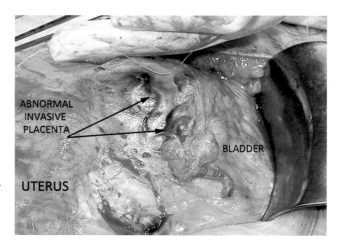

Figure 6 Superior view of anterior placental invasion. Black arrows show evident and thick newly formed vessels between the placenta and the bladder

Uterine anastomotic system

The uterus has two anastomotic systems: an upper one, supplied by the ovarian arteries; and a lower one, supplied by the vaginal arteries (see Chapter 1)[13]. Of the two, the lower or vaginal pedicle is the only one that can maintain uterine vascular integrity when both uterine arteries have been occluded or ligated. It is necessary to be aware, that simultaneous occlusion of the uterine arteries and the inferior vaginal artery (lower anastomotic pedicle) could produce uterine necrosis by over devascularization. This lower anastomotic system supplies collateral blood flow through vessels of a higher caliber than the uterine artery, and it has been shown that it is the major vascular supplementary system when the uterine arteries have been occluded.

The one-step surgery described below makes use of the occlusion of the uterine arteries, since most anterior invasions are not supplied by collaterals of the uterine artery.

ONE-STEP CONSERVATIVE SURGERY

Stage 1: invasion area

Even though ultrasound represents an accurate method to diagnose placenta accreta, pMRI is the most useful technique to establish the exact area (topography) of the invasion. Certain aspects related to the specific location of the invasion are essential when resective surgery is performed, such as parametrial invasion, and presence and location of newly formed vessels.

From a vascular point of view, the blood supply of the female generative tract can be divided into two clearly defined areas. One involves the uterine body itself, labelled sector one (S1), and the other involves the lower uterine segment, cervix and vagina, labelled sector two (S2)[13] (see also Chapter 1). S1 receives its blood supply mainly from the respective bilateral uterine and ovarian arteries; S2, in contrast, is supplied by a series of subperitoneal vessels originating primarily from internal pudendal arteries, secondarily from collaterals of the internal iliac artery and, to a lesser extent, by the uterine arteries. Precise knowledge of the location of the area of invasion makes it possible to plan efficient vascular control. For example, the occlusion of the uterine arteries or ligature of the anterior branch of the internal iliac artery in invasions in the S2 area implies a high possibility of continued bleeding, because their branches arise from the posterior division of the internal iliac artery. This trunk connects the internal iliac system with collaterals of the external iliac and the femoral arteries; therefore, this circumstance leaves only two alternatives to control bleeding: a proximal vascular control at the level of the infrarenal aorta or a specific hemostatic control over tissue and prior to fascial dissection of the pelvis.

Both areas can be identified using images of a mediosagittal pMRI slice[12]. If a perpendicular line is drawn in the medial sector of the posterior side of the bladder, two areas can be delineated, an upper one corresponding to S1 invasions and a lower one, corresponding to S2 invasions. The sagittal plane also provides information on the healthy myometrium above the cervix. In general, abnormal placental invasion near the cesarean scar promotes an anterior bulge. This determines that healthy myometrium will move in a cephalic and caudal direction. The myometrium superior to the placental invasion is easily shown with ultrasound, but this is not the case with the lower myometrium. This detail is essential when planning a conservative procedure, since the absence of a healthy myometrium below the area of invasion – minimum 2 cm – technically reduces the possibility of resecting the invaded myometrium and of performing a safe reconstruction.

Stage 2: surgical scheduling

The literature on the ideal moment to perform elective surgery in placenta accreta is contradictory. Despite this, tacit consensus exists to operate between weeks 35 and 38. This time interval is governed by the possibility of additional fetal lung maturation. There is a statistical increase in complications after week 35 related to placenta percreta; however, it is not always clear whether the authors used the same criteria to define invasion (clinical or histological). The most common complication in placenta accreta is bleeding, which is related to the disruption of the invaded area (uterine distension) attached to the placenta. In cases of anterior invasions, from week 35 the upper edge of the invasion extends beyond the upper wall of bladder. This phenomenon causes a lack of anterior parietal support, producing (spontaneously or through uterine dynamics) an additional disruption in the myometrium with higher risk of bleeding. Also, the dynamic traction on the invaded myometrium could produce variable activation of the coagulation system and, therefore, activate fibrinolysis. This phenomenon may go completely unnoticed and cause marked hypofibrinogenemia during the cesarean surgery. If this alteration is not detected through the quantification of fibrinogen and its degradation products after removing the placenta or performing the hysterectomy, a capillary and continuous hemorrhage occurs. This type of bleeding is very hard to treat, by either compression sutures or endovascular treatment. For this reason, if plasma fibrinogen reaches levels near 200 or 250 mg/dl before surgery, 1 U of cryoprecipitate per 10 kg body weight must be provided, thawed and infused before the surgery begins. This precaution is vital, because both hysterectomy and placental removal generally cause a decrease in fibrinogen levels to between 100 and 200 mg/dl. If fibrinolysis already has begun, a further postpartum physiological reduction would bring the fibrinogen level below its minimum hemostatic level to maintain a stable clot in the placental bed[17]. Because lyophilized fibrinogen is not available in all centers, it is necessary to take into consideration that the time required to use cryoprecipitate (request, defrost, transport and administer) is not usually less than 45 minutes to 1 hour. Under such circumstances, it would require an excessively and dangerously long time to correct the defibrination associated hemorrhage in conjunction with other technical problems during surgery (see Chapter 4).

The presence of a moderate, profuse or recurrent hemorrhage, as well as active labor, is an indication for termination of pregnancy. Nevertheless, and in spite of the urgency, the best clinical, hematologic and hemostatic control must be provided before surgery commences, as well as the most experienced surgical team.

Emergency

Whether in the presence of an ultrasound diagnosis or diagnostic suspicion due to clinical record and history, it is advisable to start the surgery with four or more units of red cells and plasma available 'in the surgical room'. Promises of immediate supply 'when called' are not acceptable, since the time to request, prepare and transport these agents may be excessive in the presence of bleeding of more than 500 ml per minute which is the norm in this type of abnormal placental invasion.

Basic hemostatic evaluation is recommended, as well as investigation of fibrinogen levels. However, factor-1 quantification is not always available, and in many centers it is only available after significant delays. In order to avoid this inconvenience, a 5 ml blood sample must be obtained prior to the start of surgery and placed in a dry test tube. The tube can be placed in a liquid bath at 37°C or under an assistant's armpit. The sample is examined after 15–20 min; if it produces a clot which remains firm when the tube is shaken, the fibrinogen level is correct. If the clot breaks up when moved, the fibrinogen level is near 100–150 mg%, and it is necessary to request cryoprecipitate immediately. On the other hand, if the blood does not coagulate, its level is below 50 mg%, a fact that indicates a severe fibrinolytic process. In such cases, it is advisable to administer lyophilized fibrinogen or cryoprecipitates and also to request immediately the supply of an equivalent dose to administer during surgery[19].

Although better fluid and blood replacement is under current discussion, we prefer to use two well placed large-bore venous accesses to administer crystalloids or Ringer's lactate solution on a 3:1 ratio with respect to estimated blood loss. Volumetric replacement maintains peripheral oxygenation, protects the microcirculation and avoids multisystemic damage. Administration of fluids and blood replacement must be accomplished early, according to the basic clinical signs and before the development of arterial hypotension, because the compensating mechanisms of the pregnant woman could maintain acceptable levels with blood losses of up to 30–40% of total volume. Since the contents of the circulatory system represent approximately 7% of body weight, the risk of shock is higher in women with a small body mass and in those

with previous anemia or bleeding. Common mistakes associated with management of bleeding from placenta accreta include deficiency in recognizing bleeding severity, insufficient fluid administration during resuscitation and delay in stopping the bleeding[19].

Besides the clinical signs of shock, it is absolutely necessary to check the patient's acid–base status using an arterial sample in order to assess the efficacy of resuscitation.

Presurgical measures

Standard blood tests are recommended, including a complete coagulation profile. In normal conditions, this type of surgery is performed under epidural or spinal anesthesia; however, the presence of clinical or subclinical coagulation disorders contraindicates either technique.

Two large-caliber venous accesses are recommended, and the blood bank and laboratory service must be warned of the singular characteristic of this surgery. Because abnormal placentation is a possible cause of exsanguinating hemorrhage, before starting surgery four cross-matched units of packed red blood cells (pRBC) and four bags of fresh frozen plasma (FFP) should be on hand in the surgical room. An additional amount of pRBC, FFP, cryoprecipitate and platelets should be on reserve and ready for immediate use[20]. During surgery, communication between the anesthesiologists and the surgeon must be directed to assessing the estimated volume, the speed of blood loss and avoiding any predictable hemodynamic or hemostatic deterioration.

Stage 3: laparotomy and initial evaluation

Pfannenstiel incision may provide sufficient access if the location of the invasive adherence is known and the surgeon is experienced. However, when vascular control either is or may be required at the aortic level, the essential incision must be median infraumbilical with cephalic extension. Regardless of incision type, the primary objective at this stage will consist of widely exposing the retrovesical space. When this area is apparently adherent to and fused with the placenta, it is not as technically difficult as might be thought (Figure 7). In order to identify the correct place for dissection, the bladder must be elevated with two Allis clamps, a maneuver which will noticeably simplify dissection, repair, ligature and section of the newly formed vessels between bladder-invaded uterus and the placenta. Dissection should start immediately inside the round ligament, from which a small buttonhole can be made, which will include the peritoneum and newly formed vessels, which always must be ligated between double ligatures. The poor muscular layer of the newly formed vessels often allows them to go unnoticed during the pulling maneuvers, since they collapse as veins. If they are inadvertently cut, this can be a cause of postsurgery rebleeding and secondary morbidity.

This stage is slow and requires care, and dissection of the new vessels must be made meticulously, since they are fragile and have high blood flow. On occasions, there is not much tissue between the two ligatures; in this case, an incision on the vesical side is preferred. If the ligature moves or if bleeding occurs, a stitch can be made, which includes the vesical muscular layer with polyglactin 000. On occasions, dissection may be hindered by tissue fibrosis, which makes it difficult to identify a well-defined anatomical plane. In these circumstances, dissecting the vesical surgical plane makes it possible to make a bridge, pass a finger and then exert upward traction. This maneuver, described as a retrovesical bypass, is of great use and allows access to the posterior-lower sector of bladder.

Retrovesical dissection is finished when all newly formed vessels between bladder, uterus and placenta are ligated, and the upper portion of the vagina is accessible. At this moment, hysterectomy must be considered if repair is not considered possible, as might occur when there is segmental tissue destruction of greater than 50% of the organ's axial circumference, or when tissue loss in the distal uterine segment leaves less than 2 cm of healthy segment above the uterine cervix.

Stage 4: hysterotomy

Once the anterior side of the uterus has been exposed and the newly formed vesico–uterine–placental vessels have been interrupted, control of the colpouterine pedicle remains when the placenta has been removed. This is the reason why there is no risk of hemorrhage during hysterotomy. Several authors are very careful not to make an incision in the placenta during hysterotomy, and many use intraoperative ultrasound to this aim. Hysterotomy can be performed in the upper sector of the invasive area in a completely safe manner. Even though there is placenta in this area, its insertion is normal and the newly formed vessels have been ligated; therefore, bleeding is not a problem. At this stage, it is advisable to apply the hysterotomy method described for placenta previa[21]. When hysterotomy is performed, only the muscular layer is cut (Figure 8). Next, the hand is introduced between the myometrium and the placenta until the sac is reached. After that, the baby is gently extracted and the uterus exteriorized for better handling.

Stage 5: resection and hemostasis

Once the uterus has been exteriorized, the dissection of the posterior side of the bladder can be completed if necessary. This maneuver allows clean access to the upper side of the vagina and uterine cervix, and is essential to obtain hemostasis of the colpouterine vessels. The inferior edge of the invasion can be trimmed with scissors, in order manually to remove the placenta with the invaded myometrium in one piece. Next, the cavity is cleaned with a gauze pad or a Pinard curette (Figure 9). After fetal delivery and placental

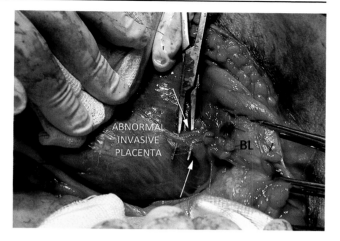

Figure 7 Superior view of anterior placental invasion. After ligature of newly formed vessels the posterior bladder wall is easily dissected. BL, bladder

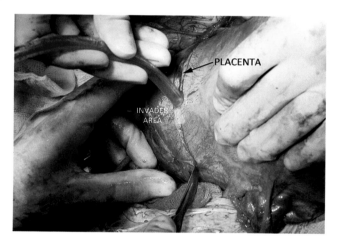

Figure 8 Cutting of the myometrium above the abnormal invasive placenta. Notice that the hysterotomy is performed over the placenta, but not over the newly formed vessels, which were ligated in a previous step

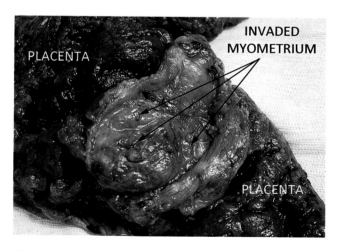

Figure 9 The entire placenta and invaded myometrium are removed in one surgical piece. In this way, uterine reconstruction is performed using healthy tissues

extraction, uterotonic drugs are administered, such as oxytocin (Syntocinon™, Novartis, Brazil) 20 IU i.v. after fetal extraction, plus 20 IU i.v. within the first 24 h, or carbetocin (Duratocin™, Ferring, Argentina) 100 mg i.v. in a single dose.

The colpouterine hemostasis component of the operation is performed with a pair of square stitches following the technique described by Cho *et al.*[16]. With the aim of preventing hematometra, a Hegar's bougy dilator #10 is placed in the uterine cervix, which will move towards one of the sides (Figure 10). In this manner the application of a square stitch is easier, and the potential for accidental closure of the internal cervical os is minimized. The advantage of using Cho's suture relies on the fact that the surgeon works on a surface instead of a specific pedicle. In addition, this procedure prevents inadvertent ureteral injury, since it is applied on uterine tissue. When the hemostatic suture has been placed, any additional bleeding can be checked. Due to the fragility of the newly formed vessels, it is preferable to apply U-stitches in order to minimize the suture cutting effect.

Stage 6: repair

Once hemostasis has been achieved, it is necessary to check that the fibrinogen level is higher than 200 mg%. The repair is performed in two stages. In the first, U-stitches are made with polyglactin suture 1 cm from the myometrial border. The aim with these stitches is to coapt the borders and reduces tension on the primary suture. In the first years of performing this surgery, a reabsorbable net was applied with excellent results; however, the net was not always available. For this reason, another anti-tension mechanism was designed (Vicryl™ mesh (polyglactin 910) Ethicon, USA), which yielded identical results. The second stage is to use a continuous suture with polyglactin 1, which closes the borders and provides secure hemostasis. On occasion, small muscular defects are observed in some areas of the posterior wall of bladder. Such defects as well as any residual focal bleeding are sutured with polyglactin 000 (Figure 11).

When the repair has been completed, the incision and dissection surfaces are inspected one more time, and a sheet of regenerated cellulose is placed as an anti-adhesion barrier between the bladder and the uterine repair.

Stage 7: postoperative care

Special attention must be paid to pain after one-step surgeries, as this type of surgery involves far more tissue disruption than is the case with a cesarean delivery. A useful plan includes morphine administration together with other painkillers starting in the immediate postsurgery period, modified depending on demand, and reduced on the second or third postoperative day.

One additional but important aspect of postoperative care is deep venous thrombosis prophylaxis.

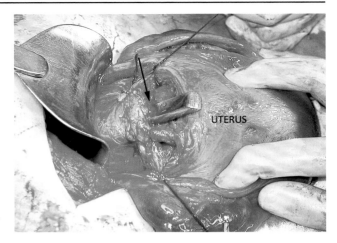

Figure 10 Superior viewing of lower uterus, a Hegar bougy (black arrow) is placed in cervical canal to avoid unwanted lochia occlusion during placement of Cho's hemostatic sutures

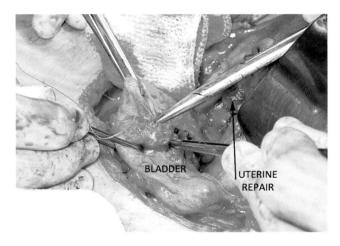

Figure 11 Superior viewing of lower uterus, on the left, the muscular bladder defects is sutured with 000 polyglactin. Repaired uterus (black arrow)

Pregnancy, pelvic surgery and bed rest should be regarded as risk factors[22]. From an ideal point of view, it is advisable to use intermittent pneumatic compressors[23]. Low-molecular weight heparin can be administered when the platelet count is over $100,000/mm^3$, and until there is effective ambulation.

FOLLOW-UP

Control uterine studies were performed between 5 and 10 months after repair. The first 100 patients who underwent one-step conservative surgeries subsequently had hysteroscopy to explore the cavity and scar characteristics. The study showed only two cases of uterine synechiae, which were related to the use of chromic catgut. This follow-up procedure was later replaced by uterine T2-weighted MRI performed between 5 and 6 days before patient menses. Uterine MRI makes it possible to observe the repaired area clearly. Prior to the study, moderate urinary retention is requested, which renders a whitish color on T2. This contrast, added to the whitish color of the premenstrual endometrium, makes it possible to define precisely the repaired myometrium.

SUBSEQUENT PREGNANCIES

To date, 106 subsequent pregnancies have been reported following this type of surgery, two cases of anterior placenta previa coincided with both cases of partial recurrence.

GENERAL OVERVIEW

Placenta accreta is a leading cause of emergency post-partum hysterectomy. Although hysterectomy can be a life-saving operation, it is associated with high maternal mortality and subsequent morbidities[24]. On other hand, conservative treatment leaving the placenta *in situ* has fewer complications of hemorrhage but more of an infectious nature including septic shock, sepsis, infection, endometritis, wound infection, peritonitis, pyelonephritis, vesicouterine fistula and uterine necrosis[25] among other medical complications.

One-step conservative surgery eliminates uterine damage and the entire placenta in the same surgical act. Its technical complexity can be learned with supervised instruction, as was the case with laparoscopy some years ago. Collaboration between countries could help to introduce this procedure as standard treatment for abnormal invasive placenta in the years to come.

References

1. Clark SL, Koonings PP, Phelan JP. Placenta previa/accreta and prior cesarean section. Obstet Gynecol 1985;66:89–92

2. Miller DA, Chollet JA, Goodwin TM. Clinical risk factors for placenta previa/placenta accreta. Am J Obstet Gynecol 1997; 177:210–4

3. Usta IM, Hobeika EM, Musa AA, Gabriel GE, Nassar AH. Placenta previa-accreta: risk factors and complications. Am J Obstet Gynecol 2005;193:1045–9

4. Shih JC, Liu KL, Shyu MK. Temporary balloon occlusion of the common iliac artery: new approach to bleeding control during cesarean hysterectomy for placenta percreta. Am J Obstet Gynecol 2005;193:1756–8

5. Andoh S, Mitani S, Nonaka A, et al. Use of temporary aortic balloon occlusion of the abdominal aorta was useful during cesarean hysterectomy for placenta accreta. Masui 2011;60: 217–9

6. Dubois J, Garel L, Grignon A, Lemay M, Leduc L. Placenta percreta: balloon occlusion and embolization of the internal iliac arteries to reduce intraoperative blood losses. Am J Obstet Gynecol 1997;176:723–6

7. Palacios-Jaraquemada JM, Pesaresi M, Nassif JC, Hermosid S. Anterior placenta percreta: surgical approach, hemostasis and uterine repair. Acta Obstet Gynecol Scand 2004;83:738–44

8. Pijnenborg R, Vercruysse L. Shifting concepts of the fetal-maternal interface: A historical perspective. Placenta 2008;29 (Suppl A):S20–5

9. Tantbirojn P, Crum CP, Parast MM. Pathophysiology of placenta creta: the role of decidua and extravillous trophoblast. Placenta 2008;29:639–45

10. Khong TY, Werger AC. Myometrial fibers in the placental basal plate can confirm but do not necessarily indicate clinical placenta accreta. Am J Clin Pathol 2001;116:703–8

11. Jacques SM, Qureshi F, Trent VS, Ramirez NC. Placenta accreta: mild cases diagnosed by placental examination. Int J Gynecol Pathol 1996;15:28–33

12. Palacios-Jaraquemada JM, Bruno CH. Magnetic resonance imaging in 300 cases of placenta accreta: surgical correlation of new findings. Acta Obstet Gynecol Scand 2005;84: 716–24

13. Palacios-Jaraquemada JM, García Mónaco R, Barbosa NE, Ferle L, Iriarte H, Conesa HA. Lower uterine blood supply: extrauterine anastomotic system and its application in surgical devascularization techniques. Acta Obstet Gynecol Scand 2007;86:228–34

14. Palacios-Jaraquemada JM. Abnormal Invasive Placenta, 1st edn. Berlin: DeGruyter, 2012

15. Pelosi MA 3rd, Pelosi MA. Modified cesarean hysterectomy for placenta previa percreta with bladder invasion: retrovesical lower uterine segment bypass. Obstet Gynecol 1999;93: 830–3

16. Cho JH, Jun HS, Lee CN. Hemostatic suturing technique for uterine bleeding during cesarean delivery. Obstet Gynecol 2000;96:129–31

17. Palacios-Jaraquemada JM, Bruno CH, Clavelli WA. Morbid adherent placenta: prediction, diagnosis and management. Fetal Matern Med Rev 2007;18:357–81

18. de Lloyd L, Bovington R, Kaye A, et al. Standard haemostatic tests following major obstetric haemorrhage.Int J Obstet Anesth 2011;20:135–41

19. Lombaard H, Pattinson RC. Common errors and remedies in managing postpartum haemorrhage. Best Pract Res Clin Obstet Gynaecol 2009;23:317–26

20. Snegovskikh D, Clebone A, Norwitz E. Anesthetic management of patients with placenta accreta and resuscitation strategies for associated massive hemorrhage. Curr Opin Anaesthesiol 2011;24:274–81

21. Ward CR. Avoiding an incision through the anterior previa at cesarean delivery. Obstet Gynecol 2003;102:552–4

22. Davis SM, Branch DW. Thromboprophylaxis in pregnancy: who and how? Obstet Gynecol Clin North Am 2010;37: 333–43

23. Casele H, Grobman WA. Cost-effectiveness of thromboprophylaxis with intermittent pneumatic compression at cesarean delivery. Obstet Gynecol 2006;108:535–40

24. Varras M, Krivis Ch, Plis Ch, Tsoukalos G. Emergency obstetric hysterectomy at two tertiary centers: a clinical analysis of 11 years experience. Clin Exp Obstet Gynecol 2010;37:117–9

25. Sentilhes L, Kayem G, Ambroselli C, et al. Fertility and pregnancy outcomes following conservative treatment for placenta accreta. Hum Reprod 2010;25:2803–10

Section 6

Misoprostol

32

Misoprostol: Theory and Practice

M. B. Bellad and S. S. Goudar

INTRODUCTION

Prostaglandins have revolutionized obstetric practice. In particular, the advent of misoprostol has precipitated an enormous amount of innovative research as well as controversy. At present, misoprostol is being simultaneously investigated for its role in the management of postpartum hemorrhage (PPH), induction of labor, cervical ripening and termination of pregnancy. Initially, this drug was only approved by the US Food and Drug Administration (FDA) in 1988 for oral administration for the prevention and treatment of peptic ulcers associated with the use of non-steroidal anti-inflammatory drugs (NSAIDs). Since the early 1990s, however, misoprostol has been viewed with increasing interest by obstetricians and gynecologists because of its uterotonic and cervical ripening activity. The multiple off-label uses for misoprostol, supported by a literature comprising thousands of individual articles, underlie its description as 'one of the most important medications in obstetrical practice'[1]. Even as recently as 2005, misoprostol was not approved by the FDA for use in pregnant women, a stand strangely and yet strongly supported by its manufacturer[2].

MISOPROSTOL

Misoprostol is a synthetic prostaglandin (PG) E1 analogue. Naturally occurring PGE1 is not orally sustainable, as it is unstable in acid media and is also not suitable for parenteral use because of its rapid degradation in the blood. Misoprostol, the synthetic PGE1 analogue, is produced by bringing about an alteration in the chemical structure of the naturally occurring compound, thereby making it orally stable and clinically useful. Misoprostol is otherwise called alprostadil and its chemical formula is $C_{22}H_{38}O_5$ ((±)-methyl(13E)-11,16-dihydroxy-16-methyl-9-oxo-prost-13-enoate), as shown in Figure 1[3].

Misoprostol is manufactured as oral tablets of 200 μg scored and 100 μg unscored. It possesses three major advantages – stability at ambient temperature, long shelf-life and low cost – that have made it a central focus of research in obstetrics and gynecology for the past 25 years[4]. Misoprostol is rapidly absorbed via the oral route and, although not formulated for parenteral use, can also be administered sublingually (buccally), rectally and vaginally[5–7].

Pharmacokinetics, physiology and teratogenicity profile

Misoprostol is extensively absorbed and undergoes rapid de-esterification to misoprostol acid; this latter compound is responsible for its clinical activity and, unlike the parent compound, it is detectable in plasma. After oral administration, the peak level of misoprostol acid is reached within 9–15 min, with a terminal half-life of 20–40 min. Plasma levels of misoprostol acid vary considerably between and within studies, but mean values after single doses show a linear relationship with the dose over the range of 200–400 μg. No accumulation of misoprostol acid was noted in multiple dose studies and a plasma steady state was achieved within 2 days. The bioavailability of misoprostol is decreased when administered with food or antacids[8].

Misoprostol is primarily metabolized in the liver, and less than 1% of its active metabolite is excreted in the urine[9]. Patients with hepatic disease should receive smaller doses, whereas dose adjustment is not necessary for patients with renal disease not requiring dialysis. Misoprostol has no known drug interactions and does not induce the hepatic enzyme systems[9].

Pharmacokinetic studies of misoprostol in pregnant women show that sublingual and oral doses used for first-trimester termination of pregnancy produce earlier and higher peak plasma concentrations than vaginal or rectal doses, resulting in earlier, more pronounced uterine tonus (oral misoprostol 7.8 ± 3.0 min vs. vaginal misoprostol 20.9 ± 5.3 min)[6,7,10]. These findings also have been validated in women after delivery[11]. The effects of misoprostol on the reproductive tract are increased and gastrointestinal adverse effects are decreased when it is administered vaginally[10,12,13].

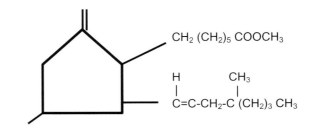

Figure 1 Chemical structure of misoprostol[3]

When misoprostol tablets are placed in the posterior fornix of the vagina, plasma concentrations of misoprostol acid peak in 1–2 h and then decline slowly (Figure 2)[5]. Vaginal application of misoprostol results in slower increases and lower peak plasma concentrations of misoprostol acid than does oral administration, but overall exposure to the drug is increased (indicated by the increased area under the curve in Figure 2)[5]. The peak plasma levels of misoprostol are sustained for up to 4 h after vaginal administration[5] (Figure 2). Among women who were 9–11 weeks pregnant and given misoprostol before a surgical termination of pregnancy, intrauterine pressure began to increase an average of 8 min after oral and 21 min after vaginal administration.

Pressure was maximal 25 min after oral administration and 46 min after vaginal administration. Uterine contractility initially increased and reached a plateau 1 h after oral administration, whereas it increased on a continuous basis for 4 h after vaginal administration. Maximal uterine contractility was significantly higher after vaginal administration[10]. Maximum serum concentration was achieved 23 min later in rectal administration, and peak levels were lower compared with oral administration of misoprostol (Figure 2)[7].

In the pharmacokinetic study by Tang and colleagues, the peak plasma level of misoprostol acid was highest and earliest after administration of misoprostol by the sublingual route[6]. Misoprostol tablets dissolved in water and taken orally also have been shown to produce a faster onset and stronger uterotonic effect than either oral or rectal tablet administration[14,15]. However, no significant difference was present when misoprostol was used in the form of moistened compared with dry tablets for first-trimester termination of pregnancy[16].

Adverse effects

Common side-effects of misoprostol include shivering, diarrhea and abdominal pain. Less common side-effects include headache, abdominal cramps, nausea and flatulence, chills and fever, all of which are dose dependent. Interestingly, before its use in pregnant women, chills, shivering and fever were not commonly reported side-effects, suggesting that these are dose dependent.

Package warnings prepared by the manufacturer and based on the original indication for which this drug was marketed clearly state that misoprostol is not to be taken by pregnant women, and that non-pregnant women should use contraceptives while taking misoprostol and should be warned about the effects of misoprostol if taken by pregnant women. Misoprostol should also be avoided in nursing mothers because of concern over causing diarrhea in the baby[8,11].

Congenital anomalies sometimes associated with fetal death have been reported subsequent to the unsuccessful use of misoprostol for termination of pregnancy, but the drug's teratogenic mechanism has

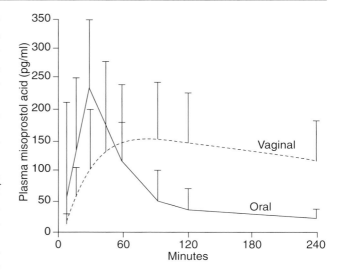

Figure 2 Mean (standard deviation) plasma concentrations of misoprostol acid after oral and vaginal administration of misoprostol in 20 women. Reprinted from Zieman M, et al.[5], with permission

not been elucidated[17,18]. Several reports associate the use of misoprostol during the first trimester of pregnancy with skull defects, cranial nerve palsies, facial malformations (Mobius syndrome) and limb defects[19]. Misoprostol is listed as a pregnancy category X drug.

Toxic doses of misoprostol have not been determined; however, pregnant women have tolerated cumulative doses up to 2200 µg administered over a period of 12 h without any serious adverse effects[20]. A dose of 6000 µg of misoprostol (which is far greater than necessary), taken orally to induce termination of pregnancy (with trifluoperazine), resulted in abortion with hyperthermia, rhabdomyolysis, hypoxemia and a complex acid–base disorder[21].

MISOPROSTOL IN THE FIRST TRIMESTER

For first-trimester medical termination of pregnancy, misoprostol has been used most extensively in conjunction with mifepristone or methotrexate. Both regimens are effective. In the initial studies of mifepristone and misoprostol for medical termination of pregnancy, both drugs were administered orally. Only regimens of mifepristone in combination with oral misoprostol have been licensed for abortion in many countries. Administration of 600 mg of oral mifepristone followed 48 h later by 400 µg of oral misoprostol resulted in 91–97% complete abortion in women who were no more than 49 days pregnant, compared with 83–95% of women who were no more than 56 days pregnant[22–25].

Lowering the dose of mifepristone to 200 mg and increasing the dose of oral misoprostol to 600 µg increases the efficacy, with abortion rates of 96–97% among women no more than 49 days pregnant and 89–93% among women 50–63 days pregnant[26,27]. The dose of mifepristone can be lowered to 200 mg without significantly decreasing efficacy[28].

A combined regimen of mifepristone and misoprostol results in complete abortion in 94–95% of women who are 9–13 weeks pregnant but is associated with high incidence of heavy bleeding[29,30]. The timing of administration of misoprostol after mifepristone for medical termination of pregnancy ranges from 6 to 48 h. Studies report high efficacy with shorter intervals of 24 h, 6–8 h and even the simultaneous administration of mifepristone and misoprostol, although one study carried out in Scotland showed reduced efficacy with a shorter interval of 6 h compared with a 36–48 h interval[31,32]. Complete abortion rates improve with one or two additional doses of misoprostol.

Vaginal administration of misoprostol was more effective and better tolerated than oral administration for the induction of first trimester abortion[33,34]. However, some studies concluded that both oral and vaginal misoprostol were of similar efficacy. Sublingual administration of misoprostol had a success rate of 92%[35].

A single dose of intramuscular or oral methotrexate (50 mg/m² body-surface area) followed 5–7 days later by 800 μg of vaginal misoprostol resulted in complete abortion in 88–100% of women provided with this regimen; 53–60% of women aborted within 24 h after one dose of misoprostol was administered[36–42]. If complete abortion did not occur within that interval, however, repeating the misoprostol dose resulted in complete termination of pregnancy in 19–32% of women within 24 h after the second dose[36,37]. The remaining 10–30% of women who aborted successfully had a delayed response, with the abortion completed over an average period of 24–28 days[36,37]. This regimen is presently not commonly used, as safer regimens with other drugs are available.

Misoprostol has also been used alone for medical termination of pregnancy, albeit with variable efficacy. The earliest studies of misoprostol induced termination of pregnancy in the first trimester and reported complete abortion rates of 5–11% among women given a total dose of 400 μg of oral misoprostol[43,44]. Up to three 800 μg doses of vaginal misoprostol given every 48 hours resulted in complete termination of pregnancy in up to 96% of women who were no more than 63 days pregnant[45].

Misoprostol alone was almost equally effective as combined mifepristone plus misoprostol. However, in a randomized trial comparing methotrexate plus vaginal misoprostol with vaginal misoprostol alone, only 47% of the women given misoprostol alone had complete termination of pregnancy, as compared with 90% of the women given methotrexate plus misoprostol ($p < 0.001$)[46]. With regard to the use of misoprostol as a cervical-priming agent before vacuum aspiration of the uterus, numerous randomized, controlled studies have shown that misoprostol is more effective than placebo and vaginal PGE2 in terms of the degree of cervical dilatation achieved[47,48]. As cervical priming facilitates surgical vacuum aspiration, the risks of dilatation and evacuation of the uterus are therefore minimized.

These results were replicated by numerous randomized, controlled trials involving a large number of participants. The best regimen for cervical ripening in the first trimester is 400 μg of vaginal misoprostol given 3–4 h before suction curettage[47,49,50]. In one study, misoprostol, when administered with mifeprostone for termination of early pregnancy in scarred uteri, was safe and effective, but further randomized trials are essential to confirm this[51]. Sublingual misoprostol was effective in facilitating cervical dilatation before surgical abortion, and its use significantly decreased the time of surgical evacuation and minimized blood loss during the procedure[52,53].

MISOPROSTOL IN EARLY PREGNANCY FAILURE

Single or repeated doses of misoprostol result in complete expulsions with minimal side-effects and complications in evacuation of first trimester missed abortions[54,55]. Vaginal misoprostol is more effective than oral administration[56]. Misoprostol is also effective in incomplete termination of pregnancy, and it is safer than the surgical method[57,58].

Based on a review, a single dose of 800 μg vaginal or 600 μg sublingual misoprostol is an effective, safe and acceptable alternative to the traditional surgical treatment for missed abortion. Bleeding may last up to or more than 14 days with additional days of light bleeding or spotting. However, in case of excessive bleeding or any evidence of infection the woman should report to her provider. A follow-up is recommended after 1–2 weeks for confirmation of complete expulsion of products of conception[59].

MISOPROSTOL IN THE SECOND TRIMESTER

Indications for second trimester termination of pregnancy include chromosomal and structural fetal abnormalities as well as social reasons. Surgical evacuation of the uterus, still being practiced in some centers, is associated with greater morbidity, mortality and complications. Intra-amniotic hypertonic saline/urea instillation, intra-amniotic PGF2 infusion, extra-amniotic ethacridine lactate, oxytocin infusion and vaginal PGE2 all were practiced before the introduction of misoprostol.

Intravaginal misoprostol in the dose of 400 μg is effective and associated with fewer side-effects[56]. Vaginal misoprostol was as effective as or more effective than PGE2. Misoprostol was equally as effective as extra-amniotic prostaglandins[60–64]. Misoprostol in the dose of 400 μg every 3 hours was more effective in terms of a significantly shorter drug administration-to-abortion interval and a higher percentage of successful abortion within 48 h compared with misoprostol 400 μg every 6 hours, and the incidence of side-effects was similar in both groups except for that of fever. However, the fever returned to normal within 24 h after the last dose of misoprostol[65]. In late second trimester, it is safer to use the less frequent dosage regimen. Vaginal misoprostol was significantly more effective as judged by drug administration-to-abortion interval and the need to augment therapy with oxytocin infusion when compared with oral misoprostol[66].

It is paradoxical that a greater dose (800 μg) of vaginal misoprostol is essential for abortion in the first trimester, whereas doses in the range of 25–50 μg induce labor in the third trimester. The optimal dose of vaginal misoprostol for induction of labor in the second trimester probably lies somewhere between 50 and 800 μg. Within this range, higher doses may be needed to cause termination of pregnancy early in the second trimester, whereas lower doses may be sufficient later in the second trimester. Higher and more frequent doses are associated with shorter drug administration-to-abortion interval compared with lower and less frequent doses (Figure 3)[1,67].

MISOPROSTOL IN THE THIRD TRIMESTER

Induction of labor

Labor induction is one of the common obstetric interventions primarily performed with the aim of reducing maternal and perinatal morbidity and mortality. The success of induction of labor not only lies with replication of physiological mechanisms, but also depends upon cervical status. An unfavorable cervix presents the greatest challenge to successful induction. The development of effective, safe (to both mother and fetus) and less expensive pharmacological agents to accomplish this task has been the focus of much clinical research.

The results of the first study (1993) in this area suggested that misoprostol was a cost-effective and safe alternative for induction of labor at term. Later studies, including randomized trials, not only confirmed this finding, but also documented that misoprostol is more effective than placebo or other prostaglandins; moreover, it is associated with a higher rate of vaginal delivery within 24 h, a shorter induction-to-delivery interval and significantly lower cesarean section rates than pooled figures for the control groups[68–71].

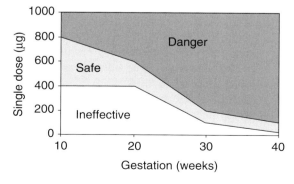

Figure 3 Safe single doses of misoprostol for producing uterine contractions at various gestations[67]

Studies of different routes of misoprostol administration (oral, vaginal, intracervical and sublingual) were conducted for induction of labor[72–77]. Although all were successful, vaginal misoprostol is associated with a shorter induction-to-delivery interval, lower number of doses and diminished oxytocin use[72,74]. Misoprostol gel is associated with fewer uterine contraction abnormalities and longer induction-to-labor and delivery interval when compared with misoprostol tablets[75].

The safety of misoprostol is crucial, as some studies have shown a high frequency of uterine tachysystole and hyperstimulation, including some reports of uterine rupture during the induction of labor with misoprostol[78–80]. A vaginal dose of 25 μg is often recommended as the more prudent dose, as it is associated with lower incidence of uterine hyperstimulation and is comparable with the 50 μg dose in achieving delivery within 24 hours[68,81–85]. Doses higher than 50 μg have been associated with increased risk of complications. The interval of administration of misoprostol ranges from every 3 to 6 h. It is better to use 6-h dosing intervals to avoid the possible risk of tachysystole[86]. Misoprostol is also effective as a cervical ripening agent for prelabor rupture of the membranes[87]. Oral misoprostol not only induced labor, but also resulted in delivery within 24 h without increasing maternal or neonatal complications[70,88].

Misoprostol is not recommended for induction in cases of previous cesarean section, as it is associated with higher frequency of disruption of prior uterine incisions compared with use of PGE2 or oxytocin. Misoprostol use is associated with a 5.6% rate of uterine scar rupture compared with 0.2% in patients attempting vaginal birth after cesarean delivery without stimulation, as shown by meta-analysis[89]. Misoprostol use in grand multiparas is not associated with adverse maternal or neonatal outcome. However, its use in such patients warrants strict vigilance[90,91]. The use of prostaglandins including misoprostol increases the uteroplacental resistance but does not affect the umbilical blood flow in a Doppler velocimetry study of umbilical, uterine and arcuate arteries immediately before and 2–3 h after the administration of vaginal misoprostol or cervical PGE2, thus suggesting misoprostol is as safe as PGE2 gel[92]. Available data suggest that vaginal misoprostol in a dose of 25 μg every 6 h is as safe as PGE2 in patients with a live fetus for induction of labor.

Induction of labor after fetal death

Misoprostol is an ideally suited agent for induction of labor after fetal death, as there is no concern about the adverse effects of uterine hyperstimulation on the fetus. For fetal death at term, a dose as low as 50 μg every 12 h may be adequate for induction of labor, whereas higher doses are necessary in patients with fetal death in the second trimester and early in the third trimester[93,94]. *It is safer to use the lowest effective dose.*

THIRD STAGE OF LABOR

PPH is a major cause of maternal morbidity and mortality. It is sudden, dramatic and unpredictable. In developing countries, approximately 28% of total maternal deaths are caused by PPH each year. Based on the uterotonic effects of misoprostol, the drug has been evaluated for both prevention and treatment of PPH. The WHO misoprostol multicenter trial concluded that use of an oral tablet of 600 µg was associated with a higher risk of severe PPH, the need for additional uterotonic agents, shivering and pyrexia compared with intramuscular or intravenous oxytocin[95]. However, the dose of misoprostol used in these trials varied from 400 to 600 µg (orally and rectally). Moreover, the frequency of PPH (blood loss more than 1000 ml) was not lower in the misoprostol group than in the control group in any of the trials. Nonetheless, there was higher use of oxytocin in the control groups. In many reports, misoprostol 600 µg oral or 400 µg rectal is significantly less effective than injectable uterotonics in preventing PPH[95–106]. Misoprostol at the dose of 400–600 µg is associated with risk of shivering, and doses more than 400 µg also significantly increase the risk of pyrexia. *At present, oral or rectal misoprostol is not as effective as conventional injectable uterotonic agents, and the high rates of shivering and fever associated with its use make it undesirable for routine use to prevent PPH, especially for low-risk women, when injectable oxytocics (oxytocin or methylergometrine) are available.* There is some evidence of increased uterotonic effect with the administration of misoprostol, either by the sublingual route or as an oral solution[6,14,15]. Use of buccal misoprostol in a placebo-controlled trial to prevent hemorrhage at cesarean delivery was not associated with a significant difference between the two groups, both in the incidence of PPH and a difference in pre- and postoperative hemoglobin level. However, misoprostol reduced the need for additional uterotonic agents during cesarean delivery[107]. In all of these studies, it is important to note that misoprostol was compared with conventional uterotonics. It is tragic but true, however, that these latter drugs are not available in many parts of the world where women deliver with no medical assistance whatsoever.

Despite the reduced efficacy of misoprostol compared with conventional injectable oxytocics and the potential to cause side-effects, several factors – ease of use, stability in field conditions, longer shelf-life and less expense – underlie its continued evaluation as a uterotonic agent. It remains of great interest, especially for use in home deliveries by traditional birth attendants and minimally qualified nurse midwives in less developed areas where administration of injectable uterotonics may not be feasible or may not be available. It offers a plausible preventive strategy in such areas for reducing maternal mortality related to PPH[108–110]. Trials with misoprostol versus placebo for prevention of PPH showed superiority of misoprostol[111,112].

Oral misoprostol in the dose 600 µg was associated with lower incidence of measured blood loss 500 ml or more and lower incidence of reduced postpartum hemoglobin (reduction of hemoglobin by 2 g/dl or more was 16.4% with misoprostol and 21.2% with ergometrine), but this difference was not statistically significant. Shivering was significantly more common with misoprostol, whereas vomiting was more common with ergometrine in a randomized, controlled trial with misoprostol 600 µg and ergometrine (0.5 mg, four tablets) in home delivery settings of rural Gambia[113].

In a randomized, double-blind, placebo-controlled trial with sublingual misoprostol (600 µg) at a primary health center in Bissau, Guinea-Bissau, West Africa, the incidence of PPH was not significantly different between the two groups. However, significantly fewer women in the misoprostol group experienced a blood loss of 1000 ml or more or 1500 ml or more. The decrease in hemoglobin concentration tended to be less in the misoprostol group, the mean difference between the two groups being 0.16 mmol/l (−0.01 to 0.32 mmol/l). From this study, it was concluded that sublingual misoprostol reduces the frequency of severe PPH[114]. *[Editor's note: These clinical finding, even without statistical differences, are of great practical importance in areas where blood supplies are insufficient or totally lacking. L.G.K.]*

Misoprostol for treatment of PPH

Current evidence suggests that misoprostol is less effective than injectable oxytocics especially versus oxytocin[115]. However, misoprostol was almost equally effective in the treatment of PPH where oxytocin was used for prophylaxis compared with when oxytocin was not used earlier[116]. It is reasonable to ask why misoprostol is effective for women with PPH, but has little effect on normal bleeding (in contrast to oxytocin). Oral misoprostol is absorbed more slowly than intramuscular oxytocin, and by the time it reaches its peak at 20 min, the third stage is over for most women (see Figure 4)[117]. Thus, the more prolonged the bleeding (i.e. the PPH), the more effective is misoprostol[117].

Hence, it is important to note that the injectable oxytocin acts more rapidly than misoprostol, so this latter agent in reality cannot be as effective as oxytocin. Future research with misoprostol must address this issue, as currently available misoprostol is recommended for oral use and takes more time to act. Newer formulations with sublingual/buccal route may probably act equal to oxytocin or injectable oxytocics. *It is also important to note that in an emergency like PPH it is important to use the sublingual rather than rectal route (least plasma concentration compared with other routes) to have earlier effective concentrations.*

OTHER USES

Cervical priming with misoprostol facilitates transcervical procedures and reduces side-effects[118].

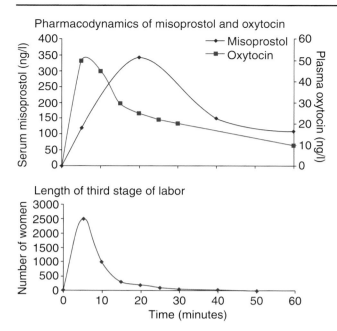

Figure 4 Comparison of concentrations of misoprostol and oxytocin in blood with duration of physiological third stage in 12,979 women[117]

Cervical priming is recommended by several evidence-based guidelines prior to surgical abortion, dilatation and curettage, hysteroscopy and intrauterine device insertion[118]. It is effective in pregnant as well as in non-pregnant women, whereas the results in post-menopausal women are conflicting[118]. Various doses, routes and time intervals between misoprostol application and the intervention have been evaluated. A single dose of 400 μg given sublingually or vaginally 3 h before the intervention has given the best efficacy with the least side-effects. Higher doses or longer intervals do not improve the effect on the cervix. Pain is a frequent side-effect, but usually responds well to NSAIDs. Other side-effects are rare[118].

Its use in cervical pregnancy is documented with one case report; however, extreme caution is recommended with this approach and methotrexate is favored by most authorities[119].

CONCLUSION

Misoprostol is one of the most important medications in obstetric practice. As of the time of writing, its use in pregnant women remains unapproved by the US FDA, except in conjunction with mifepristone (or, in some cases, methotrexate) for first-trimester medical termination of pregnancy. Despite this, the international literature is replete with innumerable favorable reports in many languages of off-label uses. For example, there is strong and consistent evidence to support the use of misoprostol for cervical ripening before surgical abortion in the first trimester and for induction of labor in the second and third trimesters. Whereas lower dose and strict vigilance are required for use of misoprostol for induction of labor with a live fetus,

it is ideal for induction of labor in patients with intrauterine fetal death.

Misoprostol may also prevent PPH when injectable uterotonic agents are either impractical or unavailable. On the other hand, misoprostol should not be the preferred uterotonic for prevention of PPH where injectable oxytocics are readily available. Its use in the treatment of PPH in regions of the world where the standard of care is delivery without uterotonic agents (i.e. delivery with no uterotonic medication) needs further evaluation. The oral route is associated with faster effect and with more side-effects. The other routes, such as vaginal and rectal, have sustained and longer effects with less side-effects. The sublingual and buccal routes and doses need further evaluation.

Finally, after considerable discussions between the American College of Obstetricians and Gynecologists (ACOG) and Searle, the manufacturer of misoprostol, the FDA has approved a new label for the use of misoprostol during pregnancy. The new labeling revises the contraindications and the precaution that misoprostol should not be used in pregnant women by stating that the contraindication is only for pregnant women who are using the medication to reduce the risk of NSAIDs. Misoprostol is now a legitimate part of the FDA-approved regimen for use with mifepristone to induce abortion in early abortion and the label warns of the complications/risks of its use for induction and augmentation of labor[120]. Uses in obstetrics and gynecology continue to be off-label.

WHO has also approved misoprostol for the prevention of PPH where oxytocin is not available or cannot be safely used and included the drug in the Model List of Essential Medicines[122]. Currently, misoprostol is registered by the national regulatory agencies of 17 countries for prevention and/or treatment of PPH. Consequently, several non-USA manufacturers are now marketing the drug with this indication included in the label.

References

1. Goldberg AB, Greenberg MB, Darney PD. Misoprostol and pregnancy. N Engl J Med 2001;344:38–47
2. Friedman MA. Manufacturer's warning regarding unapproved uses of misoprostol. N Engl J Med 2001;344:61
3. Barik S, Datta S, Gupta K. Misoprostol: pharmacology. In Barik S, Datta S, Gupta K, eds. Misoprostol in Obstetrics and Gynecology. New Delhi: Jaypee Brothers, 2003:8–15
4. Yap-Seng Chong, Lin Lin Su, Arulkumaran S. Misoprostol: a quarter century of use, abuse, and creative misuse. Obstet Gynecol Surv 2004;59:128–40
5. Zieman M, Fong SK, Benowitz NL, et al. Absorption kinetics of misoprostol with oral or vaginal administration. Obstet Gynecol 1997;90:88–92
6. Tang OS, Schweer H, Seyberth HW, et al. Pharmacokinetics of different routes of administration of misoprostol. Hum Reprod 2002;17:332–6
7. Khan RU, El-Refaey H. Pharmacokinetics and adverse-effect profile of rectally administered misoprostol in the third stage of labor. Obstet Gynecol 2003;101:968–74
8. Searle: Cytotec (misoprostol) (information package). Chicago: GD Searle & Co, 1995 9. Foote EF, Lee DR, Karim A, et al. Disposition of misoprostol and its active metabolite in patients with normal and impaired renal function. J Clin Pharmacol 1995;35:384–9

9. Foote EF, Lee DR, Karim A, et al. Disposition of misoprostol and its active metabolite in patients with normal and impaired renal function. J Clin Pharmacol 1995;35:384–9

10. Danielsson KG, Marions L, Rodriguez A, et al. Comparison between oral and vaginal administration of misoprostol on uterine contractility. Obstet Gynecol 1999;93:275–80

11. Abdel-Aleem H, Villar J, Gulmezoglu AM, et al. The pharmacokinetics of the prostaglandin E1 analogue misoprostol in plasma and colostrum after postpartum oral administration. Eur J Obstet Gynecol Reprod Biol 2003; 108:25–8

12. Creinin MD, Darney PD. Methotrexate and misoprostol for early abortion. Contraception 1993;48:339–48 [Erratum, Contraception 1994;49:99]

13. Toppozada MK, Anwar MY, Hassan HA, el-Gazaerly WS. Oral or vaginal misoprostol for induction of labor. Int J Gynaecol Obstet 1997;56:135–9

14. Chong YS, Chua S, Arulkumaran S. Sublingual misoprostol for first trimester termination of pregnancy: safety concerns. Hum Reprod 2002;17:2777–8

15. Chong YS, Chua S, Shen L, et al. Does the route of administration of misoprostol make a difference? The uterotonic effect and side effects of misoprostol given by different routes after vaginal delivery. Eur J Obstet Gynecol Reprod Biol 2004;113:191–8

16. Creinin MD, Carbonell JL, Schwartz JL, Varela L, Tanda R. A randomized trial of the effect of moistening misoprostol before vaginal administration when used with methotrexate for abortion. Contraception 1999;59:11–16

17. Pastuszak AL, Schuler L, Speck-Martins CE, et al. Use of misoprostol during pregnancy and Mobius' syndrome in infants. N Engl J Med 1998;338:1881–5

18. Gonzalez CH, Marques-Dias MJ, Kim CA, et al. Congenital abnormalities in Brazilian children associated with misoprostol misuse in first trimester of pregnancy. Lancet 1998; 351:1624–7

19. Orioli IM, Castilla EE. Epidemiological assessment of misoprostol teratogenicity. Br J Obstet Gynaecol 2000;107: 519–23

20. el-Refaey H, Templeton A. Induction of abortion in the second trimester by a combination of misoprostol and mifepristone: a randomized comparison between two misoprostol regimens. Hum Reprod 1995;10:475–8

21. Bond GR, Van Zee A. Overdosage of Misoprostol in pregnancy. Am J Obstet Gynecol 1994; 171:561–2

22. Wu YM, Gomex-Alzugaray M, Haukkamaa M, et al. Task force on Post ovulatory Methods of Fertility Regulation (WHO). Comparison of two doses of mifepristone in combination with misoprostol for early medical abortion: a randomised trial. Br J Obstet Gynaecol 2000;107:524–30

23. Peyron R, Aubeny E, Targosz V, et al. Early termination of pregnancy with mifepristone (RU 486) and the orally active prostaglandin misoprostol. N Engl J Med 1993;328: 1509–13

24. Spitz IM, Bardin CW, Benton L, Robbins A. Early pregnancy termination with mifepristone and misoprostol in the United States. N Engl J Med 1998;338:1241–7

25. Winikoff B, Sivin I, Coyaji KJ, et al. Safety, efficacy, and acceptability of medical abortion in China, Cuba, and India: a comparative trial of mifepristone–misoprostol versus surgical abortion. Am J Obstet Gynecol 1997;176:431–7

26. McKinley C, Thong KJ, Baird DT. The effect of dose of mifepristone and gestation on the efficacy of medical abortion with mifepristone and misoprostol. Hum Reprod 1993; 8:1502–5

27. Baird DT, Sukcharoen N, Thong KJ. Randomized trial of misoprostol and cervagem in combination with a reduced dose of mifepristone for induction of abortion. Hum Reprod 1995;10:1521–7

28. Kulier R, Gulmezoglu AM, Hofmeyr GJ, et al. Medical methods for first trimester abortion. Cochrane Database Syst Rev 2004;(2):CD002855

29. Ashok PW, Flett GM, Templeton A. Termination of pregnancy at 9–13 weeks' amenorrhoea with mifepristone and misoprostol. Lancet 1998;352:542–3

30. Gouk EV, Lincoln K, Khair A, Haslock J, Knight J, Cruickshank DJ. Medical termination of pregnancy at 63 to 83 days gestation. Br J Obstet Gynaecol 1999;106:535–9

31. Creinin MD, Schreiber CA, Bednarek P, et al. Mifepristone and misoprostol administered simultaneously versus 24 h apart for abortion: a randomized controlled trial. Obstet Gynecol 2007;109:885–94

32. Guest J, Chien PFW, Thomson MAR et al. Randomised controlled trial comparing the efficacy of same-day administration of mifepristone and misoprostol for termination of pregnancy with the standard 36 to 48 h protocol. Br J Obstet Gynaecol 2007;114:207–15

33. el-Refaey H, Rajasekar O, Abdalla M, et al. Induction of abortion with mifepristone (RU486) and oral or vaginal misoprostol. N Engl J Med 1995;332:983–7

34. Carbonell JL, Velazco A, Rodriguez Y, et al. Oral versus vaginal misoprostol for cervical priming in first-trimester abortion: a randomized trial. Eur J Contracept Reprod Health Care 2001;6:134–40

35. Tang OS, Ho PC. Pilot study on the use of sublingual misoprostol for medical abortion. Contraception 2001;64: 315–17

36. Creinin MD, Vittinghoff E, Galbraith S, Klaisle C. A randomized trial comparing Misoprostol three and seven days after methotrexate for early abortion. Am J Obstet Gynecol 1995;173:1578–84

37. Creinin MD, Vittinghoff E, Keder L, Darney PD, Tiller G. Methotrexate and misoprostol for early abortion: a multicenter trial. I. Safety and efficacy. Contraception 1996;53: 321–7

38. Creinin MD, Vittinghoff E, Schaff E, Klaisle C, Darney PD, Dean C. Medical abortion with oral methotrexate and vaginal misoprostol. Obstet Gynecol 1997;90:611–16

39. Creinin MD. Oral methotrexate and vaginal misoprostol for early abortion. Contraception 1996;54:15–18

40. Carbonell Esteve JL, Varela L, Velazco A, Tanda R, Sanchez C. 25 mg or 50 mg of oral methotrexate followed by vaginal misoprostol 7 days after for early abortion: a randomized trial. Gynecol Obstet Invest 1999;47:182–7

41. Hausknecht RU. Methotrexate and Misoprostol to terminate early pregnancy. N Engl J Med 1995;333:537

42. Carbonell JL, Varela L, Velazco A, Cabezas E, Fernandez C, Sanchez C. Oral methotrexate and vaginal misoprostol for early abortion. Contraception 1998;57:83–8

43. Lewis JH. Summary of the 29th meeting of the Gastrointestinal Drugs Advisory Committee, Food and Drug Administration, June 10, 1985. Am J Gastroenterol 1985;80: 743–5

44. Norman JE, Thong KJ, Baird DT. Uterine contractility and induction of abortion in early pregnancy by misoprostol and mifepristone. Lancet 1991;338:1233–6

45. Carbonell JL, Varela L, Velazco A, Fernandez C. The use of misoprostol for termination of early pregnancy. Contraception 1997;55:165–8

46. Creinin MD, Vittinghoff E. Methotrexate and misoprostol vs misoprostol alone for early abortion: a randomized controlled trial. JAMA 1994;272:1190–5

47. Bugalho A, Bique C, Almeida L, et al. Application of vaginal misoprostol before cervical dilatation to facilitate first-trimester pregnancy interruption. Obstet Gynecol 1994;83:729–31

48. Ngai SW, Yeung KC, Lao T, et al. Oral Misoprostol versus vaginal gemeprost for cervical dilatation prior to vacuum aspiration in women in the sixth to twelfth week of gestation. Contraception 1995;51:347–50

49. Singh K, Fong YF, Prasad RN, Dong F. Randomized trial to determine optimal dose of vaginal misoprostol for preabortion cervical priming. Obstet Gynecol 1998;92: 795–8

50. Singh K, Fong YF, Prasad RN, Dong F. Evacuation interval after vaginal Misoprostol for preabortion cervical priming: a randomized trial. Obstet Gynecol 1999;94:431–4

51. Xu J, Chen H, Ma T, et al. Termination of early pregnancy in the scarred uterus with mifepristone and misoprostol. Int J Gynaecol Obstet 2001;72:245–51

52. Saxena P, Salhan S, Sarda N. Role of sublingual misoprostol for cervical ripening prior to vacuum aspiration in first trimester interruption of pregnancy. Contraception 2003; 67:213–17

53. Vimala N, Mittal S, Kumar S. Sublingual Misoprostol for preabortion cervical ripening in first trimester pregnancy termination. Contraception 2003;67:295–7

54. Herabutya Y, O-Prasertsawat P. Misoprostol in the management of missed abortion. Int J Gynaecol Obstet 1997;56: 263–6

55. Wakabayashi M, Tretiak M, Kosasa T, et al. Intravaginal misoprostol for medical evacuation of first trimester missed abortion. Prim Care 1998;5:176

56. Creinin MD, Moyer R, Guido R. Misoprostol for medical evacuation of early pregnancy failure. Obstet Gynecol 1997; 89:768–72

57. Henshaw RC, Cooper K, el-Refaey H, et al. Medical management of miscarriage: nonsurgical uterine evacuation of incomplete and inevitable spontaneous abortion. Br Med J 1993;306:894–5

58. Chung TK, Lee DT, Cheung LP, et al. Spontaneous abortion: a randomized, controlled trial comparing surgical evacuation with conservative management using misoprostol. Fertil Steril 1999;71:1054–9

59. Gemzell-Danielsson K, Ho PC, Gómez Ponce de León R, Weeks A, Winikoff B. Misoprostol to treat missed abortion in the first trimester Int J Gynecol Obstet 2007;99: S182–S185

60. Bugalho A, Bique C, Almeida L, et al. The effectiveness of intravaginal misoprostol (Cytotec) in inducing abortion after eleven weeks of pregnancy. Stud Fam Plann 1993;24: 319–23

61. Nuutila M, Toivonen J, Ylikorkala O, et al. A comparison between two doses of intravaginal misoprostol and gemeprost for induction of second- trimester abortion. Obstet Gynecol 1997;90:896–900

62. Dickinson JE, Godfrey M, Evans SF. Efficacy of intravaginal misoprostol in second-trimester pregnancy termination: a randomized controlled trial. J Matern Fetal Med 1998;7: 115–9

63. Wong KS, Ngai CS, Wong AY, et al. Vaginal misoprostol compared with vaginal gemeprost in termination of second trimester pregnancy: a randomized trial. Contraception 1998;58:207–10

64. Munthali J, Moodley J. The use of Misoprostol for mid-trimester therapeutic termination of pregnancy. Trop Doct 2001;31:157–61

65. Wong KS, Ngai CS, Yeo EL, et al. A comparison of two regimens of intravaginal Misoprostol for termination of second trimester pregnancy: a randomized comparative trial. Hum Reprod 2000;15:709–12

66. Gilbert A, Reid R. A randomised trial of oral versus vaginal administration of misoprostol for the purpose of mid-trimester termination of pregnancy. Aust N Z J Obstet Gynaecol 2001;41:407–10

67. Fiala C, Weeks A. Misoprostol in obstetrics and gynaecology, summary of evidence. www.misoprostol.org

68. Hofmeyr GJ. Vaginal misoprostol for cervical ripening and labour induction in late pregnancy (Cochrane review). Cochrane Library, Issue 4, Oxford: Update Software, 1999

69. Hofmeyr GJ, Gulmezoglu AM, Alfirevic Z. Misoprostol for induction of labour: a systematic review. Br J Obstet Gynaecol 1999;106:798–803

70. Sanchez-Ramos L, Chen AH, Kaunitz AM, et al. Labor induction with intravaginal Misoprostol in term premature rupture of membranes: a randomized study. Obstet Gynecol 1997;89:909–12

71. Sanchez-Ramos L, Kaunitz AM, Wears RL, et al. Misoprostol for cervical ripening and labor induction: a meta-analysis. Obstet Gynecol 1997:89:633–42

72. Toppozada MK, Anwar MY, Hassan HA, et al. Oral or vaginal misoprostol for induction of labour. Int J Gynaecol Obstet 1997;56:135–9

73. Adair CD, Weeks JW, Barrilleaux S, et al. Oral or vaginal misoprostol administration for induction of labor: a randomized, double-blind trial. Obstet Gynecol 1998;92:810–3

74. Nopdonrattakoon L. A comparison between intravaginal and oral misoprostol for labor induction: a randomized controlled trial. JObstet Gynaecol Res 2003;29:87–91

75. Liu HS, Chu TV, Chang YK, et al. Intracervical misoprostol as an effective method of labor induction at term. Int J Gynaecol Obstet 1999;64:49–53

76. Shetty A, Mackie L, Danielian P, et al. Sublingual compared with oral misoprostol in term labour induction: a randomized controlled trial. Br J Obstet Gynaecol 2002;109:645–50

77. Shetty A, Daliellan P, Templeton A. Sublingual misoprostol for the induction of labour at term. Am J Obstet Gynecol 2002;186:72–6

78. Wing DA, Tran S, Paul RH. Factors affecting the likelihood of successful induction after intravaginal misoprostol application for cervical ripening and labor induction. Am J Obstet Gynecol 2002;186:1237–40

79. Bennett BB. Uterine rupture during induction of labor at term with intravaginal misoprostol. Obstet Gynecol 1997; 89:832–3

80. Wing DA, Lovett K, Paul RH. Disruption of prior uterine incision following misoprostol for labor induction in women with previous caesarean delivery. Obstet Gynecol 1998;91:828–30

81. Farah LA, Sanchez-Ramos L, Rosa C, et al. Randomized trial of two doses of the prostaglandin E1 analog misoprostol for labor induction. Am J Obstet Gynecol 1997;177:364–9; discussion 369–71

82. Srisomboon J, Tongsong T, Tosiri V. Preinduction cervical ripening with intravaginal prostaglandin E1 methyl analogue misoprostol: a randomized controlled trial. J Obstet Gynaecol Res 1996;22:119–24

83. Wing DA, Paul RH. A comparison of differing dosing regimens of vaginally administered misoprostol for preinduction cervical ripening and labor induction. Am J Obstet Gynecol 1996;175:158–64

84. Diro M, Adra A, Gilles JM, et al. A doubleblind randomized trial of two dose regimens of misoprostol for cervical ripening and labor induction. J Matern Fetal Med 1999;8:114–8

85. Meydanli MM, Caliskan E, Burak F, et al. Labor induction post-term with 25 micrograms vs. 50 micrograms of intravaginal misoprostol. Int J Gynaecol Obstet 2003;81: 249–55

86. Wing DA, Paul RH. A comparison of differing dosing regimens of vaginally administered misoprostol for preinduction cervical ripening and labor induction [Erratum]. Am J Obstet Gynecol 1997;176:1423

87. Ngai SW, To WK, Lao T, et al. Cervical priming with oral misoprostol in pre-labor rupture of membranes at term. Obstet Gynecol 1996;87:923–6

88. Shetty A, Stewart K, Stewart G, et al. Active management of term prelabour rupture of membranes with oral misoprostol. Br J Obstet Gynaecol 2002;109:1354–8

89. Plaut MM, Schwartz ML, Lubarsky SL. Uterine rupture associated with the use of Misoprostol in the gravid patient with a previous cesarean section. Am J Obstet Gynecol 1999;180:1535–42

90. Bique C, Bugalho A, Bergstrom S. Labor induction by vaginal misoprostol in grand multiparous women. Acta Obstet Gynecol Scand 1999;78:198–201

91. ACOG. Induction of labor. ACOG Practice Bulletin 10. Washington, DC: American College of Obstetricians and Gynecologists, 1999

92. Urban R, Lemancewicz A, Urban J, et al. Misoprostol and dinoprostone therapy for labor induction: a Doppler

comparison of uterine and fetal hemodynamic effects. Eur J Obstet Gynecol Reprod Biol 2003;106:20–4

93. Bugalho A, Bique C, Machungo F, Faundes A. Induction of labor with intravaginal Misoprostol in intrauterine fetal death. Am J Obstet Gynecol 1994;171:538–41

94. Bugalho A, Bique C, Machungo F, Bergstrom S. Vaginal misoprostol as an alternative to oxytocin for induction of labor in women with late fetal death. Acta Obstet Gynecol Scand 1995;74:194–8

95. Gulmezoglu AM, Villar J, Ngoc NT, et al. WHO multi-centre randomised trial of Misoprostol in the management of the third stage of labour. Lancet 2001;358:689–95

96. Hofmeyr GJ, Nikodem VC, de Jager M, et al. A random-ized placebo controlled trial of oral misoprostol in the third stage of labour. Br J Obstet Gynaecol 1998;105:971–5

97. Hofmeyr GJ, Nikodem C, de Jager M, et al. Oral miso-prostol for labour third stage management: randomised assessment of side effects (part 2). Proceedings of the 17th Conference on Priorities in Perinatal Care in South Africa, 1998:53–4

98. Surbek DV, Fehr PM, Hosli I, et al. Oral Misoprostol for third stage of labor: a randomized placebo-controlled trial. Obstet Gynecol 1999;94:255–8

99. Hofmeyr GJ, Nikodem VC, de Jager M, et al. Side-effects of oral misoprostol in the third stage of labour – a randomised placebo controlled trial. S Afr Med J 2001;91:432–5

100. Lumbiganon P, Hofmeyr J, Gulmezoglu AM, et al. Miso-prostol dose-related shivering and pyrexia in the third stage of labour. WHO Collaborative Trial of Misoprostol in the Management of the Third Stage of Labour. Br J Obstet Gynaecol 1999;106:304–8

101. Cook CM, Spurrett B, Murray H. A randomized clinical trial comparing oral Misoprostol with synthetic oxytocin or syntometrine in the third stage of labour. Aust N Z J Obstet Gynaecol 1999;39:414–19

102. Amant F, Spitz B, Timmerman D, et al. Misoprostol compared with methylergometrine for the prevention of postpartum haemorrhage: a double-blind randomised trial. Br J Obstet Gynaecol 1999;106:1066–70

103. el-Refaey H, Nooh R, O'Brien P, et al. The misoprostol third stage of labour study: a randomised controlled compar-ison between orally administered misoprostol and standard management. Br J Obstet Gynaecol 2000;107:1104–10

104. Ng PS, Chan AS, Sin WK, et al. A multicentre randomized controlled trial of oral Misoprostol and 1M syntometrine in the management of the third stage of labour. Hum Reprod 2001;16:31–5

105. Kundodyiwa TW, Majoko F, Rusakaniko S. Misoprostol versus oxytocin in the third stage of labor. Int J Gynaecol Obstet 2001;75:235–41

106. Caliskan E, Oilbaz B, Meydanli MM, et al. Oral misoprostol for the third stage of labor: a randomized controlled trial. Obstet Gynecol 2003;101:921–8

107. Hamm J, Russel Z, Botha T, et al. Buccal misoprostol to prevent hemorrhage at caesarean delivery: a randomized study. Am J Obstet Gynecol 2005;192:1404–6

108. Joy SD, Sanchez-Ramos L, Kaunitz AM. Misoprostol use during the third stage of labor. Int J Gynaecol Obstet 2003;82:143–52

109. Chong YS, Chua S, Arulkumaran S. Severe hyperthermia following oral misoprostol in the immediate postpartum period. Obstet Gynecol 1997;90:703–4

110. Chong YS, Chua S, El-Refaey H, et al. Postpartum intrauterine pressure studies of the uterotonic effect of oral misoprostol and intramuscular syntometrine. Br J Obstet Gynaecol 2001;108:41–7

111. Derman RJ, Kodkany BS, Goudar SS, et al. Oral Miso-prostol in preventing postpartum haemorrhage in resource-poor communities: A Randomized Controlled Trial. Lancet 2006;368:1248–53

112. Mobeen N, Durocher J, Zuberi NF, et al. Administration of misoprostol by trained traditional birth attendants to prevent postpartum haemorrhage in homebirths in Pakistan: a randomised placebo-controlled trial. BJOG 2011;118:353–61

113. Walraven G, Blum J, Dampha Y, et al. Misoprostol in the management of the third stage of labor in the home delivery setting in rural Gambia: a randomized controlled trial. Br J Obstet Gynaecol 2005;112:1277–83

114. Høj L, Cardoso P, Nielsen BB, Hvidman L, Nielsen J, Aaby P. Effect of sublingual Misoprostol on severe postpartum haemorrhage in a primary health centre in Guinea–Bissau: randomised double blind clinical trial. Br Med J 2005;331:723–8

115. Winikoff B, Dabash R, Durocher J, et al. Treatment of post-partum haemorrhage with sublingual misoprostol ver-sus oxytocin in women not exposed to oxytocin during labour: a double-blind, randomised, non-inferiority trial. Lancet 2010;375:210–6

116. Blum J, Winikoff B, Raghavan S, et al. Treatment of post-partum haemorrhage with sublingual misoprostol versus oxytocin in women receiving prophylactic oxytocin: a double-blind, randomised, non-inferiority trial. Lancet 2010;375:217–23

117. Weeks A. Oral misoprostol for postpartum haemorrhage. Lancet 2006;368:2123

118. Fiala C, Gemzell-Danielsson K, Tang OS, von Hertzen H. Cervical priming with misoprostol prior to transcervical procedures. Int J Gynecol Obstet 2007;99:S168–S171

119. Mendilcioglu I, Zorlu CG, Simsek M. Successful termina-tion of cervical pregnancy with misoprostol. Eur J Obstet Gynecol Reprod Biol 2003;106:96

120. New US Food and Drug Administration Labeling on Cytotec (Misoprostol) Use and Pregnancy. ACOG Com-mittee Opinion 283. Washington, DC: American College of Obstetricians and Gynecologists, 2003

121. World Health Organization unedited Report of the 18th Expert Committee on the Selection and Use of Essential Medicines 21–25 March 2011, Accra, Ghana: WHO

122. World Health Organization. Model List of Essential Medi-cines. WHO: Geneva, http://www.who.int/medicines/publications/unedited_trs/en/index.html

Editorial note: A randomized controlled trial by Bellad et al. comparing sublingual misoprostol and intramuscular oxytocin for the prevention of postpartum hemorrhage demonstrates that a relatively low dose of sublingual misoprostol is more effec-tive than standard intramuscular administration of oxytocin for vaginal deliveries. This is the first study to demonstrate sublingual misoprostol's superiority over intramuscular oxytocin and it is easier to administer. (Bellad M, Tara D, Ganachari M, et al. Prevention of postpartum haemorrhage with sublingual misoprostol or oxytocin: a double-blind randomised controlled trial. BJOG 2012;119:975–86). M.K.

33

Misoprostol in Practice

C. E. Henderson, H. El-Refaey and M. Potts

In the early 1990s, misoprostol was virtually unknown amongst obstetricians and gynecologists. Today, it has become an essential drug used in every part of the world by all those involved in women's health. It has gone from a limited role in gastric ulcer disease to the focus of obstetric care and an essential part of fertility regulation. As a low-cost, easy-to-administer, powerful uterotonic with an excellent safety profile and long shelf-life, misoprostol has the revolutionary potential to reduce death and morbidity from postpartum hemorrhage (PPH) in precisely those situations where it is most common – among the 40–50 million women who deliver at home without a skilled birth attendant.

The different obstetric uses of misoprostol are inextricably mixed. Misoprostol can be used for the prevention and treatment of PPH, for the treatment of incomplete abortion, and for induced abortion, as well as for labor induction, cervical dilation and the treatment of intrauterine fetal death. Millennium Development Goal (MDG) 5, to reduce maternal deaths by three-quarters between 1990 and 2015, is unlikely to be achieved in many low resource settings without the widespread distribution of misoprostol. The drug has performed superbly, but availability, accurate knowledge regarding its correct use and the regulatory framework for its approval have lagged behind the potential of misoprostol to save the lives of women on a large scale.

Women have searched for botanical uterotonics for thousands of years. In 1932, Moir reported the use of ergometrine to control PPH[1]. During that same decade, Von Euler isolated the first prostaglandins[2], but it was another 30 years before the systematic study of the obstetric and gynecological uses of various prostaglandins began. Ravenholt proposed the use of prostaglandins as an emmenagogue in 1968[3] and in 1970, Karim and Filshie demonstrated that prostaglandin F2α could be used to induce abortion[4]. However, therapeutic options were limited by high cost, the need for injection and refrigeration requirements. This changed in 1988 when the Upjohn Company began clinical trials of a synthetic prostaglandin E1 analogue called misoprostol (Cytotec®) for the treatment of gastric ulcers[5]. With the potential of a large market for long-term daily use, the company invested in developing a thermostable oral tablet. Typically, 200 μg four times per day was – and still is – prescribed for gastric ulcers. The United States Food and Drug Administration label for Cytotec states that, 'cumulative total daily doses of 1600 μg have been tolerated, with only symptoms of gastrointestinal discomfort being reported'[6].

The off-label use of misoprostol as a uterotonic began in the 1990s[7]. By 2001, over 300 papers had been published in peer-reviewed journals on the obstetric and gynecological uses of misoprostol[8]. Research has demonstrated that misoprostol can be delivered orally, vaginally, rectally, buccally and sublingually. *In utero* exposure to misoprostol, as in cases of attempted abortion, has been associated with congenital defects, but the absolute risk is low[9]. Side-effects, including pyrexia and shivering have been reported with misoprostol use, but these are often resolved with conservative treatment. In a 2010 review of 46 randomized controlled trials of misoprostol, involving more than 40,000 patients, only 11 deaths were reported; eight of these were reported as deaths associated with PPH, while the other three deaths were from causes unrelated to PPH or causes were not provided[10].

The uterotonic effect of misoprostol varies greatly over the course of gestation. Misoprostol dosages as low as 25 μg are safe and effective in the induction of labor when given orally or vaginally. The drug is also effective, when administered sublingually or rectally, for intractable PPH in single doses of 800 μg or 1000 μg, respectively[11–13]. Misoprostol is an unusually powerful drug, and some of the doses now in clinical practice may be lowered as more clinical experience is gained.

CLINICAL USE IN POSTPARTUM HEMORRHAGE

Delivery with a trained birth attendant

When active management of the third stage of labor (AMTSL) with oxytocin is compared to expectant management, the relative risk of losing 1000 ml of blood at the time of birth is 0.34 (CI 0.14–0.87)[14]. In 2001, the World Health Organization (WHO) co-ordinated a randomized controlled trial testing 600 μg of oral misoprostol against 10 units of oxytocin in well resourced hospitals. It was found that oxytocin was marginally more effective than misoprostol (RR 1.39, 95% CI 1.19–1.63), although there was only 1%

difference in the frequency of blood loss of 1000 ml or more between participants in each arm of the study[15]. Shannon and Winikoff, while accepting the statistical significance of this difference, question its clinical relevance[16].

In a randomized controlled placebo trial in Belgaum, India, 600 μg of oral misoprostol was associated with a significant reduction in severe PPH compared to placebo (RR risk 0.20, 95% CI 0.04–0.91)[17]. A pre- and postintervention comparison of the use of misoprostol and standard of care with other uterotonics, including oxytocin, was conducted in a busy hospital setting in Egypt and found that misoprostol performed consistently better than oxytocin (Figure 1)[18].

Use in low resource settings

The 1987 Nairobi Safe Motherhood Conference drew attention to the unacceptably high maternal mortality ratios (MMR) around the world. As noted, MDG 5 is not being achieved in low resource settings, where the highest death rates occur during home births that take place farthest from hospitals and without trained birth attendants. Based on a study from Zimbabwe, which found the total MMR to be 725 per 100,000, and of which 14.4% were due to PPH alone, it can be calculated that the MMR due to PPH is approximately 104/100,000 live births[19]. WHO and the International Federation of Gynecology and Obstetrics (FIGO) have emphasized the need to extend the reach of emergency obstetric care, and this should be a long-term goal for all countries. However, for the foreseeable future, lack of trained staff, reluctance to work in deep rural areas and migration from countries of the south to those of the north, will continue to stall the extension of emergency obstetric care[20].

The first national drug regulatory authority to approve the use of misoprostol for PPH was that of Nigeria in 2006, facilitated by Venture Strategies for Health and Development. Prior to the availability of misoprostol, it was impossible to do anything to significantly reduce mortality associated with PPH among the most vulnerable women, many of whom live on less than one or two US dollars per day. Most efforts to

train traditional birth attendants have failed to show a significant positive impact on the MMR[21]. PPH is difficult to predict, a traditional birth attendant may miss diagnosing pre-eclampsia, and exhorting traditional birth attendants to wash their hands, while a good idea, does not have a measurable impact on the MMR. Misoprostol changes this dynamic. It is the first life-saving technology that can be used during home delivery without a trained birth attendant[22]. Operations research in Tanzania has demonstrated that trained birth attendants can diagnose and treat PPH with 1000 μg of misoprostol given rectally[23]. In Nepal, Afghanistan, Bangladesh and elsewhere, tens of thousands of women have been taught to self-administer 600 μg of misoprostol orally after delivering their babies without serious side-effects or systematic misuse[24–26].

Induction of labor

All over the world, the induction of labor is an integral part of the management of serious conditions such as pre-eclampsia, diabetes and chorioamninotis. Even in middle income countries, prior to the introduction of vaginal misoprostol, women endured long hours of induction of labor with a Syntocinon® infusion because the available prostaglandins were too expensive (costing the equivalent of a month's disposable income) to use. The arrival of misoprostol removed this inequity. Clinicians around the world have learnt to divide misoprostol tablets into one-eighth parts, though this can be difficult, and certain manufacturers are now producing 25 μg tablets. An optimal method of delivery is to prepare a solution with 200 μg tablets and administer it orally for smaller divided doses[27].

ABORTION AND EVACUATION OF THE PREGNANT UTERUS IN THE FIRST TRIMESTER

Abortion remains illegal in most of the world to date, inaccessible to millions of women around the globe. The unmet demand for abortion is often met illicitly and is criminalized. Of the estimated 43.8 million abortions that occurred globally during 2008, nearly half of those were unsafe. The proportion of unsafe abortion is even higher in certain regions of the world, with an estimated 65% and 97% of all abortions being unsafe in South Central Asia and Africa, respectively, in 2008[28].

Where abortion is illegal, unsafe procedures to interrupt pregnancy are commonly one of the most frequent causes of maternal death after PPH. The estimated 47,000 abortion deaths in 2008 accounted for nearly 13% of all maternal deaths[29]. Women who try to achieve abortion themselves have resorted to herbal medications, the use of sharp needles and jumping from stairs. Many of these women suffer physical and mental trauma as a result, and many also end up seeking medical or paramedical help to achieve the abortion. Such help is often only available in clandestine fashion. The surgery for termination of pregnancy

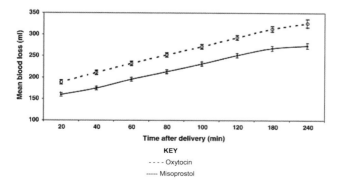

Figure 1 Cumulative mean blood loss and 95% confidence intervals. From Prata *et al.*, 2006[18], with permission

was, and is, performed in suboptimal circumstances. Anesthetics and sterilization of instruments are compromised and doctors may or may not have received proper training in the procedure. The morbidity of illegal and illicit abortion on hospital admissions is very well documented.

The rise of misoprostol in women's health around the globe led to a substantial drop in abortion morbidity on two fronts. First, it changed the nature of illicit abortion from a surgical procedure to a semi-medical procedure. A failed illicit abortion that started with misoprostol is arguably a safer intervention than a surgical one. In those same countries where abortion is illegal, but misoprostol is available to replace the use of more dangerous traditional methods, admissions for complicated incomplete abortions fall, as has been recorded in the Dominican Republic[30]. Second, the development of mifepristone, and subsequently medical induction of abortion, was a landmark in reproductive freedom. Originally, the regimen involved the use of mifepristone and a prostaglandin analogue. Two of the most widely used prostaglandin analogues available prior to misoprostol included sulprostone and gemeprost. The former is administered parenterally, while the latter is a vaginal pessary. Neither of these were appropriate technologies for use in developing countries, as both required cold chain transfer and specific storage requirements. The introduction of misoprostol as a thermostable agent heralded yet another chapter of equality in reproductive freedom around the world. Where abortion is legal, as in Ethiopia, a pilot project using community health extension workers to offer medical abortion using misoprostol in the first 9 weeks of pregnancy led to hospital admissions for abortion complications plummeting from the number one most common reason for hospital admission to the tenth reason[31].

INTRAUTERINE FETAL DEATH IN THE SECOND AND THIRD TRIMESTER

Intrauterine fetal death is a tragedy for any pregnant mother and a cause of concern to all involved. Evacuating a pregnant uterus in the second or third trimester is a biological challenge since the cervix is not ripe and the myometrial receptors are not primed for uterine contractility. Prior to misoprostol this biological challenge had no clear or pharmacological answer. In North America, dilation and evacuation or hysterectomy were widely practiced with significant physical and psychological morbidity. In Europe, the use of prostaglandins replaced the use of high dosages of Syntocinon regimens in the 1980s. Extra-amniotic administration of prostaglandins compared with intra-amniotic prostaglandins or vaginal pessaries were also explored as alternative technologies. Again, misoprostol has ushered in a new era for women throughout the world. The drug has proved effective and well tolerated in the management of fetal death in advanced pregnancies.

WHERE NEXT?

Over the past decade, misoprostol has moved from an exciting new drug to one which is widely thought can revolutionize obstetrics and reproductive health worldwide. While it takes time to assimilate this remarkable expansion of research and clinical practice, the life-saving potential of misoprostol has been unnecessarily hindered by a mixture of medical conservatism and controversy over abortion. Regulatory approval has been slow and policies for community distribution have been resisted.

Despite many years of advocacy by groups, such as FIGO, the International Confederation of Midwives, Venture Strategies Innovations, Jhpiego, Gynuity and experienced obstetricians with clinical experience with PPH, WHO delayed placing misoprostol on the Essential Medicines List for PPH until 2011. One reason for the delay was that the WHO Department for Making Pregnancy Safer imposed the 'gold standard' of randomized clinical trials to assess the strength of the evidence base for making the recommendations. However, randomized clinical trials involving misoprostol for prevention of PPH cannot be implemented during home births without a trained birth attendant. It would be ethically unacceptable to randomize misoprostol against a placebo where no alternative to save the life of a hemorrhaging woman is available, especially when we know that misoprostol is an effective uterotonic and can and does save lives.

Governments such as those of Nigeria and Bangladesh have already approved community distribution of misoprostol to pregnant women for self-administration after delivery. Prata et al.[32] demonstrate that reducing deaths from PPH and unsafe abortion will result in the greatest gains in maternal deaths averted in low resource settings (Figure 2). Their models also demonstrate that the most cost-effective interventions to reduce maternal mortality in low resource settings include family planning and safe abortion services, as well as antenatal care with misoprostol. Safe delivery, eclampsia and standard antenatal care services, which do not include the distribution of misoprostol, were found to be the least cost-effective interventions. There is an order of magnitude difference in cost per death averted between the provision of safe deliveries in a facility with trained health

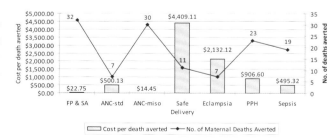

Figure 2 Average cost and number of maternal deaths averted in low infrastructure setting. ANC, antenatal care; FP, family planning; SA, safe abortion. From Prata et al., 2010[32], with permission

professionals plus emergency obstetric care, estimated at $4410 per death averted, compared to the distribution of misoprostol for home deliveries without a trained birth attendant, estimated at $15 per death averted[32].

The power of misoprostol reaches beyond medical practice into many communities. It is a potentially low cost medicine, with a wholesale price ranging from 15 to 90 US cents per tablet. However, while life-saving, any one woman may need misoprostol perhaps only once in a life time, and a low-volume, low-cost medicine is not commercially attractive to many retailers. Most women will recognize the power of a self-administered means of bringing on a delayed period, whether abortion is legal or illegal in the country where they live. Consequently, where misoprostol is difficult to obtain, as in parts of Sub-Saharan Africa, the retail price can exceed $10 US dollars per tablet.

For misoprostol to reach its full potential, women need access to a low cost or free product supported by correct information on doses and side-effects. In Bangladesh, the government purchases misoprostol tablets from local manufacturers and distributes them to women in free birthing kits to control PPH. In Nigeria, the government is buying misoprostol tablets from China and plans to distribute them at the community level. Misoprostol can also be delivered through social marketing of a branded product and it is also possible that women's groups will have the ability to distribute misoprostol in low resource settings.

Perhaps the least explored aspect of the use of misoprostol is how women who obtain this medicine through informal channels can find the information they need on its correct and safe use, and on its side-effects. For prevention of PPH, options include training front line health workers, community volunteers and the use of media. Mobile phones are now ubiquitous even in many relatively remote parts of Africa and Asia, and can be used to distribute reproductive health information.

There will always be different perspectives on abortion, even when completed early in pregnancy. However, there is consensus that in situations where abortion is illegal and a woman undergoes an unsafe abortion, she should still be given the best possible clinical care, treated with respect and offered contraceptive advice if she wants it. Every obstetrician and gynecologist knows that once a woman decides to end a pregnancy, she may go as far as risking her own life to do so. Does the ethical responsibility of professionals extend to thinking of ways to spread correct knowledge about the use of misoprostol, even where access to legal abortion is constrained?

CONCLUSIONS

Misoprostol is the 'penicillin' of reproductive health. Just as penicillin introduced a new era of large scale antibiotic use with a measurable impact on global death rates, so too can misoprostol begin to lower maternal mortality ratios worldwide. No other

medicine crosses the divide between the joy of a safe delivery of a wanted child and the despair of an unintended pregnancy. The fact that misoprostol is also the first uterotonic that women can self-administer to control PPH, bring on a late period, or induce an early abortion, is also the reason it is certain to remain controversial. The self-administration of misoprostol by lay people is not ideal, but it is an order of magnitude safer than the absence of any therapy for PPH or the alternative of highly unsafe traditional methods of bringing on a late period or inducing abortion.

The first full decade of widespread use of misoprostol has been marked by a revolution in the treatment of PPH and the spread of medical abortion. The next decade is likely to see a further scaling up of use. For the hundreds of million fertile women living on a dollar a day or less, the International Conference on Population and Development (ICPD) and MDG targets to reduce maternal mortality remain as remote today as they were when each was set. Unless technologies and distribution systems to control PPH during home births in the absence of trained birth attendants can be set up, then taking into account the rapid increase in the number of women of fertile age in the poorest countries, it is possible that more women living on a dollar or two a day will die in childbirth each year in the current decade, than died around the time of the 1987 Nairobi Safe Motherhood Conference. Bringing the use of misoprostol to scale has the power to reverse this most tragic of outcomes.

References

1. Moir C. The action of ergot preparations on the puerperal uterus. BMJ 1932;2:1199–22
2. Von Euler U. On the specific vasodilating and plain muscle stimulating substances from accessory genital glands in man and certain animals. J Physiol (Lond) 1936;88:213–34
3. Ravenholt R. Abortion in a Changing World. Hall RE, ed. New York: Columbia University Press, 1968;2:49–52
4. Karim S, Filshie G. Therapeutic abortion using prostaglandin F2-alpha. Lancet 1970;1:157–9
5. Garris R, Kirkwood C. Misoprostol: a prostaglandin E1 analogue. Clin Pharm 1989;8:627–44
6. United States Food and Drug Administration. United States Department of Health and Human Services. Cytotec® (Misoprostol) Prescribing Information. 2002. http://www.accessdata.fda.gov/drugsatfda_docs/label/2002/19268slr037.pdf
7. El Refaey H, Hinshaw K, Templeton A. The abortifacient effect of misoprostol in the second trimester. A randomized comparison with gemeprost in patients pre-treated with mifepristone (RU486). Hum Reprod 1993;8:1744–6
8. Goldberg A, Greenberg M, Darney P. Misoprostol and pregnancy. N Engl J Med 2001;344:38–47
9. Population Council. Philip N, Shannon C, Winikoff B, eds. Misoprostol and Teratogenicity: Reviewing the Evidence. New York: The Population Council, Inc., 2003. http://www.popcouncil.org/pdfs/ebert/Misoterat.PDF
10. Hofmeyr J, Gulmezoglu A, Novikova N, et al. Misoprostol to prevent and treat postpartum haemorrhage: a systematic review and meta-analysis of maternal deaths and dose-related effects. Bull World Health Organ 2009;87:666–77
11. Blum J, Winikoff B, Raghavan S, et al. Treatment of postpartum haemorrhage with sublingual misoprostol versus oxytocin in women receiving prophylactic oxytocin: a

double-blind, randomised, non inferiority trial. Lancet 2010; 375:217–23

12. Winikoff B, Dabash R, Durocher D, et al. Treatment of post-partum haemorrhage with sublingual misoprostol versus oxytocin in women not exposed to oxytocin during labour: a double-blind, randomised, non inferiority trial. Lancet 2010; 375:210–6

13. Prata N, Mbaruku G, Campbell M, Potts M, Vahidnia F. Controlling postpartum hemorrhage after home births in Tanzania. Int J Gynecol Obstet 2005;90:51–5

14. Begley C, Gyte G, Devane D, McGuire W, Weeks A. Active versus expectant management for women in the third stage of labor (review). Cochrane Database Syst Rev 2011;(11): CD007412

15. Gulmezoglu AM, Vilar J, Ngoc NN, et al. for the WHO Collaborative Group to Evaluate Misoprostol in the Management of the Third Stage of Labour. The WHO multicenter double-blind randomized controlled trial to evaluate the use of misoprostol in the third stage of labour. Lancet 2001;358: 689–95

16. Shannon C, Winikoff B. Use of misoprostol in the third stage of labour. Lancet 2002;359:709

17. Derman RJ, Koudkany BS, Goudar SS, et al. Oral misoprostol in preventing postpartum haemorrhage in resource-poor communities: a randomised controlled trial. Lancet 2006;368:1248–53

18. Prata N, Hamza S, Gypson R, et al. Misoprostol and active management of the third stage of labor. Intl J Gynecol Obstet 2006;94:149–55

19. Munjanja S. Ministry of Health and Child Welfare Zimbabwe. Maternal and Perinatal Mortality Study. 2007. http:// www.unicef.org/zimbabwe/ZMPMS_report.pdf

20. Gessessew A, Barnabas G, Prata N, et al. Task shifting and sharing in Tigray, Ethiopia, to achieve comprehensive emergency obstetric care. Int J Gynecol Obstet 2011;113:28–31

21. Sibley L, Sipe T. What can a meta-analysis tell us about traditional birth attendant training and pregnancy outcomes. Midwifery 2004;20:51–60

22. Wiknjosastro G, Sanghvi H. Preventing PPH among women living in areas where a high proportion of births are not attended by skilled providers: Safety, acceptability, feasibility and program effectiveness (SAFE) demonstration project of community-based distribution of misoprostol for prevention of PPH in rural Indonesia. Proceedings of Preventing Postpartum Hemorrhage: From Research to Practice. Bangkok, Thailand. January 20–24, 2004:31–7

23. Prata N, Mbaruka G, Campbell M, Potts M, Vahidnia F. Controlling postpartum hemorrhage after home births in Tanzania. Int J Gynaecol Obstet 2005;90:51–5

24. Rajbhandari S, Hodgins S, Sanghvi H, McPherson R, Pradhan YV, Baqui AH, and Misoprostol Study Group. Expanding uterotonic protection following childbirth through community-based distribution of misoprostol: operations research study in Nepal. Int J Gynecol Obstet 2010;108:282–8

25. Sanghvi H, Ansari N, Prata JVN, Gibson H, Ehsan A, Smith J. Prevention of postpartum hemorrhage at home birth in Afghanistan. Int J Gynecol Obstet 2010;108:276–81

26. Nasreen HE, Nahar S, Mamun M, Afsana K, Byass P. Oral misoprostol for preventing postpartum haemorrhage in home births in rural Bangladesh: how effective is it? Glob Health Action 2011;4

27. Misoprostol in Obstetrics and Gynaecology. Recommended Doses of Misoprostol (Cytotec®). 2009. www.misoprostol.org

28. Sedgh G, Singh S, Henshaw S, Bankole A. Induced abortion: incidence and trends worldwide from 1995 to 2008. Lancet 2012;379:625–32

29. World Health Organization. Unsafe Abortion: Global and Regional Estimates of the Incidence of Unsafe Abortion and Associated Mortality in 2008, 6th edn. 2011. http:// whqlibdoc.who.int/publications/2011/9789241501118_eng. pdf

30. Miller S, Lehman T, Campbell M, et al. Misoprostol and declining abortion-related morbidity in Santo Domingo, Dominican Republic: a temporal association. Int J Obstet Gynaecol 2005;112:1291–6

31. Prata N, Gessessew A, Campbell M, Potts M. A new hope for women: medical abortion is a low-resource setting in Ethiopia. J Fam Plann Reprod Health Care 2011;37: 196–7

32. Prata N, Sreenivas A, Greig F, Walsh J, Potts M. Setting priorities for safe motherhood interventions in resource-scarce settings. Health Policy 2010;94:1–13

34

Overview of Misoprostol Studies in Postpartum Hemorrhage

A. Hemmerling

INTRODUCTION

A series of tables of peer-reviewed misoprostol studies have been compiled to provide the reader with a set of comprehensive references since 1997 to the use of misoprostol for both prevention and treatment of postpartum hemorrhage (PPH). The tables include both randomized and non-randomized trials, and they represent a diversity of situations.

Table 1 provides an overview of 52 studies on the prevention of PPH (including number of participants, dosage and route of administration, and control agents). Table 2 gives an overview of 11 studies on the treatment of PPH (including number of participants, dosage and route of administration, and control agents). Table 3 lists nine reviews and meta-analyses published on the topic.

SUMMARY

Misoprostol greatly reduces severe PPH[1], but is less effective than injectable oxytocin for the prevention and treatment of PPH[2,3].

Although the use of injectable uterotonics is preferred in hospital settings, misoprostol has effectively been used in community and home settings[3–8] (see Chapter 42).

For prevention of PPH, misoprostol should be administered during the third stage of labor at any point after the anterior shoulder is delivered[9].

Currently the dose most commonly used for PPH is 600 µg of oral or sublingual misoprostol. Rectal administration may offer similar benefits, and causes fewer side-effects[9]. Newer studies show that a dose of 400 µg of oral misoprostol is as effective as 600 µg, but with fewer side-effects[10,11].

Existing evidence continues to grow regarding the use of misoprostol in treatment of PPH. A single dose of 600 µg oral or 800 µg sublingual misoprostol is recommended in instances when other treatments have either failed to work or are not available[12–14]. A Cochrane review found no significant reduction in mortality or decreased need for further blood transfusion and use of more uterotonics when comparing misoprostol with a combination of injectable uterotonics (oxytocin and ergometrine)[15].

Administering misoprostol in addition to the normal regimen with injectable uterotonics showed no added benefit[16–18].

Pyrexia and shivering were more common side-effects with misoprostol than with injectable uterotonics, and seem to be dose related[1,2,7,11,15,18,19]. Although frequently mentioned as a limitation associated with use of misoprostol, neither is life threatening or bothersome for an inordinate period of time.

In the event of continued hemorrhage, a minimum of 2 hours waiting period is recommended before the application of a second dose. In case of pyrexia or marked shivering, at least 6 h should pass[3,20].

Table 1 Misoprostol for prevention of postpartum hemorrhage (PPH)

Author	Site(s)	Study title	Journal	Total number of participants	Participants in misoprostol group(s)	Dosage of misoprostol (µg)	Route of administration	Participants in control group(s)	Control agent(s)
Hashima-E-Nasreen	Bangladesh	Oral misoprostol for preventing postpartum haemorrhage in home births in rural Bangladesh: how effective is it?	Glob Health Action 2011; Epub 2011 Aug 10	2017	1009	400 µg	Oral	1008	Placebo
Mobeen et al.	Pakistan	Administration of misoprostol by trained traditional birth attendants to prevent postpartum haemorrhage in homebirths in Pakistan: a randomised placebo-controlled trial.	BJOG 2011;118:353–61	1119	534	600 µg	Oral	585	Placebo
Hofmeyr et al.	South Africa, Nigeria, Uganda	Administration of 400 µg of misoprostol to augment routine active management of the third stage of labor	Int J Gynaecol Obstet 2011;112:98–102	1103	547	400 µg [plus 10 IU oxytocin I.M. or 0.2–0.5 mg ergometrine I.M. as routine AMTSL]	Sublingual	556	Placebo. All participants received 10 IU oxytocin I.M. or 0.2–0.5 mg ergometrine I.M. as routine AMTSL
Fawole et al.	Nigeria	A double-blind, randomized, placebo-controlled trial of misoprostol and routine uterotonics for the prevention of postpartum hemorrhage	Int J Gynaecol Obstet 2011;112:107–11	1345	672	400 µg [plus 10 IU oxytocin I.M. or 0.2–0.5 mg ergometrine I.M. as routine AMTSL]	Sublingual	673	Placebo. All participants received 10 IU oxytocin I.M. or 0.2–0.5 mg ergometrine I.M. as routine AMTSL
Mansouri et al.	Saudi Arabia	Rectal versus oral misoprostol for active management of third stage of labor: a randomized controlled trial	Arch Gynecol Obstet 2011;283:935–9	658	[1] 331 [2] 327	600	[1] Oral [2] Rectal		
Sanghvi et al.	Afghanistan	Prevention of postpartum hemorrhage at home birth in Afghanistan	Int J Gynaecol Obstet 2010;108:276–81	3187	1421	600	Oral	1148	Placebo
Afolabi et al.	Nigeria	Oral misoprostol versus intramuscular oxytocin in the active management of the third stage of labour	Singapore Med J 2010; 51:207	200	100	400	Oral	100	10 IU oxytocin I.M.
Singh et al.	India	Comparison of sublingual misoprostol, intravenous oxytocin, and intravenous methylergometrine in active management of the third stage of labour	Int J Gynaecol Obstet 2009;107:130–4	300	[1] 75 [2] 75	[1] 400 [2] 600	Sublingual	[3] 75 [4] 75	[3] 5 IU oxytocin I.V. [4] 0.2 mg methylergometrine I.V.
Vaid et al.	India	A randomized controlled trial of prophylactic sublingual misoprostol versus intramuscular methyl-ergometrine versus intramuscular 15-methyl PGF2-Alpha in active management of third stage of labor	Arch Gynecol Obstet 2009;280:893–987	200	66	400	Sublingual	[1] 67 [2] 67	[1] 0.2 mg methylergometrine I.M. [2] 125 µg 15-methyl PGF2-Alpha I.M.
Nasr et al.	Egypt	Rectal misoprostol versus intravenous oxytocin for prevention of postpartum hemorrhage	Int J Gynaecol Obstet 2009;105:244–7	514	257	800	Rectal	257	5 IU oxytocin I.V.
Harriott et al.	Jamaica	A randomized comparison of rectal misoprostol with syntometrine on blood loss in the third stage of labour	West Indian Med J 2009;58:201–6	140		400	Rectal		Syntometrine I.M. (10 IU syntocinone and 0.5 mg ergometrine)
Haque et al.	Bangladesh	Comparative study between rectally administered misoprostol as a prophylaxis versus conventional intramuscular oxytocin in post partum hemorrhage	Mymensigh Med J 2009;18(1 Suppl):S40–4	200	100	600	Rectal	100	10 IU oxytocin I.M.

Study	Country	Title	Reference	n	Misoprostol n	Dose (µg)	Route	Comparison n	Comparison
Al-Harazi et al.	Yemen	Sublingual misoprostol for the prevention of postpartum hemorrhage	Saudi Med J 2009;30:912–6	215	[1] 118 [2] 97	600	[1] Sublingual [2] Rectal	481	Current AMTSL practices
Prata et al.	Ethiopia	Prevention of postpartum hemorrhage: options for homebirths in rural Ethiopia	Afr J Reprod Health 2009;13:87–95	966	485	600	Oral	481	0.5 mg methylergometrine I.M.
Enakpene et al.	Nigeria	Oral misoprostol for the prevention of primary post-partum hemorrhage during third stage of labor	J Obstet Gynaecol Res 2007;33:810–7	864	432	400	Oral	432	
Ng et al.	China	A double-blind randomized controlled trial of oral misoprostol and intramuscular syntometrine in the management of the third stage of labor	Gynecol Obstet Invest 2007;63:55–60	355	178	400	Oral	177	1 ml syntometrine I.M. (5 IU syntocinone and 0.5 mg ergometrine)
Baskett et al.	Canada	Misoprostol versus oxytocin for the reduction of postpartum blood loss	Int J Gynaecol Obstet 2007;97:2–5	622	311	400	Oral	311	5 IU oxytocin I.V.
Parsons et al.	Ghana	Rectal misoprostol versus oxytocin in the management of the third stage of labour	J Obstet Gynaecol Can 2007;29:711–8	450		800	Rectal		10 IU oxytocin I.M.
Parsons et al.	Ghana	Oral misoprostol versus oxytocin in the management of the third stage of labour	J Obstet Gynaecol Can 2006;28:20–6	450		800	Oral		10 IU oxytocin I.M.
Derman et al.	India	Use of oral misoprostol in the prevention of PPH	Lancet 2006;368:1248–53	1620	812	600	Oral	808	Placebo
Prata et al.	Egypt	Misoprostol and active management of the third stage of labor	Int J Gynaecol Obstet 2006;94:149–55	2532	1189	600	Oral	1343	Current AMTSL practices
Nellore et al.	India	Rectal misoprostol vs. 15-methyl prostaglandin F2(alpha) for the prevention of postpartum hemorrhage	Int J Gynaecol Obstet 2006;94:45–6	120	60	400	Rectal	60	125 µg 15-methyl prostaglandin F2α I.M.
Chandhiok et al.	India	Oral misoprostol for prevention of postpartum hemorrhage by paramedical workers in India	Int J Gynaecol Obstet 2006;92:170–5	1200	600	600	Oral	600	Current government guidelines for PPH prevention
Zachariah et al.	India	Oral misoprostol in the third stage of labor	Int J Gynaecol Obstet 2006;92:23–6	2023	730	400	Oral	[1] 617 [2] 676	[1] 10 IU oxytocin I.M. [2] 2 mg ergometrine I.V.
Garg et al.	India	Oral misoprostol versus injectable methylergometrine in management of the third stage of labor	Int J Gynaecol Obstet 2005;91:160–1	200	100	600	Oral	100	0.2 mg methylergometrine I.V.
Ozkaya et al.	Turkey	Placebo-controlled randomized comparison of vaginal with rectal misoprostol in the prevention of postpartum hemorrhage	J Obstet Gynaecol Res 2005;31:389–93	150	[1] 50 [2] 50	400	[1] Rectal [2] Oral	50	Placebo
Hoj et al.	Guinea-Bissau	Effect of sublingual misoprostol on severe postpartum haemorrhage in a primary health centre in Guinea-Bissau: randomised double blind clinical trial	BMJ 2005;331:723	661	330	600	Sublingual	331	Placebo
Walraven et al.	The Gambia	Misoprostol in the management of the third stage of labour in the home delivery setting in rural Gambia: a randomised controlled trial	BJOG 2005;112:1277–83	1229	630	600	Oral	599	2 mg ergometrine oral

Continued

Table 1 Continued

Author	Site(s)	Study title	Journal	Total number of participants	Participants in misoprostol group(s)	Dosage of misoprostol (μg)	Route of administration	Participants in control group(s)	Control agent(s)
Vimala et al.	India	Sublingual misoprostol versus methylergometrine for active management of the third stage of labor	Int J Gynaecol Obstet 2004;87:1–5	120	60	400	Sublingual	60	0.2 mg methylergometrine I.V.
Lam et al.	China	A pilot-randomized comparison of sublingual misoprostol with syntometrine on the blood loss in 3rd stage of labor	Acta Obstet Gynecol Scand 2004;83:647–50	60	30	600	Sublingual	30	1 ml syntometrine I.V. (5 IU syntocinone and 0.5 mg ergometrine)
Caliskan et al.	Turkey	Oral misoprostol for the 3rd stage of labor: a randomized controlled trial	Obstet Gynecol 2003; 101:921–8	1574	388	600	Oral	[1] 404 [2] 384 [3] 398	[1] 600 μg misoprostol plus 10 IU oxytocin I.V. [2] 10 IU oxytocin I.V. [3] 10 IU oxytocin I.V. plus 0.2 mg methylergonovine
Oboro et al.	Nigeria	A randomised controlled trial of misoprostol versus oxytocin in the active management of the third stage of labour	Obstet Gynaecol 2003; 23:13–6	496	247	600	Oral	249	10 IU oxytocin I.M.
Lumbiganon et al.	Thailand	Side effects of oral misoprostol during the first 24 hours after administration in the third stage of labour	BJOG 2002;109:1222–6	1686	843	600	Oral	843	10 IU oxytocin I.M. or I.V.
Quiroga Diaz et al.	Mexico	Vaginal misoprostol in the prevention of PPH	Ginecol Obstet Mex 2002;70:572–5	400	208	800	Vaginal	192	Current AMTSL practices
Caliskan et al.	Turkey	Is rectal misoprostol really effective in the treatment of third stage of labor? A randomized controlled trial	Am J Obstet Gynecol 2002;187:1038–45	1606	396	600	Rectal	[1] 401 [2] 407 [3] 402	[1] 10 IU oxytocin I.V. plus 600 μg misoprostol rectal [2] 10 IU oxytocin I.V. [3] 10 IU oxytocin I.V. plus 1 ml methylergometrine I.M.
Karkanis et al.	Canada	Randomized controlled trial of rectal misoprostol versus oxytocin in third stage management	J Obstet Gynaecol Can 2002;24:149–54	214	110	400	Rectal	113	5 IU oxytocin I.V. or 10 IU oxytocin I.M.
Kundodyiwa et al.	Zimbabwe	Misoprostol versus oxytocin in the third stage of labor	Int J Gynaecol Obstet 2001;75:235–41	499	243	400	Oral	256	10 IU oxytocin I.M.
Benchimol et al.	France	Role of misoprostol in the delivery outcome	J Gynecol Obstet Biol Reprod 2001;30:576–83	600	200	600	Oral	[1] 200 [2] 200	[1] 2.5 IU oxytocin I.V. [2] placebo
Gerstenfeld et al.	USA	Rectal misoprostol versus intravenous oxytocin for the prevention of PPH after vaginal delivery	Am J Obstet Gynecol 2001;185:878–82	325	159	400	Rectal	166	20 IU oxytocin I.V.

Author	Country	Title	Reference	Dose	n	n	Route	n	Comparison
Gulmezoglu et al.	Argentina, China, Egypt, Ireland, Nigeria, South Africa, Switzerland, Thailand, Vietnam	WHO multicentre randomised trial of misoprostol in the management of the third stage of labour	Lancet 2001;358:689–95	18530	9264	600	Oral	9266	10 IU oxytocin I.M. or I.V.
Hofmeyr et al.	South Africa	Side-effects of oral misoprostol in the third stage of labour – a randomised placebo-controlled trial	S Afr Med J 2001;91:432–5	600	300	600	Oral	300	placebo
Bugalho et al.	Mozambique	Misoprostol for prevention of PPH	Int J Gynaecol Obstet 2001;73:1–6	663	324	400	Rectal	339	10 IU oxytocin I.M.
Ng et al.	China	A multicentre randomized controlled trial of oral misoprostol and I.m syntometrine in the management of the third stage of labour	Hum Reprod 2001;16:31–5	2058	1026	600	Oral	1032	1 ml syntometrine I.V. (5 IU syntocinone and 0.5 mg ergometrine)
Walley et al.	Canada	A double-blind placebo controlled randomised trial of misoprostol and oxytocin in the management of the third stage of labour	BJOG 2000;107:1111–5	401	203	400	Oral	198	10 IU oxytocin I.M.
El-Refaey et al.	UK	The misoprostol third stage of labour study: a randomised controlled comparison between orally administered misoprostol and standard management	BJOG 2000;107:1104–10	1000	501	500	Oral	499	Standard oxytocic regimens (10 IU oxytocin or 0.5 mg ergometrine or 1 ml syntometrine)
Cook et al.	Australia	A randomized clinical trial comparing oral misoprostol with synthetic oxytocin or syntometrine in the third stage of labour	Aust NZ J Obstet Gynaecol 1999;39:414–9	863	424	400	Oral	439	Standard oxytocic regimens (10 IU oxytocin I.M. or 1 ml syntometrine I.M.)
Amant et al.	Belgium	Misoprostol compared with methylergometrine for the prevention of postpartum haemorrhage: a double-blind randomised trial	Br J Obstet Gynaecol 1999;106:1066–70	200	100	600	Oral	100	0.2 mg methylergometrine I.V.
Surbek et al.	Switzerland	Oral misoprostol for the 3rd stage of labor: a randomized placebo-controlled trial	Obstet Gynecol 1999;94:255–8	65	31	600	Oral	34	Placebo
Bamigboye et al.	South Africa	Rectal misoprostol in the prevention of postpartum hemorrhage: a placebo-controlled trial	Am J Obstet Gynecol 1998;179:1043–6	546	271	400	Rectal	275	Placebo
Hofmeyr et al.	South Africa	A randomised placebo controlled trial of oral misoprostol in the third stage of labour	Br J Obstet Gynaecol 1998;105:971–5	500	250	400	Oral	250	Placebo
Bamigboye et al.	South Africa	Randomized comparison of rectal misoprostol with Syntometrine for management of third stage of labor	Acta Obstet Gynecol Scand 1998;77:178–81	491	241	400	Rectal	250	1 ml syntometrine I.M. (5 IU syntocinone and 0.5 mg ergometrine)
El-Refaey et al.	UK	Use of oral misoprostol in the prevention of PPH	BJOG 1997;104:336–9	237	237	600	Oral	0	–

Table 2 Misoprostol for treatment of postpartum hemorrhage (PPH)

Authors	Site(s)	Study title	Journal	Total participants	Participants in misoprostol group	Dosage of misoprostol	Route of administration	Participants in control group	Control agent(s)
Widmer A et al.	Argentina, Egypt, South Africa, Thailand, Vietnam	Misoprostol as an adjunct to standard uterotonics for treatment of post-partum haemorrhage: a multicentre, double-blind randomised trial	Lancet 2010;375: 1808–13	1422	705	600 μg [+ standard uterotonic regimen of 10 IU oxytocin I.V. or I.M.]	Sublingual	717	Placebo [+ standard uterotonic regimen of 10 IU oxytocin I.V. or I.M.]
Winikoff B et al.	Ecuador, Egypt, Vietnam	Treatment of post-partum haemorrhage with sublingual misoprostol versus oxytocin in women not exposed to oxytocin during labour: a double-blind, randomised, non-inferiority trial	Lancet 2010;375: 210–6	978	440	800 μg	Sublingual	490	40 IU oxytocin I.V.
Blum J et al.	Burkina Faso, Egypt, Turkey, Vietnam	Treatment of post-partum haemorrhage with sublingual misoprostol versus oxytocin in women receiving prophylactic oxytocin: a double-blind, randomised, non-inferiority trial	Lancet 2010;375: 217–23	809	407	800 μg	Sublingual	402	40 IU oxytocin I.V.
Zuberi N et al.	Pakistan	Misoprostol in addition to routine treatment of postpartum hemorrhage: A hospital-based radomized-controlled trial in Karachi, Pakistan	BMC Pregnancy Childbirth 2008;8:40	61	29	600 μg [+ standard uterotonic regimen]	Sublingual	32	Placebo [+ standard uterotonic regimen of 15–110 IU oxytocin I.V. and 0.2–0.4 mg methylergometrine I.V.]
Prata N et al.	Tanzania	Controlling PPH after home births in Tanzania.	Int J Gynaecol Obstet 2005;90:51–5	849	454	1000 μg	Rectal	395	Current practices
Walraven G et al.	The Gambia	Misoprostol in the treatment of PPH in addition to routine management: a placebo randomised controlled trial.	BJOG 2004;111: 1014–7	160	79	600 μg	200 μg oral and 400 μg sublingual	81	Placebo
Hofmeyr GJ et al.	South Africa	Misoprostol for treating postpartum haemorrhage: a randomized controlled trial	BMC Pregnancy Childbirth 2004;4:16	238	117	1000 μg	200 μg oral and 400 μg sublingual and 400 μg rectal	121	Placebo
Shojai R et al.	France	[Rectal misoprostol for postpartum hemorrhage]	Gynecol Obstet Fertil 2004;32:703–7	41	41	1000 μg	Rectal	0	–
Lokugamage AU et al.	UK	A randomized study comparing rectally administered misoprostol versus Syntometrine combined with an oxytocin infusion for the cessation of primary post partum hemorrhage	Acta Obstet Gynecol Scand 2001;80: 835–9	64	32	800 μg	Rectal	32	1 ml syntometrine I.M. (5 IU syntocinone and 0.5 mg ergometrine) plus 10 IU oxytocin I.V.
Abdel-Aleem H et al.	Egypt	Management of severe postpartum hemorrhage with misoprostol	Int J Gynaecol Obstet 2001;72:75–6	18	18	600 μg or 1000 μg	Rectal	0	–
O'Brien P et al.	UK	Rectally administered misoprostol for the treatment of postpartum hemorrhage unresponsive to oxytocin and ergometrine: a descriptive study	Obstet Gynecol 1998;92:212–4	14	14	1000 μg	Rectal	0	–

Table 3   Reviews of misoprostol use in postpartum hemorrhage (PPH)

Author	Institution	Study title	Journal
Sloan *et al.*	Gynuity New York, USA	What measured blood loss tells us about postpartum bleeding: a systematic review	*BJOG* 2010;117:788–800
Rajan *et al.*	University of California, Irvine, USA	Postpartum hemorrhage: evidence-based medical interventions for prevention and treatment	*Clin Obstet Gynecol* 2010;53:165–81
Hofmeyr *et al.*	University of Witwatersrand, South Africa	Misoprostol to prevent and treat postpartum haemorrhage: a systematic review and meta-analysis of maternal deaths and dose-related effects	*Bull World Health Organ* 2009;87:666–77
Elati *et al.*	University of Liverpool, UK	The use of misoprostol in obstetrics and gynaecology	*BJOG* 2009;116(Suppl 1):61–9
Hofmeyr *et al.*	University of Witwatersrand, South Africa	Misoprostol for the prevention and treatment of postpartum haemorrhage	*Best Pract Res Clin Obstet Gynaecol* 2008;22:1025–41
Alfirevic *et al.*	University of Liverpool, UK	Prevention of postpartum hemorrhage with misoprostol	*Int J Gynaecol Obstet* 2007;99:S198–201
Blum *et al.*	Gynuity New York, USA	Treatment of postpartum hemorrhage with misoprostol	*Int J Gynaecol Obstet* 2007;99:S202–5
Mousa *et al.*	University of Nottingham, UK	Treatment for primary postpartum haemorrhage	*Cochrane Database Syst Rev* 2007;(1):CD003249
Gulmezoglu *et al.*	WHO Geneva, Switzerland	Prostaglandins for preventing postpartum haemorrhage	*Cochrane Database Syst Rev* 2007;(3):CD000494

References

1. Gülmezoglu AM, Forna F, Villar J, Hofmeyr GJ. Prostaglandins for preventing postpartum haemorrhage. Cochrane Database Syst Rev 2007;(3):CD000494
2. Hofmeyr GJ, Gülmezoglu AM. Misoprostol for the prevention and treatment of postpartum haemorrhage. Best Pract Res Clin Obstet Gynaecol 2008;22:1025–41
3. Alfirevic Z, Blum J, Walraven G, Weeks A, Winikoff B. Prevention of postpartum hemorrhage with misoprostol. Int J Gynaecol Obstet. 2007;99(Suppl 2):S198–201
4. Derman RJ, Kodkany BS, Goudar SS, et al. Oral misoprostol in preventing postpartum haemorrhage in resource-poor communities: a randomised controlled trial. Lancet 2006;368:1248–53
5. Høj L, Cardoso P, Nielsen BB, Hvidman L, Nielsen J, Aaby P. Effect of sublingual misoprostol on severe postpartum haemorrhage in a primary health centre in Guinea-Bissau: randomised double blind clinical trial. BMJ. 2005;331:723
6. Walraven G, Blum J, Dampha Y, et al. Misoprostol in the management of the third stage of labour in the home delivery setting in rural Gambia: a randomised controlled trial. BJOG 2005;112:1277–83
7. Mobeen N, Durocher J, Zuberi N, et al. Administration of misoprostol by trained traditional birth attendants to prevent postpartum haemorrhage in homebirths in Pakistan: a randomised placebo-controlled trial. BJOG 2011;118:353-61
8. Hashima-E-Nasreen, Nahar S, Al Mamun M, Afsana K, Byass P. Oral misoprostol for preventing postpartum haemorrhage in home births in rural Bangladesh: how effective is it? Glob Health Action 2011 Epub 2011 Aug 10
9. Rajan PV, Wing DA. Postpartum hemorrhage: evidence-based medical interventions for prevention and treatment. Clin Obstet Gynecol 2010;53:165–81
10. Hofmeyr GJ, Gülmezoglu AM. Misoprostol for the prevention and treatment of postpartum haemorrhage. Best Pract Res Clin Obstet Gynaecol 2008;22:1025–41
11. Hofmeyr GJ, Gülmezoglu AM, Novikova N, et al. Misoprostol to prevent and treat postpartum haemorrhage: a systematic review and meta-analysis of maternal deaths and dose-related effects. Bull World Health Organ 2009;87:666–77
12. Blum J, Alfirevic Z, Walraven G, Weeks A, Winikoff B. Treatment of postpartum hemorrhage with misoprostol. Int J Gynaecol Obstet 2007;99(Suppl 2):S202–5
13. Winikoff B, Dabash R, Durocher J, et al. Treatment of post-partum haemorrhage with sublingual misoprostol versus oxytocin in women not exposed to oxytocin during labour: a double-blind, randomised, non-inferiority trial. Lancet 2010;375:210-6
14. Blum J, Winikoff B, Raghavan S, et al. Treatment of post-partum haemorrhage with sublingual misoprostol versus oxytocin in women receiving prophylactic oxytocin: a double-blind, randomised, non-inferiority trial. Lancet 2010;375:217-23
15. Mousa HA, Alfirevic Z. Treatment for primary postpartum haemorrhage. Cochrane Database Syst Rev 2007;(1):CD003249
16. Widmer M, Blum J, Hofmeyr GJ, Carroli G, et al. Misoprostol as an adjunct to standard uterotonics for treatment of post-partum haemorrhage: a multicentre, double-blind randomised trial. Lancet 2010;375:1808–13
17. Fawole AO, Sotiloye OS, Hunyinbo KI et al. A double-blind, randomized, placebo-controlled trial of misoprostol and routine uterotonics for the prevention of postpartum hemorrhage. Int J Gynaecol Obstet 2011;112:107-11
18. Hofmeyr GJ. Oral misoprostol reduces the risk of postpartum haemorrhage in home births assisted by trained traditional birth attendants in Pakistan. Evid Based Med 2011;16:180-1
19. Durocher J, Bynum J, León W, Barrera G, Winikoff B. High fever following postpartum administration of sublingual misoprostol. BJOG 2010;117:845-52
20. Elati A, Weeks AD. The use of misoprostol in obstetrics and gynaecology. BJOG 2009;116(Suppl 1):61–9

35

Sublingual Misoprostol for the Treatment of Postpartum Hemorrhage

R. Dabash, I. Dzuba and B. Winikoff

INTRODUCTION

The current gold standard for treating postpartum hemorrhage (PPH) due to atony is intravenous (IV) oxytocin[1]. However, access to this specific drug and the capacity for its timely intravenous administration are lacking in settings with limited resources, especially at lower levels of the health care system.

Misoprostol, a tablet that requires no additional supplies and/or specialized skills to administer, has the potential to play an important role as a first-line treatment for PPH in such settings. Interest in its use for both prevention and treatment of PPH has a decades-long history, and in 2011 misoprostol was added to the World Health Organization's (WHO) Model List of Essential Medicines for PPH prevention[2]. Recent research demonstrates misoprostol's safety and efficacy as compared with oxytocin.

Prior to 2010, the published literature on misoprostol for the treatment of PPH consisted of several small non-randomized trials that examined various doses and routes of administration as either a first-line treatment or an adjunct to standard uterotonics, a handful of case reports (treating 82 women) and one community-based intervention study[3–14]. Although these studies were insufficient to recommend a specific regimen for treatment with misoprostol, they provided a rationale for further investigation. Perhaps of greater import, health care providers worldwide have been using the drug for *ad hoc* treatment of PPH, despite the absence of conclusive evidence and consensus on an optimal regimen.

In 2010, three seminal studies provided evidence on the utility of sublingual misoprostol in the treatment of PPH. Two large multicenter, double-blind, placebo-controlled, randomized trials compared the effectiveness, safety and acceptability of 800 μg sublingual misoprostol with 40 IU intravenous oxytocin[15,16]. Another large multicenter, double-blind, randomized trial assessed 600 μg sublingual misoprostol when used as an adjunctive treatment for PPH (i.e. when given at the same time as the standard uterotonic treatment)[17]. The sublingual route of administration of misoprostol was chosen in all these trials because of its rapid uptake, long-lasting duration of effect and high bioavailability compared with other routes of misoprostol administration[18].

SUBLINGUAL MISOPROSTOL VERSUS OXYTOCIN AS FIRST-LINE TREATMENT OF PPH

Two non-inferiority trials compared treatment of PPH with sublingual misoprostol to intravenous oxytocin[15,16]. These trials were designed as companion studies and were implemented at tertiary and secondary hospitals in five countries. The first trial enrolled women who had received routine oxytocin prophylaxis in the third stage of labor at hospitals in Burkina Faso, Egypt, Turkey and Vietnam. The second trial enrolled only women who had not received oxytocin prophylaxis and was implemented in hospitals in Ecuador, Egypt and Vietnam where the norms did not call for routine oxytocin prophylaxis. The latter study was meant to reflect the clinical context in many lower level facilities where oxytocin is not available or feasible to administer, and where the need for alternative treatment options is greatest.

The dose of 800 μg misoprostol was carefully chosen giving consideration to expert opinion and published reports of elevated body temperatures of 40.0°C or higher following doses ranging from 600 to 1000 μg[10–12]. Expert consensus was that the optimal dose to be tested should be sufficiently high to be effective but with an acceptable side-effects profile. The 800 μg dose had been tested previously in a small randomized controlled trial without reports of excessive side-effects[10].

Over 41,000 women were screened for PPH in these two studies, and 1786 women were randomized to one of two placebo-controlled double-blind treatment arms: 800 μg sublingual misoprostol or 40 IU intravenous oxytocin (Figure 1). Women were enrolled if PPH due to uterine atony was suspected after vaginal delivery either by clinical diagnosis or when blood loss reached 700 ml on a calibrated delivery drape within 1 hour after delivery, whichever occurred first. The primary outcome of interest was cessation of active bleeding within 20 min. Additional outcomes included mean total blood loss after treatment, average time to bleeding cessation, change in

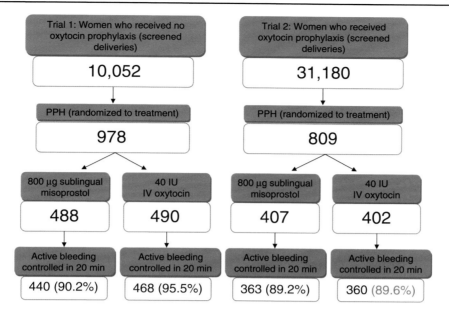

Figure 1 Enrollment and treatment allocation in the two non-inferiority trials of sublingual misoprostol versus intravenous oxytocin for treatment of atonic PPH[15,16]

hemoglobin and recourse to any additional interventions. The frequency and severity of side-effects was also recorded, as was the acceptability to women of each treatment.

Efficacy of treatment

In both trials, median blood loss at time of treatment was 700 ml for women treated. Treatment of PPH with either IV oxytocin or 800 μg sublingual misoprostol successfully controlled bleeding within 20 min of administration in nine out of ten women (Figure 1). Among women who received oxytocin prophylaxis during the third stage of labor and then went on to be diagnosed with PPH, treatment with sublingual misoprostol stopped bleeding as rapidly as IV oxytocin (mean 19 min) and with a similar quantity of additional blood lost (Table 1).

Among women who did not receive a prophylactic uterotonic, both sublingual misoprostol and IV oxytocin were very effective in controlling postpartum bleeding within 20 min, although IV oxytocin was somewhat better (96% vs. 90%; *p* = 0.001), and it stopped active bleeding on average 2 min faster than sublingual misoprostol, resulting in approximately 60 ml less blood loss.

As IV oxytocin is injected directly into the bloodstream, a patient may experience its benefits almost immediately. Pharmacokinetic data on sublingual misoprostol administration show that peak serum concentrations are achieved at around 20 min[18], so there may be a short delay in maximum benefit. In order to avoid treatment delays, study teams made great efforts to administer all medications quickly, which may have diluted the very different logistical burdens of these two treatments. In routine clinical practice, the time from diagnosis to treatment-effect of each of the two drugs may prove to be quite different.

This reality may potentially reduce the advantages of oxytocin over misoprostol in the time to bleeding cessation, especially when an intravenous line is not in place and where IV supplies are not readily available.

A cross-study comparison shows that both treatments (sublingual misoprostol or IV oxytocin) performed better and faster in stopping bleeding among women not exposed to oxytocin prophylaxis. This finding suggests that women who develop PPH despite oxytocin prophylaxis have a diminished response to an additional dose of uterotonic for treatment or have worse, more refractory, hemorrhages.

Other indicators of drug efficacy

In the trial of women who had received oxytocin prophylaxis, a similar proportion of women in each treatment group experienced a drop of 2 g/dl or more in hemoglobin concentration. Also, the proportion of women with a drop of 3 g/dl or who received a blood transfusion did not differ by treatment group. Among women in the other trial who had not received prophylactic oxytocin, median hemoglobin changes from pre-delivery to post-treatment (data not shown) were similar in women treated with IV oxytocin and those treated with sublingual misoprostol, as was the proportion of women who had a drop in hemoglobin of 2 g/dl or more (Table 1). However, hemoglobin drops of 3 g/dl or receipt of blood transfusion (40.8 % with sublingual misoprostol vs. 30.2% with IV oxytocin) were significantly more common among women who received sublingual misoprostol than among those who received IV oxytocin.

Recourse to additional interventions is an important indicator of the potential program costs associated with these two uterotonics when used as first-line treatment. In women who had received oxytocin prophylaxis but went on to have PPH, the frequency of

Table 1 Bleeding cessation, blood loss, hemoglobin change and additional intervention outcomes in women treated for PPH with sublingual misoprostol or IV oxytocin in the two non-inferiority trials. Data are expressed as numbers with percentages in parentheses unless otherwise specified

	Women not exposed to oxytocin prophylaxis[16]				Women who received prophylactic oxytocin[15]			
	Misoprostol (n = 488)	Oxytocin (n = 490)	RR (95% CI)	P value	Misoprostol (n = 407)	Oxytocin (n = 402)	RR (95% CI)	P value
Active bleeding controlled within 20 min of initial uterotonic treatment	440 (90.2%)	468 (95.5%)	0.94 (0.91–0.98)	0.001	363 (89.2%)	360 (89.6%)	0.99 (0.95–1.04)	0.867
Minutes to active bleeding controlled mean (SD)	13.4 (8.2)	11.8 (6.6)	–	0.001	19.3 (15.0)	19.1 (14.6)	–	0.854
Additional blood loss (ml) median (IQR)	200 (110–300)	150 (100–225)	–	<0.0001	200 (100–350)	200 (100–300)	–	0.199
Drop in Hb ≥2 g/dl or blood transfusion	250 (51.2%)	230 (46.9%)	1.09 (0.96–1.24)	0.101	152 (37.6%)	142 (35.7%)	1.06 (0.88–1.27)	0.567
Drop in Hb ≥3 g/dl or blood transfusion	199 (40.8%)	148 (30.2%)	1.35 (1.14–1.60)	<0.0001	104 (25.7%)	90 (22.6%)	1.14 (0.89–1.46)	0.301
Additional uterotonics	61 (12.5%)	31 (6.3%)	1.98 (1.31–2.99)	0.001	40 (9.8%)	46 (11.5%)	0.86 (0.58–1.28)	0.260
Blood transfusion	41 (8.4%)	26 (5.3%)	1.58 (0.98–2.55)	0.036	24 (5.9%)	18 (4.5%)	1.32 (0.73–2.39)	0.229
Hysterectomy/other surgery	0 (0.0)	0 (0.0)	–	–	4 (1.0%)	2 (0.5%)	1.98 (0.36–10.73)	0.350
Maternal death	0 (0.0)	0 (0.0)	–	–	1 (0.2%)	1 (0.2%)	0.99 (0.06–15.74)	0.747

RR, relative risk; Hb, hemoglobin

recourse to additional interventions was similar following initial treatment with oxytocin or misoprostol. The most common intervention was administration of additional uterotonics in approximately 1 in 10 women regardless of treatment group (Table 1).

In women not given prophylaxis before their PPH, additional interventions were more frequently used in the misoprostol group, including administration of additional uterotonics and blood transfusion (Table 1). Women treated with misoprostol were twice as likely to receive additional uterotonic drugs as those in the oxytocin group (12.5% vs. 6.3%; $p = 0.001$, RR 1.98, 95% CI 1.31–2.99; Table 1). As blood loss data suggest, all women in this study bled faster on average than those in the study with routine prophylaxis (mean blood loss within 20 min of 279 ml vs. 249 ml, respectively, in the misoprostol arms and 252 ml vs. 190 ml in the oxytocin arms). This factor, coupled with the slightly slower response time with misoprostol may have contributed to the higher rates of additional uterotonic use in women treated with misoprostol. The availability of additional drugs, as well as preference to use more than one intervention when PPH is diagnosed, may have contributed to provider choices in these hospital settings that were not necessarily based on patient needs; such choices might not be as likely in lower levels of the health care system.

Six hysterectomies (including two deaths) occurred in the study of women who received prophylaxis, while none occurred among women who received no prophylaxis. No differences were present in the rates of these events in the two treatment arms (Table 1). These findings again suggest that women who experience a PPH following prophylaxis may represent a different group of women to those who experience excessive bleeding with no prior prophylaxis. The significant difference in adverse outcomes suggests that women with PPH following prophylaxis failure have a PPH that is more difficult to treat and is less responsive to first-line treatment with additional uterotonics alone. No invasive surgeries, hysterectomies, or deaths were reported in the study of women with no prior prophylaxis.

Side-effects

Women in both studies experienced side-effects regardless of the type of uterotonic treatment received, although fever and shivering were more commonly reported in women treated with sublingual misoprostol. Prior oxytocin prophylaxis did not affect the frequency of side-effects following either treatment. Gastrointestinal side-effects, such as nausea, vomiting and diarrhea, are known effects of misoprostol, but they were also commonly reported in women treated with oxytocin. Of these side-effects, nausea was the most commonly reported, affecting 12.1% of women who took misoprostol and 12.3% of women who received oxytocin. The frequency of vomiting was low, but higher among those women treated with misoprostol (Table 2). In all cases, these side-effects

were transient and did not result in any life-threatening complications. The vast majority of study participants reported that the side-effects experienced were tolerable.

The most notable features of the side-effects following treatment with sublingual misoprostol are the rates of fever and shivering. These two side-effects were reported after both oxytocin and misoprostol, but were more likely to occur when women were treated with misoprostol (Table 2). High fever following sublingual administration of misoprostol was infrequent except for in one site in Quito, Ecuador, where a disproportionately high percentage of women receiving misoprostol treatment (35.6%) experienced high fever. In contrast, the rate of high fever in the other hospitals participating in these studies ranged from 0 to 10%[19]. Prior to these two studies, the published literature included four cases (in 146 women) of high fever ($\geq 40°C$) following use of misoprostol for treatment of PPH[11,13]. Shivering and fever following misoprostol administration are related events and known to be dose and route dependent[20–22] with higher rates following oral and sublingual administration. Pharmacokinetic research on misoprostol demonstrates a higher plasma concentration and a more rapid rise to peak concentration when it is taken by these routes[18,22,23]. For these reasons, a higher incidence of shivering and fever in studies that employ higher-dose sublingual misoprostol regimens is not unexpected.

Analysis of the reported cases of high fever that occurred in Ecuador showed that they followed a predictable and consistent pattern. They were typically characterized by a sharp increase in temperature within 1 hour of treatment, which peaked 1–2 hours after treatment, and gradually declined over the course of several hours. Average temperatures remained above 40.0°C for less than 2 hours, and measured below 38.0°C approximately 6 hours after receiving misoprostol. Temperature elevation and decline followed the rise and fall of sublingual misoprostol blood plasma concentration (Figure 2). Women with high fever were treated by nurses with oral acetaminophen, cool compresses and IV aspirin, and all women recovered with no sequelae[19].

Table 2 Side-effects following PPH treatment with misoprostol and oxytocin[15,16]. Data are expressed as numbers with percentages in parentheses unless otherwise specified

Side-effect	Misoprostol (n = 895)	Oxytocin (n = 892)	Relative risk (95% CI)
Nausea	108 (12.1)	110 (12.3)	0.98 (0.76–1.27)
Vomiting	43 (4.8)	17 (1.9)	2.52 (1.41–4.57)
Fainting or feeling faint	62 (6.9)	62 (7.0)	1.00 (0.70–1.42)
Diarrhea	7 (0.78)	5 (0.56)	1.40 (0.40–5.03)
Shivering	381 (42.6)	141 (15.8)	2.69 (2.27–3.20)
Fever	305 (34.1)	86 (9.6)	3.54 (2.83–4.44)
Temp ≥40.0°C	71 (7.9)	1 (0.11)	70.76 (9.85–508.21)

It is unclear why some women develop high fever while others do not and why the thermoregulatory response to misoprostol among Ecuadorian women was so notably different from that of participants in other study sites[19]. Despite these uncertainties, the variable responses in some populations raises the question of whether a lower treatment dose (i.e. 600 μg) would be as effective as 800 μg sublingual misoprostol and reduce the incidence of high fever. Currently, the literature does not support a lower dose or other routes of administration for first-line PPH treatment. While it is possible that a lower dose or administration by another route may reduce the occurrence of fevers, it may also reduce efficacy. Given the infrequent nature of this side-effect in most settings and the benign course of these fevers, such a trade-off may not be universally advantageous. Indeed, a rigorous comparative randomized trial to explore the potential of a reduced dose would of necessity be very large and require tremendous time and resources to address a question that may only be relevant to some settings.

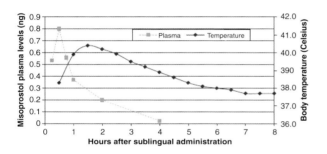

Figure 2 Mean misoprostol plasma concentrations after sublingual administration of misoprostol (800 μg), and mean temperatures over time of 58 cases of high fever following treatment with 800 μg sublingual misoprostol in Quito, Ecuador[24]. Reproduced with permission from Durocher *et al.* High fever following postpartum administration of sublingual misoprostol. BJOG 2010;117:845–52. John Wiley and Sons Ltd

MISOPROSTOL AS AN ADJUNCT TO OXYTOCIN FOR TREATMENT OF PPH

Since providers in many service delivery settings respond to life-threatening PPH with multiple treatment interventions, including more than one uterotonic, practitioners have wondered whether simultaneous administration of both oxytocin and misoprostol confers any additional advantages. A large multicenter, double-blind, placebo-controlled, randomized trial evaluated whether a regimen of 600 μg sublingual misoprostol administered at the same time as routine injectable oxytocin offered any clinical advantage[17]. Secondary outcomes in this trial included additional blood loss, recourse to additional interventions, change in hemoglobin and blood transfusion (Table 3).

The results showed no difference in postpartum blood loss among women who received misoprostol in combination with standard uterotonics and those who received placebo with standard treatment (Table 3). Furthermore, consistent with other reports of side-effects following use of misoprostol, women receiving misoprostol were more likely to experience shivering and fever (Table 3).

This study suggests that the addition of misoprostol to the initial treatment regimen is not more effective than administration of a standard uterotonic alone and is associated with more side-effects. As such, the adjunct use of sublingual misoprostol and conventional uterotonics simultaneously is not recommended. Yet, it remains possible that there could be benefits to the sequential administration of misoprostol following oxytocin or as a last-ditch effort before recourse to more invasive procedures.

PROGRAM IMPLICATIONS AND FUTURE RESEARCH

The results of the two large treatment trials evaluating first-line treatment options for PPH, along with other

Table 3 Outcomes of usual treatment with uterotonic plus concurrent addition of sublingual misoprostol or placebo[17]. Data are expressed as numbers with percentages in parentheses unless otherwise indicated

	Misoprostol + standard uterotonics (n = 705)	Placebo + standard uterotonics (n = 717)	RR (95% CI)
Blood loss of ≥500 ml within 60 min after randomization	100 (14.2)	100 (13.9)	1.02 (0.79–1.32)
Blood loss of ≥1000 ml within 60 min after randomization	9 (1.3)	9 (1.3)	1.02 (0.41–2.55)
Any uterotonic after randomization	188 (26.7)	203 (28.3)	0.94 (0.79–1.11)
Hemoglobin concentration of <8 g/dl within 24 h postpartum or need for blood transfusion*	121 (17.2)	139 (19.4)	0.89 (0.72–1.11)
Blood transfusion after randomization	103 (14.6)	117 (16.3)	0.89 (0.7–1.14)
Maternal death	2 (0.3)	0 (0)	–
Severe morbidity	8 (1.1)	10 (1.4)	0.81 (0.32–2.00)
Shivering			
Any	455 (64.6)	230 (32.1)	2.01 (1.79–2.27)
Severe	80 (11.4)	7 (1.0)	11.64 (5.41–25.03)
Fever			
≥38°C	303 (43)	107 (14.9)	2.88 (2.37–2.5)
≥40°C	18 (2.6)	3 (0.4)	6.11 (1.81–20.65)

*Data recorded for 691 patients receiving misoprostol and 710 patients receiving placebo; outcomes could not be measured in remaining patients

available literature, suggest that both sublingual misoprostol and IV oxytocin are very effective alone in controlling PPH. The broader implications of these study results depend on the context in which PPH occurs and what treatment options are available (Table 4). For women who receive prophylactic oxytocin in the third stage of labor, 800 μg sublingual misoprostol is clinically equivalent to 40 IU of IV oxytocin for treatment of primary atonic PPH, and either drug can be used to control bleeding. It is also clear that when both misoprostol and oxytocin are available, their simultaneous administration confers no advantages and is only associated with an increase in side-effects.

Where women do not receive any prophylaxis, on the other hand, oxytocin is better than misoprostol as first-line treatment. Unfortunately, the present day realities that limit access to oxytocin prophylaxis are likely also to limit its feasibility for intravenous use for PPH treatment, particularly in limited-resource settings and at the lowest level of the health care system, including the many home births in developing countries[24]. Furthermore, governmental policies commonly limit the authority of certain types of providers to offer on-site treatment. These providers, while expected to be able to diagnose PPH for referral, are infrequently authorized to administer treatment, including injections and intravenous treatments. In these settings, misoprostol appears to be a suitable alternative. Given the evidence, future research should examine the programmatic implications of introducing misoprostol as an on-site treatment option where few or no alternatives currently exist. Community-level research should focus on developing simple models that facilitate diagnosis of PPH based on clinical indicators aside from measured blood loss, which is both costly and difficult to implement.

Sublingual misoprostol and IV oxytocin may prove to be more similar treatments in real-life contexts, especially given the differences in logistical burdens, level of staff able to use the drugs, conditions of storage, etc. In addition, while the studies described above compared sublingual misoprostol to the highest recommended dose of IV oxytocin (40 IU), many country protocols and supplies only allow for lower doses, such as 5 or 10 IU of oxytocin[1]. To complicate matters, in many settings oxytocin may only be available in intramuscular (IM) administration. While the efficacy of IV oxytocin is clear, information about treatment of PPH with IM oxytocin is not yet available. Future research is critical to understanding how the current data on efficacy of misoprostol and oxytocin translate into programmatic effectiveness when service delivery realities come into play.

As misoprostol is increasingly being used for PPH prophylaxis at the community level, it is also important to understand how such prophylaxis interacts with the efficacy and safety of misoprostol for treatment. Decisions about resource allocation would benefit from information about the relative advantages of universal prophylaxis or implementation of more targeted strategies, such as treatment as needed. For example, new comparative studies are underway to assess the programmatic effectiveness of secondary prevention models, whereby the treatment dose of 800 μg sublingual misoprostol is selectively administered to women who bleed slightly more than average (around 350 ml). Novel approaches that medicate fewer women, reduce costs and still achieve comparable outcomes might be developed using new hybrid service delivery strategies

CONCLUSION

At least, two-thirds of PPH occurs in women with no known risk factors[25]. The largely unpredictable nature of PPH makes it a challenge to service delivery, especially in low-resource or remote areas. While universal prophylaxis significantly reduces the incidence of PPH, it does not eliminate the need to treat some women. In many settings, treatment only occurs after referral to higher levels of care, which can take hours to days. Since hemorrhage from uterine atony can cause death in 2 hours or less, the availability of simple treatment options where women deliver is critical.

Evidence suggests sublingual misoprostol should be used for treatment whenever oxytocin is not available. It can also be used as the first choice treatment for hemorrhages occurring after women have received oxytocin as prophylaxis. Misoprostol is an important weapon in the arsenal of methods to combat PPH in sites that for the most part have oxytocin but face logistical challenges to its IV use, for example, no stock, loss of refrigeration, or absence of a provider trained/confident in IV administration. Moreover, misoprostol may prove to be most useful in settings where few if any alternatives exist. Given the very small differences in efficacy between sublingual misoprostol and IV oxytocin, it is clear why misoprostol is being promoted for use by less skilled attendants and at lower levels of the health care system. Data on program effectiveness will be critical in better understanding the health impact of these technologies and interventions when used on a wide scale.

Table 4 Implications of research evidence on first-line treatment options for PPH in different service delivery contexts

	No prophylactic oxytocin	*Prophylactic oxytocin*
IV Oxytocin feasible	Oxytocin preferred	Either drug
IV Oxytocin not feasible	Misoprostol	Misoprostol

References

1. Mousa HA, Alfirevic Z. Treatment for primary postpartum haemorrhage. Cochrane Database Syst Rev 2007;(1): CD003249
2. WHO. Unedited Report of the 18th Expert Committee on the Selection and Use of Essential Medicines. Accra, Ghana: WHO, 2011:1–211
3. O'Brien P, El-Refaey H, Gordon A, Geary M, Rodeck CH. Rectally administered misoprostol for the treatment of

postpartum hemorrhage unresponsive to oxytocin and ergometrine: a descriptive study. Obstet Gynecol 1998;92:212–4

4. Ozan H, Bilgin T, Ozsaraç N, Ozerkan K, Cengiz C. Misoprostol in uterine atony: A report of 2 cases. Clin Exp Obstet Gynecol 2000;27:221–2

5. Abdel-Aleem H, El-Nashar I, Abdel-Aleem A. Management of severe postpartum hemorrhage with misoprostol. Int J Gynecol Obstet 2001;72:75–6

6. Shojai, R., Piéchon L, d'Ercole C, Boubli L, Pontiès JE. [Rectal administration of misoprostol for delivery induced hemorrhage. Preliminary study]. J Gynécol Obstét Biol Reprod 2001;30:572–5

7. Adekanmi O, Purmessur S, Edwards G, Barrington JW. Intrauterine misoprostol for the treatment of severe recurrent atonic secondary postpartum haemorrhage. BJOG 2001;108: 541–2

8. Oboro V, Tabowei T, Bosah J. Intrauterine misoprostol for refractory postpartum hemorrhage. Int J Gynecol Obstet 2003;80:67–8

9. Shojai R, Desbrière R, Dhifallah S, et al. [Rectal misoprostol for postpartum hemorrhage]. Gynécol Obstét Fertil 2004;32: 703–7

10. Lokugamage AU, Sullivan KR, Niculescu I, et al. A randomized study comparing rectally administered misoprostol versus Syntometrine combined with an oxytocin infusion for the cessation of primary post partum hemorrhage. Acta Obstet Gynecol Scand 2001;80:835–9

11. Hofmeyr GJ, Ferreira S, Nikodem VC, et al. Misoprostol for treating postpartum haemorrhage: a randomized controlled trial. BioMed Central Pregnancy and Childbirth 2004;4:1–7

12. Walraven G, Dampha Y, Bittaye B, Sowe M, Hofmeyr J. Misoprostol in the treatment of postpartum haemorrhage in addition to routine management: a placebo randomised controlled trial. BJOG 2004;111:1014–7

13. Zuberi NF, Durocher J, Sikander R, Baber N, Blum J, Walraven G. Misoprostol in addition to routine treatment of postpartum hemorrhage: a hospital-based randomized-controlled trial in Karachi, Pakistan. BMC Pregnancy Childbirth 2008;8:40

14. Prata N, Mbaruku G, Campbell M, Potts M, Vahidnia F. Controlling postpartum hemorrhage after home births in Tanzania. Int J Gynaecol Obstet 2005;90:51–5

15. Blum J, Winikoff B, Raghavan S, et al. Treatment of post-partum haemorrhage with sublingual misoprostol versus oxytocin in women receiving prophylactic oxytocin: a double-blind, randomised, non-inferiority trial. Lancet 2010; 375:217–23

16. Winikoff B, Dabash R, Durocher J, et al. Treatment of post-partum haemorrhage with sublingual misoprostol versus oxytocin in women not exposed to oxytocin during labour: a double-blind, randomised, non-inferiority trial. Lancet 2010;375:210–6

17. Widmer M, Blum J, Hofmeyr GJ, et al. Misoprostol as an adjunct to standard uterotonics for treatment of post-partum haemorrhage: a multicentre, double-blind randomised trial. Lancet 2010;375:1808–13

18. Tang OS, Schweer H, Seyberth HW, Lee SW, Ho PC. Pharmacokinetics of different routes of administration of misoprostol. Hum Reprod 2002;17:332–6

19. Durocher J, Bynum J, León W, Barrera G, Winikoff B. High fever following postpartum administration of sublingual misoprostol. BJOG 2010;117:845–52

20. Hofmeyr GJ, Gülmezoglu AM, Novikova N, Linder V, Ferreira S, Piaggio G. Misoprostol to prevent and treat postpartum haemorrhage: a systematic review and meta-analysis of maternal deaths and dose-related effects. Bull World Health Organ 2009;87:666–77

21. Lumbiganon P, Hofmeyr J, Gülmezoglu AM, Pinol A, Villar J. Misoprostol dose-related shivering and pryexia in the third stage of labour. BJOG 1999;106:304–8

22. Khan RU, El-Refaey H. Pharmacokinetics and adverse-effect profile of rectally administered misoprostol in the third stage of labor. Obstet Gynecol 2003;101:968–74

23. Zieman M, Fong SK, Benowitz NL, Banskter D, Darney PD. Absorption kinetics of misoprostol with oral or vaginal administration. Obstet Gynecol 1997;90:88–92

24. WHO. Coverage of Maternity Care: A Listing of the Available Information, 4th edn. Geneva, WHO, 1997:1–71

25. Mousa HA, Cording V, Alfirevic Z. Risk factors and interventions associated with major primary postpartum hemorrhage unresponsive to first-line conventional therapy. Acta Obstet Gynecol Scand 2008;87:652–61

Section 7

Hospital Preparation

36

Labor Ward Drills

M. K. Tipples and S. Paterson-Brown

INTRODUCTION

As massive obstetric hemorrhage is the leading cause of maternal mortality worldwide and a major contributor to maternal morbidity, this subject deserves center stage in the training of midwifery and obstetric staff. That this training need is global is highlighted by instances of substandard care with deaths as a result of postpartum hemorrhage (PPH) in recent UK confidential reports (CEMACH)[1]. Although much knowledge can be gained at the bedside, practical teaching with a structured approach to this unique life-threatening emergency provides a sense of security and preparedness that cannot be obtained in any other manner. Several well-established courses focus on practical emergency teaching, and further information is available through the websites of many professional organizations. Some of the courses run in the UK and abroad are listed in Addendum A at the end of this chapter. These courses present a structured approach to resuscitation with skills, drills and scenarios taught and applied to the seriously ill patient. As good as such courses may be, however, they cannot begin to train everyone in all things, and there remains a need for strong local supplementation in the form of multi-disciplinary training. Indeed, the latter has been shown to be effective in improving knowledge[2,3] and clinical outcomes[4,5] (see Chapters 40 and 41).

The recipe for successful local training is not simple and involves a local commitment with incentives to train, multiprofessional training of all staff, teamwork training combined with clinical teaching and use of high fidelity models, but it works[4,5]. Currently multidisciplinary emergency drills and scenarios are a requirement for clinical negligence scheme for trusts (CNST) ratings, a factor which promotes their establishment within UK maternity departments.

It is axiomatic that all functioning obstetric units possess a multidisciplinary massive hemorrhage protocol, which should be updated and rehearsed regularly. Running these sessions as a local drill helps to test the systems in place to deal with obstetric hemorrhage as well as the clinical staff's knowledge of these systems[6], thus making them particularly useful to local staff. Clinical scenario and skills training add detail and depth to this training, but efficiency in the system is an essential prerequisite to effective care. This chapter describes how various practical training techniques (drills, skills and scenarios) work and how such programs can be set up locally.

GENERAL PRINCIPLES OF ADULT EDUCATION

Adult learning

When adults approach the process of learning something new, they often are not satisfied with the acquisition of new facts alone, but also wish to understand and be able to apply the knowledge they acquire. Three different processes are involved in adult learning, all of which are complementary and can be featured in practical teaching sessions.

(1) *Visual* Visual learning may occur through reading in which the reader develops his/her mental picture of a situation, but it is greatly enhanced by watching a person or people doing the process of interest. Being able to recall the scene and actions that were taken enables one to better carry them out when a similar situation presents itself.

(2) *Auditory* In addition to listening, the process of auditory learning includes dialogue, questions and discussions with others with similar interests and knowledge.

(3) *Kinesthetic* Kinesthetic learning involves obtaining knowledge through hands-on practice and role play. Hands-on practice is especially useful for practical skills, whereas role play encourages the individual to work logically through a sequence of events in a clinical scenario.

All three forms of learning are variably suited to different educational objectives. For example, learning to tie a knot can be visualized and explained, but one needs to do it to finally obtain the skill. Of importance, different individuals tend to gain more from one approach compared with another: some prefer watching what is going on, others benefit most from open discussion and feedback, and still others relish the challenge of being the doers in the practical teaching demonstration. Finally, some individuals utilize all three learning techniques to gain new knowledge. Appreciating these differences and staying sensitive to the particular needs of those being taught helps keep practical teaching fun and effective while, at the same time, avoiding what can be extremely stressful for some individuals.

Practical teaching

The same preparations should be made whether teaching skills, drills or scenarios are to be used (see below).

Knowledge

A sound knowledge base is required before practical teaching can be undertaken successfully. An initial lecture/workshop/discussion should be organized if staff are unfamiliar with practical teaching or if new material is to be taught, as this allows staff to prepare themselves. It also helps reinforce the idea that practical teaching is an opportunity to put what one knows into practice.

Environment

A suitable location should be found that is conducive to the teaching that has been planned. The layout of the room should allow those involved to access the patient (if the teaching is patient oriented) and those watching to see clearly. Heating and ventilation should be considered, but acoustics are vital and can sometimes conflict (e.g. noise from an open window). When teaching about obstetric hemorrhage, a delivery room or an operating theater makes for a very realistic teaching environment, but it occasionally conflicts with clinical needs. To avoid this, one can plan impromptu teaching when the delivery suite is quiet. Impromptu or 'unannounced' teaching also is good for testing how the systems are working (i.e. drills), but, as it does not allow prior planning in terms of who or how many people can be taught, it may be less useful when running clinical scenarios. Another alternative is to consider reducing elective surgery to facilitate training in an operating theater at a given time, remembering, of course, that labor ward workloads are totally unpredictable and a back-up teaching location needs to be available (for example, a seminar room or antenatal classroom).

Setting the tone

The instructor should give a general explanation at the beginning of the teaching session in order to establish the mood and motivate the learners by outlining the usefulness of the content. A simple introduction is all that is required. For example, 'Obstetric hemorrhage is the leading cause of maternal death globally, and today we are going to run through a simulated case of placental abruption. The aim is for you to consolidate and apply your knowledge in this area, a process which should assist you when you face a similar situation in a real emergency'. At this stage, it also may be useful to introduce the clinical problem in the context of recent events either locally or something that may have been reported in the lay press.

The specific objectives of the session should then be explained along with what is expected of everyone in terms of who is going to do what, and whether questions can be asked throughout or be kept till the end. It is extremely useful to allow questioning throughout, as many people will forget if asked to wait till the end. However, this process can spoil the momentum of a scenario and role play session and must be judged anew in each session.

Dialogue

The actual 'doing' in practical teaching and role play works through the simulation that come from starting from very specific instructions. Progress can vary according to what the learner does, and the instructor needs to stay alert and flexible in order to remain in control, to cover all intended teaching points and to guide the session to an appropriate conclusion.

Feedback

This is sometimes known as critique or debriefing and is an essential part of the learning process as it promotes retention of important points. A number of techniques can be used, but the main idea is to identify and promote the good (salient) points (remembering others in the teaching group may not have known these beforehand) and to identify in a sensitive fashion, any deficiencies (lack of knowledge or errors).

One form of systematic feedback, described by Pendleton and known as Pendleton's rules[7], comprises four stages: the learner says what she/he did well; then what she/he could improve upon; this is followed by the trainer stating what the learner did well; followed by what could be improved upon. Allowing the learner to comment first provides the instructor an opportunity to assess the candidate's insight into her or his own ability and behavior. The instructor then has the opportunity to highlight both good practice and areas for improvement not already covered by the learner in order to stress and reinforce learning points to all present.

Another method of feedback involves debriefing as a learning conversation. This is less rigid in style compared with the above and involves:

(1) Making an opening gambit (individualized start to the conversation depending on how things went, such as 'That seemed to go well, what do you think?' or 'That was rather difficult, let's see if we can work out what was going on' etc.);

(2) Jointly exploring any issues that emerge (listening and responding, and involving the whole group to widen the conversation as needed);

(3) Share thoughts of whole group and the instructor considering the learning of the whole group, while being careful not to overload the practice candidate.

Closure

Bearing in mind that adults need to understand something before they change their behavior, it is crucial that questions and discussion be encouraged. A summary of the key learning points from the session should then be provided, so that everyone leaves the teaching/learning with a clear message of the most important issues.

DRILLS, SKILLS AND SCENARIOS

These three styles of teaching differ in their aims. Each requires and tests different skills and knowledge, the features of which are summarized in Table 1, together with examples of suitable teaching material.

Drills

These are practice or 'dummy' runs and are comparable to fire practices in testing local systems. Running a drill not only allows local scrutiny (i.e. what actually happens when the alarm is put out), but also can be a very effective test of local arrangements and services as well as staff knowledge of them.

Preparations for a drill

When running drills, the staff should be faced with the drill in a normal clinical area, unprepared, in order to receive a realistic idea of what would happen in a true situation. Clearly, a drill should not conflict with patient care, and timing must depend to some extent on existing workload. The lead clinician for the teaching session should, however, have informed the lead midwife and, in the case of an obstetric hemorrhage, the transfusion hematologist and other necessary individuals, such as transportation staff. This is not only as a matter of courtesy, but also to plan timings in order to avoid clashes of interests. The transfusion hematologist may prepare spare serum for grouping and make empty blood bags available for the 'dummy run'.

Running the drill

Figure 1 illustrates an example of an assessment sheet for a massive obstetric hemorrhage drill, suggesting things that can usefully be monitored including:

- Who responds to the initial emergency buzzer?

- Time emergency buzzer pulled [ ]
- Staff responding to the initial buzzer [ ]
- Time switchboard received emergency call [ ]
- Staff responding to the emergency bleep [ ]

Name	Grade	Time

- Initial treatment of ABC (airway, breathing and circulation) resuscitation instituted quickly and effectively — Yes / No

If no – comments ....

- Time transportation person arrives in blood transfusion [ ]
- Time blood samples received in the laboratory [ ]
- Time appropriate blood arrives at patient's bedside [ ]
- Time patient transferred to the operating theater [ ]

Other comments:

Figure 1 An assessment sheet for massive obstetric hemorrhage drill. This assessment sheet can be expanded to include the response times for individual doctors, and their reactions and actions

Table 1 Key features and differences in skills, drills and scenario teaching

	Skill	*Drill*	*Scenario*
Definition	Acquisition of a skill	A chain of events in response to a problem	Improvized clinical role play
Aim of the teaching	Ensure correct technique	Test the local emergency system	Apply and practice clinical care in a improvized set-up
Teaching environment	Seminar room	Throughout hospital in day-to-day environment	Seminar room, operating theater or delivery room
Examples of things suitable for teaching and testing in relation to obstetric hemorrhage	Brace suture Rusch balloon Aortocaval compression CPR Bimanual uterine compression IV cut down	Response to the emergency massive obstetric hemorrhage call	APH – abruption – placental previa PPH – atony – trauma – RPOC
Skill mix	Doctors and midwives	All delivery suite staff and laboratory staff, hematologists and porters	Multidisciplinary: obstetricians, midwives, anesthetists, pediatricians

CPR, cardiopulmonary resuscitation; APH, antepartum hemorrhage; PPH, postpartum hemorrhage; RPOC, retained products of conception

- Is the appropriate emergency call put out?

- How effective is the emergency bleeping system?

- Is transportation alerted and respond?

- Do transfusion staff receive any communication?

- How quickly does blood arrive at the bedside?

- How quickly is the patient transferred to the operating theater?

- When does the anesthetist/consultant/hematologist arrive?

Such analyses can help to illustrate system failures and modify local policies. The identification of problems stimulates and informs development of appropriate guidelines. Clarifying the roles of diverse staff and streamlining activity can also improve future responses and improve care. Such developments can be monitored at future drills and improvements in the system should be fed back to staff. Having run drills for obstetric hemorrhage at Queen Charlotte's and Chelsea Hospital for many years, the following are examples of problems identified and system changes made in response.

Communication problems and how they were addressed As identified in numerous Confidential Enquiries, problems in communication often hamper emergency responses. We found that we struggled with instructions from clinicians to blood transfusion staff regarding what was needed and when it was needed: Was it possible to wait for group-compatible blood or even cross-matched blood? How long to wait to have blood at the bedside? What clotting products were needed when? These are some examples of questions that are often not clarified 'over the phone'.

It soon became obvious that this job was normally delegated to someone very junior on the delivery suite and misunderstandings were common.

Our response was first, to install a red phone in the obstetric operating theater based on the delivery suite that linked exclusively with a red phone in the transfusion laboratory. This enabled blood requirements to be discussed by the anesthetist directly with transfusion staff without having to leave the patient to go outside the theater. Second, we then identified time limits for transfusing blood at the bedside (for example, 'We need 4 units of blood within 30 minutes'), rather than discussing whether to wait for blood to be cross-matched or not. This left the laboratory in no doubt of the clinical needs and has minimized delay in blood arriving at the bedside when needed.

Problems with transportation and how they were addressed In the past, the transportation person arrived in the delivery suite when a hemorrhage call was put out to take blood samples to the laboratory for grouping/cross-matching; however, this was deemed inefficient and delayed blood being brought to the bedside in the most urgent cases.

Our solution was first to change the process so that the transportation person went straight to the laboratory in readiness for the urgent need of collecting O-negative blood. Second, a pneumatic chute was installed for samples to be sent to the laboratory which has also helped in this context. If the clinical condition of the patient can wait for group-compatible blood, the transportation person stays in the transfusion laboratory until the sample has arrived by chute and has been grouped, ultimately bringing the appropriate blood to the delivery suite. This type of thinking is especially relevant in large modern hospitals where clinical and laboratory services are not only on different floors but in different, often widely separated, buildings.

Skills

The teaching of practical skills is of great importance in obstetric hemorrhage teaching sessions. The need for specific teaching often becomes apparent during the discussion and questioning when running a scenario. Things may have been mentioned which are not fully understood, and such circumstances illustrate how important it is for scenario teaching to be constructive (see below for examples). Staff must feel able to question what something is or how it is done. In obstetric hemorrhage, the following skills may be highlighted and need to be taught:

- Medical skills
  - bimanual uterine compression
  - aortic compression
  - cardiopulmonary resuscitation
- Surgical skills
  - insertion of an inflatable uterine balloon
  - insertion of a Brace suture
  - intravenous cut-down for venous access.

Preparation for skills teaching

Teaching any practical skill that may be required in an emergency, should be executed slowly and calmly, giving ample time for reflection, questions and practice. The use of manikins and surgical aids works well, but one must remember to point out the differences to be expected when working *in vivo* (such as the need to keep an inflatable uterine balloon well into the cavity while inflating it, or how to deal with the tendency for the brace suture to slip off the uterine cornual areas ('the shoulders') while pulling it tight).

Running the skills teaching

This teaching process is best performed in four steps:

Step 1 The instructor demonstrates the skill in silence. The skill is performed at normal speed so that the candidates appreciate the ultimate aim.

Step 2 The instructor then demonstrates the skill slowly with a commentary. Providing the commentary and breaking the technique down adds understanding to the process and can highlight points of caution and safety as well as adding helpful hints.

Step 3 The learner provides the commentary, which the instructor follows while demonstrating the skill for the third time. The instructor must be careful not to assume knowledge on the learner's part during this process and stop in mid-flow if errors are made. This step is crucial in terms of surgical safety, as the instructor can tell what the learner understands. Any errors or omissions can be addressed immediately. This step may need to be repeated.

Step 4 Once step 3 is completed satisfactorily, the learner is allowed to perform the skill while providing a commentary under direct supervision.

Scenario teaching

These practical teaching sessions describe a clinical picture and facilitate role play to manage the problem. The aim of such teaching is to demonstrate appropriate clinical behavior, including not only whether an individual has the requisite level of clinical knowledge and how it is applied, but also how individuals work together as a team and communicate. Such interactions can be complex and are worth describing further before illustrating massive hemorrhage scenarios.

Teamwork

The ability to work together as a team is absolutely requisite to good clinical care. Individuals possess differing levels of expertise, and the group's ability to carry out specific tasks depends upon the interpersonal skills of all team members. Watching a group working together can highlight its problems and help focus remedial action in terms of teamwork (or lack thereof) and occasionally individual behavior.

Every team needs a leader, and deciding who the leader is to be can sometimes be difficult. It is important to recognize that the team leader need not be the most senior person and, as the scenario develops, sometimes the leader will need to change. In any event, the leader should have appropriate knowledge and skills, be a good communicator and motivator, be able to maintain situation awareness (see the whole picture) and distribute the workload. At the same time, watching staff adapt to each other can be hugely instructive, and discussing these issues afterwards can help them understand each other, as well as individual needs and stresses.

Communication

The process of asking for and providing information and of listening to what other people are trying to say should be simple. It clearly is not, however, and is repeatedly raised as a problem area in Confidential Mortality Reports. In the Confidential Enquiry Report of 1997–1999[6], the greatest (and recurrent) cause of substandard care in maternal deaths was failure of communication and team working between

professionals. When running practical teaching sessions, communication within the team can be witnessed and discussed afterwards. Generally speaking, when dealing with any emergency, single precise commands should be addressed to specific individuals.

Voices should not be raised and an air of calm control ideally should be apparent. Unfortunately, some individuals tend to become overexcited, and noise levels can build up in emergency situations, all of which can affect everyone's behavior, as well as make it exceedingly difficult to hear what is being said without resorting to shouting. Pointing out such behavioral features under stress during mock emergencies can only help to raise awareness.

Preparing for scenario teaching

When preparing for role play, it is important to try to make things as realistic as possible.

The patient Depending on the subject, either a manikin or a live person is appropriate. Manikins tend to be good for collapse and cardiopulmonary resuscitation, whereas live models are better when responses are needed (for example, the model can pretend to fit in eclampsia, or can groan and describe pain with an abruption). Either can suit massive obstetric hemorrhage. However, the advantage of a live model is that everyone usually learns a great deal with regard to how all levels of staff communicate with a patient in such emergencies

The equipment Running clinical scenarios is more realistic if appropriate equipment is available. This may be quite simple (e.g. lateral tilt and oxygen, but using it helps to illustrate what important features have been dealt with and what omissions have occurred (e.g. intravenous access or urinary catheter). Table 2 suggests a minimum equipment list for a massive hemorrhage scenario.

Table 2 Basic equipment list for practical obstetric hemorrhage training

Airway and breathing
Guedel airway
Oxygen mask with bag and tubing
Stethoscope

Circulatory
Wedge (to provide lateral tilt for the pelvis)
Tape
Two large-bore intravenous cannulae (14 F)
20-ml syringe
Blood tubes for full blood count (FBC), cross-match (XM), clotting studies
2-liter bags of crystalloid run through administration sets
Catheter

Specific equipment for massive obstetric hemorrhage
Intrauterine inflatable balloon and bladder syringe

Running the scenario

Who should be involved? It is often difficult to decide who should be involved in the role play and who is better left to watch quietly. If staff members are inexperienced with scenario teaching, it is best initially to ask for volunteers. Lack of volunteers may be due to simple factors such as being shy, but it may result from fear of ignorance being exposed or raising issues of competency. It is for this reason that didactic teaching is absolutely required prior to running scenario training, so that the theoretical material has already been covered. If this has taken place, those previously unsure of the theory behind the problem can build on their newly acquired knowledge in a practical way. Indeed, once members of staff become used to this method of teaching, more will come forward. Occasionally, someone may need to be invited to join in, but this should be done sensitively and with support.

Give people defined roles People need to be given a defined role and told what they can or cannot expect in terms of back-up. For example, 'You are the senior house officer who has just answered the emergency buzzer to this multiparous patient. She has just bled briskly following spontaneous vaginal delivery. The midwife is here, but all other staff are busy with an emergency in theater and you should not expect help for at least 10 minutes. Please carry on as you would in real life. I will give you any observations you request.'

Keeping the scenario going The patient can be primed to give certain responses, and monitors can be prepared with readings (cardiotocograph paper sticking out of a machine/blood pressure recordings on a monitor, etc.), but it is the instructor's role to keep the scenario flowing and give as much or as little information as is requested. The scenario needs to progress, however, and gentle encouragement and occasional subtle prompts can assist the learner in achieving an understanding of the key treatment points. The aim of running scenarios is not to demonstrate ignorance on the part of one or more individuals, but to empower them to apply their knowledge in a logical and timely manner. Depending on the performance and ability of the candidate(s), the scenario can be resolved early or become more complex. This should be anticipated by the instructor well in advance. If the candidate is becoming stressed, but has done all the basic key treatment points, then the scenario can resolve and the candidate can be congratulated. If the key treatment points have not been achieved, on the other hand, then help can be at hand in the form of a registrar or consultant arriving to help. If the learner is doing a fantastic job, then the scenario can progress and more complex features can be added.

Prompting This can be difficult if it is to be done sensitively without demoralizing or embarrassing the learner; in reality, it requires skill and tact to make this form of teaching constructive. The following examples may be useful in the massive hemorrhage situation:

- Lateral tilt can be forgotten in the pregnant woman and a prompt asking whether there is 'anything else that could improve the circulation?' may jog a response

- If the candidate has not registered or responded to worrying observations such as a tachycardia or hypotension then these can be repeated and made worse, e.g. 'the tachycardia has now increased to xxx or the blood pressure is now yy/zz or unrecordable'

- Comment that uncross-matched blood is now available if staff have lost their train of thought and had already mentioned they would request blood but then forgotten about it

- Providing the patient's physiological responses can slow down/speed up the action as required. For example, once intravenous fluids have commenced, inform the candidate that the blood pressure is improving but that vaginal bleeding is still brisk. This will encourage the candidate to move on to assess the cause

- If the candidate moves away from the intravenous access without taking any bloods for laboratory investigation, the instructor may slow things down by asking if she/he would do anything else before moving on to assess the cause of the bleeding. The candidate could also be prompted with an empty syringe and blood tubes, if necessary, to make a teaching point.

Drawing things to a logical conclusion When the scenario has run its course, all people who have been involved in the role play should be congratulated and thanked for their participation, and then encouraged to engage in the feedback process as described above. Questions and discussion should then be encouraged before closure, with particular emphasis given to the key treatment points.

Examples of possible massive obstetric hemorrhage scenarios are provided, together with their key treatment points in Addenda B and C.

SUMMARY

Setting up practical teaching locally improves local processes, builds on teamwork, aids with communication, and improves clinical knowledge and its application in the emergency situation. It is best kept simple and, because it can be stressful to those involved in role play, it must be introduced sensitively and conducted within an encouraging atmosphere. Staff need to know what style of teaching will be used, and what it aims to accomplish. Advertising the planned content of the session in advance will encourage staff to prepare and capitalize on enthusiasm and learning. Good luck.

References

1. Confidential Enquiry into Maternal and Child Health. Saving Mothers' Lives 2003–2005. London: RCOG Press, 2007
2. Grady K, Howell C, Cos C. Managing Obstetric Emergencies and Trauma: The MOET Course Manual. London: RCOG, 2007
3. Sen R, Paterson-Brown S. Prioritisation on the labour ward. Curr. Obstet Gynaecol 2005;15:228–36
4. Crofts JF, Ellis D, Draycott TJ, Windter C, Hunt LP, Akande VA. Change in knowledge of midwives and obstetricians following obstetric emergency training: a randomised controlled trial of local hospital, simulation centre and teamwork training. Br J Obstet Gynaecol 2007;114:1534–41
5. Ellis D, Croft JF, Hunt LP, Read M, Fox R, James M. Hospital, simulation centre, and teamwork training for eclampsia management. Obstet Gynecol 2008;111:723–31
6. Confidential Enquiry into Maternal Deaths in the UK. Why Mothers Die 1997–1999. London: RCOG Press, 2001
7. Pendleton D, Scofield T, Tate P, Havelock P. The consultation: an approach to learning and teaching. Oxford: Oxford University Press, 1984

Further reading

Mackway-Jones K, Walker M. Pocket Guide to Teaching for Medical Instructors. London: BMJ Books, 1999

Firth-Cozens J. Teams, culture and managing risk. In Vincent C, ed. Clinical Risk Management: Enhancing Patient Safety. London: BMJ Books, 2001:355–68

Gaba DM, Fish KJ, Howard SK. Crisis Management in Anesthesiology. New York: Churchill Livingstone, 1994

Glavin R, Maran N. Simulation and non-technical skills. In Greaves JD, Dodds C, Kumar C, Mets B, eds. Clinical Teaching: a Guide to Teaching Practical Anaesthesia. Lisse: Swets & Seitlinger, 2003:219–29

Helmreich RL, Schaefer HG. Team performance in the operating room. In Bogner MS, ed. Human Error in Medicine. Hillsdale, New Jersey: Lawrence Erlbaum Associates, 1994:225–53

Addendum A: Websites for practical emergency training

ALSO (advanced life support organisation) at www.also.org.uk

MOET (Managing Obstetric Emergencies and Trauma) at www.moet.org.uk

RCOG Essential Obstetric Care and Newborn Care Course at www.rcog.org.uk/what-we-do/international/partnerships/life-saving-skills

UK based MOSES (Managing obstetric scenarios and emergency simulations) at blsimcentre@bartsandthelondo.nhs.uk

Addendum B: Sample scenario for PPH due to atonic uterus

Instructor's information

This scenario is one of PPH due to uterine atony. You are looking for rapid resuscitation of the woman at the same time as diagnosing and treating the problem (uterine compression, evacuation of clots, administration of uterotonic drugs and checking for trauma). Depending on how the scenario flows you can allow for rapid recovery, or not – if bleeding persists there can be discussion about other causes of hemorrhage and you are looking for an early decision to go to theater for an examination under anesthetic to exclude trauma/retained products.

Candidate information

A 34-year-old grand multipara delivered a healthy baby boy weighing 4.00 kg 40 minutes ago. She had physiological management of her third stage, and the placenta was delivered 10 minutes ago. The midwife has noticed fresh and brisk vaginal bleeding and accosts you as you were walking past the delivery room.

Initial observations

The patient is talking but very pale; pulse 110/min; blood pressure 120/80 mmHg; large volume of blood on bed and floor. Please proceed as you would in real life together with the midwife who called you. I will give you any observations you request. (The candidate can be obstetric or midwifery as either should be able to manage this emergency. If further progress to theater is needed, more senior help can arrive as requested.)

Instructor's notes/Key treatment points to be achieved

- Call for help and initiate the massive obstetric hemorrhage drill
- Recognize that this is a circulatory problem: progress rapidly through airway and breathing and attach face mask for oxygen
- Establish intravenous access
- Send blood for full blood count, cross-match, coagulation and U&Es
- Commence warmed intravenous fluids
- Do clinical examination and diagnose uterine atony
- Administer transabdominal uterine massage
- Administer a uterotonic agent
- Perform a vaginal examination and evacuate clots
- Check for obvious vaginal or cervical lacerations
- Do bimanual uterine compression
- Go through medication cascade logically and give intravenous fluids and blood appropriately
- Consider examination under anesthetic if patient fails to respond and consider other causes of PPH
- Knowledge of surgical techniques to control hemorrhage, i.e. Rüsch balloon, brace suture, etc.

Addendum C: Sample scenario for PPH not due to atony

This scenario is more complex – a precipitate labor with the possibility of a concealed abruption or genital tract trauma. The focus will be on distinguishing between abruption, genital tract trauma and retained products/membranes with/without disseminated intravascular coagulation (DIC). How this scenario will unfold will depend on the learner's experience and ability. You are looking for rapid resuscitation of the woman at the same time as diagnosing and treating the problem (uterine compression, evacuation of clots, administration of uterotonic drugs and checking for trauma). On this occasion bleeding persists and you are looking for an early decision to go to theater for an examination under anesthetic. For a junior trainee you may choose to let them find and repair a vaginal or cervical tear, but for a senior trainee you can take them further with DIC, blood and clotting products, checking for acidosis and need for ventilation, etc.

Candidate information

A 24-year-old primipara is induced at 42 weeks' gestation. She is having intermittent abdominal pain when the prostaglandin is inserted. One hour later she is transferred to the delivery suite in extreme pain and 20 minutes later she delivers a 3.8 kg baby boy rapidly followed by the placenta.

Initial observations

Talking; pulse is 100/min; blood pressure 115/70 mmHg; steady trickle of blood vaginally.

Please proceed as you would in real life and I will give you any observations you request.

Instructor's notes/Key treatment points achieved

- Call for help and institute massive hemorrhage call
- Recognize circulatory problem. Move swiftly through airway and breathing. Administer face mask oxygen
- Insert intravenous access
- Send blood for full blood count, cross match and coagulation screen
- Commence warmed intravenous fluids
- Abdominal examination to confirm uterus well contracted
- Vaginal examination to check for vaginal lacerations
- Transfer to theater for analgesia and examination
- Catheterize
- Full EUA: check vagina, cervix and uterine cavity
- If trauma found – timely repair?
- If products membranes remaining – evacuation performed?
- If DIC – knowledge of blood products, significance of acidosis, need for ITU

37

Preparedness for Postpartum Hemorrhage: an Obstetric Hemorrhage Equipment Tray

T. F. Baskett

Only in a minority of cases does postpartum hemorrhage (PPH) occur in women who are clearly at increased risk for the condition. In contrast, most women with PPH have no identifiable risk factors. PPH, unlike many other obstetric conditions, is therefore a predictably unpredictable life-threatening emergency. Thus, every maternity unit should know that PPH will be the most common emergency it has to deal with, and that the majority of cases will occur in women without obvious risk factors[1–3].

In the past decade, the principles of medical emergency preparedness[4], education and guidelines[5], and simulation training as pre-emptive responses to obstetric emergencies have been proposed and gained increasing acceptance from the profession[6–9]. Part of this preparation should include clear identification and availability of the equipment and resources needed to deal with the emergency.

Primary PPH is most often as a result of uterine atony which usually responds to the appropriate application of oxytocic agents. In a minority of cases, however, the atonic uterus will not contract with administration of any uterotonic agents, particularly in those cases of prolonged and augmented labor with an exhausted and infected uterus. In such circumstances, a variety of surgical techniques may be necessary, including uterine tamponade with packing[10] or balloon devices[11–13], uterine compression sutures[14–17], major vessel ligation[18,19] and hysterectomy. All such procedures are described in other chapters of this book (see Chapters 46–48 and 51–55).

That said, in addition to uterine atony unresponsive to oxytocic agents, numerous other causes of PPH may require surgical intervention using equipment that is not available in the standard vaginal delivery or cesarean section packs. These include high vaginal or cervical lacerations with poor exposure, placenta previa and/or placenta accreta at the time of cesarean section and uterine rupture. In most obstetric units, and for the individual obstetrician and nursing personnel who work there, the additional equipment and instruments for these surgical techniques are rarely used. Thus, when needed they may not be readily available and valuable time will be lost searching for them. For these reasons, every obstetric unit should

have a readily available, sterile 'obstetric hemorrhage equipment tray' upon which is placed all the necessary material for surgical management of PPH. In a sense, the tray becomes the equivalent of a 'crash cart' for cardiopulmonary resuscitation. Experience from a large Canadian maternity unit shows that the tray is used in about 1 in 250 cesarean deliveries and 1 in 1000 vaginal deliveries[20]. The most common surgical techniques used were uterine compression sutures, uterine tamponade, uterine and ovarian artery ligation, and suture of cervical and/or vaginal lacerations. The commonest predisposing causes were placenta previa, with or without partial accreta, and uterine atony refractory to oxytocic agents[20].

The contents of an obstetric hemorrhage tray are shown in Table 1. As individual obstetric units undoubtedly have varying availability of supplies, local conditions may modify these contents. Three vaginal retractors are necessary for access to and exposure of high vaginal and/or cervical lacerations. Heaney or

Table 1 Contents of obstetric hemorrhage equipment tray

Access/exposure
- Three vaginal retractors (Heaney, Breisky-Navratil)
- Four sponge forceps

Eyed needles
- Straight 10 cm
- Curved 70–80 mm, blunt point

Sutures
- No. 1 polyglactin (Vicryl)
- O and No. 2 chromic catgut with curved needle
- Ethiguard curved, blunt point monocryl

Uterine/vaginal/pelvic tamponade
- Vaginal packs
- Kerlix gauze roll
- Uterine balloon (depending on local availability):
  Sengstaken-Blakemore, Rüsch urological balloon, Bakri balloon, surgical glove and catheter, condom and catheter
- Plastic bag for pelvic pressure pack

Diagrams (Figures 1–4)
Pages with diagrams and instructions
- Uterine and ovarian artery ligation
- Uterine compression suture techniques: B-Lynch, square and vertical

Non-pneumatic anti-shock garment (selected units)

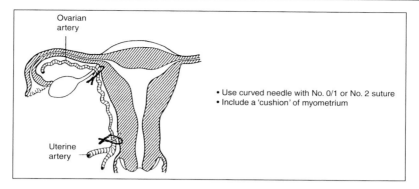

Figure 1 Uterine and ovarian artery ligation

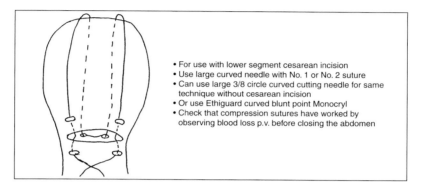

Figure 2 Uterine compression sutures: B–Lynch technique. p.v., per vagina

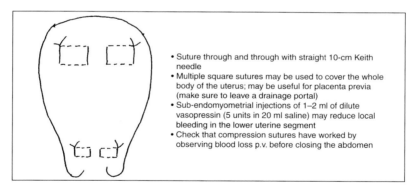

Figure 3 Uterine compression sutures: square. p.v., per vagina

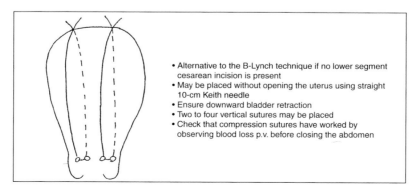

Figure 4 Uterine compression sutures: vertical. p.v., per vagina

Breisky-Navratil vaginal retractors are suitable for this purpose. Four sponge forceps are useful to identify and compress cervical lacerations, to provide compression to the edges of extensive vaginal lacerations, or to uterine edges at the time of laparotomy for uterine rupture. Standard packaged suture material often contains needles that are too small for the placement of uterine compression sutures. Thus, two-eyed needles, preferably blunt point, one straight 10 cm and one 70–80 mm curved, are advisable. A number of standard sutures should be included: No. 1 polyglactin (Vicryl) has a small needle but the Vicryl can be cut off and inserted into the eyed needles. For the full B-Lynch compression suture, two of the standard suture lengths of Vicryl may need to be tied together. If available, Ethiguard poliglecaprone (Monocryl) on a curved blunt point 90 mm needle is ideal for the B-Lynch compression suture[21]. The standard 0 and No. 2 chromic needles are suitable for uterine and ovarian artery ligation. For vertical uterine compression sutures and square uterine compression sutures, the straight 10-cm needle threaded with No. 1 Vicryl is appropriate.

Material and equipment for uterine and vaginal tamponade should be provided. For vaginal tamponade, which may be necessary to prevent hematoma formation following suture of extensive vaginal lacerations, standard vaginal packing should suffice, although it may be necessary to tie more than one of these packs together. For packing the uterine cavity, standard vaginal packing tied together can be adequate, but the ideal is the Kerlix gauze roll which has a thicker six-ply gauze than the four-ply of the usual vaginal pack.

In recent years, balloon tamponade has been used for uterine atony unresponsive to oxytocic drugs following vaginal delivery. Originally, balloon devices that were available for other medical conditions, such as the Sengstaken-Blakemore[11] and Rusch[13] balloons, were adopted for uterine tamponade. In addition, the commercially available custom-made Bakri balloon, which is really just a large Foley-type catheter, has been widely adopted for this purpose. If it is not available, because of expense or other reasons, one can improvize using a surgical glove tied at the wrist around a plain urethral catheter which, when filled with water or saline, will mould to the contour of the uterus[20]. A condom has also been adapted for this purpose, using the same technique as the surgical glove[22]. Depending on local availability, one or more of these balloon tamponade kits should be provided on the tray.

Another worthwhile addition to the tray is the material to make the pelvic pressure pack[23]. This only requires a sterile plastic bag and a lot of Kerlix gauze roll. (You really can't have too much Kerlix gauze roll on the obstetric hemorrhage tray!) The details of how to use this pack and its application to provide tamponade to the bleeding pelvic basin following hysterectomy for obstetric hemorrhage is covered in Chapter 54.

Because uterine compression sutures and major vessel ligation will rarely be used by an individual obstetrician the techniques may be forgotten, it is therefore useful to have laminated diagrams which can be easily sterilized and included in the tray (Figures 1–4)[20].

In maternity units where only limited surgical procedures are available to stem the bleeding, transfer of the woman to a hospital with more sophisticated surgical and interventional radiological resources may be necessary. In such cases the non-pneumatic anti-shock garment (NASG) can have life-saving application[24] and, as such, it should be kept beside the obstetric hemorrhage tray in selected units. The application of the NASG is covered in Chapter 39.

For PPH due to uterine atony refractory to oxytocic agents, or secondary to trauma of the genital tract, the rapid application of surgical techniques for hemostasis is essential to reduce or mitigate the need for blood transfusion, with its inherent potential morbidity. Often, hysterectomy is the final definitive treatment and may be necessary as a life-saving maneuver (see Chapter 55). However, in one hospital using an obstetric hemorrhage tray on nine occasions in 1 year, hysterectomy was avoided in all cases[20]. Thus, if the instruments and equipment are readily available for the prompt application of alternative surgical methods, one is less likely to have to resort to hysterectomy with its attendant morbidity and fertility-ending implications.

References

1. Baskett TF. Epidemiology of obstetric critical care. Best Pract Res Clin Obstet Gynaecol 2008;22:763–74
2. Cameron CA, Roberts CL, Olive EC, Ford JB, Fischer WE. Trends in postpartum haemorrhage. Aust NZ J Public Health 2006;30:151–6
3. Joseph KS, Rouleau J, Kramer MS, Young DC, Liston RM, Baskett TF. Investigation of an increase in postpartum haemorrhage in Canada. Br J Obstet Gynaecol 2007;114: 751–9
4. American College of Obstetricians and Gynecologists. Committee Opinion No.353. Medical emergency preparedness. Obstet Gynecol 2006;108:1597–99
5. Rizvi F, Mackay R, Barrett T, McKenna P, Geary M. Successful reduction of massive postpartum haemorrhage by use of guidelines and staff education. Br J Obstet Gynaecol 2004;10:495–8
6. Guise JM. Anticipating and responding to obstetric emergencies. Best Pract Res Clin Obstet Gynaecol 2007;21: 625–38
7. Upadhyay K, Scholefield H. Risk management and medico-legal issues related to postpartum haemorrhage. Best Pract Res Clin Obstet Gynaecol 2008;22:1149–69
8. Clark EA, Fischer J, Araleb J, Druzin M. Team training/simulation. Clin Obstet Gynecol 2010;53:265–77
9. Ennen CS, Satin AJ. Training and assessment in obstetrics: the role of simulation. Best Pract Res Clin Obstet Gynaecol 2010;24:747–58
10. Maier RC. Control of postpartum hemorrhage with uterine packing. Am J Obstet Gynecol 1993;169:17–23
11. Chan C, Razvi K, Tham KA, Arulkumaran S. The use of the Sengstaken-Blakemore tube to control postpartum haemorrhage. Int J Gynaecol Obstet 1997;58:251–2

12. Bakri YN, Amri A, Jabbar FA. Tamponade balloon for obstetrical bleeding. Int J Gynaecol Obstet 2001;74: 139–42

13. Johanson R, Kumar M, Obhari M, Young P. Management of massive postpartum haemorrhage: use of hydrostatic balloon catheter to avoid laparotomy. Br J Obstet Gynaecol 2001;108: 420–2

14. B-Lynch C, Cocker A, Lowell AH, Abu J, Cowan MJ. The B-Lynch surgical technique for control of massive haemorrhage: an alternative to hysterectomy? Five cases reported. Br J Obstet Gynaecol 1997;104:372–5

15. Hayman RC, Arulkumaran S, Steer PJ. Uterine brace sutures – a simple modification of the B-Lynch surgical prodedure for the management of postpartum hemorrhage. Obstet Gynecol 2002;99:502–6

16. Cho JH, Jun HS, Lee CN. Hemostatic suturing technique for uterine bleeding during Cesarean delivery. Obstet Gynecol 2000;96:129–31

17. Baskett TF. Uterine compression sutures for postpartum hemorrhage: efficacy, morbidity and subsequent pregnancy. Obstet Gynecol 2007;110:68–71

18. Fahmy K. Uterine artery ligation to control postpartum haemorrhage. Int J Gynaecol Obstet 1987;25:363–7

19. Joshi VM, Otiv SR, Majunder R, Nikam YA, Shrivastava M. Internal iliac artery ligation for arresting postpartum haemorrhage. Br J Obstet Gynaecol 2007;114:356–61

20. Baskett TF. Surgical management of severe obstetric haemorrhage: experience with an obstetric haemorrhage equipment tray. J Obstet Gynaecol Can 2004;26:805–8

21. Price N, B-Lynch C. Technical description of the B-Lynch brace suture for treatment of massive postpartum haemorrhage and review of published cases. Int J Fertil Womens Med 2005;50:148–63

22. Akhter S, Begum MR, Kebir Z, Rashid M, Laila TR, Zabean F. Use of a condom to control massive postpartum hemorrhage. Med Gen Med 2003;5:38

23. Dildy GA, Scott JR, Saffer CS, Belfort MA. An effective pressure pack for severe pelvic hemorrhage. Obstet Gynecol 2006;108:1222–6

24. Miller S, Martin JL. Anti-shock garment in postpartum haemorrhage. Best Pract Res Clin Obstet Gynaecol 2008;22: 1057–74

38

Non-pneumatic Anti-Shock Garments: Clinical Trials and Results

S. Miller, J. L. Morris, M. M. F. Fathalla, O. Ojengbede, M. Mourad-Youssif and P. Hensleigh (deceased)

INTRODUCTION

The International Federation of Gynecology and Obstetrics (FIGO)/International Confederation of Midwives (ICM) recommendations for active management of third-stage labor, including uterotonic prophylaxis with additional uterotonic treatment when necessary, clearly reduce the incidence of severe postpartum hemorrhage (PPH) due to uterine atony[1]. Despite this, many women suffer intractable PPH from atony or other obstetric etiologies, including genital lacerations, ruptured uterus, ruptured ectopic pregnancies, as well as placenta previa, accreta and abruption. Multiple blood transfusions are often required to resuscitate and stabilize these individuals, and the institution of hemostasis may require surgical interventions or procedures only available at tertiary levels with skilled providers. Until the time when quality comprehensive emergency obstetric care (CEmOC), including surgery and/or blood transfusions, is readily available for all women in all locations, strategies and technologies for treatment of hemorrhage and hypovolemic shock are of exceptional value, especially those that can be readily provided and easily applied, even by persons with little or no medical training. Among the most promising of technologies to reduce maternal mortality is the non-pneumatic anti-shock garment (NASG), a first-aid device that when appropriately used may reduce the mortality and morbidity associated with obstetric hemorrhage[2–8].

THE NON-PNEUMATIC ANTI-SHOCK GARMENT

The NASG is a simple device, proposed as the immediate first-aid treatment for reversing hypovolemic shock and decreasing blood loss secondary to obstetric hemorrhage, by application of lower body counter pressure. The NASG also has the potential to keep women alive during long transports from lower level facilities or home to the CEmOC facilities and during delays while waiting for definitive therapies at these facilities.

The NASG is a lightweight, washable and reusable (at least 40 times), neoprene compression garment that resembles the lower part of a wet suit. The NASG, manufactured by the Zoex Company, received a United States Food and Drug Administration (FDA) 510(k) medical device regulations number (FDA device # K904267/A, Regulatory Class: II, January 17, 1991) (Section 510(k) Medical Device Amendment, FDA, Office of Device Evaluation, 1991) and can be exported to countries outside the United States. The NASG is designed in horizontal segments, with three segments for each leg, a segment to be placed over the pelvis, and a segment over the abdomen that contains a small, foam compression ball (Figure 1).

Unlike the pneumatic anti-shock garment (PASG), or medical anti-shock trousers (MAST), both of which preceded the development of the NASG, there are no pumps, tubing, or gauges to add either complexity or risk of malfunction. Using the three-way elasticity of neoprene and the tight grip of the Velcro fasteners, the garment applies circumferential counter pressure to the lower body from the ankles all the way up to the level of the diaphragm (Figure 2). Excess pressure and

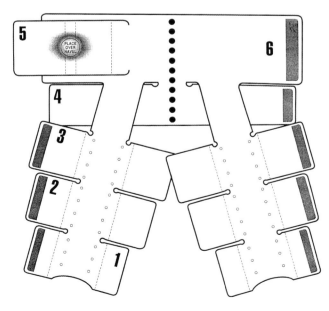

Figure 1 Schematic diagram of the non-pneumatic anti-shock garment (NASG)

resultant tissue ischemia, reported complications with the pneumatic PASG, are not an issue with the NASG.

Application of the garment requires about 2 minutes; about 10 minutes after application, most patients with severe shock regain consciousness and vital signs begin to recover. With the bleeding slowed and the blood pressure restored, clinicians' panic levels decrease, and there is time to deliberately assess the situation. The patient and her family can be given emotional support and prepared for transport to a referral-level facility. In addition, patients can remain in a stable condition for hours while blood transfusions are initiated and arrangements made for surgery or other required therapies.

Development of the NASG

The modern NASG is a non-pneumatic refinement of the PASG. The PASG was adapted from a device developed by George Crile in the early 1900s before the advent of technologies for blood transfusions. Crile, a surgeon who wrote textbooks on blood pressure and shock, designed the first inflatable pressure suit to maintain blood pressure during surgery. This pneumatic suit underwent multiple modifications and was further refined for use as an anti-gravity suit (G-suit) for the Army Air Corps in 1942. During the Vietnam War, the G-suit was modified for stabilizing and resuscitating soldiers with traumatic injuries before and during transport. The G-suit was then modified to a half-suit, which became known as military anti-shock trousers (MAST).

The PASG: pneumatic predecessor of the NASG

The MAST/PASG has been used since the 1970s by emergency rescue squads in the United States to stabilize patients with a variety of disorders: pelvic and lower limb fractures, hypovolemic shock, septic shock, and to control intra-abdominal, pelvic, thigh and obstetric–gynecological hemorrhages[9,10]. More recently, Andrea and colleagues reported using MAST devices to stabilize two women with intractable uterine bleeding while preparations were made for transcatheter embolization[11].

The PASG requires inflation and careful management of pressure levels, both to maintain adequate pressure and to prevent over-inflation which could result in compartment syndromes, ischemia and necrosis. Moreover, the valves and manometers that maintain inflation are subject to leak and malfunction. In addition, specialized training for safe and effective usage is necessary, which makes widespread application of the PSAG in developing countries problematic. The high cost (596–1099 US$ plus potential costs for maintenance and replacement parts) further restricts utilization[12].

Efficacy of the PASG for pre-hospital trauma care

In 1988 McSwain reviewed the physical principles responsible for the physiologic effects of lower-body counter pressure with application of the PASG[9]. Numerous studies in hypovolemic animals and humans demonstrated that the PASG increased blood

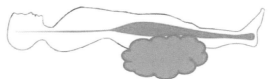

In decompensatory shock, the heart, lungs and brain are deprived of oxygen as blood accumulates in the lower part of the body

In obstetric hemorrhage, blood also leaves the body through the vagina or pools in the retroperitoneum

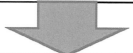

The NASG reverses shock by increasing blood volume in the upper body, heart, brain and lungs

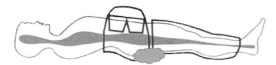

It reduces blood loss because it compresses the blood vessels. When the radius of a blood vessel is decreased, blood flow through the vessel is decreased

Figure 2 Possible mechanisms of action of the non-pneumatic anti-shock garment

pressure by decreasing the vascular volume and increasing vascular resistance within the compressed region of the body. When blood flow or arterial vascular size is measured above the device, the flow is greater and vessels are larger. In the compressed region, the radius of blood vessels is decreased, thus diminishing blood flow. In the hypovolemic model, the PASG increases venous return and the increase in preload is associated with increased cardiac output[13].

Although animal studies show improved survival rates except for thoracic injuries[14,15], it is uncertain if the rapid, positive changes in vital signs and blood loss affect survival in humans. Despite widespread acceptance of the PASG for use in military and civilian trauma injuries, including being required on ambulances in the late 1970s and 1980s[16], and the appearance of reports of small series demonstrating successful treatment of various bleeding conditions in adults and children, no definitive prospective randomized treatment trials show improvement in survival. The three United States-based, prospective, alternate-day, randomized treatment trials of civilian trauma cases failed to find consistent results and are confounded by inclusion of injuries to the upper body, a contraindication to use of the PASG[17-19]. In some studies, the pH on hospital admission was lower with PASG use; at the same time, intensive care unit and hospital stays were longer and survival worse. A factor confounding the interpretation of these reports is that these studies were all conducted in a metropolitan setting where high-level hospital care was available within minutes; in such circumstances, even a brief delay in applying the PASG may have been a detriment to the benefits of early hospital care.

Current status of PASG for trauma and other indications

Although it is no longer required as essential equipment for ambulances, the PASG remains on the curriculum and in the textbooks for emergency medical technicians in the US[20,21]. A position paper on the PASG by the National Association of EMS Physicians cited the lack of controlled trials, but, on the basis of other reports, deemed the PASG as 'Class I usually indicated and effective for hypotension due to ruptured aortic aneurysm, but of uncertain efficacy for other emergency situations'. Its use for uncontrolled gynecologic hemorrhage, urologic hemorrhage and ruptured ectopic pregnancy was described as 'Class IIb acceptable, but uncertain efficacy, may be helpful, probably not harmful'. PASG proponents particularly recommend its use for bleeding in the abdomen, retroperitoneum, pelvis, or thighs[22]. The current recommendations in the US are that, while its effects on survival are unknown, it is probably indicated in patients with bleeding in the very areas (abdomen, retroperitoneum and pelvis) that are the bleeding sites for women with obstetric hemorrhage. Research on euvolemic female volunteers demonstrated that the PASG decreases aortic blood flow over a small area

immediately distal to the renal arteries by up to 90%, but has little or no effect above this point[23]. This finding provides support for PASG use to decrease uncontrollable hemorrhage from the iliac, pelvic and leg vessels, but not for injuries above them[8]. In France, use of the 'pantalon antichoc' is questioned for widespread use, but its use for PPH, disseminated intravascular coagulopathies (DIC) associated with pregnancy and labor, and other obstetric and gynecological bleeding is endorsed[24].

It is not known whether outcomes might be different if the PASG (or the NASG) were to be used in low-resource settings with longer transport times, slower responses at the hospital level and longer delays in obtaining definitive therapy such as blood transfusions and/or surgery.

POTENTIAL BENEFITS OF THE NON-PNEUMATIC ANTI-SHOCK GARMENT FOR OBSTETRIC HEMORRHAGE IN LOW-RESOURCE SETTINGS

In 1971, a team working on technology spin offs at the National Aeronautics and Space Administration (NASA)/Ames Research Center developed a prototype pressure suit designed to protect hemophiliac children from bleeding into elbow and knee joints by straightening and compressing the joint until medical attention was available[25]. This pressure suit, the NASG, was adapted from PASG/MAST garments. Both PASG and NASG provide circumferential counter pressure in the lower body, but the NASG is simpler in design, more quickly and easily applied, less expensive and avoids the risk of over-inflation and excessive pressure[26] (Figure 3).

The NASG is particularly suited for use in low-resource settings. It is lighter and more flexible than the PASG, is more comfortable for a woman to wear for long periods of time, something which is necessary with the long transport times and delayed treatment conditions of low-resource settings. As with the PASG, within minutes of being placed in the NASG, a patient's vital signs are restored and, if confused or unconscious, their sensorium generally clears[3]. Women can remain in the NASG for as long as is required to restore their circulatory volume with crystalloids and to replace blood. In many prior reports

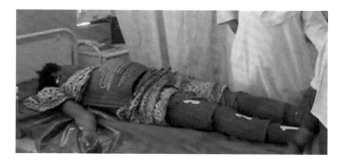

Figure 3 Patient wearing the non-pneumatic anti-shock garment in hospital. Reproduced with kind permission of Dawn Shapiro, 2010

of cases where blood transfusions were not readily available, this has often required 18–24 hours and, in one case, a woman remained safely in the NASG for almost 60 hours[27]. In Egypt, the mean time documented in the NASG was 269 minutes (more than 4 hours) ($n = 554$), and in Nigeria mean times documented were 690 minutes (more than 10 hours) ($n = 273$)[28].

A second benefit of the NASG for obstetric indications is that the design of the garment permits complete perineal access. Genital lacerations can be repaired, speculum or bimanual examinations performed, and manual removal of placenta or emptying of the uterus with vacuum aspiration or curettage can be accomplished with the NASG *in situ*. Stated another way, the source of most obstetric hemorrhages can be located and attended to while the garment maintains vital signs.

A third benefit of the NASG is that it significantly reduces further blood loss. When the NASG is applied, the external circumferential counter pressure is distributed evenly throughout the abdominal cavity and to the outside of the circulatory vessels, thereby tamponading venous bleeding. In the event of an arterial injury, continued bleeding results from the tension in the wall of the artery keeping the defect open. However, the NASG compresses all the intra-abdominal vessels including the internal iliac and uterine arteries. This compression reduces the radius of the arteries and reduces the transmural pressure (the difference between the pressure inside the artery and the pressure outside the artery) which, in turn, reduces the tension in the arterial wall, closing the defect and reducing blood loss[13]. Because the applied pressures could interfere with uterine blood flow, the NASG is not recommended for obstetric bleeding when the fetus is still viable, such as might be the case with placenta previa or abruption at more than 28 weeks. Post-delivery, however, or very early pregnancy (abortion, ectopic, trophoblastic disease of pregnancy) or when the fetus is not viable or is dead, the NASG can be used for any obstetric hemorrhage.

Another potential benefit for the use of the NASG for obstetric hemorrhage in low-resource settings is that persons with no medical background can learn to apply the garment rapidly and safely with minimal training. Hands-on practice in application and removal of the NASG takes approximately 1 hour. Once the garment has been properly applied, patients can be safely transported and/or await definitive treatment in a more stable physical condition. This final point is critical, as the majority of maternal deaths due to obstetric hemorrhage occur in areas where skilled birth and critical care attendance are limited or absent.

Decreased blood loss and reduced need for emergency hysterectomy, as well as diminished maternal morbidity and mortality, have currently been documented in case series, pilot studies and pre-intervention phase/NASG-intervention phase comparative studies in tertiary care centers in Pakistan, Nigeria and Egypt[28–37]. As of May, 2012, we have documented care with the NASG on over 5500 women.

SUGGESTED PROTOCOL FOR USING THE NON-PNEUMATIC ANTI-SHOCK GARMENT

The NASG is recommended for cases of obstetric hemorrhage meeting the American College of Surgeons' criteria for class II hypovolemic shock: more than 750 ml blood loss, pulse more than 100 bpm and blood pressure normal or slightly decreased[38]. The NASG is not recommended for use with a viable fetus, for patients with mitral stenosis, congestive heart failure, pulmonary hypertension, or in clinical conditions where bleeding sites are supra- diaphragmatic. It is axiomatic that the availability of the NASG does not negate the importance of preventive measures such as the active management of the third stage of labor or administration of uterotonics to treat uterine atony. Rather, the NASG can be part of the resuscitation measures aimed at 'damage control', that is, non-definitive control of the source of bleeding[39]. The authors recommend cardiovascular resuscitation using limited crystalloid infusion with the goal of 'permissive hypotension'[40–46]. This means infusing 1000–1500 ml of saline rapidly followed by a slower rate of infusion, 150 ml/h, to achieve a systolic blood pressure of 80–100 mmHg and urine output of at least 30 ml/h. Supplemental oxygen should be given until the patient is resuscitated, hemorrhage arrested and circulation fully normalized.

NASG application

The technique for application is for one person to stretch the neoprene panels with all their strength and fasten them with the Velcro as tightly as possible. The lowest (ankle) segment is applied first and the abdominal segment last. Anyone, at any level of the health care system or community, can be trained to apply the NASG rapidly and correctly. On the other hand, management of the women in the NASG requires more complex skills and training.

After application, if the woman experiences difficulty breathing, the abdominal panel should be loosened slightly, but not removed. However, if dyspnea continues, the NASG should be removed and the cause of the respiratory problem evaluated. A woman with normal cardiorespiratory function should experience no problems with ventilation. If there is no prompt response in terms of vital signs with placement of the NASG, the application should be checked for adequate tightness, and additional saline infusion given promptly. As soon as the patient is stable, there must be a diligent evaluation for the specific source and cause of the blood loss.

Timing of NASG application in resuscitation protocol

The ideal time to apply the NASG in the course of hypovolemic shock resuscitation depends largely on the capacity of the facility level and the respective staff who are applying it and whether the woman can rapidly receive definitive therapy. In the lowest levels of the health care system, or even at the highest levels, if blood and/or surgery will be delayed, the NASG should be one of the first measures taken. Application can help in filling the blood vessels of the arms, thus making IV resuscitation more rapid, easy and, perhaps, not requiring surgical cut-down. In more highly resourced settings, the NASG has been applied when medical therapies have failed to stop bleeding, and during delays in obtaining surgery, or, when surgery has been tried, but bleeding continues or when awaiting arterial embolization (interventional radiology) teams[11,47].

Management of patient in the NASG

Care for the women in a NASG should proceed depending on her condition and the level of facility or health care system. The source of bleeding should be ascertained and measures taken to stop it depending on its origin, i.e., massage and uterotonics for uterine atony, repair of lacerations, etc. If the patient needs transportation, at a minimum she should receive IV fluids and oxygen, with close monitoring of vital signs. Vaginal procedures, such as speculum exam, manual removal of tissue (vacuum or curettage), can all be performed with the NASG in place. If laparotomy is necessary, the abdominal segments can be opened, but only immediately prior to making the incision, all other segments should remain closed. Often there will be a drop in blood pressure when this panel is removed; this should respond to additional crystalloid infusion. The abdominal panel should then be closed immediately after surgery; the NASG can be closed over the bandage. It does not seem to increase pain in the incision area, but seems to serve a splinting function.

NASG removal

The NASG is left in place as long as needed to achieve hemostasis and replace red blood cell volume with transfusions of blood and blood products. The NASG can be removed when the hemoglobin level is more than 7 g/dl or hematocrit 20%, pulse of less than 100 bpm and the systolic pressure more than 100 mmHg. Removal of the NASG begins with the lowest segment (#1) and proceeds upwards, allowing 15 min between removing each segment for redistribution of blood. If the blood pressure falls by 20 mmHg or the pulse increases by 20 bpm after a segment is removed, replace the NASG and consider the need for more saline or blood transfusions. If recurrent bleeding becomes apparent, replace the NASG and determine the source of bleeding.

STUDIES OF THE NON-PNEUMATIC ANTI-SHOCK GARMENT FOR OBSTETRIC HEMORRHAGE

Early examples of the potential benefits of using the NASG in obstetric hemorrhage in resource-challenged settings were documented in two published reports based on a series of 20 obstetric cases from one hospital in Sialkot, Pakistan[3,27]. These reports documented rapid resuscitation from hypovolemic shock, as well as an extended period of stabilization while awaiting definitive treatment for patients treated with the NASG. A combined analysis of data contained in these reports[48] showed no adverse effects of a prolonged time spent in the NASG. On the basis of these case series, NASG pilot studies were conducted (John Snow Inc., Egypt and University of California, San Francisco) and comparative pre-intervention/NASG intervention studies in CEmOC facilities in Nigeria* and Egypt† undertaken.

Comparative design used in Egypt and Nigeria studies

These studies compare the outcomes of a standardized protocol of shock and hemorrhage management in a pre-intervention (observational) phase with the same protocol plus the NASG in the intervention phase). The primary outcome was volume of measured blood loss after initiation of treatment with or without the NASG. To obtain a relatively objective measure of blood loss, maternal bleeding was measured using a specially designed, closed-end, calibrated plastic blood collection drape. Prior investigations with the use of this drape indicate that it is more accurate than visual assessment in measuring postpartum blood loss[49]. Other outcomes included mortality, severe acute maternal morbidities (SAMMs) associated with obstetric hemorrhage (acute respiratory distress syndrome, cardiac deficiency, central nervous system damage and renal failure)[50], and the need for emergency hysterectomy for intractable bleeding associated with uterine atony. The standardized, evidence-based protocol included active management of third-stage labor, immediate use of uterotonics for suspected postpartum uterine atony, training in administration of intravenous crystalloid fluid[51,52], thorough assessment for the source of bleeding, manual procedures such as bimanual compression, vaginal procedures, surgery, replacement of lost blood and, in the intervention phase, prompt application of the NASG.

Inclusion criteria for study enrollment included obstetric hemorrhage with hypovolemic shock (estimated blood loss ≥750 ml, systolic blood pressure <100 mmHg and/or pulse >100 bpm). All obstetric hemorrhage etiologies were included, *early pregnancy hemorrhage* (ectopic pregnancy, molar pregnancy, complications of abortion, retained placenta/tissue,

*Dr Oladosu Ojengbede, University of Ibadan, Principal Investigator, Nigeria.
†Dr Mohamed M.F. Fathalla, Assiut, Dr Mohammed Mourad Youssif, El Galaa, Principal Investigators, Egypt.

DIC), *antepartum hemorrhage* (placenta previa, abruption, ruptured uterus, DIC), and *postpartum hemorrhage* (placenta accrete, uterine atony, retained placenta/tissue, lacerations, DIC).

Results from Egyptian pilot study

The four study sites in Egypt comprised high-volume referral CEmOC teaching facilities (El Galaa, Alexandria, Assiut and Al Minya)[30]. All were staffed by senior obstetricians and obstetric residents with immediate access to banked donor blood and surgery if required. In the pilot assessment, pre-intervention data, including measured blood loss, were collected for 3 months, after which all providers were trained in the use of the NASG. The only change to the pre-intervention clinical management was the use of the NASG. NASG-intervention data were collected for another 3 months.

The sample comprised 158 hypovolemic shock patients in the pre-intervention phase and 206 hypovolemic shock patients in the NASG-intervention phase. A range of primary diagnoses was present with no statistically significant differences between pre-intervention phase and NASG-intervention phase patients. Women in the NASG-intervention phase had more severe signs of shock ($p < 0.001$) than those in the pre-intervention phase. Despite this, NASG-intervention phase patients had 50% less median measured blood loss after study entry ($p < 0.001$). There was a non-statistically significant, but clinically important (69%) lower incidence of SAMMs and mortalities, which were combined as 'extreme adverse outcomes' (EAO). Specifically, the EAO rate was 1.0% (2/206) in the NASG-intervention phase patients compared to 3.2% (5/158) in the pre-intervention patients) (OR 0.31, 95% confidence interval (CI) 0.06–1.56). In larger study samples, this difference could well attain statistical significance and serve as a marker of the utility of the technology, considering the recent moves worldwide to diminish EAO.

Decreased shock recovery times

A post-hoc analysis of the Egyptian pilot study data was conducted to examine the lengths of recovery time from shock. Results indicated that median recovery times were nearly twice as rapid (1.6–2.0 times) for women treated during the NASG-intervention phase compared to time to recovery of women in the pre-intervention phase. The reduction in recovery times was even greater when adjustments were made for severity of the woman's condition at study entry[28].

Expanded comparative studies in Egypt and Nigeria

These pilot results were judged promising, but thought to require a larger sample over a longer period of time in order to demonstrate differences in EAO. Therefore a year later a larger pre-intervention/NASG-intervention study in two of the four facilities in Egypt[32] and at four facilities in Nigeria was

conducted[31,35]. The methods described above for the Egyptian pilot study were replicated in Nigeria. The Nigerian NASG program was carried out in 12 urban, referral hospitals throughout Northern and Southern Nigeria. Some of these secondary and tertiary CEmOC facilities were teaching hospitals, and the others were state hospitals. Many facilities had high numbers of obstetric deliveries, a high proportion of un-booked patients, and a large number of high-risk complications. A total of 756 women were enrolled in Nigeria from 2004 to 2008. (By design, eight of the facilities were NASG-intervention use only, without a pre-intervention phase.)

A number of reports have examined data from women in both countries with all etiologies of bleeding[34] as well women from both countries where PPH was the etiology of the hemorrhage[33]. Egypt-only analyses include data from all obstetric hemorrhage etiologies[32], uterine atony only[53], and non-atonic etiologies only[37]. Nigeria-only analyses include data for all obstetric hemorrhage etiologies in one facility[31], for PPH etiologies in the four facilities[35], and for uterine atony only in 12 facilities[54]. Results demonstrated similar trends for all studies, except for the Egyptian non-atonic hemorrhage only, with better outcomes for women in the NASG-intervention phase including statistically significant reduced rates of morbidity, mortality, emergency hysterectomy (for uterine atony) and reduced blood loss.

In the remainder of this chapter, we discuss outcomes for women in both countries with all hemorrhagic etiologies, with PPH etiologies only, and the non-atonic etiologies in Egypt; in addition we discuss a post-hoc analysis of the effect of NASG for ameliorating negative outcomes specifically associated with delays[36] and the results of some qualitative studies of provider and patient acceptance[55–57].

Analysis of data on 1442 women with obstetric hemorrhage in Nigeria and Egypt

These results derive from data on 1442 women with hypovolemic shock secondary to obstetric hemorrhage (607 pre-intervention and 835 NASG-intervention phase). As shown in Table 1[34], there were no significant differences in demographic characteristics, but etiologies were different with significantly more ectopic pregnancy, ruptured uteri and placenta previa during the pre-intervention phase and more uterine atony, complications of abortion and lacerations during the NASG-intervention phase use. During the pre-intervention phase, significantly more women entered the study who had started bleeding at home or at another facility rather than having begun their bleeding in the hospital ($p < 0.001$). Women in the NASG-intervention phase were in worse condition on study entry (38.5% had mean arterial pressure (MAP) less than 60 mmHg vs. 29.9% in the pre-intervention phase, $p = 0.001$). Regarding treatment, significantly fewer women in the NASG phase received either 1500 ml or more crystalloid fluids or a

Table 1 Egypt and Nigeria combined etiologies: diagnoses and condition on entry (*n* = 1442). Data are expressed as numbers with percentages in parentheses. From Miller *et al.*, *BMC Pregnancy and Childbirth* 2010;10:64, with permission

	Pre-intervention phase (n = 607)	NASG-intervention phase (n = 835)	p Value
Primary definitive diagnosis			
Uterine atony	190 (33.0)	319 (38.2)	0.007
Ectopic pregnancy	95 (15.7)	85 (10.2)	0.002
Complications of abortion	45 (7.4)	93 (11.1)	0.02
Abruption of placenta	79 (13.0)	98 (11.7)	0.47
Vaginal, cervical or genital lacerations	25 (4.1)	65 (7.8)	0.004
Retained placenta or tissue	71 (11.7)	83 (9.9)	0.29
Ruptured uterus	46 (7.6)	32 (3.8)	0.002
Placenta previa	40 (6.6)	31 (3.7)	0.01
Placenta accreta	6 (1.0)	9 (1.1)	1.000*
Molar pregnancy	7 (1.2)	11 (1.3)	1.000*
Condition on study entry			
Where hemorrhage began			<0.001
Transferred in bleeding	382 (72.9)	333 (56.4)	
Began bleeding in hospital	142 (27.1)	258 (43.6)	
Estimated revealed blood loss at study entry[†]			—
Mean ml (SD)	1210.0 (507.7)	1327.5 (480.7)	
Median ml (IQR)	1000 (1000–1500)	1200 (1000–1500)	<0.0001
Women with MAP <60 mmHg or non-palpable BP[‡]	181 (29.9)	321 (38.5)	0.001

NASG, non-pneumatic anti-shock garment
Tests of significance of differences by study phase were c^2 for categorical variables, *t* tests (assuming unequal variances) for normally distributed continuous variables and Wilcoxon rank-sum tests for non-normal distributions
★Fisher's exact test used
[†]Data missing for 250 patients
[‡]MAP (mean arterial pressure) <60 category includes those with non-palpable blood pressure (BP). Data missing for two patients

blood transfusion in the first hour (*p* < 0.001); by the end of the second hour from study admission, however, 87.5% in the pre-intervention phase and 86.6% in the NASG phase had received more than 1500 ml (*p* = 0.62).

Despite being in worse condition on study entry and receiving the recommended treatment fluids and blood more slowly, negative outcomes were significantly reduced in the NASG phase. Mean measured blood loss decreased from 444 to 240 ml (*p* < 0.001), maternal mortality decreased from 6.3% to 3.5% (RR 0.56, 95% CI 0.35–0.89), severe morbidities declined from 3.7% to 0.7% (RR 0.20, 95% CI 0.08–0.50), and the rate of emergency hysterectomy (for intractable uterine atony) fell from 8.9% to 4.0% (RR 0.44, 0.23–0.86).

As shown in Table 2, in a multiple logistic regression model, women with a MAP less than 60 mmHg had over eight times the odds of mortality (OR 8.42, 95% CI 3.13–22.66) relative to those with MAP 60 mmHg or more. No other control variables (parity, primary diagnosis or facility) were significantly associated with mortality, but NASG intervention was

associated with 55% lower odds of mortality (OR 0.45, 95% CI 0.27–0.77). In the model of factors associated with severe maternal morbidity, women with a MAP less than 60 mmHg had almost five times the odds of morbidity (OR 4.83, 95% CI 1.80–12.94) relative to those with MAP 60 mmHg or more. Those with a parity of five or more had 2.4 times the odds of morbidity (OR 2.43, 95% CI 1.06–5.58), but where the bleeding began and the type of facility were not associated with the outcome. The NASG intervention was significantly associated with 80% lower odds of a morbidity (OR 0.20, 95% CI 0.07–0.56).

Because the odds of morbidity and of mortality were so high for women in severe shock, independent of the study phase, a stratified analysis by severity of condition (MAP <60 mmHg vs. MAP ≥60 mmHg) was conducted for each of the two outcomes, using the same model specification from the multiple logistic regression. An ameliorative effect of the intervention for reduced morbidity was seen in both women with MAP less than 60 (aOR 0.20, 95% CI 0.05–0.80,) and MAP 60 mmHg or more (aOR 0.18, 95% CI 0.04–0.90). For the stratified mortality model, the NASG intervention was significantly associated with a reduced odds of death in women with MAP less than 60 mmHg (aOR 0.46, 95% CI 0.26–0.80), but not in women with MAP 60 mmHg or more (aOR 0.68, 95% CI 0.14–3.22).

Analysis of data from Nigeria and Egypt of PPH etiologies

An analysis was conducted on data from 854 women (343 pre-intervention and 511 NASG-intervention phase) with diagnoses of PPH, uterine atony, retained placenta, ruptured uterus, vaginal or cervical lacerations or placenta accreta; all were selected from the total of 1442 women with hypovolemic shock from obstetric hemorrhage. Study design, study definitions, entry criteria, clinical and study protocol were the same; analyses were performed on the outcomes of measured blood loss, emergency hysterectomy, mortality, morbidity (each individually) and a combined variable, adverse outcomes, defined as severe morbidity and mortality. Approximately 36% of women in both phases were in severe shock. See Table 3 for etiologies and condition on study entry[33].

Measured blood loss decreased by 50% between phases; women lost 400 ml of blood after study entry during the pre-intervention phase and 200 ml in the NASG-intervention phase (*p* < 0.001). Mortality (as an individual outcome) decreased from 9% (*n* = 31) in the pre-intervention phase to 3.1% (*n* = 16), (RR 0.35, 95% CI 0.19–0.62), while the combined adverse outcomes of mortality and morbidity decreased from 12.8% (*n* = 44) to 4.1% (*n* = 21), (RR 0.32, 95% CI 0.19–0.53). Rates of emergency hysterectomy for hemostasis of intractable PPH from uterine atony (only) decreased from 9% (*n* = 20) to 4% (*n* = 14) (RR 0.44, 95% CI 0.23–0.86).

A multiple logistic regression model was used to estimate the independent association between the

Table 2 Egypt and Nigeria combined etiologies: multiple logistic regression (*n* = 1442). From Miller *et al.*, *BMC Pregnancy and Childbirth* 2010;10:64, with permission

	Dependent variable: mortality				*Dependent variable: morbidity*			
Factor	*aOR*	*p Value*	*95% CI*		*aOR*	*p Value*	*95% CI*	
Severity of shock								
MAP <60 mmHg (or non-palpable BP)	8.42	<0.001	3.13	22.66	4.83	0.002	1.80	12.94
MAP 60 mmHg or higher	*1*				*1*			
Parity								
5 or more live births	1.33	0.35	0.73	2.42	2.43	0.04	1.06	5.58
0–4 live births	*1*				*1*			
Primary diagnosis								
Uterine atony	1.44	0.19	0.83	2.49	2.68	0.07	0.93	7.76
Other condition	*1*				*1*			
*Where bleeding began**								
Transferred in bleeding	—	—	—	—	1.82	0.51	0.30	10.93
Began bleeding in hospital	—	—	—	—	*1*			
Study phase								
NASG-intervention phase	0.45	0.004	0.27	0.77	0.20	0.002	0.07	0.56
Pre-intervention phase	*1*				*1*			

NASG, non-pneumatic anti-shock garment

Reference groups for categorical variables shown in italics. Hospital facility included as control variable in both models but not shown here The number of observations in Table 4 is less than 1442 because of missing data; *n* = 1038 for the morbidity model, and *n* = 1442 for the mortality model. Robust standard errors used to adjust for clustering at the facility level

*Where bleeding began was not a significant predictor of mortality, but it was associated with morbidity, in bivariate analysis. Therefore it is included in the multiple logistic regression model of factors predictive of morbidity only

Table 3 Egypt and Nigeria PPH only: diagnoses and condition on entry (*n* = 854). Data are expressed as numbers with percentages in parentheses unless otherwise stated. The denominator is the entire population, unless otherwise noted. From Mourad-Youssif *et al.*, *Reprod Health* 2010;7:24, with permission

	Pre-intervention phase (n = 343)	*NASG-intervention phase (n = 511)*	*p Value*
*PPH Diagnoses**			
Uterine atony	197 (57.4)	324 (63.4)	0.079
Vaginal, cervical or genital lacerations	24 (7.0)	65 (12.7)	0.007
Retained placenta or tissue	69 (20.1)	80 (15.7)	0.092
Ruptured uterus	45 (13.1)	32 (6.3)	0.001
Placenta accrete	8 (2.3)	10 (2.0)	0.809†
Condition on study entry			
Where hemorrhage began			<0.001
Transferred in bleeding	145 (51.4)	104 (29.1)	
Began bleeding in hospital	137 (48.6)	253 (70.9)	
Estimated revealed blood loss at study entry‡			
Mean ml (SD)	1223.8 (509.5)	1288.7 (447.9)	—
Median ml (IQR)	1000 (1000–1500)	1000 (1000–1500)	0.008
Women with MAP <60 or non-palpable BP**	123 (35.9)	183 (35.9)	0.995

NASG, non-pneumatic anti-shock garment

Tests of significance of differences by study phase were χ^2 for categorical variables, *t* tests (assuming unequal variances) for normally distributed continuous variables and Wilcoxon rank-sum tests for continuous variables with non normal distributions

*PPH diagnosis includes primary or secondary diagnosis of any of the following >24 weeks with uterine atony, rupture, placenta accreta, vaginal/cervical lacerations, retained placenta or tissue

†Two-side Fisher's exact test used

‡Data missing for 37 patients

**MAP, mean arterial pressure <60 category includes those with non-palpable blood pressure (BP). Data missing for 1 patient

NASG and the combined outcome of mortality and severe morbidity. Findings suggested that severity of condition upon study admission was strongly associated with mortality after controlling for other variables in the model (MAP <60 mmHg had 19 times the odds of suffering the combined adverse outcomes variable (adjusted odds ratio (aOR) 19.1, 95% CI 6.95–52.65, *p* < 0.001). High parity and where bleeding began were not significantly associated with mortality/morbidity in the adjusted model. Importantly, being in the NASG phase remained significantly associated with reduced odds of adverse outcome (aOR 0.42, 95% CI 0.18–0.99, *p* = 0.046) (Table 4).

Ameliorating effect of NASG on delays in women with PPH and PAH

One post-hoc analysis examined the effects of delays on adverse outcomes in both phases for women with postabortion hemorrhage and PPH in Egypt and Nigeria[36]. This analysis was conducted to determine whether the NASG ameliorated effects of delays in transport to and treatment at hospitals and whether the NASG affected the timing of delivery of other interventions necessary for recovery. This analysis included 349 women from the facility in Cairo, 274 from Assiut, 57 from Southern Nigeria and 124 from Northern Nigeria and compared associations of delays with extreme adverse outcomes (EAO). The analysis showed that 20% of women in the pre-intervention phase who experienced a delay more than 60 minutes from the beginning of their hemorrhage to study admission experienced an adverse outcome compared to only 6% of those in the NASG-intervention phase

Table 4 Egypt and Nigeria PPH only: multiple logistic regression models of factors predictive of combined outcome severe maternal morbidity and mortality ($n = 639$). From Mourad-Youssif *et al.*, *Reprod Health* 2010;7:24, with permission

Factor	Dependent variable: combined severe morbidity and mortality		
	Adjusted OR	p Value	95% CI
Severity of shock			
MAP <60 mmHg (or non-palpable BP)	19.1	<0.001	6.95 52.65
MAP 60 mmHg or higher	1		
Parity			
5 or more live births	2.29	0.050	1.00 5.26
0–4 live births	1		
*Where bleeding began**			
Transferred in bleeding	1.88	0.222	0.68 5.15
Began bleeding in hospital	1		
Study phase			
NASG-intervention phase	0.42	0.046	0.18 0.99
Pre-intervention phase	1		

NASG, non-pneumatic anti-shock garment; MAP, mean arterial pressure; BP, blood pressure

Reference groups for categorical variables shown in italics. The number of observations in Table 4 is less than 854 because of missing data. Hospital facility was used as a control variable in the model but not shown in Table 4

$\chi^2 = 13.71$, $p = 0.000$), despite more women in the NASG-intervention phase experiencing in-hospital delays in receiving IV fluids and blood. The conclusion was drawn that use of the NASG reduces the adverse impact of delays, but that stabilization with the NASG does not replace treatment, and that delays in fluid/blood administration with the NASG must be avoided.

NASG for non-atonic etiologies: Egypt

Only one analysis from these pre-intervention phase/NASG-intervention phase studies on a variety of etiologies had different outcomes. This was an analysis of 434 non-atonic hemorrhage etiologies from the Egypt sites (226 pre-intervention phase and 208 NASG-intervention phase) with non-atonic etiologies, ectopic gestation, trophoblastic disease of pregnancy, placenta previa, accreta or abruption, ruptured uterus, or vaginal or cervical lacerations[37]. These etiologies comprised 44% of the 1442 women in the combined two-country database. Women were similar in age and parity, but more women in the NASG-intervention phase were in severe shock, (15.6% pre-intervention phase vs. 24.5% NASG-intervention phase had MAP less than 60 mmHg on study entry ($p = 0.020$)). Despite their worse condition on study entry, significantly fewer women in the NASG-intervention phase received 1500 ml or more fluid in the first study hour (93.4% pre-intervention vs. 64.9% NASG-intervention phase, $p < 0.0001$) and fewer received a blood transfusion in the first hour after study admission (96.5% pre-intervention vs. 86.5% NASG-intervention phase, $p < 0.0001$). Outcomes by phase were significantly lower only for measured blood loss, those in the

NASG-intervention phase having lost 257.7 ml during treatment, while those in the pre-intervention phase lost 370.4 ml ($p < 0.0001$). Other outcomes, mortality, morbidity and the combined EAO outcomes were not reduced for the NASG-intervention phase. In fact, mortality actually increased, from 0.4% (1/226) pre-intervention phase to 1.9% (4/208) in the NASG-intervention phase (RR for mortality 4.35, 95% CI 0.49–38.57). Possible explanations for these outcomes, which are different to the other outcomes of NASG analyses to date, might be the smaller sample size, rarity of adverse outcomes, the worse condition of the women on admission to the study, or the less timely use of resuscitation measures (IV fluids and blood). It cannot be determined from this analysis whether the NASG does not work as well for non-atonic etiologies; indeed, it would require a much larger study powered for these etiologies and in which treatment begin similarly in both phases.

Study limitations for all NASG comparative pre-intervention/intervention phase studies

All analyses conducted on the Nigeria and/or Egypt comparative data are limited by the study design. The effect of time and experience in managing women in hypovolemic shock could have worked in favor of the NASG phase, as it followed the pre-intervention phase. Selection bias, always present in a nonrandomized trial where not every patient in a facility is enrolled, could have also played a part. The participating hospitals were very busy and had limited staff; it is thus possible that not all patients who met study criteria were enrolled. There were also imbalances in the numbers of patients with different hemorrhage etiologies: more patients in the NASG phase[33,34] had uterine atony. Finally, NASG phase patients tended to enter the study in worse condition, yet received less timely and appropriate care. A possible explanation for this observation is that the rapid and visible effect of the NASG (blood loss slows down and vital signs return to normal) decreased panic among providers. If so, this must be prevented with better training and monitoring.

NASG qualitative studies

Berdichevsky and colleagues conducted a qualitative study to explore responses to the NASG in rural health facilities in Mexico[55]. The study included in-depth, semi-structured interviews with clinical and administrative staff ($n = 70$) involved in pilot studies of the NASG at primary health care facilities and rural hospitals. Researchers found that staff response to the garment fell into four categories: owning, doubting, resisting and rejecting. Overall, however, positive reactions were voiced regarding the garment as a relevant technology for saving women's lives. These findings may guide future implementation of the garment and other new technologies. In addition to the Berdichevsky study, three health sciences/public health students have conducted research on the NASG for master's theses in Nigeria and Zambia. These young authors documented challenges and opportunities for diffusion of innovation with the NASG[56,57].

NASG mechanisms of action studies

Studies have been conducted on the mechanisms of action of the NASG (see Chapter 39).

THE NASG HAS A UNIQUE ROLE IN HEMORRHAGE TREATMENT

Because the NASG plays a unique role in reversing shock, maintaining vital signs and keeping the heart, lung and brains perfused with oxygen, it can be used with all other maternal hemorrhage therapies. The NASG does not compete with other technologies, pharmacological or surgical, in obstetric hemorrhage and shock management. It is meant to be used with, not instead of other approaches. For example, for PPH, medical management with uterotonics is the first line of treatment and it is not suggested to use an NASG *instead* any uterotonic medication. Rather, if uterotonics fail to stop atonic hemorrhage, the NASG can be used with uterotonics to decrease blood loss. Furthermore, even if a woman with atonic hemorrhage stops bleeding, if she has lost so much blood that she is in shock, the NASG can be applied to reverse shock and stabilize the woman until she can have a blood transfusion. For other obstetric hemorrhage etiologies that do not respond to uterotonics (such as rupture, abruption, accreta), the NASG is the only technology to use while awaiting definitive therapy. Similarly the NASG can be used with balloon tamponade. The balloon tamponade can often be used as definitive therapy of atonic uterus, but its application does not reverse shock. Only the NASG reverses shock. Therefore, the two devices could be used together, the balloon to treat the cause of the bleeding and the NASG to reverse shock.

Summary of pre-intervention phase/NASG-intervention phase studies to date

Data from these pre-intervention phase/NASG-intervention phase studies are promising for use of NASG for most obstetric hemorrhage etiologies, including PPH care level. The Egypt pilot was adequately powered to demonstrate a statistically significant difference in measured blood loss for women suffering obstetric hemorrhage, with symptoms of hypovolemic shock treated with the NASG and a standardized hemorrhage and shock protocol compared with women with similar diagnoses and clinical symptoms treated only with the standardized hemorrhage protocols. The Nigeria and Egypt analyses, either alone or as a combined database, except for the one analysis of non-atonic hemorrhage etiologies in Egypt, demonstrate stronger evidence of effectiveness

at the tertiary level, although the study design has potential biases and is not as rigorous as a randomized control trial. The lack of statistical significant differences in the small, single country non-atonic hemorrhage etiology analysis certainly warrants more follow-up. Further, little is known about the efficacy, effectiveness and acceptability of the NASG at lower levels where women deliver at the community and at home; guidelines on obtaining the maximum efficacy of the garment have also yet to be established.

FUTURE DIRECTIONS

Randomized cluster trial of the NASG for transport from midwifery-led primary care centers to CEmOC facilities

In order to demonstrate that the NASG not only decreases blood loss, but also facilitates resuscitation from shock and decreases mortality and morbidity from PPH at the primary health care level, a much larger trial with a strong experimental design set at the community level is needed. An international collaborative between the University of California, San Francisco, the University of Zambia, University Teaching Hospital, Lusaka, and the University of Zimbabwe-University of California, San Francisco Reproductive Health Research Collaborative in Zimbabwe and the World Health Organization (Department of Reproductive Health and Research) is currently conducting such a trial in two sites in Zambia (Lusaka and the Copperbelt region) and one site in Zimbabwe (Harare): Clinicaltrials.gov: NCT00488462. This randomized cluster trial has been designed to demonstrate the efficacy of the NASG with a more rigorous research design, to investigate any potential side-effects associated with its use, and importantly, to determine whether the NASG provides even greater effect when implemented at a lower-level in the health system. Initiated in 2007, the research is in the final stage in which clinics in each cluster have been randomized, with half of the clinics using the NASG for immediate first-aid and transport and the other half providing the control cases. Control women will receive the NASG when they arrive at the referral facility. Further, the sample should be large enough that when looking at different etiologies, for example, the non-atonic etiologies, there may be enough power to see differences in outcomes if they exist. Significant differences in outcomes may lead to the inclusion of the NASG onto the World Health Organizations list of essential devices, which would enable bilateral and multilateral organizations to invest in the NASG and scale up its implementation. In 2012, FIGO published guidelines for PPH management and included the NASG as a 'potentially life-saving procedure' to be considered if uterotonic treatment fails[58]. In March 2012, when WHO convened a panel of experts to update their guidelines on PPH, they recommended the use of NASGs 'as temporizing measures until substantive care is available'[59].

Manufacture

A frequently raised issue about the NASG is its cost and sole manufacturing source. Until 2011, the NASG was only produced by Zoex, and only distributed by Stork Medical Company (URL: storkmedical.com). Stork sells three sizes of NASG: small, medium and large.

Having a sole manufacturer makes it difficult to procure for those countries that require competitive bids from more than one source. Further, the cost (US$295.00) may also be too high for some extremely low resource settings.

To reduce costs, a team at PATH established a package of quality standards, engineering documents and quality inspection procedures, and identified a list of potential manufacturers in India and China. PATH met with prospective manufacturers and, using a quantitative assessment tool, negotiated affordable pricing with a manufacturer in China for the large size garment and a manufacturer in India for the small size garment. PATH worked with the Chinese and Indian manufacturers to source raw materials and manufacture a pre-production batch of NASG garments. Verification testing was performed on the pre-production batch to establish that all performance and quality requirements were met prior to commercial distribution. Procurement, distribution and access remain a challenge, so PATH is working with third parties and governments to facilitate the availability and accessibility of the NASG to mothers everywhere (personal communication with Rick Kearns, PATH).

As of May, 2012, Maternova, a global marketplace for ideas and technologies for mothers and newborns (www.maternova.net), serves as an online distributor for the Chinese made NASG.

Understanding mechanisms of action and physiological effects

Further research is also required to examine the mechanisms of action of the NASG to establish a direct way to measure intra-abdominal pressure, gauge the ideal amount of pressure that should be exerted and thus provide guidelines for obtaining optimal effect (see Chapter 39).

NASG for use in developed countries

The possibility of exploring potential uses of the NASG in countries with well developed health care also exists. The US and the UK, for example, presently are seeing increased rates of placenta accreta, presumably as a result of scar tissue from prior cesarean section[60]. Some facilities in California, USA, keep NASGs in their labor suites[47]; as such, the NASG could be used to reduce blood loss and stabilize these patients for surgery if required. The NASG could also be used for women with complications in rural communities ill equipped to deal with complications; patients from such locations normally experience lengthy transport time to urban tertiary care facilities. Another potential use could be for women awaiting specialized equipment and expertise for uterine artery embolization, which might save them from having a hysterectomy. Finally, for women who refuse blood transfusions despite massive hemorrhage, such as Jehovah's Witnesses, the NASG might also provide benefit. Outcomes in terms of cost (number of transfusions, IVs, number of days in hospital or ICU for example) should be examined also to see whether the NASG can prove a cost-effective intervention in developed countries.

The NASG is lightweight, reusable, relatively inexpensive and can be used at the lowest level of the health care system; it has the potential to make a great contribution to reducing maternal mortality and morbidity from obstetric hemorrhage and hypovolemic shock if it proves efficacious in clinical trials.

PRACTICE POINTS

- The PASG for pre-hospital treatment of lower body trauma in high-resource urban settings fell out of use due to lack of difference or negative outcomes in randomized controlled trials; in contrast, the NASG shows promise for obstetric hemorrhage first aid in low-resource settings

- Application of the NASG could be part of a standardized hemorrhage and shock management algorithm; the timing of NASG application in the algorithm depends on patient acuity, level of staff available, level of health care facility level and the capacity for definitive treatment

- The NASG is segmented; it is applied sequentially on a woman in hypovolemic shock starting at the ankle segment and is removed in the same sequence. Removal should not be initiated until the woman has been hemodynamically stable for at least 2 hours. Removal is then performed incrementally every 15 minutes; vital signs must remain stable throughout removal or the NASG should be replaced and the source of bleeding re-examined

- Results from comparative pre-intervention phase/ NASG-intervention phase trials in tertiary facilities in Egypt and Nigeria show the NASG may significantly reduce rates of hysterectomy for intractable uterine atony, and decrease morbidity, mortality, and decrease further blood loss for many obstetric hemorrhage etiologies

- A strong experimental design trial set at the community/primary health care level is necessary to determine whether the NASG will be effective in reducing maternal mortality and morbidity.

References

1. ICM/FIGO. Joint Statement: Prevention and Treatment of Post-partum Haemorrhage. New Advances for Low

Resource Settings. 2006 www.figo.org/files/figo-corp/docs/PPH Joint Statement 2 English.pdf

2. Tsu VD, Coffey PS. New and underutilised technologies to reduce maternal mortality and morbidity: what progress have we made since Bellagio 2003? BJOG 2009;116:247–56

3. Hensleigh PA. Anti-shock garment provides resuscitation and haemostasis for obstetric haemorrhage. BJOG 2002;109: 1377–84

4. Tsu VD, Langer A, Aldrich T. Postpartum hemorrhage in developing countries: is the public health community using the right tools? Int J Gynaecol Obstet 2004;85(Suppl 1): S42–51

5. Lalonde A, Daviss BA, Acosta A, Herschderfer K. Postpartum hemorrhage today: ICM/FIGO initiative 2004–2006. Int J Gynaecol Obstet 2006;94:243–53

6. Pathfinder International. Continuum of Care: Addressing Postpartum Hemorrhage in India, Nigeria, Bangladesh, Peru and Tanzania. Watertown, MA, USA 2010 www.pathfind.org/site/PageServer?pagename=Major_Projects_Continuum_of_Care www.pathfind.org/site/PageServer?pagename=Major_Projects_Continuum_of_Care.

7. Geller SE, Adams MG, Miller S. A continuum of care model for postpartum hemorrhage. Int J Fertil Womens Med 2007; 52:97–105

8. Kerr N, Dresang LT. Does the non-pneumatic anti-shock garment (NASG) have a role in the management of postpartum hemorrhage? Evidence-Based Practice, Family Physicians Inquiries Network, Inc. 2010;13:6

9. McSwain NE Jr. Pneumatic anti-shock garment: state of the art 1988. Ann Emerg Med 1988;17:506–25

10. Pelligra R, Sandberg EC. Control of intractable abdominal bleeding by external counterpressure. JAMA 1979;241: 708–13

11. Andrae B, Eriksson LG, Skoog G. Anti-shock trousers (MAST) and transcatheter embolization in the management of massive obstetrics hemorrhage. A report of two cases. Acta Obstet Gynecol Scand 1999;78:740–1

12. Life Medical Supplier. Trauma Air Pants. 2010 www.lifemedicalsupplier.com/immobilization-extrication-trauma-air-pants-c-16_131.html

13. McSwain MJ, McSwain N.E. Pneumatic antishock garment: state of the art at the turn of the century. Trauma 2000;2: 63–75

14. Ali J, Duke K. Pneumatic antishock garment decreases hemorrhage and mortality from splenic injury. Can J Surg 1991; 34:496–501

15. Gardner WJ. Hemostasis by pneumatic compression. Am Surg 1969;35:635–7

16. Schwab CW, Gore D. MAST: medical antishock trousers. Surg Ann 1983;15:41–59

17. Bickell WH, Pepe PE, Bailey ML, Wyatt CH, Mattox KL. Randomized trial of pneumatic antishock garments in the prehospital management of penetrating abdominal injuries. Ann Emerg Med 1987;16:653–8

18. Mattox KL, Bickell W, Pepe PE, Burch J, Feliciano D. Prospective MAST study in 911 patients. J Trauma 1989;29: 1104–11; discussion 11–2

19. Chang FC, Harrison PB, Beech RR, Helmer SD. PASG: does it help in the management of traumatic shock? J Trauma 1995;39:453–6

20. Johnson M, Bruce D, Gilbertson J, Murkowski F. Alaska EMS Goals: A Guide for Developing Alaska's Emergency Medical Services System. Juneau: Alaska Department of Health and Social Services – Section of Community Health & Emergency Medical Services, 2003

21. Stoy W. Mosby's Emt-Basic Textbook: C.V. Mosby, 1995

22. Domeier RM, O'Connor RE, Delbridge TR, Hunt RC. Use of the pneumatic anti-shock garment (PASG). National Association of EMS Physicians. Prehosp Emerg Care 1997, reaffirmed 2002;1:32–5

23. Hauswald M, Greene ER. Regional blood flow after pneumatic anti-shock garment inflation. Prehosp Emerg Care 2003;7:225–8

24. Quinot J, Cantais E, Kaiser E. Le pantalon antichoc: A-ti-il reelement une place dans le traitement du choc? Med d'urgence 2001:119–26

25. Haggerty J. Anti Shock Garment. National Aeronautical Space Administration, Office of Space Access and Technology, Commercial Development and Technology Transfer Division, 1996; http://www.sti.nasa.gov/tto/spinoff1996/28.html

26. Pelligra R. Non-pneumatic antishock garment use. Emergency 1994;26:53–6

27. Brees C, Hensleigh PA, Miller S, Pelligra R. A non-inflatable anti-shock garment for obstetric hemorrhage. Int J Gynaecol Obstet 2004;87:119–24

28. Miller S, Turan J, Dau K, et al. Use of the non-pneumatic anti-shock garment (NASG) to reduce blood loss and time to recovery from shock for women with obstetric haemorrhage in Egypt. Global Public Health 2007;2:110–24

29. Miller S, Turan JM, Ojengbede A, et al. The pilot study of the non-pneumatic anti-shock garment (NASG) in women with severe obstetric hemorrhage: Combined results from Egypt and Nigeria. Int J Gynecol Obstet 2006;94(Suppl 2): S154–S6

30. Miller S, Hamza S, Bray E, Gipson R, Nada K, Fathalla MF, et al. First Aid for Obstetrical Haemorrhage: The Pilot Study of the Non-pneumatic Anti-Shock Garment (NASG) in Egypt. BJOG 2006;113:424–9

31. Miller S, Ojengbede O, Turan JM, Morhason-Bello IO, Martin HB, Nsima D. A comparative study of the non-pneumatic anti-shock garment for the treatment of obstetric hemorrhage in Nigeria. Int J Gynaecol Obstet 2009;107: 121–5

32. Miller S, Fathalla MM, Youssif MM, et al. A comparative study of the non-pneumatic anti-shock garment for the treatment of obstetric hemorrhage in Egypt. Int J Gynaecol Obstet 2010;109:20–4

33. Mourad-Youssif M, Ojengbede OA, Meyer CD, et al. Can the Non-pneumatic Anti-Shock Garment (NASG) reduce adverse maternal outcomes from postpartum hemorrhage? Evidence from Egypt and Nigeria. Reprod Health 2010;7: 24

34. Miller S, Fathalla M, Ogengbede O, et al. Obstetric hemorrhage and shock management: using the low technology non-pneumatic anti-shock garment in Nigerian and Egyptian tertiary care facilities. BMC Pregnancy Childbirth 2010;10:64

35. Ojengbede OA, Morhason-Bello IO, Galadanci H, et al. Assessing the role of the non-pneumatic anti-shock garment (NASG) in reducing mortality from postpartum hemorrhage in Nigeria. Gynecol Obstet Invest 2011;71:66–72

36. Turan J, Ojengbede O, Fathalla M, et al. Positive effects of the non-pneumatic anti-shock garment on delays in accessing care for postpartum and postabortion hemorrhage in Egypt and Nigeria. J Womens Health 2011;20:91–8

37. Fathalla MF, Mourad Youssif MM, Meyer C, et al. Nonatonic obstetric haemorrhage: effectiveness of the non-pneumatic anti-shock garment in Egypt. ISRN Obstet Gynecol 2011;2011:179349

38. ACOG. Educational Bulletin #243: Postpartum Hemorrhage. Washington, DC: American College of Obstetricians and Gynecologists, 1998

39. Johansson PI, Ostrowski SR, Secher NH. Management of major blood loss: an update. Acta Anaesthesiol Scand 2010; 54:1039–49

40. Harbrecht BG, Alarcon LH, Peitzman AB. Management of Shock. In: Moore EE, Feliciano DV, Mattox KL, eds. Trauma, 5th edn. New York, Chicago, San Francisco: McGraw - Hill Med Publ Div, 2004:220–5

41. Pepe PE, Eckstein M. Reappraising the prehospital care of the patient with major trauma. Emerg Med Clin North Am 1998;16:1–15

42. Jacobs LM. Timing of fluid resuscitation in trauma. N Engl J Med 1994;331:1153–4

43. Capone AC, Safar P, Stezoski W, Tisherman S, Peitzman AB. Improved outcome with fluid restriction in treatment of

uncontrolled hemorrhagic shock. J Am Coll Surg 1995;180: 49–56

44. Soucy DM, Rude M, Hsia WC, Hagedorn FN, Illner H, Shires GT. The effects of varying fluid volume and rate of resuscitation during uncontrolled hemorrhage. J Trauma 1999;46:209–15

45. Li T, Zhu Y, Hu Y, et al. Ideal permissive hypotension to resuscitate uncontrolled hemorrhagic shock and the tolerance time in rats. Anesthesiology 2011;114:111–9

46. Marietta M, Pedrazzi P, Girardis M, Busani S, Torelli G. Posttraumatic massive bleeding: a challenging multidisciplinary task. Intern Emerg Med. 2010;5:521–31

47. El-Sayed Y, Brodzinsky L, Collins J, Munro I, Helmer A, Miller S, editors. Incorporation of the Non-Pneumatic Anti-Shock Garment (NASG) in the Management of Postpartum Haemorrhage and Shock at a Tertiary Level Hospital. International Federation of Gynecology and Obstetrics (FIGO) World Congress; 2006 November 5–10; Kuala Lumpur.

48. Miller S, Lester F, Hensleigh P. Prevention and treatment of postpartum hemorrhage: new advances for low-resource settings. J Midwifery Womens Health 2004;49:283–92

49. Patel A, Goudar SS, Geller SE, et al. Drape estimation vs. visual assessment for estimating postpartum hemorrhage. Int J Gynaecol Obstet 2006;93:220–4

50. Mantel GD, Buchmann E, Rees H, Pattinson RC. Severe acute maternal morbidity: a pilot study of a definition for a near-miss. Br J Obstet Gynaecol 1998;105:985–90

51. Bickell WH, Wall MJ Jr, Pepe PE, et al. Immediate versus delayed fluid resuscitation for hypotensive patients with penetrating torso injuries. N Engl J Med 1994;331:1105–9

52. Pope A, French G, Longnecker D. Fluid resuscitation. State of the science for treating combat casualties and civilian injuries. Washington, DC: National Academy Press, 1999

53. Morris J, Meyer C, Fathalla M, et al. Treating uterine atony with the NASG in Egypt. African J Midwifery Womens Health 2011;5:37–42

54. Ojengbede O, Galadanci H, Morhason-Bello I, et al. The non-pneumatic anti-shock garment for postpartum haemorrhage in Nigeria. African J Midwifery Women's Health 2011; 5:135–9

55. Berdichevsky K, Tucker C, MartÃnez A, Miller S. Acceptance of a new technology for management of obstetric hemorrhage: a qualitative study from rural Mexico. Health Care Women Int 2010;31:444–57

56. Oshinowo A, Galadanci H, Awwal M, et al., eds. Overcoming Delays in Childbirth due to Hemorrhage: A Qualitative Study of the Non-pneumatic Anti-Shock Garment (NASG) in Nigeria. American Publich Health Association (APHA) 135th Annual Meeting and Exposition, November 3–7; 2007; Washington, DC

57. Liu L. A mixed methods study of the implementation of two interventions to reduce maternal mortality in Ibadan, Oyo state, Nigeria. [dissertation for MIPH degree].2009

58. FIGO Safe Motherhood and Newborn Health Committee. FIGO Guidelines: Prevention and Treatment of Postpartum Hemorrhage in Low Resource Settings. IJGO 2012;117: 108-18

59. Souza JP. WHO Guidelines for Prevention and Treatment of PPH. 2012 http://www.scribd.com/doc/92342526/Souza-New-WHO-PPH-Guidelines

60. Miller DA, Chollet JA, Goodwin TM. Clinical risk factors for placenta previa-placenta accreta. Am J Obstet Gynecol 1997; 177:210–4

39

The Mechanisms of Action of the Non-Pneumatic Anti-Shock Garment

A. L. Stenson, S. Miller and F. Lester

INTRODUCTION

Globally, severe obstetric hemorrhage is the leading cause of maternal death, largely due to delays in accessing life-saving services such as surgery or blood transfusion[1-4]. Effective, reliable means of stabilizing patients during delays in obtaining effective treatment would save many mothers' lives. This simplistic statement represents the premise underlying the use of the non-pneumatic anti-shock garment (NASG) in low resource settings. Preintervention phase/NASG phase studies in tertiary care facilities in Egypt and Nigeria have shown a 50% reduction in measured blood loss from a median of 400 ml to 200 ml (p <0.0001); at the same time, mortality was reduced from 9% to 3.1% (RR 0.35, 95% CI 0.19–0.62)[5]. For details of clinical trials evaluating the NASG see Chapter 38. In this chapter, we discuss the mechanisms of action underlying the NASG, both what is known and the deficiencies where additional research is needed.

The NASG is an articulated neoprene and Velcro® first-aid compression device designed to reverse shock by shunting blood from the lower extremities and pelvis to the vital organs[6,7]. The NASG is comprised of five articulated segments; the abdominal segment contains a foam ball for extra compression on the abdomen (Figure 1). It is *assumed* that the NASG increases circulating blood volume by compressing (and thus depleting) venous reservoirs in the abdomen and legs, and it is further *hypothesized* that blood flow in the pelvis and lower abdomen is diminished by the uterine compression ball. The NASG has had FDA 510K certification for over 20 years; however, until recently few studies evaluating the mechanisms underlying device effectiveness have been published. The work presented in this chapter is preliminary and far from complete, but it represents a thorough discussion of the ongoing efforts at obtaining a better understanding of how the NASG affects human physiology, particularly that of the pregnant/postpartum woman.

HISTORY OF ANTI-SHOCK GARMENTS

The use of anti-shock garments dates back to the early 1900s, when Dr George Crile created the first pneumatic suit to sustain blood pressure, decrease bleeding and increase peripheral resistance[7]. In 1942, this was modified into what became the anti-Gravity suit, or G-suit, for the Army Air Corps in order to prevent syncope during rapid ascent[7]. During the Vietnam War, this same G-suit was used to stabilize patients suffering from shock and was modified from a full-body suit to a half-suit. As such, it became known as the Military/Medical® Anti-Shock Trousers (MAST suit) or pneumatic anti-shock garment (PASG)[8,9]. Based on reported success in the field, this device was used more widely for emergency medicine and trauma patients in the 1970s[10,11]. Recommendations for use of the garment and limited supportive anecdotal reports continued into the 1980s; however, by the late 1980s and into the 1990s several published studies raised questions regarding the efficacy and safety of the PASG[12-16]. A Cochrane database review in 2000 failed to find sufficient evidence to support the continued use of the garment, based in part on the increased mortality seen in patients with penetrating thoracic injuries[17]. Further, reports were published of side-effects, including compartment syndrome and ischemia, from over inflation[12-16,18-21].

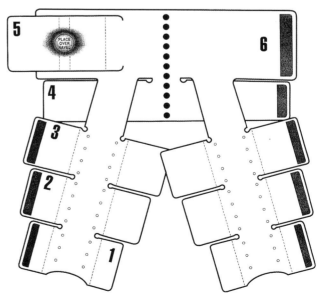

Figure 1 Schematic diagram of the non-pneumatic anti-shock garment

Despite these less than salutary findings when used in the area of general trauma, the PASG gained recognition as a possible first aid device for obstetric hemorrhage based on several case reports documenting favorable outcomes in cases of severe hemorrhage and shock[22]. Because obstetric hemorrhage results from blood loss from vessels that are branches of the internal iliac arteries (and ultimately the aorta), these findings are consistent with the thinking that the PASG has differential effectiveness depending on whether blood loss is from injuries below the waist or above[22]. The favorable findings of these case reports were further supported by studies of the hemodynamic impact of the PASG showing a significant decrease in aortic blood flow below the level of the renal arteries, suggesting that the device would be particularly useful for stemming uterine blood flow which is supplied by the internal iliac artery[23,24].

The NASG was adapted from the PASG by a team at the National Aeronautics and Space Administration (NASA). It was commercialized and is currently manufactured as the Non-Inflatable Anti-Shock Garment™ (ZOEX, Coloma, CA, USA). The first published report on NASG use for obstetric hemorrhage was a case series with six women in hypovolemic shock in Pakistan[25]. The NASG has now been evaluated in comparative trials in Egypt[26,27] and Nigeria[5,28], and qualitative studies have been conducted in Mexico[29] and Nigeria[30,31]. An ongoing randomized clinical trial is being conducted in Zambia and Zimbabwe, with results expected in 2013. For details of the clinical trials see Chapter 38.

ANATOMY AND PHYSIOLOGY

Cardiovascular physiology of hypovolemic shock

Shock is a physiological state characterized by a decrease in tissue perfusion resulting in insufficient delivery of oxygen to the tissues. Deprivation of oxygen at the cellular level leads to a derangement of biochemical processes that result in systemic effects[32]. At the cellular level, the cell membrane ion pump begins to fail, leading to intracellular edema, leakage of intracellular contents into the extracellular space and changes in intracellular pH[33]. These cellular changes then lead to alterations in the serum pH, endothelial dysfunction and the stimulation of inflammatory and anti-inflammatory cascades. If the tissue oxygen deprivation continues, the result is cellular death, end-organ damage, multisystem failure and ultimate demise[34].

Tissue perfusion is determined by cardiac output (stroke volume x heart rate) and systemic vascular resistance. Stroke volume is related to preload, myocardial contractility and afterload, while systemic vascular resistance is determined by vessel length and diameter and blood viscosity. Hypovolemic shock is a consequence of decreased preload due to intravascular volume loss, which in the case of obstetric hemorrhage results from severe uterine blood loss. The decrease in blood volume (decreased preload) results in a diminished cardiac output, while the systemic vascular resistance increases initially to compensate and maintain perfusion.

Shock progresses along a physiological continuum that begins with preshock when the patient is compensating for the blood loss through increased heart rate, peripheral vasoconstriction and minimal changes to systemic vascular resistance[35]. As the situation progresses, however, the compensatory mechanisms become overwhelmed, and the patient experiences tachycardia, dyspnea, restlessness, metabolic acidosis and oliguria. If shock continues to progress, organ damage may become irreversible with renal failure, acidemia and severe alterations in cellular metabolism. At this stage, the patient may rapidly evolve from an agitated to an obtunded and, finally, to a comatose state. It is therefore axiomatic that early identification of hypovolemic shock with cessation of bleeding, replacement of intravascular volume and supportive measures (such as oxygen supplementation) are critical to preventing end-organ damage and death.

Anatomy of blood flow to the pelvis

The descending aorta bifurcates into the right and left common iliac arteries at the level of the fourth lumbar vertebrae. The common iliac then divides into the internal (sometimes called the hypogastric) and external iliac arteries. The external iliac artery provides the blood supply primarily to the lower extremities as the femoral arteries, while the internal iliac supplies the walls and internal organs of the pelvis, the gluteal muscles and the medial compartment of the thigh. The uterine blood supply is derived primarily from the uterine artery, which is a branch of the internal iliac artery. About 15–20% of the uterine blood supply comes from the ovarian artery, which branches directly from the aorta just below the renal arteries. The uterine artery anastomoses the ovarian artery superiorly and the vaginal artery inferiorly also supplying a portion of the blood to the ovary and vagina, respectively. In hypovolemic shock due to uterine atony, if uterotonics and tamponade (either balloon or manual) (see chapters in Section 8) fail to control hemorrhage, the next step generally involves surgical intervention for vessel ligation (uterine, ovarian or internal iliac) or to place uterine compression sutures (B–Lynch or one of its modifications see Chapter 51). The O'Leary stitch is performed by ligating the ascending branch of the uterine artery; in contrast, the internal iliac artery ligation involves placing a stitch just after the posterior division has branched off (see Chapters 52 and 53). Both result in cessation of blood flow and a cessation of the arterial pulse pressure beyond the point of ligation.

Urban et al. have evaluated blood flow to the uterus during labor and delivery using Multigate spectral Doppler analysis and have demonstrated that uterine contractions following delivery result in absent flow in the arcuate artery (Chapter 12).

THEORETICAL MODEL OF NON-PNEUMATIC ANTI-SHOCK GARMENT FUNCTION

At least two main theoretical mechanisms of action underlie the effectiveness of the NASG. The first involves the shunting of blood from the lower extremities and pelvis back to the central circulation in order to improve perfusion of vital organs. The second involves the pressure exerted by the abdominal compression ball onto the uterus and surrounding vasculature in order to decrease blood flow to the pelvis and diminish uterine blood loss. A model of these proposed mechanisms of action is shown in Figure 2.

Physical laws

Circumferential compression of the abdomen and lower extremities, leading to a reduction in total vascular volume, is thought to be the main mechanism accounting for ASG efficacy[15,27]. Preload, peripheral resistance and cardiac output are increased as a result of the expansion of the central circulation. Three laws of physics underlie these changes. First, Poiseuille's law ($F = (P1 - P2) R^4/8NL$) states that the flow rate (F) through a blood vessel is related to the vessel's radius (R) to the 4th power, the length of the vessel (L) and to viscosity (N), where P1 is the entrance pressure and P2 is the exit pressure. Therefore, reduction in the vessel radius should lead to exponential reductions in blood flow. Second, Laplace's law ($T = PR$) relates the tension (T) across a blood vessel to the vessel radius (R) and the transmural pressure (P). External pressure exerted on the lower body by the ASG reduces the transmural pressure and the radius of the vessel, thereby reducing both tension and blood flow. Finally, Bernoulli's principle [$Q = (AP + 2V)/E$] describes how the rate of bleeding (Q) depends on the area of the torn vessel wall (A) and the transmural pressure (P), where E is the density of blood and V is the velocity of blood flow (Figure 3). External pressure from the ASG compresses vessels, leading to diminished vascular volume in the compressed area, an exponential decrease in flow and, ultimately, reduced blood loss[15,27].

PHYSIOLOGIC STUDIES OF THE PNEUMATIC ANTI-SHOCK GARMENT

Animal studies

Several animal studies have demonstrated decreased bleeding, increased systolic blood pressure and improved survival after placement of a PASG/sleeve. The first study, a case series using eight dogs treated with a pneumatic abdominal sleeve after having had their intra–abdominal aorta transected, had a sustained mean systolic blood pressure of 74 mmHg. After removal, six of eight dogs died within 5 minutes, but two dogs survived 30 and 40 minutes and showed sealing of the aortic incision[36]. Subsequently, in 1969 a comparative study was performed using 16 dogs (eight controls, eight PASG) that had undergone lacerations

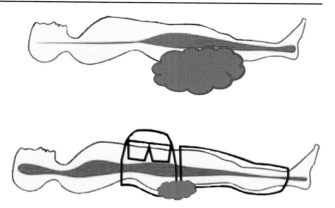

Figure 2 The NASG reverses the effects of shock by decreasing the container of the circulatory system as it compresses the lower extremities and abdomen. This increases the circulating volume in the uncompressed upper body. Thus, there is more blood circulating to the brain, heart and lungs, elevating blood pressure and increasing preload and cardiac output. Further, the circumferential pressure of the tight neoprene and the additional pressure exerted by the abdominal compression ball decreases the radius of the blood vessels in the pelvis; decreasing blood flow and reducing uterine blood loss

Poiseuille's Law
$F = (P1-P2) R^4/8N*L$
F, flow; P1, entrance pressure; P2, exit pressure; R, radius; N, viscosity; L, length
Laplace's Law
$T = P*R$
T, tension inside blood vessel; P, transmural pressure; R, vessel radius
Bernoulli's Principle
$Q= (A*P + 2V)/E$
Q, rate of leakage; A, area of laceration/tear/opening; P, transmural pressure; E, density of blood; V, speed or velocity of blood flow

Figure 3 Laws and principles governing the mechanisms of action underlying ASGs

of the iliac artery. All controls died within minutes; however, the dogs with the PASG survived until it was deflated, after which 75% expired within 5 minutes[37].

Subsequently, another group of researchers studied 30 rats with lethal hepatic and vena caval injury. Animals were allocated as follows: five controls, five with PASG alone, ten with saline infusion alone and ten with PASG and saline infusion. The PASG group demonstrated improved median survival compared to controls (120 min vs. 10 min). The group that received saline infusion alone showed no survival improvement, and fulminant pulmonary edema developed in 90% of the rats that received both the PASG and saline[38].

In a study of 12 dogs (six controls, six PASG) with splenic crush injuries, the PASG group effectively sustained systolic blood pressure after 1 hour (100 mmHg vs. 0 mmHg in controls), survived twice as long as controls (2 h vs. <1 h) and bled significantly less (1.6 ml/min vs. 9.4 ml/min)[39].

The effect of the PASG on the cerebral function of 29 rats with severe hepatic injury was examined in another murine study. The PASG prolonged the time before the EEG amplitude began to decrease, the time during which a sensory response could be observed and increased survival time[40].

The hemodynamic effect of the PASG was studied using 20 anesthetized dogs (10 controls and 10 PASG) with hemorrhagic hypotension[41]. Carotid artery blood flow increased by 50% and femoral artery decreased tenfold in the PASG group; this was accompanied by a transient increase in cardiac output (2.4 l/min to 2.7 l/min; $p < 0.05$), which later fell to 1.9 l/min. The authors concluded that an initial increase in cardiac output due to compression of the venous system was followed by an emptying of the blood into the central circulation; however, this combination of events later led to a reduction of cardiac output due to further venous compression and an increase in afterload, without an increase in preload.

Subsequently, using three groups of piglets, it was shown that with a small (2.5 mm) injury to the descending aorta, hemorrhage and mortality were increased with the PASG[42]. In group 1, the animals did not have the garment applied and 100% survived; the hemorrhage rate was 22.5 ml/min, and bleeding stopped after 18–24 min. In group 2, a PASG was inflated to maintain 15 torr below the piglet's normal baseline carotid artery pressure; in this group, survival was 50% and the animals bled at a rate of 32.5 ml/min, stopping after 26–35 min. In the third group, the PASG was inflated to maintain the normal baseline pressure of the carotid artery. The pigs bled at 107.5 ml/min and none survived, with expiration after 10–18 min being the norm. This finding led the authors to conclude that with thoracic injury, PASG inflation increases mortality and hemorrhage. Their conclusion is not surprising given the discussion presented above showing that its use is more effective when the source of the blood loss was lower in the trunk.

In summary, animal studies of the PASG to date have demonstrated significantly deceased bleeding and increased survival time after aortic or internal iliac laceration, and lethal hepatic or vena cava injury; however, when injuries occurred in the thoracic region, the PASG resulted in increased mortality. The PASG has been shown in animal studies to decrease femoral artery blood flow (10 times), increase carotid artery blood flow (50%) and transiently increase cardiac output as well as improve cerebral function.

Human studies

The hemodynamic effects of PASGs have been examined in several human studies. In 1981, Gaffney *et al.* demonstrated with 10 healthy normovolemic male patients who were not bleeding placed in the supine position that the PASG raised blood pressure and increased peripheral resistance but slightly decreased cardiac output and stroke volume[43]. When these patients were examined with a 60-degree head up tilt (which leads to venous pooling in the lower extremities and more closely approximates hypovolemia), PASG application induced a 30% increase in cardiac output, a 52% increase in stroke volume and a 40% increase in total peripheral resistance.

Two dimensional echo was used to evaluate the effect of the PASG on end diastolic volume, stroke volume, cardiac output and blood pressure in eight supine healthy non-bleeding males using two different inflation protocols (50 and 100 mmHg)[44]. Both protocols resulted in a rise in end diastolic volume and blood pressure. In the 50 mmHg protocol, the stroke volume and end diastolic volume decreased over time, whereas with the 100 mmHg protocol, the cardiac output was increased and maintained, likely through the mechanism of increased peripheral resistance. A second study by the same research group reported that the optimal inflation sequence to produce the greatest increase in end diastolic volume, stroke volume and cardiac output was to inflate the legs simultaneously, followed by the abdominal segment[45].

The effects of different pressure levels (2, 4 and 6 psi) on 10 healthy male volunteers in supine and standing position were also investigated[46]. Again, while supine, the men experienced increased blood pressure with all three pressures, but cardiac output and end diastolic volume did not increase. In the standing protocol, however, mean arterial pressure, end diastolic volume, stroke volume and cardiac output rose at all three inflation pressures ($p < 0.05$). This observation suggests that increases in blood pressure are caused by increased cardiac preload and cardiac output in the standing position, which more closely approximates hypovolemia, and suggests utility of using the PASG for hypovolemic patients. This study further demonstrated that the effects of the PASG differ depending on the amount of pressure applied/ level of inflation.

More recently, the effect of the PASG inflated to 90 mmHg was studied in 10 healthy adults[23]. Cardiac output and blood flow in several major arteries including the left carotid, left subclavian, superior mesenteric, left renal and distal aorta were measured. The authors demonstrated no change in cardiac output (5.45 vs. 5.83 l/min; $p = 0.26$), or left subclavian or left carotid blood flow, whereas aortic blood flow distal to the renal artery was markedly decreased in all subjects (1.01 vs. 0.11 l/min, $p < 0.001$). The authors concluded that the PASG has a dramatic effect on aortic blood flow distal to the renal arteries, but does not significantly affect flow above that point, and suggested that the garment may result in decrease in bleeding from injuries distal to this point (iliac, pelvic and lower extremity vessels) (Figure 4).

A subsequent case documenting use of the PASG in a woman with pelvic trauma supports the findings of the study reported above[24]. The patient presented in a severe state of shock with a Glasgow coma scale of 6, systolic blood pressure of 60 mmHg and pulse of 80 beats/min with suspicion of pneumothorax. The PASG was inflated to a pressure of 60 mmHg in the extremities and 50 mmHg abdominally. After placement, blood pressure rose to 72 mmHg and her pulse became 121 bpm. The patient then was taken to angiography for possible embolization. The PASG was deflated to place the embolization catheters, and the internal iliac artery visualized. Once the abdominal segment of the PASG was re-inflated the internal iliac was no longer visualized on angiography, and blood flow through the vessel had effectively stopped. The patient then received embolization to control the hemorrhage permanently, along with multiple blood products to correct her deficiencies[24].

The studies of the PASG in human subjects to date have documented increased blood pressure, but have found mixed results on the effect of the PASG on cardiac output, stroke volume and end diastolic volume. These parameters appear to vary with inflation pressure and/or patient position (supine versus standing or 60-degree head tilt). The PASG significantly decreases blood flow in the distal aorta.

External aortic compression device

An external abdominal compression device, made of a strong metal spring that is cylindrical in shape and covered with leather, also has been studied for use in PPH[47,48] (Figure 5). The device is set to exert 103.5 mmHg/cm^2 and is placed just above the compressed fundus over the umbilicus with the objective of compressing the distal aorta. Use of this compression device reduces the time to cessation of bleeding (36.8 vs. 118.6 min; $p < 0.001$), the number of blood transfusions (200 vs. 302 units) and the amount of uterotonics used ($p < 0.001$)[47]. The investigators also studied femoral artery blood flow using Doppler velocimetry analysis with the device in place, showing that flow to the lower extremities is reduced, but remains sufficient to maintain tissue perfusion[48].

PHYSIOLOGIC STUDIES OF NON-PNEUMATIC ANTI-SHOCK GARMENT

For each of the studies described below, IRB approval was obtained from the University of California, Los Angeles, and/or the University of California, San Francisco and all participants/volunteers underwent an informed consent process.

Measured blood loss

Data from the NASG clinical trials conducted in Egypt and Nigeria demonstrated a significantly diminished blood loss (50%) with application of the NASG in pre-intervention phase/NASG intervention phase studies ($p < 0.0001$)[5]. A further analysis of Egyptian women with uterine atony revealed that even

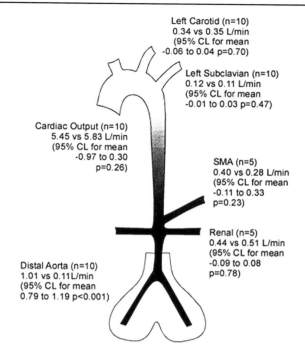

Figure 4 A diagram of blood flow before and after ASG inflation. CL, confidence limit; SMA, superior mesenteric artery. From Hauswald M, Greene R. Regional blood flow after pneumatic anti-shock garment inflation. *Prehospital Emergency Care* 2003;7: 225–8, with permission

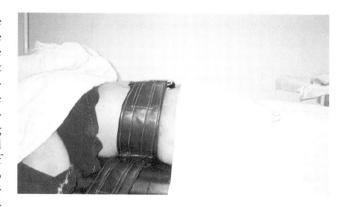

Figure 5 External aortic compression device. From Soltan *et al.* Assessing changes in flow velocimetry and clinical outcome following use of an external aortic compression device in women with postpartum hemorrhage. *Int J Gynecol Obstet* 2010;110:257–61, with permission

after controlling for the amount of administered uterotonics, women treated with the NASG had 303 ml less measured blood loss (299 ml) compared with the women who did not have the NASG available (602 ml)[27].

Shock index

The time to recovery of a normal pulse was faster for women with hypovolemic shock in the NASG-intervention phase (90 min) than for women in the pre-intervention phase (180 min) in Egypt[26]. This difference also held when the pulse at study entry was controlled for[26]. The shock index (SI) is a better clinical indicator of hypovolemia than either the pulse or the blood pressure alone, because it simultaneously accounts for both pulse (P) and systolic blood pressure (SBP). The formula[49] for the SI is $SI = P/SBP$. A higher shock index is associated with a greater risk of severe morbidity and mortality. When the data from the Egyptian NASG study were analysed, the median recovery times for the SI were significantly shorter in the NASG-intervention phase (75 min) than in the pre-intervention phase (120 min) (log rank 8.99, $p = 0.003$); this effect persisted even after stratifying for SI at study entry as well as blood transfusion and IV fluids received[26] (Figure 6).

External abdominal pressure

The effect of the NASG on the pressure exerted on the external abdominal wall underneath the NASG abdominal compression ball was studied in 10 healthy non-pregnant, non-postpartum female volunteers[50]. No participant reported any side-effects during NASG application and vital signs remained stable throughout. Mean pressures were low at baseline (1.1 mmHg, SD 1.9), with a significant rise upon full application after 5 min (66.6 mmHg, SD 11.2), and a rapid return to near baseline levels upon complete removal (−1.9 mmHg, SD 3.8). Pressure at full application after 5 min was significantly greater than pressure immediately before application (Wilcoxon matched-pairs signed-rank test; $p = 0.005$) and upon removal ($p < 0.001$) (Figure 7)[50].

The effect of body mass index and applier strength

Ten healthy non-pregnant, non-postpartum volunteers with varied body mass indexes (BMIs) were evaluated in a separate study to evaluate the effect of BMI and applier strength during application[50]. Average age of study participants was 33 years, the majority were nulligravid (8/10), and two had delivered two children each. Mean BMI by category were as follows: three underweight (mean BMI 18.3), four normal weight (mean BMI 21.0) and three overweight (mean BMI 30.3). Two appliers of different self-reported strength (one strong and one weak) were recruited to apply the NASG to each of the volunteers. There were a total of 20 applications, with each volunteer having a 'strong' and a 'weak' application of the NASG.

For all participants, application of the NASG resulted in a significant increase in pressure at the level of the abdominal wall. There were no changes in vital signs with application of the NASG and no reported side-effects. A high degree of correlation existed between the pressure generated immediately after application and after 5 min with both strong (Spearman correlation 0.963, $p = 0.001$) and weak appliers (Spearman correlation 0.854, $p = 0.002$). Application of the NASG by the strong applier versus the weak applier for all three BMI groups resulted in higher mean pressure (Figure 8). The difference between the pressure generated by a strong applier in an

underweight patient and a weak applier in an overweight patient was statistically significant (Wilcoxon rank sum test; $p = 0.05$)[50].

An inverse relationship existed between pressure and BMI, which was statistically significant for

Cox regression results for the effects of study group on shock index recovery time, controlling for initial SI value and other resuscitative measures						
	B	Wald	Sig.	Exp(B)	95.0% CI for Exp(B)	
					Lower	Upper
Blood transfusion (n = 222)						
NASG	0.651	19.337	0.000	1.918	1.435	2.563
Initial SI value	-1.199	15.809	0.000	0.301	0.167	0.544
Blood transfusion for resuscitation	0.856	26.131	0.000	2.353	1.695	3.266
Volume of IV fluids given in the first hour (n = 196)						
NASG	0.454	8.519	0.004	1.575	1.161	2.136
Initial SI value	-1.841	37.367	0.000	0.159	0.088	0.286
More than >1000 ml of IV fluids in first hour	0.154	0.829	0.363	1.167	0.837	1.625

Figure 6 Egyptian NASG study data, the median recovery times for the shock index (SI) were significantly shorter in the NASG-intervention phase (75 min) than in the pre-intervention phase (120 min) (log rank 8.99, $p = 0.003$); this effect persisted even after stratifying for SI at study entry as well as blood transfusion and IV fluids received. B, beta (the estimated regression coefficient); Wald, Wald statistic; Sig., significance of the Wald statistic; Exp(B), predicted change in the hazard for a unit increase in the predictor. From Miller *et al.* Use of the non-pneumatic anti-shock garment (NASG) to reduce blood loss and time to recovery from shock for women with obstetric haemorrhage in Egypt. *Global Public Health J* 2007;2;110–24, with permission

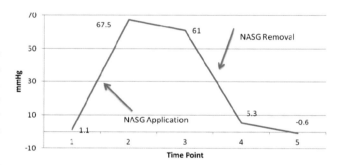

Figure 7 The effect of NASG on mean external abdominal wall pressure ($n = 10$)

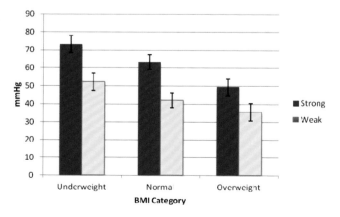

Figure 8 Mean pressure during NASG application by strong and weak appliers for each BMI category with standard error bars ($n = 10$)

the strong applier (Spearman correlation −0.905, $p = 0.0003$), but not significant for the weak applier (Spearman correlation −0.232, $p = 0.5182$). Placement of the NASG abdominal segment for 5 min resulted in a rapid rise in mean pressure on the external abdomen below the NASG abdominal compression ball in both the strong and weak applier groups (see Figure 4). The mean pressure generated by the strong applier was significantly greater than that generated by the weak applier (ANOVA; $p < 0.001$) (Figure 9). Pressure rapidly returned to baseline after removal of the NASG. Vital signs in these euvolemic female volunteers did not change with NASG application[50].

Pelvic blood flow

Because NASG users have a decrease in uterine bleeding after garment application, investigators considered how the NASG affects blood flow to the uterus specifically. Two recent studies investigated the effect of the NASG on lower abdominal or pelvic blood flow.

Hauswald *et al.* studied the effect of the NASG on distal aortic blood flow in 12 healthy adults (male or female not-specified)[51]. Using an Acuson Sequoia 512 Ultrasound and 4VI probe operating at 2–3 MHz (Siemens, Mountain View, CA, USA), measurements were obtained of heart rate, apparent artery diameter, Doppler-to-vessel angle and blood flow velocity at the abdominal aorta below the superior mesenteric artery (SMA). These data then were used to calculate flow rate (volume per time). Placement of the NASG resulted in a mean decrease in blood flow in the distal aorta of 33% or 0.65 l/min. This result then was compared to an improvized pneumatic anti-shock device made out of three bicycle tubes and sheets, which decreased flow by 56% or 1.11 l/min.

A study by Lester *et al.* examined the impact of the NASG on internal iliac resistive indices (RI) of healthy postpartum volunteers[52]. The RI is defined as the peak of systole divided by the sum of systole (S) and diastole (D): $RI = S/(S + D)$. A higher RI is correlated with decreased blood flow to a given vessel. A value less than 1.0 indicates forward flow, whereas a value of greater or equal to 1.0 indicates absent or reverse flow. All 10 patients evaluated in this study had delivered vaginally at term without complications. The majority (9/10) had received prophylactic IV oxytocin after delivery; one did not. The mean time from delivery to study inclusion was 12 h (range 2–18 h). Mean maternal age was 25 (range 18–37), and the patients had delivered an average of 2.4 babies (range 1–6). The majority were normal weight; none were underweight, and four were overweight.

The median internal iliac RI was evaluated using transabdominal Doppler ultrasound at nine time points before, during and after application of the NASG. Little change was observed in RI from baseline (0.83, SD 0.11) with application of leg panels alone (0.84, SD 0.12). When the abdominal panel was applied, however, the median value rose significantly (1.05, SD 0.15) and stayed elevated after full application for

10 min (1.00, SD 0.15). The RI rapidly returned to baseline with removal of the abdominal segment (0.82, SD 0.04), and remained low and near baseline after the removal of the entire garment (0.81, SD 0.11). There was a significant change in RI from baseline to full application (Wilcoxon matched-pairs signed-rank test; $p = 0.02$), as depicted in Figure 10. Vital signs in these euvolemic women remained stable throughout the application with little change noted in any of the parameters[50].

Several methods are available for analysing Doppler blood flow including flow volume or velocity measurement, resistance indices and waveform analysis[53]. Flow volume analysis most closely approximates true blood flow; however, it is difficult to perform and prone to error, as accurate measurement is dependent on the angle of insonation, vessel diameter measurement and vessel tortuosity. Most ultrasound machines used in routine obstetrics are not able to calculate flow volume due to the high analytic requirements of these calculations. Resistance indices are indirect measures of flow volume; however, they are angle independent and are considered to be useful for estimating blood flow in vessels distal to the point of the examination. One drawback of RI calculation is that it may not be as accurate in cases when blood flow is not continuous throughout the cardiac cycle. Waveform analysis is more complicated; however, it may provide a more accurate estimate of blood flow in conditions of

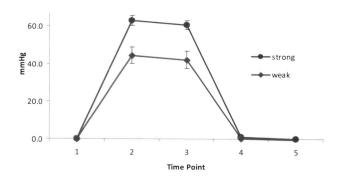

Figure 9 The effect of applier strength on mean pressure with NASG application ($n = 10$)

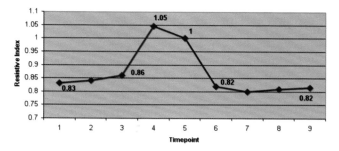

Figure 10 Median internal iliac resistive index with application of NASG. (Timepoint 1 is baseline, 2 is application of the leg segments, Timepoint 4 is full application of the NASG. Timepoint 6 represents removal of the abdominal panel. Timepoint 8 is after full removal of the garment.) Lester *et al.* Impact of the non-pneumatic antishock garment on pelvic blood flow in healthy postpartum women. *Am J Obstet Gynecol* 2011;204:409.e1–5

non-continuous blood flow during the cardiac cycle[53]. In the study cited above, the blood flow to the pelvis was measured transabdominally using Doppler ultrasound. Due to the location of the NASGs abdominal/pelvic segment and uterine compression ball in relationship to where the transabdominal ultrasound probe should be placed to image the uterine artery, an accurate measurement of the RI in these vessels was not possible.

The authors of this chapter have now conducted a transvaginal ultrasound study of uterine blood flow with the NASG in 18 non-pregnant, normal, healthy female volunteers of reproductive age. Using Doppler ultrasound to identify both the internal iliac artery and the uterine artery, RIs were calculated as an approximation of uterine blood flow before, during and after placement of the NASG. The preliminary results demonstrate an increase in the RIs of both vessels. The RI of the uterine artery increased an average of 0.33 (SD 0.15, $n = 18$) from a mean of 0.72 (SD 0.094, $n = 18$) to 1.04 (SD 0.15, $n = 18$). Similarly, in the internal iliac artery, the RI increased 0.13 (SD 0.09, $n = 18$) from 0.91 (SD 0.06, $n = 18$) to 1.04 (SD 0.16, $n = 17$). These studies are ongoing. In addition to recruiting more volunteers, future studies will focus on postpartum patients and better delineating the pelvic blood flow in parturient patients.

Intra-abdominal pressure

The sole manufacturer of the NASG is Zoex (Coloma, CA, USA). The manufacturer's brochure states that the pressure exerted by the NASG is between 20 and 40 mmHg; however, published studies of the impact of the NASG on intra-abdominal pressure, whether in male or female volunteers, are not available[54].

In the absence of such information, the authors conducted preliminary investigations of the intra-abdominal pressure generated by NASG placement on 20 healthy female volunteers of reproductive age. Standard urodynamic equipment and minimally invasive techniques routinely performed in clinical gynecologic evaluations were employed. A 2.3 mm rectal pressure catheter (7 Fr, aircharged™ abdominal catheter; T-DOC® Company, Wilmington DE) placed transrectally was used to approximate intra-abdominal pressure. Measurements were performed using the Triton urodynamic monitor (Laborie Medical Technologies, Inc, Williston, VA) attached to the rectal pressure catheter. This technique provided a minimally invasive, accurate approximation of intra-abdominal pressure and allowed measurements to be taken continuously throughout the study. Preliminary results demonstrated a mean increase of 15.3 mmHg (SD 5.60).

DISCUSSION AND CLINICAL IMPLICATIONS

The evidence presented in this chapter supports the theoretical model of NASG function. Compression of capacitance vessels in the lower extremities appears to produce a shifting of pooled blood back into the central circulation. The rapid recovery of the shock index and vital sign recovery times reported in clinical trials to date suggest that this may occur. An evaluation of the impact of the NASG on cardiac output and central venous return is needed.

In the pelvic vasculature, the distal aorta branches into the common iliac artery which in turn branches into the external iliac which proceeds to become the femoral in the leg and the internal iliac artery, which supplies the majority of blood flow to the uterus via the uterine arteries. Three studies have now evaluated lower abdominal and pelvic blood flow with NASG placement; all demonstrated decreased flow in the distal aorta and increased resistive indices in the internal iliac and uterine arteries. These findings are consistent with the decrease in blood loss from PPH that has been reported in published studies of the NASG[26–28]. The observed increase in the RI of the internal iliac and uterine arteries with NASG application provides a physiologically plausible mechanism to explain how hemorrhage is reduced by NASG application.

Both NASG efficacy and potential side-effects (oliguria and/or dyspnea) probably depend on the circumferential compression of vessels from pressure exerted by the device; therefore, understanding how pressure varies in individual applications is of critical importance. The studies cited above demonstrate that both internal and external abdominal pressure increase with NASG application, and that the pressure generated likely varies with applier strength and patient BMI. The NASG has no pressure gauge or mechanism to inform appliers that the appropriate pressure is being exerted. This initial evaluation of pressure variation among patients and appliers provides critically important baseline information that can inform development of means to ensure that appropriate pressure is exerted with each application of the NASG.

Severe PPH affects a diverse cohort of over 100,000 women annually throughout the world[2,55]. In pre-intervention phase/NASG-intervention phase studies in tertiary facilities, use of the NASG enhanced maternal outcomes for women, including a significantly reduced blood loss. The initial blood flow studies seem to indicate that NASG application increases RI and helps explain how the NASG decreases blood loss. Although the science behind the success of the NASG has advanced compared to the available knowledge even a decade ago, much remains to be learned about this device. The available pressure studies indicate that body size and strength of the person applying the garment are important.

The garment could affect outcomes. Because the body habitus of a woman affected by PPH in rural India may be very different than a woman in peri-urban Nigeria or in the Peruvian highlands, it is important to consider height, weight, BMI and habitus of prospective patients. Similarly, health care providers vary in size and strength; the maximal pressure generated by a taller, stronger applier is likely to be significantly different than a smaller, shorter, weaker applier. It may be that individualized training methods could be developed to better standardize the amount of pressure generated. Alternatively, it may be beneficial to develop a simple pressure gauge, or other means of ensuring appropriate garment placement in patients with different body habitus.

FUTURE DIRECTIONS

The ideal amount of pressure that should be generated with NASG application is not known. Moreover, the current sole manufacturer of the device provides no information regarding the necessity or lack thereof to apply more or less pressure dependent on the size of the patient. Studies to more fully elucidate the impact of the NASG on intra-abdominal vascular flow would clarify the relationship between pressure applied and perfusion of intra-abdominal organs (e.g. uterus, intestines, kidney). It would also be important to correlate the pressure exerted by the NASG with the cardio-vascular impact on the central circulation, namely central venous pressure, systemic vascular resistance and cardiac output.

Future studies should expand the sample size and recruit a larger number of participants with different body habitus, including height, weight, BMI, abdominal circumference and ethnicity. It may also be useful to conduct this study in a postpartum cohort, as the physiology of pregnancy and the puerperium may result in some important differences in pressure outcomes. Similarly, the effect of applier size and strength should be further explored by evaluating a more diverse cohort of appliers with varied height, weight, strength, gender and ethnicity, and using a standardized method of strength testing to evaluate applier strength and its correlation to pressure. It is also likely that differences in effect exist based on the intravascular volume status of the patients. The effect of the NASG on cardiac output may be greater or different in a severely hypovolemic patients. It would be useful to conduct studies in patients who have experienced PPH and shock to evaluate the cardiovascular impact of the NASG in this cohort.

Understanding how pressure, vascular flow and cardiovascular function are related in a diverse cohort of patients and health care providers is an important step towards optimizing NASG application. Future studies should endeavor to define this relationship and to more clearly elucidate the individual characteristics that affect NASG application. If significant variation persists in future studies, modification of NASG design (e.g. simple pressure gauge) or improved training protocols may result in improved individual application.

The goal of these future studies would be to ensure that each placement of the NASG will result in optimal results: immediate diminished uterine bleeding, resuscitation from shock, and survival without adverse effects. Achieving this objective may improve obstetric shock management and reduce deaths from obstetric hemorrhage, the world's leading cause of maternal mortality.

PRACTICE POINTS

- The NASG reduces the time to recovery from shock as demonstrated by improvement in vital signs and the shock index, as well as improved survival

- The NASG decreases blood loss by increasing the resistive index in the internal iliac and uterine arteries, which indicates decreased blood flow through these vessels

- The NASG increases both external and internal abdominal pressure; preliminary data suggest that the amount of increase in intra-abdominal pressure is 10–20 mmHg

- There may be variability in effectiveness of the NASG depending on individual patient characteristics such as BMI and abdominal circumference. This area warrants additional research.

References

1. Gabrysch S, Campbell OM. Still too far to walk: Literature review of the determinants of delivery service use. BMC Pregnancy Childbirth 2009;9:34.
2. Hogan MC, Foreman KJ, Naghavi M, et al. Maternal mortality for 181 countries, 1980–2008: a systematic analysis of progress towards Millennium Development Goal 5. Lancet 2010;375:1609–23
3. Thaddeus S, Maine D. Too far to walk: maternal mortality in context. Soc Sci Med 1994;38:1091–110
4. WHO/UNICEF/UNFPA/TheWorldBank. Trends in maternal mortality: 1990 to 2008: Estimates developed by WHO, UNICEF, UNFPA and The World Bank. Geneva: WHO, 2010
5. Mourad-Youssif M, Ojengbede OA, Meyer CD, et al. Can the Non-pneumatic Anti-Shock Garment (NASG) reduce adverse maternal outcomes from postpartum hemorrhage? Evidence from Egypt and Nigeria. Reprod Health 2010;7:24
6. Miller S. Anti-Shock Garments: Non-Pneumatic Anti-Shock Garment (NASG) And Pneumatic Anti-Shock Garment (PASG). California Maternal Quality Care Collaborative (CMQCC), 2009 www.cmqcc.org/resources/ob_hemorrhage/anti_shock_garments
7. Miller S, Martin HB, Morris JL. Anti-shock garment in postpartum haemorrhage. Best Pract Res Clin Obstet Gynaecol 2008;22:1057–74
8. Kaplan B, Poole F, Flagg J, David Clark Company Inc assignee. Medical pneumatic trouser for emergency autotransfusion. United States Patent 3933150. USA1976 02/08/1974
9. Cutler BS, Daggett WM. Application of the "G-suit" to the control of hemorrhage in massive trauma. Annals Surg 1971;173:511–4
10. Kaplan BC, Civetta JM, Nagel EL, Nussenfeld SR, Hirschman JC. The military anti-shock trouser in civilian pre-hospital emergency care. J Trauma 1973;13:843–8
11. McSwain MJ, McSwain N.E. Pneumatic antishock garment: state of the art at the turn of the century. Trauma 2000;2:63–75
12. Bickell WH, Pepe PE, Bailey ML, Wyatt CH, Mattox KL. Randomized trial of pneumatic antishock garments in the prehospital management of penetrating abdominal injuries. Ann Emerg Med 1987;16:653–8
13. Chang FC, Harrison PB, Beech RR, Helmer SD. PASG: does it help in the management of traumatic shock? J Trauma 1995;39:453–6

14. Mattox KL, Bickell W, Pepe PE, Burch J, Feliciano D. Prospective MAST study in 911 patients. J Trauma 1989;29: 1104–11; discussion 11–2

15. McSwain NE, Jr. Pneumatic anti-shock garment: state of the art 1988. Ann Emerg Med 1988;17:506–25

16. Pepe PE, Bass RR, Mattox KL. Clinical trials of the pneumatic antishock garment in the urban prehospital setting. Ann Emerg Med 1986;15:1407–10

17. Dickinson K, Roberts I. Medical anti-shock trousers (pneumatic anti-shock garments) for circulatory support in patients with trauma. Cochrane database Syst Rev 2000;(2): CD001856

18. Maull KI, Capehart JE, Cardea JA, Haynes BW, Jr. Limb loss following Military Anti-Schock Trousers (MAST) application. J Trauma 1981;21:60–2

19. Aprahamian C, Gessert G, Bandyk DF, Sell L, Stiehl J, Olson DW. MAST-associated compartment syndrome (MACS): a review. J Trauma 1989;29:549–55

20. Vahedi M, Ayuyao A, Parsa M, Freeman H. Pneumatic Antishock Garment-Associated Compartment Syndrome in Uninjured Lower Extremities. J Trauma 1995;384:616–8

21. Brotman S, Browner BD, Cox EF. MAS trousers improperly applied causing a compartment syndrome in lower-extremity trauma. J Trauma 1982;22:598–9

22. Miller S, Ojengbede A, Turan JM, Ojengbede O, Butrick E, Hensleigh P. Anti-Shock Garments for Obstetric Hemorrhage. Curr Women's Health Rev 2007;3:3–11

23. Hauswald M, Greene ER. Regional blood flow after pneumatic anti-shock garment inflation. Prehosp Emerg Care 2003;7:225–8

24. Laplace C, Martin L, Rangheard AS, Menu Y, Duranteau J. [Pneumatic anti-shock garment use leading to non-visualization of pelvic arterial bleeding on angiography]. Ann Fr Anesth Reanim 2004;23:998–1002

25. Hensleigh PA. Anti-shock garment provides resuscitation and haemostasis for obstetric haemorrhage. BJOG 2002;109: 1377–84

26. Miller S, Turan J, Dau K, et al. Use of the non-pneumatic anti-shock garment (NASG) to reduce blood loss and time to recovery from shock for women with obstetric haemorrhage in Egypt. Global Public Health 2007;2:110–24

27. Miller S, Hamza S, Bray E, et al. First Aid for Obstetrical Haemorrhage: The Pilot Study of the Non-pneumatic Anti-Shock Garment (NASG) in Egypt. BJOG 2006;113:424–9

28. Miller S, Ojengbede O, Turan JM, Morhason-Bello IO, Martin HB, Nsima D. A comparative study of the non-pneumatic anti-shock garment for the treatment of obstetric hemorrhage in Nigeria. Int J Gynaecol Obstet 2009;107: 121–5

29. Berdichevsky K, Tucker C, Martinez A, Miller S. Acceptance of a New Technology for Management of Obstetric Hemorrhage: A Qualitative Study From Rural Mexico. Health Care Women Int 2010;31:444–57

30. Oshinowo A, Galadanci H, Awwal M, et al., editors. Overcoming Delays in Childbirth due to Hemorrhage: A Qualitative Study of the Non-pneumatic Anti-Shock Garment (NASG) in Nigeria. American Publich Health Association (APHA) 135th Annual Meeting and Exposition, November 3–7; 2007; Wasington, DC

31. Liu L. A mixed methods study of the implementation of two interventions to reduce maternal mortality in Ibadan, Oyo state, Nigeria. [dissertation for MIPH degree]. 2009; in press

32. Barber AE, Shires GT. Cell damage after shock. New Horiz 1996;4:161–7

33. Kristensen SR. Mechanisms of cell damage and enzyme release. Danish Med Bull 1994;41:423–33

34. Rodgers KG. Cardiovascular shock. Emerg Med Clin North Am 1995;13:793–810

35. Abboud F. Pathophysiology of hypotension and shock. In: Hurst J, ed. The Heart. New York: McGraw-Hill, 1982:452

36. Gardner WJ, Storer J. The use of the G-Suit in control of intra-abdominal bleeding. Surg Gynecol Obstet 1966;123: 792–8

37. Gardner WJ. Hemostasis by pneumatic compression. Am Surg 1969;35:635–7

38. Aberg T, Steen S, Othman K, Norgren L, Bengmark S. The effect of pneumatic antishock garments in the treatment of lethal combined hepatic and caval injuries in rats. J Trauma 1986;26:727–32

39. Ali J, Duke K. Pneumatic antishock garment decreases hemorrhage and mortality from splenic injury. Can J Surg. 1991;34:496–501

40. Aberg T, Rosen I, Walther B, Steen S. Cerebral function monitoring in rats with a critical hepatic injury treated with pneumatic antishock garment and infusion. J Trauma 1989; 29:168–74

41. Ali J, Duke K. Timing and interpretation of the hemodynamic effects of the pneumatic antishock garment. Ann Emerg Med 1991;20:1183–7

42. Ali J, Vanderby B, Purcell C. The effect of the pneumatic antishock garment (PASG) on hemodynamics, hemorrhage, and survival in penetrating thoracic aortic injury. J Trauma 1991;31:846–51

43. Gaffney FA, Thal ER, Taylor WF, et al. Hemodynamic effects of Medical Anti-Shock Trousers (MAST garment). J Trauma 1981;21:931–7

44. Jennings TJ, Seaworth JF, Tripp LD, Howell LL, Goodyear CD, Kennedy KW. The effects of inflation of antishock trousers on hemodynamics in normovolemic subjects. J Trauma 1986;26:544–8

45. Jennings TJ, Seaworth JF, Howell LL, Tripp LD, Goodyear CD. The effects of various antishock trouser inflation sequences on hemodynamics in normovolemic subjects. Ann Emerg Med 1986;15:1193–7

46. Seaworth JF, Jennings TJ, Howell LL, Frazier JW, Goodyear CD, Grassman ED. Hemodynamic effects of anti-G suit inflation in a 1-G environment. J Appl Physiol 1985;59: 1145–51

47. Soltan MH, Faragallah MF, Mosabah MH, Al-Adawy AR. External aortic compression device: the first aid for postpartum hemorrhage control. J Obstet Gynaecol Res 2009;35: 453–8

48. Soltan MH, Imam HH, Zahran KA, Atallah SM. Assessing changes in flow velocimetry and clinical outcome following use of an external aortic compression device in women with postpartum hemorrhage. Int J Gynaecol Obstet 2010;110: 257–61

49. Birkhahn RH, Gaeta TJ, Van Deusen SK, Tloczkowski J. The ability of traditional vital signs and shock index to identify ruptured ectopic pregnancy. Am J Obstet Gynecol 2003;189:1293–6

50. Stenson A, Miller S, Lester F, et al. NASG: Validation of Pressures and Hemodynamic Flow. Seattle, WA: Report Prepared by UCSF Team for PATH International, 2010

51. Hauswald M, Williamson M, Baty G, Kerr N, Edgar-Mied V. Use of an improvised pneumatic anti-shock garment and a non-pneumatic anti-shock garment to control pelvic blood flow. Int J Emerg Med 2010;3:173–5

52. Lester F, Stenson A, Meyer C, Morris J, Vargas J, Miller S. Impact of the Non-pneumatic Antishock Garment on pelvic blood flow in healthy postpartum women. Am J Obstet Gynecol 2011;204:409e1–5

53. Dickey RP. Doppler ultrasound investigation of uterine and ovarian blood flow in infertility and early pregnancy. Hum Reprod Update 1997;3:467–503

54. ZOEX NIASG. How do you apply the ZOEX NIASG http://www.zoexniasg.com/video/

55. Khan KS, Wojdyla D, Say L, Gulmezoglu AM, Van Look PF. WHO analysis of causes of maternal death: a systematic review. Lancet 2006;367:1066–74

40

Building Hospital Systems for the Care of Women with Major Obstetric Hemorrhage

D. W. Skupski, G. S. Eglinton and I. P. Lowenwirt

Here we describe a proven program of changes within a hospital setting designed to decrease morbidity and mortality of women with major obstetric hemorrhage[1]. This program hinges on building, developing and improving all existing hospital systems that are necessary for the care of women with major obstetric hemorrhage.

BACKGROUND

In the US, the incidence of major obstetric hemorrhage and cesarean hysterectomy have increased in recent years, most likely due to the increase in the rates of cesarean and repeat cesarean delivery[2–4]. Repeat cesarean delivery, in particular, has been associated with a marked increase in the rate of placenta previa and accreta[2–4]. In the setting of intractable obstetric hemorrhage, emergency peripartum hysterectomy often is used as a life-saving procedure (see also Chapter 55), and additional techniques are also available for use in such circumstances (see Chapters 46–58 and 51–54). According to one recent article, the incidence of emergency peripartum hysterectomy is approximately 2.5 per 1000 births[3], and hemorrhage associated with uterine atony is the most frequent indication, followed by placenta accreta[5]. Apart from whether hysterectomy is necessary, maternal death is a known complication of major obstetric hemorrhage[6].

TACKLING THE PROBLEM OF MAJOR OBSTETRIC HEMORRHAGE

Recently developed programs[1,7,8] to improve outcomes for women with major obstetric hemorrhage have focused on at least two important factors: the initial response to the hemorrhage and the prevention of hemorrhage in those patients who can be identified as being at high risk for hemorrhage. This latter effort is in recognition of the fact that two of the three most common causes of hemorrhage (uterine atony, placenta previa and placenta accreta) cannot be identified in advance[4]. Only placenta previa is reliably able to be diagnosed in advance.

Programs aimed at improving outcomes from major obstetric hemorrhage must also consider the interface between individuals and departments not traditionally thought of as being important in the process of caring for women with obstetric hemorrhage, including hospital administration and the department of surgery. This chapter describes in detail these hospital systems and how they have undergone changes at a major New York teaching hospital, with a corresponding decrease in morbidity and mortality.

IMPORTANCE OF COMMUNICATION AND EDUCATION

Two extremely important processes (communication and education) underpin the success of any program aimed at improving outcomes related to obstetric hemorrhage. Clear and open channels of communication must be developed between all personnel and departments involved in caring for women with major obstetric hemorrhage. These include the rapid and coordinated communications that are inevitably necessary for any rapid response team to work at maximum capacity. Communication must be comprehensive and include a far wider field than the members of the obstetric department. In order for communication to be truly effective it must include hospital administration, the emergency department, anesthesiology, the labor and delivery suite, nursing administration, the operating rooms, neonatology and the blood bank.

Basic education is equally important. It is imprudent (and indeed dangerous) to believe that attending physicians or house staff will know (*a priori*) all the component parts of the program in place based on their past experience and training. All care providers who evaluate bleeding patients and institute therapy must possess requisite knowledge of the pathophysiology of hemorrhagic shock in order to identify the presence and assess the severity of this problem, and to begin the process of treatment. It cannot be overemphasized to all levels of staff that the diagnosis of major obstetric hemorrhage is not always as easy as training manuals might suggest. The involvement of departmental leaders who are experienced with the management of obstetric hemorrhage and who are available 24 hours a day for all 365 days each year is key. Training for less experienced care providers must be developed and be repeated on a regular basis. Such training must be thought of as a continuous and never-ending process – something that has to be repeated to every new rotation of house staff and attending consultants.

EVENTS AT NEW YORK HOSPITAL MEDICAL CENTER OF QUEENS

The New York Hospital Medical Center of Queens (NYHQ), an acute care 480 bed hospital in Flushing, New York, is affiliated with the Weill Medical College of Cornell University as well as the New York Presbyterian Healthcare System. The hospital serves an urban community of great ethnic diversity whose care is paid for by both commercial and governmental health insurance. The hospital is designated for the highest level (level III) of neonatal intensive and maternal care, and has been afforded the highest designation for a trauma center (level I). Separate critical care units are dedicated to surgical, medical and cardiac services.

Two maternal deaths following major obstetric hemorrhage, one each in the years 2000 and 2001, prompted the creation of a patient safety team that worked to improve all hospital systems at NYHQ caring for women at risk for, or suffering from, major obstetric hemorrhage. This patient safety team created a mission involving an improved management scheme (clinical pathway) for the identification and management of major obstetric hemorrhage, with the express intent of reducing maternal deaths due to hemorrhage. The team was very successful in this mission, so much so that the New York State Assembly proposed legislation mandating the management pathway in other hospitals in the State of New York and the management pathway in various modified forms is now in widespread use in Illinois and California.

Patient safety teams

Beginning in 2001, a multidisciplinary patient safety team was established that included individuals from obstetric anesthesiology, maternal fetal medicine, neonatology, the blood bank, nursing, communication and administration. Over the course of 6–12 months, meeting usually every week for 1–2 hours, this patient safety team evaluated the totality of the medical center's care of the two women who died from major obstetric hemorrhage, considered both the proximate and systems-related causes of these unfortunate outcomes, discussed possible recommended changes in management, and decided on the best manner in which to change the systems at NYHQ that were then present for the care of these women.

Objective of our study

In order to assess the impact of the patient safety team's proposed changes in hospital systems on the future outcomes of our patients, we carefully recorded outcomes prospectively from that point (2001) forward, and looked back retrospectively to record the same outcomes for the 2 years in which the deaths had occurred. The team was of the opinion that the accurate recording of outcomes was essential to demonstrate any effect of changes in management over time. *Specifically, we hypothesized that the changes we implemented in our hospital systems would lead to improved outcomes for women with major obstetric hemorrhage.*

Methods

Our multifaceted approach included the following:

(1) We formed an obstetric rapid response team (Team Blue) modeled after the cardiac arrest team, and included quarterly mock drills on all shifts for various emergency clinical scenarios.

(2) We developed clinical pathways – guidelines and protocols – specifically designed to provide for early diagnosis of patients at risk for major obstetric hemorrhage and for streamlined care in emergency situations.

(3) In response to a marked increase in the volume of gynecologic emergency cases and births at NYHQ, we separated the in-house obstetric and gynecologic responsibilities by adding an additional in-house attending physician at all times. This allowed the in-house obstetrician to focus on obstetrical emergencies without fear of neglecting gynecological emergencies.

(4) We revised the duties of the 24-hour in-house attending obstetrician to include continuous and frequent monitoring of all patients on the labor and delivery unit. This monitoring included those patients who had private obstetricians who might or might not be present on a continuous basis.

(5) We empowered all obstetric care providers (including physician assistants, nurses, resident physicians and the in-house attending physician) to immediately involve senior members of the Department whenever there was disagreement with or concern about the management scheme (particularly when there was a possible delay in recognition of the severity of hemorrhage). A senior member of the Department was then required to discuss the issue immediately with the attending physician to avoid delay.

(6) Through weekly didactic sessions, we educated all of our staff to recognize the severity of hemorrhage described in the Advanced Trauma Life Support Manual of the American College of Surgeons[9], and disseminated information regarding the new protocols for patient care. The attending, nursing and ancillary staffs were all also informed regarding the intent of the changes (i.e. to improve patient safety) and the importance of early diagnosis of major hemorrhage.

(7) We established a role for the Trauma Team of the Surgical Department, with the full agreement of the Director of Trauma Services, which was to respond and assist in cases of severe obstetrical hemorrhage. We chose the Trauma Team because they were the most experienced in resuscitation of patients with hemorrhagic shock within our institution. The Trauma Team includes surgical house officers working under the direction of the surgical trauma attending physician. These team members are expert in the placement of large bore intravenous lines (by venous cutdown if necessary), knowledgeable about the physiology of volume resuscitation, ready to assist in obtaining adequate amounts of blood products for massive blood replacement, and are the most experienced in inserting intraluminal lines directly into the major vessels for monitoring and obtaining requisite samples.

The creation of new protocols and guidelines

The following protocols and guidelines were created to enhance the identification of women at risk for major obstetric hemorrhage, the reception of new patient safety activities and the perpetuation of these activities.

(1) We prepared for major hemorrhage in patients with known placenta previa (Figure 1). This preparation included antenatal consultation with maternal fetal medicine, obstetric anesthesiology and senior gynecologic surgeons; liberal use of ultrasound to identify placenta accreta in patients with prior uterine surgery and/or placenta previa. When such patients were identified, they underwent twice weekly type and screen of blood to allow for more rapid availability of blood products if major hemorrhage were to occur. Amniocentesis for fetal lung maturity was performed at 36 weeks of gestation followed by planned cesarean delivery if the fetal lungs were shown to be mature.

(2) We prepared for major hemorrhage in patients in whom we suspected placenta accreta (Figure 1). This included autologous blood donation as often as every week for a period of 4–5 weeks before the planned cesarean delivery; erythropoietin, iron and vitamin therapy in an effort to boost red blood cell production; consultation with interventional radiology regarding consideration of placement of ports preoperatively, so that embolization of major pelvic blood vessels could occur rapidly in the event of substantial hemorrhage during the operation; judicious placement of additional

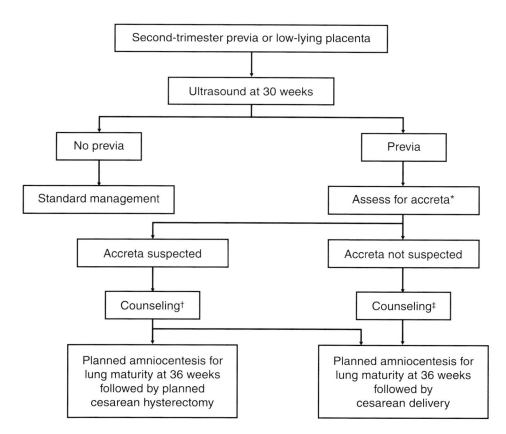

Figure 1   Proposed management scheme for patients at risk for major obstetric hemorrhage. *Suspicion for accreta is markedly increased with prior cesarean delivery and anterior placenta; ‡includes bed rest, pelvic rest, preparation for cesarean delivery, serial complete blood count, consider erythropoietin, iron and vitamin supplements and serial autologous blood donation; †includes the counseling above and a recommendation for cesarean hysterectomy. Low parity may decrease the strength of the recommendation if future child bearing is desired

intravenous lines and a 7.5 Fr internal jugular cordis for invasive monitoring and volume replacement; intraoperative monitoring with an arterial line and central venous pressure; and transfer to the surgical intensive care unit as needed. In addition, we used the cell saver (see Chapter 70), but only after delivery of the fetus and after copious peritoneal irrigation had been performed[4]. Weekly autologous blood donation was used not only to prevent the introduction of blood-borne infection by transfusion, but also to help resolve any potential shortage of blood in our area.

(3) We obtained consultation with the trauma team as necessary.

(4) For patients with suspected placenta accreta, we discussed the likely decreased maternal mortality of planned cesarean hysterectomy[10]. Planned cesarean hysterectomy was then performed for those who agreed.

(5) For patients with suspected placenta accreta, cesarean delivery and cesarean hysterectomy were scheduled in the main operating room under the direction of senior gynecologic surgeons (Figure 1), because the staff and facilities of the main operating room are better equipped to perform hysterectomy than is the case with the labor and delivery suite. This procedural change also avoided the problem of consuming staff and resources on labor and delivery that were considered necessary for the care of other patients.

Table 1 shows the hospital systems and individual changes involved, along with an assessment of the impact on improving outcomes in women with major obstetric hemorrhage and the relative amount of work involved in each change.

In addition to the changes in systems detailed above, data on obstetric volume, mode of delivery, occurrence of major obstetric hemorrhage and outcomes important in identifying improvements were collected from 2000 to 2005. Cases were identified prospectively for the entire patient cohort (2000–2005). Demographic and outcome data on each patient were recorded retrospectively during the time period of January of 2000 to May of 2001 and prospectively beginning in June 2001.

The data collection program also involves monitoring by senior departmental leaders who receive reports on a daily basis from care providers regarding all cases of major obstetric hemorrhage. These cases were highlighted and included in the database as they occurred. Outcomes analysed included maternal deaths, lowest documented maternal pH, lowest documented maternal temperature and the occurrence of coagulopathy.

Our definition of major obstetric hemorrhage included one or more of the following: estimated blood loss of 1500 ml or more, need for blood transfusion, need for uterine packing, performance of uterine artery ligation, and performance of cesarean hysterectomy. Admittedly, this definition is different from that of postpartum hemorrhage (PPH) that is detailed in other chapters of this volume. Accordingly, the rate of major obstetric hemorrhage by our definition was expected to be lower than the known incidence of PPH. Data were compared between the 2 years before and the 3 years after the systemic changes were implemented, 2000–2001 versus 2002–2005.

Results

During each successive year of the study the following important changes occurred simultaneously: increasing obstetrical volume, increasing rate of cesarean delivery, an increasing rate of repeat cesarean delivery, and an increasing number of cases of major obstetric hemorrhage (Table 2). The increases in cesarean delivery, repeat cesarean delivery and cases of major obstetric hemorrhage were all significant when comparing the time period of 2000–2001 to that of 2002–2005, but no difference was shown in the rate of cesarean hysterectomy (Table 2).

Table 1 Impact of hospital system changes on the outcomes of women with major obstetric hemorrhage

System	Specific change	Impact	Amount of work involved
Administrative	Patient safety team	Critical	Extensive
	Trauma team involvement	Minor	Moderate
Departmental	Obstetric rapid response team	Critical	Extensive
	Development of clinical pathways or guidelines	Major	Moderate
	Dissemination of clinical pathways or guidelines	Major	Moderate
	Separation of in-house obstetrician and gynecologist	Minor	Moderate
	Culture change to proactive attending physician	Major	Moderate
	Care provider empowerment	Major	Moderate
	Didactic teaching about physiology and treatment of hemorrhagic shock	Major	Moderate
Clinical pathways or guidelines	Antenatal management of known placenta previa	Major	Moderate
	Preparation for hemorrhage in suspected placenta accreta	Minor	Moderate
	Counseling about planned cesarean hysterectomy	Minor	Minimal
	Scheduled cesarean delivery for previa and accreta in the main operating room	Minor	Minimal
Nursing	Culture change to team participation	Major	Extensive
	Empowerment of nurses	Major	Moderate

Clinical characteristics, measures of severity of hemorrhage and outcomes are shown in Table 3. The patient groups from the two time periods (2000–2001 versus 2002–2005) were similar in demographics as measured by age, parity and incidence of prior cesarean delivery. The severity of obstetric hemorrhage also appeared to be similar between the time periods. The severity measures were APACHE II scores[11], occurrence of placenta accreta and estimated blood loss (Table 3).

The major result of this combined effort was that maternal deaths were significantly reduced in the time period following the systemic changes ($p = 0.036$). This was supported by the additional findings of significant differences (improvement) in lowest pH ($p = 0.004$) and lowest temperature ($p < 0.0001$). There also was a trend toward less coagulopathy ($p = 0.09$). These findings were very important because it is known that a triad of physiologic derangements occurs in hemorrhagic shock that can lead to death. This triad comprises acidemia, hypothermia and coagulopathy. The presence of this triad confirms that our major finding of reduced maternal death is not a statistical chance event, and also argues that our response to the event of a major obstetric hemorrhage became better as time passed and as care providers became more experienced and knowledgeable.

The two time periods were also analysed according to other characteristics: need for cesarean hysterectomy, volume of transfusion, operative time, need for intubation for more than 24 hours, and number of hours intubated (Table 3). No significant differences were seen in these measures between 2000–2001 and 2002–2005. The incidence of peripartum hysterectomy was 1.3/1000 (24/18,723) during the entire study period (2000–2005). Placenta accreta with prior cesarean delivery accounted for 14/24 (58.3%) cases of cesarean hysterectomy; we suspected accreta in seven cases and confirmed it in four cases at delivery. The operative characteristics, morbidity and mortality of patients undergoing peripartum hysterectomy are shown in Table 4. The numbers here are different from those in Table 3, because the data in Table 3 show all patients during the entire study period, and the data in Table 4 are confined to those patients who underwent cesarean hysterectomy. A significant difference was also present in the lowest pH in patients

Table 2   Major obstetric hemorrhage 2000–2005

Year	Births	Total cesarean births*	Repeat cesarean births†	Cases of major obstetric hemorrhage‡	Cesarean hysterectomy§	Mortality
2000	2705	516	217	3	1	1
2001	3106	801	287	8	5	1
2002	3323	903	332	8	5	0
2003	3395	932	326	14	4	0
2004	3648	1053	374	18	5	0
2005 (8 months)	2546	759	275	12	4	0
Total	18,723	4964	1811	63	24	2

*2000–2001 compared to 2002–2005, $p < 0.0001$
†2000–2001 compared to 2002–2005, $p = 0.002$
‡2000–2001 compared to 2002–2005, $p = 0.02$
§Rate of cesarean hysterectomy as a function of the total number of major obstetric hemorrhage cases 2000–2001 compared to 2002–2005, $p = 0.37$

Table 3   Major obstetric hemorrhage: comparison of demographics, measures of severity and outcomes

	2000–2001 (n = 12)	2002–2005 (n = 49)	P value
Demographics			
Age, mean (SD)	36.5 (6.0)	34.2 (5.9)	0.23
Parity, median (range)	1 (0–3)	1 (0–5)	0.70
Prior cesarean delivery, n (%)	6 (50.0)	32 (65.3)	0.33
Severity measures			
Occurrence of placenta accreta, n (%)	4 (33.3)	11 (22.4)	0.46
APACHE score, median (range)	11.5 (7–31)	10 (6–18)	0.07
Estimated blood loss in ml, mean (SD)	2725 (1289)	2429 (1214)	0.46
Outcomes			
Maternal death, n (%)	2 (16.7)	0 (0.0)	0.036*
Lowest pH, median (range)	7.23 (6.8–7.39)	7.34 (7.08–7.44)	0.004*
Lowest temperature (°C), median (range)	35.2 (30.2–35.8)	36.1 (35.2–37.8)	<0.0001*
Coagulopathy, n (%)	7 (58.3)	15 (30.6)	0.09
Cesarean hysterectomy, n (%)	6 (50.0)	18 (36.7)	0.51
Volume of transfusion in ml , mean (SD)	1313 (1029)	1194 (1547)	0.80
Operative time, mean (SD)	185 (91)	184 (79)	0.99
Intubation >24 h, n (%)	7 (58.3)	16 (32.7)	0.18

*Significant difference

undergoing cesarean hysterectomy between the time periods of 2000–2001 versus 2002–2005. This observation underscores the likelihood that our response to women with hemorrhagic shock from blood loss improved over the course of time.

Deciphering the data

The response to major obstetric hemorrhage must be multifaceted and rapid in order to be successful. A quality assurance committee would be the traditional departmental or institutional response to a poor outcome such as a maternal death from hemorrhage, and after this peer review, specific physician education would occur regarding the components of early identification and 'best' treatment, as determined by departmental leaders. However, this traditional response ignores the lessons learned from the Institute of Medicine report regarding errors that lead to morbidity and mortality during hospital stays[12]. When clinical judgment fails and hemorrhagic shock is not recognized or when a patient presents in an advanced state of hemorrhagic shock, hospital systems need to improve in order to provide a safety net for patients; this is as important as is the education of a specific

physician or group of physicians after an adverse outcome.

Our findings indicated that significant improvements in outcomes occurred after we introduced systemic changes at our institution; improvements were noted in maternal deaths, frequency of low pH and frequency of low temperature. There were no differences in measures of severity of obstetric hemorrhage in spite of significant increases in the number of cases of major obstetric hemorrhage between the study time periods, leading us to the conclusion that this improvement in outcomes is a true finding. When comparing the time periods before and after the systemic changes, the significant differences in lowest temperature and in lowest pH (Table 3) suggest that the team's response to massive hemorrhage improved after the system-wide interventions. The reduction in maternal mortality, however, cannot be considered a robust observation, because this observation is hospital-based and may not be replicated in a population-based sample. This caveat in no way diminishes the value of our findings in terms of their broad applicability in other hospitals throughout the US and other countries.

The process of implementing the systemic changes required considerable effort by many individuals and

Table 4 Peripartum hysterectomy 2000–2005. All data are expressed as number of cases unless otherwise designated. Incidence 24/18,723 (1.3/1000)

	2000–01[†]	2002–05[‡]	Total[§]
Etiology			
Placenta accreta	4	10	14
Placenta accreta with prior CD	4	10	14
Uterine atony	2	6	8
Morbidity			
Cystotomy	1	1	2
Pulmonary embolus	1	0	1
Coagulopathy	5	8	13
Acute tubular necrosis	0	0	0
ARDS	0	0	0
Myocardial infarction	0	0	0
Pneumonia	0	0	0
Mortality			
Placenta percreta	1	0	1
Other characteristics			
Operative time in min, mean (SD)	259 (52.3)	250 (66.6)	252 (62.4)
EBL in ml, median (range)	3500 (2500–5200)	3000 (1000–7000)	3250 (1000–7000)
Transfusion total volume in ml, mean (SD)	2125 (847.8)	2292 (2076.4)	2250 (1829.9)
FFP/platelets given (*n*)	5	10	15
Lowest pH, mean (SD)	7.15* (0.17)	7.27* (0.07)	7.24 (0.12)
Intubated	5	12	17
Intubated >24 h	3	3	6
Days to discharge, median (range)	6 (4–7)	4 (3–11)	5 (3–11)
Anesthetic management			
Regional anesthesia only	1	3	4
Conversion to general	2	12	14
General anesthesia only	3	3	6

*Significant difference $p = 0.02$
[†]2000–2001 hysterectomy *n* = 6, total births *n* = 5811
[‡]2002–2005 hysterectomy *n* = 18, total births *n* = 12,912
[§]2000–2005 (total) hysterectomy *n* = 24, total births *n* = 18,723
CD, cesarean delivery; ARDS, adult respiratory distress syndrome; EBL, estimated blood loss; FFP, fresh frozen plasma; SD, standard deviation

was very time intensive. The patient safety team met numerous times and deliberated on the specifics of our response. These efforts included repeated education of care providers on the diagnosis and management of hypovolemic shock. It is of considerable interest that the entire staff accepted these additional time expenditures as a part of their ongoing self-education and were proud of the outcome and the results (Table 1).

This study design does not allow a determination of which of several interventions may have accounted for improvements in outcome. We strongly believe that the data presented in this chapter support the conclusion that a well reasoned, carefully constructed and multifaceted program focusing on patient safety can improve outcomes, although we cannot attribute any specific improvement to any specific change that was undertaken. We also strongly believe that our experience demonstrates that focusing on the problem of obstetric hemorrhage by the medical and administrative departments in a given hospital can and does lead to improved outcomes. The effort involved is substantial, but rewarding.

CONCLUSION

Prospective data[14,15] corroborate retrospective data[13] on the substantial risk of accreta associated with previa and prior cesarean[16]. Placenta previa is a detectable condition, allowing for a preventive clinical pathway such as that developed in Figure 1 to be implemented. We believe that the preparation that takes place after the early identification of patients at risk is an important component in the ability to improve outcomes in our program.

When confronted with adverse outcomes, principles of quality improvement require that 'systems' thinking takes place. It is tempting to attempt to correct the proximate cause (e.g. an individual physician's lack of attention to detail or suboptimal clinical judgment on an individual case) without addressing the 'systems'. We believe these data support a clear need for a systemic response and hope they are useful to others faced with the task of improving safety in obstetric suites. The specific series of changes in systems at our institution was uniquely adapted to the circumstances we encountered. It is possible that these changes may not be as important or as easily achievable in other areas of the world. However, in any institution's response to major obstetric hemorrhage it is important to keep in mind the numerous and

potentially changing nature of obstacles to system changes and the need to put together a multidisciplinary response to overcome these obstacles. Though this is a challenging task, the result of improvements in outcomes for women with obstetric hemorrhage remains rewarding and, most importantly, achievable.

References

1. Skupski DW, Lowenwirt IP, Weinbaum FI, Brodsky D, Danek MM, Eglinton GS. Improving hostpial systems for the care of women with major obstetric hemorrhage. Obstet Gynecol 2006;107:977–83
2. Kastner ES, Figueroa R, Garry D, Maulik D. Emergency peripartum hysterectomy: Experience at a community teaching hospital. Obstet Gynecol 2002;99:971–5
3. Miller DA, Chollet JA, Goodwin TM. Clinical risk factors for placenta previa-placenta accreta. Am J Obstet Gynecol 1997; 177:210–4
4. ACOG Committee on Obstetric Practice. ACOG Committee Opinion No. 266: Placenta accreta. Obstet Gynecol 2002; 99:169–70
5. Forna F, Miles AM, Jamieson DJ. Emergency peripartum hysterectomy: a comparison of cesarean and postpartum hysterectomy. Am J Obstet Gynecol 2004;190:1440–4
6. Frieden TR, Novello AC, King J. Health Alert: Prevention of maternal deaths through improved management of hemorrhage. Letter from State of New York Department of Health and The New York City Department of Health and Mental Hygiene, August 9, 2004
7. Warshak CR, Ramos GA, Eskander R, et al. Effect of predelivery diagnosis in 99 consecutive cases of placenta accreta. Obstet Gynecol 2010;115:65–9
8. Hull AD, Resnik R. Placenta accreta and postpartum hemorrhage. Clin Obstet Gynecol 2010;53:228–36
9. American College of Surgeons Committee on Trauma. Advanced Trauma Life Support for Doctors. Chapter 3. Shock. Chicago, IL: American College of Surgeons, 1997
10. Sheiner E, Levy A, Katz M, Mazor M. Identifying risk factors for peripartum cesarean hysterectomy. A population-based study. J Reprod Med 2003;48:622–6
11. Knaus WA, Draper EA, Wagner DP, Zimmerman JE. APACHE II: a severity of disease classification system. Crit Care Med 1985;13:818–29
12. Kohn LT, Corrigan JM, Donaldson M. To err is human: building a safer health system. Washington, DC: Institute of Medicine, 1999
13. Greene MF. Vaginal Birth after Cesarean Revisited. N Engl J Med 2004;351:2647–9
14. Silver RM for the MFMU Network of the NICHD. The MFMU cesarean section registry: maternal morbidity associated with multiple repeat cesarean delivery. Abstract. Am J Obstet Gynecol 2004:191:S17
15. Rashid M, Rashid RS. Higher order repeat caesarean sections: how safe are five or more? BJOG 2004;111:1090–4
16. Clark SL, Koonings PP, Phelan JP. Placenta previa/accreta and prior cesarean section. Obstet Gynecol 1985;66:89–92

41

State Mandated Training in Obstetric Hemorrhage: the Illinois Model

R. Malapati, A. Patel and E. S. Linn

INTRODUCTION

Obstetric hemorrhage remains one of the leading causes of maternal morbidity and mortality in the United States as well as in countries that have less abundant resources[1,2]. The death rate has increased according to recent statistics. In the state of Illinois, 20 maternal deaths were recorded during the period of 2001–2006 as a direct result of hemorrhage[3]. Of these, 90% were deemed to be potentially avoidable, as the majority occurred in hospitalized women. The deaths occurred at every level of care throughout the state and affected women from all socioeconomic backgrounds[3].

BACKGROUND

Based on the Maternal Mortality Review Committee (MMRC) report 2007[4], the Illinois Department of Public Health (IDPH) implemented mandatory state-wide training in obstetric hemorrhage in 2009. The main purpose of this project was to reduce maternal mortality and morbidity secondary to hemorrhage through the combined processes of education and simulation drills. The Obstetric Hemorrhage Education Project (OHEP) was then developed and implemented by IDPH. This was based on the hemorrhage project that has been in place in New York[5]. All providers in obstetric care including physicians, nurses, midwives and anesthesia personnel were targeted.

This chapter reports the implementation of this project at a major teaching hospital in the City of Chicago that caters for under-insured and impoverished women, many of whom do not speak English as their first language.

The project focus included:

(1) Risk assessment and preparation for possible hemorrhage;

(2) Estimation of blood loss;

(3) Recognition and treatment of hemorrhage/hypovolemia;

(4) Development of a rapid response team.

COMPONENTS OF THE OBSTETRIC HEMORRHAGE EDUCATION PROJECT

The project was initiated in 2008. All hospitals were given 1 year to implement the curriculum and report to the IDPH. The components of the project were developed by the OHEP workgroup which consisted of ten members, physicians and nurses, representing the perinatal centers across the state. The components were as follows:

(1) Benchmark assessment validation (30 min);

(2) Didactic lecture and discussion (90 min);

(3) Skill stations (30 min);

(4) Simulation drills (30 min each);

(5) Debriefing (60 min).

RESULTS FROM OUR INSTITUTION

Our hospital embarked on the project as mandated. Physicians, midwives, nurses and anesthesia staff were included.

Benchmark assessment

A 25 question pre-test was administered prior to the education session. Questions involved issues related to estimating blood loss, recognizing hemorrhage and hypovolemia, recognizing risk factors for postpartum hemorrhage (PPH) and, finally, detailed knowledge of blood volume replacement. This was followed by didactics and simulation drills.

Six months after the drill, a post-test consisting of exactly the same questions was administered. The results are illustrated in Figure 1, and clearly demonstrate improved provider knowledge and perspectives on obstetric hemorrhage after the training and retention of this knowledge.

Didactic lecture and discussion

A PowerPoint presentation was provided by the state for educating the providers. The presentation consisted of statistics, the basis for the project and each of the objectives of the OHEP. Case scenarios were

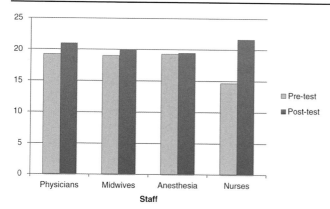

Figure 1 Benchmark test results across providers at a perinatal center. Results are the average scores across providers (maximum score of 25). There was a significant improvement in knowledge and retention among the nurses (36%) compared to physicians (16%), midwives (8%) and anesthesia staff (4%)

presented and discussions focused on steps involved in care of obstetric hemorrhage. A plan to improve care was put forward and discussed.

Skill stations

Skills stations included estimating blood loss, introducing intrauterine balloon tamponade and discussion of surgical techniques, especially the B-Lynch suture. For the first station, providers were expected to visually estimate blood loss. Grape jelly and juice was used to simulate blood and clots on laparotomy sponges, sanitary pads and under-buttock drapes. Providers were then educated on the individual variation of blood loss estimation and how under- or overestimation can influence decision making. Station 2 demonstrated techniques for uterine tamponade. Station 3 demonstrated the B-Lynch suture, where providers were shown how to place the suture using tissue simulation (bovine tongue).

Simulation drill

As the purpose of the drill was to educate all providers on the importance of team work and communication, several different scenarios of obstetric hemorrhage were enacted, and teams were video recorded for subsequent review. The drill was also used to help clarify the potential shortcomings of hospital systems.

Our institution developed a PPH protocol incorporating a rapid response team (Figure 2). A large volume transfusion protocol was initiated in conjunction with the blood bank that when activated allows providers to access blood products within 10 min (Figure 3).

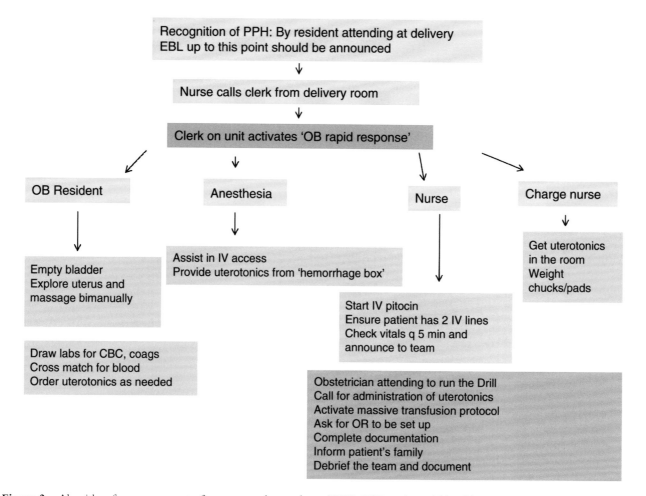

Figure 2 Algorithm for management of postpartum hemorrhage (PPH). EBL, estimated blood loss; OB, obstetric; CBC, complete blood count; coags, coagulation profile; OR, operating room

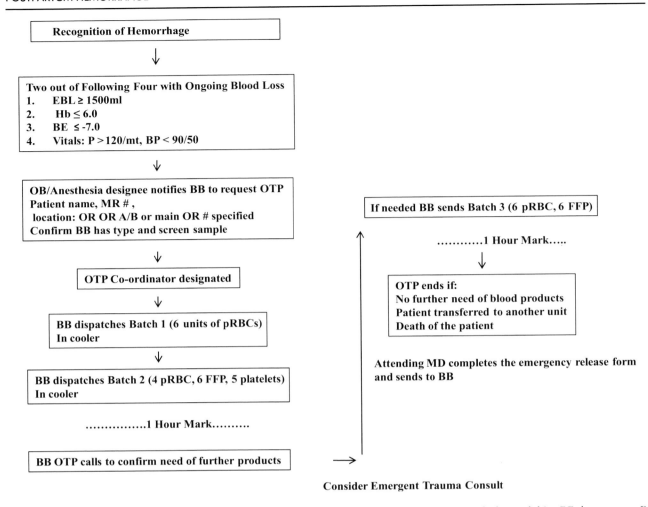

Figure 3 Obstetric hemorrhage large volume transfusion protocol. EBL, estimated blood loss; Hb, hemoglobin; BE, base excess; P, pulse; BP, blood pressure; OB, obstetric; BB, blood bank; OTP, obstetric transfusion protocol; MR, medical record number; OR, operating room; RBC, red blood cells; FFP, fresh frozen plasma

CONCLUSION

Following the initial drill and education, each hospital is currently mandated to perform the drills annually. Every obstetric center has an identified physician and nurse 'champion' who go through the 'train the trainers' session. These trainers are then responsible for carrying out the drills at their individuals centers. Providers who practice at multiple centers have to go through the education session, skills station and drill at one institution, but are required to go through the skills station at each of the centers in order to become familiar with each center's rapid response and emergency protocols.

Currently IDPH is in the process of receiving the results of the OHEP project from all the obstetric centers and evaluating the results to determine whether this has had an impact on maternal morbidity and mortality secondary to hemorrhage.

A similar initiative has been undertaken by the California Maternal Quality Care Collaborative (CMQCC)[6]. The task force was co-chaired by both nurse and physician team leaders. The goal was to identify key priorities for action and development of a comprehensive hemorrhage guideline. The obstetric hemorrhage care guideline is presented in three formats: a comprehensive bedside checklist to guide team care and two cognitive aids (a table and a flowchart) that present the most critical points in different formats for ease of use by clinicians.

References

1. World Health Organization. Maternal mortality in 2005 : estimates developed by WHO, UNICEF, UNFPA, and the World Bank. Geneva: WHO, 2005
2. Berg CJ, Callaghan WM, Syverson C, Henderson Z. Pregnancy-related mortality in the United States, 1998 to 2005. Obstet Gynecol 2010;116:1302–9
3. Illinois Department of Public Health. Hemorrhage Education Project 2008. Illinois Department of Public Health, 2008
4. Hoyert DL. Maternal mortality and related concepts. National Center for Health Statistics. Vital Health Stat 2007;(33):1–13
5. Novello A. Health Advisory: Prevention of Maternal Deaths Through Improved Management of Hemorrhage. State of New York Department of Health, 2004
6. Bingham D, Lyndon A, Lagrew D, Main EK. A state-wide obstetric hemorrhage quality improvement initiative. MCN Am J Matern Child Nurs 2011;36:297–304

Section 8

Therapy for Atonic Bleeding

42

Management of Postpartum Hemorrhage at the Community Level at Home

N. Prata

The ability to manage postpartum hemorrhage (PPH) at the community level should be an essential element in programs aiming to address PPH, the main cause of maternal mortality[1]. In this regard, the efficacy, safety and importance of misoprostol use for PPH management has been established (see Chapters 32–35), with a recommended dose of 600 µg orally immediately after delivery[2]. Misoprostol's most significant impact is at the household level, where most deliveries occur in many parts of the world[3].

Three randomized controlled trials[4–6] (Table 1) and seven intervention trials have successfully tested such technology in home births, with self administration by the delivering woman[7,8] or by a traditional birth attendant (TBA)[9]. The differences in PPH reduction when misoprostol is used at the community level (Table 1) are not unexpected, because these studies use different methods of measuring and collecting blood after delivery. Such differences can influence the outcome of interest, blood loss of 500 ml or more. Nevertheless, in all three studies, the 95% confidence intervals around the relative risk overlap, indicating a clinically important range in PPH reduction in community studies, but not necessarily statistically significant differences between studies.

Scant data exist on the use of misoprostol for treatment of PPH at the community level. In one intervention study conducted in Tanzania, Prata and colleagues demonstrated that TBAs, who assist in most deliveries, were able to diagnose PPH and effectively and safely administer 1000 µg of rectal misoprostol to control PPH[10]. This study took place in rural Kigoma, an area in Tanzania where TBAs were trained to administer 1000 µg (5 tablets) of misoprostol rectally using gloves after visual identification of PPH using the blood loss collection garment the kanga. TBAs in the control areas were similarly trained to diagnose PPH and refer the patient to the nearest facility. Of the 454 women recruited in the treatment areas, 2% were referred to the nearest facility for additional interventions after being diagnosed with PPH and receiving misoprostol at home. In the control areas, 395 women were recruited and 19% required transfer and additional interventions for PPH management.

Three years after the study, Prata and colleagues returned to the original sites and reported continued use of misoprostol by TBAs in a safe and effective manner[11]. The second study on long-term community-based use of misoprostol by TBAs assessed knowledge, use, effectiveness and acceptability of the drug for PPH management in home births. Using a cluster design, women delivering between July 2004 and May 2007 were interviewed. This assessment found 239 women who were diagnosed with PPH. Of these, 71.5% were administered 1000 µg of misoprostol at home, while only 1.8% needed additional interventions.

Overall, published studies show that the ability to manage PPH in home births resulted in significant reductions in the number of women with PPH, the number of referrals and the need for additional interventions, all of which represent crucial issues in low resource settings.

Having said this, it is important to remember that effective community level interventions for PPH management constantly face the challenge of accurate blood loss measurement. Despite this, however, blood loss measurement can be standardized by employing local tools. Similar to the 'kanga' in Tanzania[12], other garments/tools have been used with similar success.

Table 1 Summary of studies showing efficacy of misoprostol for postpartum hemorrhage (PPH) prevention at community level

Author, location	Study type	Misoprostol administered at home by	Blood loss ≥500 ml	
			RR	95% CI
Mobeen et al., 2011[4], Pakistan	Placebo controlled RCT	TBAs	0.76	0.59–0.97
Derman et al., 2006[5], India	Placebo controlled RCT	Auxiliary nurse midwives	0.53	0.39–0.74
Walraven et al., 2005[6], Gambia	RCT ergomethrine vs. misoprostol	TBAs	0.77	0.60–0.98

RCT, randomized controlled trial; TBA, traditional birth attendant

These include the 'mat' in Bangladesh, the 'chittengue' in Zambia and the 'moda' in northern Nigeria, amongst others. The mat is a square piece of cotton fabric of pink color covered on the bottom side with a plastic sheet. The plastic sheet is of the same size and is stitched in the borders of the fabric. The size of the mat is standardized so that it collects 500 ml of blood when soaked. The chittengue is a piece of local fabric, similar to the kanga, but it is called different names in different countries, for example, it is called 'kapulana' in Mozambique. The moda is a local name for a plastic container (shaped like a cup) used to gather water by women, which holds exactly 500 ml of liquid.

Misoprostol should be available to all women delivering at home. It will be many decades before all women in low resource settings can receive skilled attention at delivery. In the meantime, misoprostol has the potential to make a significant impact in reducing PPH associated morbidity and mortality.

References

1. Khan KS, Wojdyla D, Say L, et al. WHO analysis of causes of maternal death: a systematic review. Lancet 2006;367: 1066–74
2. Alfirevic Z, Blum J, Walraven G, et al. Prevention of postpartum hemorrhage with misoprostol. Int J Gynaecol Obstet 2007;99(Suppl 2):S198–201
3. Prata N, Sreenivas A, Vahidniaa F, et al. Saving maternal lives in resource-poor settings: Facing reality. Health Policy 2008; 89:131–48
4. Mobeen N, Durocher J, Zuberi N, et al. Administration of misoprostol by trained traditional birth attendants to prevent postpartum haemorrhage I home births in Pakistan: a randomized placebo controlled trial. BJOG 2011;118:353–61
5. Derman RJ, Kodkany BS, Goudar SS, et al. Oral misoprostol on preventing pastpartum haemorrhage inresource poor communities: a randomized controlled trial. Lancet 2006; 368:1248–53
6. Walraven G, Blum J, Dampha Y, et al. Misoprostol in the management of the third stage of labour in the home setting in rural Gambia: a randomized controlled trial. BJOG 2005; 112:1277–83
7. Sanghvi H, Ansari N, Prata N, et al. Prevention of postpartum hemorrhage at home birth in Afghanistan. Int J Gynaecol Obstet 2010;108:276–81
8. Rajbhandari S, Hodgins S, Sanghvi H, et al. Misoprostol Study Group. Expanding uterotonic protection following childbirth through community-based distribution of misoprostol: operations research study in Nepal. Int J Gynaecol Obstet 2010;108: 282–8
9. Prata N, Gessessew A, Abraha AK, et al. Prevention of postpartum hemorrhage: options for home births in rural Ethiopia. Afr J Reprod Health 2009;13:87–95
10. Prata N, Mbaruku G, Campbell M, et al. Controlling postpartum hemorrhage after home births in Tanzania. Int J Gynaecol Obstet 2005;90:51–5
11. Prata N, Mbaruku G, Grossman AA, et al. Community-based availability of misoprostol: is it safe? Afr J Reprod Health 2009;13:117–28
12. Prata N, Mbaruku G, Campbell M. Using the kanga to measure postpartum blood loss. Int J Gynaecol Obstet 2005; 89:49–50

43

Standard Medical Therapy for Postpartum Hemorrhage

J. Unterscheider, F. Breathnach and M. Geary

INTRODUCTION

Failure of the uterus to contract and retract following childbirth has for centuries been recognized as the most striking cause of postpartum hemorrhage (PPH) and complicates up to 10% of pregnancies globally. In the developing world, PPH is responsible for one maternal death every 7 minutes[1].

In the 19th century, uterine atony was treated by intrauterine placement of various agents with the aim of achieving a tamponade effect. 'A lemon imperfectly quartered' or 'a large bull's bladder distended with water' were employed for this purpose, with apparent success. Douching with vinegar or iron perchloride was also reported[2,3]. Historically, the first uterotonic drugs were ergot alkaloids, followed by oxytocin and, finally, prostaglandins.

Ergot, the alkaloid-containing product of the fungus *Claviceps purpurea* that grows on rye, was recognized for centuries as having uterotonic properties and is the substance referred to by John Stearns in 1808 as '*pulvis parturiens*' (a powder [for] childbirth), at which time it was used as an agent to accelerate labor[4]. By the end of the 19th century, however, recognition of the potential hazards associated with ergot use in labor, namely its ability to cause uterine hyperstimulation and stillbirth, had tempered enthusiasm for its use. Focus was diverted toward its role in preventing and treating PPH at a time when, according to an 1870 report, maternal mortality in England approached one in 20 births[5].

Attempts to isolate the active alkaloids from ergot were not successful until the early 20th century, when Barber and Dale isolated ergotoxine in 1906[3]. Initially thought to be a pure substance, this agent was subsequently found to comprise four alkaloids, and in 1935 Moir and Dudley were credited with isolating ergometrine, the active aqueous extract 'to which ergot rightly owes its long-established reputation as the pulvis parturiens'[6,7]. Moir reported on its clinical use in 1936, stating[7]:

'. . . the chief use of ergometrine is in the prevention and treatment of postpartum haemorrhage. Here the ergometrine effect is seen at its best. If after the delivery of the placenta the uterus is unduly relaxed, the administration of ergometrine, 1 mg by mouth or 0.5 mg by injection, will quickly cause a firm contraction of the organ. If severe haemorrhage has already set in, it is highly recommended that the drug should be given by the intravenous route. For this purpose one-third of the standard size ampoule may be injected or, for those who wish accurate dosage, a special ampoule containing 0.125 mg is manufactured. An effect may be looked for in less than one minute.'

Another uterotonic agent, oxytocin, the hypothalamic polypeptide hormone released by the posterior pituitary, was discovered in 1909 by Sir Henry Dale[8] and synthesized in 1954 by du Vigneaud[9]. The development of oxytocin constituted the first synthesis of a polypeptide hormone and gained du Vigneaud a Nobel Prize for his work.

The third group of uterotonics comprises the ever-expanding prostaglandin family. The prostaglandins were discovered in 1935 by a group led by Swedish physiologist Ulf von Euler[10] who found that extracts of seminal vesicles or of human semen were capable of causing contraction of uterine tissue and lowering blood pressure. The term 'prostaglandin' evolved from von Euler's belief that the active material came exclusively from the prostate gland. This family of 'eicosanoids', 20-carbon fatty acids, was subsequently found to be produced in a variety of tissues and capable of mediating a myriad of physiologic and pathologic processes. Prostaglandins, by virtue of their ability to cause tetanic myometrial activity, are increasingly used as adjunctive therapy to standard oxytocin and ergometrine to treat PPH resulting from uterine atony (see Section 8).

This chapter is devoted to critical evaluation of the standard pharmacological methods available to treat uterine atony, with particular focus on agent selection based on effectiveness, safety profile, ease of administration, cost and applicability in low resource settings.

UTERINE ATONY

Powerful efficient contractions of the myometrium are essential to arrest blood loss after delivery. The resultant compression of the uterine vasculature serves to halt the 800 ml/min blood flow in the placental bed. Recognition of a soft, boggy uterus in the setting of a postpartum bleed alerts the attendant to uterine atony.

The particular contribution that uterine atony makes toward PPH is so well known that a universal reflex action when faced with excessive postpartum bleeding is to induce uterine contraction using bimanual massage. Prompt recognition of this condition and institution of uterotonic therapy will effectively terminate the majority of cases of hemorrhage. Once effective uterine contractility is established, persistent bleeding should prompt the search for retained placental fragments, genital tract trauma or a bleeding diathesis.

Astute risk assessment is crucial in identifying women at increased risk of uterine atony, thereby allowing preventive measures to be instituted and for delivery to take place where transfusion and anesthetic facilities are available. That having been said, one must remember that the majority of parturients with one or more risk factors do not bleed excessively and, conversely, large numbers of women with no risk factors experience true hemorrhage.

The established risk factors associated with uterine atony are outlined in Table 1. It is worth noting that multiparity, hitherto believed to be a significant risk factor, has not emerged as having an association with uterine atony in recent studies[11-13]. Whereas previous PPH confers a 2–4-fold increased risk of hemorrhage compared to that in women without such a history[13,14]. The presence of leiomyomata may result in more than a two-fold increase in the risk for PPH[15].

It is appropriate that women with these predisposing risk factors should deliver in a hospital with adequate facilities to manage PPH. Prophylactic measures include appropriate hospital booking for women at risk and correction of anemia before delivery, active management of the third stage of labor, ensuring the availability of cross-matched blood and access to interventional radiology services and critical care.

Table 1 Risk factors for uterine atony

Factors associated with uterine overdistension
Multiple pregnancy
Polyhydramnios
Fetal macrosomia

Labor-related factors
Induction of labor
Prolonged labor
Precipitate labor
Augmented labor
Instrumental delivery
Manual removal of placenta

Use of uterine relaxants
Deep anesthesia (especially halogenated anesthetic agents)
Magnesium sulfate
Nitroglycerin

Intrinsic factors
Previous postpartum hemorrhage
Previous cesarean section
Antepartum hemorrhage (abruptio or previa)
Chorioamnionitis
Obesity
Uterine fibroids
Age > 35 years

Recognizing the risks of pulmonary embolus and alloimmunization associated with blood transfusion, intraoperative cell salvage has recently been introduced into obstetric practice in cases where massive obstetric hemorrhage is anticipated or in the management of patients who decline blood transfusion (see Chapter 72). The fact that uterine atony occurs unpredictably in women with no identifiable predisposing risk factors underpins the need for strict protocols for PPH management to be in place in every unit that provides obstetric care (see Chapters 40 and 41).

OXYTOCIN

With timely and appropriate use of uterotonic therapy, the majority of women with uterine atony can avoid surgical intervention. Stimulation of uterine contraction is usually achieved in the first instance by bimanual uterine massage and the injection of oxytocin (either intramuscularly or intravenously), with or without ergometrine. The mode of action of oxytocin involves stimulation of the upper uterine segment to contract in a rhythmical fashion. Owing to its short plasma half-life (mean 3 min), a continuous intravenous infusion is required in order to maintain the uterus in a contracted state[16]. The usual dose is 40 IU in 500 ml of saline, with the dosage rate adjusted according to response (typical infusion rate 10 IU/h or 2 ml/min). When administered intravenously, the onset of action is almost instantaneous and plateau concentration is achieved after 30 minutes. By contrast, intramuscular administration results in a slower onset of action (3–7 min) but a longer lasting clinical effect (up to 60 min).

Metabolism of oxytocin is via the renal and hepatic routes. Its antidiuretic effect, amounting to 5% of the antidiuretic effect of the endogenous peptide hormone vasopressin, can result in water toxicity, especially if administered in large volumes of electrolyte-free solutions. This degree of water overload can manifest itself with headache, vomiting, drowsiness and convulsions. On the other hand, rapid intravenous bolus administration of undiluted oxytocin results in relaxation of vascular smooth muscle, which can lead to hypotension. The intravenous route is contraindicated in known hypersensitivity or profound hypotension. It is therefore best given intramuscularly or by dilute intravenous infusion. Oxytocin is stable at temperatures up to 25°C, but refrigeration is recommended if stored for extended periods to prolong its shelf-life.

Disadvantages of oxytocin are its short half-life, the requirement for parenteral administration, and the need for refrigeration for storage. The use and re-use of syringes in low resource settings carry the risk of spreading infectious diseases such as HIV and hepatitis. Uniject injection devices have been proposed for some clinical circumstances, whereby 10 IU of oxytocin is administered in prefilled, disposable and non-reusable vials[17]. The long-acting oxytocin analog carbetocin with a more sustained action, similar to that of ergometrine but without its associated side-effects, may offer advantages over standard oxytocic therapy[18]. Comparative studies of carbetocin for the prevention of PPH have identified enhanced effectiveness of this analog when compared with an oxytocin infusion[19,20] (see Chapter 44).

Whether the administration of oxytocin infusion (40 IU/h over 4 hours) after cesarean delivery is beneficial was the subject of the Elective Caesarean Section Syntocinon Infusion Trial (ECSSIT), a multicenter randomized trial. Over 2000 patients, who underwent elective cesarean delivery at term, were randomized to either oxytocin bolus or oxytocin bolus and infusion. Results showed no difference in the occurrence of major hemorrhage between the groups (bolus and infusion 15.7% versus bolus only 16.0%). However, oxytocin infusion was found to be beneficial in patients who were delivered by a junior obstetrician[22].

ERGOMETRINE

In contrast to oxytocin, the administration of ergometrine results in a sustained tonic uterine contraction via stimulation of myometrial α-adrenergic receptors. Both upper and lower uterine segments are stimulated to contract in a tetanic manner[16]. Intramuscular injection of the standard 0.25 mg dose results in an onset of action of 2–5 min. Metabolism is via the hepatic route, and the mean plasma half-life is 30 min. Nonetheless, the clinical effect of ergometrine persists for approximately 3 h. The co-administration of ergometrine and oxytocin results in a complementary effect, with oxytocin achieving an immediate response and ergometrine a more sustained action.

Common side-effects of ergometrine include nausea, vomiting and dizziness; all are more striking when the intravenous route is used. As a result of its vasoconstrictive effect via stimulation of α-adrenergic receptors, hypertension can occur. Contraindications to the use of ergometrine therefore include hypertension (including pre-eclampsia), heart disease and peripheral vascular disease. If given intravenously, where its effect is almost immediate, it should be administered over 60 s with careful monitoring of pulse and blood pressure. Its heat lability is relevant to the developing world in particular. Ergometrine is both heat and light sensitive, and should be stored at temperatures below 8°C and away from light.

The product Syntometrine® (5 units oxytocin and 0.5 mg ergometrine) combines the rapid onset of oxytocin with the prolonged effect of ergometrine. The mild vasodilatory property of oxytocin may counterbalance the vasopressor effect of ergometrine.

First-line treatment of uterine atony, along with bimanual massage, therefore involves administration of oxytocin or ergometrine as an intramuscular or diluted intravenous bolus, followed by repeat dosage if no effect is observed after 5 min and complemented by continuous intravenous oxytocin infusion. Atony that is refractory to these first-line oxytocics warrants prostaglandin (PG) therapy from a medical point of view, the institution of bimanual massage at the bare minimum, inspection of the vulva, vagina and cervix, assessment of the presence of retained tissues, and other modalities mentioned in this text.

CARBOPROST

Carboprost (15-methyl PGF2α) acts as a smooth muscle stimulant and is a recognized second-line agent for use in the management of postpartum uterine atony unresponsive to oxytocin or ergometrine. It is an analog of PGF2α (dinoprost) with a longer duration of action than its parent compound, which is attributed to its resistance to inactivation by oxidation at the 15-position. Available in single-dose vials of 0.25 mg, it may be administered by deep intramuscular injection or, alternatively, by direct intramyometrial injection. The latter route of administration is achieved either under direct vision at cesarean section or transabdominally or transvaginally following vaginal delivery and has the advantage of a significantly quicker onset of action[23,24]. Peripheral intramuscular injection yields peak plasma concentrations at 15 min in contrast to less than 5 min for the intramyometrial route. Using a 20-gauge spinal needle, intravascular injection can be avoided by pre-injection aspiration, and intramyometrial rather than intracavitary placement of the needle can be confirmed by observing resistance on injection, as described by Bigrigg and colleagues[25]. The dose may be repeated every 15 min up to a maximum cumulative dose of 2 mg (eight doses), although, in reported case series, the majority of patients require no more than one dose.

Reported efficacy is high. Successful arrest of atonic hemorrhage was reported in 13/14 patients by Bigrigg and colleagues[25]. The largest case series to date[24], by Oleen and Mariano, involved a multicenter surveillance study of 237 cases of PPH refractory to standard oxytocics and reported an efficacy of 88%. The majority of women in this study required a single dose only.

Owing to its vasoconstrictive and bronchoconstrictive effects, carboprost can result in nausea, vomiting, diarrhea, pyrexia and bronchospasm. Contraindications therefore include cardiac and pulmonary disease. The cost of carboprost makes it unsuitable for consideration in low resource settings. Furthermore, it is both light and heat sensitive and must be kept refrigerated at 4°C.

MISOPROSTOL

Misoprostol is a synthetic analog of prostaglandin E1 which selectively binds to myometrial EP-2/EP-3 prostanoid receptors, thereby promoting uterine contractility. (Its use and clinical efficacy are discussed in Section 6) It is metabolized via the hepatic route. It may be given orally, sublingually, vaginally, rectally or via direct intrauterine placement. The rectal route of administration is associated with a longer onset of action, lower peak levels and a more favorable side-effect profile when compared with the oral or sublingual route. The results of an international multicenter, randomized trial of oral misoprostol as a prophylactic agent for the third stage of labor showed it to be less effective at preventing PPH than parenteral oxytocin[26]. Fifteen per cent of women in the misoprostol arm required additional uterotonics compared with 11% in the oxytocin group. This may be due to its longer onset of action (20–30 min to achieve peak serum levels compared to 3 min for oxytocin). However, owing to the fact that its more prolonged time interval required to achieve peak serum levels may make it a more suitable agent for protracted uterine bleeding, there is mounting interest in its role as a therapeutic rather than a prophylactic agent.

The use of rectal misoprostol for the treatment of PPH unresponsive to oxytocin and ergometrine was first reported by O'Brien and colleagues[27] in a descriptive study of 14 patients. Sustained uterine contraction was reported in almost all women within 3 min of its administration. However, no control group was included for comparison. A single-blinded, randomized trial of misoprostol 800 µg rectally versus Syntometrine intramuscularly plus oxytocin by intravenous infusion found that misoprostol resulted in cessation of bleeding within 20 min in 30/32 cases (94%) compared to 21/32 (66%) for the comparative agents[28]. A Cochrane review supports these findings, suggesting that rectal misoprostol in a dose of 800 µg could be a useful 'first-line' drug for the PPH[29].

Although oxytocin is the drug of choice in the management of obstetric hemorrhage, misoprostol is an excellent and widely used alternative when the use of oxytocin is not possible. The latter has the significant advantage of low cost (US$ 0.10/ tablet), thermostability, long shelf life, light stability and lack of requirement for sterile needles and syringes for administration. The optimal dosage of misoprostol is the subject of ongoing debate (see Chapter 34). Physiological studies have shown uterotonic effects with doses as low as 200 µg. In their systematic review, Hofmeyr et al. state that 400 µg misoprostol may be safer than and just as effective as 600 µg for PPH prophylaxis[30]. For treatment, doses lower than 800 µg may be as effective. The same review describes that 8/11 maternal deaths occurred in women receiving more than 600 µg misoprostol which raises concern over its safety or the accuracy in ascribing the cause of hemorrhage to atony. Further research needs to address the smallest dose of the drug that is effective and safe.

The need to evaluate the effectiveness of misoprostol is ongoing in settings where other standard uterotonic agents are not available. Recently the community-based distribution of misoprostol has been proposed as a means of reducing maternal mortality rates in regions where home births are prevalent. In many countries, women are currently empowered to self-administer 600 µg misoprostol orally to prevent PPH (see Chapter 42). WHO initially welcomed this approach[31], but more recently due to the unresolved concern regarding a possible increase in the risk of maternal mortality concluded that its use should not be extended to distribution on a community level[32]. There is an urgent need for FIGO and WHO to release a joint statement for the use of misoprostol in developing countries and the circumstances under which it is best used.

Side-effects of misoprostol are mainly gastrointestinal and are dose and route dependent. The commonly reported side-effects of shivering and pyrexia are usually self-regulating and certainly not life threatening. Moreover, shivering occurs commonly even when misoprostol has not been administered. Oral and sublingual routes of administration achieve a higher and quicker maximum plasma concentration than vaginal or rectal administration, which results in higher rates of shivering and high grade fever[33].

OTHER PROSTAGLANDINS

Dinoprost (prostaglandin F2α) is used via intramyometrial injection at doses of 0.5–1.0 mg with good effect[34]. Low-dose intrauterine infusion via a Foley catheter has also been described, consisting of 20 mg dinoprost in 500 ml saline at 3–4 ml/min for 10 min, then 1 ml/min. Bleeding was arrested in all but one of 18 patients and no adverse outcome was reported. As mentioned earlier, however, this agent has a shorter duration of activity than carboprost and indeed has been unavailable in the US since the 1980s where its withdrawal was attributed to financial considerations.

Prostaglandin E2 (dinoprostone), in spite of its vasodilatory properties, causes smooth muscle contraction in the pregnant uterus, thus making it a potentially suitable uterotonic agent. Its principal indication is in pre-induction cervical priming, but intrauterine placement of dinoprostone has been successfully employed as a treatment for uterine atony[35]. The vasodilatory effect of dinoprostone, however, renders it unsuitable for use in the hypotensive or hypovolemic patient. It may, however, be of use in women with cardiorespiratory disease in whom carboprost is contraindicated.

Experience with gemeprost, a prostaglandin E1 analog, in pessary formulation delivered directly into the uterine cavity or placed in the posterior vaginal fornix, is largely anecdotal[36–38]. Its mode of action resembles that of PGF2α. Rectal administration has also been reported. A retrospective series of 14 cases in which rectal gemeprost 1 mg was used for PPH unresponsive to oxytocin and ergometrine reported prompt cessation of bleeding in all cases, with no apparent maternal adverse sequelae[39].

HEMOSTATICS: TRANEXAMIC ACID AND RECOMBINANT ACTIVATED FACTOR VII

The antifibrinolytic agent, tranexamic acid, prevents binding of plasminogen and plasmin to fibrin; as such, it may well have a role in the control of intractable PPH, particularly where coagulation is compromised. A recent review[40] suggests that tranexamic acid reduces the amount of blood loss at cesarean and

Table 2 Medical uterotonic therapy

Agent	Dose	Cautions
Oxytocin (Pitocin®, Syntocinon®)	5 or 10 IU im/iv followed by iv infusion of 40 IU in 500 ml crystalloid titrated versus response (e.g. 10 IU/h)	Hypotension if given by rapid iv bolus. Water intoxication with large volume
Ergometrine (Ergonovine®)	0.25 mg im/iv	Contraindicated in hypertensive patients. Can cause nausea/vomiting/dizziness
Carboprost (15-methyl PGF2α) (Hemabate®)	0.25 mg im repeat every 15 min to maximum dose of 2 mg (8 doses)	Bronchospasm (caution in patients with asthma, hypertension, cardiorespiratory disease)
Dinoprost (PGF2α) (Prostin F2α®)	0.5–1 mg intramyometrial or 20 mg in 500 ml N/saline infused via Foley catheter into uterine cavity	Bronchospasm, nausea, vomiting and diarrhea can occur
Dinoprostone (Prostin®/Prepidil®)	2 mg pr 2-hourly	Hypotension
Gemeprost (Cervagem®)	1–2 mg intrauterine placement/1 mg pr	Gastrointestinal disturbance
Misoprostol (Cytotec®)	0.6–1 mg pr/intracavitary 0.6–0.8 mg orally/sublingually	Gastrointestinal disturbance, shivering, pyrexia
Tranexamic acid (Cyclokapron®)	1 g 8-hourly iv	May increase risk of thrombosis
rFVIIa (Novoseven®)	60–90 μg/kg iv	Fever, hypertension

im, intramuscularly; iv, intravenously; pr, per rectum

vaginal deliveries, and reduces the requirement for blood transfusion. Tranexamic acid (1 g) is cheap and appears to be safe and effective in the prevention and management of bleeding during pregnancy. The currently ongoing World Maternal Antifibrinolytic Trial (WOMAN)[41], a randomized double-blind placebo-controlled trial, aims to determine the effect of early administration of tranexamic acid on mortality, hysterectomy and other morbidities (surgical interventions, blood transfusion, risk of non-fatal vascular events) in 15,000 women with clinically diagnosed PPH.

The use of recombinant activated factor VII (rFVIIa, Novoseven®) as a hemostatic agent for refractory PPH is described elsewhere in this volume. The mode of action of this agent involves enhancement of the rate of thrombin generation, leading to formation of a fully stabilized fibrin plug that is resistant to premature lysis. Currently, recombinant factor VIIa (60–90 μg/kg) is advocated only after failure of other conventional therapies including embolization or conservative surgery, but prior to peripartum hysterectomy[42]. A recent review of 272 published cases showed that Novoseven arrested or reduced bleeding in 85% of cases[43]. Prospective randomized controlled trials are highly desirable, but may not be forthcoming because of the reluctance of clinicians to enter their patients in such trials. A full discussion can be found in Chapter 50 of this textbook.

CONCLUSIONS

Although the decline in the number of deaths from obstetric hemorrhage in the developed world is impressive, the developing world has benefited little from the many medical advances of the past two decades, especially when one considers deaths directly related to PPH. Even in the UK, the 2006–2008 triennial report[44] recorded five maternal deaths from PPH. In 60% of these deaths, there was a concern over substandard care; in particular, routine observation in the postpartum period was lacking, or it was not appreciated that bleeding was occurring. Regular observations of pulse and blood pressure should be

made postdelivery. The use of modified early obstetric warning score (MEOWS) charts should alert caregivers to abnormal trends in hemodynamic measurements that require further action. Obstetricians, midwives and hospital management staff need to be vigilant and ensure that care is optimized through use of regular drills and skills (see Chapter 36) and adherence to national guidelines to further reduce hemorrhage-related maternal deaths[44]. Integral to any protocol on management of PPH will be a stepwise approach to achieving effective uterine contractility.

The successful management of uterine atony depends on staff being thoroughly familiar with the pharmacologic agents available to them with respect to dosage, route of administration and safety profile (Table 2). Application of such protocols achieves a successful reduction in the morbidity associated with PPH[45]. It is tempting to credit the second- or third-line agent with successfully controlling a PPH; however, it is certainly plausible that a synergistic effect is observed where a combination of uterotonics is used.

The global quest for an 'ideal' uterotonic agent must take into account the fact that what is applicable in one setting may have no relevance in another. The cost and instability of standard oxytocic drugs are prohibitive in many low resource settings. *Safety and parallel efficacy should therefore suffice as parameters by which an agent such as misoprostol is judged rather than demonstration of clinical superiority over established uterotonics.* There is an urgent need for a consensus statement to be issued by FIGO and WHO to make misoprostol available in communities where home births are prevalent. The self-administration of misoprostol is practiced in many developing countries and may be the single most efficient way to reduce maternal mortality.

References

1. Potts M, Prata N, Sahin-Hodoglugil NN. Maternal mortality: one death every 7 min. Lancet 2010;375:1762–3
2. Davis DD. The Principles and Practice of Obstetric Medicine. London: Rebman, 1896:602
3. De Costa C. St Anthony's fire and living ligatures: a short history of ergometrine. Lancet 2002;359:1768–70

4. Thoms H. John Stearns and pulvis parturiens. Am J Obstet Gynecol 1931;22:418–23
5. Edgar JC. The Practice of Obstetrics. Philadelphia: Blakiston, 1913:475–7
6. Dudley HW, Moir C. The substance responsible for the traditional clinical effect of ergot. BMJ 1935;1:520–3
7. Moir C. Clinical experiences with the new alkaloid, ergometrine. BMJ 1936;ii:799–801
8. Dale HH. The action of extracts of the pituitary body. Biochem J 1909;4:427–47
9. du Vigneaud V, Ressler C, Swan JM, et al. The synthesis of an octapeptide amide with the hormonal activity of oxytocin. J Am Chem Soc 1954;75:4879–80
10. von Euler U, Adler E, Hellstrom H, et al. On the specific vasodilating and plain muscle stimulating substance from accessory genital glands in man and certain animals (prostaglandin and vesiglandin). J Physiol (London) 1937;88:213–34
11. Stones RW, Paterson CM, Saunders NJ. Risk factors for major obstetric haemorrhage. Eur J Obstet Gynaecol Reprod Biol 1993;48:15–8
12. Tsu VD. Postpartum haemorrhage in Zimbabwe: a risk factor analysis. BJOG 1993;100:327–33
13. Waterstone M, Bewley S, Wolfe C. Incidence and predictors of severe obstetric morbidity: case-control study. BMJ 2001;322:1089–94
14. Hall MH, Halliwell R, Carr-Hill R. Concomitant and repeated happenings of complications of the third stage of labour. BJOG 1985;92:732–8
15. Qidwai GI, Caughey AB, Jacoby AF. Obstetric outcomes in women with sonographically identified uterine leiomyomata. Obstet Gynecol 2006;107:376–82
16. Dollery C, ed. Therapeutic Drugs, 2nd edn. Edinburgh: Churchill Livingstone, 1999
17. Tsu VD, Sutanto A, Vaidya K, Coffey P, Widjaya A. Oxytocin in prefilled Uniject injection devices for managing third-stage labor in Indonesia. Int J Gynaecol Obstet 2003;83:103–11
18. Hunter DJ, Schulz P, Wassenaar W. Effect of carbetocin, a long-acting oxytocin analog on the postpartum uterus. Clin Pharmacol Ther 1992;52:60–7
19. Boucher M, Nimrod CA, Tawagi GF, et al. Comparison of carbetocin and oxytocin for the prevention of postpartum hemorrhage following vaginal delivery: a double-blind randomized trial. J Obstet Gynaecol Can 2004;26:481–8
20. Dansereau J, Joshi AK, Helewa ME, et al. Double-blind comparison of carbetocin versus oxytocin in prevention of uterine atony after caesarean section. Am J Obstet Gynecol 1999;180:670–6
21. Murphy DJ, Carey M, Montgomery AA, Sheehan SR and The ECSSIT Study Group. Study Protocol. ECSSIT-Elective Caesarean Section Syntocinon® Infusion Trial. A multi-centre randomised controlled trial of oxytocin (Syntocinon ®) 5IU bolus and placebo infusion versus oxytocin 5IU bolus and 40IU infusion for the control of blood loss at elective caesarean section. BMC Pregnancy and Childbirth 2009;9:36
22. Sheehan SR, Montgomery AA, Carey M, McAuliffe FM, Eogan M, Gleeson R, Geary M, Murphy DJ; ECSSIT Study Group. Oxytocin bolus versus oxytocin bolus and infusion for control of blood loss at elective caesarean section: double blind, placebo controlled, randomised trial. BMJ 2011;343:4661
23. Jacobs M, Arias F. Intramyometrial PGF2α in treatment of severe postpartum hemorrhage. Obstet Gynecol 1980;55:665–6
24. Oleen MA, Mariano JP. Controlling refractory postpartum hemorrhage with hemabate sterile solution. Am J Obstet Gynecol 1990;162:205–8
25. Bigrigg A, Chui D, Chissell S, et al. Use of intramyometrial 15-methyl prostaglandin F2α to control atonic postpartum

haemorrhage following vaginal delivery and failure of conventional therapy. BJOG 1991;98:734–6
26. Gülmezoglu AM, Villar J, Ngoc NT, et al. WHO multicentre randomised trial of misoprostol in the management of the third stage of labour. Lancet 2001;358:689–95
27. O'Brien P, El-Refaey H, Geary M, et al. Rectally administered misoprostol for the treatment of postpartum haemorrhage unresponsive to oxytocin and ergometrine: a descriptive study. Obstet Gynecol 1998;92:212–4
28. Lokugamage AU, Sullivan KR, Niculescu I, et al. A randomized study comparing rectally administered misoprostol versus syntometrine combined with an oxytocin infusion for the cessation of primary postpartum haemorrhage. Acta Obstet Gynecol Scand 2001;80:835–9
29. Mousa HA, Alfirevic Z. Treatment for primary postpartum haemorrhage. Cochrane Database Syst Rev 2003;(1): CD003249
30. Hofmeyr GJ, Gülmezoglu AM, Novikova N, Linder V, Fereirra S, Piaggio G. Misoprostol to prevent and treat postpartum haemorrhage: a systematic review and meta-analysis of maternal deaths and dose-related effects. Bull World Health Organ 2009;87:666–77
31. Department of Making Pregnancy Safer, WHO. WHO recommendation for the prevention of postpartum haemorrhage. 2007. http://whqlibdoc.who.int/hq/2007/WHO_MPS_07.06_eng.pdf
32. Department of Reproductive Health and Research, WHO. WHO statement regarding the use of misoprostol for postpartum haemorrhage prevention and treatment. 2009. http://whqlibdoc.who.int/hq/2009/WHO_RHR_09.22_eng.pdf
33. Durocher J, Bynum J, Leon W, Barrera G, Winikoff B. High fever following postpartum administration of sublingual misoprostol. BJOG 2010;117:845–52
34. Kupferminc MJ, Gull I, Bar-Am A, et al. Intrauterine irrigation with prostaglandin F2α for management of severe postpartum haemorrhage. Acta Obstet Gynecol Scand 1998;77:548–50
35. Peyser MR, Kupferminc MJ. Management of severe postpartum hemorrhage by intrauterine irrigation with prostaglandin E2. Am J Obstet Gynecol 1990;162:694–6
36. Barrington JW, Roberts A. The use of gemeprost pessaries to arrest postpartum haemorrhage. BJOG 1993;100:691–2
37. El-Lakany N, Harlow RA. The use of gemeprost pessaries to arrest postpartum haemorrhage. BJOG 1994;101:277
38. Bates A, Johansen K. The use of gemeprost pessaries to arrest postpartum haemorrhage. BJOG 1994;101:277–8
39. Craig S, Chau H, Cho H. Treatment of severe postpartum haemorrhage by rectally administered gemeprost pessaries. J Perinat Med 1999;27:231–5
40. Peitsidis P, Kadir RA. Antifibrinolytic therapy with tranexamic acid in pregnancy and postpartum. Expert Opin Pharmacother 2011;12:503–16
41. Shakur H, Elbourne D, Gülmezoglu M, Alfirevic Z, Ronsmans C, Allen E, Roberts I. The WOMAN Trial (World Maternal Antifibrinolytic Trial): tranexamic acid for the treatment of postpartum haemorrhage: an international randomised, double blind placebo controlled trial. Trials 2010;11:40
42. Mercer FJ, Bonnet MP. Use of clotting factors and other prohemostatic drugs for obstetric hemorrhage. Curr Opin Anaesthesiol 2010;23:310–6
43. Franchini M, Franchi M, Bergamini V, Montagnana M, Salvagno GL, Targher G, Lippi G. The use of recombinant activated FVII in postpartum hemorrhage. Clin Obstet Gynecol 2010;53:219–27
44. Saving Mothers' Lives: Reviewing maternal deaths to make motherhood safer: 2006–2008. BJOG 2011;118(Suppl 1):71–6
45. Rizvi F, Mackey R, Geary M, et al. Successful reduction of massive postpartum haemorrhage by use of guidelines and staff education. BJOG 2004;111;495–8

44

Carbetocin for the Prevention of Postpartum Hemorrhage

D. Cordovani, J. C. A. Carvalho, M. Boucher and D. Farine

INTRODUCTION

Considering the physical and emotional costs of postpartum hemorrhage (PPH) worldwide, it is not surprising that institutions as diverse as the World Health Organization, the International Confederation of Midwives (ICM) and the International Federation of Gynecology and Obstetrics (FIGO) all recommend active management of the third stage of labor (AMTSL) even for patients with low risk for PPH[1,2] (see Chapters 14 and 15). Their consensus is understandable given that numerically more women without risk factors for PPH suffer from it than do women with obvious risk factors[2].

The administration of a uterotonic medication soon after the delivery of the fetus is an essential part of the AMTSL[2] that is capable of decreasing the incidence of PPH by 40%[3,4]. However, these medications pose some challenges, in that individually and collectively they have side-effects, contraindications and problems with storage and administration. As such, the search for the ideal uterotonic continues, and today the main uterotonic agents are oxytocin, ergonovine, carboprost, carbetocin and misoprostol. This chapter focuses on carbetocin.

Oxytocin is the most widely available and used uterotonic agent[3,5] (see Chapter 43). It binds to the myometrial oxytocin receptors and stimulates contraction of the uterine muscle by increasing the intracellular concentration of calcium[6,7]. However, its use is not without some limitations. Oxytocin has a short half-life of 3–17 minutes, and a continuous intravenous (IV) infusion is necessary to achieve sustained uterotonic activity[3,5,7]. Moreover, large doses or boluses of oxytocin are associated with adverse effects in the form of hypotension, nausea, vomiting, dysrhythmias, ST-T changes, pulmonary edema and severe water intoxication with convulsions[3,8,9].

In contrast, carbetocin (1-deamino-1-carba-2-tyrosine(O-methyl)-oxytocin) is a synthetic oxytocin analogue that binds to the same oxytocin receptors in the myometrium with an affinity similar to that of oxytocin[6,7]. Its main advantage over oxytocin is a four-fold longer uterotonic activity, a fact which precludes the necessity of a continuous infusion[10,11].

PHARMACOLOGY

As noted above, carbetocin is a synthetic oxytocin analogue that binds to the same myometrium receptors as oxytocin with similar affinity[7,12]. Despite a similar affinity, its potency in animal models is about one-tenth that of oxytocin on a mole per mole basis[13]. At the same time, its plasma half-life is approximately 40 minutes after IV injection, which is 4–10 times longer than that of oxytocin[10]. Similarly to oxytocin, it causes an increase in the intracellular concentration of calcium that promotes uterine contractility, through the generation of inositol phosphates[14].

Oxytocin and vasopressin are neurohypophysial hormones with a short half-life in plasma. By removing the primary amino group from the vasopressin molecule, a prolongation of the half-life was achieved, something which did not happen when the same alteration was made in the oxytocin molecule. A further alteration of the molecule was necessary in order to achieve this same goal. The disulfide bond had been proven not to be important in the mechanism of action of oxytocin[6]. By removing the amino group (1-deamino), and replacing the sulfur atom at position 1 with a carba group ($-CH_2-$), a prolonged myometrial action was observed[6,7]. Carbetocin is the carba analogue being used clinically in order to prevent and/or treat PPH. The deamination protects carbetocin from aminopeptidase cleavage, and the replacement of the disulfide bond by CH_2S protects the analogue from disulfidase cleavage[15] (Figure 1). This is the suggested explanation for the protracted half-life of carbetocin in plasma. Another suggested explanation for the prolonged activity of carbetocin is its higher lipophilicity that can alter its tissue distribution[7,13]. Atke *et al.* suggested that this increased lipophilicity was responsible for an increased half-life in the receptor compartment[7].

The structural differences between the molecules of oxytocin and carbetocin could also explain the decreased potency of the latter when compared with the former. The current recommended dose of carbetocin for the prevention of PPH is 100 μg, which is roughly equivalent to 10 μg (5 IU) of oxytocin[13]. However, it is important to highlight that these figures are derived from animal data. Human myometrium

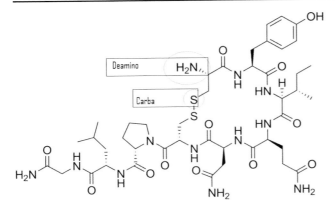

Figure 1 Oxytocin molecule. The amino group and the disulfide bond, which were altered in order to create carbetocin, are indicated. The amino group was removed and the sulfur atom was replaced by a carba group

receptors might have higher affinity to carbetocin than rat receptors; therefore, it is not clear if the decreased potency found in animal models can be extrapolated to humans[7,13].

In a study, performed on 40 women, carbetocin was administered either IV in doses varying from 8 to 30 μg or intramuscularly (IM) in doses varying from 10 to 70 μg, 24–48 h postpartum. After IV administration, tetanic contraction was achieved in a mean time (± SD) of 1.2 ± 0.5 min. Uterine tetany lasted for 6.9 ± 2.1 min followed by rhythmic contraction for 60 ± 18 min. After IM administration, the onset was 1.9 ± 0.6 min, with tetanic contractions lasting for 11.3 ± 3 min, followed by rhythmic contractions that lasted for 119 ± 69 min[13]. According to these findings, the onset is not affected by the route of administration, but the uterotonic activity is significant longer (two-fold) after IM injection when compared with IV. After IM injection, carbetocin reaches peak plasma levels in 30 min and its bioavailability is 80%[5,10,16,17].

Small amounts of carbetocin can cross over from plasma to breast milk, with a mean peak concentration in breast milk that is 50 times lower than in plasma[11]. This small amount is not of clinical concern, as carbetocin would be rapidly degraded by peptidases in the infant's gastrointestinal tract.

CARBETOCIN AT CESAREAN DELIVERY

To the best of our knowledge, only nine studies have used carbetocin for prevention of PPH after cesarean delivery. These are presented in Table 1 in chronological order.

The first study was published in abstract form. It was a dose-finding study with a total of 18 patients who underwent elective cesarean section under epidural anesthesia. This study established the recommended dose of 100 μg. There was a 0% response in terms of uterine contractility with doses below 60 μg, and 83% (5 out of 6) response with a dose of 100 μg[18].

Barton et al. published in abstract form their findings comparing carbetocin 100 μg versus placebo[19].

Although carbetocin is in fact more efficient than placebo, 28% of the women in the placebo group did not require any uterotonic therapy.

Boucher et al. conducted a double-blind randomized control trial to compare carbetocin 100 μg IV bolus after placental delivery with oxytocin 2.5 IU IV bolus followed by a 16 h infusion of oxytocin for a total of 30 IU[20]. Their primary outcome was blood loss as calculated by means of aspiration from the surgical field from the time the study drug was administered until skin closure. Although not statistically significant, women in the carbetocin group bled 29 ml less (p = 0.3). More important, significantly fewer women had blood loss greater than 200 ml with carbetocin (p = 0.0041). In addition, the three study participants that required additional uterotonic intervention were all in the oxytocin group.

Similarly, Dansereau et al. also compared carbetocin as a single 100 μg bolus IV with oxytocin IV bolus followed by 8 h infusion of oxytocin after cesarean delivery for women with low risk for PPH[9]. This Canadian multicenter double-blind randomized controlled trial is the largest study to date, with 694 participants. The major finding was a 50% decrease in the necessity of additional uterotonic therapy in patients treated with carbetocin when compared with oxytocin.

Del Angel-Garcia et al. published in abstract form their findings comparing carbetocin 100 μg IV with oxytocin 5 IU IV after elective cesarean delivery in patients with at least one risk factor for PPH[21]. Uterine atony was reported in 8% of the patients in the carbetocin group versus 19% in the oxytocin arm. This Mexican study included a cost analysis. According to the authors, allocation of patients to carbetocin therapy resulted in lower cost than those treated with oxytocin (US dollars 3525 vs. US dollars 4054).

Borruto et al. also compared carbetocin as a single IV bolus with oxytocin infusion. Their study included both elective and emergency cesarean delivery among patients who had at least one risk factor for PPH[22]. Similar to the previous studies, the odds ratio (OR) for uterotonic intervention was 1.83 (95% CI 0.9–2.6) times higher in the oxytocin group compared with the carbetocin group.

Attilakos et al., in a double-blind randomized controlled trial compared carbetocin 100 μg single IV bolus with oxytocin 5 IU single IV bolus after low risk cesarean deliveries[23]. Additional uterotonics were necessary in 33.5% of patients in the carbetocin group patients compared with 45.5% in the oxytocin group (p = 0.023). This study included 377 patients. Although the need for additional uterotonics was decreased, not dissimilar to other studies mentioned above, this study did not demonstrate a decrease in blood loss or in the incidence of PPH. Of interest, both arms of the study had a high failure rate.

Triopon et al., in a French two-phase observational study[24], compared the outcomes of a cohort of 155 patients who received oxytocin with the outcomes of a subsequent cohort of 155 patients who received carbetocin after cesarean delivery (after the

Table 1 Studies with carbetocin after cesarean delivery

Author	Year	Type of study	Population	Intervention	Outcomes
Boucher et al.[18]	1991	Dose-ranging	Low-risk, elective C/S under epidural (n = 18)	Carbetocin IV ranging from 10 to 100 μg after delivery of placenta	0% response with doses ≤60 μg 83% (5/6) with tetanic contraction with 100 μg
Barton et al.[19] (abstract)	1996	Double-blind RCT	Low-risk elective C/S under regional anesthesia (n = 119)	100 μg carbetocin (n = 62) vs. saline (n = 57)	Uterine tone significantly increased in carbetocin treated women (p <0.05) Use of additional uterotonic therapy 8/62 vs. 41/57, RR 0.18 (CI 95% 0.09–0.35)
Boucher et al.[20]	1998	Double-blind RCT	Low-risk, elective C/S under epidural (n = 57)	Carbetocin 100 μg IV (n = 29) vs. oxytocin 2.5 IU IV bolus + 16 h infusion of 30 IU after delivery of placenta	Mean intraoperative blood loss was 159 vs. 188 ml (p = 0.3) Significantly fewer women had blood loss ≥200 ml with carbetocin (33%) vs. oxytocin (79%) (p = 0.0041) Comparable vital signs and hematologic values
Dansereau et al.[9]	1999	Canadian multicenter double-blind RCT	Low-risk elective C/S under regional anesthesia (n = 694)	Carbetocin 100 μg IV (n = 317) vs. oxytocin 5 IU IV bolus 8 h infusion of 20 IU (n = 318)	Additional oxytocic intervention was 4.7% vs. 10.1% (p <0.05) OR for treatment failure was 2.03 times higher with oxytocin vs. carbetocin (95% CI 1.1–2.8) Similar safety profile
Del Angel-Garcia et al.[21] (abstract)	2006	Randomized pragmatic clinical trial	At least 1 risk factor for PPH, elective C/S (n = 152)	Carbetocin 100 μg IV (n = 77) vs. oxytocin 5 IU IV (n = 75)	Uterine atony in 8% vs. 19 % (p <0.0001) Blood loss ≥500 ml only observed with oxytocin Cheaper mean cost per patient treated with carbetocin (USD 3525 vs. USD 4054)
Borruto et al.[22]	2009	Randomized controlled clinical trial	Singleton, at least 1 risk factor for PPH, elective or emergency C/S (n = 104)	Carbetocin 100 μg (n = 52) vs. oxytocin 2 h infusion of 10 IU (n = 52) after placental delivery	Uterotonic intervention in 3.8% vs. 9.6% (p <0.01) OR for treatment failure was 1.83 (95% CI 0.9–2.6) Mean blood loss 30 ml less with carbetocin (p = 0.05)
Attilakos et al.[23]	2010	Double-blind RCT	Low-risk, elective or emergency C/S (n = 377)	Carbetocin 100 μg IV (n = 188) vs. oxytocin 5 IU IV (n = 189)	Additional oxytocic 33.5% vs. 45.5% (RR 0.74, 95% CI 0.57–0.95, p = 0.023) No difference in estimated blood loss, side-effects, or hematologic values
Triopon et al.[24]	2010	Two-phase observational study	Elective or emergency C/S (n = 310)	Use of carbetocin as a sentinel event separating the 2 groups. Data from 155 who received oxytocin 5 IU compared with 155 women who received carbetocin 100 μg after fetal delivery	Significant decrease in postoperative IV iron administration in the carbetocin group (6.5% vs. 14.5%, p = 0.03) Fewer compression sutures (although not significant) in the carbetocin group (0.6% vs. 4.5%, p = 0.06) No difference in the incidence of vascular sutures, necessity of additional uterotonic, and blood transfusion
Cordovani et al.[25]	2012	Double-blind, randomized dose-finding study	Low-risk, elective C/S under spinal anesthesia (n = 80)	Carbetocin 80, 90, 100, 110 or 120 μg IV after fetal delivery	Similar failure rate among all dose groups. Not possible to calculate ED95 Similar incidence of side-effects and blood loss in all groups Overall, uterus was boggy at 2 min in 10/80 (12.5%) Additional uterotonic given to 9/80 (11.25%) 6/10 (60%) with boggy uterus at 2 min 3/70 (4.3%) with firm uterus at 2 min

RCT, randomized controlled trial; C/S, cesarean section; USD, US dollars

department's drug of choice for prevention of PPH was converted from oxytocin to carbetocin). In contrast to the previous studies, there was no significant decrease in the need for additional uterotonics. On the other hand, there was a significant decrease in postoperative IV iron administration in the carbetocin group (6.5% vs. 14.5%, $p = 0.03$) and fewer compression sutures were necessary (although not significant) in the carbetocin group (0.6% vs. 4.5%, $p = 0.06$).

A recent dose-finding study performed by Cordovani et al. attempted to calculate the ED95 of carbetocin for elective cesarean delivery in low-risk patients for PPH[25]. The authors were unable to calculate the ED95 of carbetocin, as the failure rate was evenly distributed across all dose groups (80, 90, 100, 110 and 120 μg). Overall, 12.5% of patients failed to present a firm uterus after 2 min of drug administration, and 11.25% of women required additional uterotonic therapy within 4 h. It is important to point out that, three of the women requiring additional uterotonics in fact had a firm uterus after 2 min of carbetocin administration.

In general, the studies on cesarean deliveries have shown a decrease in the necessity of additional uterotonic intervention, although none demonstrated a decrease in either the incidence of PPH or the mean blood volume loss, as the study design practically eliminated such end points. At the same time, fewer patients in the carbetocin arms of the studies lost larger amounts of blood[21,22]. The optimal dose of carbetocin is yet to be determined, but recent data suggest that doses as low as 80 μg are as effective as the current recommended dose of 100 μg[25].

CARBETOCIN IN VAGINAL DELIVERY

Six studies on carbetocin therapy used in vaginal deliveries are presented in Table 2 in chronological order.

Van Dongen et al. performed an ascending dose-tolerance study with IM carbetocin administered after low risk vaginal deliveries[10]. Their findings revealed a maximum tolerated dose of 200 μg due to the presence of limiting side-effects, namely retained placenta, blood loss of 1000 ml or more and blood transfusion. Optimal results were within the 75–125 μg dose range in keeping with the 100 μg dose determined in the original dose-finding study[19].

Boucher et al., in a double-blind randomized controlled trial involving 160 patients with at least one risk factor for PPH, compared carbetocin 100 μg IM with oxytocin 10 IU IV infusion over a 2 h period[26]. Their findings showed no difference in the requirement of additional uterotonics or in the presence of PPH. However, significantly fewer women in the carbetocin arm required uterine massage compared with in the oxytocin arm.

Leung et al. compared carbetocin 100 μg IM ($n = 165$) with Syntometrine®, a combination of oxytocin and ergometrine, IM ($n = 164$) given after low risk vaginal deliveries[17]. No significant difference was observed in hemoglobin drop or use of additional uterotonics, but women treated with Syntometrine had a significantly higher incidence of nausea, vomiting and hypertension.

Ngan et al., in a retrospective study involving 118 low risk patients, found that carbetocin was associated with less blood loss compared with a combination of oxytocin and ergometrine[27].

Nirmala et al. studied 120 women at high risk for PPH who delivered vaginally in another randomized controlled trial which compared carbetocin 100 μg IM with Syntometrine IM[16]. In contrast to the findings observed in a low risk population[17], these authors found a significant decrease in the mean blood loss as well as a significant smaller decrease in hemoglobin drop in the carbetocin group. However, there was no difference in the necessity of additional uterotonic agents or blood transfusion. Interestingly, also in contrast to the findings of Leung et al.[17], there was no difference in the incidence of side-effects.

Su et al. performed yet another comparison of carbetocin with Syntometrine[28] evaluating 370 women with low risk for PPH. Similar to previous findings[17], no differences were found in the requirements for additional uterotonic agents, in blood loss or in the incidence of PPH. On the other hand, side-effects were noticeably more prevalent in the Syntometrine group.

In general, studies of vaginal deliveries found no difference in the requirement for additional uterotonic medication when compared with oxytocin or with a combination of oxytocin and ergometrine. However, when compared with oxytocin alone, carbetocin-treated patients with at least one risk factor for PPH required less uterine massage. The findings regarding decrease in blood loss are conflicting. The most consistent finding was a decrease in the incidence of nausea and vomiting when compared with a combination of oxytocin and ergometrine.

SIDE-EFFECTS AND CONTRAINDICATIONS

Oxytocin and carbetocin are without differences regarding either the types of side-effects or their frequency[9,20,22,23]. The incidence of side-effects in three reports is presented in Table 3[9,20,22]. Although not shown in the table, Borruto et al. described 28.8% of arrhythmias after oxytocin injection, but none for carbetocin[22]. Similarly, Boucher et al. found a 3.6% incidence of premature ventricular contraction after oxytocin administration, but none after carbetocin[20]. The safety of carbetocin in patients with severe cardiovascular disease has not yet been determined.

As carbetocin should not be administered prior to fetal delivery, under no circumstances should it be used for induction of labor or labor augmentation. It should be administered as an IM injection or slow IV bolus over 1 min after fetal or placental delivery[1,11]. The following is an extract from the product leaflet provided by its manufacturer:

Table 2 Studies with carbetocin after vaginal delivery

Author	Year	Type of study	Population	Intervention	Outcomes
Van Dongen et al.[10]	1998	Ascending dose tolerance	Low-risk, vaginal delivery (n = 45)	Carbetocin IM (15, 30, 50, 75, 100, 125, 150, 175, 200 μg) immediately after birth of infant	Maximum blood loss at the upper and lower dose levels. Lowest in the 70–125 μg range. Maximum tolerated dose calculated to be 200 μg (4/18 retained placenta, 3/18 blood transfusion, 4/18 additional oxytocics)
Boucher et al.[26]	2004	Double-blind RCT	At least 1 risk factor for PPH (n = 160)	Carbetocin 100 μg IM + IV placebo (n = 83) vs. placebo IM + oxytocin 10 IU 2 h IV infusion (n = 77) after delivery of placenta	No difference in requirement for additional uterotonic medication, nor in laboratory PPH indicators. Uterine massage required in 43.4% vs. 62.3% (p <0.025)
Leung et al.[17]	2006	Double-blind RCT	Low-risk, vaginal delivery (n = 329)	Carbetocin 100 μg IM (n = 165) vs. Syntometrine IM (n = 164) after delivery of infant	No difference in drop of hemoglobin (1.4 vs. 1.5 g/dl), or additional uterotonic agents (8.7% vs. 6.7%). Significant lower incidence of nausea (RR 0.18, 95% CI 0.04–0.78), vomiting (RR 0.1, 95% CI 0.01–0.74), hypertension at 30 min (p <0.01) and 60 min (p <0.05). Higher incidence of tachycardia (RR 1.68, 95% CI 1.03–3.57)
Ngan et al.[27]	2007	Retrospective study	Low-risk, vaginal delivery (n = 118)	Carbetocin 100 μg IM vs. IM combination of oxytocin 5 IU and ergometrine 0.2 mg immediately after infant delivery	Mean blood loss 388 vs. 551 (p = 0.01). Blood loss ≥500 ml was 21.4% vs. 43.5% (p = 0.01) and blood loss ≥1000 ml was 1.8 % vs. 14.5% (p = 0.02)
Nirmala et al.[16]	2009	Randomized controlled study	High-risk for PPH, vaginal delivery (n = 120)	Carbetocin 100 μg IM (n = 60) vs. Syntometrine IM (n = 60) immediately after infant delivery	No difference in requirement for additional oxytocic agent, time interval to well contracted uterus, blood transfusion, adverse effect or complications. Significantly lower mean blood loss in carbetocin group (244 ± 114 ml vs. 343 ± 143 ml, 95% CI 52–146 ml). Significant reduced drop in hemoglobin in carbetocin group (0.3 ± 0.2g/dl vs. 0.4 ± 0.2 g/dl, 95% CI 0.1–0.2)
Su et al.[+28]	2009	Double-blind RCT	Low-risk, vaginal delivery (n = 370)	Carbetocin 100 μg IM (n = 185) vs. Syntometrine IM (n = 185) immediately after infant delivery	No difference in requirement for additional oxytocic agent, blood loss or incidence of PPH. Women who had Syntometrine were four times more likely to experience nausea (RR 4.2, 95% CI 2.2–7.8) and vomiting (RR 4.3, 95% CI 1.9–9.5). Tremor, sweating, retching and uterine pain were also more likely in the Syntometrine group (p <0.05)

RCT, randomized controlled trial

Table 3 Side-effects associated with carbetocin and frequency of occurence

>20%	<20% and >10%	<10% and >5%	<5%
Abdominal pain	Feeling of warmth	Pruritus	Back pain
Nausea	Headache	Shortness of breath	Sweating
Flushing	Tremors	Vomiting	Dizziness
		Metalic taste	

'Because of its long duration of action relative to oxytocin, uterine contractions produced by carbetocin cannot be stopped by simply discontinuing the medication. Therefore, carbetocin should not be administered prior to delivery of the infant for any reason, including elective or medical induction of labour. Inappropriate use of carbetocin during pregnancy could theoretically mimic the symptoms of oxytocin over-dosage, including hyperstimulation of the uterus with strong (hypertonic) or prolonged (tetanic) contractions, tumultuous labour, uterine rupture, cervical and vaginal lacerations, postpartum hemorrhage, utero-placental hypoperfusion and variable deceleration of fetal heart, fetal hypoxia, hypercapnia, or death. Carbetocin should not be used in patients with a history of hypersensitivity to oxytocin or carbetocin. Carbetocin should not be used in patients with vascular disease, especially coronary artery disease, except with extreme caution. Carbetocin is not intended for use in children.'

CARBETOCIN TODAY

In email correspondence with Ferring Pharmaceuticals in July 2011, the authors were informed that carbetocin has been available for clinical use since the year of 2000. Today, carbetocin is approved in 23 countries for the prevention or treatment of uterine atony[5]. Of these, Canada has undertaken a leading role in carbetocin research, including the largest randomized controlled trial executed to date[9]. As a consequence, the Society of Obstetricians and Gynaecologists of Canada (SOGC) in their 2009 guidelines on the active management of the third stage of labor[1], released the following recommendations:

'6. Carbetocin, 100 μg given as an IV bolus over 1 minute, should be used instead of continuous oxytocin infusion in elective Caesarean section for the prevention of PPH and to decrease the need for therapeutic uterotonics. (I-B)
7. For women delivering vaginally with 1 risk factor for PPH, carbetocin 100 μg IM decreases the need for uterine massage to prevent PPH when compared with continuous infusion of oxytocin. (I-B)'

This means that, for cesarean delivery performed in Canada under regional anesthesia, carbetocin is the first choice as a uterotonic agent. It is also recommended for vaginal deliveries with increased risk for PPH. How frequent these recommendations are being followed is yet to be assessed, as it is recognized that the practice varies across the country.

COST-EFFECTIVENESS

British data from 2010 states that one ampoule of carbetocin 100 μg costs £17.64, whereas one ampoule of oxytocin 10 IU costs £0.86[23]. Although it is significantly more expensive, other factors must be considered. Among these, only one ampoule of carbetocin would be used in a successfully treated patient, whereas an average of 2–4 ampoules of oxytocin would be necessary to supply a continuous infusion.

A Mexican study from 2006 analysed the overall cost to treat women with carbetocin compared with oxytocin[21]. The use of resources was obtained from a clinical trial involving 152 women with high risk for PPH who underwent cesarean delivery. The cost was calculated using the financial information provided by the Mexican Institute of Social Security, which is the third party payer. Their finding was that women treated with carbetocin cost less to the health care system than those treated with oxytocin (US dollars 3525 vs. US dollars 4054)[21]. One could infer that this is due to a decrease in the necessity for additional uterotonic, blood products and faster hospital discharge. However, at this point this inference cannot be confirmed. These data were accurate for Mexico at the time of the study, but a similar benefit with carbetocin in other settings could be expected.

The ease of administration and the potentially lower overall cost with a greater efficacy could become the basis of a wider use of carbetocin for the prevention of PPH, especially in low-resource areas. However, because the manufacturer recommends carbetocin to be stored at temperatures of 2–8°C, this requirement may preclude its more widespread use in poorly resourced areas where 24 h access to reliable sources of electricity is problematic. Carbetocin in a room temperature formulation would potentially increase its usefulness in such countries. To date, no data have been published on drug stability at room temperature

REMAINING QUESTIONS

Although current data suggest that carbetocin can be more effective than oxytocin in the prevention of PPH, studies to date have not focused on the hemodynamic effects of this agent. The practice of administering oxytocin as a bolus has been discouraged due to its hemodynamic effects[3,8,9]. At the same time, current recommendations of carbetocin, which is an oxytocin analogue with agonistic properties at the same receptors, state that this drug should be given as a single IV bolus. The only caveat is that the recommendation is for a slow IV bolus administered over a 1 min duration. This is not based on clinical data, but presumably on extrapolation from findings with oxytocin[29,30].

The safety of carbetocin for use in patients with vascular disease as well as coronary disease has not been tested. Similarly, no studies were performed on patients under general anesthesia. Although there is no clear reason that would preclude the use of carbetocin in women under a general anesthetic, the lack of clinical trials accounts for the manufacturer's recommendation of using this drug only in women who are not anesthetized or who are only under regional or local anesthesia[11].

Further analysis is warranted to assess the cost-effectiveness of carbetocin. Should the Mexican study findings[21] be replicated in different settings, this will further justify the use of carbetocin as a first choice of uterotonic agent. In addition, the drug stability at room temperature remains unclear.

Finally, the optimal dose of carbetocin is still to be determined. In the case of oxytocin, initial IV doses as low as 0.5 IU are effective in providing adequate uterine contractility at elective cesarean delivery[31]. Extrapolating the findings for carbetocin, it is reasonable to assume that 100 μg, which is equivalent to 5 IU of oxytocin according to animal data[13], is considerably more than the minimum necessary. This is especially true if the suggestions that the human uterus is more sensitive to carbetocin than the rat myometrium are accurate[7,13]. In addition, similarly to oxytocin, carbetocin will have to be evaluated in different clinical scenarios, namely non-laboring elective cesarean section, urgent/emergent cesarean section on laboring women and vaginal delivery. Its usefulness in the area of medical interruptions of pregnancy remains to be investigated.

CONCLUSIONS

Carbetocin is a synthetic oxytocin analogue. It combines the quick onset of oxytocin with the long-acting effect of ergometrine. Compared with oxytocin, it reduces the necessity of uterotonic intervention with similar incidence of side-effects; compared with a combination of oxytocin and ergometrine, it is as effective with fewer side-effects, namely nausea, vomiting and hypertension. According to the Society of Obstetricians and Gynaecologists of Canada, it should be the first choice of uterotonic agent to prevent PPH at elective cesarean delivery under regional anesthesia. It is also suggested that it should be used in women at risk for PPH after vaginal delivery.

References

1. Leduc D, Senikas V, Lalonde A, et al. Active management of the third stage of labour: prevention and treatment of postpartum hemorrhage. J Obstet Gynaecol Can 2009;31:980–93
2. World Health Organization. Recommendations for the Prevention of Postpartum Haemorrhage. WHO/MPS/07.06. Geneva: WHO, 2007
3. Peters NCJ, Duvekot JJ. Carbetocin for the prevention of postpartum hemorrhage: a systematic review. Obstet Gynecol Surv 2009;64:129–35
4. Vercauteren M, Palit S, Soetens F, Jacquemyn Y, Alahuhta S. Anaesthesiological considerations on tocolytic and uterotonic therapy in obstetrics. Acta Anaesthesiol Scand 2009;53:701–9
5. Rath W. Prevention of postpartum haemorrhage with the oxytocin analogue carbetocin. Eur J Obstet Gynecol Reprod Biol 2009;147:15–20
6. Barth T, Krejci I, Kupkova B, Jost K. Pharmacology of cyclic analogues of deamino-oxytocin not containing a disulphide bond (carba analogues). Eur J Pharmacol 1973;24:183–8
7. Atke A, Vilhardt H. Uterotonic activity and myometrial receptor affinity of 1-deamino-1-carba-2-tyrosine(O-methyl)-oxytocin. Acta Endocrinol (Copenh) 1987;115:155–60
8. Moran C, Ni Bhuinneain M, Geary M, Cunningham S, McKenna P, Gardiner J. Myocardial ischaemia in normal patients undergoing elective Caesarean section: a peripartum assessment. Anaesthesia 2001;56:1051–8
9. Dansereau J, Joshi K, Helewa ME, et al. Double-blind comparison of carbetocin versus oxytocin in prevention of uterine atony after cesarean section. Am J Obstet Gynecol 1999;180:670–6
10. van Dongen PWJ, Verbruggen MM, Groot AN de, Roosmalen J van, Sporken JM, Schulz M. Ascending dose tolerance study of intramuscular carbetocin administered after normal vaginal birth. Eur J Obstet Gynecol Reprod Biol 1998;77:181–7
11. Ferring Inc. Product monograph: Duratocin (Carbetocin Injection). 2006
12. Dyer RA, Dyk D van, Dresner A. The use of uterotonic drugs during caesarean section. Int J Obstet Anesth 2010;19:313–9
13. Hunter DJS, Schulz P, Wassenaar W. Effect of carbetocin , a long-acting oxytocin analog on the postpartum uterus. Clin Pharmacol Ther 1992;52:60–7
14. Engstrøm T, Barth T, Melin P, Vilhardt H. Oxytocin receptor binding and uterotonic activity of carbetocin and its metabolites following enzymatic degradation. Eur J Pharmacol 1998;355:203–10
15. Sweeney G, Holbrook AM, Levine M, et al. Pharmacokinetics of carbetocin, a long-acting oxytocin analogue, in nonpregnant women. Curr Ther Res 1990;47:528–40
16. Nirmala K, Zainuddin AA, Ghani NAA, Zulkifli S, Jamil MA. Carbetocin versus syntometrine in prevention of post-partum hemorrhage following vaginal delivery. J Obstet Gynaecol Res 2009;35:48–54
17. Leung SW, Ng PS, Wong WY, Cheung TH. A randomised trial of carbetocin versus syntometrine in the management of the third stage of labour. BJOG 2006;113:1459–64
18. Boucher M, Durocher F, Schulz P, Wassenaar W. Carbetocin to produce uterine contraction during Cesarean-section. A dose-ranging study. Proceedings of the 11th Annual Meeting – Society of Perinatal Obstetricians; 1991 Jan 28-Feb 02; San Francisco, CA, USA. Abstract #556
19. Barton SR, Jackson A. The safety and efficiency of carbetocin to control uterine bleeding following caesarean section. Prenat Neonat Med 1996;1:185
20. Boucher M, Horbay GL, Griffin P, et al. Double-blind, randomized comparison of the effect of carbetocin and oxytocin on intraoperative blood loss and uterine tone of patients undergoing cesarean section. J Perinatol 1998;18:202–7
21. Del Angel-Garcia G, Garcia-Contreras F, Constantino-Casas P. Economic evaluation of carbetocine for the prevention of uterine atony in patients with risk factors in Mexico. Value Health 2006;9:A254
22. Borruto F, Treisser A, Comparetto C. Utilization of carbetocin for prevention of postpartum hemorrhage after cesarean section: a randomized clinical trial. Arch Gynecol Obstet 2009;280:707–12
23. Attilakos G, Psaroudakis D, Ash J, et al. Carbetocin versus oxytocin for the prevention of postpartum haemorrhage following caesarean section: the results of a double-blind randomised trial. BJOG 2010;117:929–36
24. Triopon G, Goron A, Agenor J, et al. Use of carbetocin in prevention of uterine atony during cesarean section. Comparison with oxytocin. Gynecol Obstet Fertil 2010;38:729–34
25. Cordovani D, Balki M, Seaward G, Farine G, Carvalho JCA. Carbetocin at elective cesarean delivery: a randomized controlled trial to determine the effective dose. Can J Anesth 2012;in press
26. Boucher M, Nimrod CA, Tawagi GF, Meeker TA, Rennicks White RE, Varin J. Comparison of carbetocin and oxytocin for the prevention of postpartum hemorrhage following

vaginal delivery: a double-blind randomized trial. J Obstet Gynaecol Can 2004;26:481–8

27. Ngan L, Keong W, Martins R. Carbetocin versus a combination of oxytocin and ergometrine in control of postpartum blood loss. Int J Gynaecol Obstet 2007;97:152–3

28. Su LL, Rauff M, Chan YH, et al. Carbetocin versus syntometrine for the third stage of labour following vaginal delivery—a double-blind randomised controlled trial. BJOG 2009;116:1461–6

29. Thomas JS, Koh SH, Cooper GM. Haemodynamic effects of oxytocin given as i.v. bolus or infusion on women undergoing Caesarean section. Br J Anaesth 2007;98:116–9

30. Tsen LC, Balki M. Oxytocin protocols during cesarean delivery: time to acknowledge the risk/benefit ratio? Int J Obstet Anesth 2010;19:243–5

31. Carvalho JC, Balki M, Kingdom J, Windrim R. Oxytocin requirements at elective cesarean delivery: a dose-finding study. Obstet Gynecol 2004;104:1005–10

45

Intraluminal Pressure Readings whilst Achieving a Positive 'Tamponade Test' in the Management of Postpartum Hemorrhage

C. Georgiou

INTRODUCTION

Whereas pharmacological agents such as oxytocin, ergometrine, prostaglandin F2α and misoprostol used in the treatment of postpartum hemorrhage (PPH) normally result in a generalized contraction of uterine size[1,2], the use of uterine tamponade results in a temporary enlargement of the uterine cavity. Uterine packing as a method of tamponade was described as early as 1856, and is still used throughout the world today[3]. Sterilized cotton gauze is commonly used to pack the uterus, and although considered effective by those who have used the method regularly over the years, one of the arguments against this methodology was the 'unphysiological' nature of expanding the uterus[4], as the uterus normally is expected to 'contract down'[5]. This paradoxical concept of expanding the uterine cavity, together with the possibilities of causing trauma and/or infection, ineffective packing and the coincidental development of effective pharmacological uterotonic agents, resulted in a gradual decline in its use[6,7].

More recently, a marked resurgence of interest in the use of uterine tamponade for the management of PPH has occurred using balloon technology[8]. A variety of balloons are available, including the purpose designed uterine balloons (Figure 1) such as the Bakri balloon, Ebb™ balloon and BT-Cath® as well as the Foley and condom catheters[9–14]. In addition, other non-uterine specific types of balloons, previously used in other body cavities where bleeding can be problematic, have also been used in the therapy of PPH. Two examples are the Sengstaken–Blakemore tube (esophagus) and the Rusch balloon (bladder)[15,16].

Despite publication of recent guidelines recommending the use of balloon tamponade in the management of PPH, the mechanism by which these balloons provide their effect remains controversial[17,18]. In practice, the term 'tamponade' is often used to explain the effect of the balloon. One proposed mechanism by which balloons provide tamponade effect is by

'exerting an inward-to-outward pressure' within the uterine cavity 'that is greater than the systemic arterial pressure'[17].

Variations exist with respect to how balloons are insufflated; some authors place a fixed or predetermined volume in the balloon, whereas others suggest titrating the volume to clinical effect[8]. However, none of the published methods describe measuring intra-uterine pressures. Furthermore, although the term 'tamponade test' has been used to characterize the process with respect to using balloon tamponade in the management of PPH, studies do not specifically relate to this terminology during balloon insufflation[8,19].

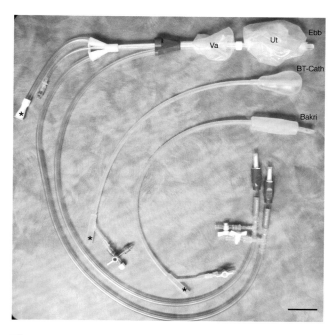

Figure 1 Uterine specific balloons. The Bakri balloon and the BT-Cath are single balloon devices. The Ebb balloon is designed for one balloon in the uterine cavity (Ut) and the other within the vagina (Va). *Drainage channel for each balloon system. Bar = 5 cm

This chapter describes a prospective study that was designed to investigate the hypothesis that it was necessary for the intraluminal pressure (ILP) to exceed the patient's systolic blood pressure in order to achieve a positive tamponade test. The study describes the measurement of intrauterine ILPs whilst achieving a positive tamponade test in a series of seven cases.

Ethics approval was granted for the study from the University of Wollongong/South Eastern Sydney Illawarra Area Health Service and Medical Human Research Ethics Committee (HE09/240 and HE09/241). Cases 1 and 2 have been previously published[20].

IN VITRO INTRALUMINAL PRESSURES OF THE BAKRI, BT-CATH AND EBB BALLOONS

ILP recordings were determined for the various uterine-specific balloons and the condom catheter in the laboratory setting. These readings were obtained using a DigiMano (Netech Corporation, New York, USA) pressure recorder (Figure 2) as previously described[20].

Briefly, the ILP was recorded after 50-ml aliquots of normal saline were used to insufflate the various

balloons. This was continued until a final volume of 500 ml was reached for all balloons. Each 50-ml aliquot series was repeated three times using a single balloon (Figure 3).

For the Bakri balloon, the readings demonstrate that, in the absence of any external restrictions, the ILP reaches a peak of approximately 85 mmHg at 50 ml insufflation. This pressure does not vary by more than 10–25 mmHg despite the balloon being incrementally filled to a volume of 500 ml. The pattern is similar for the BT-Cath and the condom catheter, with initial peak pressures of approximately 25–30 and 10 mmHg, respectively, at volumes of 100 ml normal saline. Pressures varied by 1–5 mmHg as these latter balloons were subsequently insufflated. In contrast, the ILPs were not recordable on the Digimano manometer device from the Ebb balloon even when insufflated to 500 ml.

In contrast to these experiments, external compressive forces, such as squeezing the balloons by hand, increase the ILP for all balloons (Figure 2)[20].

METHODOLOGY

Case selection

Seven cases of women who experienced a PPH and were unresponsive to first-line uterotonic agents were included in this study (Table 1). Prior to insertion of the balloon, retained products of conception and genital tract trauma were excluded as a primary cause of the PPH.

Tamponade test

In this case series, a tamponade test was performed once first-line uterotonics (Syntocinon®, syntometriene, ergometrine, misoprostol and PGF2α) had been used and bleeding continued. A positive tamponade test was demonstrated in all cases.

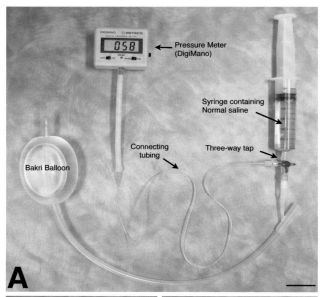
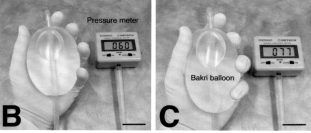

Figure 2 Intraluminal pressure recording apparatus. (A) The Bakri balloon is connected via a three-way tap to a pressure meter (DigiMano, Netech Corporation, Farmingdale, NY, USA). This enables the intraluminal pressures to be measured independent of insufflation of the balloon with normal saline. (B) and (C) By clasping the balloon the intraluminal pressure increases and is recorded by the pressure meter device. Bar = 4 cm. Reproduced from Figure 1 in reference 20, with permission

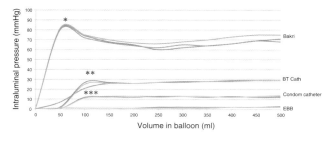

Figure 3 Intraluminal pressure readings (*in vitro*). Aliquots of 50 ml of normal saline were used to insufflate each of the uterine specific balloons and the condom catheter to a final volume of 500 ml. The corresponding intraluminal pressure was then recorded after each 50 ml aliquot. Only the uterine balloon component (Ut in Figure 1) of the Ebb balloon was insufflated with normal saline. *Pressure at initial 50 ml normal saline in the Bakri balloon. ** Pressure reading at 100 ml in the BT-Cath. ***Pressure reading at 100 ml in the Ebb balloon (uterine component). Note the differences in recorded intraluminal pressures despite similar volumes in each balloon from 50 to 500 ml saline

Table 1   Patient demographics, details of postpartum hemorrhage (PPH) and methodological parameters when using the Bakri balloon in cases 1–7

Case	Age	Risk factors	Previous pregnancy	Gestation at delivery (weeks + days)	Mode of delivery	Time of PPH	Cause of PPH	Oxytocics	Mode of insertion (all), laparotomy not closed	Use of USS	Tamponade test positive (volume: ml)	Mechanism to ensure Bakri remains in uterus	Analgesia (insertion)	Post op care (location)	Total time duration of balloon in uterus (h)	Deflation regimen	Final PPH (l)	Placental pathology
1	31	Oxytocin augmentation FTP (2nd stage) Ruptured uterus	1 LSCS (twins)	41 + 1	Em LSCS	At LSCS	Atonic uterus	S10, S40, PGF	From vagina	No	360	Vaccum	RA (spinal)	HDU	22	50% (12 h) 50% (22 h)	2.8	Not sent
2	28	Retained placenta	–	37 + 3	SVD	SVD	Atonic uterus	S10, S40, Miso, PGF	From vagina	No	350	Vaccum	GA	HDU	18	50% (14 h) 50% (18 h)	2.5	Normal
3	40	Prev PPH	1 SVD	37 + 4	SVD	During perineal tear repair	Atonic uterus	S10, S40, Ergo, Miso	From vagina	Yes*	350	Vaccum	GA	LW–PNW	23	50% (17 h) 50% (23 h)	1.3	Not sent
4	28	Retained placenta	3 SVD 2 TOP 1 Misc	37 + 2	SVD	Following manual removal	Atonic uterus	S10, S40, Ergo, Miso	From vagina	No	400	Vaccum	GA	LW–PNW	21	50% (18 h) 50% (21 h)	1	Not sent
5	39	Augmented labor	–	41 + 5	Em LSCS	At LSCS	Atonic uterus	S10, S40, Ergo, PGF	From vagina	No	450	Vaccum	GA	LW–PNW	19	50% (11 h) 50% 192 h)	2.5	Not sent
6	16	Pre-eclampsia IOL oxytocin augmentation	–	35 + 6	SVD	SVD	Atonic uterus	S10, S40, Miso	From vagina	No	500	Vaccum	GA	LW–PNW	27	30% (11 h) 20% (15 h) 50% (27 h)	2	Not sent
7	23	Twins	–	38 + 1	El LSCS	At LSCS	Atonic uterus	S10, S40, Ergo	From vagina	No	300	None required	RA (spinal)	LW–PNW	20	33% (8 h) 67% (20 h)	2.5	Not sent

El LSCS, elective lower segment cesarean section; Em LSCS, emergency lower segment cesarean section; Ergo, ergometrine 250–500 µg; FTP, failure to progress; GA, general anesthetic; HDU, high dependency unit; IOL, induction of labor; LW–PNW, labor ward–postnatal ward; Misc, miscarriage; Miso, misoprostol (800 µg per rectum); PGF, prostaglandin PGF2α; PP, placenta previa; Prev. PPH, previous PPH; SVD, spontaneous vaginal delivery; S10, 10 IU syntocinon (oxytocin); S40, 40 IU syntocinon (oxytocin infusion, over 4 h); TOP, termination of pregnancy; RA, regional anesthetic; *ultrasound scan (USS) used for teaching technique of balloon placement

Balloon selection

At the time that these patients were cared for, the Bakri balloon was the only uterine-specific balloon available in Australia. As such, it was used in all cases.

Using the Bakri balloon

The method of insertion, maintenance and removal of the Bakri balloon is described in Chapter 48. Briefly, the balloon is inserted digitally or using a Rampley's forceps together with a speculum, and the balloon is initially insufflated with 200 ml normal saline. The drainage channel and the cervix are then assessed for ongoing blood loss. If bleeding continues, a further 50 ml of normal saline is added, and blood loss is reassessed. This is repeated until bleeding has ceased. This tamponade method determined the final volume of normal saline insufflated in to the balloon.

Discharge and follow-up

All women were discharged within 3–7 days of their PPH. A follow-up appointment with a pelvic ultrasound scan was arranged 6–8 weeks following discharge. All endometrial cavities of these scans were reported as normal.

RESULTS

Demographics and pregnancy details

Table 1 outlines the demographic and pregnancy details in this series of seven cases. Case 1 and 2 have been previously published and cases 1 and 3–5 have been previously included as part of a poster on Bakri balloon methodology[20,21].

The average age of the women in this study was 29 years (range 16–40), with an average gestation of 38 weeks + 3 days (range 35 weeks + 6 days to 41 weeks + 5 days). Four of the seven women were in their first pregnancy (cases 2 and 5–7). Risk factors as noted in the recent Royal College of Obstetricians and Gynaecologists guidelines were present in all cases[22]. These included previous PPH (case 3), labor augmentation (cases 1 and 5) and twins (case 7). Both elective (cases 1 and 5) and emergency (case 7) cesarean sections, together with vaginal deliveries (cases 2–4 and 6) were represented.

The cause of PPH in all instances was uterine atony in accordance with the inclusion criteria of this study. However, the atony may have been secondary to manual removal of retained products (case 4), or subsequent to delivering the placenta at cesarean section during an elective (case 7), or emergency (cases 1 and 5) procedure. The remaining cases occurred after vaginal delivery following the delivery of the placenta (cases 2, 3 and 6)

First-line uterotonics

First-line oxytocics comprising oxytocin 10 IU IM and an oxytocin infusion (40 IU over 4 hours) were administered to all women (Table 1). In addition, some cases received in addition: 800 μg misoprostol per rectum (cases 2–4 and 6), 250 μg ergometrine iv/im (cases 3–5 and 7) or prostaglandin PGF2α intramyometrial (cases 1, 2 and 5).

Bakri insertion

All Bakri balloons were inserted transvaginally manner (see Chapter 48). At cesarean section, balloons were inserted following a two-layer closure of the lower uterine segment and only after observing ongoing vaginally bleeding from the cervix. An ultrasound scan was used during the insertion of the balloon in case 3 to aid in teaching of the technique of balloon insertion/insufflation.

Tamponade test final volume

The tamponade test was positive at volumes of 300–500 ml normal saline (average 387 ml). The tamponade 'method' was used to clinically assess the effectiveness of balloon filling (see Chapter 48). There were no assumptions made as to the capacity of the uterine cavity and, therefore, no prior estimation of volume required to reach a positive tamponade test.

Intraluminal pressure

The ILPs are shown in Table 2. ILPs that resulted in a positive tamponade test varied from 43 to 154 mmHg. When the ILPs were plotted against the volume of normal saline used to achieve a positive tamponade test, there was no direct correlation (Figures 4 and 5). However, in cases 2, 4 and 5, the final ILP resulting in a positive tamponade test was lower than the initial ILP produced by 50 ml normal saline. The remaining cases (cases 1, 3, 6 and 7) had a positive tamponade test at ILPs greater than the initial ILP produced at 50 ml normal saline.

Correlation to patient's systolic pressure

Whether an average systolic blood pressure or a range of such readings was used, in the majority of cases (cases 1–3 and 6–7) the final ILP was lower than the systolic blood pressure. The two exceptions were cases 4 and 5 (Table 2).

Following the immediate resuscitation and subsequent stabilization of the patient, the normal saline within the balloon was removed over the next 11–27 h (average 21.4 h). Antibiotics (metronidazole and cephazolin) and an ongoing oxytocin infusion were used for the duration of balloon placement.

Table 2 Intraluminal pressures and corresponding blood pressure readings when a positive tamponade test was achieved in cases 1–7. *Data from intraoperative anesthetic charts

Case	Final volume (ml) in balloon-positive tamponade test	Corresponding intraluminal pressure (mmHg)	Range of patient's blood pressure* (systolic/diastolic – mmHg)	Average blood pressure* (mmHg)	Average mean arterial pressure* (mmHg)
1	360	83	80–110/40–65	92/46	61
2	350	43	90–140/50–60	110/55	73
3	350	76	75–110/45–60	87/49	62
4	450	118	90–120/45–60	103/52	69
5	350	154	80–140/40–85	117/63	81
6	500	90	90–130/45–90	98/59	72
7	300	81	95–130/55–100	121/62	82

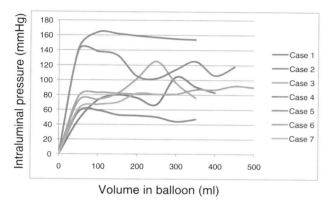

Figure 4 Intraluminal pressure readings (cases 1–7). In each case the pressure initially increases when 50 ml saline is insufflated into the Bakri balloon. These pressures vary as further saline is insufflated until a positive tamponade test is achieved. Note that similar volumes in each case result in variable corresponding intraluminal pressure readings

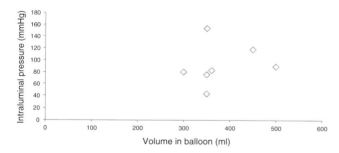

Figure 5 Correlation between final volume of saline required to achieve a positive tamponade test (using the tamponade 'method') and the corresponding intraluminal pressures (correlation coefficient = 0.18)

Final PPH volumes and placental pathology

The final volume of blood loss was estimated to be between 1 and 2.8 l. *The decision to use a balloon was not based on the estimated blood loss per se, but after recognition that the first-line uterotonics were ineffective.* Placental pathology was reported as normal for the retained placenta.

DISCUSSION

The management of PPH involves a stepwise series of physical, pharmacological and possibly surgical procedures to stop uterine bleeding[23]. Once retained products and genital tract trauma have been excluded, ongoing bleeding is assumed to be from an atonic uterus. Previous literature commonly describes the uterus as 'hypotonic', implying some residual ability to contract[24]. However, the commonly used term 'atonic' implies that the uterus is unable to initiate or maintain contractions in order to achieve hemostasis. This is paradoxical because, in the majority of cases of PPH secondary to uterine 'atony', uterotonic agents are clinically successful[1,2].

The primary goal of the interventions used in the management of PPH is to cause uterine contraction and a corresponding reduction in the volume of the uterine cavity. In contrast, uterine tamponade using balloon technology involves a fundamentally different approach, that is, temporarily expanding the uterine cavity[8]. A balloon made of rubber or silicone is introduced into the uterine cavity and incrementally inflated with normal saline, thereby increasing the uterine cavity volume. This tamponade test is considered 'positive' if the bleeding ceases[19].

Currently, one proposed mechanism of action by which these intrauterine balloons act is by exerting an inward-to-outward pressure 'that is greater than the systemic arterial pressure'[17,25]. An analogy to the 'first aid technique to stop a vessel from bleeding' has also been made. The technique works because the pressure on the blood vessel is greater than the pressure within the vessel[26]. This case series investigates the hypothesis that the mechanism by which an intrauterine balloon exerts a tamponade effect on the uterus is via exceeding the patient's systolic blood pressure.

In non-uterine systems where bleeding is successfully counteracted by balloon tamponade, relatively low ILPs are required. For example, based on pressures required to collapse the coronary–esophageal circuit, 25–30 mmHg is required when using the Sengstaken–Blakemore tube in the esophagus[27]. In the bladder, 75–80 mmHg, is required 'equal to the diastolic arterial pressure' to 'induce a reduction of blood circulation'[28,29].

Although the original description of the Bakri balloon stated it could 'withstand 300 mmHg', there do not appear to be any experimental recordings of intraluminal postpartum pressures required to stop uterine bleeding from an atonic uterus in the literature[30].

Pressure–volume relationships

The case series reported in this chapter demonstrates that, as the balloon is insufflated with normal saline in order to achieve a clinically effective positive tamponade test, the numerical relationship between this volume and the resulting ILP is curvilinear (Figure 4). Furthermore, uterine bleeding is controlled with ILPs that range from 43 mmHg (case 2) to 154 mmHg (case 5). The broad range of ILPs observed arise from similar volumes of normal saline in the Bakri balloon (Tables 1 and 2, Figures 4 and 5).

The intraluminal volumes used to obtain a positive tamponade test ranged from 300 to 500 ml (Tables 1 and 2). However, a larger volume did not necessarily produce a higher ILP (Figures 4 and 5). For example, a relatively small volume of 350 ml resulted in the highest pressures recorded (cases 2 and 5), whereas the greatest volume used (500 ml) resulted in a moderate ILP of 90 mmHg (case 6), similar to the lowest volume used (300 ml) in case 7 (81 mmHg). Furthermore, a twin pregnancy in which the resulting uterine cavity might be considered larger than a singleton cavity resulted in an ILP of 81 mmHg (case 7). This compares to the other singleton pregnancies that ranged from 43 to 154 mmHg.

As previously noted and as demonstrated in these cases, when the volume of fluid increases within the balloon, the ILP also gradually increases (Figure 4)[20]. However, subsequent ILP readings rise and fall during the establishment of a positive tamponade test (Figure 3). In some cases the final ILP, when the tamponade test is positive, is lower than previously recorded readings when bleeding was ongoing (cases 1–5). In other cases, the final ILP when the tamponade test is positive, is eventually higher than the initial ILPs (cases 6 and 7).

Relationship to systolic blood pressure

Based on the proposed mechanism of exerting an inward-to-outward pressure that is greater than the 'systolic arterial pressure', one might have expected that the final ILPs would have exceeded those of the patient's systolic pressure[17]. However, in some cases the ILPs were actually lower (cases 2 and 7), similar (cases 1, 3 and 6) or higher (cases 4 and 5) than the range of systolic blood pressures. With respect to the diastolic blood pressure, the final ILP was greater than (cases 1 and 3–5), similar (cases 6 and 7), or less than (case 2) the range of these documented values, respectively (Table 2).

As the relationship in this case series between ILP, intraluminal volume, systolic/diastolic blood pressures and bleeding cessation is inconsistent and variable, alternative explanations are proposed. On the assumption that the resulting ILP represents a cumulative effect in achieving a positive tamponade test, the following contributing factors are considered: uterine wall structure/compliance, balloon–uterine interface, stretching of the uterine cavity and distal effects on the uterine arteries.

Uterine wall structure/compliance

In order to achieve a tamponade effect during the management of bleeding, a relatively non-compliant surface serves as a semi-rigid barrier preventing further expansion of an enlarging collection of blood. This phenomenon should be reflected in the ILPs as the balloon is being insufflated with normal saline and the bleeding ceases.

During a PPH, if the uterus is considered completely 'atonic', it may be considered unable to counteract an increase in the uterine cavity volume (UCV) as hemorrhage ensues within the cavity. Provided that the inherent structure of the uterine wall does not limit this expansion, thereby acting as the semi-rigid surface described above, the *in vivo* ILP would be expected to be similar to the *in vitro* experiments where there were no external restrictions to balloon expansion (Figure 3). In other words, the uterine structure would be relatively inert to the expanding uterine cavity volume. Conversely, if during a given PPH the uterus is again considered 'atonic', but now able to withstand a *defined* increase in uterine cavity volume, the ILP would be expected to initially plateau as the balloon volume approximated that of the uterine cavity (Figure 3). However, as the expanding balloon becomes subsequently restricted from the non-compliant uterus, the pressure would be expected to rise again in a linear fashion.

Both of these hypothetical models, however, involve an assumption of the compliance characteristics of the uterine wall, the point at which the tamponade test becomes positive must be taken into account. The volume–ILP profiles in Figure 4 suggest that the uterine cavity expands to a point at which bleeding ceases but that this is not associated with a secondary rise in ILPs.

In the 'physiological contracting-down' postpartum uterus, a currently accepted mechanism that stops bleeding involves the structural arrangement of the uterine muscle fibers in relation to the intervening blood vessels[18]. Helie described a figure of eight arrangement of muscle fibers around the vasculature. When the uterus contracts, the effect is referred to as 'living sutures'[31]. Images of the uterine wall thickness following balloon placement and insufflation with normal saline demonstrate a thinning of the uterine wall (Figure 6a and c). It could be hypothesized that one of the mechanisms by which the balloon functions is by compressing the intervening vascular supply within the uterine wall (Figure 6b and d).

Balloon–uterine interface

Studies using condom catheters also result in a positive tamponade test at similar volumes to other balloons[13,14]. From the *in vitro* pressures described in this chapter, it can be seen that compared with those of the other uterine specific balloons, these pressures are relatively low: 12–15 mmHg (Figure 3). If, *in vivo*, such low pressures are sufficient to generate a positive tamponade test, it may be that it is not the magnitude

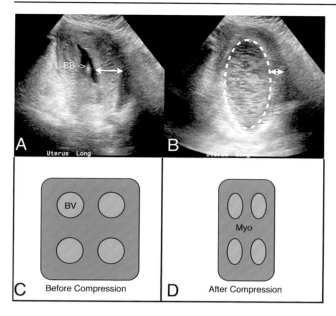

Figure 6 Ultrasound images of Bakri balloon within uterine cavity (A) and (B), and proposed mechanism of action involving myometrial compression (C) and (D). At commencement of insufflation with saline of Bakri balloon (BB), note the myometrial thickness (arrows in (A)). Compare the myometrial thickness (arrows in (B)) after a positive tamponade test. A schematic diagram of the hypothesized compressive effect of intrauterine balloons on the blood vessels (BV) within the myometrium (Myo). (C) represents 'before compression' corresponding to the ultrasound images (A) above. (D) represents 'after compression' corresponding to the ultrasound images in (B) above. Arrowheads in (B) represent a 50% reduction in wall thickness compared with arrowheads in (A). Adapted from Figure 5 in reference 20, with permission

of the pressure exerted which is important, but the effect of balloon contact at the uterine surface that elicits a clinical response.

A similar observation is made in the use of an 'OAT patch' when used to stop the bleeding from a vascular bed or a large vessel such as the aorta or inferior vena cava[32,33]. Here the approximation of a piece of autologous tissue, such as a piece of rectus sheath prevents ongoing bleeding. Again, minimal external pressures are required to stop bleeding. The authors of this method propose mechanisms which include: (1) lamina flow within the damaged vessel creates suction on the overlying patch (Venturi effect); (2) resistance to flow between the large patch and the vessel wall beyond the defect may be sufficient impedance to stop flow completely; and (3) that the Patch provides a framework for the deposition of fibrin and platelets[32,33].

Finally, low intracavity pressures obtained in the Sengstaken–Blakemore tube and the Rusch balloons are also sufficient to control bleeding[27].

Stretching of uterine cavity

An undulating pattern of ILPs during the establishment of a positive tamponade test may be interpreted as the uterus exhibiting an inherent contractile ability

(Figure 4). Thus, the rising and falling pressures may represent phases of uterine contractile activity and relaxation, respectively. Clearly the initial phases of uterine activity are insufficient to result in hemostasis, as the tamponade test is still negative at this initial time (Figure 4). However, as the uterus distends to accommodate the increasing intraluminal volume, hemostasis is achieved. In fact this undulating pattern is also seen after a positive tamponade test is achieved[20].

Therefore, regardless of the pressure exerted in the uterine cavity, a hemostatic effect may be facilitated by stimulating a contractile response of the uterine musculature secondary to stretching of the uterine musculature by insufflating the balloon with normal saline. It is noteworthy that, in addition to the known association of polyhydramnios and uterine activity, stretching of human myometrial cells *in vitro* results in an increase in the oxytocin receptor synthesis/mRNA[34]. Therefore, the uterus itself should not be considered an inert component as the term 'atonic' implies.

Distal effects on the uterine arteries

One study has suggested that the tamponade effect acts distally by compressing the uterine arteries, 'a mechanism akin to mechanical uterine artery embolization or ligation'[18]. This is based on a single case of PPH managed with a Sengstaken–Blakemore tube that was insufflated with normal saline within the lower uterine segment following a vaginal delivery[18]. In addition studies demonstrate that an extensive collateral circulation may redirect blood from the uterine arteries resulting in a lowering of the internal iliac/uterine arterial pressures, thereby facilitating clotting and therefore hemostasis. Of note, however, are the descriptions of using balloon tamponade technology in patients who have impaired coagulopathies[35].

SUMMARY

These seven cases suggest that although insufflating an intrauterine balloon with normal saline within a postpartum uterus is correlated with a rise in ILP, this pressure does not need to exceed the patient's systolic blood pressure to result in a tamponade effect.

Furthermore, the uterus does not appear to be entirely 'atonic', and the tamponade effect of the resulting ILPs may represent a combination of factors elicited by the distended balloon. These may involve endometrial–balloon interface interactions, alterations of vascular flow patterns within the uterine arteries, uterine activity secondary to myometrial stretching, and an occlusive effect on compressed vascular structures secondary to uterine wall attenuation.

PRACTICE POINTS

- Intraluminal pressures vary with different volumes in different uteri

- Specific intraluminal pressures do not necessarily reflect the volume used and vice versa

- Other factors may contribute to the resulting 'tamponade' effect of the balloons including:
  - Balloon-endometrial interface
  - Alterations of the uterine muscular wall
  - Local effects on the uterine artery blood flow
  - Uterine activity following stretching of the uterine cavity.

ACKNOWLEDGMENTS

The author would like to acknowledge the excellent and efficient library staff at the Wollongong Hospital (Christine Monie, Sharon Hay, Vivienne Caldwell and Jill Brady). In addition, the author would like to thank the Department of Biomedical Engineering at Wollongong Hospital (Gary De Lucia and Marcus Poplawski) that provided the 'DigiMano' pressure transducer.

ETHICS APPROVAL

The intraluminal pressure measurements were obtained as the balloons were inflated and did not result in any delay in establishing the tamponade test. Ethics committee approval was granted from the University of Wollongong/South Eastern Sydney Ilawarra Area Health Service and Medical Human Research Ethics Committee (HE09/240 and HE09/241).

References

1. Mousa HA, Alfirevic Z. Treatment for primary postpartum haemorrhage (Review). Cochrane Database Syst Rev 2007;(1):CD003249
2. Lombaard H, Pattinson RC. Common errors and remedies in managing postpartum haemorrhage. Best Prac Res Clin Obstet Gynaecol 2009;23:317–26
3. Ramsbotham PH. The Principles and Practice of Obstetrical Medicine and Surgery. Philadelphia: Blanchard and Lea, 1856:371:415–6
4. Williams JW. Changes in the maternal organism resulting from pregnancy. In: Obstetrics: A Textbook for the Use of the Student and Practitioner, reprint of 1st edn. Stanford, Connecticut: Appleton and Lange, 1997;Chapter VI:145–8
5. Cosgrove SA. Obstetric haemorrhage and its management. South Med J 1936;29:1219–25
6. Douglass LH. The passing of the pack. Bull Soc Med (Baltimore, MD) 1955;40:37–9
7. Maier RC. Control of postpartum haemorrhage with uterine packing. Am J Obstet Gynecol 1993;169:317–23
8. Georgiou C. Balloon tamponade in the management of postpartum haemorrhage: a review. BJOG 2009;116:748–57
9. Utah Medical Products Inc. BT-Cath. http://www.utahmed.com/btcath.htm 2011
10. Glenveigh Medical. Ebb—The Complete Tamponade Solution for Postpartum Hemorrhage. http://www.glenveigh.com/products/ebb.html 2011
11. Bakri YN. Uterine tamponade-drain for hemorrhage secondary to placenta previa-accreta: Int J Gynecol Obstet 1992;37:302–3
12. De Loor JA, van Dam PA. Foley catheters for uncontrollable obstetric or gynecologic hemorrhage. Obstet Gynecol 1996;88:737–8
13. Akhter S, Begum MR, Kabir Z, Rashid M, Laila TR, Zabeen F. Use of a condom to control massive postpartum hemorrhage. MedGenMed 2003;5:38
14. Akhter S, Begum MR, Kabir, J. Condom hydrostatic tamponade for massive postpartum hemorrhage. Int J Gynecol Obstet 2005;90:134–5
15. Katesmark M, Brown R, Raju KS. Successful use of a Sengstaken-Blakemore tube to control massive postpartum haemorrhage. BJOG 1994;101:259–60
16. Johanson R, Kumar M, Obhrai M, Young P. Management of massive postpartum haemorrhage: use of a hydrostatic balloon catheter to avoid laparotomy: BJOG 2001;108:420–2
17. Arulkumarah S, Condous G. The "tamponade test" in the management of massive postpartum hemorrhage. Obstet Gynecol 2003;102:641–2
18. Cho Y, Rizvi C, Uppal T, Condous G. Ultrasonographic visualization of balloon placement for uterine tamponade in massive primary postpartum hemorrhage. Ultrasound Obstet Gynecol 2008;32:711–3
19. Condous GS, Arulkumarah S, Symonds I, et al. The "tamponade test" in the management of massive postpartum hemorrhage. Obstet Gynecol 2003;101:767–72
20. Georgiou C. Intraluminal pressure readings during the establishment of a positive "tamponade test" in the management of postpartum haemorrhage. BJOG 2010;117:295–303
21. Georgiou C. Practical guidelines for using the Bakri balloon in the management of postpartum haemorrhage. Poster presented at RANZCOG Meeting, Adelaide, 21–24 March, 2010
22. Royal College of Obstetricians and Gynaecologists. Green top Guideline No.52. Prevention and management of postpartum Haemorrhage. London: RCOG, 2009
23. Doumouchtsis SK, Papageorghiou AT, Arulkumaran S. systematic review of conservative management of postpartum hemorrhage: what to do when medical treatment fails: Obstet Gynecol Surv 2007;62:540–7
24. Salacz P. The treatment of post-partum hemorrhage due to atony. J Obstet Gynaecol 1935;476–89
25. Danso D, Reginald PW. Internal uterine tamponade. In: Lynch CB, Keith LG, Lalonde AB, Karoshi M, eds. A Textbook of Postpartum Hemorrhage. Duncow, UK: Sapiens Publishing, 2006:263–7
26. Vitthala S, Tsoumpou I, Anjum ZK, Aziz NA. Use of Bakri balloon in post-partum hemorrhage: A series of 15 cases. Aust NZ J Obstet Gynaecol 2009;49:191–4
27. Sengstaken R.W, Blakemore AH. Balloon tamponage for the control of hemorrhage from esophageal varices: Sengstaken and Blakemore: Ann Surg 1950;131:781–9
28. Harrison,J. Tumors of the bladder. In: Hartwell, ed. Campbell's Urology, 4th edn. Philadelphia: W.B. Saunders Company,. 1978;2:1064
29. Helmstein K. Treatment of bladder carcinoma by a hydrostatic pressure technique. Br J Urol 1972;44:434–50
30. Bakri YN, Amri A, Abdul Jabbar F. Tamponade balloon for obstetrical bleeding. Int J Gynecol Obstet 2001;74:139–42
31. Helie PT. In: Willams' Obstetrics: A Textbook for the Use of the Student and Practitioner, reprint of 1st edn., 1903. Stanford, CT: Appleton and Lange, 1997:147
32. Hammond IG, Obermair A, Taylor JD, Lawrence-Brown M. The overlay autogenous tissue (OAT) patch to control major intraoperative vascular injury in an ovine model. Gynecol Oncol 2004;94 560–3
33. Hammond IG, Obermair A, Taylor JD, Lawrence-Brown M. The control of severe intraoperative bleeding using an overlay autogenous tissue (OAT) patch: case reports. Gynecol Oncol 2004;94:564–6
34. Terzidou V, Sooranna SR, Kim LK, et al. Mechanical stretch up-regulates the human oxytocin receptor in primary human uterine myocytes. J Clin Endocrinol Metab 2005;90:237–46
35. Bagga R, Jain V, Sharma S, Suri V. Postpartum haemorrhage in two women with impaired coagulation successfully managed with condom catheter tamponade. Ind J Med Sci 2007;61:157–8

46

Internal Uterine Tamponade

D. Danso and P. W. Reginald

INTRODUCTION

The origin of the word tamponade appears to have come from an old French word for tampon, which carries the connotation of a plug, a bung or a stopper inserted into an open wound or a body cavity to stop the flow of blood[1]. Today, the common usage of this term includes the collection of menstrual effusion by insertion of a preformed sanitary pledget into the vagina.

In the context of postpartum hemorrhage, tamponade refers to plugging the uterus with some type of device to stop the flow of blood. Normally, this is in the form of a gauze pack or a balloon catheter. Internal tamponade procedures have been used successfully alone[2–5] or in combination with the Brace suture[6] to reduce or arrest massive postpartum hemorrhage.

PRINCIPLES OF UTERINE TAMPONADE

Uterine tamponade requires developing intrauterine pressure to stop bleeding. This can be accomplished in two ways:

(1) By insertion of a balloon that distends in the uterine cavity and occupies the entire space, thereby creating an intrauterine pressure that is greater than the systemic arterial pressure. In the absence of lacerations, the blood flow into the uterus should stop the moment the pressure in the tamponade balloon is greater than that of the systemic arterial pressure.

(2) By insertion of a uterine pack consisting of a gauze roll that is tightly packed into the uterus in such a manner that pressure is applied directly on capillary/venous bleeding vessels or surface oozing (of the deciduas) from within the uterus, thereby resulting in either a significant reduction or stoppage of uterine bleeding.

BASIC GENERAL PRINCIPLES

After failure of medical intervention to stop or reduce postpartum hemorrhage, one should consider performing internal uterine tamponade. This should be carried out in the operating theater with anesthetic and nursing staff present as well as blood transfusion service back-up. The woman should be placed in the Lloyd Davies or lithotomy position with an indwelling urethral catheter. Examination under anesthesia should be carried out to exclude lacerations, retained placenta, and to empty the uterus of clots. Only then should tamponade procedures be attempted. Uterotonics and hemostatics are advised as adjunct therapy and may be given simultaneously. Any of the internal uterine tamponade methods described below can be embarked upon before resorting to surgical interventions.

The following is a description of the 'tamponade test' and various other methods of tamponade with their potential advantages and disadvantages.

THE TAMPONADE TEST

This test, first described in 2003 by Condous and colleagues[7], was proposed as a prognostic index as to whether laparotomy would be needed in patients with major postpartum hemorrhage unresponsive to medical therapy. In the original description, a Sengstaken–Blakemore esophageal catheter was inserted into the uterine cavity via the cervix, using ultrasound guidance when possible, and filled with warm saline until the distended balloon was palpable per abdomen surrounded by the well-contracted uterus, and visible at the lower portion of the cervical canal. The position of the Sengstaken–Blakemore esophageal catheter was checked to ensure it was firmly fixed *in situ* within the uterine cavity by the application of gentle traction. If no or only minimal bleeding was observed via the cervix or there was only minimal bleeding into the gastric lumen of the Sengstaken–Blakemore esophageal catheter, the tamponade test result was considered to be positive. If this were the case, surgical intervention, with possible hysterectomy, was avoided. On the other hand, if significant bleeding continued via the cervix or the gastric lumen of the tube, the tamponade test was deemed a failure and laparotomy was performed. In this study, 14 out of 16 women (87%) with intractable hemorrhage responded positively. Of the women who did not respond, one continued to bleed because of an overlooked cervical extension of the lower transverse uterine incision at cesarean delivery. The balloon was inadequately inflated in the other. The Rüsch urological balloon has also been used successfully for the tamponade test[3]. Chapter 47 describes in more detail a longitudinal study still in progress to determine the effectiveness of the Rüsch urological balloon for the tamponade test.

SENGSTAKEN–BLAKEMORE TUBE

The Sengstaken–Blakemore esophageal catheter was originally designed for the treatment of esophageal variceal bleeds and the introduction of contrast media. It is a three-way catheter tube with stomach and esophageal balloon components (see Figure 1). It can be inflated to volumes greater than 500 ml. Several reports on its successful use to arrest major postpartum hemorrhage are available[2,7,8–11]. Before insertion of the tube, the distal end of the tube beyond the stomach balloon is severed to minimize the risk of perforation. The main advantage is its simplicity of use and, therefore, junior residents can easily learn and perform the test while waiting for help.

The main disadvantages are that it is not purpose-designed for postpartum hemorrhage and may not easily adapt to the shape of the uterine cavity. Moreover, it contains latex and may not be affordable in resource-poor settings.

RÜSCH HYDROSTATIC UROLOGICAL BALLOON

This is a two-way Foley catheter (simplastic 20 ch, 6.7 mm, 30 ml), which can also be used for postpartum hemorrhage. It has a capacity greater than 500 ml (see Figure 2)[3]. The technique of insertion is similar to the description already given for the Sengstaken–Blakemore esophageal catheter. A 60-ml

bladder syringe can be used for inflating the balloon with warm saline via the drainage port. It is a simple technique and therefore junior residents can easily learn and become adept in its use, especially if practised after a manual removal of the placenta.

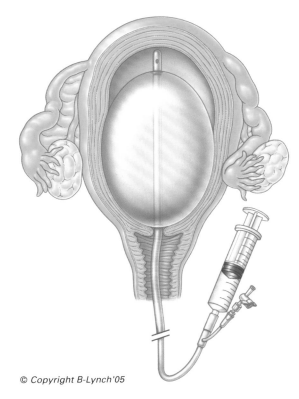

Figure 2   Rüsch hydrostatic balloon catheter

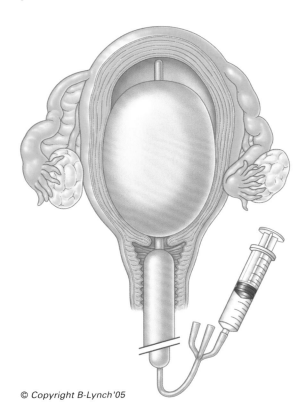

Figure 1   Sengstaken–Blakemore tube

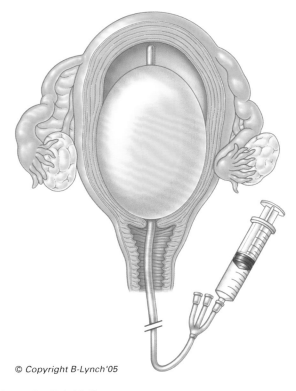

Figure 3   Bakri balloon

BAKRI BALLOON

The SOS Bakri tamponade balloon catheter (Cook Ob/Gyn) is marketed as 100% Silicon (no latex), purpose-designed two-way catheter, to provide temporary control or reduction of postpartum uterine bleeding when conservative management is warranted (see Figure 3)[4]. Again, the insertion technique is simple. Insert the balloon portion of the catheter in the uterus, making sure that the entire balloon is inserted past the cervical canal and internal os, under ultrasound guidance if possible. At cesarean delivery, the tamponade balloon can be passed via the cesarean incision into the uterine cavity with the inflation port passing into the vagina via the cervix. An assistant pulls the shaft of the balloon through the vaginal canal until the deflated balloon base comes into contact with the internal cervical os. The uterine incision is closed in the usual fashion, taking care to avoid puncturing the balloon while suturing. A gauze pack soaked with iodine or antibiotics can then be inserted into the vaginal canal to ensure maintenance of correct placement of the balloon and maximize the tamponade effect. The balloon is then inflated with sterile fluid to the desired volume for tamponade effect. Gentle traction on the balloon shaft ensures proper contact between the balloon and the tissue surface and may enhance the tamponade effect. Success can be judged by the declining loss of blood seen through the drainage port and the fluid connecting bag.

The main disadvantage of this method is that it may not be affordable in resource-poor countries because of the expense.

FOLEY CATHETER

The successful use of the Foley catheter balloon for internal uterine tamponade is also described[12,13]. A Foley catheter with a 30-ml balloon capacity is easy to acquire and may routinely be stocked on labor and delivery suites. Using a No. 24F Foley catheter, the tip is guided into the uterine cavity and inflated with 60–80 ml of saline (anecdotally, a volume of 150 ml can be reached before it bursts). Additional Foley catheters can be inserted, if necessary, until bleeding stops. As attractive, easy and cheap as this method is, some concerns have been raised regarding the use of the Foley catheter for uterine tamponade. First, the capacity of the immediate postpartum uterine cavity, especially if term, is too large for effective tamponade to be achieved with one inflated balloon, and the risk of one balloon falling out of the uterus is increased[14]. Second, significant bleeding may occur above the Foley bulb, as it may not fill the entire uterine cavity. Even the use of multiple Foley catheters cannot ensure a complete compression effect on the entire uterine surface.

HYDROSTATIC CONDOM CATHETER

This innovative approach from Bangladesh uses a sterile rubber catheter fitted with a condom as a tamponade balloon device[14]. The sterile catheter is inserted within the condom and tied near the mouth of the condom with a silk thread, and the outer end of the catheter is connected to a saline set. In its original description, after placement in the uterus, the condom is inflated with 250–500 ml normal saline according to need, and the outer end of the catheter was folded and tied with thread after bleeding had stopped[14]. Vaginal bleeding is observed and further inflation is stopped when bleeding has ceased. To keep the balloon *in situ*, the vaginal cavity is packed with roller gauze and sanitary pads. Success is gauged by the amount of blood loss per vaginum. Hemorrhage was arrested within 15 min in all 23 cases in the original series[14]. Although the sample size was small, this method represents a cheap, simple and quick intervention which may prove invaluable in, especially, resource-poor countries.

UTERINE PACKING

Uterine packing entails placing, carefully and systematically, several yards of gauze inside the uterine cavity to occlude the whole intrauterine space and, thus, control major hemorrhage. The technique fell out of favor in the 1950s, as it was thought to conceal hemorrhage and cause infection. It re-emerged in the 1980s and 1990s after these concerns were not verified[15]. The main disadvantages of this technique are:

(1) Experience is required to pack properly and tightly and therefore junior residents may not be able to perform proficiently, especially if they have large hands. Speed is also necessary because the intrauterine/vaginal hand becomes numb rapidly;

(2) Delay in recognizing continual hemorrhage as blood needs to soak through yards of gauze before it becomes evident;

(3) Success of the procedure will not be known immediately, as the blood must soak through the pack to reveal itself;

(4) The tightness of the pack is difficult to determine, especially if blood soaks through, leading to a loss of the tamponade effect;

(5) Potential risk of trauma and infection;

(6) Removing the pack may often require a separate surgical procedure to dilate and extract the intrauterine material, thus falling short of an ideal option.

Notwithstanding, uterine packing remains an option, especially, if balloon catheters or balloons are not available. The risk of intrauterine infection can be minimized by prophylactic antibiotics.

CARE AFTER SUCCESSFUL UTERINE TAMPONADE

All patients should be managed in a high-dependency or intensive care unit with very close monitoring of their vital signs, fluid input/output, fundal height and vaginal blood loss. Continued oxytocin infusion may be necessary to keep the uterus contracted over 12–24 h. Prophylactic broad-spectrum antibiotic cover should be administered. The mean time for leaving tamponade balloons or uterine packs ranges from 8 to 48 h[2,7,9–12]. A graduated deflation of the balloon is advised to reduce the potential risk of further bleeding.

In summary, tamponade procedures are simple, cheap, easy to use, and effective measures that should be considered in women with intractable postpartum hemorrhage, especially when other options may be unavailable.

References

1. Collins English Dictionary, 5th edn. London: Collins, 2000:1563
2. Katesmark M, Brown R, Raju KS. Successful use of a Sengstaken–Blakemore tube to control massive postpartum haemorrhage. Br J Obstet Gynaecol 1994;101:259–60
3. Johanson R, Kumar M, Obrai M, Young P. Management of massive postpartum haemorrhage: use of a hydrostatic balloon catheter to avoid laparotomy. Br J Obstet Gynaecol 2001; 108:420–2
4. Bakri YN, Amri A, Abdul Jabbar F. Tamponade-balloon for obstetrical bleeding. Int J Gynaecol Obstet 2001;74:139–42
5. Ferrazzani S, Guariglia L, Caruso A. Therapy and prevention of obstetric haemorrhage by tamponade using a balloon catheter. Minerva Ginecol 2004;56:481–4
6. Danso D, Reginald P. Combined B-Lynch suture with intrauterine balloon catheter triumphs over massive postpartum haemorrhage. Br J Obstet Gynaecol 2002;109: 963
7. Condous GS, Arulkumaran S, Symonds I, Chapman R, Sinha A, Razvi K. The 'Tamponade test' in the management of massive postpartum hemorrhage. Obstet Gynecol 2003;101: 767–72
8. Condie RG, Buxton EJ, Paynes ES. Successful use of Sengstaken–Blakemore tube to control massive postpartum haemorrhage. Br J Obstet Gynaecol 1994;101:1023–4
9. Chan C, Razvi K, Tham KF, Arulkumaran S. The use of a Sengstaken–Blakemore tube to control postpartum hemorrhage. Int J Gynaecol Obstet 1997;58:251–2
10. Japaraj RP, Raman S. Sengstaken–Blakemore tube to control massive postpartum haemorrhage. Med J Malaysia 2003;58: 604–7
11. Frenzel D, Condous GS, Papageorghiou AT, McWhinney NA. The use of the 'tamponade test' to stop massive obstetric haemorrhage in placenta accreta. Br J Obstet Gynaecol 2005; 112:676–7
12. De Loor JA, van Dam PA. Foley catheters for uncontrollable obstetric or gynaecologic hemorrhage. Obstet Gynecol 1996; 88:737
13. Marcovici I, Scoccia B. Postpartum hemorrhage and intrauterine balloon tamponade. A report of three cases. J Reprod Med 1999;44:122–6
14. Akhter S, Begum MR, Kabir Z, Rashid M, Laila TR, Zabeen F. Use of a condom to control massive postpartum hemorrhage. Med Gen Med 2003;115:38
15. Maier RC. Control of postpartum hemorrhage with uterine packing. Am J Obstet Gynecol 1993;169:317–21

47

Balloon Internal Uterine Tamponade: Experience with 39 Patients from a Single Institution

S. Ferrazzani, A. Perrelli, C. Piscicelli and S. De Carolis

INTRODUCTION

During the past several years, a number of new and simple techniques have been developed in the attempt to avoid major surgical procedures for treatment of postpartum hemorrhage (PPH). In addition, a variety of surgical and radiological options have been proposed to avoid hysterectomy. Unfortunately, a suitable conservative technique is still lacking for all situations[1], and it is well recognized that all proposed options have risks as well as advantages. A practice bulletin from the American College of Obstetricians and Gynecologists (ACOG)[2] suggests that tamponade of the uterus can be effective in decreasing hemorrhage secondary to uterine atony, and that procedures such as uterine artery ligation or B-Lynch suture may be used to obviate the need for hysterectomy.

In general, four types of procedures can summarize all the conservative interventions in PPH: balloon tamponade, compression sutures, arterial embolization and pelvic devascularization. Among these, the uterine balloon tamponade has the advantage of simplicity and safety so that it can be easily carried out by doctors with minimal training and/or experience. Of interest, balloon tamponade has been used to control hemorrhage in other obstetric conditions in which bleeding is of a serious nature, for example, following first- and second-trimester termination of pregnancy[3,4], cervical pregnancy[5–7] as well as to control PPH from vaginal lacerations[8].

THEORETICAL PRINCIPLE OF ACTION

The effect of the balloon tamponade is such that temporary and steady mechanical compression of the bleeding surface of the placental site can be accomplished while waiting for the natural hemostatic mechanisms of the blood to take effect. The balloon, inflated inside the uterine cavity in order to stretch the myometrial wall, provides an intrauterine pressure that overcomes the systemic arterial pressure, thus resulting in cessation of the intrauterine blood flow[9]. More recently, an alternative mechanism of action has been proposed, which involves the hydrostatic pressure effect of the balloon on the uterine arteries[10].

In all probability, a quite different mechanism can be proposed for the efficacy of a balloon in the case of uterine atony. With separation of the placenta, the numerous uterine arteries and veins that carry blood to and from the placenta are severed abruptly. Elsewhere in the body, hemostasis in the absence of surgical ligation depends upon intrinsic vasospasm and formation of blood clots locally. At the placental implantation site, however, the most important factors for achieving hemostasis are contraction and retraction of the myometrium in order to compress the vessels and obliterate their lumens. Uterine atony from any origin can prevent this physiological mechanism, leading to massive hemorrhage.

The most common approach to atony is based on the use of uterotonic agents and mechanical stimulation by massage of the uterus. In such situations, the efficacy of the tamponade balloon may derive from the mechanical stimulation of myometrial contraction caused by the balloon's elasticity pressing against the myometrial wall. The simultaneous and continuous stimulation of myometrial contraction and the tamponade effect on the open vessels, reached with the contraction, explain its efficacy. However, the uterus must be empty for the tamponade to be successful.

THE BALLOON TAMPONADE TEST

To date, there is no diagnostic test to identify which patients with intractable hemorrhage will require surgery. Condous and colleagues[9] proposed the use of an inflated Sengstaken–Blakemore balloon catheter as a test to create tamponade and identify those patients who will or will not need surgery ('tamponade test'). With positive results, the tamponade test not only halts the blood loss and preserves the uterus, but also gives an opportunity to reverse and correct any consumptive coagulopathy. More than 87% of their patients (14/16) with intractable PPH responded to the tamponade test. Seror and colleagues[11] reported that, in a series of 17 cases, tamponade treatment prevented surgery in 88% of patients; furthermore, Doumouchtsis et al.[12] showed that hemostasis was achieved in 22/27 (81%) women who had placement of the balloon catheter. From these clinical experiences, it is possible to state that early use of the balloon catheter may reduce total blood loss, and, in all probability, any type of inflatable balloon with high fluid-filling capacity could be used for the same purpose[13].

The experience at the Catholic University of Rome, Italy

A longitudinal study is currently continuing at the Obstetrics and Gynaecology Department of the Catholic University of Holy Heart in Rome, Italy; it started in January 2002 and was approved by the Institutional review board. The study's aim is to evaluate the efficacy of the balloon tamponade, its advantages in terms of subsequent hysterectomy (not only in terms of fertility loss, but also of blood loss and maternal morbidity), and the medium- and long-term reproductive follow-up of the patients.

Patients and methods

Between January 1 2002 and June 30 2010, a total of 25,918 patients delivered in the maternity department. During this time, 39 women who experienced PPH underwent treatment by intrauterine tamponade. PPH was defined as a blood loss of more than 500 ml after vaginal delivery quantified with a collection pouch placed after delivery or more than 1000 ml of blood loss during a cesarean section. Additionally, the blood loss was defined as persisting and not responding to conventional uterotonic therapy.

The initial medical treatment included the use of oxytocic agents, prostaglandin analogues and ergometrine. According with our hospital's protocol, every woman had an intramuscular prophylactic dose of oxytocin (5 IU) (Syntocinon®) and ergometrine (0.2 mg) (Methergin®, only in normotensive women) after spontaneous delivery and an intramyometrial dose of oxytocin in case of cesarean section. If bleeding persisted, oxytocin was administered at a dose of 10–20 IU in 500 ml of glucose 5% solution; sometimes, intravenous sulprostone (Nalador®, 0.5 mg in 250 ml of saline solution) was infused; seldom, five intrarectal tablets (1 mg total) of misoprostol (Cytotec®, tablets 200 μg) were used. Other obstetric measures included uterine massage to stimulate uterine contraction and evaluation for the presence of retained placental tissue or vaginal/cervical lacerations under regional or general anesthesia. When present, retained placental tissue was removed and lacerations were sutured. Coagulation studies were carried out simultaneously to exclude coagulopathy as the first or the complementary cause of the hemorrhage.

In those patients delivering by the vaginal route who showed no response to these measures, a sterile hydrostatic (bladder distension) balloon catheter size 5.3 mm, Rüsch balloon (Rüsch (UK), High Wycombe, UK), was inserted into the uterine cavity via the cervix. This was achieved using minimal analgesia or regional anesthetics. Insertion was facilitated by grasping the anterior and lateral margins of the cervix with sponge forceps and placing the empty balloon into the uterine cavity with another sponge forceps. The balloon catheter was then filled with warm saline solution until a contracted uterus was palpable through the abdomen. Applying gentle traction at this stage confirmed that the filled balloon was firmly fixed in the uterine cavity. If no or minimal bleeding was observed through the cervix, laparotomy was avoided and gauze packing was placed in the vagina to avoid expulsion of the balloon from the dilated cervical os. If significant bleeding continued through the cervix, the 'tamponade test' had failed and laparotomy was performed.

In patients delivering by cesarean section, the problem of abnormal placental insertion or suspicion of morbid adhesions was confirmed by ultrasound scan before surgery. The placenta was delivered by firmly controlled cord traction, or by manual removal if it was abnormally attached to the uterine wall. According to Benirschke and Kaufmann[14], the histological diagnosis of accreta can be made only when the uterus is removed with the attached placenta remaining in situ; in case of removal of the placenta from the uterus, the diagnosis of placenta accreta was necessarily based on clinical criteria consisting of the inability to remove the placenta by controlled cord traction because of a adherence to the underlying myometrium and the failure to develop a cleavage plane between the placenta and uterus.

If severe bleeding persisted despite a contracted uterus after local intramyometrial and intravenous infusion of oxytocin and prostaglandin analogues, the hydrostatic balloon catheter filled with warm saline solution, was inserted intra-abdominally (Figure 1) through the uterine incision and the lower end brought through the cervical canal by a sponge forceps, thus leaving the balloon in the uterine cavity.

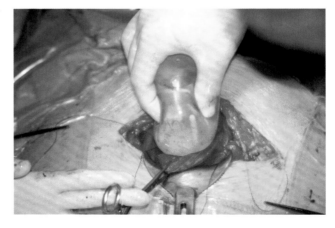

Figure 1 Intra-abdominal insertion of the hydrostatic balloon catheter into the uterine cavity (surgery drill)

Tamponade was achieved by pulling the distal end of the catheter shaft out of the vagina. Uterine contraction over the balloon was maintained after the uterine closure by a slow oxytocin infusion (20–40 IU) that was administered over the next 24 h. A single-layer closure of the uterine incision was performed, taking care not to include the balloon in the suture line. Only when the bleeding was adequately controlled was the abdominal wall closed.

Patients who responded to the balloon catheter therapy, irrespective of route of delivery, were stabilized in the labor and delivery unit for ongoing management. In all cases, intravenous broad-spectrum antibiotics were administered for at least the first 24 h. The balloon catheter was left *in situ* until the next day. During this time interval, blood transfusion and coagulopathy correction were possible. Once the above parameters were within acceptable limits, the balloon catheter was slowly deflated and withdrawn, and the patient observed for any active bleeding.

A second sample of 30 patients was randomly extracted from 79 historical cases of postpartum hysterectomy performed as first-line treatment for PPH from 1985 to 2001 before the introduction of the use of the balloon in January 2002. This second group (hysterectomy sample) was compared to the balloon sample in order to observe differences in co-morbidity (in addition to fertility loss) between the historical aggressive method and the conservative approach of recent years.

Normally distributed continuous variables were compared using a two-sample Student t test. Cross-tabulation and χ^2 (with Yates' continuity correction) were used to examine the relationship between nominal variables. All p values less than 0.05 were considered statistically significant. Patients, treated successfully with the balloon were subsequently contacted by phone in order to evaluate the subsequent fertility, pregnancy rates and possible medium- and long-term complications.

Results

The mean patient age was 34.6 years (26–46 years), and the mean gestational age at delivery was 35.9 weeks (21–42 weeks). Seventeen patients were multiparous (44%). The mean parity was 1.29 ± 0.6. Ten patients had a vaginal delivery and 29 underwent cesarean section (of which 15 were planned). In 17 instances, an atonic uterus caused PPH, whereas placenta previa/accreta was diagnosed in 22, of which four were associated with uterine atony.

Table 1 displays the results of the study. The 'tamponade test' was successful in 31 out of 39 cases; the hydrostatic catheter immediately arrested hemorrhage in 9/10 (90%) cases of vaginal delivery and in 22/29 (75%) cases of cesarean section.

The mean volume of saline solution used to inflate the balloon was 318 ± 163 ml; if bleeding ceased, the balloon was maintained in place for a median of 21.3 ± 10 h. Twenty-five patients required blood

transfusions during the acute episode of hemorrhage; six patients received fresh frozen plasma (FFP). No platelet transfusions were required.

Additional surgery was deemed necessary in eight cases (20%) where the tamponade procedure failed. One patient with placenta previa and accreta, one patient with placenta accreta and uterine atony, one patient with placenta previa, accreta and uterine atony, and one patient with placenta previa, uterine atony and abruptio placentae required immediate hysterectomy. In a case of uterine atony following cesarean section, a B-Lynch compression suture was performed after the balloon application. However, the B-Lynch suture was unsuccessful and hysterectomy was necessary. In another case of atony, Hayman compression suture was able to stop bleeding where the balloon had been unsuccessful. Bilateral O'Leary ligation was performed successfully in one case of emergency cesarean section for hemorrhage in placenta previa and in one case of elective cesarean section for placenta previa and accreta.

The comparison between the balloon and the hysterectomy samples is shown in Table 2. A statistically significant difference was found between the two samples in terms of blood loss, transfused units of red blood cells and days of postpartum admission.

Two patients experienced postpartum sepsis, both commencing after balloon removal. The first patient had a cesarean section for vaginal bleeding after a failed labor induction. Because of severe anemia (Hb 6.1 g/dl) 48 hours after delivery, a transfusion of 1 unit of red blood cells (RBC) was started but soon after stopped because of fever (38°C). Five days later, the patient presented with dyspnea, chest pain, cough, apprehension, tachycardia and leg pain. Doppler ultrasonography revealed a superficial thrombophlebitis of the left leg; computed tomographic pulmonary angiography showed lung embolism and bilateral pleural effusion. Anticoagulant therapy was initiated with subcutaneous enoxaparin (Clexane®) 6000 IU two times daily. As blood cultures were positive for *Staphylococcus* spp, intravenous therapy consisting of tazobactam plus piperacillin (Tazocin®) 4.5 g three times daily and teicoplanin (Targosid®) 400 mg daily was administered. The clinical condition gradually improved and the patient was discharged 15 days after cesarean section with oral antibiotic therapy and subcutaneous enoxaparin.

The second postpartum sepsis was observed in a woman who underwent an emergency cesarean section for placenta previa. In this case, however, fever began the first day after surgery, and blood cultures were positive for *Klebsiella pneumoniae*. She was treated with antibiotic therapy and discharged well 10 days later.

Twenty-five of the 31 women who underwent successful balloon tamponade were available for a follow-up; 18 did not wish to have any further children, three had pregnancies at term without incident, two had early spontaneous abortion, one had a tubal pregnancy and one suffered sterility.

Table 1 Causes of PPH, success rate of the intervention and results

Causes of PPH	Estimated blood loss (ml) (mean ± SD)	Hemoglobin (g/dl) (mean ± SD) Antepartum	> 24 h	Replaced blood (units) RBC median (range)	FFP median (range)	Total (n)	Successful treatment n	Rate (%)	Surgery
Uterine atony	1618 ± 588	11.4 ± 1.7	7.4 ± 0.9	2 (0–7)	0 (0–13)	17	15/17	88.2	1 case B-Lynch suture + hysterectomy; 1 case Hayman suture
Uterine atony + placenta previa and/or accreta	2925 ± 1680	11.1 ± 1.2	7.6 ± 2.6	6 (0–11)	2 (0–13)	4	1/4	25	3 cases hysterectomy
Placenta previa	1520 ± 590	10.7 ± 1.2	8.3 ± 1.6	2.5 (0–2)	0	10	9/10	90	1 case O'Leary ligation
Placenta accreta	2000 ± 1080	10.7 ± 0.7	7.5 ± 1.7	3 (0–5)	0 (0–3)	4	4/4	100	None
Placenta previa and accreta	1875 ± 942	11.2 ± 0.8	7.8 ± 1.6	1 (0–11)	0 (0–5)	4	2/4	50	1 case O'Leary ligation; 1 case hysterectomy
Total	1792 ± 886	11.1 ± 1.4	7.7 ± 1.4	1 (0–11)	0 (0–13)	39	31/39	80	8 cases

FFP, fresh frozen plasma; RBC, red blood cells

Table 2 Comparison between the historical hysterectomy and the balloon samples

	Cases of hysterectomy (n = 30)	Cases of balloon (n = 39)	P value
Age (years; mean ± SD)	37 ± 3.9	34 ± 3.6	0.003
Gestational age (weeks; mean ± SD)	36 ± 3.7	36 ± 5	NS
Number of placenta previa (%)	8 (27)	10 (25)	NS
Number of placenta accreta (%)	2 (6)	4 (10)	NS
Number of placenta previa and accreta (%)	9 (30)	4 (10)	NS
Number of uterine atony (%)	11 (37)	21 (53)	NS
Units of RBC median (range)	4 (0–11)	1 (0–11)	0.013
Hemoglobin prepartum (mean ± DS)	10.9 ± 1.4	11.1 ± 1.4	NS
Hemoglobin postpartum (mean ± DS)	7.8 ± 1.6	7.7 ± 1.4	NS
Blood loss (ml; mean ± DS)	2443 ± 1452	1792 ± 886	0.03
Day of postpartum admission (mean ± DS)	9.9 ± 8.3	6.1 ± 2.8	0.02
Maternal death	0	0	NS

NS, not significant

Discussion

PPH is the major cause of maternal death in Italy[15]. In the majority of cases, relatively simple methods that could be used to avert a disaster are not always employed[16]. Among these techniques, one of the most simple and effective is tamponade using intrauterine balloons. Successful use of tamponade has been reported in case reports and retrospective case series using the Bakri balloon[3], a condom[20], a Foley catheter[21], the Sengstaken-Blakemore tube[9,11] and the Rüsch urological hydrostatic balloon[22–24].

Because these studies primarily have been retrospective in nature, they may have been influenced by selection, reporting and publication bias[11,23,25]. As such, the conclusions that can be drawn from such data are limited by the study design. The strength of the current study is the prospective identification of cases and method of data collection. Our results are similar to other prospective figures, suggesting that the true effectiveness of balloon tamponade approximates 80%[9,20]. Doumouctsis et al. performed a systematic review of observational studies[1] that showed comparable success rates among the different conservative measures in the management of PPH unresponsive to medical treatment.

CONCLUSIONS

An ideal study design to investigate these various management options would be prospective, randomized and controlled. Unfortunately, such a study design may be difficult for a number of reasons: the urgency of the condition including the degree of on-going bleeding and the hemodynamic status of the woman, the low frequency of severe PPH needing surgical intervention, the staff skills required for each intervention, and the debate on how to perform randomized studies in a field such as PPH. When all these issues are considered, the ethics of undertaking such an investigation would not be considered in a favorable light.

Despite the absence of evidence from randomized studies, the internal balloon tamponade has several obvious advantages over arterial embolization and surgical procedures: simplicity, rapidity of application and removal (no or minimal anesthesia), availability (surgical approach needs laparotomy and technical expertise), safety (the shorter list of complications compared to surgical procedures and arterial embolization) and, finally, low cost. Given that the technology is simple to deploy and has minimal adverse effects, a balloon tamponade method should become a familiar component of existing guidelines for the management of

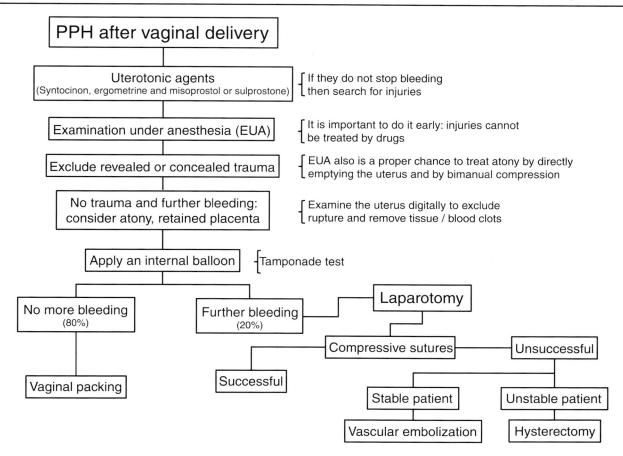

Figure 2 Proposed flowchart about the use of the uterine internal balloon as first-line conservative technique in case of postpartum hemorrhage (PPH) after vaginal delivery.

PPH, although not as an isolated form of therapy. In Figure 2 a flow chart is proposed on balloon application in case of PPH after vaginal delivery.

The RCOG guidelines of 2009[26] on PPH suggested that the intrauterine balloon tamponade is an appropriate first-line 'surgical' intervention for most women where uterine atony is the only or main cause of hemorrhage. As proposed in Figure 2 and from the results of the present study, we also found this technique very helpful in case of abnormal insertion of the placenta. The RCOG guidelines of 2011 on placenta previa and accreta begin to consider the balloon tamponade for these indications[27].

In most studies published to date, the fertility data are either not mentioned or very limited. A single pregnancy is reported following the use of the Rüsch balloon[22] along with two pregnancies following the use of a Bakri balloon in combination with a B-Lynch suture[28]. In our series, pregnancy following balloon insertion occurred in three instances, but among 25 women only seven wanted another child. This may be due to the small duration of follow-up or the patients' reluctance to experience a subsequent pregnancy after having undergone the trauma of a PPH.

In conclusion, the internal tamponade balloon was evaluated prospectively and found effective as a management option for intractable PPH due to both uterine atony and placenta previa/accreta. We believe it should be a first-line treatment in women in whom

uterotonic agents fail to arrest bleeding. The procedure can be easily carried out and may stop hemorrhage in around 80% of women. When it fails, the bleeding may be treated with further conservative measures before performing a hysterectomy. The use of the uterine internal balloon could be expected to result in reduced total blood loss and a lower rate of maternal morbidity in addition to preservation of fertility.

References

1. Doumouchtsis SK, Papageorghiou AT, Arulkumaran S. Systematic review of conservative management of postpartum hemorrhage: what to do when medical treatment fails. Obstet Gynecol Surv 2007;62:540–7
2. American College of Obstetricians and Gynecologists. Postpartum, haemorrhage. ACOG Practice Bulletin No 76. Obstet Gynecol 2006;108:1039–47
3. Bakri YN, Amri A, Jabbar FA. Tamponade-balloon for obstetrical bleeding. Int J Gynaecol Obstet 2001;74:139–42
4. Olamijulo JA, Doufekas K. Intrauterine balloon tamponade for uncontrollable bleeding during first trimester surgical termination of pregnancy. J Obstet Gynaecol 2007;27:441–2
5. Thomas RL, Gingold BR, Gallagher M. Cervical pregnancy. J Reprod Med 1991;36:459–62
6. De La Vega GA, Avery C, Nemiroff R, Marchiano D. Treatment of early cervical Pregnancy with cerclage, carboprost, curettage and balloon tamponade. Obstet Gynecol 2007;109:505–7
7. Ferrazzani S, Guariglia L, Caruso A. Therapy and prevention of obstetric hemorrhage by tamponade using a balloon catheter. Minerva Ginecol 2004;56:481–4

8. Tattersall M, Braithwaite W. Balloon tamponade for vaginal lacerations causing severe postpartum haemorrhage. BJOG 2007;114:647–8

9. Condous GS, Arulkumaran S, Symonds I, Chapman R, Sinha A, Razvi K. The 'tamponade test' in the management of massive postpartum hemorrhage. Obstet Gynecol 2003;101:767–72

10. Cho Y, Rizvi C, Uppal T, Condous G. Ultrasonographic visualization of balloon placement for uterine tamponade in massive primary postpartum hemorrhage. Ultrasound Obstet Gynecol 2008;32:711–3

11. Seror J, Allouche C, Elhaik S. Use of Sengstaken-Blakemore tube in massive postpartum hemorrhage: a series of 17 cases. Acta Obstet Gynecol Scand 2005;84:660–4

12. Doumouchtsis SK, Papageorghiou AT, Vernier C, Arulkumaran S. Management of postpartum hemorrhage by uterine balloon tamponade: Prospective evaluation of effectiveness. Acta Obstet Gynecol 2008;87:849–55

13. Georgiou C. Balloon tamponade in the management of postpartum haemorrhage: a review. BJOG 2009;116:748–57

14. Benirschke K, Kaufmann P, eds. Pathology of the Human Placenta, 4th edn. New York: Springer, 2000:554

15. Biaggi A, Paradisi G, Ferrazzani S, De Carolis S, Lucchese A, Caruso A. Maternal mortality in Italy, 1980–1996. Eur J Obstet Gynecol Reprod Biol 2004;114:144–9

16. Knight M. On behalf of UKOSS. Peripartum hysterectomy in the UK: management and outcomes of the associated haemorrhage. BJOG 2007;114:1380–7

17. Dildy GA 3rd. Postpartum hemorrhage: New management options. Clin Obstet Gynecol 2002;45:330–44

18. Grotegut CA, Larsen FW, Jones MR, Livingston E. Erosion of a B-Lynch suture through the uterine wall: A case report. J Reprod Med 2004;49:849–52

19. Porcu G, Roger V, Jacquier A, et al. Uterus and bladder necrosis after uterine artery embolization for postpartum haemorrhage. BJOG 2005;112:122–3

20. Akhter S, Begum MR, Kabir Z, Rashid M, Laila TR, Zabeen F. Use of a condom to control massive postpartum hemorrhage. MedGenMed 2003;5:38

21. Goldrath MH. Uterine tamponade for the control of acute uterine bleeding. Am J Obstet Gynecol 1983;147:869–72

22. Johanson R, Kumar M, Obhrai M, Young P. Management of massive postpartum haemorrhage: use of a hydrostatic balloon catheter to avoid laparotomy. BJOG 2001;108:420–2

23. Keriakos R, Mukhopadhyay A. The use of the Rusch balloon for management of severe postpartum haemorrhage. J Obstet Gynaecol 2006;26:335–8

24. Majumdar A, Saleh S, Davis M, Hassan I, Thompson PJ. Use of balloon catheter tamponade for massive postpartum haemorrhage. J Obstet Gynaecol 2010;30:586–93

25. Dabelea V, Schultze PM, McDuffie RS. Intrauterine balloon tamponade in the management of postpartum hemorrhage. Am J Perinatol 2007;24:359–64

26. RCOG Prevention and Management of Postpartum Haemorrhage. Green-top Guidelines 52. London, UK: Royal College of Obstetricians and Gynaecologists, 2009

27. RCOG Placenta praevia, placenta praevia accreta and vasa praevia: diagnosis and management. Green-top Guidelines 27. London, UK: Royal College of Obstetricians and Gynaecologists, 2011

28. Nelson WL, O'Brien JM. The uterine sandwich for persistent uterine atony: combining the B-Lynch compression suture and an intrauterine Bakri balloon. Am J Obstet Gynecol 2007;196:e9–10

48

Using the Uterine-Specific Bakri Balloon in the Management of Postpartum Hemorrhage: Case Series and Conceptual/Practical Guidelines

C. Georgiou

INTRODUCTION

Various approaches have been advocated for the management of postpartum hemorrhage (PPH) due to uterine atony[1,2]. These range from massage of the uterine fundus, to the use of pharmacological agents, embolization procedures, compression sutures, vascular occlusion and ultimately hysterectomy[3]. Many of these approaches, however, require the availability of specialized equipment and/or personnel (embolization procedures), a degree of surgical dexterity (compression sutures/vascular occlusion by surgical ligation), or the presence of a hemodynamically stable patient (embolization procedures)[4,5].

In contrast, studies that use the recently introduced uterine balloon tamponade technology suggest that it is easily used, rapidly deployed, has minimal complications, may avoid a laparotomy and, in conjunction with the 'tamponade test', can serve as an orderly stepwise approach to the management of PPH[6-8].

Although the Bakri balloon (Cook Medical, Bloomington, IN, USA) has been specifically designed for use in the uterus, in 168 published cases where the balloon type is specified, 76% use other non-uterine-specific (NUS) balloons (Figure 1)[7,9-11]. These balloons may have been otherwise used in other cavities where bleeding is problematic (i.e. esophagus and bladder)[12,13]. Furthermore, studies of evaluations of effectiveness, prospective trials and feasibility studies of balloon tamponade in the management of PPH are not only based on NUS devices, but also these balloons require modification prior to usage (such as folding or removing a potentially perforating drainage tip), possess no drainage channel and may require prior sterilization[6-8,14].

Assuming genital tract trauma, retained products of conception and device damage prior to placement are excluded, one might expect 100% success if the balloons were effective regardless of how they were used in the management of an atonic uterus. However, data from confidential enquiries and from peripartum hysterectomies suggest that using balloon tamponade in the management of PPH is not always effective[15,16]. One of the reasons why this is the case may be the methodological variation used for uterine-specific and NUS balloons[9].

Despite methodological variation, the paucity of data in the literature and a reporting bias toward NUS devices, recent PPH management guidelines call for the use/availability of tamponade balloons in the management of PPH[3,17] without any recommendation regarding which one(s) should be used and how they should be applied in the clinical situation.

The primary aim of this chapter is to provide a conceptual and practical guide to the use of a uterine-specific tamponade balloon based on a personal case series that utilizes a consistent method of balloon placement and insufflation that relates to the clinical outcome of the so-called tamponade test.

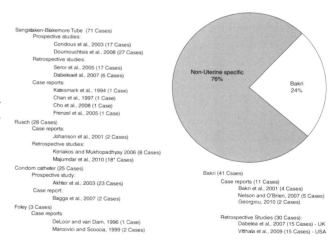

Figure 1 Reporting bias of non-uterine-specific balloons. In 168 published cases of using a specified balloon in the management of PPH, 127 cases are non-uterine-specific and 41 cases involve the uterine-specific Bakri balloon. *Cases greater than 20 weeks' gestation

METHODS

Ethics approval was obtained from the University of Wollongong/Wollongong Hospital Human Research Ethics Committee (HE/09/374) in order to review the medical records of patients in whom a Bakri balloon was used in the management of PPH in which the author was involved

Fifteen cases were identified over a 4-year period from three hospitals within the same area health region in which the author has/had a clinical appointment (Table 1). The medical records of these cases were reviewed with respect to demographic data (maternal age, gestational age and previous pregnancies), risk factors, mode of delivery, cause of PPH and the specific methodology used (mode of insertion, use of ultrasound scan, mechanism used to prevent balloon displacement, total duration of use and deflation regimen (Table 1)). The Bakri balloon was used in all cases, as this was the only uterine-specific balloon available in Australia at the time of the study.

DEFINITIONS

Postpartum hemorrhage

Although PPH was defined as greater than 500 ml estimated blood loss (regardless of mode of delivery or whether the PPH was primary or secondary), the actual amount of estimated blood loss was not an indication for the use the Bakri balloon. The decision to use a Bakri balloon was based on the 'failure' of first-line uterotonics to arrest hemorrhage (see below).

First-line uterotonics

First-line uterotonics were used in all cases described ('oxytocics' in Table 1). These included 10 IU Syntocinon® following the delivery of the baby (IV or IM), a 40 IU Syntocinon infusion, misoprostol 800 μg PR and intramyometrial injection of prostaglandin F2α (PGF2α) (1–3 mg). 'Failure' was defined as continued bleeding following the use of first-line uterotonics after retained placenta and genital tract trauma were excluded.

Tamponade test

The tamponade test involved insufflating the Bakri balloon with normal saline within the uterine cavity and assessing whether this was successful in stopping uterine bleeding. The test was considered 'positive' if the bleeding was successfully minimized or stopped (Figure 2).

The tamponade method

The tamponade method is the methodology by which the tamponade test is applied. It is based on a clinical outcome. It involves initially filling the balloon with 200 ml normal saline and then assessing blood loss from around the cervix as well as from the drainage channel of the Bakri balloon. If bleeding continues, a further 50 ml normal saline is insufflated into the balloon and blood loss is re-assessed. This cycle is continued until bleeding has stopped or is significantly reduced[13]. If 500 ml of normal saline (the recommended capacity of the balloon) is insufflated and the bleeding is still ongoing, the tamponade test is considered negative (Figure 2).

RESULTS (CASE SERIES)

Postpartum hemorrhage incidence

During the 4-year retrospective audit period (April 2007–April 2010), 12,229 deliveries occurred across the three hospital sites. These deliveries included 1272 cases (9.6%) of PPH, 90 cases (0.7%) of which were accompanied by greater than 1500 ml estimated blood loss. In addition, three cases underwent peripartum hysterectomy for PPH after first-line uterotonics were unsuccessful. In two of these, a clinical decision to proceed with hysterectomy was made with no attempt at balloon tamponade. In the remaining case, the Bakri balloon had not yet been introduced at that site. The author was not involved in these three cases.

During the study period, one case was noted in which a Bakri balloon was used after a B-Lynch suture was found to be unsuccessful in managing the PPH. This case is included despite the balloon being used following a failed surgical intervention (B-Lynch) and not immediately following the failure of first-line uterotonics. There were no other cases during the study period in which another procedure, other than balloon insertion, was attempted when first-line uterotonics failed.

There were no maternal deaths during this period and incidence data on secondary PPH was not available from any of the hospital sites.

Bakri balloon insertions

In total, 15 Bakri balloon insertions were made during this period (Table 1). All cases resulted in a positive tamponade test. In one case, the balloon was forcibly removed following extubation by the agitated patient. A second balloon was subsequently reinserted. This was not considered a failure of balloon tamponade, although it did result in a subsequent PPH and required a second Bakri balloon to be inserted (case 8).

Demographics

Maternal and gestational age

Patients' ages ranged from 20 to 43 years with a median of 32 years. The gestational age at delivery ranged from 33 weeks and 6 days to 40 weeks and 6 days.

Table 1 Patient demographics, details of PPH and methodological parameters when using the Bakri balloon

Case	Age	Risk factors	Previous pregnancy	Gestation at delivery (weeks + days)	Mode of delivery	Time of PPH	Cause of PPH	Oxytocics	Use of USS	Tamponade test positive (volume: ml)	Mechanism to ensure remains in uterus	Analgesia (insertion)	Postoperative care (location)	Total time duration of balloon in uterus (h)	Deflation regimen	Final PPH (l)	Placental pathology
1	34	Augmentation of labor	1 MISC	40 + 2	Em LSCS/ failed B-Lynch	At LSCS	Atonic uterus	S10, S40, Miso, PGF	No	300	None mentioned	RA→GA	HDU	24	33% (13 h), 33% (22 h), 33% (30 h)	3.5	Not sent
2	43	–	1 MISC, 2 SVD	39 + 6	SVD	Return to theater (+4 h)	Atonic uterus	S10, S40, Miso, PGF	No	500	Vaginal pack	GA	HDU	24	50% (14 h), 50% (18 h)	2.8 (including primary repair)	Not sent
3	43	Prev. placenta, placenta; augmentation of labor	1 TOP, 1 LSCS (breech)	36 + 5	EL LSCS	At LSCS	Placenta previa/accreta/atonic uterus	S10, S40, Miso, PGF	No	400	None mentioned	GA	HDU	24	50% (14 h), 50% (18 h)	3	Not sent
4	36	Pre-eclampsia	–	40 + 6	Em LSCS	At LSCS	Atonic uterus	S10, S40, PGF	No	450	None mentioned	RA	HDU	30	33% (13 h), 33% (22 h), 33% (30 h)	3	Accreta
5	33	Prev PPH, low placenta, augmentation of labor	1 SVD, 1 MISC, 1 LSCS (PP)	37 + 4	Em LSCS	At LSCS	Atonic uterus	S10, S40	No	500	None required	RA (spinal)	HDU	40	33% (15 h), 67% (40 h)	4	Normal
6	31	FTP (2nd stage), ruptured uterus	1 LSCS (twins)	41 + 1	Em LSCS	At LSCS	Atonic uterus	S10, S40, PGF	No	360	Vaccum	RA (spinal)	HDU	22	50% (12 h), 50% (22 h)	2.8	Not sent
7	28	Retained placenta	–	37 + 3	SVD	SVD	Atonic uterus	S10, S40, Miso, PGF	No	350	Vaccum	GA	HDU	18	50% (14 h), 50% (18 h)	2.5	Normal
8	20	Secondary Prev PPH	1 TOP, 1 MISC	39 + 5	SVD	8 days	Atonic uterus	S40	Yes	450/500	Vaccum, vaginal packs	GA	HDU	30	25% (20 h), 25% (24 h), 25% (28 h), 25% (30 h)	3.5 and 2.3	Not sent
9	35	Placenta previa IV, APH	–	35	Em LSCS	At LSCS	Atonic uterus	S10, S40	No	400	None required	GA	PNW	18	50% (13 h), 50% (18 h)	2	Not sent
10	31	Placenta previa IV, APH	–	33 + 6	Em LSCS	At LSCS	Atonic uterus	S10, S40, Ergo	No	500	Vaccum	GA	PNW	19	30% (12 h), 30% (16 h), 40% (19 h)	3.5	Normal
11	30	–	4 SVD	38 + 5	EL LSCS	Return to theater (+9 h)	Atonic uterus	S10, S40, Ergo, Miso, PGF	Yes	300	Vaccum	GA	PNW	20	50% (13 h), 50% (20 h)	2.4	Not sent
12	36	None	–	38 + 2	EL LSCS	2 weeks	Atonic uterus/endometritis	S40	Yes	400	Vaccum	GA	NDU	34	25% (16 h), 75% (34 h)	2.3	Endometritis in uterine curretings
13	22	Prev PPH	1 SVD	40 + 6	SVD	SVD	Atonic uterus	S10, S40, Ergo, Miso, PGF	No	400	Vaccum	GA	LW-PNW	30	25% (14 h), 25% (22 h), 50% (30 h)	3.6	Normal
14	24	None	–	39 + 5	SVD	SVD	Atonic uterus	S10, S40, Ergo, Miso, PGF	No	500	Vaccum	GA	LW-PNW	26	50% (18 h), 50% (26 h)	2.3	Not sent
15	31	None	3 TOP EDIU (16 weeks), 1 SVD	39 + 4	SVD	Ongoing (6 h)	Retained products, atonic uterus	S10, S40, Ergo, Miso, PGF	No	250	Vaccum	GA	PNW	22	50% (12 h), 50% (22 h)	2.5	Normal retained products

APH, antepartum hemorrhage; EL LSCS, elective lower segment cesarean section; Em LSCS, emergency lower segment cesarean section; Ergo, ergometrine 250–500 μg; FDIU, fetal death in utero; FTP, failure to progress; GA, general anesthetic; HDU, high dependency unit; IOL, induction of labor; LW-PNW, labor ward-postnatal ward; MISC, miscarriage; Miso, misoprostol (800 μm per rectum); MOD, mode of delivery; PGF, prostaglandin PGF2 α; PP, placenta previa; Prev PPH, previous PPH; SVD, spontaneous vaginal delivery; S10, 10 IU Syntocinon (oxytocin); S40, 40 IU Syntocinon (oxytocin infusion, over 4 h); TOP, termination of pregnancy; RA, regional anesthetic
*Ultrasound scan used for teaching technique of balloon placement

Parity

Two women (cases 1 and 8) experienced PPH following the birth of their first pregnancy, six women had had previous pregnancies (cases 4, 7, 9, 10, 12 and 14).

Mode of delivery

Six cases of PPH followed vaginal deliveries (cases 2, 7, 8 and 13–15), three followed elective cesarean section (cases 3, 11 and 12) and six were subsequent to emergency cesarean section (cases 1, 4–6, 9 and 10).

Risk factors

Although some cases had identifiable risk factors (cases 1, 3, 5, 10 and 13), others had none (cases 2, 11, 12, 14 and 15).

Timing of PPH

Primary PPH was diagnosed at delivery in ten out of the 13 cases (cases 1, 3–7, 9, 10, 13 and 14). Two cases were diagnosed at 4 and 6 h, respectively, after a vaginal delivery (cases 2 and 15) and one case was diagnosed 9 h after following an elective cesarean section (case 11). The remaining two cases represented secondary PPH at 8 days and 2 weeks postpartum (cases 8 and 12, respectively).

Cause of PPH

Uterine atony was considered the cause in all primary PPH, whereas the secondary PPH was attributed to endometritis. In one of these cases *Proteus mirabilis* infection was demonstrable from uterine curettings (case 12).

Uterotonics used

Most cases received all available first-line uterotonics (Table 1). However, relative contraindications such as the presence of hypertension occasionally restricted their use (e.g. case 4).

PPH volumes

Although the actual PPH volume was not an absolute indication for insertion of the Bakri balloon, the final PPH volumes ranged from 2 to 4 l of blood (average of 3.1 l).

Site of placement

In the majority of cases, the Bakri balloon was inserted in the operating room. In one case (case 8), an attempt was made to insert the balloon in the high dependency unit (HDU). However, the amount of bleeding obscured the view and the patient's discomfort with the procedure (vaginal and speculum examination), resulted in this attempt being abandoned. The balloon was then successfully inserted in the operating room.

Mode of insertion

In all cases the Bakri balloon was inserted via a transvaginal (anterograde) direction, i.e. from the vagina into the uterine cavity (Figure 3). In cases of PPH that occurred during a cesarean section, the lower segment incision was closed in two layers and the bleeding reassessed from the vaginal aspect *before* the final decision was made to insert the balloon.

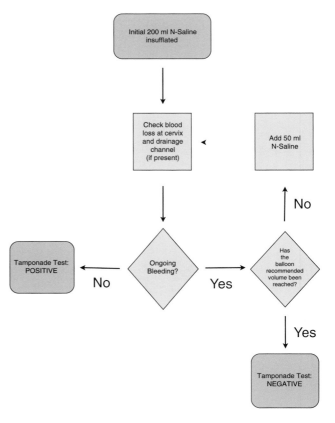

Figure 2 The tamponade method in relation to the tamponade test in the management of PPH. N-Saline, normal saline

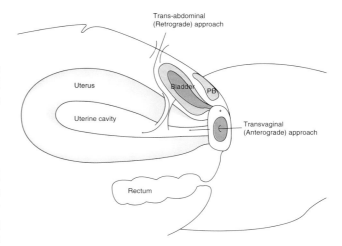

Figure 3 Transvaginal (anterograde) and transabdominal (retrograde) approaches to the uterine cavity for balloon placement. PB, pubic bone

Tamponade test

A tamponade test was performed in all cases involving the 'tamponade method' (Figure 2). The volume of normal saline insufflation that resulted in a positive tamponade test ranged from 250 to 500 ml (average 410 ml). The manufacturer's recommended maximal volume of 500 ml was not exceeded.

Preventing balloon displacement

Of the patients with a dilated cervix, vacuum drainage was used in the majority of cases (9/12) to prevent caudal migration of the insufflated balloon[18]. However, in one case (case 8), the patient forcibly displaced an intact fluid-filled Bakri balloon into the vagina by pulling on the balloon shaft whilst being agitated following extubation. No cervical trauma was evident during the reinsertion of a second Bakri balloon, suggesting that the balloon was able to re-mould itself with the original quantity of fluid during expulsion. Following the subsequent positive tamponade test, a vaginal pack was used in addition to the vacuum method in this patient.

Analgesia

Regional and general anesthesia was used to insert the balloon, particularly if the PPH occurred during an ongoing cesarean delivery. One case was converted from a regional to a general anesthetic because of patient discomfort secondary to the prolonged operating time (case 1).

In another case (case 5), 50 ml of the balloon volume was removed in the recovery area as the patient experienced significant cyclical period-type discomfort. The cyclical discomfort was more tolerable following this reduction in balloon volume.

Location of postinsertion care

Initially all cases were managed in the high dependency units (HDU) (cases 1–7). As familiarity of using the balloon in the management of PPH occurred with hospital staff at different locations, the postinsertion management migrated transiently via the labor ward and eventually directly to the postnatal ward (cases 9–11 and 13–15). However, some cases required specific HDU or intensive care unit (ICU) management (e.g. intubation or coagulopathic issues, in cases 8 and 12, respectively).

Duration of balloon insertion

Factors such as the time of day/night of initial placement and management of other co-morbidities affected the total duration of the balloon placement. This ranged from 18 to 40 h (average 25 h).

Deflation regimen

Depending on the time of insertion and other co-morbidities, various regimens were used. The main emphasis was to ensure the initial and final balloon volumes of normal saline were removed during 'working hours' rather than at times when staff availability was reduced.

Placental pathology

Of the five placentas that were sent for histologic examination in the 13 cases of primary PPH, only one case of placenta accreta was identified (case 4).

Success rate

In this series, all cases in which a Bakri balloon was used were successful.

COMMENTS

The management of PPH invariably involves the use of physical and pharmacological agents to facilitate uterine contraction while excluding genital tract trauma and retained products of conception[3]. Although evidence-based data on the use of uterotonics recommends them as first-line management, it is not clear which of the multitude of secondary approaches are to be used first when uterotonics prove to be ineffective for the commonest cause of PPH, namely uterine atony[19]. Specifically, there is no evidence for a hierarchy of use in relation to arterial ligation, compression sutures or hysterectomy. The subsequent course of action is usually dependent on operator preference and the facilities available within the respective units.

Although placenta accreta/previa was the initial circumstance in which the uterine-specific Bakri balloon was used[20], this technology can be used for a variety of other PPH scenarios including endometritis and secondary PPH in the presence of coagulopathy (cases 8 and 12, respectively). Therefore, the case mix in this series reiterates the reality that balloon tamponade in the management of PPH is broadly applicable to a variety of atonic bleeding situations. It also has the advantage of not requiring specialized personnel or equipment other than the balloon itself.

Limitations of this study

Although other studies involving the Bakri balloon report an overall success rate of 80–90%[10,14], the 100% success rate in this case series must be viewed with caution. In this particular series, the author was involved as soon as the first-line uterotonics were considered ineffective and the Bakri was inserted in a timely manner. This early intervention is likely to have contributed significantly to the high success rate[15].

Additional limitations include the small sample size and patient selection. With respect to the latter, three cases within the study period had a peripartum hysterectomy. Although the decision to proceed with this was not based on a failed tamponade test, it is unclear whether these cases would have been successfully managed with the Bakri balloon alone.

UTERINE-SPECIFIC BALLOON GUIDELINES

As previously mentioned, a number of NUS balloons have successfully been used in the management of PPH and contribute to the majority of the published literature (Figure 1). However, there are no comparative studies between these NUS balloons and the uterine-specific balloons to enable a direct comparison of the various balloons or methodologies used. Although 'failures' of the tamponade balloons are mentioned in prospective studies of peripartum hysterectomies and audits of PPH, the reasons for failure are not always discussed or explained[15,16]. This knowledge deficit makes it difficult to determine whether there are any specific methodological contributions to the success, or failure, of balloon tamponade technology. Therefore, it is possible that the success rates reported for each balloon device may be attributed to the methodology used in that particular study.

Published recommendations exist for the NUS Rusch balloon, and these may be considered applicable to the uterine-specific Bakri balloon[8]. However, a few noteworthy points pertain to the *method* by which the NUS balloon is filled. The principle of insufflating the balloon until 'a resistance (is) felt' with 'the pressure required (being) equivalent to that used when inflating a Foley catheter balloon' is ambiguous[8].

Unfortunately, similar methodological ambiguity exists in published case series using the Bakri balloon. For example 'the amount of saline instilled…(depends) on the size and capacity of the uterus'[10], and the 'procedure was successful, if the bleeding is stopped after the balloon was inflated' without defining how an effective final volume is reached[10]. In another series using the Bakri balloon, the balloon was inflated 'until the uterine fundus was firmly palpable or bleeding was controlled'[14]. Furthermore, the product information supplied from Cook Medical (J-SOS1106) states the intraluminal volume is to be 'determined by direct examination or ultrasound scan'.

THE TAMPONADE TEST

The tamponade test is based on a clinical outcome[6]. This outcome is likely to be dependent on a specific insufflated volume of normal saline for the individual uterus concerned. Since it is the clinical outcome that is paramount, and not the volume used or pressure generated, it is imperative that the amount of fluid used is directly correlated to the tamponade test and not estimated or predetermined[18]. Surprisingly, the NUS (Rusch) balloon guidelines, Cook Medical information leaflets and published cases involving the Bakri balloon, do not mention the tamponade test[8,10,14].

Stages of use

In an attempt to consolidate the methodological variations that exist within various studies, a series of stages is described in relation to the use of tamponade

Table 2 Five 'stages' in the use of balloon tamponade technology in the management of PPH

Stage	Description
1	Risk factors, indication for use and location of insertion
2	Patient positioning and access to the uterine cavity
3	Tamponade test and prevention of balloon displacement
4	Postinsertion observation and supportive treatment
5	Removal of balloon and follow-up

balloons (Table 2). It is envisioned that these stages may be universally implemented for both uterine- and non-uterine-specific balloons, to provide a consistent reference for usage, regardless of the methodologies used.

In particular, the use of these stages may serve to enhance training in order to identify factors that result in balloon tamponade failure or success. It is anticipated that others will publish not only their successful cases, but also complications and reasons for failure with respect to these stages, so that a consistent method of usage can be established, thereby allowing comparisons and improvements in the methodologies used.

The five stages are described with a series of 'consider', 'preparation' and 'potential complications' comments. In clinical practice these stages are continuous and conceptually overlap.

Stage 1: Risk factors, indications for use and location of insertion

Consider

- Risk factors (emergency box)
- Timing (early recourse to theater)
- Indications (cause of bleeding)

Risk factors may not always be present for PPH, but their presence should help to alert the care giver that there may be a need to use a tamponade balloon.

Timing is also likely to be a significant contributor to the eventual outcome of the uterine tamponade technique. Therefore, the inclusion of a Bakri balloon in the labor ward 'emergency/PPH box' or the 'obstetric emergencies' theater box will help to minimize the decision-to-tamponade test interval.

Indications for using balloon tamponade should be for ongoing bleeding after failure of first-line uterotonics in the management of an atonic uterus. Exclusion of retained products and genital tract trauma is paramount to a successful tamponade test.

Preparation

Although the balloon can be inserted on the birthing unit, postnatal ward or recovery bay, it is important to be able to exclude genital tract trauma and retained products of conception. The operating theater environment provides excellent lighting conditions, a table that can be put into the Trendelberg position, appropriate instruments and the opportunity to proceed to laparotomy if the tamponade test is negative (see stage 3, Figure 2).

Potential complications

Although the balloon has been used for vaginal lacerations[21], examples in the literature demonstrate that a failure of uterine tamponade occurs if genital tract trauma is overlooked[6,22]. In addition, if the uterine cavity contains retained products or collections of blood clots, correct placement of the balloon may prove to be difficult.

Stage 2: Patient positioning and access to the uterine cavity

Consider

- Patient positioning

- Transvaginal (anterograde) placement of the balloon

- Ultrasound to assist/monitor balloon placement

If the use of a Balloon is anticipated prior to the beginning of a cesarean section, for example in placenta previa, the patient can be initially positioned, and draped, in a lithotomy position with the thighs in a horizontal position. If the balloon is going to be inserted, the legs may be subsequently flexed to improve exposure to the vagina. This preoperative positioning will minimize re-draping with potentially breaching of the sterile field as the balloon is placed prior to closure of the laparotomy site. If the PPH occurs unexpectedly during a cesarean section, the 'frog-leg' position is useful once the uterus is closed and the laparotomy site is covered with a sterile drape.

Alternatively, if the PPH follows a vaginal delivery, or as a secondary PPH, a lithotomy position is preferable.

Access to the uterine cavity for balloon placement will depend on whether the uterine cavity has already been exposed, e.g. at cesarean section. Although transabdominal (retrograde) placement, i.e. from the uterine cavity to the vagina, has been advocated, practical problems may arise. These include trauma to the undilated cervix, damage to the balloon device on subsequent uterine cavity closure and suboptimal uterine closure. Conversely, inserting the balloon from the vagina to the uterine cavity (transvaginal) involves a 'smoother' conical passage of the device and is preferred (Figure 3). Furthermore, a two-layer closure of the lower segment incision may alleviate the need for balloon insertion when bleeding is subsequently re-assessed from the cervix.

The routine use of ultrasound is controversial. In the absence of a recent uterine scar or the necessity to curette the uterine cavity (as in secondary PPH), ultrasound is not necessary for balloon placement. However, confirming the position following the insertion of the balloon device may be useful if the tamponade test is negative when the maximal balloon volume is reached. Furthermore, the use of ultrasound provides a visual guide to balloon placement, and is therefore a valuable teaching tool in balloon placement (Figure 4).

Preparation

Balloon access to the uterine fundus can be challenging in the presence of PPH. Use of a Rampley's forceps on the cervical lip provides gentle counter-traction when inserting the balloon via the vagina (transvaginal placement). This helps to ensure the tip of the balloon reaches the fundus.

When a speculum cannot provide adequate visual access to the cervix, consider using fingers to not only guide the balloon into the uterus, but also to maintain the balloon in position (See stage 3 and Figure 4).

If PPH occurs during a cesarean section and the cervix is not dilated sufficiently to pass the balloon device, Hagar dilators may be used to dilate the cervix from below prior to transvaginal (anterograde) placement. Alternatively, a finger may be used to dilate the cervical canal from within the uterus if a transabdominal (retrograde) approach is being contemplated (Figure 3).

Potential complications

If the balloon is placed in a transabdominal manner with subsequent uterine incision closure, damage to the balloon may occur or uterine closure may be compromised in an attempt to avoid balloon damage. In addition, the transabdominal (retrograde) approach has the potential to cause cervical trauma when attempted in the presence of a closed cervix. Although the collapsed diameters of the Bakri balloon at the proximal and distal ends are approximately 2 cm, the transvaginal (anterograde) approach results in a smoother, more conical entry through the cervix due to the shape of the drainage tip. It is assumed that the detachable two-way tap is removed prior to insertion when

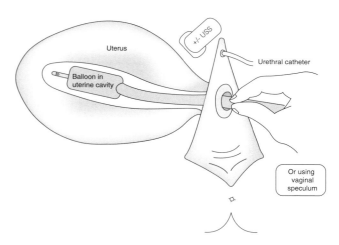

Figure 4 Ensuring the balloon is inserted and maintained at the fundus as the balloon is insufflated. +/– USS, with or without the use of ultrasound scanning (to demonstrate/ensure appropriate placement)

contemplating the transabdominal (retrograde) approach.

Finally, inadequate visualization of access to the cervix can lead to suboptimal placement and an inability to perform the tamponade method (Figures 2 and 5).

Stage 3: Tamponade test and prevention of balloon displacement

Consider

- The tamponade test and the tamponade method
- Maintenance of the balloon at the uterine fundus
- Additional surgical methods (e.g. B-Lynch)

The tamponade *test* is a clinical indicator of successful tamponade and formalizes the need to resort to other procedures such as laparotomy or hysterectomy. The tamponade test can only be effectively applied if the balloon is in the correct location within the uterine cavity and the cervix around the balloon shaft can be visualized to assess blood loss (Figure 5).

The tamponade *method* involves a cyclical assessment of bleeding following sequential insufflation of the balloon with normal saline within the uterine cavity (Figure 2). This method of uterine filling is based on a clinical outcome (ongoing blood loss) and does not depend on 'estimating' or guessing the amount of

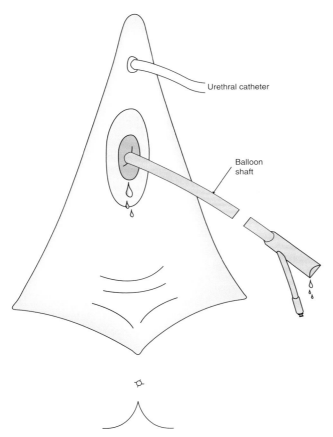

Figure 5 Monitoring blood loss from the cervix and drainage channel (if present) in order to determine a clinical outcome in relation to balloon insufflation

fluid required. If the balloon maximum is reached and bleeding is ongoing, the tamponade test is negative and subsequent steps to control bleeding must be taken (Figure 2).

Maintaining the balloon in the uterus can be problematic during placement. Furthermore, using traction as originally described by Bakri, may result in displacement of the balloon into the vagina despite successful intrauterine placement following a vaginal delivery[20].

If the cervix is fully/partially dilated prior to placement of the balloon, a number of options can be used to maintain the balloon in the correct position. For example, placing a gauze pack in the vagina is useful, but it is imperative that the tamponade test is positive prior to packing the vagina, as ongoing blood loss may not be detected due to the absorbent quality of the gauze. Another option is to connect the drainage channel to a suction drain[18]. The vacuum generated thus maintains the balloon within the cavity.

Finally, once a positive tamponade test has been achieved, ensure the input valve of the balloon is secured, perhaps with tape, so that it is not inadvertently opened during patient transfer.

Preparation

As the balloon in insufflated with normal saline, it expands within the area of least resistance. Following a vaginal delivery this area is generally through the cervical canal and into the vagina (Figure 6). Therefore, the balloon should be maintained at the uterine fundus during insufflation with saline. This may be achieved by using a Rampley's forceps gently applied at the base of the balloon. Alternatively, the balloon can be maintained in place by maintaining the shaft at the base of the balloon within the vagina using fingers as an assistant insufflates the balloon with saline (Figure 4).

Potential complications

To date there have been no reports of perforation of the balloon devices through the uterus following placement. However, such examples have been reported for the Sengstaken–Blakemore tube in the esophagus[23]. One particular advantage of using the Bakri balloon is in eliminating the need to 'trim' the rather long drainage stalk of the Sengstaken–Blakemore tube, which potentially could result in uterine perforation[7].

Although, the postpartum uterine cavity is compliant, it is difficult to determine how much volume is required to achieve a positive tamponade test. 'Guesstimating' the volume required does not constitute a tamponade test and underfilling the balloon may result in a negative tamponade test. The test should not involve estimations of required volumes. The endpoint of the tamponade test is a clinical one (Figure 2). The bleeding either stops (test positive) or continues at an unacceptable rate (test negative). Conversely, overdistending the uterine cavity may result in uterine scar dehiscence following a cesarean section or subsequent adverse effects on the endometrium.

If the Bakri balloon is used in conjunction with other surgical approaches, other 'complications' may occur[24]. An example would be failing to gain access to the uterine cavity when a B-Lynch suture is used[14]. According to the original B-Lynch publication, a cavity should exist after suture placement to allow drainage[25]. It is in this area that the Bakri balloon will enter. Therefore, modifications of the B-Lynch suture that eliminate this cavity resulting in approximation of the anterior and posterior uterine walls will not allow placement of the Bakri balloon[26].

The Bakri balloon can theoretically be used in combination with uterine artery embolization and selective devascularization. However, there are no data to support a hierarchy when using these surgical approaches.

Stage 4: Postinsertion observation and supportive treatment

Consider

- Resuscitation

- Assessment of blood loss

- Ongoing oxytocin infusion, antibiotics and analgesia

Assessing any ongoing blood loss following a positive tamponade test is critical in determining whether balloon tamponade is successful.

Following balloon insertion, and after the first aliquot of saline is removed after 8–12 h (Figure 7) perineal pads should be collected at 15 min intervals over the first hour period ('golden hour'). This will give a visual estimation of blood loss. Alternatively, these pads may be weighed.

Although blood loss from the balloon's drainage channel will also give an indication of ongoing bleeding, normal/corrected coagulation usually results in clot formation within this channel. Flushing the channel, as suggested by the Bakri instruction leaflet (J-SOS1106), will not prevent this.

The patient should be resuscitated following a positive tamponade test, as the cessation of bleeding is only one component of the patient's management. Therefore, multidisciplinary involvement including hematology, anesthetics and ICU/HDU staff is usually necessary to re-establish normal parameters once the bleeding has been controlled (Figure 7).

Preparation

The location of the patient postoperatively is paramount. Whether this is in ICU/HDU owing to other medical problems or a postnatal ward, the 'golden hour' must be emphasized to minimize the delay of diagnosing failure of the balloon tamponade technique.

Antibiotic cover with a broad-spectrum antibiotics such as a cephalosporin with or without metronidazole

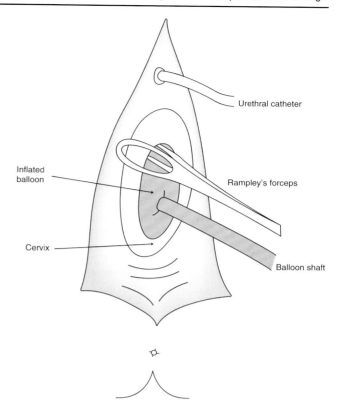

Figure 6 Using a Rampley's forceps to provide counter traction of the cervix when inserting the balloon. If the balloon is not maintained in position within the uterine cavity, the balloon is seen extruding from the cervical canal as it is being insufflated with normal saline

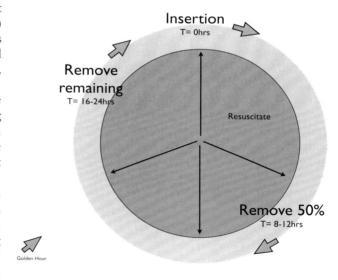

Figure 7 Using a 24-hr clock to manage when to resuscitate the patient and plan removal of the saline within the balloon following the achievement of a positive tamponade test. T, time from successful tamponade test

is advisable to minimize iatrogenic infection secondary to the balloon placement method[9].

Ongoing oxytocin infusion is logical but not empirical. Therefore, if the risk of fluid overload is to be minimized secondary to the crossreaction of oxytocin with vasopressin receptors, sodium ion concentrations should be assessed throughout this time period, particularly in the presence of reduced urine output.

Analgesia may need to be provided, as uterine distension may give rise to spasmodic uterine pain.

Potential complications

Unidentified ongoing bleeding may occur by not checking the perineal pads and being falsely reassured by minimal blood loss from an occluded balloon drainage channel.

Failure to consider other co-morbidities such as acute renal failure as well as iatrogenic infection, hyponatremia and inadequate analgesia are also possible complications of this stage.

Stage 5: Removal of balloon and follow-up

Consider

- Timing of removal
- Monitor blood loss and systemic parameters
- Follow-up

There is considerable variation as to when, and how, the balloon should be removed[9]. One method is to remove 50% of the balloon volume within 12–18 h of insertion during office hours in case bleeding restarts (Figure 7). The balloon can always be re-inflated at this stage to allow consideration of subsequent management options if bleeding ensues. Otherwise, the remaining balloon volume can then be removed within 24 h of insertion. Sometimes this time scale may need to be extended, but there is no evidence that leaving the balloon longer improves the outcome (Table 1). Furthermore, any deleterious effect on the endometrial function such as menstruation, synechae formation and subsequent implantation is as yet unknown. However, two pregnancies following the use of a Bakri 'sandwich' (balloon with a B-Lynch suture) have been reported[24].

Preparation

Ensure that clear instructions are provided to the staff looking after the patient postinsertion with respect to the potential of re-bleeding. The meticulous observation of blood loss in the golden hour following any fluid removal is paramount in determining the success or otherwise of using the balloon in the postinsertion period (Figure 7).

Provide adequate opportunity to discuss/review with the patient the recent course of events prior to discharge and encourage follow-up in 6–8 weeks or when menses return. The experience can be quite overwhelming. An ultrasound scan at this follow-up stage may serve to reassure the patient of subsequent normal appearances of uterine anatomy.

Potential complications

Removing the balloon too soon may result in bleeding recurrence. There are no data on the shortest time that a balloon needs to be *in situ* to exert its effect. Conversely, maintaining the balloon for prolonged periods may potentiate uterine necrosis and ulceration, both of which have been reported in the esophagus when balloon tamponade technology was used[23].

PRACTICE POINTS

- Balloon tamponade technology can be successfully used for a variety of conditions that are associated with an atonic uterus

- Using defined stages, teaching concepts of balloon placement, insufflation and postoperative care can be facilitated

- Complications regarding the use of balloon tamponade technology in the management of PPH may be reported in relation to these stages to enable comparisons to be made between studies.

ACKNOWLEDGMENTS

The author would like to thank the labor wards, ICU/HDU, postnatal and theater staff from the participating hospitals involved in these cases (St George Hospital, Shoalhaven Hospital and Wollongong Hospital of the South Eastern Sydney and Illawarra Area Health Service, Australia)

Some of this work has been presented as an abstract/poster at the Royal Australian and New Zealand College of Obstetricians and Gynaecologist Annual Scientific Meeting as a poster in Adelaide, 21–24 March 2010.

References

1. Lalonde A, Daviss BA, Acosta A, Herschderfer K. Postpartum haemorrhage today: ICM/FIGO initiative 2004–2006. Int J Gynecol Obstet 2006;94:243–53

2. World Health Organization. Attending to 136 million births, every year: Make every mother and child count: Chapter 4: Risking death to give life. The World Health Report 2005. Geneva, Switzerland: WHO, 2005

3. Royal College of Obstetricians and Gynaecologists. Green-top Guideline No. 52. Prevention and Management of Postpartum Haemorrhage. London: RCOG, 2009

4. Doumouchtsis SK, Papageorghiou AT, Arulkumaran S. Systematic review of conservative management of postpartum hemorrhage: what to do when medical treatment fails. Obstet Gynecol Surv 2007;62:540–7

5. American College of Obstetricians and Gynecologists. ACOG Practice Bulletin No.76. Obstet Gynecol 2006;108: 1039–47

6. Condous GS, Arulkumarah S, Symonds I, et al. The "tamponade test" in the management of massive postpartum hemorrhage. Obstet Gynecol 2003;101:767–72

7. Doumouchtsis SK, Papageorghiou AT, Vernier C, Arulkumaran S. Management of postpartum haemorrhage by uterine balloon tamponade: prospective evaluation of effectiveness. Acta Obstet Gynecol Scand 2008;87:849–55

8. Keriakos R, Mukhopadhyay A. The use of the Rusch balloon for management of severe postpartum haemorrhage. J Obstet Gynaecol 2006;26:335–8

9. Georgiou C. Balloon tamponade in the management of postpartum haemorrhage: a review. BJOG 2009;116:748–57

10. Vitthala S, Tsoumpou I, Anjum ZK, Aziz NA. Use of Bakri balloon in post-partum hemorrhage: A series of 15 cases. Aust N Z J Obstet Gynaecol 2009;49:191–4

11. Majumdar A, Saleh H, Davis M, Hassan I, Thompson P. Use of balloon catheter tamponade for massive postpartum haemorrhage. J. Obstet Gynaecol 2010;30:586–93

12. Katesmark M, Brown R, Raju KS. Successful use of a Sengstaken-Blakemore tube to control massive postpartum haemorrhage. BJOG 1994;101:259–60

13. Johanson R, Kumar M, Obhrai M, Young P. Management of massive postpartum haemorrhage: use of a hydrostatic balloon catheter to avoid laparotomy. BJOG 2001;108:420–2

14. Dabelea V, Schultze PM, McDuffie RS. Intrauterine balloon tamponade in the management of postpartum hemorrhage. Am J Perinatol 2007;24:359–64

15. Knight M, on behalf of UKOSS. Peripartum hysterectomy in the UK: management and outcomes of the associated haemorrhage. BJOG 2007;114:1380–7

16. Brace V, Kernaghan D, Penney G. Learning from adverse outcomes: major obstetric haemorrhage in Scotland, 2003–05. BJOG 2007;114:1388–96

17. Condous G. Re – Vitthala et al. Use of Bakri balloon in post-partum hemorrhage: a series of 15 cases. Aust N Z J Obstet Gynecol 2009;49:445–6

18. Georgiou C. Intraluminal pressure readings during the establishment of a positive "tamponade test" in the management of postpartum haemorrhage. BJOG 2010;117:295–303

19. Mousa HA, Alfirevic Z. Treatment for primary postpartum haemorrhage. Cochrane Database Syst Rev 2007;(1): CD003249

20. Bakri YN, Amri A, Jabbar FA. Tamponade-balloon for obstetrical bleeding. Int J Gynecol Obstet 2001;74:139–42

21. Tattersall M, Braithwaite W. Balloon tamponade for vaginal lacerations causing severe postpartum haemorrhage. BJOG 2007;114:647–8

22. Seror J, Allouche C, Elhaik S. Use of Sengstaken – Blakemore tube in massive postpartum hemorrhage: a series of 17 cases. Acta Obstet Gynecol Scand 2005;84:660–4

23. Conn HO, Simpson JA. Excessive mortality associated with balloon tamponade of bleeding varices. JAMA 1967;202:135–9

24. Nelson WL, O'Brien JM. The uterine sandwich for persistent uterine atony: combining the B-Lynch compression suture and an intrauterine Bakri balloon. Am J Obstet Gynecol 2007;196:e9–10

25. B-Lynch C, Coker A, Lawal AH, Cowen MJ. The B-Lynch surgical technique for the control of massive post partum haemorrhage: an alternative to hysterectomy? Five cases reported. BJOG 1997;104:372–5

26. Cho JH, Jun HS, Lee CN. Hemostatic suturing technique for uterine bleeding during cesarean delivery. Obstet Gynecol 2000;96:129–31

49

Embolization and Balloon Catheter Placement

K. Choji and T. Shimizu

INTRODUCTION: OVERVIEW

Embolization is a technique in which a plastic catheter is inserted into the target artery through which small particles or other embolic materials are infused to occlude the artery. The objective of embolization is to stop active hemorrhage. Embolization is valid in both primary (i.e. within 24 hours of delivery) and secondary (i.e. after 24 hours from delivery) postpartum hemorrhage (PPH). When embolization is successful, the patient recovers without undergoing additional surgery. Embolization saves not only the life of the patient and provides quick recovery, but also the uterus and adnexal organs, thus ensuring future fertility, if this be desired.

The report of successful embolization to treat PPH published by Heaston et al. in 1979[1] was followed by others in the 1980s[2–10]. By the 1990s the technique was used in maternity units around the world[11–25]. In an extensive review of the literature by Vedantham and colleagues in 1997[19], cessation of hemorrhage was reported in 100% of 49 cases after vaginal delivery and 89% of 18 cases after cesarean section. More recent reports include 70–79%[26–28], 83–89%[24,29], 91–97%[25,30–33] and 100%[7,11,34–36] cessation of hemorrhage rates. The clinical success is believed not to be related to mode of delivery, cause of PPH, transfusion requirements or time from delivery to embolization[28]. Rather, success depends on reducing the perfusion pressure of the source arteries of hemorrhage to allow coagulation and healing of the injured arteries. The degree of pressure reduction necessary varies according to the coagulation status of the patient. If complete occlusion of an artery with embolic material is achieved, it will result in null perfusion pressure, which will be followed by coagulation and healing of the artery. In practice, not all the source arteries can be identified. As a result, there is frequently a degree of arbitrariness in the amount of embolic material infused and the site of infusion. This could lead to insufficient infusion (underembolization) or excessive embolization (overembolization)[28]. The former indicates unsuccessful hemostasis, while the latter increases the risk of ischemic complications. Prior hysterectomy makes the embolization more difficult and, if possible, this should be avoided[28,37].

Virtually no contraindications to embolization are thought to exist. In contrast to surgery, even severe coagulopathy does not present a contraindication. Coagulopathy is frequently encountered in PPH due to a number of factors, including disseminated intravascular coagulation (DIC), depletion of clotting factors ('wash-out phenomenon') and dilution of clotting factors with crystalloid fluid that is administered as part of the resuscitation process as well as the lack of clotting factors in stored blood[7,38,39]. The likely mechanism of rapid recovery following embolization is as follows. If emboli successfully occlude the breached arterial branches, the acute and continuous washout effect ceases. This is followed by the reinforcement of depleted coagulation factors produced by the patient's body or through transfusion. The result is rapid recovery from both blood loss and coagulation abnormality. Embolization can lead to hemostasis in cases with known coagulopathy[31]. In addition, hemostasis and correction of acquired coagulopathy has also been reported[25].

Complications occur but only in a relatively small proportion of cases[1–3,7,11,17,24–29,31,32,35,36,40–43], and, in view of the data obtained from cases where radiation doses were measured, it appears unlikely that the patients suffer from significant radiation effects[24,33,36,40,44].

In hospitals where embolization is available, it should be the procedure of choice for PPH that fails to respond to initial intraoperative maneuvers including B-Lynch sutures and following conventional medical treatment, leaving hysterectomy as the last resort. In obstetric units where an in-house radiology team is unavailable to undertake appropriate interventions, reliable access to such a team should be sought. Once established, the means by which this collaboration can be activated must be widely available to staff and posted prominently in nursing and clerical stations.

In some cases, particularly with placental abnormalities, higher risk of PPH is foreseen prior to planned surgery[45–51]. Prophylactic intra-arterial balloon catheter placement for cases with high risk of PPH such as placental abnormalities has been proposed[14,20,24,27,33,40–42,52,53] and is discussed in other chapters.

VASCULAR ANATOMY ON IMAGING

General anatomy

The internal iliac artery is the first major branch of the common iliac artery, which descends from the bifurcation of the aorta and proceeds into the pelvis. There may be some variation in the distance between the aortic and the iliac bifurcations. Normally, there should be little difficulty in identification of the internal iliac artery because of its substantial size and its inward (inferomedial) direction compared with the external iliac artery which courses laterally after the bifurcation of the common iliac trunk. The proximal bifurcation of the internal iliac artery produces two trunks that are officially termed the anterior and posterior branches. The posterior branch supplies the gluteal region, whilst the anterior branch supplies the remainder of the pelvis. In the majority of instances, the branches of this anterior trunk include the uterine, vaginal, superior cystic, middle rectal, obturator, internal pudendal and inferior gluteal arteries (Figure 1a). In fact, a number of variations in the distribution of the branches of the internal iliac artery are possible[54,55]. In 30% of patients, however, some of these arteries have more proximal origins at the level of the bifurcation of the anterior and posterior branches (Figure 1b). This is especially true in the case of the obturator and uterine arteries. In addition,

the internal pudendal artery may arise from the posterior branch. A recent article from Kenya has shown that the actual anatomy differs from that seen in classical descriptions in as many as 20% of cases[56]. To avoid confusion as a result of such anatomical variation, we advise referring to the anterior and posterior branches as the inferior and superior gluteal trunks, respectively. This nomenclature becomes more appropriate when performing angiography.

On an angiographic image, the inferior gluteal artery is seen as descending relatively laterally and extending lower than the bony pelvis. The importance of this artery is to give off the sciatic branch which supplies the sciatic nerve. Therefore, the accidental embolization of the inferior gluteal artery could result in transient or long-term injury to the sciatic nerve. Furthermore, heavy embolization of the branches of the superior gluteal trunk (posterior branch) could result in ischemia of the nerves and gluteal muscles, which could cause pain in the gluteal region.

The uterine artery is identified from the distribution in the enlarged prenatal or immediately postnatal uterus. Note that the characteristic coiling appearance of the intramural branches of the uterine artery in the normal sized uterus have disappeared in the enlarged near natal uterus. Identifying the origin of the uterine artery on the usual frontal projection in fluoroscopy

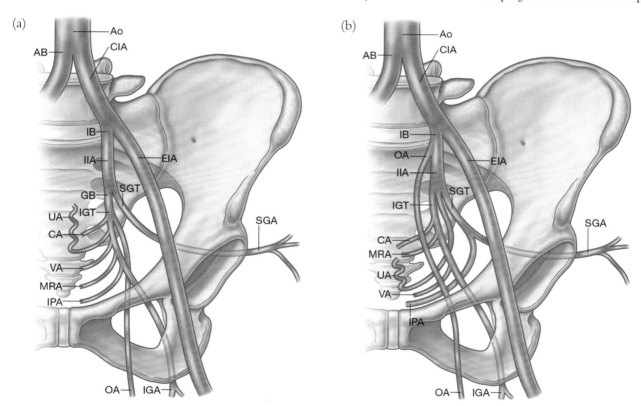

Figure 1 Branch patterns of the arteries to the uterus and the birth canal. (a) The most frequent pattern of branching. The internal iliac artery (IIA) is initially divided into the posterior and anterior divisions, which are hereafter termed as superior and inferior gluteal trunks (SGT and IGT, respectively). The point of division is termed the gluteal bifurcation (GB). The uterine, vaginal and internal pudendal arteries (UA, VA and IPA, respectively) are the branches of the IGT together with the obturator and cystic arteries (OA and CA, respectively). (b) Less common patterns include the uterine artery (UA) arising at the gluteal bifurcation (GB), the obturator artery (OA) arising directly from the internal iliac artery (IIA) proximal to the gluteal bifurcation (GB), the internal pudendal artery (IPA) arising from the superior gluteal trunk (SGT). Ao, aorta; AB, aortic bifurcation; IB, iliac bifurcation; CIA, common iliac artery; EIA, external iliac artery; MRA, middle rectal artery; SGA, superior gluteal artery; IGA, inferior gluteal artery

can be difficult. This is because it lacks any characteristic appearance and the image of the artery is often overlapped by other branches of the internal iliac artery on the usual frontal projection in fluoroscopy. As a result, oblique views of the inferior gluteal trunk (anterior branch) are frequently required to clarify the origin of the uterine artery.

The superior cystic artery can be identified by superselective catheterization and manual contrast injection; these techniques demonstrate the distal network of the artery in the bladder wall and occasionally the cystic artery on the opposite side. The pudendal artery, usually a branch from the inferior gluteal trunk (anterior branch), is harder to confirm, and often requires some guesswork. Further difficulties may arise from the presence of a hematoma which can alter the appearance and distribution of all these arteries.

The middle and inferior rectal arteries originate from the inferior gluteal and the internal pudendal arteries, respectively. These supply the middle and lower portions of the rectum, anal canal and the perianal skin. *Theoretically*, superselective embolization of the middle or inferior rectal artery may result in necrosis of these areas. However, such complications have not been reported thus far, presumably due to the prominent collateral network of other arteries.

The vaginal artery may originate from either the uterine artery at the level of the cervix or the inferior gluteal trunk (anterior branch). In addition, the vagina is also supplied by branches of the internal pudendal artery. These arteries are important and often not thought of when it is necessary to reduce blood flow to the pelvis.

Collateral pathways

Abundant collateral networks of blood vessels exist throughout the pelvis. This is of particular importance when performing embolization or related radiological interventional procedures. Stated another way, embolization of the uterine artery exclusively may not be sufficient to achieve satisfactory cessation in major life-threatening hemorrhage because of the existence of collaterals. The major potential collateral arteries to the uterus include the ovarian arteries, which directly branch off from the abdominal aorta, as well as the vaginal and pudendal arteries. There are reported cases where it was necessary to perform embolization of such small arteries with superselective catheterization into the ovarian artery[30], vaginal artery[25,30] and pudendal artery[30]. In addition, lower lumbar arteries can occasionally be the main feeding artery for the retractable intrapelvic hemorrhage[2], as well as branches of the external iliac artery and femoral arteries, particularly medial circumflex femoral artery[1,2], but such circumstances are not common.

EMBOLIC MATERIALS

Table 1 summarizes embolic materials, including particles (including pledgets), coils and liquids. Figure 2

illustrates the theoretical mechanism and arterial positions for each embolic material, and also for temporary balloon occlusion.

Among the potential particles (Figure 2a), gelatin sponge is the material of first choice. The main reason why gelatin sponge is deemed most appropriate for PPH is that it dissolves within approximately 3 weeks, thus preserving the peripheral microarterial circulation[11]. In contrast, particles of permanent embolic materials, including polyvinyl alcohol (PVA) particles, tend to remain in the blood vessels and soft tissue[57]. On embolization, peripheral tissue survives when crucial collateral circulation is spared or new collaterals are developed. The common wisdom is that using gelatin sponge lowers the risk of serious ischemic complications. Nevertheless, such complications are not as rare as previously described, suggesting that the benefit of using gelatin sponge particles compared with truly permanent particles is a higher probability, but not a certainty, of avoiding ischemic complications.

In practice, gelatin sponge is supplied in the plate form which is normally used in the operating theater as hemostatic material. The gelatin sponge plate must be either cut into small pieces such as pledgets or grated into particles. The majority of authors reporting embolization for PPH used pledgets of gelatin sponge, which were handcut during the emergency treatment. The typical sizes of gelatin sponge particles and pledgets appear to be between 1 mm × 1 mm × 1 mm and 1 mm × 1 mm × 10 mm, they are usually cut using fine scissors or razor. However, making gelatin sponge pledgets is a time-consuming and tedious process. The authors' choice is grated gelatin sponge particles; a sterilized stainless steel grater is used for grating (Figure 3). This has the advantage of short preparation time, in addition to the inherent advantages of gelatin sponge including availability, effect, safety and cost. We recommend grated gelatin sponge as the first choice of embolic material.

Although the sizes of the grated particles vary in each case, the principle is that the size of the grated particles depends on the force exerted on grating; the greater the grating force exerted, the larger the particles and vice versa. The authors tend to use grated particles approximately 5 mm in diameter. When they are mixed with fluid such as saline or radiological contrast, the particles become softer and easily pass through 4 and 5 Fr catheters. Slightly smaller (2–3 mm) particles are more appropriate for 3 Fr catheters. However, it should be noted that there are reports warning about the risk of using small sized particles[7]. Where calibrated gelatin sponge particles are commercially available, some authors have recommended avoiding the usage of those smaller than 1 mm × 1 mm × 10 mm[58].

Although the use of gelatin sponge is popular in practice and is recommended by authors, no evidence is available to contraindicate the use of permanent embolic materials, such as polyvinyl alcohol (PVA) particles, except for the warning of the risk using small particles as mentioned above. Successful use of

Table 1 Embolic materials

Materials	Duration of effect	Approximate size	Mechanism of effect	Advantages	Disadvantages
Particles					
Gelatin sponge (cut)	Temporary	1–5 mm	Blockage of blood vessel, inflammatory occlusion (partly)	Economic, safe	Cutting is time-consuming
Gelatin sponge (grated)	Temporary	0.3–5 mm	Blockage of blood vessel, inflammatory occlusion (partly)	Economic, safe, easy to make	Smaller particles (<1 mm) cannot be prevented, proximal embolization could occur
Polyvinyl alcohol (PVA)	Permanent	100–700 μm	Blockage of blood vessel, inflammatory occlusion (partly)	Readily available	Could be expensive, proximal embolization could occur
Autologous blood clot	Temporary	1–5 mm	Blockage of blood vessel, inflammatory occlusion (partly)	Available by adding thrombin *in vitro*	Duration of effect is unreliable
Autologous blood clot (degenerate)	Permanent	<1–5 mm	Blockage of blood vessel, inflammatory occlusion (partly)	Available by heating or exposing to alcohol or its derivatives	Usually not readily available, smaller particles cannot be prevented
Liquid					
Alcohol	Permanent		Destruction of blood vessel by ablating the intima, producing degenerate thrombi	Economic and ultrapotent	Painful, hazardous as unwanted vessels could be affected
Ethanolamine oleate	Permanent		Similar to alcohol but milder effect	Similar to alcohol but milder effect, the effect could be stabilized when combined with gelatin sponge	Similar to alcohol but milder effect
Glues such as cyanoacrylate and tris–acryl gelatin ('Biosphere', Merit Medical)	Permanent		Blockage of blood vessel	Readily available, stable	Requires expertise in the use of materials, adherence of the delivery catheter could occur
Coils such as Granturco coils	Permanent	From microsize to large ones	Mechanical blockage with or without thrombosis limited at the deployed site	No ischemic complications on their own. Protects distal portions in non-targeted particle embolization	Weak embolization effect if not accompanied by particles

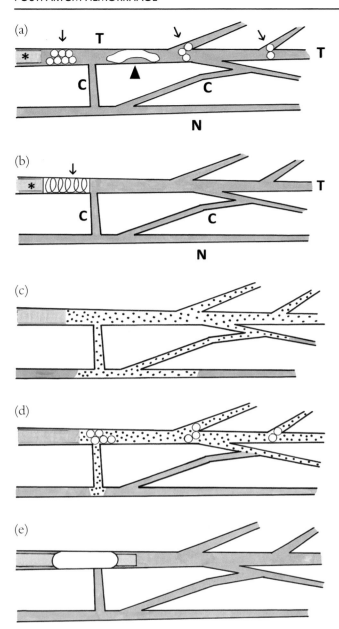

Figure 2 Mechanism of each embolic material. (a) Particles. Particles (arrows) including pledgets (arrowhead) are infused through the delivery catheter (*) and flow to more peripheral sites. Good obstruction including that of the peripheral circulation can be achieved. Gelatin sponge particles/pledgets are degradable within 2–3 weeks after delivery, although a substantial proportion of blood vessels will be occluded with inflammation. Peripheral tissue will survive when crucial collateral circulation is spared or new collaterals are developed. (b) Coils. Coils (or microcoils if a 3 Fr gauge microcatheter is used) are deployed at the tip of the delivery catheter, when it is pushed out with guidewire. Coils (arrow) occlude the artery at the point of deployment; peripheral circulation is preserved. Coils are generally used as an adjunct to other embolic materials (mainly particles) to increase the embolization effect. Similar to ligation, coils, once deployed, cannot be moved and preclude further intervention at the periphery of the deployment site. Because of this, coils can be placed to prevent particles from reaching the periphery to the coils in order to preserve peripheral arteries supplying the nerves. Other indications for coils include sites of vascular injury. (c) Liquids. Alcohol (stippled zones), when it replaces blood in the vessels, causes intimal damage and formation of permanent embolic material from degenerated blood cells. Glues occlude the vessels by filling the lumina with a hard cast of the glue material/products. Liquid of low viscosity (e.g. alcohol) tends to go through collaterals even to larger blood vessels beyond the collaterals, potentially resulting in extensive occlusion and vascular injury. (d) EGGS. Ethanolamine oleate containing grated gelatin sponge particles (EGGS) is a mixture of 5% ethanolamine oleate solution (stippled zones) and gelatin sponge particles (circles) to the consistency of soft paste. This is more potent than simple particles, as it acts as a half liquid material, while the gelatin sponge prevents washout. Only a small amount (e.g. 0.5 ml) can be infused into a targeted artery which is profusely hemorrhagic. (e) Balloon. When inflated, a temporary balloon (white area) occludes the proximal portion only, usually at a single site on each side. The effects may be similar to ligation or coil deployment, although the balloon will be deflated subsequently and removed; intervention beyond the balloon is also a possibility. Balloons must not be continuously inflated prior to delivery or fetal distress could occur. T, target artery of embolization; C, collaterals; N, nearby artery which is not the target of embolization

PVA[15,24,25,42,53,59] and cyanoacrylate[25], mainly as an adjunct to gelatin sponge, has been described in several reports. The size of commercially available synthetic particles varies from 20 μm to larger than 1 mm. For intrapelvic use, particles smaller than 300 μm (i.e. 0.3 mm) should not be used; 500–900 μm (0.5–0.9 mm) particles are safer and effective in producing good obstruction including in the peripheral circulation. Larger particles tend to clog the small caliber catheters. When PVA particles are used, caution is needed as they tend to gather together and stay in the proximal sites more than would be expected (proximal embolization). Among the commercially available permanent embolic particles, tris-acryl collagen-coated microspheres appear to have a reduced effect of proximal embolization.

Larger embolic materials such as coils occlude or reduce the blood flow significantly at the point of

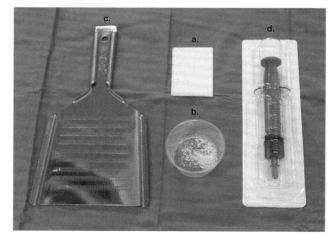

Figure 3 Typical embolization particles. (a) Gelatin sponge; (b) grater for gelatin sponge; (c) grated gelatin sponge particles; and (d) polyvinyl alcohol (PVA) particles in a bottled syringe

deployment (Figure 2b). Coils act by proximal obstruction; peripheral circulation will be preserved. Because of this, ischemic complications rarely occur with coil deployment only; on the other hand, the hemostatic effect is often suboptimal, although a report exists of successful hemostasis following the deployment of several coils in the bilateral inferior gluteal trunks (anterior divisions) in a case with a large arteriovenous shunt[60]. As the peripheral networks of collateral small arteries are not occluded, the effect of coil deployment is similar to that of ligation. After the deployment, radiological intervention using catheters and guidewire cannot be achieved in the peripheral part of the artery beyond the coil. Owing to these limitations, coils should be used as an adjunct to the primary embolic materials such as gelatin sponge: the role of the coils is to reduce perfusion pressure and flow within the target artery so that the embolization effect

of the particles will be increased. Other roles of coils include preservation of the peripheral branches of the superior gluteal trunk (posterior branch) and inferior gluteal trunk (anterior branch). Following the deployment of coil(s) in the branches of either (or both) of the superior and inferior gluteal arteries, the peripheral branches of each artery will be guarded from any further embolization; infusion of embolic particles to the proximal portion to the coil is unlikely to compromise the flow in these arteries, thus avoiding ischemic complications to the nerves and muscles[7,58] (Figure 4). When there is injury to relatively large vessels, deployment of the coil at the injury site is also effective (Figure 5), where the physical size and immobility of the coils are advantageous factors.

Liquid materials (Figure 2c) are divided into alcohols and glues. Alcohol damages the arterial wall, particularly the intima, resulting in stenosis and occlusion.

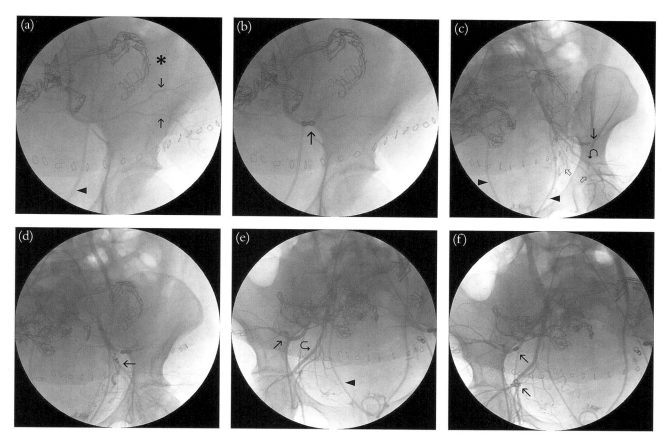

Figure 4 Coil deployment to avoid nerve injury in the superior and inferior gluteal trunks prior to non-targeted embolization. The patient was a 31-year-old Caucasian with prenatally diagnosed placenta increta/percreta at the lower anterior myometrium. The patient had previously undergone four cesarean sections. Primary PPH occurred on the 5th cesarean section. Despite hysterectomy, hemorrhage persisted, resulting in disseminated intravascular coagulation. Nephrocystic stents to reduce hydronephrosis had been placed. (a) Superselective arteriogram of the left superior gluteal trunk (posterior division). Its peripheral branches (arrows) were shown. Packed gauze (*), surgical staples of lower abdominal wound and the left sided nephrocystic stent (arrowhead) were noted. (b) A coil (Azur, Terumo) was placed in the superior gluteal trunk (arrow). Immediate reduction of the flow distal to the coil was observed. (c) Left internal iliac arteriogram following coil placement in the superior gluteal trunk. Arrowheads indicate nephrocystic stents. The practically occluded superior gluteal trunk at the coil (arrow), patent inferior gluteal trunk (curved arrow) and its branches were demonstrated. Bilateral nephrocystic stents (arrowheads) were *in situ*. (d) A coil (Azur) was deployed (arrow) in the inferior gluteal trunk. Non-targeted embolization of the internal iliac artery using grated gelatin sponge particles was then performed. (e) Right internal iliac arteriogram. Superior gluteal (arrow) and inferior gluteal (curved arrow) trunks were shown. Nephrocystic stent (arrowhead) was present. (f) Deployed coils (Azur) in the superior and inferior gluteal trunks (arrows). The flow in the distal portions to the coils was reduced greatly several minutes later, when non-targeted embolization of the internal iliac artery was undertaken. Grated gelatin sponge particles were used. The hemodynamics soon stabilized without the signs of ischemic complications; the patient recovered fully

This is coupled by degeneration of blood cells acting as permanent embolic particles, which are formed when the blood cells are exposed to alcohol. Glue fills in the arterial lumina; cyanoacrylate incorporates blood as it polymerizes with water, while other glues, such as Onyx®, replace the blood within the lumen and hardens. Most liquid materials are not viscous. Liquids, especially alcohol, carry the risk of damaging the arteries of adjacent organs by reversely traversing collaterals, when infused in sufficient amount to ablate the target artery. Glues can solidify within the blood vessels earlier than expected. This may result in fixation of the catheter. Because of these risks, liquids should be used as adjuncts to gelatin sponge, and only in cases where hemostasis is not achieved with gelatin sponge only.

Ethanolamine oleate, a type of alcohol, can be absorbed in gelatin sponge materials. Grated gelatin sponge can be soaked in 5% ethanolamine oleate to form a soft paste consistency. This combined material (ethanolamine in grated gelatin sponge (EGGS)) is a very potent embolic material, as gelatin sponge particles will hold ethanolamine oleate to prevent early wash-out. At the same time, the viscosity due to the addition of gelatin sponge particles reduces the risk of significant penetration through the collaterals to the adjacent organ arteries (Figure 2d). EGGS should be used only in small amounts, e.g. up to 0.5 ml into the uterine artery with overt extravasation, or, in extremely severe cases 1–1.5 ml (Figure 6). Deep insertion of the catheter tip into the target artery before injecting EGGS would be safer to prevent injury to organs adjacent to the uterus.

Racker and Braithwaite reported the fine arterial communication between the uterine artery and arteries to the lower ureters[61]. This is one of the examples explaining why particles which are too small or liquid materials are theoretically more hazardous as embolic materials than larger sized particles. It is, therefore, strongly recommended to use non-microscopic sized gelatin sponge. Liquid materials including EGGS are to be considered only when it is highly suspected that it may be difficult to achieve hemostasis using larger sized gelatin sponge. The amount of liquid material should be limited to as little as possible to prevent complications.

Catheters with an inflatable balloon achieve temporary occlusion at relatively proximal sites, from the internal iliac to uterine arteries (Figure 2e). They are used mainly in the prophylaxis of PPH in cases with adhesive or invasive placenta as described below and in Chapters 25–29. The advantages of balloon catheter placement are: (1) it can be planned during normal working hours, changing possible emergency cases to elective ones; (2) the balloon is removable, resuming normal flow when hemostasis is confirmed; (3) peripheral circulation is untouched, and ischemic complications do not occur; and (4) if used prophylactically, quick conversion to embolotherapy is possible, in case balloon placement is of suboptimal effect. The disadvantage of balloon placement is that the preservation of the peripheral circulation also means that the collateral circulation is untouched, and therefore, persisting hemorrhage via collaterals is still a possibility. In fact, there is no consensus that balloon occlusion of the internal iliac arteries and their branches only effectively reduces PPH. From a technical perspective, balloons are of two types, occlusion or dilation. The former is softer and shorter in length, whereas the latter has a stronger structure with variable length (e.g. 4–26 cm). Either type can be used for the prophylaxis of PPH. Appropriate balloon diameters are 10–11 mm

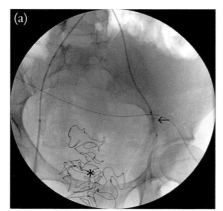
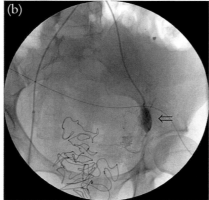
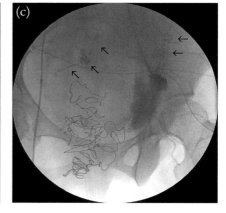

Figure 5 Non-targeted embolization of the internal iliac artery with repair of injured artery in primary PPH on a 39-year-old patient of a Chinese origin. Despite hysterectomy, the patient suffered from persistent per vaginal hemorrhage. (a) Contralateral cannulation to the left inferior gluteal trunk (anterior division). The catheter tip is shown with an arrow. Gauze pack in the vagina noted (*). (b) Extravasation (open arrow) was encountered immediately on test injection. Non-targeted embolization using grated gelatin sponge particles was performed, followed by the deployment of a 5 mm × 5 cm Gianturco coil (Cook, UK). (c) A more gentle test injection of a small amount of radiological contrast, after shifting the catheter tip to a slightly more proximal location, resulted in another immediate extravasation. Thus proving that with the fragile arterial wall, surgical repair and ligation would have been difficult. Demonstration of several branches of the inferior gluteal trunk (arrows), including branches of intrauterine arteries. A further focus of extravasation occurred in the more proximal portion in the internal iliac artery. These sites of arterial injury were again treated with the deployment of Gianturco coils of the same size. Hemostasis was successfully achieved following embolization

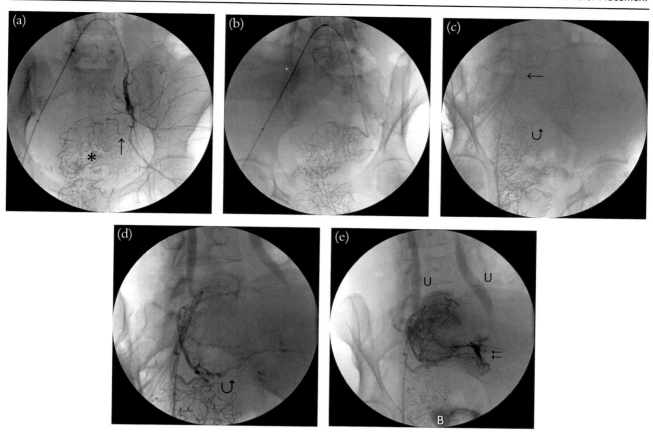

Figure 6 Uterine artery embolization in primary PPH on a 28-year old of Arabic origin with postvaginal delivery and uterine atony. (a) Contralateral cannulation to the left internal iliac artery and selective arteriogram was obtained (frontal views). The uterine artery (arrow) was detected. Gauze pack in the vagina shown (*). (b) The uterine artery was cannulated and superselective arteriograms were obtained. No extravasation was disclosed. This artery was embolized using grated gelatin sponge particles only. (c) Ipsilateral cannulation. The catheter tip (arrow) was in the right internal iliac artery. The uterine artery (curved arrow) was detected without the signs of extravasation. Arteriograms on this side were obtained in the right anterior oblique position. (d) Superselective cannulation to the uterine artery and arteriogram in the early phase. The uterine artery (curved arrow) was clearly identified. (e) The late phase of the uterine arteriogram. Extravasation appeared (arrows). The uterine artery was embolized using a small amount of EGGS (5% ethanolamine oleate containing grated gelatin sponge particles) in addition to simple grated gelatin sponge particles. Hemorrhage stopped and the patient recovered. Ureters (U) and bladder (B) containing balloon catheter

for internal iliac artery, 6–9 mm for inferior gluteal trunk and 5–7 mm for uterine artery. The amount of fluid to fill the balloon differs with the site of placement and balloon size. For example, it will be 2–3 ml, if a 10 mm × 6 cm balloon is inflated at the boundary between the internal iliac artery and inferior gluteal trunk. However, this quantity must be tested and confirmed under fluoroscopy when the catheter is inserted. It is preferable to use a pressure meter when the balloon is inflated. The necessary pressure to temporally occlude the artery is 1 atm or less, which is far smaller than the pressure required in balloon angioplasty of the iliac arteries which is at least 6 atm, typically between 10 and 12 atm. The length of the balloon and its placement position need to be decided by the radiologist on a case by case basis: there is no clear consensus on these issues. It is of note that the catheter/balloon must be deflated when the balloon is removed or repositioned, which is a procedure to prevent damaging the intima of the artery possibly resulting in subsequent stenosis or occlusion where the balloon is placed.

TECHNICAL ASPECTS

Preparation

Unless working in an absolute emergency, it is worthwhile to obtain a coagulation panel including platelet count and prothrombin time (international normalized ratio (INR)). Although dysfunctional coagulation does not contraindicate embolization[3,39,44], its correction may help in preparation for postprocedural hemostasis and the prevention of complications relating to it. Because embolization is an invasive procedure, obtaining informed consent from the patient is essential, provided the patient retains her consciousness. This process must include a full explanation of the procedure and a discussion of the possible complications, effect on future fertility and potential effects of the radiation. In cases where the patient has lost consciousness, however, such as in a shock or semi-shock status, consent is not practical. In such situations, explanations must be provided to the direct family, if present, particularly regarding possible complications.

Ideally the patient is kept nil by mouth for an appropriate duration prior to procedure, in order to avoid complications from vomiting. Bladder catheterization is not essential, although it is helpful in preventing the bladder from filling with contrast, containing urine that could obscure angiographic findings during the procedure.

Cross-sectional imaging

Antenatal diagnosis of placenta abnormalities

Ultrasonography is the principal means used to assess conditions of placental abnormality including placenta accreta, increta and percreta[45,62,63]. However, results are inconclusive in some cases and magnetic resonance imaging (MRI) has been proposed for detailed analysis of adjacent deep organs[46–51]. Placenta accreta, increta and percreta are demonstratable when bulging of the uterine boundary towards the adjacent organs such as bladder is present on both modalities, hypervascularity of the placenta is detected in the suspected areas, normal myometrial appearances are absent, and dark intraplacental bands are present on MRI. In cases where such abnormalities are present and which are regarded as high risk for hemorrhage, the placement of a balloon catheter in the internal iliac or uterine arteries can and should be considered.

Estimation of hematoma size

Localization and measurement of the size of the hematoma prior to arteriography and embolization is extremely useful, although not essential, and, in some cases, impractical. Confirming whether the hematoma is within or outside the uterus and its relationship to pelvic structures dictates the course of the embolization procedure[64] (Figure 7). Plain MRI is a useful method to examine the pelvis, as it requires a small number of examinations with different radiofrequency signal maneuvers (sequences) to demonstrate the objective images in the sagittal, coronal and axial (transverse) cross-sections. On the other hand, high speed arterial phase computer tomography (CT) is advantageous in the detection of active hemorrhagic sites[65].

Premedication

The interventional radiologist needs to decide the type and quantity of agents used for premedication, unless the patient is under anesthetic control as would be the case for those in shock status. If no interacting drugs have been administered, the authors recommend a combination of opiate and sedative antihistamines such as pethidine 50–100 mg i.m. (in two divided doses, if more than 50 mg is given) and promethazine hydrochloride 25–50 mg i.m.

Location for embolization and arterial puncture

The ideal location for embolization is the interventional radiology suite where vascular procedures routinely take place. In reality, however, interventional radiologists may be requested to perform procedures in surgical theaters in emergency situations. The obvious advantage in performing the embolization or related procedures in theaters is that the patient requiring the hemostatic procedure is already under anesthesia. The disadvantages are that the imaging system is usually suboptimal in image quality and functions, and the range of available devices and consumables including catheters may be limited. As described below, there is usually sufficient time for the patient to be transferred to the interventional radiology suite without undergoing extremely urgent procedures in the vast majority of cases, and the authors strongly recommend this if at all possible.

Targets of embolization

The prime target of embolization is the arterial source of the bleeding. Commonly, this is the uterine artery, when the source of hemorrhage is in the myometrium, cervix or endometrium (Figure 6). On the other hand, if the hemorrhage is as a result of a laceration of the birth canal below the level of the uterus, the source is likely to be a smaller vessel such as the vaginal or internal pudendal artery. If branches other than the uterine artery are the source of hemorrhage, superselective catheterization and arteriogram of each branch are required to assess the extent of extravasation (Figure 7). Fortunately, the availability of smaller diameter catheters and hydrophilic coated guidewires makes such superselective catheterization less challenging. Extravasation is unlikely to be demonstrated on non-superselective angiograms such as the global pelvic arteriogram and internal iliac arteriogram.

When extravasation is confirmed, embolic material is infused to occlude the artery. If extravasation is not proven, embolization of each of the branches supplying the suspected area of hemorrhage may be performed; alternatively, non-targeted embolization of slightly proximal arteries (or the internal iliac artery in extreme cases) can be performed. In such cases, protection of the distal branches of the inferior gluteal trunk and the superior gluteal trunk with coils is a safe option (Figure 4).

The most accurate demonstration of the flow distribution of transcatheterally infused material is obtained with combined arteriographs, using a combination of dedicated angiography table and CT equipment. Unfortunately, such complex equipment is available only in highly specialized institutions. More often than not, the interventional radiologist judges the vascular anatomy and the distribution of the embolic material on the basis of simple two-dimensional arteriograms in the frontal or oblique projections.

The order of arteriogram and catheter maneuvers

All procedures should be performed using aseptic technique. Unilateral or bilateral groin puncture(s) is

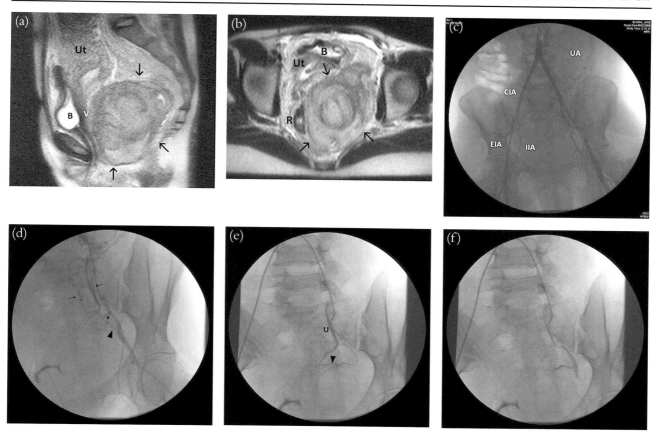

Figure 7 Extrauterine artery embolization in primary PPH from the birth canal on a 23-year-old Caucasian after vaginal delivery. The patient had a double uterus, double vagina and previous removal of the right uterus. Hemorrhage per vagina was only of a moderate degree. (a) and (b) T2-weighted magnetic resonance images (MRI) in the sagittal and axial (horizontal) cross-sections, respectively. A 9 cm hematoma (arrows) was demonstrated inferior to the uterus (Ut), left lateral to the rectum (R), posterior to the bladder (B) and vaginal zone (V). From these views and the information of the anatomical variation, it was anticipated that left-sided embolization only would achieve hemostasis. (c) Whole pelvic arteriography. The right common femoral artery was punctured and a 5 Fr gauge modified hook catheter was inserted into the distal aorta where radiological contrast was infused. The outline of the common, internal and external iliac arteries (CIA, IIA and EIA, respectively) and their major branches were shown. The intramural branches of the uterine artery (UA) distributed both above and within the pelvis. On this distant arteriogram, general vascular anatomy of the pelvis was demonstrated, although the suspected hemorrhagic lesion was not detected. (d) Left internal iliac arteriography in the left anterior oblique position. Both uterine artery (arrows) and vaginal artery (arrowhead) were identified. The superior gluteal trunk (*) was superimposed by the inferior gluteal trunk. This falls into the category of vascular anatomy shown in Figure 1b. A 5 Fr gauge cobra-shaped catheter was used. (e) Left vaginal arteriography. Tiny extravasation was confirmed (arrowhead) on hand injection of radiological contrast through the 3 Fr gauge microcatheter (arrow). Embolization was performed using particles of grated gelatin sponge particles until the extravasation was barely detectable. U, ureter. (f) Left vaginal arteriography postembolization. Compared with the image prior to embolization (e), the disappearance of small arterial branches around the extravasation was evident. Following embolization, the hemoglobin level increased to 11 g/dl on the next day and 12 g/dl on the following day. The patient was discharged 2 days after embolization without undergoing any other intervention. Her outpatient follow-up was uneventful

performed. An introducer sheath is used to stabilize the arterial entrance at the puncture site(s) in the groin(s). The standard diameter of the sheath is 5 Fr gauge; a 6 Fr gauge (or larger) sheath is usually necessary for 8–11 mm diameter balloon occlusion.

Hook shaped catheters are the first choice to enter the contralateral iliac arteries from either the aorta or the common iliacs on either side. We recently modified our technique with bilateral groin punctures, changing from a 5 Fr hook catheter to a 4 Fr soft J-curved catheter. Although the 5 Fr catheter works for relatively larger arteries such as the internal iliac, proximal portions of the inferior and superior gluteal trunks (anterior and posterior branches), and for superselective catherization of the uterine arteries, a 4 Fr appears to be a better size. The 3 Fr microgauge catheters may be required to go into smaller branches, which then can be inserted through the aforementioned 4 or 5 Fr catheters. For the catheter maneuvers, hydrophilic coated guidewires with angled tips are used. In principle, the performing interventional radiologist should choose the combination of catheters, with which the radiologist feels comfortable and familiar. Catheters made of soft polyurethane appear to be less irritating to the arterial wall. Once the arterial wall is irritated, spasm may supervene, resulting in a difficult maneuver and increasing the risk of arterial wall damage. Spasm can be prevented and treated by the intra-arterial infusion of nitrate vasodilators, such as isosorbide dinitrate 0.05–0.25 mg per branch. A

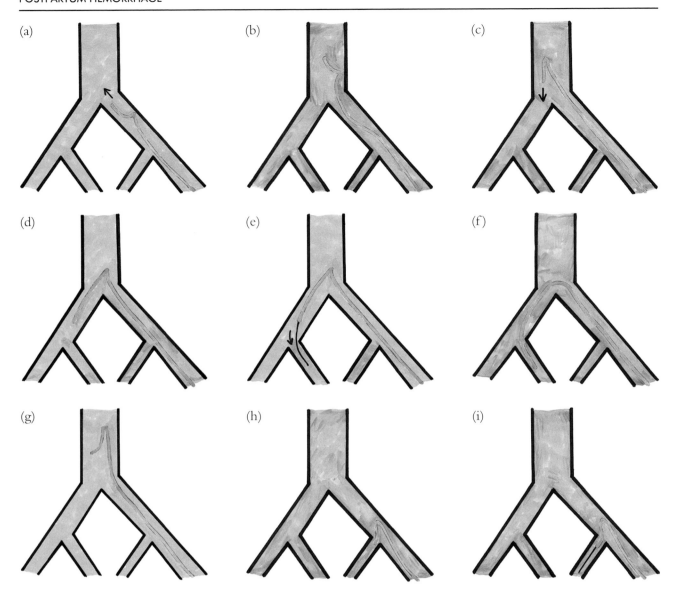

Figure 8 Routes of catheterization. (a) Cannulation to the contralateral internal iliac artery with a hook type catheter. The first step is to insert the catheter into the common iliac artery on the ipsilateral side. (b) The catheter is advanced to the lower aorta. (c) The catheter tip is turned downwards. Then the catheter is pulled down. (d) The catheter tip is inserted into the contralateral common iliac artery. Guidewire is often necessary. (e) Angled tip guidewire with hydrophilic coating is inserted into the internal iliac artery. (f) The catheter is pushed into the internal iliac artery lumen over the guidewire. If the catheter is a soft 4 Fr one, it will enter distal branches of the internal iliac artery by gently maneuvering the hydrophilic coated wire. (g) Cannulation into the ipsilateral internal iliac artery with the same hook type catheter. The hook shape of the catheter head is formed within the aorta. (h) The catheter is pulled down to the ipsilateral common iliac artery. The catheter is further pulled down, keeping the catheter tip facing inferiorly and medially, so that the tip enters the internal iliac artery. (i) Using hydrophilic coated guidewire, the catheter can be advanced to distal portions of the internal iliac artery. If the catheter is unlikely to go deeper into the internal iliac artery, the catheter should be then be replaced by a softer one at this point over guidewire

hydrophilic coated guidewire with a small J-shape tip is often useful to advance the catheter in tortuous and branching arteries.

The first arteriogram to be obtained should be an image of the pelvis from the aortic bifurcation to the groins; this provides a global view of the pelvic arteries. In reality, either common or internal iliac arteriograms often provide this view. Following this, the catheter should be advanced to the areas closer to the target of embolization. Frontal views are the basic projection; oblique views aid in the demonstration of the origins of the target areas and facilitate catheterization.

BALLOON CATHETER PLACEMENT AND EMBOLIZATION IN ADHESIVE AND ADHERENT PLACENTATION

Among the placental abnormalities, the adhesive and invasive forms, namely placenta accreta, increta and percreta, represent the second largest cause of PPH after atony. High success rates for embolization techniques have been reported in cases with these abnormalities in terms of cessation of bleeding[14,27,29,31,36,41,42,53]. At the same time, difficulties in obtaining hemostasis after embolization or cases with hemorrhagic complications following initial

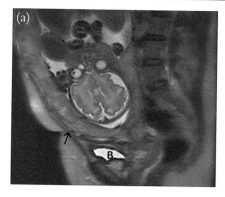
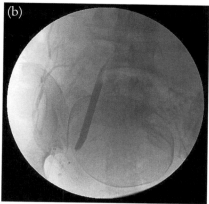
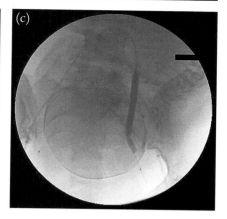

Figure 9 Prophylactic placement of balloon catheters in a case with antenatally diagnosed placenta increta. (a) A sagittal cross-section of antenatal MRI (T2-weighted). Cephalic presentation of the fetus, placenta previa, thin and disrupted lower anterior myometrium with placental invasion (arrow) were detected, consistent with placent increta. The bladder (B) was preserved. (b) Contralateral cannulation of a 9 mm × 10 cm dilation balloon catheter to the right internal iliac artery and its inferior gluteal trunk (anterior division). Test inflation of the balloon proved satisfactory filling within the artery as shown on this image, which was immediately deflated so that no distress of the fetus would occur. (c) Likewise, the same type of catheter was inserted into the left boundary area between the internal iliac artery and the inferior gluteal trunk. Test inflation of the balloon was repeated

hemostasis by embolization also have been reported[29,42,53]. One report noted that coils were necessary in addition to standard gelatin sponges in more than 80% of placenta accreta cases[41].

In cases where such placental abnormalities are suspected or confirmed on prenatal imaging, prophylactic catheterization can be achieved by the placement of catheters in the internal iliac, inferior gluteal trunk (anterior branch) or uterine arteries[20,27,40,42,44,52] (Figure 9). The choice of balloon catheters and advantages of the method using balloon catheters are described in the section on 'embolic materials' of this chapter. This process is neither complicated nor time consuming. The best timing for catheter placement is immediately prior to the delivery. However, for logistical reasons, we tend to place the catheters one day prior to planned delivery by section. Caution is necessary to prevent thrombosis mainly of the femoral artery, if catheters and sheaths are placed for more than several hours. As only one balloon can be placed on each side in practice, balloon catheters are inserted from both groins via the common femoral arteries on both sides through sheaths. The sheaths inserted and catheters placed can inflict irritation and intimal injury at the sites of placement. The authors flush the catheters and sheath slowly and continuously using four infusion pumps independently to prevent such injuries. An example regimen would be for each sheath to be infused with 1 liter of normal saline containing heparin 100 IU at an infusion rate of 40 ml/h, and for each catheter to be infused with 1 liter only of normal saline at an infusion rate of 40 ml/h.

Some reported series state that balloon inflation only was not useful in reducing hemorrhage during cesarean delivery[40,44], whereas others reported successful outcomes. In view of the mechanism of hemostasis depicted in Figure 2e, it is understandable that hemostasis is not achievable with balloon occlusion of the proximal arteries only as a result of the presence of well-developed peripheral collateral arteries such as the ovarian, femoral circumflex and lumbar arteries. Regardless, prophylactic catheter placement in cases of placental abnormality has the distinct advantage of prompt commencement of embolization, if hemostasis is difficult to achieve[42].

Figure 10 shows a reasonable protocol involving prophylactic balloon placement and therapeutic embolization in cases with suspected or diagnosed placenta accreta, increta or percreta. Several authors have reported no major complications in their series[11,14,24,30,33,34].

COMPLICATIONS

Numerous complications have been described[1–3,7,11,17,24–29,31,32,35,36,39–42] and major complications range from 0%[14,24,30,33,34] up to 18%[27,32]. It is rare, however, that these complications contribute directly to the death of a patient.

The causes of complications include:

(1) *Technical errors* These are rather uncommon, including hematoma at the puncture site[12,28], pseudoaneurysm formation[35] and vascular injury[7,28,29,31].

(2) *Systemic reactions* Pulmonary edema[1,26,29,40] and allergy to iodine[29] have been reported.

(3) *Pre-existing hypovolemia related complications* Cardiac ischemia[26], renal impairment[2,25,26] and retroperitoneal hemorrhage[28,29,65] have been described, as has necrosis of small bowel loops[7,31], which are more likely due to prolonged hypervolemia than embolization. Serious complications as a result of prolonged hemorrhage and hypervolemia occurred in four cases including death from brain hypoxia[28], panpituitary necrosis resulting in diabetes insipidus owing to prolonged hypoxia[28] and

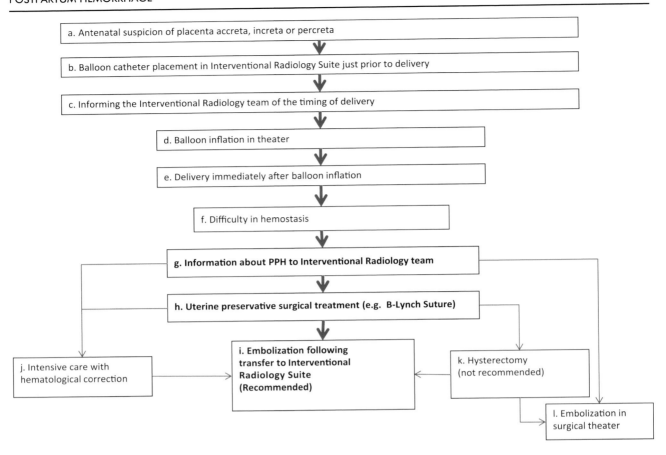

a. Antenatal suspicion of placenta accreta, increta or percreta

b. Balloon catheter placement in Interventional Radiology Suite just prior to delivery

c. Informing the Interventional Radiology team of the timing of delivery

d. Balloon inflation in theater

e. Delivery immediately after balloon inflation

f. Difficulty in hemostasis

g. Information about PPH to Interventional Radiology team

h. Uterine preservative surgical treatment (e.g. B-Lynch Suture)

j. Intensive care with hematological correction

i. Embolization following transfer to Interventional Radiology Suite (Recommended)

k. Hysterectomy (not recommended)

l. Embolization in surgical theater

Figure 10 Recommended protocol in cases with antenatal diagnosis of placenta accreta, increta or percreta

deaths from brain hemorrhage despite successful genital hemostasis[25,26]. It should be noted that these factors which are not direct consequences of embolization could pose a serious threat to patient prognosis.

(4) *Postembolic ischemia* Necrosis of the uterus has been reported sporadically[27,28,31,42,43,57]. Adjacent organs such as vagina[27], bladder[43] and ureters[40] are also prone to ischemic necrosis. Fistula formation following necrosis between the bladder and vagina has been described[32], as has atrophy of the endometrium, adhesion of the uterus and scarring within the uterus[42].

(5) *Sciatica and nerve injury* Symptoms owing to ischemia of the lumbar nerve plexus have been described[3,7,26,27,31,34–36].

(6) *Infection* Intrapelvic abscess formation[10,13] and endometrial infection[28,36] have been reported.

(7) *Acute thromboembolism of the lower limb arteries* This has been reported in a small number of cases[25,27,31,32] and has been attributed to overflow of gelatin sponge products from the internal iliac artery to the external iliac circulation. Surgical intervention of leg arteries may become necessary.

(8) *Deep venous thrombosis* This is a rather uncommon complication. Only one case with deep ipsilateral

femoral vein thrombosis without any particular cause was reported in a series of 36 cases[35].

(9) *Other abdominal or systemic symptoms* Pyrexia is commonly encountered and is usually of a self-limiting nature, unless an abscess results[1,11,17,24,34,41]. Abdominal pain is also common[11] and ileus has been reported[2,28].

(10) *Multiple organ damage* This report followed embolization of a wide range of arteries within the pelvis for PPH from a ruptured uterus[2] in which renal failure, ileus, surgical wound abscess, perforated sigmoid colon resulting in fistula to skin surface, subphrenic abscess, pneumonia and ulcer of the flank occurred.

(11) *Radiation* The biological effect of radiation only has been measured in two studies[33,36]. Doses to the ovaries measured in six cases averaged 586 mGy ranging between 204 and 729 mGy[36], whereas the skin dose averaged 34 mGy, ranging from 11 to 80 mGy[33]. These figures are consistent with measured absorption doses of skin and estimated doses to the ovaries in a series of 20 cases of uterine artery embolization[66]. In this latter study, fluoroscopy was performed for a maximum of 52.5 min with the mean value of 21.9 min, resulting in a maximum skin dose of 304 cGy (mean 162 cGy); the estimated maximum ovarian dose was 65 cGy (mean 22.3 cGy). These figures were

greater than the doses of other image examinations of the pelvis such as hysterosalpingography (0.04–0.55 cGy), recanalization of the Fallopian tube (0.2–2.75 cGy), or CT of the body trunk (0.1–1.9 cGy); on the other hand, they were smaller than the dose in radiotherapy for intra-pelvic Hodgkin's lymphoma (263–3500 cGy). On the basis of the known risks of pelvic irradiation administered for Hodgkin's disease, the dose associated with uterine artery embolization is unlikely to result in acute or long-term radiation injury to the patient or to a measurable increase in the genetic risk to the patient's future children. In embolization cases for PPH, there may be instances where longer fluoroscopy time is required than in uterine artery embolization for fibroids. Nevertheless, it would still be similar to that of uterine artery embolization, and, therefore, injury from irradiation is unlikely. In cases where catheter insertion to the intrapelvic arteries was undertaken, radiation doses to the fetus have been estimated in at least three studies. These estimates were 100–160 mGy[24], 40–200 mGy (median 6 mGy)[40] and 32 mGy[44]. Although it is commonly held that there exists no threshold dose below which no excess risk to the fetus arises, the doses to the fetus are supposed to be unlikely to cause injury based on available data[67,68].

(12) *Menstruation* Recovery of menstruation occurred in the vast majority of patients who underwent follow-up, excluding those undergoing hysterectomy, having natural menopause or who developed malignancy and received chemotherapy[14,17,29–31,33,42]. In a study of a subgroup consisting of 23 patients, 91% resumed regular menstruation, whereas 8.7% suffered from dysmenorrhea[35].

(13) *Fertility* All series assessing fertility following embolotherapy of the intrapelvic arteries for PPH conclude that fertility and pregnancy do not appear affected by embolotherapy[21,30,31,33,35,36,69]. In these reports, the majority of the patients who wished to conceive were successful; most delivered a healthy child. In one series, the authors noted a high frequency of PPH (100% four cases) as a result of adhesive placenta in patients who had previously undergone embolization for PPH in the preceding delivery[70]. This issue requires further examination.

In summary, the complications of embolotherapy for PPH have occurred in a relatively small proportion of patients undergoing the procedure. The vast majority of these were owing to ischemic damage to the uterus and nearby organs. It is important to view the complications against the backdrop of the circumstances wherein the operations are performed on seriously and sometimes critically ill patients, some of whom are literally and figuratively at 'death's door'. Under such circumstances, those who perform embolization on patients with serious PPH need to seek the best point of compromise between embolization effect and prevention of tissue ischemia. At the same time, there is no evidence that embolotherapy in PPH patients or prophylactic catheter placement in patients with antenatally diagnosed placental abnormalities will result in significant radiation injury to the patients or fetus. The majority of the patients who undergo embolization and preservation of the uterus retain menstruation and fertility potential.

LOGISTICS

In order to provide embolotherapy for PPH in an efficient manner, it is essential to establish a network that allows reliable access to an interventional radiology team; it is neither realistic nor necessary for all sites providing obstetric care to have such a team. This is because cases of PPH that require embolization are relatively uncommon and generally there is a relatively long time interval between the onset of PPH and the need for radiological interventions.

In a 54-month study in Jerusalem[37], the authors encountered 636 cases of PPH among 20,255 births (3.1%). Among these, only nine required embolization (1.4% of the PPH cases, but 0.045% of the entire cohort).

In the majority of instances, a relatively long time interval ensued during which obstetricians performed the first lines of treatment including transfusion and when the preparation by the interventional radiology team took place simultaneously. Indeed, extremely urgent (e.g. in less than 60 min) radiological intervention is rarely requested. The time interval between delivery and intervention averages 263 min, ranging from 90 to 750 min[29] or a mean of 11 h and median of 6 h[28]. This fact, while somewhat reassuring, must be considered in light of knowledge that delays in performing embolization can result in death or necrosis of critical organs. Such events follow prolonged organ ischemia, hypoxia or depletion of coagulation materials[25,26,28].

In view of this, it is logical to set up a system whereby an early warning and request is issued to the interventional radiology team. A recommended protocol involving embolotherapy is shown in Figure 11.

Similarly, prophylactic balloon catheter placement should be considered in cases where placenta accreta, increta or percreta is suspected or diagnosed on prenatal imaging such as ultrasonography or MRI. Although such procedures increase the number of irradiated cases among pregnant women and their fetuses, the radiation dose is not high and the procedure is not time consuming. Implementation of such a system would reduce the level of urgency to a semielective procedure, from otherwise possible emergency situations; thus further reducing the number of truly emergency cases. A recommended protocol involving prophylactic placement of balloon catheters is shown in Figure 10 as previously described in this chapter.

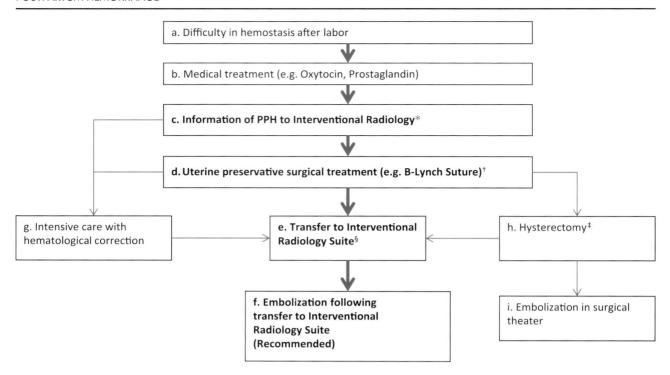

Figure 11 Recommended protocol in unexpected primary and secondary PPH. *Including the interventional radiology team of a nearby center, if embolization is to take place in that center. If this is the case, the team involved in the patient's transfer needs to be informed. †Only valid in primary PPH; in cases with secondary PPH, go straight to either (e) or (g). ‡Preferably avoid hysterectomy and extensive ligation of the arteries including the uterine arteries. §Including the interventional radiology suite of nearby center, if embolization is not available in the original hospital

EMBOLIZATION FOR ECTOPIC PREGNANCIES

In addition to PPH, ectopic pregnancies, especially cervical pregnancies, also can result in fatal hemorrhage. Using prenatal ultrasonography, these abnormal pregnancies can be readily diagnosed. Bilateral uterine artery embolization has been reported to be effective for hemostasis in cases with life-threatening hemorrhage after the evacuation of ectopic pregnancies[58,71–74], other forms of abortion[14,33,75] and hemorrhage after abortion due to retained placenta increta[76]. Either gelatin sponge or polyvinyl alcohol particles have been used successfully.

CONCLUSION

Embolization of the hemorrhagic source arteries in cases with intractable PPH is a highly feasible, decisive, relatively safe and beneficial procedure, which can preclude laparotomy and hysterectomy. The majority of the patients will retain fertility following the procedure.

Embolization should be implemented in the treatment strategy for PPH. It is indicated when conventional medical and surgical (non-hysterectomy) treatments fail in hemostasis. In principle, it should be performed prior to hysterectomy. Prophylactic balloon catheter placement is an option in cases where placenta accreta, increta or percreta is diagnosed or suspected antenatally.

ACKNOWLEDGMENT

The authors are grateful to Professor Louis G. Keith for a thorough review of this chapter, to Dr K. Envar, T. Choji and H. Choji for correction, and to Mrs S. Monsen-Fry for typing the manuscript.

References

1. Heaston DK, Mineau DE, Brown BJ, Miller FJ Jr. Transcatheter arterial embolization for control of persistent massive puerperal hemorrhage after bilateral surgical hypogastric artery ligation. Am J Roentgenol 1979;133:152–4
2. Pais SO, Glickman M, Schwartz P, Pingoude E, Berkowitz R. Embolization of pelvic arteries for control of postpartum hemorrhage. Obstet Gynecol 1980;55:754–8
3. Heffner LJ, Mennuti, MT, Rudoff JC, McLean GK. Primary management of postpartum vulvovaginal hematomas by angiographic embolization. Am J Perinatol 1985;2:204–7
4. Rosenthal DM, Colapinto R. Angiographic arterial embolization in the management of postoperative vaginal hemorrhage. Am J Obstet Gynecol 1985;151:227–31
5. Itol M, Matsui K, Mabe K, Katabuchi H, Fujisaki S. Transcatheter embolization of pelvic arteries as the safest method for postpartum hemorrhage. Int J Gynaecol Obstet 1986;24:373–8
6. Minck RN, Palestrant A, Chemey WB. Successful management of postpartum vaginal hemorrhage by angiographic embolization. Ariz Med 1984;41:537–8
7. Greenwood LH, Glickman MG, Schwartz PE, Morse SS, Denny DF. Obstetric and nonmalignant gynecologic bleeding: treatment with angiographic embolization. Radiology 1987;164:155–9.
8. Feinberg BB, Resnik E, Hurt WG, Bump RC, Kubota R, Cho SR. Angiographic embolization in the management of

late postpartum hemorrhage. A case report. J Reprod Med 1987;32:929–31

9. Shweni PM, Bishop BB, Hansen JN, Subrayen KT. Severe secondary postpartum haemorrhage after Caesarean section. S Afr Med J 1987;72:617–9

10. Chin HG, Scott DR, Resnick R, Davis GB, Lurie AL. Angiographic embolization of intractable puerperal hematomas. Am J Obstet Gynecol 1989;160:434–8

11. Yamashita Y, Takahashi M, Ito M, Okamura H. Transcatheter arterial embolization in the management of postpartum hemorrhage due to genital tract injury. Obstet Gynecol 1991;77:160–3

12. Bakri YN, Linjawi T. Angiographic embolization for control of pelvic genital tract hemorrhage. Report of 14 cases. Acta Obstet Gynecol Scand 1992;71:17–21

13. Gilbert WM, More TR, Resnick R, Doemeny J, Chin H, Brookstein JJ. Angiographic embolization in the management of hemorrhagic complications of pregnancy. Am J Obstet Gynecol 1992;166:493–7

14. Mitty HA, Sterling KM, Alvarez M, Gendler R. Obstetric hemorrhage: prophylactic and emergency arterial catheterization and embolotherapy. Radiology 1993;188:183–7

15. Abbas FM, Currie JL, Mitchell S, Osterman F, Rosenshein NB, Horowitz IR. Selective vascular embolization in benign gynecologic conditions. J Reprod Med 1994;39:492–6

16. Joseph JF, Mernoff D, Donovan J, Metz SA. Percutaneous angiographic arterial embolization for gynecologic and obstetric pelvic hemorrhage. A report of three cases. J Reprod Med 1994;39:915–20

17. Yamashita Y, Harada M, Yamamoto H, et al. Transcatheter arterial embolization of obstetric and gynecological bleeding: efficacy and clinical outcome. Br J Radiol 1994;67:530–4

18. Merland JJ, Houdart E, Herbreteaux D, et al. Place of emergency arterial embolization in obstetrics hemorrhage about 16 personal cases. Eur J Obstet Gynecol Reprod Biol 1996;65:141–3

19. Vedantham S, Goodwin SC, McLucas B, Mohr G. Uterine artery embolization: an underused method of controlling pelvic hemorrhage. Am J Obstet Gynecol 1997;176:938–48

20. Dubois J, Garel, Grignon A, Lemay M, Leduc L. Placenta percreta: balloon occlusion and embolization of the internal iliac arteries to reduce intraoperative blood losses. Am J Obstet Gynecol 1996;176:723–6

21. Stancato-Pasik A, Mitty HA, Richard HM, Eshkar N. Obstetrics embolotherapy: effect on menses and pregnancy. Radiology 1997;204:791–3

22. Hsu YR, Wan YL. Successful management of intractable puerperal hematoma and severe postpartum hemorrhage with DIC through transcatheter arterial embolization – two cases. Acta Obstet Gynecol Scand 1998;77:129–31

23. Pelage JP, Le Dref O, Mateo J, et al. Life-threatening primary postpartum hemorrhage: treatment with emergency selective arterial embolization. Radiology 1998;208:359–62

24. Hansch E, Chitkara U, McAlpine J, El-Sayed Y, Dake MD, Razavi MK. Pelvic arterial embolization for control of obstetric hemorrhage: a five-year experience. Am J Obstet Gynecol 1999;180:1454–60

25. Pelage JP, Soyer P, Repiquet D, et al. Secondary postpartum hemorrhage: treatment with selective arterial embolization. Radiology 1999;212:385–9

26. Touboul C, Badiou W, Saada J, et al. Efficacy of selective arterial embolisation for the treatment of life-threatening post-partum haemorrhage in a large population. PLoS ONE 2008;3:e3819

27. Ojala K, Perälä J, Kariniemi J, Ranta P, Raudaskoski T, Tekay A. Arterial embolization and prophylactic catheterization for the treatment for severe obstetric hemorrhage. Acta Obstet Gynecol Scand 2005;84:1075–80

28. Kirby JM, Kachura JR, Rajan DK, et al. Arterial embolization for primary postpartum hemorrhage. J Vasc. Interv Radiol 2009;20:1036–45

29. Chauleur C, Fanget C, Tourne G, Levy R, Larchez C, Seffert P. Serious primary post-partum hemorrhage, arterial embolization and future fertility: a retrospective study of 46 cases. Hum Reprod 2008;23:1553–9

30. Deux JF, Bazot M, Le Blanche AF, et al. Is elective embolization of uterine arteries a safe alternative to hysterectomy in patient's with postpartum hemorrhage? Am J Roentgenol 2001;177:145–9

31. Ornan D, White R, Pollak J, Tal M. Pelvic embolization for intractable postpartum hemorrhage: long-term follow-up and implications for fertility. Obstet Gynecol 2003;102:904–10

32. Maassen MS, Lambers MDA, Tutein Nolthenius RP, van der Valk PHM, Elgrsma OE. Complications and failure of uterine artery embolization for intractable postpartum hemorrhage. Br J Obstet Gynaecol 2009;116:55–61

33. Uchiyama D, Koganemaru M, Abe T, Hori D, Hayaduchi N. Arterial catheterization and embolization for management of emergent or anticipated massive obstetrical hemorrhage. Radiat Med 2008;26:188–97

34. Tsuang ML, Wong WC, Kun KY, et al. Arterial embolisation in intractable primary post-partum haemorrhage: case series. Hong Kong Med J 2004;10:301–6

35. Boulleret C, Chahid T, Gallot D, et al. Hypogastric arterial selective and superselective embolization for severe post-partum hemorrhage: a retrospective review of 36 cases. Cardiovasc Intervent Radiol 2004;27:344–8

36. Eriksson LG, Mulic-Lutvica A, Jangland L, Nyman R. Massive Postpartum hemorrrhage treated with transcatheter arterial embolization: technical aspects and long-term effects on fertility and menstrual cycle. Acta Radiol 2007;48:635–42

37. Bloom AI, Verstandig A, Gielchinsky Y, Nadjari M, Elchalal U. Arterial embolisation for persistent primary post-partum haemorrhage: before or after hysterectomy? Br J Obstet Gynaecol 2004;111:880–4

38. Mukherjee S, Arulkumaran S. Post-partum haemorrhage. Obstet Gynaecol Reproductive Med 2009;19:121–6

39. Porteous AOR, Appleton DS, Hoveyda F, Lees CC. Acquired haemophilia and post-partum haemorrhage treated with internal pudendal embolisation. Br J Obstet Gynaecol 2005;112:678–9

40. Levine AB, Kuhlman K, Bonn J. Placenta acreta: comparison of cases managed with and without pelvic artery balloon catheters. J Matern Fetal Med 1999;8:173–6

41. Chou MM, Hwang JI, Tseng JJ, Ho ESC. Internal iliac artery embolization before hysterectomy for placenta accreta. J Vasc Interv Radiol 2003;14:1195–9

42. Diop AN, Chabrot P, Bertrand A, et al. Placenta acreta: management with uterine artery embolization in 17 cases. J Vasc Interv Radiol 2010;21:644–8

43. Porcu G, Roger V, Jacquier A, et al. Uterus and bladder necrosis after uterine artery embolisation for post-partum haemorrhage. Br J Obstet Gynaecol 2005;112:122–3

44. Bodner LJ, Nosher JL, Gribbin C, Siegel RL, Beale S, Scorza W. Balloon-assisted occlusion of the internal iliac arteries in patients with placenta accrete/percreta. Cardiovasc Intevent Radiol 2006;29:354–61

45. Finberg HJ, Williams JW. Placenta acreta: prospective sonographic diagnosis in patients with placenta previa and prior cesarean section. J Ultrasound Med 1992;11:333–43

46. Levine D, Hulka CA, Ludmir J, Li W, Edelman RR. Placenta acreta: evaluation with color Doppler US, power Doppler US, and MR imaging. Radiology 1997;205:773–6

47. Kirkinen P, Helin-Martikainen HL, Vanninen R, Partanen K. Placenta acreta: imaging by gray-scale and contrast-enhanced color Doppler sonography and magnetic resonance imaging. J Clin Ultrasound 1998;26:90–4

48. Maldjian C, Adam R, Pelosi M, Pelosi M III, Rubellis R, Maldjian J. MRI appearance of placenta percreta and placenta acreta. Magn Reson Imaging 1999;17:965–71

49. Lam G, Kuller J, McMahon M. Use of magnetic resonance imaging and ultrasound in the antenatal diagnosis of placenta acreta. J Soc Gynecol Investig 2002;9:37–40

50. Palacios Jaraquemada JM, Bruno CH. Magnetic resonance imaging in 300 cases of placenta acreta: surgical correlation of new findings. Acta Obstet Gynecol Scand 2005;84:716–24

51. Dwyer BK, Belogolovkin V, Tran L, et al. Prenatal diagnosis of placenta acreta: sonography or magnetic resonance imaging? J Ultrasound Med 2008;27:1275–81

52. Kidney DD, Nguyen AM, Ahdoot D, Bickmore D, Deutsch LS, Majors C. Prophylatic perioperative hypogastric artery balloon occlusion in abnormal placentation. Am J Roentgenol 2001;176:1521–4

53. Soyer P, Morel O, Fargeaudou Y, et al. Value of pelvic embolization in the management of severe postpartum hemorrhage due to placenta accreta, increta or percreta. Eur J Radiol 2010;doi:10.1016/j.ejrad.2010.07.018

54. Ito T. The Pelvis. In: Kaibougaku kougi Lectures in Anatomy, (in Japanese) 1st edn. Tokyo: Nanzando, 1983:475–84

55. Lippert H, Pabst R. Arterial Variations in Man: Classification and Frequency, 1st edn. Munich: Bergmann, 1985

56. Obimbo MM, Ogeng'o JA, Saidi H. Variant anatomy of the uterine artery in a Kenyan population. International J Gynecol Obstet 2010;111:49–52

57. Cottier JP, Fignon A, Tranquart F, Herbreteau D. Uterine necrosis after arterial embolization for postpartum hemorrhage. Obstet Gynecol 2002;100:1074–7

58. Hare WSC, Holland CJ. Paresis following internal iliac artery embolization. Radiology 1983;146:47–51

59. Has R, Balci NC, Ìblahimoğlu L, Rozanas Ì, Topuz S. Uterine artery embolization in a 10-week cervical pregnancy with coexisting fibroids. Int J Gynecol Obstet 2001;72:253–8

60. Kumar S, Souza JD, Indrajit IK, Mohindra V. Internal iliac artery embolization in post LSCS haemorrhage. Med J Armed Forces India 2006;62:198–9

61. Racker DC, Braithwaite JL. The blood supply to the lower end of the ureter and its relation to Wertheim's hysterectomy. J Obstet Gynaecol 1951;58:608–13

62. Chou MM, Ho ESC, Lee YH. Prenatal diagnosis of placenta previa accreta by transabdominal color Doppler ultrasound. Ultrasound Obstet Gynecol 2000;15:28–35

63. Comestock CH, Love JJ Jr, Bronsteen RA, et al. Sonographic detection of placenta accreta in the second and third trimesters of pregnancy. Am J Obstet Gynecol 2004;190:1135–40

64. Boulton H, Choji K, Pandit M. Embolization as first-line treatment in the management of puerperal haematoma in a case of congenital urogenital anomaly. Congenit Anom 2008;48:48–50

65. Lee NK, Kim S, Kim CW, Lee JW, Jeon UB, Suh DS. Identification of bleeding sites in patients with postpartum hemorrhage: MDCT compared with angiography. Am J Roentgenol 2010;194:383–90

66. Nikolic B, Spies JB, Lundsten MJ, Abbara S. Patient radiation dose associated with uterine artery embolization. Radiology 2000;214:121–5

67. Wagner LK, Lester RG, Saldana LR. Exposure of the pregnant patient to diagnostic radiations: a guide to medical management, 2nd edn. Madison, WI: Medical Physics Publishing, 1997:88

68. Hunda W, Stone R. Review of Radiation Physics. Baltimore, MD: Williams & Williams, 1995:85

69. Descargues G, Mauger Tinlot F, Douvrin F, Clavier E, Lemoine JP, Marpeau L. Menses, fertility and pregnancy after arterial embolization for the control of postpartum haemorrhage. Human Reproduction 2004;19:339–43

70. Salomon LJ, de Tayrac R, Castaigne-Meary V, et al. Fertility and pregnancy outcome following pelvic arterial embolization for severe post-partum haemorrhage. A cohort study. Hum Reprod 2003;18:849–52

71. Lobel SM, Meyerovitz MF, Benson CC, Goff D, Bengtson JMB. Preoperative angiographic uterine artery embolization in the management of cervical pregnancy. Obstet Gynecol 1990;76:938–41

72. Simon P, Donner C, Delcour C, Kirkpatrick C, Rodesch F. Selective uterine artery embolization in the treatment of cervical pregnancy: two case reports. Eur J Obstet Gynecol 1991;40:159–61

73. Ryu KY, Kim SR, Cho SH, Song SY. Preoperative uterine artery embolization and evacuation in the management of cervical pregnancy: report of two cases. J Korean Med Sci 2001;16:801–4

74. Ratnam LA, Gibson M, Sandhu C, Torrie P, Chandraharan E, Belli AM. Transcatheter pelvic arterial embolisation for control of obstetric and gynaecological haemorrhage. J Obstet Gynaecol 2008;28:573–9

75. Takeda A, Koyama K, Imoto S, Mori M, Nakano T, Nakamura H. Conservative management of placenta increta after first trimester abortion by transcatheter chemo-embolization: a case report and review of the literature. Arch Gynecol Obstet 2010;281:381–6

76. Soleymani Majd H, Srikantha M, Majumdar S, B-Lynch C, Choji K, Canthaboo M, Ismail L. Successful use of uterine artery embolization to treat placenta increta in the first trimester. Arch Gynecol Obstet 2009;279:713–5

50

The Use of Recombinant Factor VIIa*

S. Sobieszczyk and G. H. Breborowicz

INTRODUCTION

As described in detail in other chapters of this volume, conditions with excessive bleeding, as are seen with uterine rupture, placenta accreta, abruption and uterine atony, often require intensive resuscitation with blood components and coagulation factors. In such circumstances, blood transfusion may be life-saving, but on occasion involves exposing the patient to additional risks. Over the years, numerous efforts have been put forward to reduce these risks. One of the most spectacular is discussed in this chapter.

Recombinant activated factor VII (rFVIIa) (NovoSeven®; Novo Nordisk A/S, Bagsvaerd, Denmark) was developed for the treatment of spontaneous and/or surgical bleeding episodes in patients with hemophilia A or B with formation of allo-antibodies to FVIII or FIX after replacement therapy[1–3]. rFVIIa is currently licensed for this indication in most countries world-wide. The US Food and Drug Administration (FDA) licensed rFVIIa on March 25, 1999 for bleeding episodes in patients with hemophilia A or B and inhibitors to FVIII or FIX. The FDA approved use of rFVIIa in 2005 for additional indications such as surgical procedures in patients with hemophilia A or B and inhibitors, and treatment of bleeding episodes in patients with factor VII deficiency[4]. In Europe, it is also approved for use in bleeding episodes in patients with acquired hemophilia due to auto-antibodies against endogenous FVIII or FIX, surgical procedures in this group of patients, and Glanzmann's thrombasthenia.

Beyond its currently recognized indications, rFVIIa has been effectively used 'off label' on an empirical basis as a general hemostatic agent in a wide range of conditions associated with acute, uncontrolled, or otherwise profound bleeding, and in other clinical circumstances associated with excessive bleeding in patients without pre-existent coagulation defects[5,6]. Indeed, the early descriptions of the benefits of rFVIIa in trauma patients[7–9] were bolstered by a compassionate use study, which suggested that rFVIIa administration could reverse massive bleeding, and thus significantly decrease transfusion requirements observed in critically ill, multi-transfused trauma patients[10,11].

Recently, rFVIIa was approved for the treatment of hemorrhage associated with congenital factor VII deficiency[12,13] and Glanzmann's thrombasthenia[14,15].

PECULIARITIES OF OBSTETRIC HEMORRHAGE

Patients who develop massive, life-threatening postpartum hemorrhage often have a combination of 'coagulopathic' diffuse bleeding in addition to 'surgical bleeding'. Whereas bleeding from larger vessels may be controlled by surgeons using a variety of operations (see Chapters 49–53), the ability to control diffuse bleeding is limited and, in many cases, not feasible. Thus administration of hemostatic drugs that can control the coagulopathic component of blood loss may reduce mortality and morbidity in such patients. Clinical experience presently suggests that rFVIIa is a safe and effective hemostatic measure in severe obstetric hemorrhage, both as a adjunctive treatment to surgical hemostasis as well as a 'salvage' or 'rescue' therapy where postpartum hemorrhage is refractory to current pharmaceutical and 'uterus sparing' surgical techniques. The 'evidence' behind the preceding statement comes from three sources:

(1) Studies on its mechanism of action;

(2) Accumulating reports in the literature; and

(3) Data from clinical studies.

All suggest that rFVIIa has the potential to function as a 'universal hemostatic agent'[16] across a range of indications characterized by impaired thrombin generation in non-hemophilic patients, many of whom are critically ill and refractory to other hemostatic treatment options.

The usual manner for treating postpartum hemorrhage includes, first, non-invasive/non-surgical methods, including administration of crystalloid solutions and/or red blood cells, uterine massage, uterotonic medications (oxytocin, ergotamine, prostaglandins), and, second, invasive/surgical methods, e.g. ligation of uterine vessels, ligation of iliac arteries, angiographic embolism of uterine/iliac arteries, or the B-Lynch

*This chapter is reprinted from the first edition and a follow-up chapter will appear in the on-line edition available at www.glowm.com. L.G.K.

method. Unfortunately, the overall effectiveness of such procedures to arrest hemorrhage and prevent the need for emergency hysterectomy is estimated to be only about 50%[17,18]. Moreover, comparatively few centers world-wide have access to the physical equipment or surgical manpower resources necessary to conduct all the aforementioned procedures.

COAGULATION FACTOR VII: THE HUMAN PROTEIN AND RECOMBINANT PRODUCT

Structure of the human FVII (hFVII)

Human factor VII (eptacog alpha) is a serine protease (molecular weight 50 kDa) composed of 406 amino acid residues, belonging to the group of vitamin K-dependent coagulation glycoproteins. The primary site of FVII synthesis in humans is the liver. Factor VII is composed of four discrete domains: a γ-carboxyglutamic acid (Gla)-containing domain, two epidermal growth factor (EGF)-like domains, and a serine protease domain. All appear to be involved, to different extents, in an optimal interaction with tissue factor (TF). The Gla domain of factor VII is also essential for activation of factor X and other macromolecular substrates. The activation of factor VII to factor VIIa involves the hydrolysis of a single peptide bond between Arg152 and Ile153. The result is a two-chain molecule consisting of a light chain of 152 amino acid residues and a heavy chain of 254 amino acid residues held together by a single disulfide bond[19,20] (Figures 1 and 2).

Production of rFVIIa using recombinant DNA technique

The development of rFVIIa was undertaken to alleviate the problems associated with the use of plasma-derived factor VIIa, such as limited supply and possible

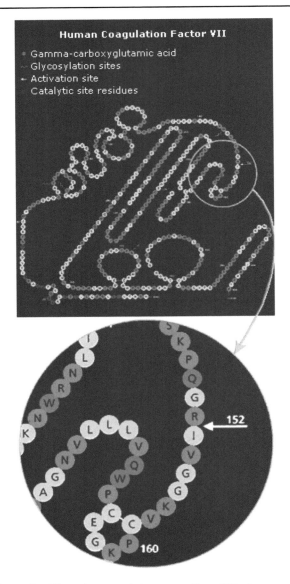

Figure 2 The active two-chain enzyme factor VIIa, is generated by specific cleavage AT Arg 152. Reproduced with permission from Novo Nordisk

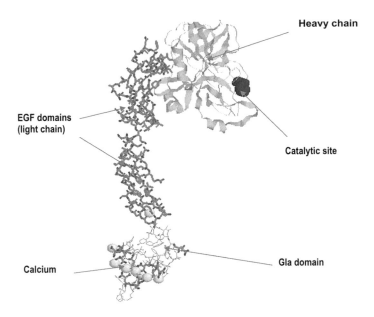

Figure 1 Three-dimensional molecular structure of factor VII. Reproduced with permission from Novo Nordisk

viral contamination. Multiple steps were involved in the development of this recombinant protein. First, the human gene for factor VII, located on chromosome 13, comprising eight exons (coding regions), was isolated from the liver gene library. After standard amplification procedures used to generate multiple copies of the hFVII gene, it was transfected into a baby hamster kidney cell line. A master cell bank of the transfected cell line that secretes factor VII in a single-chain form into the culture medium was then established. During the last steps, proteolytic conversion by autocatalysis to the active two-chain form (rFVIIa) takes place in a chromatographic purification process, which was shown to remove exogenous viruses. No human serum or other proteins are used in the production of rFVIIa (see Chapter 72). The protein backbone is identical with human purified factor VIIa. The final product (rFVIIa), despite minor differences in carbohydrate composition, is structurally similar to plasma-derived factor VIIa. The activity of rFVIIa is similar to that of natural factor VIIa present in the body[21,22] (see Table 1).

Human activated factor VII (hFVIIa) or recombinant activated factor VII (rFVIIa) is a naturally occurring initiator of hemostasis that is vital to the coagulation process, as it combines with tissue factor (TF) at the site of blood vessel damage in a natural way, stimulates thrombin generation, permits stable fibrin clot formation, and thereby the cessation of bleeding.

PHARMACOKINETIC STUDIES OF rFVIIa IN HUMANS

The pharmacokinetics of single-bolus doses of rFVIIa have been studied in various adult populations: patients with hemophilia, patients with cirrhosis, and healthy volunteers. The pharmacokinetic parameter values of rFVIIa after bolus administration were similar. The elimination half-life ($t_{1/2}$) ranged from 2.45 to 2.72 h and clearance (CL) ranged from 32.8 to 34.9 ml/h/kg[23]. Lindley and colleagues investigated the single-dose pharmacokinetics of rFVIIa, evaluated in three dose levels (17.5, 35.0, 70 µg/kg) in hemophilic A/B patients with inhibitors. The results of these investigations demonstrate that the mean $t_{1/2}$ of recombinant factor VIIa is independent of dose level[24].

Pharmacokinetic evaluations suggest the elimination of rFVIIa follows linear kinetics with a faster clearance rate and shorter $t_{1/2}$ when rFVIIa is administered for bleeding episodes (medians: 2.70 and 2.41 h, respectively) compared to non-bleeding indications

(medians: 3.44 and 2.89 h, respectively). Therefore, the duration of action may by shorter when rFVIIa is used to control bleeding episodes. The average percentage of the preparation found in plasma was significantly lower after administration of rFVIIa in a dose of 70 µg/kg (42.7%) compared to doses of 17.5 µg/kg (50.1%) or 35 µg/kg (49.0%) ($p = 0.0067$). Additional doses for specific patient populations are warranted however[23,24]. An increased elimination rate and lower recovery of rFVIIa during bleeding may be related to consumption through complex formation with TF exposed at the site of vessel damage and on the phospholipids exposed on the activated platelet surface. The volume of distribution at steady state (V_{ss}), is two to three times that of plasma and similar to the half-life of recombinant factor VIIa[24].

MECHANISM OF HEMOSTATIC ACTION OF rFVIIa
(see Figure 3)

Recombinant factor VIIa induces hemostasis at the site of injury. The mechanism of action includes the binding of factor VIIa to the exposed tissue factor-dependent pathway and, independently of tissue factor, activation of factor X directly on the surface of activated platelets localized to the site of injury[25,26].

The formation of the TF/FVIIa or TF/rFVIIa complex at the site of injury is necessary to initiate hemostasis. TF is a membrane-bound glycoprotein, which normally is expressed on cells in the subendothelium and is only exposed following injury. Tissue injury disrupts the endothelial cell barrier that normally separates TF-bearing cells from the circulating blood. Once exposed to the blood, TF serves as a

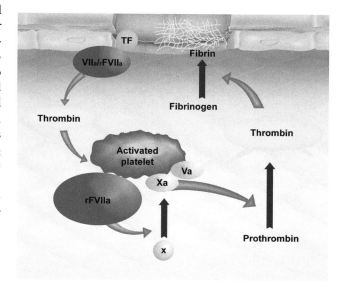

Table 1 Recombinant vs. plasma-derived FVIIa[21]

Amino acid sequence	identical
Amino acid composition	identical
Gamma-carboxylation	identical
Peptide map	identical
Biological activity	identical
Carbohydrate composition	similar

Figure 3 Mode of action of Eptacog alfa (activated) (with permission Novo Nordisk). (1) Tissue factor (TF)/FVIIa, or TF/rFVIIa interaction, is necessary to initiatiate hemostasis. (2) At pharmacological concentrations, rFVIIa directly activates FX on the surface of locally activated platelets. This activation will initiate the 'thrombin burst' independently of FVIII and FIX. This step is independent of TF. (3) The thrombin burst leads to the formation of a stable clot

high-affinity receptor for FVIIa. FVIIa is found in the circulation, comprising about 1% of the total circulating FVII protein mass in the plasma. It is endowed with very weak enzymatic activity, which only becomes fully realized upon binding to its cofactor, TF, at a site of vascular injury[25,26]. Factor VIIa alone shows very little proteolytic activity, only attaining its full enzymatic potential when complexed to TF.

In studies using TF incorporated into lipid vesicles, van't Veer and colleagues demonstrated that zymogen FVII acts as an inhibitor of FVIIa:TF-initiated thrombin generation. The addition of FVIIa at a concentration of 10 nmol/l in hemophilic conditions overcomes this inhibition and results in a thrombin generation equivalent to normal. These data suggest that the therapeutic effect of rFVIIa is due in part to its ability to overcome the inhibitory effect of physiologic FVII on FVIIa:TF-initiated thrombin generation[27].

However, if TF is no longer available or exposed to the clotting factors in the bloodstream, e.g. when a platelet plug covers the TF-containing subendothelial space, or when TF activity is inhibited by TFPI (tissue factor pathway inhibitor), then rFVIIa-mediated large-scale thrombin generation could take place on the activated platelet surface independently of TF[28].

The initial formation of a TF/FVIIa or TF/ rFVIIa complex allows activation of FIX and FX, and is crucial in generating the initial conversion of small amounts of prothrombin into thrombin (on the TF-bearing cells), which is essential to the amplification and propagation phase of coagulation. FXa cannot move to the platelet surface because of the presence of normal plasma inhibitors, but instead remains on the TF-bearing cell and activates a small amount of thrombin. Thrombin leads to the activation of platelets and FV and FVIII at the site of injury.

This small amount of thrombin is not sufficient for fibrinogen cleavage, but is critical for hemostasis, as it can activate platelets, activate and release FVIII from von Willebrand factor (vWF) or activate platelet and plasma FV, and FXI. FIXa moves to the platelet surface, where it forms a complex with FVIIIa and activates FX on the platelet surface. The activated platelets provide for further thrombin generation. Platelet-surface FXa is relatively protected from normal plasma inhibitors and can complex with platelet-surface FVa, where it activates thrombin in quantities sufficient to provide for fibrinogen cleavage.

FIXa, FVIIIa and FVa bind efficiently to the surface of the activated platelet and further activation of FX into FXa occurs via the complex between FIXa and FVIIIa. During amplification, FXa complexes with FVa to generate thrombin and subsequently activate FV, FVIII and platelets.

At pharmacological concentrations (supraphysiological doses), rFVIIa also directly activates FX on the surface of locally activated platelets, helping to generate thrombin and fibrin (platelet-dependent TF-independent pathways). rFVIIa does not bind to resting platelets. Instead, the effect of high-dose rFVIIa (which only activates FX on activated platelets) is

localized to the sites of vessel injury where TF is exposed and platelets are activated[29,30]. This results in the conversion of prothrombin into large amounts of thrombin. The full thrombin burst mediated by FXa in complex with FVa is necessary for the formation of a fully stabilized and solid fibrin hemostatic plug.

rFVIIa works by producing a stable fibrin clot directly at the site of vascular injury, both dependently and independently of TF. This reaction provides an extremely strong activation of thrombin at the site of tissue damage, leading to the formation of a stable fibrin network. Administration of rFVIIa might result in formation of a more stable hemostatic plug by a variety of mechanisms, including enhancement of activation of thrombin activatable fibrinolysis inhibitor[31], improvement of the physical properties of the fibrin clot, enhancement of platelet activation[32], and possibly enhancement of FXIII activation.

Lisman and colleagues observed that the enhanced thrombin generation from FVIIa not only accelerates clot formation, but also inhibits fibrinolysis by activation of thrombin activatable fibrinolytic inhibitor (TAFI) in factor VIII-deficient plasma[28]. rFVIIa binding to thrombin- activated platelets provides extra thrombin and thus ensures both full activation of TAFI and FXIII, and the formation of a dense fibrin structure. The full thrombin burst generated converts fibrinogen into a firm plug that is resistant to premature lysis, thereby facilitating full hemostasis.

MONITORING THE CLINICAL EFFECT OF rFVIIa

Currently, there is no good and/or satisfactory laboratory method for monitoring the clinical effectiveness of rFVIIa. Administration of rFVIIa results in shortening of the prothrombin time (PT) and the activated partial thromboplastin time (APTT). The PT generally shortens to around 7–8 s except in FV- or FX-deficient plasma, suggesting that patients completely deficient in FV and/or FX will not benefit from therapy with this product[33]. PT may not adequately reflect coagulation function. The APTT shortening is due to the direct activation of FX by circulating FVIIa on the phospholipids used in the partial thromboplastin time test. Data indicate that clinical improvement during rFVIIa treatment is associated with a shortening of APTT of 15–20 s[33]. Post-rFVIIa coagulation parameters normalize as early as 20 min after infusion. Thus, the shortening of these two screening tests of coagulation does not necessarily reflect clinical effectiveness, which is judged subjectively.

Coagulopathy is usually easy to recognize by the clinical assessment of ongoing bleeding, physical examination and observation of oozing from cut surfaces, intravascular catheter sites or mucus membranes. The initial evaluation during hemorrhage includes the PT, APTT, thrombin time (TT) and fibrinogen concentration, antithrombin and platelet count. In the interpretation of these tests, it is important to know the normal range and to be aware of the sensitivity of the screening tests for each coagulation factor, as these vary from laboratory to laboratory. In addition, assays of clotting parameters may provide different results with different reagents, although these parameters do not show a direct correlation to the level of hemostasis achieved. Finally, it is important to remember that laboratory coagulation parameters may be used as an adjunct to the clinical evaluation of hemostasis for monitoring the effectiveness and treatment schedule of rFVIIa[34].

Clotting parameters obtained prior to rFVIIa administration are often outside the normal range, perhaps indicating the development of dilutional or consumption coagulopathy in these patients. Post rFVIIa, clotting parameters improve, but do not normalize, and thus cannot be used as predictors of rFVIIa efficacy.

Laboratory monitoring of the efficacy of rFVIIa treatment is helpful. The effect on PT is particularly marked, but this does not always translate to clinically improved blood coagulation. Similarly, measurement of the level of FVII in plasma does not correlate with clinical efficacy. Study of the effects of rFVIIa on monitoring plasma FVIIa levels demonstrates a linear relationship between the concentration of FVIIa and FVII:C (functional clotting ability), but the therapeutic concentration range for FVIIa has not yet been established. The use of plasma VIIa levels is controversial, and is not an assay that is widely available.

Levels of functional fibrinogen and antithrombin do not change during repeated injections of rFVIIa for the treatment of hemorrhage. The minimal changes that occur postoperatively are not greater than those seen with patients who do not have coagulation disorders. Nonetheless, it is still advisable to monitor patients at risk of systemic activation.

Telgt and colleagues showed that low concentration of rFVIIa, in the absence of TF, can activate FX as assayed by the PT[33,35]. Higher concentration of rFVIIa had no additional effect on the PT. At rFVIIa doses well below the clinically therapeutic dose, a maximum shortening of the PT occurs. Thus, at doses in the clinically therapeutic range, no further effect on the PT is observed. This suggests that, at concentrations typical for clinical use, tests based on the PT are not useful for monitoring the effect of rFVIIa. Telgt and colleagues, in an experimental study, observed that rFVIIa effectively reduced PT and APTT in normal and deficient (FVIII, FIX, FXI, FXII) plasma. This reduction of both parameters (PT and APTT) has been attributed to the ability of rFVIIa to directly activate FX, even in the absence of TF[34,35].

The best available indicator of rFVIIa efficacy is the arrest of hemorrhage judged by visual evidence, hemodynamic stabilization and reduced demand for blood components[36]. There is currently no satisfactory laboratory test to monitor the clinical effectiveness of rFVIIa.

SAFETY OF rFVIIa

The complex coagulopathy and high complication rates seen in patients with intractable postpartum hemorrhage, together with the understanding of the localized mechanism of action of rFVIIa, and the low risk of thromboembolic complications following administration of the drug both in animal models and in clinical use, all suggest that rFVIIa is a useful adjunctive therapy for control of severe postpartum hemorrhage. Recombinant FVIIa is a manufactured product, does not contain any human plasma components, and therefore is free from viral contamination. Neither albumin nor any other human protein is used in its manufacturing process. This means that there is no risk of transmission of human viruses or prions. Strict quality control standards are applied to the fermentation process as well as the subsequent extensive purification measures. Genetic recombination eliminates the dependency on donors and allows for the production of unlimited amounts of the medication[20].

Safety analyses demonstrate that rFVIIa is associated with very few treatment-related adverse events and is very well tolerated. Thus, experience with recombinant factor VIIa in several thousand patients has shown that the incidence of non-serious adverse events is 13% and serious adverse events are less than 1%[37].

Aledort calculated that the risk of rFVIIa-related thrombosis is 25 per 10^5 infusions[38]. Despite the mechanism of action, use of rFVIIa in DIC and sepsis remains controversial. Several reports suggest that rFVIIa may be used safely in such situations, without induction of thrombotic complications or when conventional replacement therapy with fresh frozen plasma and red blood cell concentrates fails to provide a hemostatic response. Non-serious side-effects are rarely seen during treatment with recombinant factor VIIa; the most common being pain at the infusion site, fever, headache, vomiting, changes in the blood pressure and skin-related hypersensitivity reactions. Adverse events have not been related to dose.

OUR EXPERIENCE

Between 2000 and 2006 in the Department of Gynecology and Obstetrics, University of Medical Sciences, Poznań we used rFVIIa in almost 45 cases of postpartum hemorrhage[39–46]. According to data gathered from other areas of Poland, we estimate that it has been used in approximately 100 cases of postpartum hemorrhage.

The data presented below concern our first 18 patients in whom rFVIIa was used. Detailed information is presented in Tables 2–5. Our patient data were obtained when we were using a study protocol and were prepared to use the drug. This was not always the case in other centers (see Table 6).

Recombinant FVIIa was administered intravenously at doses of 16.6–48 µg/kg. In most cases, single administration of rFVIIa was sufficient. However, in severe coagulopathy coexisting with postpartum hemorrhage or prolonged periods of treatment (transfusions, complications of shock) and recurrent bleeding, a second dose similar to the initial dose was necessary to control the bleeding.

Table 2 Clinical details of patients with severe, recurring and uncontrollable bleeding post-delivery

	Number of patients
Number of postpartum hemorrhages	18
Cause of bleeding/complications	
Uterine atony	8
Genital tract trauma	1
Disseminated intravascular coagulation	8
Shock	18
Reoperations before rFVIIa administration	7
Obstetric hysterectomy*	2

*In six cases, hysterectomy was not performed. rFVIIa was administered after the decision to operate was made due to uncontrolled, life-threatening bleeding. After its administration, the bleeding stopped and the operation was not necessary. In two women, hysterectomy was performed in another hospital, before the patients were transported to our department

Table 3 Blood loss before and after rFVIIa administration

Blood loss	Median (range) (ml)
Before rFVIIa	3000 (1800–6800)
After rFVIIa	0.00 (0–350)

Table 4 Transfusion needed before and after rFVIIa administration

	Before rFVIIa		After rFVIIa	
	Median (range)	U/P	Median (range)	U/P
Red blood cell (IU)	6 (3–13)	6	4 (0–9)	3
Fresh frozen plasma (IU)	4 (1–8)	4	2 (0–9)	2

U/P, units per patient

Table 5 Selected laboratory tests before and after rFVIIa administration. Data are given as median (range)

Parameter	Normal range	Before rFVIIa	2 hours after rFVIIa	4 hours after rFVIIa	12 hours after rFVIIa
PT (s)	11.5–13.5	17.35 (11.9–26.7)	11.10 (9.1–18.3)	11.25 (9.1–17.6)	12.65 (11.2–17.1)
APTT (s)	25–37	55.00 (26–81)	35.00 (26–76)	36.80 (22–69)	39.10 (24–60)
PLT (Gpt/l)	140–440	76.50 (21–223)	70.00 (20–197)	69.50 (19–186)	70.50 (37–165)

PT, prothrombin time; APTT, activated partial thromboplastin time; PLT, platelets

Conclusions

The analysis of our data clearly shows that rFVIIa was an effective hemostatic drug, which significantly decreased bleeding and led to the rapid stabilization of our patients' conditions. Clearly, the early use of this agent decreases the amount of transfused preparations. An important secondary observation was the contraction of the uterus after the drug application in patients who had qualified for hysterectomy shortly before the drug was administered. We suggest that rFVIIa should be administered in every case in which embolization

of uterine arteries is being considered. Coagulation parameters showed typical shortening of PT and APTT; however, the clinical effect – control of bleeding – was the most important overall effect of the drug. There were no complications of rFVIIa administration. The dose, timing of administration after the diagnosis of postpartum hemorrhage, and the apparent ability to enhance uterine contractility will need further study in the future.

WORLD-WIDE EXPERIENCE

Tables 6–8 present the world-wide experience with rFVIIa in obstetric hemorrhage. The results reported in the literature support the benefit of rFVIIa therapy in obstetric cases with major/life-threatening hemorrhage, even in the presence of disseminated intravascular coagulopathy (DIC)-like 'coagulopathy'. They demonstrate that rFVIIa is highly effective and safe in allowing quick arrest of life-threatening postpartum hemorrhage unresponsive to conventional treatments. Treatment with rFVIIa led to a reduction in the use of blood products in this relatively large group of patients, decreasing blood product exposure for patients and sparing an expensive and limited resource. Administration of rFVIIa should be also considered before hysterectomy and as an adjunct to invasive/surgical procedures, before they are undertaken. This is particularly true in patients who wish to preserve fertility

Conclusions

Randomized controlled studies are required to determine the optimal dose and dose schedule of rFVIIa for intractable postpartum hemorrhage and to investigate whether the need for hysterectomy/surgical procedures and overall morbidity rates can be reduced by earlier treatment with higher doses of rFVIIa. In the meanwhile, clinicians caring for acutely bleeding obstetric patients should be aware of the potential of rFVIIa to arrest life-threatening postpartum hemorrhage. Although an expensive product, a trial of one to four doses of rFVIIa can be justified in cases of uncontrolled bleeding which persists despite maximal medical and surgical treatment to achieve hemostasis.

Although the limitations of anecdotal case data are recognized, in the absence of efficacy and safety data from randomized trials, voluntary registry submissions are being used to provide a preliminary insight into the scope of the low incidence of clinical problems, as well as the usefulness and adverse effects of this medication when it is used 'off-label'.

rFVIIa dose

When a rationale for using rFVIIa was stated, it was most commonly 'last-resort' therapy, after other clinical measures had failed. There was no clear correlation between the severity of bleeding and the dose of rFVII administered. Possibly the 'timing' determined the level of the dosing.

Efficacy

Bleeding either stopped, markedly decreased or decreased following rFVIIa administration in 54 of the cases. In one patient, there was no response to therapy with rFVIIa. Also only in one patient after an early significant reduction of bleeding, recurrence was observed. In general, however, the rapid onset of action means that rFVIIa can be used in the perioperative period. There was no clear correlation between the speed of response and either the type of procedure performed, the severity of the bleeding condition, or the dose of rFVIIa given.

Most patients continued to require some form of blood product replacement therapy during the 24 h following rFVIIa administration, but the need was greatly reduced compared with the 24 h prior to rFVIIa administration. No correlation existed between baseline and post-rFVIIa administration in laboratory measurements and the predictability of response to rFVIIa (data obtained from references but not presented in tables). Furthermore, of great importance, the results observed in these tables of cases of postpartum hemorrhage suggest that rFVIIa may be administered even in the presence of DIC-like 'coagulopathy'. In the patients shown in Tables 6–8, major conditions reported to be associated with postpartum hemorrhage included some individuals with HELLP syndrome and others with both laboratory and clinical signs of DIC before rFVIIa was administered. However, none of these patients developed an objectively confirmed, clinically manifest thromboembolism (deep vein thrombosis, pulmonary embolism, myocardial infarction, cerebrovascular embolism) after rFVIIa therapy, even if some patients had pre-existing signs of DIC (often severe).

Patients with HELLP syndrome who develop DIC are recognized as being at particular risk for life-threatening complications. The HELLP syndrome is a form of severe pre-eclampsia, and may be confused with the development of DIC. Data presented in Tables 6–8 suggest a high efficacy and safety profile of rFVIIa in the treatment of HELLP syndrome and/or DIC with massive bleeding. These findings are supported by clinical experiences about the therapeutic effectivity of rFVIIa in three patients with massive obstetric hemorrhage due to placenta previa, accreta, rupture of the uterus and pre-eclampsia with HELLP recently published by an Israeli group[71]. As mentioned by Segal and colleagues, these results raise the possibility that rFVIIa may be administered in obstetric cases with life-threatening bleeding episodes, even in the presence of DIC-like coagulopathy. Injection of rFVIIa should be also considered before hysterectomy in a young patient with severe bleeding, or after internal iliac artery ligation, if bleeding continues.

The series of patients reported here provides data on the safety and efficacy of rFVIIa in intractable early postpartum hemorrhage. However, as with any case series, there are difficulties in data analysis because data were collected retrospectively after the bleeding episode had occurred.

Safety

Adverse thromboembolic events were reported in one case that was considered to be directly related to the use of rFVIIa[54]. In general, rFVIIa administration was associated with an excellent safety profile.

PROPOSAL OF RECOMMENDATION FOR THE USE OF rFVIIa IN SEVERE POSTPARTUM HEMORRHAGE

Based on our own experience and data from the literature[36,72–80], we have prepared guidelines for treatment of postpartum hemorrhage that include administration of rFVIIa.

Definitions of severe hemorrhage

(1) Loss of entire blood volume within 24 h;

(2) Loss of 50% of blood volume within 3 h;

(3) Blood loss at a rate of 150 ml/min (for 20 min >50% blood volume);

(4) Blood loss at a rate of 1.5 ml/kg/min for ≥20 min;

(5) Sudden blood loss >1500–2000 ml (uterine atony; 25–35% blood volume).

Definition of insufficient standard management

The hemorrhage continues despite:

(1) All standard pharmacological and surgical treatment methods have been used;

(2) Replacement therapy was performed;

(3) Coagulopathy was confirmed by laboratory testing

    (a) PT or APTT >1.5 × times the control value

    (b) Thrombocytopenia $<50 \times 10^9/l$

    (c) Fibrinogen <0.6–0.8 g/l.

Preconditions for rFVIIa administration

(1) Hematological parameters

    Hemoglobin levels >70 g/l (4.3 mmol/l)
    International normalized ratio (INR) <1.5
    Fibrinogen levels ≥1 g/l
    Platelets levels $\geq 50 \times 10^9/l$

(2) pH correction (≥7.2) (suggest using $NaHCO_3$)

(3) Body temperature should be restored if possible to physiological values: rFVIIa retains its activity in the presence of hypothermia

Correction of the pH to ≥7.2 is recommended before rFVIIa administration (efficacy of rFVIIa decreases at a pH ≤7.1). We also suggest using bicarbonate to elevate the serum pH. It should be noted that $NaHCO_3$ has

Table 6 Clinical characteristics of patients with risk of severe, recurring and uncontrollable blood loss during delivery and postpartum: literature review

Year	Ref.	n	Provocation of bleed	Type of delivery	Surgical treatment	Blood products given pre-rFVIIa (units) (hemostatic agents)	Blood loss before rFVIIa (ml)	Timing (when rFVIIa given)	Dose of rFVIIa (µg/kg) (number of doses)	Overall bleeding response to rFVIIa (min)	Comments
2001	47	1	DIC, liver dysfunction, renal failure; severe intra-abdominal bleeding after CS	CS	HYS	NA	3000	Post hysterectomy; last resort	90 (9) 3-h intervals	Response after 2 single doses; significantly reduced	
2002	48	1	Congenital FVII deficiency (1% before application of rFVIIa)	VD	No	No	No evidence of bleeding	Prophylactic first dose at complete dilatation of the cervix	50; 35 4-h intervals	No evidence of bleeding	The first case of a pregnant woman with FVII deficiency receiving rFVIIa intrapartum
2002	49	1	Acquired hemophilia (FVIII 0.5%)	VD	HYS	RBC (65); FFP (60); CRYO (60); vWF (3 × 500); FVIII (30 × 1068); FIX (26 × 600); 18 g sandoglobulin	NA (massive)	11 days post-delivery; last resort	160	Bleeding stopped (rapidly)	
2002	50	1	2-h post CS massive vaginal bleeding; shock; DIC, HELLP	CS	No	RBC (12); FFP (10); PPTs (8); CRYO (950)	NA	Last resort	90	Bleeding stopped	Normalization of coagulation tests
2003	51	1	Bleeding from the placenta bed in lower uterine segment and cervical canal	CS	Under-running sutures in the placenta bed; application of hot packs; direct manual tamponade with surgical gauze; insertion of intra-cervical Foley's catheter balloon	RBC (1.5); FFP (500 ml)	>3000	Last resort	90	Bleeding stopped (15)	The balloon was removed on the first postoperative day
2003	52	2	(case 1) uterine rupture, shock (case 2) uterine atony	(case 1) VD (case 2) eCS	(case 1) subtotal HYS	(case 1) RBC (10); FFP (4) (case 2) RBC (5)	NA	(case 1) intraoperative (case 2) before planned hysterectomy	NA	Bleeding stopped (few minutes)	(case 2) Hysterectomy was avoided
2003	53	1	Uterine atony; shock	IVD	laparotomy: bilateral artery ligation; subtotal HYS; packing of pelvis	Before 1st administration RBC (42); FFP (31); PPTs (4); (desmopressin) before 2nd administration FFP (3); PPTs (2)	NA	Post laparotomy	60; 120 2-h interval, (2nd for consolidation)	Bleeding stopped	Cardiac arrest, resuscitation; high-pressure ventilation, pulmonary edema, pneumothorax, ARDS

Year	Ref	N	Diagnosis	Delivery	Surgical procedure	Blood products (units)	Blood loss	Indication for rFVIIa	Dose (µg/kg)	Outcome	Comments
2003	54	1	Uterine atony, pre-eclampsia	CS	HYS	RBC (3); FFP (2); CRYO (6)	NA	Intraoperative (CS) before hysterectomy	12	Bleeding significantly reduced	During general anesthesia induction, failed intubation was followed by cardiac arrest; postoperatively DIC; ARDS; transit encephalopathy, and brachial venous thrombosis (Folckmann syndrome)
2003	55	2	*(case 1)* congenital deficiency of FVII (2% before application rFVIIa) *(case 2)* liver dysfunction	*(case 1)* VD *(case 2)* CS	No	No	No evidence of bleeding	*(case 1)* Prophylactic first dose at complete dilation of the cervix *(case 2)* prophylactic before CS	*(case 1)* 60; 30 (5) every 2 h *(case 2)* 90	No evidence of bleeding	*(case 2)* No evidence of FVII deficiency
2003	56	1	AFE, DIC	CS	HYS; pelvic packing	RBC (12); FFP (8); (aprotinin)	NA	Last resort	60	Bleeding significantly reduced	MOF, died
2004	57	1	Uterine rupture; shock; DIC	IVD	3 laparotomy: 1st: HYS; 2nd: packing of pelvis; 3rd: small arteries ligated in the broad ligaments	*Before 1st* administration: RBC (26); FFP (11); PPTs (10); PCC (1200). *Total:* RBC (27); FFP (27); PPTs (10); 22 plateletpheresis; (tranexamic acid)	4000 to 2nd laparotomy; before 3rd laparotomy sudden increase of bleeding 1350 l in 1 h	Before, intra- and postoperative period; last resort	120 (19), start before 2nd laparotomy, repeated following next 2 days. First two doses (1st laparotomy) at 1-h intervals, next doses during the 2nd day 3 doses; next day two doses at 1-h intervals followed further doses every 3 h	Bleeding significantly reduced or stopped; recurrent bleeding was observed	Cardiac arrest, resuscitation before 2nd laparotomy (hyperkalemia 8.5 mmol/l, hypothermia 32°C); MOF Recurrent bleeding was observed because patient developed severe hypothermia, acidosis, hypoxia, dilution coagulopathy, all these reduced the efficacy of rFVIIa *in vivo*.

Continued

Table 6 *Continued*

Year	Ref.	n	Provocation of bleed	Type of delivery	Surgical treatment	Blood products given pre-rFVIIa (units) (hemostatic agents)	Blood loss before rFVIIa (ml)	Timing (when rFVIIa given)	Dose of rFVIIa (μg/kg) (number of doses)	Overall bleeding response to rFVIIa (min)	Comments
2004	58	2	Uterine atony, shock; severe coagulopathy	(case 1) CS (case 2) CS	(case 1) ligation of hypogastric arteries (case 2) laparotomy; ligation of hypogastric arteries	(case 1) RBC (19); FFP (3350 ml); PPTs (900 ml); fibrinogen (3 g); [aprotynin] (case 2) RBC (22); FFP (3400 ml); PPTs (3400 ml); fibrinogen (2 g); [aprotynin]	(case 1) 200 ml/h (case 2) 2000 ml, hemo-peritoneum	Last resort	(case 1) 60 (case 2) 60	Bleeding stopped (rapidly)	(case 1) 4 weeks later developed thrombosis of both ovarian veins
2004	59	1	Placenta previa; accreta; DIC	CS	No	RBC (11); FFP (4); CRYO (6)	1000 (in the drain) 5 h after CS		12 mg	Bleeding stopped (few hours)	
2004	60	1	Glanzmann's thrombasthenia	VD	No	PPTs (4)	No evidence of bleeding	Prophylactic	36 (2) 1st during vaginal delivery, 2nd 2 h after delivery	800 ml (intra- and postpartum blood loss)	rFVIIa may offer an alternative option in patients with Glanzmann's thrombasthenia during delivery
2004	61	1	AFE; DIC (developed 2 min after delivery)	CS	No	RBC (6); FFP (1); PPTs (2)	3000		90	Hemostasis was secured within 30 min	
2004	62	3	(case 1) Eclampsia; HELLP; consumptive coagulopathy; subcapsular liver hematoma with capsule rupture (case 2) placenta percreta, pre-eclampsia; HELLP (case 3) pre-eclampsia; HELLP; placenta accreta; consumptive coagulopathy; severe vaginal bleeding and uterine cramping	(case 1) CS (case 2) CS (case 3) CS	No	(case 1) RBC (16); FFP (14); PPTs (18); CRYO (10); (case 2) RBC (8); FFP (4); PPTs (6) (case 3) RBC (2); FFP (4); PPTs (6); CRYO (10)	(case 1) 2500 (case 2) 3000 (case 3) 1300	last resort	(case 1) 90 (2) (case 2) 120 (3); 90 (2) 2-h intervals (case 3) 90 (2) 2-h interval	Bleeding controlled	(case 1) patient developed anuric renal failure; cardiac arrest; patient died; no evidence of systemic thrombosis identified (case 2) no future transfusion requirement; coagulation profile stabilized

Year	Ref	n	Diagnosis	Delivery	Surgical procedures	Transfusion	Blood loss (ml)	Timing of rFVIIa	Dose (μg/kg)	Outcome	Comment
2004	63	1	Pre-eclampsia; HELLP; DIC; shock	eCS	Laparotomy 12 h after CS, because intra-abdominal hemorrhage	RBC (22); FFP (30); CRYO (20); (aprotynin)	3500 in abdominal cavity and 600 postoperatively from drains	Post laparotomy	90	Bleeding reduced (30), Bleeding stopped (180)	Improve coagulation parameters
2005	64	3	(case 1) Uterine atony, shock (case 2) placenta previa, uterine atony (case 3) laceration of vagina, atony, consumptive coagulopathy	(case 1) CS (case 2) VD (case 3) IVD	(case 1) relaparotomy with intracavitary oxytocin injected into the uterus; ligature of both uterine arteries; placement of B-Lynch sutures	(case 1) RBC (7); FFP (9); (case 2) RBC (10); FFP (13); PPTs (2); (case 3) RBC (13); FFP (16); PPTs (2)	NA	(case 1) before relaparotomy (cases 2, 3) last-resort	(case 1) 120 (2) 1-h interval (2) within 3 h (case 2) 60 (2) (case 3) 120 (2)	(case 1) Bleeding stopped (case 2) Bleeding stopped (case 3) Bleeding stopped	
2005	65	1	Uterine atony; shock; DIC	CS	HYS; packing of the pelvis	NA	NA	Before relaparotomy and ligation hypogastric artery	2.4 mg	Bleeding controlled (rapid response)	Resolution of the coagulopathy
2005	66	4	Uterine atony	VD	Uterus and vagina tamponade	NA	(case 1) 1600 (case 2) 2400 (case 3) 1100 (case 4) 2500	Before developed severe coagulopathy, surgical procedures; avoided massive transfusion	(case 1) 82 (case 2) 73 (case 3) 61 (case 4) 72	(case 1) Bleeding stopped (15) (case 2) Bleeding stopped (25) (case 3) Bleeding stopped (35) (case 4) Bleeding stopped (40)	Lower than standard doses may be effective when respect good timing, before complication develops
2005	67	3	(case 1) dehiscence of uterine scar (case 2) placenta percreta, adherent; dehiscence of uterine scar (previous CS) (case 3) NA	(case 1) eCS (case 2) VD (case 3) ieCS	(case 1) 3 laparotomy; bilateral internal iliac ligation (case 2) subtotal HYS	(case 1) WB (12); FFP (17); PPTs (2); (case 2) WB (11); FFP (7)	(case 1) 225 ml/h (case 2) 600 within 40 min (case 3) 500 hematoma		(case 1) 90 (case 2) 90 (case 3) 80	(case 1) Bleeding controlled (16) (case 2) Bleeding stopped (14) (case 3) Bleeding stopped	

RBC, red blood cell concentrates; FFP, fresh frozen plasma; PPTs, platelets; CRYO, cryoprecipitates; WB, whole blood; PCC, prothrombin complex concentrate; vWF, von Willebrand factor; CS, cesarean section (e, emergency); VD, vaginal delivery; IVD, instrumental vaginal delivery; DIC, disseminated intravascular coagulation; MOF, multiple organ failure; NA, not available; HYS, hysterectomy; laceration – uterine or vaginal; AFE, amniotic fluid embolism; HELLP, hemolysis, elevated liver enzymes, low platelets; 'last resort', therapy, after other clinical measures had failed; *n*, number of cases

Table 7 Patients with severe postpartum hemorrhage, presented by Ahonen and colleagues (2005)[68]. The authors concluded that treatment with rFVIIa may be of benefit in life-threatening postpartum hemorrhage of up to 20 l of blood in 5–8 h. For comments on this article, see reference 69

Case	Provocation of bleed	Type of delivery	Additional surgeries (number of surgery)	Blood products given pre-rFVIIa (units)	Blood loss before rFVIIa (l)	Timing (when rFVIIa administered)	Dose of rFVIIa (μg/kg) (number of doses)	Overall bleeding response to rFVIIa (min)
1	Placenta accreta	VD	HYS	RBC (42); FFP (25); PPTs (40)	25.0	After HYS	44	Partial
2	Adherent placenta	CS	HYS	RBC (35); FFP (14); PPTs (24)	20.0	After HYS	95	Good
3	Uterine atony, LAC	VD	Surgery (3)	RBC (19); FFP (8); PPTs (8)	11.0	Before HYS	78	Good
4	Laceration	VD	Surgery (2), embolization	RBC (25); FFP (16); PPTs (24)	14.0	NA	103	Partial
5	Laceration	CS	HYS (3 laparotomy)	RBC (32); FFP (20); PPTs (40)	19.0	After HYS	90	Good
6	Uterine atony	CS	Surgery, embolization	RBC (10); FFP (8); PPTs (16)	5.5	NA	116	Partial
7	Placenta accreta	VD	HYS	RBC (14); FFP (6); PPTs (4)	7.5	After HYS	42	Partial
8	Laceration	CS	Surgery (2), right uterine artery ligation	RBC (11); FFP (4); PPTs (8)	5.3	NA	120	None
9	Placenta percreta	CS	HYS (2)	RBC (25); FFP (14); PPTs (16)	14.0	After HYS	77	Good
10	Laceration	IVD	Surgery, embolization	RBC (12); FFP (10); PPTs (32)	8.8	NA	74	Partial
11	Laceration	VD	Surgery	RBC (11); FFP (6); PPTs (6)	5.5	NA	86	Good
12	Laceration	VD	Surgery, embolization	RBC (10); FFP (8); PPTs (16)	5.8	NA	96	Partial

RBC, red blood cell concentrates; FFP, fresh frozen plasma; PPTs, platelets; CS, cesarean section (e, emergency); VD, vaginal delivery; IVD, instrumental vaginal delivery; DIC, disseminated intravascular coagulation; MOF, multiple organ failure; NA, not available; HYS, hysterectomy; laceration – uterine or vaginal; AFE, amniotic fluid embolism; HELLP, hemolysis, elevated liver enzymes, low platelets; 'last resort', therapy, after other clinical measures had failed

Table 8 Patients with severe postpartum hemorrhage presented by Segal and colleagues[70,71]

Case	Provocation of bleed	Type of delivery	Additional surgeries	Blood products given pre-rFVIIa (units)	Blood loss before rFVIIa (l)	Timing (when rFVIIa administered)	Dose of rFVIIa (µg/kg) (number of doses)	Overall bleeding response to rFVIIa (min)
1	Placenta accreta	CS	HYS; ligation of internal iliac arteries; packing	RBC (44); FFP (24); PPTs (60); CRYO (54)	NA	NA	90 (2)	Bleeding stopped
2	Uterine rupture	VD	HYS; ligation of internal iliac arteries	RBC (20); FFP (16); PPTs (60); CRYO (60)	NA	NA	100	Bleeding stopped
3	Uterine atony	CS	CS, packing of uterus; laparotomy; packing of tears on liver	RBC (19); FFP (8); PPTs (8)	NA	NA	90	Bleeding reduced
4	Uterine atony	NA	Subtotal HYS; ligation of internal iliac arteries	RBC (14); FFP (12); PPTs (10); CRYO (10)	NA	NA	90	Bleeding stopped
5	Uterine rupture	NA	Ligation of internal iliac arteries; subtotal HYS	RBC (26); FFP (16); PPTs (30); CRYO (60)	NA	NA	90	Bleeding stopped
6	Placenta accreta	NA	Arterial embolization; HYS; iliac ligation; 4 laparotomies; packing	RBC (100); FFP (50); PPTs (50); CRYO (50)	NA	NA	90	Bleeding controlled
7	Uterine rupture	NA	HYS; ligation of internal iliac arteries; packing	RBC (10); FFP (6); CRYO (4)	NA	NA	90	Bleeding reduced
8	Uterus myomatosus, menorrhagia	NA	HYS	RBC (6); FFP (9)	NA	NA	60	No bleeding
9	Uterine rupture	NA	HYS	RBC (15); FFP (6); PPTs (15); CRYO (30)	NA	NA	90	Bleeding stopped
10	Placenta accreta	NA	HYS; ligation of internal iliac arteries; aortic clamp	RBC (27); FFP (30); PPTs (10); CRYO (30)	NA	NA	90	Bleeding stopped

RBC, red blood cell concentrates; FFP, fresh frozen plasma; PPTs, platelets; CRYO, cryoprecipitates; CS, cesarean section; VD, vaginal delivery; NA, not available; HYS, hysterectomy

not been shown to provide benefits to patients in hemorrhagic shock.

Recommended replacement therapy

(1) Fresh frozen plasma: 5–10 ml/kg (4–5 units);

(2) Cryoprecipitates: 1–1.5 units/10 kg (8–10 units);

(3) Platelets: 1 units/10 kg (5–8 units);

(4) Correction of acidosis (defined as pH ≥7.2);

(5) Warming of hypothermic patients (recommended, but not mandatory for administration of rFVIIa).

Dosing administration protocol proposal

(1) The recommended initial dose of rFVIIa for treatment of severe postpartum hemorrhage is ~40–60 µg/kg administered intravenously.

(2) If bleeding still continuous beyond 15–30 min, following the first dose of rFVIIa, an additional dose of ~40–60 µg/kg should be considered. Repeat 3–4 times at 15–30-min intervals if clinical signs of bleeding are still present (based on visual evidence).

(3) If the response remains inadequate following a total dose of >200 µg/kg, the preconditions for rFVIIa administration should be re-checked, and corrected as necessary before another dose is considered.

(4) Only after these corrective measures have been applied should the next dose of rFVIIa ~100 µg/kg be administered.

Recommended timing of administration

Because our experience suggests that rFVIIa permits effective control of obstetric bleeding, especially in situations of coexisting coagulopathy, we therefore recommend administration of rFVIIa as soon as possible under the following circumstances:

(1) When no blood is available;

(2) Before metabolic complications develop;

(3) In women refusing transfusions (e.g. Jehovah Witnesses) (see Chapter 72);

(4) In acquired hemophilia (see Chapter 25);

(5) Before the symptoms of severe thrombocytopathies, hypoxia and organ injury appear;

(6) If correction of INR (PT) is urgently needed;

(7) Before packing of the uterus or pelvis;

(8) Before surgical procedures such as hysterectomy, laparotomy;

(9) Before medical procedures such as embolization, ligation of the uterine and internal iliac arteries (see Chapters 52 and 53).

Information obtained from the literature allows us to summarize the advantages and disadvantages of rFVIIa as follows.

Advantages

(1) Recombinant product;

(2) Not subject to blood shortage;

(3) No viral transmission;

(4) No human protein;

(5) Localized hemostasis;

(6) Low risk of anaphylaxis;

(7) No anamnestic responses;

(8) Low thrombogenicity;

(9) Effective during and after surgery.

Disadvantages

(1) Short $t_{1/2}$ requires frequent, repetitive dosing;

(2) Not 100% effective;

(3) No measurable lab parameter for efficacy;

(4) Limited vial sizes;

(5) Venous access;

(6) Cost.

References

1. Luster JM, Roberts HR, Davignon G, et al. A randomized, double-blind comparison of two doses of recombinant factor VIIa in the treatment of joint, muscle and mucocutaneous haemorrhages in persons with haemophilia A and B, with and without inhibitors. rFVIIa Study Group. Haemophilia 1998; 4:790–8

2. Shapiro AD, Gilchrist GS, Hoots WK, Cooper HA, Gastineau DA. Prospective, randomized trial of two doses of rFVIIa (NovoSeven®) in haemophilia patients undergoing surgery. Thromb Haemost 1998;80:773–8

3. Abshire T, Kenet G. Recombinant factor VIIa: review of efficacy, dosing regimens and safety in patients with congenital and acquired factor VIII or IX inhibitors. J Thromb Haemost 2004;2:899–909

4. O'Connell KA, Wood JJ, Wise RP, Lozier JN, Braun MM. Thromboembolic adverse events after use of recombinant human coagulation factor VIIa. JAMA 2006;295:293–8

5. Michalska-Krzanowska G, Sajdak R, Stasiak-Pikula E. Effects of recombinant factor VIIa in haemorrhagic complications of urological operations. Acta Haematol 2003;109:158–60

6. Naik VN, Mazer DC, Latter DA, Teitel JM, Hare GMT. Successful treatment using recombinant factor VIIa for severe bleeding post cardiopulmonary bypass. Can J Anesth 2003;50: 599–602

7. Danilos J, Goral A, Paluszkiewicz P, Przesmycki K, Kotarski J. Successful treatment with recombinant factor VIIa for intractable bleeding at pelvic surgery. Obstet Gynecol 2003;101:1172–3

8. Martinowitz U, Kenet G, Lubetski A, Luboshitz J, Segal E. Possible role of recombinant activated factor VII (rFVIIa) in the control of haemorrhage associated with massive trauma. Can J Anaesth 2002;49:S15–20

9. Martinowitz U, Kenet G, Segal E, et al. Recombinant activated factor VII for adjunctive haemorrhage control in trauma. J Trauma 2001;51:431–9

10. Kenet G, Walde R, Eldad A, Martinowitz U. Treatment of traumatic bleeding with recombinant factor VIIa. Lancet 1999;354:1879

11. Dutton RP, Hess JR, Scalea TM. Recombinant factor VIIa for control of haemorrhage: early experience in critically ill trauma patients. J Clin Anesth 2003;15:184–8

12. Mariani G, Testa MG, Di Paolantonio T, Molskov Bech R, Hedner U. Use of recombinant, activated factor VII in the treatment of congenital factor VII deficiencies. Vox Sang 1999;77:131–6

13. Hunault M, Bauer KA. Recombinant factor VIIa for the treatment of congenital factor VII deficiency. Semin Thromb Hemost 2000;26:401–5

14. d'Oiron R, Menart C, Trzeciak MC, et al. Use of recombinant factor VIIa in 3 patients with inherited type I Glanzmann's thrombasthenia undergoing invasive procedures. Thromb Haemost 2000;83:644–7

15. van Buuren HR, Wielenga JJ. Successful surgery using recombinant factor VIIa for recurrent idiopathic nonulcer duodenal bleeding in a patient with Glanzmann's thrombasthenia. Dig Dis Sci 2002;47:2134–6

16. Hedner U. Recombinant factor VIIa (NovoSeven) as a haemostatic agent. Bloodline Rev 2001;1:3–4

17. Dildy GA 3rd. Postpartum hemorrhage: new management options. Clin Obstet Gynecol 2002;45:330–44

18. Yamamoto H, Sagae S, Nishikawa S, Kudo R. Emergency postpartum hysterectomy in obstetric practice. J Obstet Gynaecol Res 2000;26:341–5

19. Sakai T, Lund-Hansen T, Thim L, Kisiel W. The gamma-carboxyglutamic acid domain of human factor VIIa is essential for its interaction with cell surface tissue factor. J Biol Chem 1990;265:1890–94

20. NovoSeven® summary of product characteristics. Available at: http://www.novoseven.com/content/product_information/summary_of_product_characteristics/product_information_spc.asp

21. Lund-Hansen T, Petersen LC. Comparison of enzymatic properties of human plasma FVIIa and human recombinant FVIIa. Thromb Haemost 1987;58:270

22. Jurlander B, Thim L, Klausen NK, et al. Recombinant factor VII (rFVIIa): characterization, manufacturing, and clinical development. Semin Thromb Hemost 2001;27:373–84

23. Erhardtsen E. Pharmacokinetics of recombinant activated factor VII (rFVIIa). Semin Thromb Hemost 2000;26:385–91

24. Lindley CM, Sawyer WT, Macik BG, et al. Pharmacokinetics and pharmacodynamics of recombinant factor VIIa. Clin Pharmacol Ther 1994;55:638–48

25. Monroe DM, Hoffman M, Oliver JA, et al. Platelet activity of high-dose Factor VIIa is independent of tissue factor. Br J Haematol 1997;99:542–7

26. Hoffman M, Monroe DM, Roberts HR. Activated Factor VII activates Factor IX and X on surface of activated platelets: thoughts on the mechanism of action of high-dose activated Factor VII. Blood Coagul Fibrinolysis 1998;9:S61–5

27. van't Veer C, Golden NJ, Mann KG. Inhibition of thrombin generation by the zymogen factor VII: implications for the treatment of hemophilia A by factor VIIa. Blood 2000;95:1330–5

28. Lisman T, De Groot PG. Mechanism of action of recombinant factor VIIa. J Thromb Haemost 2003;1:1138–9

29. Hoffman M, Monroe DM. A cell-based model of haemostasis. Thromb Haemost 2001;85:958–65

30. Hedner U. Recombinant factor VIIa (Novoseven) as a hemostatic agent. Semin Hematol 2001;38:43–7

31. Friederich PW, Levi M, Bauer KA, et al. Ability of recombinant factor VIIa to generate thrombin during inhibition of tissue factor in human subjects. Circulation 2001;103:2555–9

32. Monroe DM, Hoffman M, Allen GA, Roberts HR. The factor VII–platelet interplay: effectiveness of recombinant factor VIIa in the treatment of bleeding in severe thrombocytopathia. Semin Thromb Hemost 2000;26:373–7

33. Telgt DS, Macik BG, McCord DM, Monroe DM, Roberts HR. Mechanism by which recombinant factor VIIa shortens the aPTT: activation of factor X in the absence of tissue factor. Thromb Res 1989;56:603–9

34. Kessler CM. Antidotes to haemorrhage: recombinant Factor VIIa. Best Pract Res Clin Haematol 2004;17:183–97

35. Gabriel DA, Carr M, Roberts HR. Monitoring coagulation and the clinical effects of recombinant factor VIIa. Semin Hematol 2004;41:20–4

36. Martinowitz U, Michaelson M, on behalf of the Israeli Multidisciplinary rFVIIa Task Force. Guidelines for the use of recombinant activated factor VII (rFVIIa) in uncontrolled bleeding: a report by the Israeli Multidisciplinary rFVIIa Task Force. J Thromb Haemost 2005;3:640–8

37. Roberts HR, Monroe DM III, Hoffman M. Safety profile of recombinant factor VIIa. Semin Hematol 2004;41:101–8

38. Aledort LM. Comparative thrombotic event incidences after infusion of recombinant factor VIIa versus factor VIII inhibitor bypass activity. J Thromb Haemost 2004;2:1700–8

39. Bręborowicz GH, Sobieszczyk S [Usefulness of recombinant active factor VIIa (rFVIIa, NovoSeven®) in obstetric practice – own experiences]. Przydatność rekombinowanego aktywnego czynnika VIIa (rFVIIa, NovoSeven®) w praktyce położniczej – doświadczenia własne. Klin Perinat Ginek 2001;34:7–12

40. Bręborowicz GH, Sobieszczyk S, Szymankiewicz M. Efficacy of recombinant activated factor VII (rFVIIa, NovoSeven®) in prenatal medicine. Arch Perinat Med 2002;8:21–7

41. Bręborowicz GH, Sobieszczyk S, Szymankiewicz M. Efficacy of recombinant activated factor VII (rFVIIa, NovoSeven®) in prenatal medicine. J Perinat Med 2003;31(Suppl 1):18

42. Bręborowicz GH, Sobieszczyk S, Szymankiewicz M. Recombinant factor VIIa in the management of major postpartum hemorrhage. Arch Perinat Med 2004;10:17–19

43. Sobieszczyk S, Bręborowicz GH. Management recommendations for postpartum hemorrhage. Arch Perinat Med 2004;10:53–6

44. Sobieszczyk S, Bręborowicz GH, Kubiaczyk B, Opala T. Efficacy of recombinant activated factor VII (r FVIIa; NovoSeven®) in obstetrical haemorrhagic shock. Crit Care 2003;7(Suppl 2): S52

45. Sobieszczyk S, Skrzypczak J, Szymankiewicz M, Kruszyński Z, Kornacki J, Bręborowicz GH. Zastosowanie rekombinowanego aktywnego czynnika VII (rFVIIa, NovoSeven®) podczas cięcia cesarskiego u ciężarnej z mechaniczną zastawką serca. [Application of recombinant activated factor VII (rFVIIa, NovoSeven®) during cesarean section of a woman with artificial heart valve]. Klin Perinat Ginek 2001;34:173–9

46. Sobieszczyk S, Bręborowicz GH, Markwitz W, Mallinger S, Adamski D, Kruszyński Z. Effect of recombinant activated factor VII (rFVIIa; NovoSeven®) in a patient in haemorrhagic shock after obstetrical hysterectomy. Ginekol Pol 2002;73:230–3

47. Moscardó F, Pérez F, de la Rubia J, et al. Successful treatment of severe, intra-abdominal bleeding associated with disseminated intravascular coagulation using recombinant activated factor VII. Br J Haematol 2001;113:174–6

48. Eskandari N, Feldman N, Greenspoon JS. Factor VII deficiency in pregnancy treated with recombinant factor VIIa. Obstet Gynecol 2002;99:935–7

49. Ciaćma A, Langie T, Zając K, Fabian W. Acquired haemophilia in parturient. Case report. Anaesthesiology Intensive Therapy 2002;34:269–70

50. Zupančić Šalek S, Sokolić V, Visković T, Šanjug J, Šimić M, Kaštelan M. Successful use of recombinant factor VIIa for massive bleeding after caesarean section due to HELLP syndrome. Acta Haematol 2002;108:162–3

51. Loo CC, Kwek Bielanom, Tan HM, Yeo SH, Tien SL, Loh Bielanom. Successful treatment of postpartum hemorrhage with recombinant activated coagulation factor VII

(NovoSeven®). 7th Novo Nordisk Symposium on Haemostasis Management. Clinical and Scientific Posters. 2003; May:23

52. Bielanow T, Sidor M, Maciejewski M, Skrzypek W. [Effectiveness of recombinant activated factor VIIA (NovoSeven) in case of severe obstetric complication with coagulopathy]. Ginekol Pol 2003;74:1055–9

53. Bouwmeester FW, Jonkhoff AR, Verheijen RH, van Geijn HP. Successful treatment of life-threatening postpartum hemorrhage with recombinant activated factor VII. Obstet Gynecol 2003;101:1174–6

54. Michalska-Krzanowska G, Stasiak-Pikula E, Sajdak R. Recombinant activated factor VII: A new treatment for obstetric haemorrhage? Anest Intens Ther 2003;35:110–12

55. Pehlivanov B, Milchev N, Kroumov G. Factor VII deficiency and treatment in delivery with recombinant factor VII. Eur J Obstet Gynecol Reprod Biol 2004;116:237–8

56. Kretzschmar M, Zahm DM, Remmler K, Pfeiffer L, Victor L, Schirrmeister W. Pathophysiological and therapeutic aspects of amniotic fluid embolism (anaphylactoid syndrome of pregnancy): Case report with lethal outcome and overview. Anaesthesist 2003;52:419–26

57. Boehlen F, Morales MA, Fontana P, Ricou B, Irion O, de Moerloose P. Prolonged treatment of massive postpartum haemorrhage with recombinant factor VIIa: case report and review of the literature. Br J Obstet Gynaecol 2004;111:284–7

58. Brice A, Hilbert U, Roger-Christoph S, et al. [Recombinant activated factor VII as a life-saving therapy for severe postpartum haemorrhage unresponsive to conservative traditional management]. Ann Fr Anesth Reanim 2004;23:1084–8

59. Gidiri M, Noble W, Rafique Z, Patil K, Lindow SW. Caesarean section for placenta praevia complicated by postpartum haemorrhage managed successfully with recombinant activated human coagulation Factor VIIa. J Obstet Gynaecol 2004;24:925–6

60. Kale A, Bayhan G, Yalinkaya A, Yayla M. The use of recombinant factor VIIa in a primigravida with Glanzmann's thrombasthenia during delivery. J Perinat Med 2004;32:456–8

61. Lim Y, Loo CC, Chia V, Fun W. Recombinant factor VIIa after amniotic fluid embolism and disseminated intravascular coagulopathy. Int J Gynaecol Obstet 2004;87:178–9

62. Merchant-Shakil H, Prasad M, Vanderjagt TJ, Howdieshell TR, Crookston P. Recombinant factor VIIa in management of spontaneous subcapsular liver hematoma associated with pregnancy. Obstet Gynecol 2004;103:1055–8

63. Price G, Kaplan J, Skowronski G. Use of recombinant factor VIIa to treat life-threatening non-surgical bleeding in a postpartum patient. Br J Anaesth 2004;93:298–300

64. Hollnberger H, Gruber E, Seelbach-Goebel B. Major postpartum hemorrhage and treatment with recombinant factor VIIa. Anesth Analg 2005;101:1886–7

65. Holub Z, Feyereisi J, Kabelik L, Rittstein T. Successful treatment of severe post-partum bleeding after caesarean section using recombinant activated factor VII. Ceska Gynekol 2005;70:144–8

66. Tanchev S, Platikanov V, Karadimov D. Administration of recombinant factor VIIa for the management of massive bleeding due to uterine atonia in the post-placental period. Acta Obstet Gynecol Scand 2005;84:402–3

67. Shamsi TS, Hossain N, Soomro N, et al. Use of recombinant Factor VIIa for massive haemorrhage: Case series and review of literature. J Pak Med Assoc 2005;55:512–15

68. Ahonen J, Jokela R. Recombinant factor VIIa for life-threatening post-partum haemorrhage. Br J Anaesth 2005;94:592–5

69. Butwick AJ, Riley ET, Ahonen J, Jokela R. Recombinant factor VIIa for life-threatening post-partum haemorrhage. Br J Anaesth 2005;95:558

70. Segal S, Shemesh IY, Blumental R, et al. The use of recombinant factor VIIa in severe postpartum hemorrhage. Acta Obstet Gynecol Scand 2004;83:771–2

71. Segal S, Shemesh IY, Blumenthal R, et al. Treatment of obstetric hemorrhage with recombinant activated factor VII (rFVIIa). Arch Gynecol Obstet 2003;268:266–7

72. Hedner U. Dosing with recombinant factor VIIa based on current evidence. Semin Hematol 2004;41(Suppl 1):35–9

73. Monroe DM, Roberts HR. Mechanism of action of high-dose factor VIIa: points of agreement and disagreement. Arterioscler Thromb Vasc Biol 2003;23:8–9;discussion 10

74. Poon MC, D'Oiron R, Von Depka M, et al. Prophylactic and therapeutic recombinant factor VIIa administration to patients with Glanzmann's thrombasthenia: results of an international survey. J Thromb Haemost 2004;2:1096–103

75. Mayer SA. Ultra-early hemostatic therapy for intracerebral hemorrhage. Stroke 2003;34:224–9

76. Dutton RPHJ, Scalea TM. Recombinant factor VIIa for the control of hemorrhage: early experience in critically ill trauma patients. Can J Anaesth 2003;50:184–8

77. Aldouri M. The use of recombinant factor VIIa in controlling surgical bleeding in non-haemophiliac patients. Pathophysiol Haemost Thromb 2002;32(Suppl 1):41–6

78. Meng ZH, Wolberg AS, Monroe DM III, Hoffman M. The effect of temperature and pH on the activity of factor VIIa: implications for the efficacy of high-dose factor VIIa in hypothermic and acidotic patients. J Trauma 2003;55:886–91

79. DeLoughery TG. Management of bleeding emergencies: when to use recombinant activated Factor VII. Expert Opin Pharmacother 2006;7:25–34

80. Friederich P, Heny C, Messelink E, et al. Effects of recombinant activated factor VII on perioperative blood loss in patients undergoing retropubic prostatectomy: a double blind placebo controlled trial. Lancet 2003;361:201–5

Section 9

Therapy for Non-atonic Bleeding

51

Conservative Surgical Management

C. B-Lynch and H. Shah

INTRODUCTION

A key factor in the surgical management of postpartum hemorrhage is the awareness of predisposing factors[1–3] and the readiness of therapeutic teams consisting of obstetric, anesthetic and hematology staff[3,4].

In the past, the surgical management of postpartum hemorrhage included use of an intrauterine pack, with or without thromboxane[5], thrombogenic uterine pack[6], ligation of uterine arteries[7], ligation of internal iliac artery[8], stepwise devascularization[9] and, finally, subtotal or total abdominal hysterectomy[10]. Most of these are discussed in detail in other chapters of this text.

A more conservative procedure, now colloquially known as the Brace suture technique, was first described by B-Lynch and colleagues in 1997[3]. Along with later modifications by Hayman and colleagues[11] and Cho and colleagues[12], this[13] may prove more effective than radical surgery for the control of life-threatening postpartum hemorrhage[3,11,12]. Although subtotal and total abdominal hysterectomy are still available and indeed useful in their own right, they should be considered as a last resort.

Common causes of postpartum hemorrhage are listed in Table 1, which is not to mean that additional causes cannot or do not exist. Most, if not all, are considered in references to postpartum hemorrhage in modern standard textbooks of obstetrics and further described in the other chapters of this volume. Three important points merit attention.

First, there is significant increase in cardiac output in pregnancy in accordance with red cell mass and plasma volume, which provides a compensative reserve for acute blood loss and hemostatic response following massive hemorrhage[14]. Second, the arrangement of the uterine muscle fibers, vis-à-vis the course of the uterine arteries, facilitates the use of compression techniques for effective control of postpartum hemorrhage and, finally, conservative treatment such as bimanual compression of the uterus may control blood loss (Figure 1), whilst intensive resuscitative measures are undertaken according to established labor ward protocols, which involve the anesthetists, hematologists, the obstetric team and intensive care support (see Chapters 36 and 40).

NEW DEVELOPMENTS IN THERAPEUTIC OPTIONS

The type of surgical intervention depends upon several factors, paramount of which is the experience of the surgeon. Other factors include parity and desire for future children, the extent of the hemorrhage, the general condition of the patient and place of confinement. Women at high risk of postpartum hemorrhage should not be delivered in isolated units or units ill-equipped to manage sudden, life-threatening emergencies. Immediate access to specialist consultant care, blood products and intensive care are essential.

Table 1 Common causes of postpartum hemorrhage

Pre-existing conditions	Uterine overdistention, atony and disseminated intravascular coagulation (DIC)	Disorders of placenta, uterine and genital tract trauma
Thrombocytopenic purpura	Polyhydramnios	Acute uterine inversion
Hypertensive disease	Multiple gestation	Lower segment cesarean section
Uterine myoma	Macrosomia	Operative vaginal delivery
Anticoagulation therapy	Prolonged labor	Precipitate delivery
Coagulation factor deficiency	Chorionamnionitis	Previous uterine surgery
Systemic disease of hemorrhagic nature	Tocolytic agents	Internal podalic version
Consumptive coagulopathy	Halogenated anesthetic agents	Breech extraction
Müllerian malfunction	High parity	Mid-cavity forceps
Anemia	Abruptio placentae	Obstructed labor
	Courvelliar's uterus	Abnormal fetal presentation
	Placenta previa	Vacuum site extraction
	Placenta accreta, increta, percreta	Placental subinvolution
		Retained products of conception
		Ruptured uterus

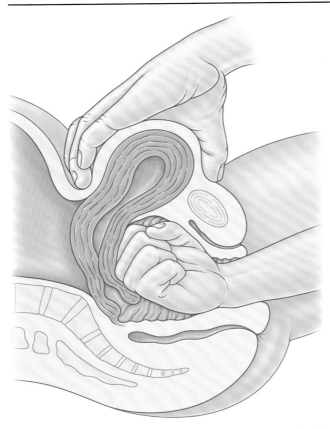

© Copyright B-Lynch '05

Figure 1 Bimanual compression of the uterus, illustrating the first-line approach to mechanical hemostasis. This in itself might control bleeding significantly by assisting the uterus to use its anatomical and physiological properties such as the cross-over interlinked network of myometrial fibers for vascular compression and bleeding control. The patient should be placed in stirrups or frog-legged position in the labor ward or in theater whilst intravenous fluid and/or appropriate blood product runs freely. In some cases and commonly so, there may be failure to achieve satisfactory and lasting hemostasis by this method

The B-Lynch suture compression technique

The procedure was first performed and described by Mr Christopher B-Lynch, a consultant obstetrician, gynecological surgeon, Fellow of the Royal College of Obstetricians and Gynaecologists of the UK and Fellow of the Royal College of Surgeons of Edinburgh, based at Milton Keynes General Hospital National Health Service (NHS) Trust (Oxford Deanery, UK), during the management of a patient with a massive postpartum hemorrhage in November 1989. This patient refused consent to an emergency hysterectomy[3]! Table 2 provides an audit summary of five case histories of other patients with severe life-threatening postpartum hemorrhage managed with this technique.

The principle

The suture aims to exert continuous vertical compression on the vascular system. In the case of postpartum hemorrhage from placenta previa, a transverse lower segment compression suture is effective.

The technique[2–4]

See Figures 2a (i and ii), 2b and 2c.

Surgeon's position In outlining the steps involved, we assume that the surgeon is right-handed and standing on the right-hand side of the patient. A laparotomy is always necessary to exteriorize the uterus. A lower segment transverse incision is made or the recent lower segment cesarean section suture (LSCS) removed to check the cavity for retained placental fragments and to swab it out.

Test for the potential efficacy of the B-Lynch suture before performing the procedure The patient is placed in the Lloyd Davies or semi-lithotomy position (frog leg). An assistant stands between the patient's legs and intermittently swabs the vagina to determine the presence and extent of the bleeding. The uterus is then exteriorized and bimanual compression performed. To do this, the bladder peritoneum is reflected inferiorly to a level below the cervix (if it has been taken down for a prior LSCS, it is pushed down again). The whole uterus is then compressed by placing one hand posteriorly with the ends of the fingers at the level of the cervix and the other hand anteriorly just below the bladder reflection. If the bleeding stops on applying such compression, there is a good chance that application of the B-Lynch suture will work and stop the bleeding.

Even in the presence of coagulopathy, bimanual compression will control diffuse bleeding points. If this test is successful, the application of the suture will also succeed. However, application of the B-Lynch suture is not a substitute for the medical treatment of coagulopathy, which should take place along with the operative intervention (see Chapter 25).

Suture application Given that the test criteria for the B-Lynch suture placement are met, the uterus remains exteriorized until application of the suture is complete. The senior assistant takes over in performing compression and maintains it with two hands during the placement of the suture by the principal surgeon.

(1) *First stitch relative to the low transverse cesarean section/hysterotomy wound.* With the bladder displaced inferiorly, the first stitch is placed 3 cm below the cesarean section/ hysterotomy incision on the patient's left side and threaded through the uterine cavity to emerge 3 cm above the upper incision margin approximately 4 cm from the lateral border of the uterus (Figure 2a(i)).

(2) *The fundus* The suture is now carried over the top of the uterus and to the posterior side. Once situated over the fundus, the suture should be more or less vertical and lie about 4 cm from the cornu. It does not tend to slip laterally toward the broad ligament because the uterus has been compressed and the suture milked through, ensuring that proper placement is achieved and maintained (Figure 2a).

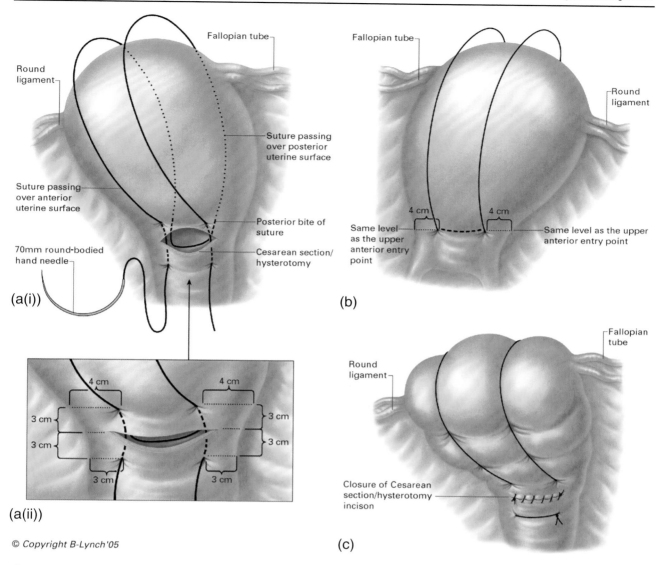

Figure 2 Summary of the application of the B–Lynch procedure

(3) *The posterior wall* The location on the posterior uterus where the suture is placed through the uterine wall is actually easy to surface mark posteriorly. It is on the horizontal plane at the level of the uterine incision at the insertion of the uterosacral ligament (Figure 2b).

(4) *Role of the assistant* As the operation proceeds, the assistant continues to compress the uterus as the suture is fed through the posterior wall into the cavity. This will enable progressive tension to be maintained as the suture begins to surround the uterus. Assistant compression will also help to pull the suture material through to achieve maximum compression, without breaking it, at the end of the procedure. Furthermore, it will prevent suture slipping and uterine trauma. The suture now lies horizontally on the cavity side of the posterior uterine wall.

(5) *The fundus* As the needle pierces the uterine cavity side of the posterior wall, it is placed over the posterior wall, bringing the suture over the top of the

fundus and onto the anterior right side of the uterus. The needle re-enters the cavity exactly in the same way as it did on the left side, that is 3 cm above the upper incision and 4 cm from the lateral side of the uterus through the upper incision margin, into the uterine cavity and then out again through 3 cm below the lower incision margin (Figure 2a(ii)).

(6) *Later role of the assistant* The assistant maintains the compression as the suture material is milked through from its different portals to ensure uniform tension and no slipping. The two ends of the suture are put under tension and a double throw knot is placed for security to maintain tension after the lower segment incision has been closed by either the one- or two-layer method.

(7) *Relation to the hysterotomy incision* The tension on the two ends of the suture material can be maintained while the lower segment incision is closed, or the knot can be tied first, followed by closure of the lower segment (Figure 2c). If the latter option

Table 2 Audit summary of five selected case histories of patients with severe life-threatening postpartum hemorrhage treated by ecbolics and the B-Lynch brace suture application in the period 1989–1995 at Milton Keynes General Hospital, UK[2]

Age (years)	Parity	GA	Presenting diagnosis	Mode of delivery	Infant sex and weight (g)	Apgar score at 5 and 10 min	Type of PPH	Treatment and volume transfused	Intensive care admission	Outcome
28	PP	39/40	placental abruption, PPH, DIC	spontaneous vertex	male (2800)	4, 7	primary	ecbolics, 20 units fresh blood, 8 units FFP	48 h; full antibiotic cover	good; 3 years later spontaneous vertex delivery; female (3890 g); no problems
22	PP	43/40	prolonged labor, persisting occipito position?, cephalopelvic disproportion	emergency CS	male (4190)	7, 10	primary	ecbolics, 13 units blood, 5 units packed cells, BSA	48 h; full antibiotic cover	good; normal CT pelvimetry 2 years later; elective CS at 39 weeks; female (3820 g); no problems
23	PP (twin)	37/40	eclampsia in labor, PPH, DIC	emergency CS	(1) female (2735), (2) female (2430)	(1) 3, 8 (2) 5, 8	primary	ecbolics, 19 units blood, 5 units FFP, BSA	72 h; full antibiotic cover	good; no complications
35	PP (IVF)	38/40	major placenta previa	elective CS	female (3370)	9, 10	secondary, 9th day readmission	ecbolics, 15 units blood, 5 units FFP, BSA	72 h; full antibiotic cover	good; no complications
30	PP	40/40	uterine atony	spontaneous vertex	female (3890)	9, 10	primary	ecbolics, 15 units blood, 7 units packed cells, BSA	48 h; full antibiotic cover	good; no complications

PP, primiparous; GA, gestational age in weeks; PPH, postpartum hemorrhage; CS, cesarean section; CT, computerized tomography; DIC, disseminated intravascular coagulations; BSA, brace suture application; IVF, *in vitro* fertilization; FFP, fresh frozen plasma
*Refused consent to emergency hysterectomy

is chosen, it is essential that the corners of the hysterotomy incision be identified and stay sutures placed before the knot is tied. This ensures that, when the lower segment is closed, the angles of the incision do not escape it. Either procedure works equally well. It is important to identify the corners of the uterine incision to make sure no bleeding points remain unsecured, particularly when most of these patients are hypotensive with low pulse pressure at the time of the B-Lynch suture application.

(8) *Post-application and hysterotomy closure* It is probable that the maximum effect of suture tension lasts for only about 24–48 h. Because the uterus undergoes its primary involutionary process in the first week after vaginal or cesarean section delivery, the suture may have lost some tensile strength, but hemostasis would have been achieved by that time. There is no need for delay in closing the abdomen after the application of the suture. The assistant standing between the patient's legs swabs the vagina again and can confirm that the bleeding has been controlled.

Application after normal vaginal delivery If laparotomy is required for the management of atonic postpartum hemorrhage, hysterotomy is necessary to apply the B-Lynch suture. Hysterotomy will also allow exploration of the uterine cavity, exclude retained products of conception, evacuate large blood clots and diagnose abnormal placentation and decidual tears, damage and

bleeding. B-Lynch suture application or any modification of it (see below) without hysterotomy or re-opening of the cesarean section wound runs the potential risk of secondary postpartum hemorrhage. Therefore, confirmation that the uterine cavity is completely empty is essential. Furthermore, hysterotomy ensures that the correct application of the suture provides maximum and even distribution of the compressive effect during and after application of the B-Lynch suture (Figures 2 and 3). Also, it avoids blind application of the suture and the possibility of obliteration of the cervical and/or uterine cavities that may lead to clot retention, infected debris, pyometria, sepsis and morbidity[3,11,12,15].

Application for abnormal placentation The B-Lynch suture may be beneficial in cases of placenta accreta, percreta and increta. In a patient with placenta previa, a figure-of-eight or transverse compression suture to the lower anterior or posterior compartment or both is applied to control bleeding. If this is not completely successful, then, in addition, the longitudinal Brace suture component may be applied for further/complete hemostasis[3].

POSTOPERATIVE FOLLOW-UP

Three patients from the original series had laparoscopy postoperatively for sterilization, suspected pelvic inflammatory disease or appendicitis. One patient who

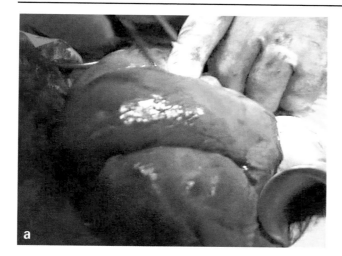

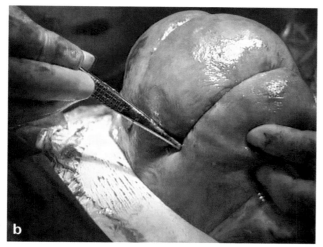

Figure 3 The *in vivo* effect of correct application of the B–Lynch surgical technique seen immediately after successful suture application. No congestion, no ischemia and no 'shouldering' of the sutures at the fundus

had a history of ileostomy for surgical reasons had laparotomy 10 days after her B–Lynch suture for suspected intestinal obstruction (unpublished data, B-Lynch). Magnetic resonance imaging and hysterosalpingography were performed on one patient, showing no intraperitoneal or uterine sequelae[16] (Figure 4a–c). No complications have been observed in the five patients of the first published series[2] (see Table 1). Moreover, all have succeeded in further pregnancy and delivery[17,18].

Tables 3–5 lists the clinical points of the B–Lynch surgical technique, the Hayman uterine compression suture (see Figure 5) and the Cho multiple square sutures (see Figure 6).

WORLD-WIDE REPORTS

The current level of application of the B–Lynch suture world-wide includes over 1300 successful cases; of these, there are only 19 failures. The Indian subcontinent has the largest number of reported successful applications, over 250, followed by Africa, South

(a)

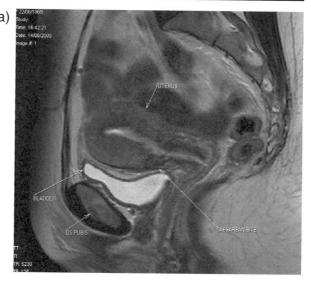

(b)

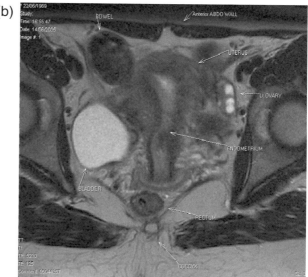

(c)

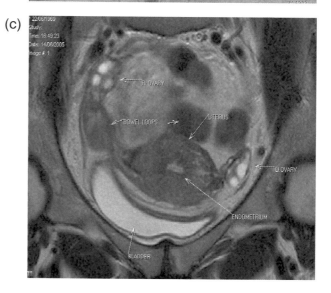

Figure 4 Normal MRI 6 months after massive postpartum hemorrhage treated by B–Lynch surgical technique followed by uneventful spontaneous vertex vaginal delivery 22 months later. (a) Sagittal view showing normal endometrial cavity and treated cesarean incision site; (b) coronal view, with no uterine cavity synechiae[19]; (c) view at level of incision for cesarean section, showing well-healed features

Table 3 The B-Lynch surgical technique: clinical points

1. User-friendly suture material monocryl No.1 mounted on 90-cm curved ethigard blunt needle (codeW3709) (Ethicon, Somerville, NJ). Other rapidly absorbable sutures can be used according to the surgeon's preference. A good length and needle are essential[19]
2. Basic surgical competence required
3. Uterine cavity checked, explored and evacuated
4. Suture bends maintain even and adequate tension without uterine trauma or 'shouldering'
5. Allows free drainage of blood, debris and inflammatory material
6. Transverse compression suture applied to the lower segment for abnormal placentation effectively controls bleeding
7. Simple, effective and cost-saving
8. Fertility preserved and proven[3]
9. Mortality avoided[3]
10. World-wide application and successful reports (> 1300) (B-Lynch, personal data base, christopherbl@aol.com)
11. Potential for prophylactic application at cesarean section when signs of imminent postpartum hemorrhage develop, e.g. placenta accreta, or where blood transfusion is declined, e.g. placenta previa surgery on a Jehovah's Witness

Table 4 The Hayman uterine compression suture: clinical points

1. Lower uterine segment or uterine cavity not opened
2. Uterine cavity not explored under direct vision
3. Probably quicker to apply
4. No feed-back data on fertility outcome
5. Morbidity feed-back data limited
6. Unequal tension leads to segmented ischemia secondary to slippage of suture – 'shouldering' with venous obstruction

Table 5 The Cho multiple square sutures: clinical points

1. Multiple full-thickness square sutures applied, probably time-consuming if many square sutures required
2. Uterine cavity drainage restriction – pyometra risk[15]
3. No feed-back data on fertility outcome
4. Morbidity feed-back data limited
5. Rhythmic contraction not facilitated and involution impeded
6. The production of multiple uterine senechiae (see Chapter 28)

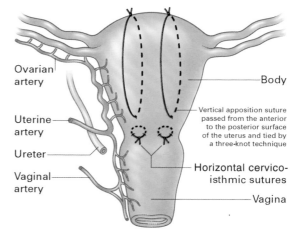

© Copyright B-Lynch'05

Figure 5 The Hayman uterine compression suture without opening the uterine cavity[11]

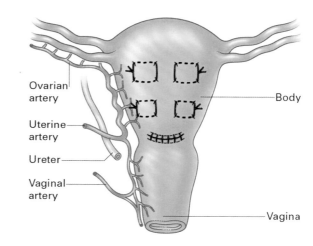

© Copyright B-Lynch'05

Figure 6 The Cho multiple square sutures compressing anterior to posterior uterine walls[12]

America, North America, Europe and other countries. The 17 reported failures were because of delay in application, poor technique, defibrination and inappropriate material. Various suture materials have been used. However, the monocryl suture (code WC3709) is recommended because it is user- and tissue-friendly with uniform tension distribution and is easy to handle[20]. Holtsema and colleagues recently opined, in a review, that the B-Lynch technique for postpartum hemorrhage should be an option for every gynecologist[21]. Wohlmuth and colleagues published outcome of a large series with a 91% success rate (world-wide cumulative success rate 98%)[22].

CONCLUSION

Of the compression suturing techniques described above, the B-Lynch procedure has been recommended by the 2000–2002 Triennial Confidential Enquiry into Maternal Deaths in the United Kingdom[23], The Royal College of Obstetricians and Gynaecologists in the UK, and the Cochrane Database of systematic reviews. To date, no serious adverse outcomes have been associated with the B-Lynch surgical technique[3,17,20,22,24]. Furthermore, the latest 2000–2002 Triennial Confidential Enquiry states that no deaths were reported in women who had had

interventional radiology or B-Lynch suture in the management of postpartum hemorrhage[23].

It is important to remember that, if a patient is a known or appreciated risk for postpartum hemorrhage, then the elective delivery should be performed in the day time, with prearranged co-operation between the imaging department and the obstetric team. Theater staff should be alerted in time so that conservative surgery can be carried out quickly if needed. Patients at particular risk are those with obesity, cardiomyopathy, coagulopathy, abnormal placentation, polyhydramnios and specific religious convictions contraindicating blood transfusion.

PLACEMENT OF LIGATURES IN STEPWISE DEVASCULARIZATION

The essential requirements are not simple and may not be available in every unit. First, there is a need for a competent obstetrician who is conversant and competent at pelvic gynecological procedures, and who has a

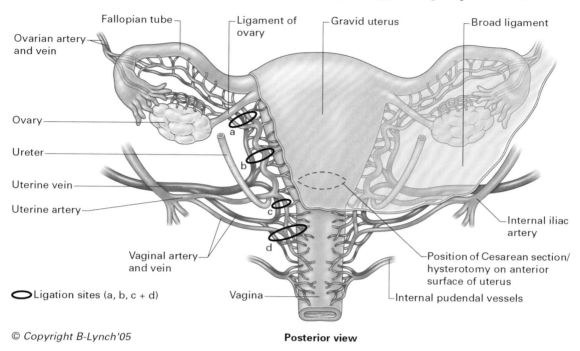

© Copyright B-Lynch'05   **Posterior view**

Figure 7   Placement of ligatures in the process of stepwise devascularization, including ligature of the descending uterine and vaginal arteries

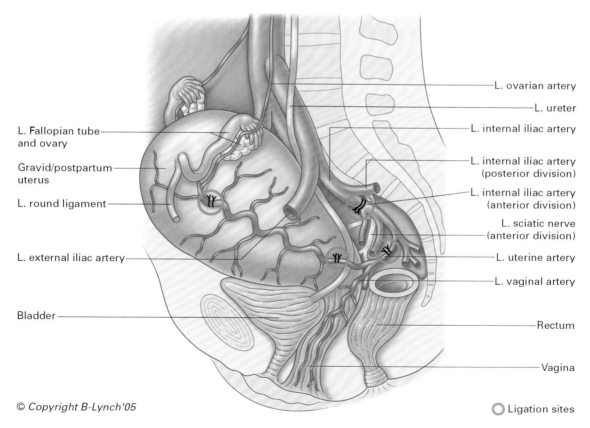

© Copyright B-Lynch'05   ○ Ligation sites

Figure 8   The complex vascular distribution to the pelvic organs. In this procedure of stepwise devascularization, the patient must be in the Lloyd Davis or modified lithotomy position, with one of the assistants able to access and swab the vagina to assess bleeding control

working knowledge of the pelvic anatomy, including the vascular and neurological supply of the pelvic organs. Second, there is a need for an obstetric anesthetist, as well as a vascular and/or gynecological cancer surgeon on standby. Finally, provisions must be available for admission postoperatively to the intensive care unit.

This set of requirements takes full account of the extraordinarily generous blood supply to the uterus and the pelvic organs (see Figure 7). The surgical approach starts with ligature of the uterine artery and its distribution to the uterus, preferably as it emerges from crossing over the ureter or as it approaches the uterine wall to penetrate and establish its division[25]. This could be carried out unilaterally or bilaterally about 2 cm from the uterine angle at cesarean section or where the lower segment is opened after conservative surgery for postpartum hemorrhage has failed (Figure 8).

It is absolutely essential to remember that the internal iliac (hypogastric artery) gives off independent branches that descend to the cervix and vagina (vaginal branch), respectively (see Chapter 52). Devascularization can be achieved by independent ligation sutures applied bilaterally to the cervix and/or vagina. The ovarian vascular supply to the uterus is also ligated, either unilaterally or bilaterally. Unilateral or bilateral ligature of the internal iliac artery may become necessary as a further step to control massive postpartum hemorrhage. A skilful surgeon should aim to ligate the anterior division of the internal iliac artery in order to achieve further devascularization of the uterus without compromising blood supply to the posterior division. However, ligation of the internal iliac directly could be done unilaterally or bilaterally without devascularizing the pelvic organs[8,26]. This may save time, life and organ.

References

1. Drife J. Management of primary post partum haemorrhage. Br J Obstet Gynaecol 1997;104:275–7
2. B-Lynch C, Coker A, Lawal AH, Cowen MJ. The B-Lynch surgical technique for the control of massive post partum hemorrhage: an alternative to hysterectomy? Five cases reported. Br J Obstet Gynaecol 1997;104:372–5
3. B-Lynch C, Cowen M.J. A new non-radical surgical treatment of massive post partum hemorrhage. Contemp Rev Obstet Gynaecol 1997; March:19–24
4. Chez RA, B-Lynch C. The B-Lynch suture for control of massive post partum hemorrhage. Contemp Obstet Gynaecol 1998;43:93–8
5. Day LA, Mussey RD, DeVoe RW. The intrauterine pack in the management of post partum hemorrhage. Am J Obstet Gynecol 1948;55:231–43
6. Bobrowski RA, Jones JB. A thrombogenic uterine pack for post partum hemorrhage. Obstet Gynecol 1995;85:836–7
7. Waters EG. Surgical management of postpartum hemorrhage with particular reference to ligation of uterine arteries. Am J Obstet Gynecol 1952;64:1143–8
8. Evans S, McShane P. the efficacy of internal iliac artery ligation in obstetric hemorrhage. Surg Gynaecol Obstet 1985; 160:250–3
9. Abdrabbo SA. Step-wise uterine devascularization: a novel technique for management of uncontrollable post partum hemorrhage with the preservation of the uterus. Am J Obstet Gynecol 1999;171:694–700
10. Baskett TF. Surgical management of severe obstetric hemorrhage: experience with an obstetric hemorrhage equipment tray. J Obstet Gynaecol Can 2004;26:805–8
11. Hayman RG, Arulkumaran S, Steer PJ. Uterine compression sutures: surgical management of post partum hemorrhage. Obstet Gynecol 2002;99:502–6
12. Cho JH, Jun HS, Lee CN. Hemostatic suturing technique for uterine bleeding during cesarean delivery. Obstet Gynecol 2000;96:129–31
13. Roman A, Rebarbar A. Seven ways to control post partum haemorrhage. Contemp Obstet Gynaecol 2003;48:34–53
14. WHO Report of Technical Working Group. The Prevention and Management of Post Partum Haemorrhage. Geneva: World Health Organisation, 1999;WHO/MCH/90–7
15. Ochoa M, Allaire AD, Stitely ML. Pyometra after hemostatic square suture technique. Obstet Gynecol 2002;99:506–9
16. Ferguson JE, Bourgeois FJ, Underwood PB, B-Lynch C. Suture for post partum hemorrhage. Obstet Gynecol 2000;95: 1020–2
17. El-Hammamy E, B-Lynch C. A worldwide review of the uses of the uterine compression suture techniques as alternative to hysterectomy in the management of severe postpartum haemorrhage. J Obstet Gynaecol 2005;25:143–9
18. Tsitpakidis C, Lalonde A, Danso D, B-Lynch C. Long term anatomical and clinical observations of the effects of the B-Lynch uterine compression suture for the management of post partum hemorrhage – ten years on. J Obstet Gynaecol 2006; in press
19. Wu HH, Yeh GP. Uterine cavity synechiae after hemostatic square suturing technique. Obstet Gynecol 2005;105: 1176–8
20. Price N, B-Lynch C. Technical description of the B-Lynch suture for treatment of massive hemorrhage and review of published case. Int J Fertil Womens Med 2005;50:148–63
21. Holtsema H, Nijland R, Huisman A, Dony J, van den Berg PP. The B-Lynch technique for post partum haemorrhage: an option for every gynaecologist. Eur J Obstet Gynaecol Reprod Biol 2004;115:39–42
22. Wohlmuth C, Gumbs J, Quebral-Ivie J. B-Lynch suture, a case series. Int J Fertil Womens Med 2005;50:164–73
23. Department of Health. Why Mothers Die: Report on Confidential Enquiries into Maternal Deaths in the United Kingdom 2000–2002 Triennial Report. London: RCOG Press, 2004: 94–103
24. Allam MS, B-Lynch C. The B-Lynch and other uterine compression suture techniques. Int J Gynaecol Obstet 2005;89: 236–1
25. O'Leary JA. Uterine artery ligation in the control of post-caesarean hemorrhage. J Reprod Med 1995;40:189–93
26. Clarke SL, Koonings P, Phelan JP. Placenta accreta and prior cesarean section. Obstet Gynecol 1985;66:89–92

52

Internal Iliac (Hypogastric) Artery Ligation

C. B-Lynch, L. G. Keith and W. B. Campbell

BACKGROUND HISTORY

The historical background of ligature of the internal iliac artery for the control of hemorrhage is not clear[1]. Numerous publications have attributed the procedure to different surgeons in diverse specialties worldwide[2–4]. In the United Kingdom and the United States, the operation was reported before 1900 and, since then, many surgeons have practiced it and found it useful.

Howard Kelly first pioneered ligation of the internal iliac (hypogastric) artery in the treatment of intra-operative bleeding from cervical cancer prior to this technique being applicable to postpartum hemorrhage[5]. Studies have shown that, in postpartum hemorrhage, the reduction of pulse pressure may only be achieved in 48% of cases. It is for this reason that other workers have advocated bilateral ligation of the internal iliac arteries to significantly improve the chances of reducing pelvic pulse pressure and facilitate hemostasis[5]. Reported complications include nerve injury, inadvertent ligature of the common iliac artery, prolonged blood loss and prolonged operative time. It has also been reported that there is a high rate of complication and low rate of success for hemostasis if the procedure is not done correctly[6]. Therefore, this procedure should be reserved for hemodynamically stable patients of low parity in whom future child-bearing itself is of paramount concern.

Unilateral or bilateral hypogastric artery ligation can be life-saving in patients with massive postpartum hemorrhage[6,7]. Although surgeons may be reluctant to perform bilateral hypogastric artery ligation for fear of injury to the pelvic viscera, there is no evidence that this is the case or that there is any significant impairment of function of the pelvic viscera. If the procedure is performed correctly, there is no morbidity, either short- or long-term[7].

Historically, the practice of internal iliac ligation was within the competency of most obstetricians and gynecologists. Today, however, subspecialization means that their training and experience may be insufficient, so pelvic floor specialists or vascular surgeons are often called upon when internal iliac artery ligation is required.

INTRODUCTION

In 1963, Lane and Aldemann reported that hemorrhage was one of the major causes of maternal mortality in the United States[8]. Eastman correlated this in an extensive review of the literature[9]. Any obstetrician who attends and experiences a case of severe postpartum hemorrhage clearly understands the risk of losing a patient from hemorrhage. The memory will last for ever. Modern methods offer the likelihood of resuscitation and survival through competent management by medical means or conservative surgery before such patients reach the point of exsanguination[10]. However, when it becomes obvious that conservative methods have failed, unilateral or bilateral internal iliac artery ligation should be considered urgently[5,11,12].

ANATOMICAL CONSIDERATIONS

The pelvic vasculature is arranged in such a manner that there is ample collateral circulation[13] (Tables 1–3). The common iliac artery bifurcates into two main branches – the external iliac artery (which becomes the femoral artery at the inguinal ligament) and the internal iliac (hypogastric) artery which descends into the true pelvis. The latter divides into anterior and posterior branches. It is essential to identify this division because the uterine artery branches off from the anterior division.

Clinical anatomy

The level of bifurcation of the common iliac artery is quite constant, and there are two easily identifiable

Table 1 Branches of the internal iliac artery

Posterior division	Anterior division
Parietal	Visceral
Iliolumbar	Umbilical
Lateral sacral	Superior vesical
Superior gluteal	Middle hemorrhoidal
Obturator	Uterine
Internal pudendal	Vaginal
Inferior gluteal	

Table 2 Anastomoses of internal iliac arteries

Branch of internal iliac	Anastomotic vessels
1. The uterine arteries	1. Right and left ovarian arteries (direct branches of the aorta)
2. Inferior and middle hemorrhoidal	2. Superior hemorrhoidal artery (branch of inferior mesenteric)
3. Pubic branches of obturator	3. Inferior epigastrics (branch of external iliac)
4. Inferior gluteal	4. Circumflex and perforating branches of the deep femoral artery
5. Superior gluteal	5. Lateral sacral (posterior branches)
6. Iliolumbar	6. Lumbar artery (from aorta)
7. Lateral sacral	7. Middle sacral
8. Vesical arteries	8. Branches of the uterine and vaginal arteries

Table 3 Major pelvic anastomoses

Vertical
1. Ovarian artery (branch of aorta) with the uterine artery
2. Superior hemorrhoidal artery (branch of inferior mesenteric) with middle hemorrhoidal artery
3. Middle hemorrhoidal artery with inferior hemorrhoidal (branch of internal pudendal from hypogastric)
4. Obturator artery with inferior epigastric artery (branch of external iliac)
5. Inferior gluteal artery with circumflex and perforating branches of deep femoral artery
6. Superior gluteal artery with lateral sacral artery (posterior branches)
7. Lumbar arteries with iliolumbar artery

Horizontal
1. Branches of vesical arteries from each side
2. Pubic branches of obturator from each side

guides. These are the sacral promontory and a line drawn between both anterior superior iliac spines. The bifurcation of the common iliac artery is found at the level of both of these landmarks in the majority of patients. Reich and co-workers in 1964[14] used dissection of fresh cadavers to show that numerous variations occur in the anatomy of these vessels. It is not always true, for example, that one or both of the internal iliac (hypogastric) branches of the common iliac artery are of similar diameter along the entire length. Therefore, visual observation alone can be misleading. Likewise, there may be some difference in the length and diameter of the right and left internal iliac arteries. Surgeons should therefore be aware of the fact that subdivision of the main internal iliac trunk may be into branches that are not significantly narrower than the main trunk.

The important anatomical relations of the internal iliac (hypogastric) artery can be summarized as follows:

(1) Anterior medial — covered by peritoneum (the internal iliac artery is entirely retroperitoneal);

(2) Anterior — the ureter (retroperitoneal and attached to the peritoneum);

(3) Posterolateral — the external iliac vein and the obturator nerve;

(4) Posteromedial — the internal iliac vein;

(5) Lateral — the psoas major and minor muscles.

Physiology of internal iliac artery ligation

Because of the excellent collateral circulation in the pelvis, vascular compromise does not occur when one or both internal iliac arteries are ligated. At one time, ligation of the hypogastric system was regarded as equivalent to shutting off all the blood to the area. Fortunately, this is not true. If it were, it is likely that the procedure would not be harmless. In reality, the hypogastric artery distal to the point of ligation is never emptied of blood because the rich anastomotic network starts to function immediately after ligation[15]. What does occur is the virtual abolition of the arterial pulse pressure. This is associated with reduced mean blood pressure and rate of blood flow in the collateral system. As a result, the trip-hammer effect of arterial pulsations is abolished. The surgeon must be aware that bilateral ligature of the internal iliac artery is more effective than the unilateral procedure in that the patient has less chance of returning to theater for secondary surgery to control hemorrhage. The reduced pressure and lack of pulsation do, however, mean that thrombosis in the vessels may remain *in situ*.

INDICATIONS FOR LIGATION OF THE INTERNAL ILIAC ARTERY

Prophylactic

Differentiation between prophylactic and therapeutic use of internal iliac artery ligation is by no means absolute. Conditions that may indicate ligation as a prophylactic measure include post-abortion bleeding, postpartum hemorrhage, atonic uterus prior to hysterectomy, abruptio placenta with uterine atony, abdominal pregnancy with pelvic implantation of the placenta, placenta accreta with intractable bleeding, and prior to total or subtotal hysterectomy when all conservative measures have failed.

Patients also considered to be at high risk for recurrent postpartum hemorrhage, those with recurrent major placenta previa, or Jehovah's Witnesses with important risk factors may be candidates for prophylactic internal iliac ligation. Good clinical judgement is essential and, if prophylactic ligation is thought to be the best course, then it should not be delayed.

Therapeutic

Therapeutic ligation may become necessary:

(1) Before or after hysterectomy for postpartum hemorrhage;

(2) Where bleeding continues from the base of the broad ligament;

(3) Where there is profuse bleeding from the pelvic side-wall;

(4) Where there is profuse bleeding from the angle of the vagina;

(5) Where areas of diffuse bleeding are present without a clearly identifiable vascular bed;

(6) In the case of ruptured uterus in which the uterine artery may be torn at the site of its origin from the internal iliac artery;

(7) When there are additional indications including atony of the uterus where conventional methods have failed;

(8) Where extensive lacerations of the cervix have occurred following difficult instrumental delivery;

(9) Where there is significant bleeding from the lower part of the broad ligament;

(10) When there are gunshot wounds to the lower abdomen;

(11) In the case of fracture of the pelvis and intraperitoneal hemorrhage.

In such circumstances, hysterectomy alone may not be sufficient to control hemorrhage. Internal iliac artery ligation, unilateral or bilateral, may become necessary and should not be delayed in such life-threatening situations.

SURGICAL TECHNIQUES

General considerations

All obstetric surgeons should be fully aware of the indications, timing and technical aspects of unilateral or bilateral hypogastric artery ligation.

Experimental evidence by Burchell has shown that it is the abolition of the 'trip-hammer effect' of arterial pulsations that allows effective clotting to take place, so that small vessels stop bleeding[2,3]. This may explain why bilateral ligation works better than unilateral ligation.

Either a mid-line or a transverse abdominal incision may be used. The surgeon should not use an unfamiliar incision. A transverse incision may take more time, especially in obese patients. Visualization is considerably better from the opposite side of the pelvis. To

work on the contralateral side, the surgeon may elect to change sides during the operation.

In most situations, bilateral ligation is preferable to unilateral ligation. Not only is hemostasis more secure, but, in addition, it allows greater confidence in making a decision not to re-explore the patient. Although it is possible to perform the operation by the extraperitoneal approach, the intra-abdominal approach is preferable except in cases of extreme obesity.

Some surgeons advocate complete transection of the internal iliac artery between two ligatures. This has no practical or physiologic advantage. On the contrary, its practice may lead to injury of the underlying veins.

The choice of material for ligating the artery depends on the preference of the surgeon. For example, 1–0 Vicryl and umbilical artery tape have been used. Two ties should be placed firmly but gently in continuity approximately 0.5 cm apart and 0.5–1 cm below the bifurcation (Figure 1).

Transabdominal approach

The abdomen is opened and the viscera packed away in the usual manner. Identification of the bifurcation of the common iliac artery is made by the two bony landmarks: the sacral promontory and an imaginary line drawn through both anterosuperior iliac spines. A longitudinal incision is made into the posterior parietal peritoneum. If the uterus is present, this incision can be started in the peritoneum on the posterior surface of the round ligament, at the junction of the middle and medial thirds. The incision is extended proximally for about 10 cm. If the uterus is absent, the incision can be started over the external iliac artery and carried proximally to the level of the bifurcation. Another method is to incise into the peritoneum directly over the bifurcation. The incision is then extended distally a few centimeters. All these incisions have one feature in common: they result in the formation of a medial and lateral peritoneal flap. The ureter is always beneath the medial flap and may be visualized, reflected, and protected with ease. The ureter normally crosses the common iliac artery from lateral to medial at a point just proximal to the bifurcation.

Once the peritoneum is opened, loose areolar tissue is separated from it by blunt dissection in the direction of the vessels, not across them to avoid unnecessary trauma. Small pieces of dental cotton ('pledgets' on long, curved forceps) are effective. The fingers also may be used. When the areolar tissue has been separated, the bifurcation comes into view. If the arteries are difficult to find, feel for a pulse (but remember that pulses may be difficult to palpate if a patient is hypotensive). The bifurcation feels like an inverted Y. The branch coming off at right angles is the hypogastric (internal iliac) artery. It courses medially and inferiorly to the palpating finger. The continuing branch is the external iliac artery. It courses laterally and superiorly out over the psoas muscles to the leg, where it becomes the femoral artery.

The surgeon must accurately identify these two branches because inadvertent ligation of the external iliac artery will produce an acutely ischemic leg, and limb loss is then a risk. If the external iliac artery is ligated, the ligature can be cut but it must then be checked for adequate flow, because the inner layer of the wall may have been disrupted. If the artery has been transected, then it needs to be formally repaired and a graft may be required. The attendance of a vascular surgeon becomes essential.

The common and internal iliac arteries are often adherent to the underlying veins which can be difficult to see, particularly beneath the origin of the internal iliac artery. This is the most hazardous part of the operation. Good retraction of the pelvic contents and displacement of the arteries are needed to visualize the veins. Meticulous dissection with scissors is required to separate the internal iliac vein from the artery if they are adherent. Once a plane has been developed between them, a Mixter or other fine right-angled forceps, or the forceps designed by Reich and colleagues[13] are gently introduced between them. This is best done onto the tip of a finger of the opposite hand, which allows gentle manipulation of the tips of the closed forceps, while feeling if there is still tissue present which requires division by sharp dissection. Simply pushing the forceps between the artery and the vein in an uncontrolled fashion is dangerous. It is also inadvisable to try separating the artery and the vein by opening the tips of the forceps forcibly until a path has been found between them.

The peritoneum should be closed with interrupted 2–0 Vicryl because a continuous suture can kink the ureter. The procedure on the left pelvic wall may be slightly more difficult because it is frequently necessary to mobilize the sigmoid flexure at the 'white line' to obtain adequate exposure.

Extraperitoneal approach

The skin incision in the inguinal area parallels the course of the external oblique muscle. It runs 10–15 cm in length in a line 3–5 cm medial to the anterosuperior iliac spine. After the fat and subcutaneous tissues are dissected away, a muscle-splitting incision exposes the peritoneum. This is gently reflected medially, together with the ureter. Ligation is performed as previously described. Closure is the same as for a herniorrhaphy and can be time-consuming if a bilateral approach is to be carried out.

Mid-line extraperitoneal approach (uncommon)

A mid-line extraperitoneal approach to the aorta has been advocated[16]. One hospital authority extended its use to bilateral ligation of the hypogastric arteries. A mid-line abdominal incision is made. After the anterior sheath of the rectus muscle is exposed and opened below the level of the umbilicus, dissection caudal to the semilunar line of Douglas is performed, and the peritoneal and preperitoneal fat are separated. The peritoneum and its contents are reflected to the right (or left), thus exposing the retroperitoneal structures[16].

ESSENTIAL SURGICAL CONSIDERATIONS

(1) The ureter crosses the common iliac artery at the level of its bifurcation;

(2) An incision is made inferolaterally and parallel to the ureter, which can be identified visually for safe identification and dissection;

(3) Following such incision, the peritoneal flap under which the ureter runs is displaced medially and retracted away (the ureter may be controlled with a sling for safety);

(4) The internal iliac at the point of its bifurcation into the anterior and posterior divisions can be seen and palpated with its vein and the obturator nerve. It is extremely important not to damage the internal iliac vein. The main arterial branch of the internal iliac is ideal for identification and ligature by passing a right angle, blunt-ended eye needle upon which is threaded a non-absorbable suture such as silk of 0 caliber or vicryl suture of the same caliber and passed between the artery and the vein.

Postoperative care

Intensive care is necessary because these women may be moribund and have required huge blood transfusion. Large hematomas or collections of serosanguineous fluid can be drained through separate stab wounds. Usually, this is unnecessary. Antibiotics are not indicated after ligation of the arteries. Their use is dictated only by the presence of infection. Early ambulation is advisable in all cases. An indwelling catheter may be necessary to facilitate adequate assessment of urinary output in women who are at risk of serious morbidity.

Special clinical considerations

The major pitfall associated with ligation of the hypogastric artery is delay. When hemorrhagic shock is irreversible, this operation will not overcome it. Inadequate transfusion is another pitfall in the therapy of patients with severe hemorrhage. Blood loss is often seriously underestimated.

Failure to remember that the vaginal artery is a separate branch of the hypogastric artery, rather than a branch of the uterine artery, may lead the surgeon into the pitfall of an unnecessary and ineffective hysterectomy for control of bleeding. Injury to the external iliac artery from retractors or mistaken ligation of this vessel can lead to lower limb amputation. Also, accidental ligature of one or both ureters would lead to renal function impairment. Accidental incorporation of the anterior division of the sciatic nerve may lead to foot drop (Figure 1b).

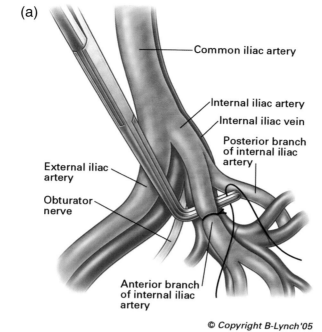

(a)

Common iliac artery

Internal iliac artery

Internal iliac vein

Posterior branch of internal iliac artery

External iliac artery

Obturator nerve

Anterior branch of internal iliac artery

© Copyright B-Lynch'05

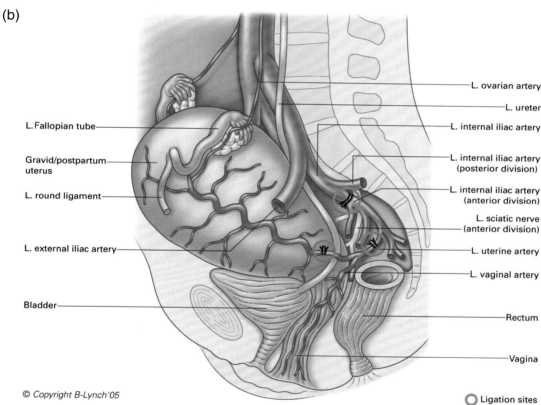

(b)

L. ovarian artery

L. ureter

L. internal iliac artery

L. internal iliac artery (posterior division)

L. internal iliac artery (anterior division)

L. sciatic nerve (anterior division)

L. uterine artery

L. vaginal artery

Rectum

Vagina

L. Fallopian tube

Gravid/postpartum uterus

L. round ligament

L. external iliac artery

Bladder

© Copyright B-Lynch'05

◯ Ligation sites

Figure 1 Ligation of the anterior branch of the internal iliac artery with its associated vein. (a) Demonstrable vulnerability of internal iliac vein and obturator nerve in close proximity; (b) A 'skeletal' anatomy, showing proximity of external iliac artery, ureter and anterior branches of sciatic nerve

Most authors consider internal iliac artery ligation to be a very safe procedure. The available data suggest that this operation does not result in necrosis of vital pelvic structures. The only report to the contrary is by Tajes[4] who cited a case of his own in which this operation resulted in necrosis of the buttocks. Tajes also reviewed two previously reported cases: in one case, the bladder mucosa sloughed, in the other, scrotal necrosis ensued. However, his report was 50 years ago.

Maintenance of reproductive function

It has not always been possible to follow young patients for whom this operation has been performed.

More important, many patients do not understand the exact nature or extent of their operation. A patient may remember only that she was sick and bleeding, that she was operated on and that she recovered.

The incidence of postoperative amenorrhea is not known. It is common for menses to resume after the operation. There have been reports of normal pregnancy and delivery occurring after bilateral hypogastric artery ligation, although it is impossible to say how frequently this occurs. It is entirely reasonable to believe that reproductive capacity is not lost after this operation, provided that the patient has a normal uterus. It is important to remember that pituitary necrosis can affect the ability to reproduce after postpartum hemorrhage, especially if blood replacement has been delayed or inadequate, hemorrhage has been severe, and shock profound. Fortunately, this is not a common occurrence in many modern and well-equipped obstetric units.

Potential failures and consequences[18]

Occasionally, ligation of the hypogastric arteries fails to stem pelvic hemorrhage. The reason for this is not clear, but some suggestions are:

(1) Massive necrosis after infection with destruction of the vessels;

(2) The presence of large, aberrant branches feeding blood to the area;

(3) Dislodgement of clots when blood pressure rises;

(4) Concomitant severe venous bleeding; however, this is rare;

(5) Coagulopathy with deranged hematological indices.

Avoiding accidental ligation of the common or external iliac artery

It is essential to identify the internal iliac artery clearly. Ligation of the common or external iliac produces an acutely ischemic leg. The classical signs are whiteness or pallor of the foot and absence of distal pulses – but these may be difficult to assess in a hypotensive, vasoconstricted patient. If there is concern that the main artery to the lower limb may have been ligated, check for a pulse in the external iliac artery above the inguinal ligament, beyond the area of ligation; the femoral pulse in the groin; or the Doppler signals at the ankle, using a hand-held Doppler. If the wrong artery has been tied, the ligature should be removed. If this fails to restore a good pulse (or if the artery has been transected), a vascular surgeon should be called to repair the vessel (either by end-to-end anastamosis or with the use of a short bypass graft of vein or synthetic material).

Damage to the ureter

Damage to either or both ureters should be avoided by careful visualization and dissection. In life-threatening surgery or delayed intervention to control massive hemorrhage, accidental damage to a ureter may occur. Ligature is more probable than transection. Prompt diagnosis and remedial surgery by a urological colleague are essential. Accidental ligature of one ureter may not lead to renal failure but increase morbidity.

Damage to other vessels

Damage to the common or iliac vein or one of its major tributaries results in brisk hemorrhage. Its source can be difficult to see and to control. It can threaten the patient's life, particularly in the context of pre-existing major blood loss from postpartum hemorrhage.

Steps to avoid damage to the iliac veins have been described in detail above: great care should be taken when dissecting in the area behind the origin of the internal iliac artery and when separating the arteries from the veins. If sudden venous bleeding does occur, the first step should be to apply firm pressure to the area. Adequate suction should be prepared – two suction tips may be helpful. Swabs mounted on sponge-holding forceps can then be applied distal and proximal to the site of damage to compress the veins and allow the defect to be visualized. If the venous defect cannot be seen, deep in the pelvis behind the iliac artery, then transaction of the iliac artery to expose the vein may solve the problem. The artery can then be re-anastamosed. When the defect in the vein has been seen, its edges can be held together using atraumatic forceps such as Stiles, before being sutured.

Repair of the vein is best performed with a non-absorbable vascular suture, such as polypropylene on a round-bodied needle. For large iliac veins, a 3/0 is a reasonable choice: needles smaller than those supplied with 4/0 sutures can be difficult to retrieve during repair of large veins and present a small danger of becoming 'lost' inside the vein. Finally, it is most important to avoid incorporating branches of the anterior division of the sciatic nerve into any ligatures[17] (Figure 1b).

USEFUL HINTS

The position of the surgeon relative to the patient

The surgeon should stand where he/she is most comfortable and this may be influenced by right- or left-handedness. The choice of the surgeon's position also depends on the ability and dexterity of the assistant. If the assistant is relatively inexperienced, then it may be particularly helpful for the surgeon to changes sides during the procedure in order to deal with each internal iliac artery from the opposite side of the operating table.

Checking for thorough control of bleeding before closure of abdomen

(1) Whilst the patient is in the frog-leg or Lloyd Davis position throughout the operation, an assistant stands between the legs and swabs the vagina to confirm bleeding has stopped.

(2) The abdomen is examined to ascertain that the ligatures have been correctly placed.

(3) The posterior abdominal wall peritoneum, which had been incised to access the posterior abdominal wall, may or may not need closure.

(4) The abdomen is checked once again thoroughly to ensure all instruments, swabs and foreign materials have been removed.

(5) The abdomen is closed according to type of the initial incision, i.e. large, pfannenstiel or mid-line. The mid-line incision is commonly closed by the mass closure technique.

(6) The sick patient should be quickly transferred directly to a high-care setting such as ITU for an appropriate length of time, to ascertain hemostasis, to ensure that pulse and blood pressure have returned to normal, and to permit surveillance of the urinary systems with a bladder catheter *in situ*.

(7) Counselling for post-traumatic stress, depression, panic attacks and flashbacks should be provided.

References

1. Burchell RC, Olson G. Internal iliac artery ligation: aortograms. Am J Obstet Gynecol 1966;94:117
2. Burchell RC. Hemodynamics of the internal iliac artery ligation. Presented at the 1964 Clinical Congress of the American College of Obstetricians and Gynaecologists
3. Burchell RC. Internal iliac artery ligation: hemodynamics. Obstet Gynecol 1964;24:737
4. Tajes RV. Ligation of the hypogastric arteries and its complications in resection of cancer of rectum. Am J Gastroenterol 1956;26:612
5. Kelly H. Ligation of both internal iliac arteries for hemorrhage in hysterectomy for carcinoma uteri. Bull John Hopkins Hosp 1894;5:53
6. Evans S, McShane P. The efficacy of internal iliac artery ligation in obstetric hemorrhage. Surg Gynecol Obstet 1985;160:250–3
7. Clark SL, Phelan JP, Yeh S-Y, et al. Hypogastric artery ligation for obstetric hemorrhage. Obstet Gynecol 1985;66:353–6
8. Lane RE, Andleman SL. Maternal mortality in Chicago, 1956 through 1960: preventable factors and cause of death. Am J Obstet Gynecol 1963;85:61–9
9. Eastman NJ. Gleanings from maternal mortality reports. Presented in a lecture at Milwaukee County Hospital and the Department of Obstetrics and Gynaecology of Marquette University, February 8, 1963
10. Lynch C, Coker Y, Abu J, et al. The B-Lynch surgical technique for the control of massive postpartum haemorrhage: an alternative to hysterectomy? Five cases reported. Br J Obstet Gynaecol 1997;104:372–5
11. Shafiroff BGP, Grillo EB, Baron H. Bilateral ligation of hypogastric arteries. Am J Surg 1959;98:34
12. O'Leary JA. Uterine artery ligation in the control of post-cesarean hemorrhage. J Reprod Med 1995;40:189–93
13. Reich WJ, Nechtow MJ, Keith L. Supplementary report on hypogastric artery ligation in the prophylactic and active treatment of hemorrhage in pelvic surgery. Int Surg 1965;44:1
14. Reich WJ, Nechtow HJ, Bogdan J. The iliac arteries: a gross anatomic study based on dissection of 75 fresh cadavers. Clinical surgical correlations. J Int Coll Surg 1964;41:53
15. Burchell RC, Mengert WF. Internal iliac artery ligation: a series of 200 patients. J Int Fed Obstet Gynecol 1969;7:85
16. Shumacker HB Jr. Midline extraperitoneal exposure of the abdominal aorta and iliac arteries. Surg Gynecol Obstet 1972;135:791–2
17. Varner M. Obstetric emergencies (postpartum haemorrhage). Crit Care 1991;7:883–97

53

Initial Interventions to Combat Hemorrhage during Cesarean Section and Internal Iliac Artery Ligation

V. P. Paily

Editorial note: The material in this chapter duplicates that of many other chapters in this book. The editors present it because each surgeon possesses a 'voice' that is based on his/her personal experience. Readers of the entire volume will soon determine that many surgical points of view are unique and worthy of consideration. This is not to say that some are better than others, but rather to suggest that the novice surgeon would do well to read more than one description of specific operations. L.G.K.

INTRODUCTION

This chapter deals with the causes of bleeding and interventions to combat the bleeding during cesarean section. Many of the topics covered herein are discussed in other chapters in greater detail.

CAUSES OF EXCESSIVE BLEEDING

The etiology of excessive bleeding during cesarean section often is similar to that after vaginal delivery, but additional causes relate to the operative procedure itself (Table 1). For convenience, these causes are considered in the sequence in which one is likely to encounter them.

Bleeding from anterior abdominal wall

Ordinarily, bleeding from the anterior abdominal wall is not significant; however, in situations where the patient is already in coagulopathy or has been placed on anticoagulants or antiplatelet agents, anterior abdominal wall bleeding can be significant. The type of incision also makes a difference; vertical midline incisions causing less blood loss than transverse incisions. Less blood is lost if the muscles are not cut. In cases of re-entry through a previous scar, sharp dissection may be required to separate the rectus sheath.

It is important to avoid injury to the inferior epigastric vessels which lie under the lateral aspect of the rectus muscle. However, in case the inferior epigastric vessels are injured, they should be tied before

proceeding further, as without ligature or coagulation, excessive blood loss and/or hematoma formation is possible.

The other usual site of abdominal wall bleeding is the lower peritoneal edge in the midline, especially if the incision is close to the apex of the bladder. Also, the median umbilical ligament (vestige of the urachus) may have a vessel with it, and bleeding is a possibility. Once the peritoneum is opened and the abdominal cavity entered, omental bands or fibrous bands from the anterior surface of uterus will have to be tied off.

Bleeding from the uterus

The most common cause of PPH during cesarean section is atony. Since that bleeding is from the placental site, it is dealt with later under placental site bleeding as is the next most common cause, laceration of the uterine vessels when the lower segment is incised for the extraction of the infant's head.

Table 1   Causes of excessive bleeding during cesarean section

---

From the anterior abdominal wall
Related to coagulopathy
   Disseminated intravascular coagulation (DIC), e.g. abruptio placenta
   Women on antiplatelet agents, e.g. aspirin or heparin
   Women on anticoagulants, e.g. coumarine for artificial heart valve
Injury of inferior epigastric vessels
Extensive adhesions from previous surgeries

Bleeding from the uterus
From the uterine incision site
   Thick lower segment
   Due to coagulopathy or anticoagulants as noted above
   Extension of incision involving uterine vessels
   Classical cesarean section
From placental site
   Atonic uterus
   Retained placental or membranous tissues
   Abnormal placental implantation
      Lower segment implantation
      Placenta invading deeper, e.g. accreta

Bleeding from uterine incision

Numerous factors influence bleeding from the uterine wound (Table 2). A thick lower segment is usually encountered in elective cesarean sections performed before the onset of labor. Proportionate to the thickness, the incision will have to be larger and hence blood loss will be greater. Trying to arrest bleeding at that point with cautery or ligation is not advisable. One has to proceed to deliver the fetus and then tackle the bleeding. A thick lower segment may demand use of forceps or ventouse to facilitate delivery of the fetus.

Increased vascularity and congestion of the lower segment is associated with various conditions such as use of prostaglandins and/or prolonged rupture of membranes with chorioamnionitis. Use of prostaglandins (both E1 and E2) also makes the lower segment, cervix and vagina more friable. In such cases, one has to anticipate excess bleeding and proceed briskly once incision on the myometrium has been made. Waiting for the assistants to clear the field with suction is an all too common mistake.

Previous scar on the lower segment can pose a challenge regarding the site of the present incision. If the scar lies in the middle of the lower segment and is within easy reach, then incision on the same scar is the ideal. If, however, the previous scar is too high in the upper part of the lower segment, one must decide whether to incise over the same scar or go lower to the middle of the lower segment. Incision on the previous scar helps reduce bleeding, whereas if the previous scar is too low or too difficult to reach with the bladder densely adherent, placing the incision at a higher level is safer.

Pelvic endometriosis leads to adhesion of the posterior wall of the lower segment to bowel, omentum, ovaries or tubes. Bleeding from the lower segment will be increased in these cases especially if the placental implantation overlies these areas. To arrest bleeding from such an open placental sinus, a simple method is to catch and lift up that part of uterine wall with an Allis forceps and take a purse string stitch around it with catgut or delayed absorbable suture material (Figure 1).

Placenta previa, either total or partial, increases the bleeding risk in several ways. This risk depends on the site (anterior or posterior), previous surgery (for example, previous cesarean scar increases risk of placenta

accreta and is dealt with separately in this and other chapters) and the technique used. When blood vessels run vertically on the lower segment, especially if there are many, it may be wiser to make a vertical incision on the upper segment. In case few vessels are seen, on the other hand, it is advisable to tie them above and below the level of proposed incision (Figure 2). While trying to take the stitches around these vessels, care should be taken not to injure them, as a hematoma can form very quickly at the puncture point.

Once the incision on the myometrium is started, the surgeon should proceed swiftly to incise it up to the decidual level and extend laterally by cutting with scissors to either side for about two inches and then tearing with fingers laterally to get the final desired length. One should take care to avoid the uterine arteries at this time.

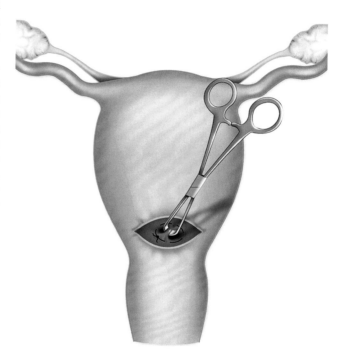

Figure 1 Purse string stitch around a bleeding sinus at the placental implantation site

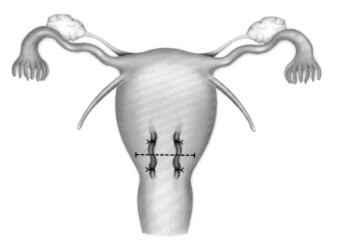

Figure 2 Underpinning vessels above and below the line of incision

Table 2 Factors that influence bleeding from uterine wound

Thickness of lower segment

Congested/inflamed lower segment – prostaglandin induction of labor or chorioamnionitis

Previous surgery – cesarean, myomectomy or surgery for pelvic endometriosis

Lower segment placental insertion

Extension of incision involving uterine arteries or veins

Presence of fibroid or adenomyosis

Classical cesarean incision

Length of incision

Proximity to placental implantation site

We do not recommend cutting through placenta to reach the amniotic cavity, unless it is a very thin, membranaceous placenta under the incision. The preoperative ultrasound scan would have given an idea about the outline of the placenta and the thickness of tissue under the incision. After reaching the placental plane, separate the placenta towards the side which is closest to the membranes, after which the membranes will bulge. On rupturing the membranes the fetal head can be delivered with forceps or ventouse.

Incision of placenta may become inevitable if the placenta is accreta or membranaceous. On the fetal surface of the placenta, fetal vessels or cord may get cut in some cases leading to rapid blood loss from the fetal circulation. Since the total blood volume of the fetus is only about 400 ml, this loss can be catastrophic. Hence, before trying to deliver the fetus, the surgeon should identify the cord and clamp it. Delivery of the fetus can be difficult because the placenta will occupy part of the space created by the incision. Use of forceps or ventouse will help in delivering the fetal head. Quick delivery of the fetus is essential in this situation. Until the uterine volume is reduced by delivering the fetus and placenta, bleeding will be excessive and difficult to control. Once the fetus is delivered, oxytocics should be promptly administered. Exteriorization of the uterus helps to identify and control bleeding. The immediate blood loss will be primarily from the angles and edges of the wound, as well as from open placental sinuses which will continue to well up because the lower segment myometrium will not contract effectively to constrict the vessels.

Persistent bleeding from the placental sinuses in the lower segment can be arrested with purse string stitches described earlier (Figure 1). However, the priority should be to tackle the bleeders at the angles of the incision and any arterial spurters present at the incision edges. These may be temporarily controlled with Green Armitage forceps and later tied separately. For control of the arterial bleeders, however, one should not depend on the running stitch used to close the uterine wound. Almost always it is the left incisional angle that becomes involved, owing to dextrorotation of the uterus making the left side become more anterior and vulnerable. Exteriorization of the uterus and upward traction helps to reduce bleeding and identify torn vessels. Removal of the placenta should be completed as quickly as possible. If the tear has extended laterally or downwards, the bladder must be pushed down first, and this maneuver will help the ureter to drop down. Clamping and ligation of the vessels without this step may inadvertently include the ureter. If the incisional angle is torn irregularly it may be safer to tie the vessels away from the edges both above and below. Keeping the bladder and ureter safely away, stitches can be placed on the side of the uterus including part of the myometrium so that both arteries and veins are tied. If unfortunately a hematoma has already formed, it should be evacuated before searching for the bleeder, as torn arteries will have receded and gone into spasm. Unless the clots are

removed and the bed of that space 'moped clean' the artery may not be visible.

As torn vessels at the angles of the uterine wound are the usual causes of excessive blood loss, we recommend securing the angles with mattress stitches before the running stitch is used to close the wound. Start at the angle on the right side and after securing the anchoring stitch, the same suture material is used to take a mattress stitch 1 cm medial to the angle to approximate the edges. The rest of the suture material can then be used for similar stitches on the left side followed by the running stitch to approximate the remaining part of the wound (Figure 3).

Fibroids and adenomyosis enhance bleeding risk. Even though submucous fibroids are not that common, intramural and subserous fibroids as well as adenomyosis are not uncommon findings. The main reason for excessive bleeding in these cases is atonicity. Subserous fibroids pose another threat. They may have large tortuous veins on their surface and may get torn while handling the uterus. Attempting to exteriorize the uterus through a small abdominal incision may lead to such trauma. Catastrophic bleeding can occur in posterior subserous fibroids if this possibility is not kept in mind and acted on. Once identified,

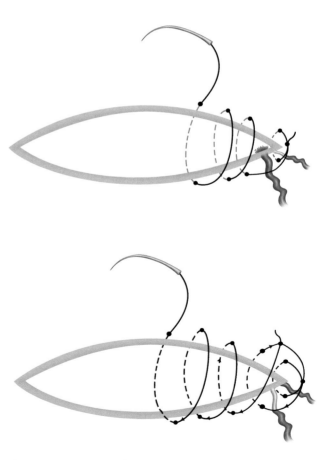

Figure 3 Mattress stitches at the angle and about 1 cm medial, to take care of the angle bleeder. Upper illustration shows usual anchoring stitch followed by running stitch, leading to ongoing bleeding from vessel joining medial to angle. Lower illustration shows the recommended additional mattress stitch 1 cm medially which includes such vessels

controlling such bleeding is easy if one tackles the base of the fibroid rather than trying to tie the vessel at the site of bleeding.

Bleeding in classical cesarean

Since classical cesarean is undertaken only in rare or special situations, many obstetricians may be unfamiliar with the technique. Both the thickness of the myometrium and the increased length of the incision lead to more blood loss. The chance of the incision extending to the placental site also is greater. Steps to tackle the hemorrhage in these circumstances will depend on the primary reason for resorting to this unusual uterine incision. For example, if it is a case of placenta previa accreta, the management described under that section may be resorted to (see section below). For other indications (fibroids or abnormal lie) the aim should be to complete the delivery of the fetus and placenta and proceed with closure of the uterine wound. The uterine wall being thick, one may need two or three layers to close it.

Bleeding from placental site

Atonic PPH

Atonic PPH during cesarean section occurs as a result of similar causes to atonic PPH during vaginal delivery or owing to factors specific to cesarean. The latter include effects of anesthesia and sedation. General anesthesia, especially if agents like halothane are used, will make the myometrium lose its tone. This is one of the reasons why regional anesthesia is preferred over general anesthesia for cesarean section. But there are some special situations (transverse lie) where relaxant general anesthesia is deliberately chosen and the obstetrician should anticipate some atonicity and bleeding after delivery of the fetus.

Once atonic PPH has developed, the management algorithm is the same as after vaginal delivery. It is well covered in other chapters, and only a few salient points pertinent to cesarean section are mentioned here. Cesarean actually provides the advantage of direct compression of the uterus by the operator or assistant. Whether the compression is effective can be ascertained directly by observing for blood welling up or the lack thereof. The first step obviously is to gently massage the uterine fundus. If the uterus remains flabby, bimanual compression can be used. Simultaneously, oxytocics should be administered, and the opportunity is present to administer methergin and prostaglandin F2α directly to the myometrium. If these measures fail, one has to consider surgical steps in a sequential manner. Our own practice is to approach in the order mentioned in Table 3 and discussed in great detail in other chapters.

Triple tourniquet Occasionally one may be forced to perform a cesarean when excess bleeding is expected. A typical case is severe degree of abruptio placenta or a patient on the verge of, or actually in coagulation

failure, as is seen in amniotic fluid embolism. The uterus in these cases will be flabby and bleeding will be profuse. The uterus may not respond to normal oxytocic administration. In many settings, neither manpower nor immediate blood transfusion facilities are readily available. In such instances and in others where resuscitative therapies are available, a triple tourniquet is a very effective first aid measure to stop the profuse bleeding. Here, the blood flow to the uterus is totally cut off by a tourniquet applied at the isthmus and to both infundibulopelvic ligaments.

For the *isthmial tourniquet*, the bladder is pushed down as a first step. Then, by transillumination an avascular area on the broad ligament lateral to the side of uterus and uterine vessels at the level of isthmus is identified. This spot is bluntly pierced with the tip of an artery forceps and the end of a sterile plastic suction catheter (size 8 or 10 Fr) pulled from back to front on the left side. The other end is pulled through similarly on the right side after cutting away the dilated proximal part of the catheter. The two ends are crossed in front of the isthmus and twisted repeatedly so that the catheter constricts the isthmus tightly. An artery forceps is clamped on the catheter close to the isthmus to prevent it from getting loose (Figure 4). A clamp applied like this rather than a knot makes it easier to compress the isthmus tightly and release the tourniquet later.

Both *infundibulopelvic ligaments also have to be constricted using a tourniquet*. For this, we keep the round ligament and infundibulopelvic ligament of each side together. A tourniquet on infundibulopelvic ligament alone tends to cause damage to the slender ovarian

Table 3 Surgical steps to arrest atonic PPH

Triple tourniquet (in exceptional situations – see notes)
Bilateral ligation of uterine and anastomosing branch of ovarian artery
Brace stitch – B-Lynch or Hayman's stitch
Bilateral internal iliac artery ligation
Hysterectomy

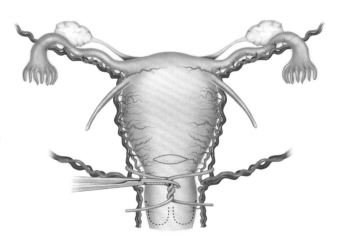

Figure 4 The technique of isthmial tourniquet. The artery clamp has to be close to the isthmus, keeping the tightness of the plastic catheter around the isthmus

veins and lead to hematoma formation. The same window created in the broad ligament for isthmial tourniquet can be used to take a catheter and tightening the tourniquet lateral to the ovary. We use a size 6 infant feeding tube. A sliding knot is placed, and a mosquito forceps applied to prevent the knot from getting loose (Figure 5).

A triple tourniquet applied as described above will totally cut off blood flow to uterus and stop the bleeding. However, a myometrium that is devoid of its oxygen supply will not contract. Hence, the tourniquet should be released as soon as IV fluids, blood and blood products are present and running, and the condition of the patient has improved. In other words, triple tourniquet in PPH is only a first aid measure. Other procedures, such as a stepwise devascularization or brace stitch should be used if needed and the tourniquet released unless one has decided to do hysterectomy.

Stepwise devascularization and brace stitch The sequence of steps, whether brace stitches should be taken before uterine and ovarian vessel ligation is debatable. Our own practice is to take uterine and ovarian vessel ligation as the first step and, if necessary, to proceed with brace stitches after that. Details of these procedures are not given in this chapter as they are described elsewhere. However, a few points worth emphasizing are mentioned here. For uterine artery ligation, we recommend taking the stitch including myometrium on lateral wall of isthmus to include uterine artery and vein as one bundle. Bladder should be pushed down for reasons mentioned above. While taking the stitch one has to be careful to avoid injury to bowel behind (Figure 6).

The ovarian vessel ligation is shown at different sites in different textbook illustrations. Some even show ligation lateral to the ovaries which will lead to atrophy of ovaries. The commonest illustration is to tie the vessel on the side of the uterus below the cornual region. This will not include the arcuate vessel that takes off near the fundus of the uterus close to the tubal implantation site. We recommend taking the stitch between the tube and the vessel running under it and taking the needle medially to include part of the side of the uterus (Figure 7). This will stop the blood flowing to the fundus of the uterus which often is the placental implantation site.

Regarding the brace stitch, we recognize and appreciate the procedure published by Christopher B-Lynch *et al.* in 1997[1]. This has revolutionized the management of atonic PPH. However, we find that the technique suggested by Hayman, Arulkumaran and Steer is simpler and achieves similar results[2]. As the tissue passage is minimal in the Hayman technique, the #1 delayed absorbable braided stitch (polyglycolic acid or polyglactin) that is readily available in any operating theater can be used. The point to be emphasized is to tighten the stitch at the fundus medial to the tubal insertion site so that the tube is not damaged (Figure 8).

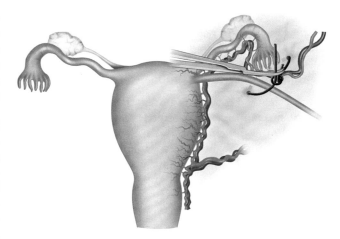

Figure 5 Tourniquet at infundibulopelvic ligament. Inclusion of round ligament helps to reduce damage to ovarian veins. The artery clamp should be applied after tightening the loop around the vessels (sliding knot) to prevent the loop from getting loose

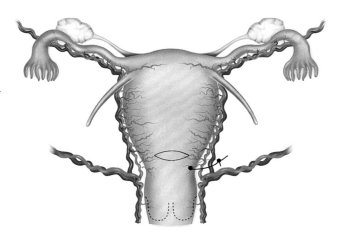

Figure 6 Uterine artery ligation at the isthmus of uterus. The stitch should include the vessels, with part of adjacent uterine wall, at the level close to where the uterine artery joins the uterus. Bladder has to be pushed down

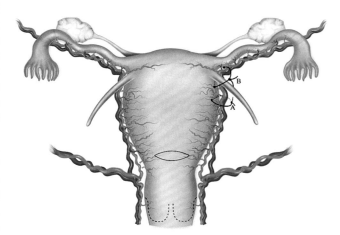

Figure 7 Tying of the anastomosing branches of uterine and ovarian arteries at the cornual region. (A) The usually seen illustration of stitch for the anastomosing branch. Blood flow to the fundus of uterus will continue unimpeded. (B) The recommended technique. The arcade of vessels on the mesosalpinx, from just under the tube to the side of the uterus, are included so that the branches supplying the fundal region are occluded

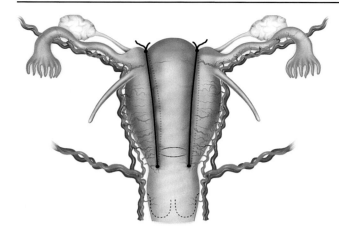

Figure 8   Hayman's uterine compression stitches

If these fail, in selected cases we proceed to bilateral internal iliac artery ligation which is described later in this chapter.

Obstetric hysterectomy   If none of the above steps work and the patient is still bleeding, hysterectomy may have to be considered. Once a decision is made to perform a hysterectomy, the next steps have to be taken quickly. What we recommend is to put clamps on both sides, cut and proceed until the uterine arteries on both sides are clamped. Only after that are the stumps to be ligated. We recommend double ligation of all pedicles, as the risk of reactionary hemorrhage from the edematous stumps is high. Unless there is a tear or pathology involving the cervix, we perform subtotal hysterectomy. Trying to remove the cervix increases the risk of bleeding from the vault and is almost always unnecessary. The cervical stump is a much easier tissue to stitch than the thin vault of vagina. Any attempt to push down the bladder to remove the entire cervix can increase the risk of bleeding from the underside of the bladder or the azygos vessels of the vagina, and the time lost in such an effort could be critical.

Retained placental tissue or membranes

In the context of a cesarean section, retained placental tissue or membranes is an unlikely cause of bleeding. However, unless one makes a habit of inspecting the placenta for its completeness as well as palpating the uterine cavity for any retained cotyledons or membranes, this can happen. Digital exploration of the upper uterine cavity and fundus should be routine before closing the uterine wound. Occasionally, one will be rewarded with the diagnosis of an unsuspected septum or submucous fibroid in addition to the retained placental tissue or membranes. Placenta accreta can occur at any part of the uterus, especially if there are scars resulting from a prior myomectomy or cesarean delivery. Another factor is presence of infection as in chorioamnionitis. If retained placental tissue is suspected, the uterine cavity can be checked through the cesarean incision and any retained tissue

removed. In case the placental bits are densely adherent, one may have to resort to sharp curettage under direct vision or local excision.

Deeper invasion of placenta (placenta accreta)

Editor's note: The surgery described herein is ideally not for the novice surgeon. If placental invasion is suspected, experienced help is mandatory. Additional material is found in Chapters 29–31. L.G.K.

Although in classical writings on the topic, conventionally morbid invasion of placenta was divided into accreta (into basal layer of endometrium), increta (into myometrium) and percreta (up to serosa and adjacent viscus, i.e. bladder); current literature uses the term accreta to include all three varieties. Placenta accreta can be present in the upper or the lower segment. The usual mechanism(s) of placental separation does not occur at these sites, leading to retention of placental tissue and bleeding from the normally implanted areas. This becomes more of a problem in the lower segment insertion, because in placenta previa accreta there is altered blood flow to the placental site. Anastomoses can occur between the lower uterine segment vessels with the vessels on the surface of the bladder which in turn can anastomose with blood vessels in the lower abdominal wall (branches of inferior epigastric artery). Similarly, the anastomosis between cervical and vaginal vessels will also be prominent, and tortuous vessels may be present under the bladder. Because of the altered blood flow described above, ligation of the internal iliac arteries alone may not control the bleeding from the placental site in cases of placenta previa accreta (Chapters 1 and 2).

Bleeding from placenta previa accreta during a cesarean can be torrential and lead to rapid exsanguination. This possibility calls for a prepared stepwise course of action. Preparations must include the availability of senior obstetricians, anesthesiologists and a urologist. Intravenous lines with wide bore cannula (two) and a central line to monitor central venous pressure are essential. Blood and blood products must be available in sufficient quantity for rapid use (see Chapters 4–6). Injury to the bladder and ureter is common, and unless the obstetrician is confident in tackling such injuries, a urologist should be on standby. It is crucial to prevent the rapid blood loss that will start once the placenta is disturbed, as tying the internal iliac artery will not be adequate in arresting the bleeding.

Many case reports describe occlusion of pelvic artery or aorta for management of placenta previa accreta (see Chapters 29–31). Ophir *et al.*[3] report their experience with preoperative balloon catheter placement in the internal iliac artery, prophylactic balloon occlusion after delivery of the fetus and resection of the invaded uterine wall conserving the rest of the uterus. After deflation of the balloon, bleeding came from branches of the uterine artery and was embolized. In their article, they reviewed the various options available for endovascular occlusion for management of placenta previa accreta (this subject is also treated in the Chapters 1, 2 and 31).

Another option is the conservative management of the placenta by leaving it *in situ*. Some authors employ methotrexate to hasten the resorption of the placental tis0sue. On the whole, the failure rate is about 20% and failure can be followed by hysterectomy[4]. Conservative management should be tried in those cases where there is a desire for fertility and adequate technical support for intervention including massive blood transfusion. About 20% of conservatively managed cases subsequently require emergency hysterectomy. When the uterus is left *in situ*, the chance of recurrence of placenta previa accreta in a subsequent pregnancy varies from 0 to 100%. Kayem et al.[5] reported a recurrence risk of 100% in conservatively managed cases. Timmermans *et al.*[4] quoted a series of 26 patients with three pregnancies of which two had recurrence. The same authors quote other case reports of patients managed with adjuvant treatment such as methotrexate and selective arterial embolization[4]. In the methotrexate group there were 22 patients out of which five treatments failed, but two had subsequent uneventful pregnancies. In the arterial embolization group treatments failed in three out of five, but another three had subsequent pregnancies without recurrence.

Considering these limitations, it may be better for centers in the developing world to consider radical treatment (hysterectomy) as the best option. Centers in the developed world, on the other hand, have established strategies to tackle the problem that include a multidisciplinary team approach, intensive care facilities and arrangements for massive blood transfusion[6]. In the setting of a developing country, however, these preparations are difficult if not impossible to arrange. In the state of Kerala in India where confidential review of maternal deaths is practiced, five maternal deaths out of a total of 307 were as a result of placenta previa (four with previous cesarean) in the years 2004–2005[7]. Hence, we developed a strategy to tackle the problem with limited resources.

The salient steps are as follows:

- Establish the diagnosis and extent of placental invasion with ultrasound scan and/or magnetic resonance imaging in the antenatal period

- Ensure that adequate blood and blood products are available

- Ensure the presence of an experienced obstetrician and urologist

- Insert bilateral ureteric catheters and leave them *in situ*

- Keep a Foley catheter in the bladder

- Use regional or general anesthesia or a combination

- Do classical cesarean section to deliver the fetus

- Decide whether to remove the placenta or leave it behind. If the decision is for the latter, tie the cord close to its placental base and close the uterine wound

- If the decision is for hysterectomy, occlude the blood flow to the uterus by temporary clamping of the common iliac arteries for about 30–40 min with specially developed atraumatic vascular clamps (clamps developed by the author; patent pending). If these clamps are not available, bilateral internal iliac artery ligation may be employed. Both infundibulopelvic ligaments may be occluded with tourniquets

- For hysterectomy, proceed until the level of the uterine artery clamps and then separate the bladder from the uterus and continue with hysterectomy. Take special care at the previous scar area to avoid injury to the bladder. A subtotal hysterectomy ensuring that the placental implantation site is removed completely may be better than trying to remove the entire cervix

- Double check all pedicles. Ensure hemostasis especially at the bladder base. Double ligation of all pedicles is recommended. Close the abdomen after leaving a wide bore drain.

- Please note that the common iliac artery should not be kept clamped for more than 30–40 min. On removal of the clamps, the vessels should be massaged to relieve local spasm. Verify re-establishment of circulation to lower limbs. Postoperative thromboprophylaxis is highly recommended.

In case placenta previa accreta is encountered unexpectedly during a cesarean, further steps should be altered in the line with the above recommendations. A classical cesarean should be done. If massive blood transfusion and the assistance of experienced personnel cannot be arranged immediately, a conservative course may be followed; deliver the fetus through classical cesarean incision and leave the placenta intact. Even if a second surgery is required after 2 or 3 days, it will be less bloody and adequate help can be organized by that time. Alternatively the patient can be moved to a center with better facilities. During transfer, the non-pneumatic antishock garment (NASG) should be used (see Chapters 38 and 39).

If the placental invasion is recognized after placing the incision on the lower segment or attempting placental removal, bleeding can be torrential. The anesthetist should put in extra lines for fluid replacement. Additional help in the form of an experienced obstetrician and urologist should be summoned. Arrangements for blood and blood products should be made. If severe bleeding starts, the common iliac artery clamps described above should be applied and both ovarian vessels occluded with tourniquet at the infundibulopelvic ligaments. If common iliac artery clamps are not available, an assistant should directly apply pressure over the aorta (see Chapter 52) and the surgeon should remove as much of the placenta as possible and try to separate the bladder and proceed with hysterectomy.

INTERNAL ILIAC (HYPOGASTRIC) ARTERY LIGATION

Background

The internal iliac arteries supply all the pelvic organs – uterus, vagina, bladder, rectum and anal canal. It is thus only natural to assume that ligation of these arteries will stop bleeding from these viscera. This applies to PPH as well. However, all the pelvic organs possess extensive collateral circulations (see below) which act both as an advantage as well as a disadvantage. On the one hand, one can ligate the internal iliac artery without fear of ischemic necrosis of the aforementioned viscera. On the other hand, because of this extensive alternative supply, the ligation of the iliacs often fails to arrest the bleeding. This is all the more true when additional collaterals develop as in placenta previa accreta (see above and Chapter 1).

Anatomic considerations (Figure 9)

The internal iliac artery arises by the bifurcation of the common iliac artery at the pelvic brim; it takes a course medially into the pelvis to give off branches to the pelvic viscera as well as the gluteal region. *Usually*, after running as a single trunk for a short distance it divides into an anterior and posterior division. The

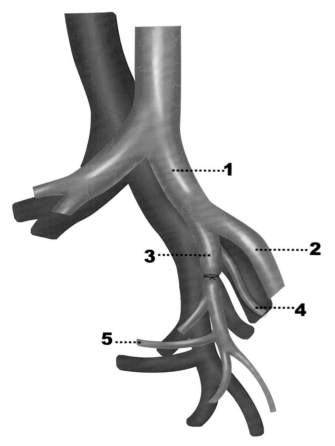

Figure 9 The internal iliac artery and its branches: (1) common iliac artery, (2) external iliac artery, (3) internal iliac artery (anterior division), (4) Internal iliac artery (posterior division) and (5) uterine artery

posterior division *usually* takes off from the posterior aspect of the internal iliac and may not be easily visible. It supplies the gluteal region.

The anterior division gives off branches to the uterus, bladder, vagina, anorectum, perineum, clitoris and vulva. *Wide variation is present in the branching pattern of the internal iliac artery*. One anatomical principle that is *usually* maintained is for the uterine artery to be at right angles to the direction of the internal iliac artery.

The proximity of the internal and external iliac veins to the internal iliac artery is *crucial*. On the left side, the external iliac vein crosses the artery posteriorly near the bifurcation of the common iliac. The internal iliac vein lies posteromedially. When circulatory collapse is present, these veins may also be collapsed and not easily visible. It is quite easy to injure them in such circumstances unless the operator is especially conscious of this issue.

The internal iliac artery is *to a greater or lesser degree* enveloped in a sheath of fibroareolar tissue called the adventitia. The lymphatic vascular tissue lies in this envelope, and often lymph nodes and fat are present on the surface of these vessels. It is better to isolate the vessel from these tissues prior to having a suture passed under the artery.

It is often recommended that the ligation should be distal to the origin of the posterior division to avoid ischemia of the gluteal region; there are case reports of gluteal pain following iliac artery ligation. In practice, however, this happens extremely rarely. Tying the ligature about 2 cm below the origin of the internal iliac will help to avoid the posterior division. *[Editorial note: This was the technique I was taught by masters of this operation during my residency, and this is the technique that is used by most surgeons with whom I have discussed this issue. L.G.K.]*

Procedure

There are two approaches to the internal iliac artery, and it is advisable to master both, as both may be needed depending on the clinical situation.

Broad ligament approach

At term, the internal iliac artery becomes easily accessible at the base of broad ligament if one opens the two leaves of it. The simplest way to achieve this is to open the uterovesical fold of peritoneum in front of the lower uterine segment (already undertaken in case of cesarean section) and extend the incision laterally up to the round ligament. The areolar tissue easily gives way allowing the surgeon to palpate the external iliac artery pulsations at the pelvic brim. It is important to avoid digging into the pelvis at this level. Follow the external iliac artery cranially by bluntly separating the tissue with fingers until the common iliac is reached. Keeping the superior leaf of the broad ligament intact helps to prevent the bowels and omentum from coming into the field. This can be achieved with the uterus exteriorized or left inside the abdomen; our preference is to keep the uterus exteriorized. *The ureter will be seen at the bifurcation of the common iliac. It is better to move the ureter medially and hold it there with the blade of a long retractor.* The internal iliac artery is then traced caudally using a long clamp with a narrow tip; the fat and areolar tissue surrounding the internal iliac artery can be separated by just running the tip of the clamp (often with a pledget of dental roll cotton 1 cm in diameter) on both sides. A right angled clamp (Mixter) can be passed under the internal iliac artery about 2 cm below its origin, taking extreme care that its tip does not injure the veins nearby. Pulling up the internal iliac artery trunk with a Babcock forceps is helpful but not essential. The operator keeps the jaws of the Mixter clamp open (Figure 10). The assistant/nurse then feeds the tip of the suture between the jaws and the thread is then pulled out under the vessel. It is essential that the suture material be held on a long clamp and taken directly to the open Mixter clamp rather than be brought into the incision with the assistant's hand because the hand will obstruct vision and coordinated action will be difficult. We even suggest that if the surgeon and the nurse/assistant are operating together for the first time, they practice this step before the Mixter clamp is taken under the internal iliac artery. The suture material we prefer is catgut or one of the delayed absorbables like polyglycolic acid or polyglactin. A non-braided material has the advantage that it does not drag the areolar tissue with it when the suture is pulled through. One tie is enough because our aim is only a temporary occlusion. [Editor's note: Other surgeons use a double tie by passing a loop to the Mixter which then is cut and makes two sutures. Silk or other non-absorbable can also be used. L.G.K.]

The procedure is then repeated on the other side. If the indication is pelvic sidewall bleeding or hematoma, unilateral ligation of that side may be enough. In all other situations, bilateral ligation is preferred.

Direct approach

In some cases, the uterus has already been removed or the pathology is such that it may not be possible to approach the artery between the two layers of broad ligament. In such instances, a direct approach over the internal iliac is essential. The vessel is identified by palpation of pulsation in either the common or external iliac. At a point about 2 cm below the bifurcation of the common iliac artery, the peritoneum is held up on Allis forceps and incised for about 2–4 cm. We prefer to incise longitudinally in relation to the vessel but lateral to the ureter. The peritoneum is separated craniocaudally and transversally, and the internal iliac artery isolated and tied as described for the broad ligament approach above. The peritoneal incision does not have to be closed.

Difference between right and left sides

Subtle differences exist between the right and left sides. The right side is more easily accessible and the venous relationship slightly different. On the left side, the root of the mesosigmoid mesentry overlies the area of the common iliac. In the direct approach, it is better to approach the vessels after keeping the sigmoid cranially. In the broad ligament approach, the sigmoid will be pushed cranially anyway.

The ureter overlies the bifurcation of the common iliac and is kept medially in the broad ligament approach as well as the direct approach.

Complications

The following complications may be encountered.

(1) *Bleeding as a result of injury to the main veins* described above is the commonest serious complication. It should be avoided by all means. If it happens, direct pressure can help to control it. Vascular clamps then have to be applied above and below, and the tears repaired. Help of a vascular surgeon is ideal. If this is not possible, attempts should be made to suture the defect with 6 '0' prolene. A tear of the internal iliac vein is less hazardous, as it can be tied off. In contrast, external iliac vein injuries have to be sutured and the circulation maintained. Otherwise, lower limb edema and eventually ischemia and necrosis will occur.

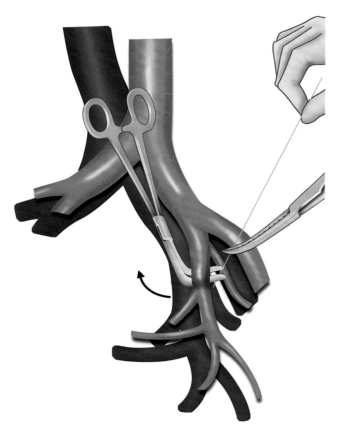

Figure 10 Taking sutures under the internal iliac artery with right angled clamp. The Mixter clamp is negotiated under the internal iliac artery without injuring the veins. The tip of the thread is fed to the open clamp with the help of a long forceps

(2) *Inadvertent ligation of the external iliac artery* should also be avoided by all means. A safety check is to make a routine of palpating the femoral pulse immediately before and immediately after the internal iliacs are tied.

(3) *Injury to ureter* – the ureter should be identified before the peritoneal incision is made. This helps in avoiding inadvertent injury to the ureter. It is not necessary to isolate the ureter or separate it from the peritoneum. Displacing it with the blunt end of the retractor is enough.

(4) *Gluteal pain/ischemia* – when the ligature is placed close to the origin of the internal iliac, the posterior division also may be involved in the ligature and ischemia to the gluteal muscle is possible. If the ligature is taken about 2 cm below the bifurcation, this eventuality is unlikely to occur. Because of the anastomoses between the branches of the gluteal artery and the lumbar arteries arising from the aorta, ischemic necrosis in the gluteus maximus is very rare.

Reproductive function after internal iliac artery ligation

Normal menstruation and fertility have been described after bilateral internal iliac artery ligation[8].

Current status of internal iliac artery ligation

After the brace stitch became popular, the use of internal iliac artery ligation for atonic PPH changed. We now use it mainly for traumatic PPH and tear of lower genital tract. The internal iliac artery ligation helps in the control of bleeding at such sites and makes suturing possible.

CONCLUSIONS

This chapter details the surgical steps that help to control bleeding during cesarean section. Internal iliac artery ligation is discussed in detail, but other surgical steps are covered in other chapters.

References

1. B-Lynch C, Cocker A, Lawal AH, Abu J, Cowen MJ. The B-Lynch surgical techniques for the control of massive postpartum haemorrhage: an alternative to hysterectomy? Five cases reported. Br J Obstet Gynaecol 1997;104:372–5
2. Hayman RG, Arulkumaran S, Steer PJ. Uterine compression sutures: Surgical management of postpartum hemorrhage. Obstet Gynecol 2002;99:502–6
3. Ophir E, Singer-Jordan J, Odeh M, et al. Abnormal placental invasion – A novel approach to treatment Case report and review. Obstet Gynecol Surv 2009;64:811–22
4. Timmermans S, van Hof AC, Duvekot JJ. Conservative management of abnormally invasive placentation. Obstet Gynecol Surv 2007;62:529–39
5. Kayem G, Clement D Goffinet F. Recurrence following conservative management of placenta previa accreta. Int J Gynecol Obstet 2007;99:142–3
6. Hull AD, Resnik R. Placenta accreta and postpartum hemorrhage. Clin Obstet Gynecol 2010;53:228–36
7. Paily VP. Why Mothers Die, Kerala 2004–05. Thrissur 5, Kerala, India: India Kerala Federation of Obstetrics & Gynaecology (KFOG), 2009:30
8. Nizard J, Barrinque L, Frydman R, Fernandez H. Fertility and pregnancy outcomes following hypogastric artery ligation for severe postpartum hemorrhage. Hum Reprod 2003;18:844–8

EDITORS' SUMMARY OF KEY POINTS

INITIAL INTERVENTIONS TO COMBAT HEMORRHAGE DURING CESAREAN SECTION

Simple measures to combat hemorrhage during cesarean section include:

- Checking the angles of the uterus to make sure there are no missed vessel(s)

- Checking the uterine cavity to rule out any retained fragments of placenta

- Considering the use of a second or third uterotonic.

If bleeding is mainly from the fundus and the mid-part of the uterine body, examine the patient in the Lloyd Davies position and perform a manual uterine compression test to assess the feasibility of uterine compression sutures. If there is no bleeding whilst compression of uterus is being performed, uterine compression sutures are appropriate.

If bleeding still continues and the source of bleeding is from the lower segment or cervical region, the balloon tamponade test can be performed and assessment of continued bleeding carried out. If the tamponade test shows no bleeding, a uterine balloon (Bakri, Rüsch, condom catheter, etc.) can be used. The balloon is inserted via the uterine end and the stem passed down the cervical canal. It is inflated after closing the uterine incision and after inserting two simple vertical compression sutures. The balloon should be inflated whilst observing the closed uterine wound for any bleeding via the cervix. If there is no bleeding from the uterine incision wound or via the cervix and if there is no herniation of the balloon, then this 'sandwich technique' can be considered to be successful. A vaginal pack may help to keep the balloon *in situ* in the uterine cavity.

In the majority of circumstances, the above measures will stop bleeding during cesarean section. In a minority of cases, however, bleeding may still continue, and, in such circumstances, advanced procedures such as internal iliac artery ligation, as mentioned above, will help to control bleeding.

54

The Pelvic Pressure Pack and the Uterovaginal Balloon System

G. A. Dildy III

When pharmacologic and conservative surgical interventions fail to correct postpartum hemorrhage (PPH), hysterectomy most often becomes the option of last resort[1]. Contemporary reports on the incidence of obstetric hysterectomy range between 0.29 and 0.77 per 1000 deliveries[2–7]. Under these circumstances, a moderately busy obstetric unit with 4000 deliveries per year may perform as many as three emergency hysterectomies annually. This is especially true for women undergoing multiple repeat cesarean deliveries. Silver and colleagues reported in the Maternal–Fetal Medicine Units Network examination of 30,132 women undergoing cesarean delivery, that hysterectomy was required in 0.65% of first, 0.42% of second, 0.90% of third, 2.41% of fourth, 3.49% of fifth, and 8.99% of sixth or greater number cesarean deliveries[8].

A systematic review of 981 cases of emergency postpartum hysterectomy reported an overall maternal mortality rate of 2.6%[9]. The maternal mortality associated with obstetric hysterectomy is higher (4–12.5%) in resource poor countries[7,10], but not unheard of (0–4%) in developed areas[4,8,11] for a number of reasons, often relating to the moribund condition of the patient when the operation commences, the difficulty of the procedure itself, particularly in the presence of factors which make the anatomy unclear, and the extent of the bleeding which may accompany the operation. Indeed, Clark and colleagues reported an average estimated blood loss of 3.5 liters during emergency obstetric hysterectomy[12]. Furthermore, as the original extent of bleeding may have been underestimated, thus delaying resuscitation, surgical intervention and administration of blood component therapy, uncontrollable hemorrhage may be the event that mandates the hysterectomy[13–15]. As recounted in several other chapters in this Textbook, severe hemorrhage and emergency hysterectomy are often accompanied by secondary coagulopathy. In the setting of acquired coagulopathy, posthysterectomy bleeding may continue despite secure surgical pedicles, much to the consternation of the surgeon and the members of the operating team.

Abdominal and pelvic postsurgical packing is an old concept and one that has been used to control hemorrhage from a variety of sources, including liver trauma[16], pre-eclampsia-induced hepatic rupture[17], rectal cancer[18], gynecologic cancer[19] and, more recently, retroperitoneal packing as a part of damage-control surgery for trauma-related pelvic fracture management[20–22]. Various packing methods have been described, such as the 'bowel bag'[19] or packing with dry laparotomy packs[23]. These methods, however, require re-laparotomy after initial stabilization to remove the packing materials. Other reported methods for packing, albeit not requiring re-laparotomy but with limited cumulative obstetric experience, include transcutaneous placement of an inflated condom over a 22-Fr catheter[24] or ribbon gauze within a Penrose drain[25].

In 1926, Logothetopoulos described a pack for the management of uncontrolled posthysterectomy pelvic bleeding[26]. This technique has subsequently been called the mushroom, parachute, umbrella, pelvic pressure, or Logothetopoulos pack. It is important to note that the pelvic pressure pack described is applied posthysterectomy, and it should not be confused, as it often is, with uterine packing[27], or with various intra-uterine balloons for treatment of PPH due to uterine atony or placental site bleeding which are described in Chapters 47, 48 and 54 of this volume[28–30].

The pelvic pressure pack controls hemorrhage from large raw surfaces, venous plexuses and inaccessible areas by exerting well distributed pressure, compressing bleeding areas against the bony and fascial resistance of the pelvis[31,32]. According to Parente and colleagues, several references to the pelvic pressure pack appeared in European medical journals during the decades following the original report[31]. The first reported cases appearing in the English literature were not until the 1960s, and these pertained specifically to gynecologic posthysterectomy hemorrhage[31,32]; since then, several case reports and a case series for obstetric posthysterectomy bleeding have been published. Table 1 summarizes these cases, 23 for control of gynecologic and 13 for control of obstetric posthysterectomy hemorrhage, with success rates of 100% and 85%, respectively. Admittedly, accurate success rates are difficult to determine based on rare cases collected retrospectively, with possible underreporting of unfavorable outcomes. Nonetheless, successful control of severe hemorrhage appears to have been achieved in the majority of cases.

As seen in Figure 1, the pack is constructed by filling a bag (we prefer a sterile X-ray cassette drape, but other materials also have been described) with gauze rolls tied end-to-end (in this case, five 11.4 cm × 2.8 m Kerlix rolls), starting at the 'dome' of the pack (A), with the 'tail' of the gauze protruding from the 'neck' of the pack (B–D). Gauze should be removed, as visually indicated, from the pack before placement, in order to fit the true pelvis.

The pack is introduced transabdominally in the posthysterectomy patient into the pelvis (Figure 2), and the 'neck' is delivered transvaginally through the introitus by passing a surgical clamp from below through the open vaginal cuff. The surgeon should avoid trapping small bowel behind the pack. Traction and resulting pressure are applied to the pack by tying intravenous (IV) tubing to the neck of the pack and

suspending a 1-liter IV fluid bag off the foot of the bed. A 1-liter glass IV bottle and mild Trendelenburg position provide additional weight and traction if needed. The IV tubing or a cord can simply be hung over the foot of the bed, or over an orthopedic pulley attached to the foot of the bed. Compression of the pack can also be maintained by placing the 'neck' of the pack through a #80 doughnut pessary (not shown) applied flush against the perineum with a surgical clamp. However, caution must be taken to avoid perineal pressure necrosis.

We advise placement of an intraperitoneal large-gauge closed-system (e.g. Jackson–Pratt) drain to

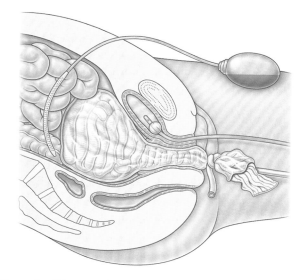

Figure 2 Diagram of the pelvic pressure pack *in situ*. See text for further explanation

Table 1 Summary of contemporary cases of the pelvic pressure pack for obstetric and gynecologic posthysterectomy hemorrhage. The success rate is defined as the pelvic pressure pack being the last intervention to control bleeding. Modified from Dildy *et al.*[37]

Series	Gynecology success rate	Obstetrics success rate
Parente, 1962[31]	14/14	–
Burchell, 1968[32]	8/8	–
Cassels, 1985[33]	–	1/1
Robie, 1990[34]	–	1/1
Hallak, 1991[35]	–	1/1
Howard, 2002[36]	–	1/1
Dildy, 2006[37]	1/1	7/9
Total	23/23 (100%)	11/13 (85%)

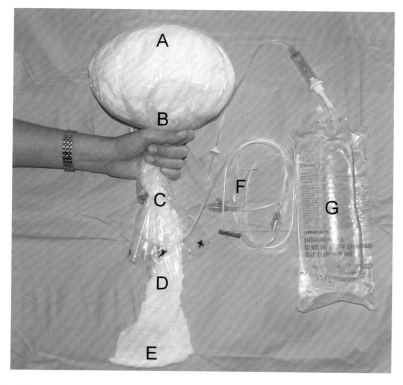

Figure 1 Photograph of a pelvic pressure pack, as constructed from an X-ray cassette drape, sterile gauze rolls and an intravenous infusion set-up. See text for further explanation

monitor for postoperative bleeding. An indwelling urinary catheter allows monitoring of urine output and avoidance of urinary outflow obstruction. After stabilization of the patient, an attempt to remove the pack transvaginally is made by slowly removing the gauze rolls under intravenous sedation, to allow gradual decompression without inciting bleeding. The optimal time to leave the pack *in situ* varies, but extended placement has certain risks (see below). Usually transvaginal pack removal is successful, but in some cases the pack will require removal by re-laparotomy or with laparoscopic assistance.

In one study of trauma patients suffering intra-abdominal hemorrhage, Garrison and colleagues found that patients who experienced hypothermia, refractory hypotension, coagulopathy and acidosis required *early packing* if they were to survive[38]. Thus, packing should be considered early on when homeostasis is significantly altered. Febrile morbidity is very common in these critically ill postoperative patients who have already received massive blood component therapy and then have a foreign body placed into a contaminated operative field[37]. Prophylactic broad-spectrum antibiotics should be administered whenever a pelvic pressure pack is placed, and this regimen should be continued after pack removal until the patient is afebrile for at least 24–48 hours. Another study of abdominal trauma patients showed those packed for up to 72 hours had lower abscess, sepsis and mortality rates than those packed for more than 72 hours[39]. Thus pack removal should be accomplished as soon as possible following stabilization.

A newly developed medical device, the Belfort-Dildy Obstetrical Tamponade System, trade named the ebb™ Complete Tamponade System (Glenveigh Medical, LLC, Chattanooga, TN)* was cleared by the US Food and Drug Administration (FDA) in 2010 for use in providing temporary control or reduction of *postpartum uterine bleeding* when conservative management is warranted[40]. The system (Figure 3) has an upper uterine balloon approved for filling to 750 ml and a lower vaginal balloon approved for filling to 300 ml. While not yet studied in, or cleared/approved for, the setting of posthysterectomy pelvic bleeding, future research may be warranted to determine whether this device may prove effective in controlling such cases.

In summary, the pelvic pressure pack is simple to construct from commonly available medical materials, and control of hemorrhage is successfully achieved in the majority of cases. If the pelvic pressure pack fails to control bleeding, other medical[41], surgical[42], or interventional radiology[43] approaches will be necessary to ultimately control bleeding. The pelvic pressure pack should be particularly useful in developing countries where more advanced surgical skills for pelvic vascular

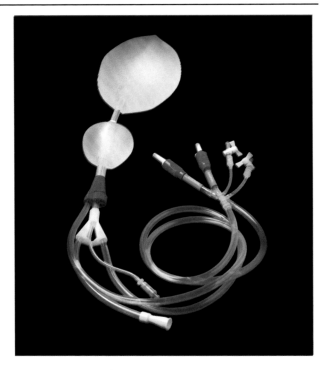

Figure 3 The Belfort-Dildy Obstetrical Tamponade System, trade named the ebb™ Complete Tamponade System (Glenveigh Medical, LLC, Chattanooga, TN)

ligation and technologies, such as selective arterial embolization, are not readily available. In developed countries, the pelvic pressure pack may serve as a temporizing measure pending transport to a tertiary care facility. In the majority of instances, the pelvic pressure pack will afford transfer of the critically ill patient to a postsurgical recovery setting, where restoration of hemodynamic, thermal, hematologic and acid–base homeostasis can be accomplished.

References

1. Dildy GA 3rd. Postpartum hemorrhage: new management options. Clin Obstet Gynecol 2002;45:330–44
2. Baskett TF. Emergency obstetric hysterectomy. J Obstet Gynaecol 2003;23:353–5
3. Eniola OA, Bewley S, Waterstone M, Hooper R, Wolfe CD. Obstetric hysterectomy in a population of South East England. J Obstet Gynaecol 2006;26:104–9
4. Kwee A, Bots ML, Visser GH, Bruinse HW. Emergency peripartum hysterectomy: A prospective study in The Netherlands. Eur J Obstet Gynecol Reprod Biol 2006;124:187–92
5. Lau WC, Fung HY, Rogers MS. Ten years experience of caesarean and postpartum hysterectomy in a teaching hospital in Hong Kong. Eur J Obstet Gynecol Reprod Biol 1997;74:133–7
6. Whiteman MK, Kuklina E, Hillis SD, et al. Incidence and determinants of peripartum hysterectomy. Obstet Gynecol 2006;108:1486–92
7. Yucel O, Ozdemir I, Yucel N, Somunkiran A. Emergency peripartum hysterectomy: a 9-year review. Arch Gynecol Obstet 2006;274:84–7

*Disclosure: As the name of the device indicates, the author of this chapter, Gary A. Dildy, MD, is one of the co-inventors (along with Michael A. Belfort, MD, PhD) of this medical device. As such, and in the interest of full disclosure, the author wishes to note that he has a personal financial interest in the device's commercialization.

8. Silver RM, Landon MB, Rouse DJ, et al. Maternal morbidity associated with multiple repeat cesarean deliveries. Obstet Gynecol 2006;107:1226–32

9. Rossi AC, Lee RH, Chmait RH. Emergency postpartum hysterectomy for uncontrolled postpartum bleeding: a systematic review. Obstet Gynecol 2010;115:637–44

10. Okogbenin SA, Gharoro EP, Otoide VO, Okonta PI. Obstetric hysterectomy: fifteen years' experience in a Nigerian tertiary centre. J Obstet Gynaecol 2003;23:356–9

11. Knight M, Kurinczuk JJ, Spark P, Brocklehurst P. Emergency postpartum hysterectomy for uncontrolled postpartum bleeding: a systematic review. Obstet Gynecol 2010;115:1306–7; author reply 7

12. Clark SL, Yeh SY, Phelan JP, Bruce S, Paul RH. Emergency hysterectomy for obstetric hemorrhage. Obstet Gynecol 1984;64:376–80

13. Dildy GA 3rd, Paine AR, George NC, Velasco C. Estimating blood loss: can teaching significantly improve visual estimation? Obstet Gynecol 2004;104:601–6

14. Stafford I, Dildy GA, Clark SL, Belfort MA. Visually estimated and calculated blood loss in vaginal and cesarean delivery. Am J Obstet Gynecol 2008;199:519 e1–7

15. Clark SL, Belfort MA, Dildy GA, Herbst MA, Meyers JA, Hankins GD. Maternal death in the 21st century: causes, prevention, and relationship to cesarean delivery. Am J Obstet Gynecol 2008;199:36 e1–5; discussion 91–2 e7–11

16. Feliciano DV, Mattox KL, Burch JM, Bitondo CG, Jordan GL Jr. Packing for control of hepatic hemorrhage. J Trauma 1986;26:738–43

17. Smith LG Jr, Moise KJ Jr, Dildy GA 3rd, Carpenter RJ Jr. Spontaneous rupture of liver during pregnancy: current therapy. Obstet Gynecol 1991;77:171–5

18. Zama N, Fazio VW, Jagelman DG, Lavery IC, Weakley FL, Church JM. Efficacy of pelvic packing in maintaining hemostasis after rectal excision for cancer. Dis Colon Rectum 1988;31:923–8

19. Finan MA, Fiorica JV, Hoffman MS, et al. Massive pelvic hemorrhage during gynecologic cancer surgery: "pack and go back". Gynecol Oncol 1996;62:390–5

20. Bach A, Bendix J, Hougaard K, Christensen EF. Retroperitoneal packing as part of damage control surgery in a Danish trauma centre–fast, effective, and cost-effective. Scand J Trauma Resusc Emerg Med 2008;16:4

21. Osborn PM, Smith WR, Moore EE, et al. Direct retroperitoneal pelvic packing versus pelvic angiography: A comparison of two management protocols for haemodynamically unstable pelvic fractures. Injury 2009;40:54–60

22. Papakostidis C, Giannoudis PV. Pelvic ring injuries with haemodynamic instability: efficacy of pelvic packing, a systematic review. Injury 2009;40 Suppl 4:S53–61

23. Ghourab S, Al-Nuaim L, Al-Jabari A, et al. Abdomino-pelvic packing to control severe haemorrhage following caesarean hysterectomy. J Obstet Gynaecol 1999;19:155–8

24. Luijendijk RW, JN IJ, Jeekel J, Bruining HA. An inflated condom as a packing device for control of haemorrhage. Br J Surg 1994;81:270

25. Awonuga AO, Merhi ZO, Khulpateea N. Abdominal packing for intractable obstetrical and gynecologic hemorrhage. Int J Gynaecol Obstet 2006;93:160–3

26. Logothetopulos K. Eine absolut sichere blutstillungsmethode bei vaginalen und abdominalen gynakologischen operationen. [An absolutely certain method of stopping bleeding during abdominal and vaginal operations.]. Zentralbl Gynakol 1926;50:3202–4

27. Maier RC. Control of postpartum hemorrhage with uterine packing. Am J Obstet Gynecol 1993;169:317–21; discussion 21–3

28. Katesmark M, Brown R, Raju KS. Successful use of a Sengstaken-Blakemore tube to control massive postpartum haemorrhage. Br J Obstet Gynaecol 1994;101:259–60

29. Johanson R, Kumar M, Obhrai M, Young P. Management of massive postpartum haemorrhage: use of a hydrostatic balloon catheter to avoid laparotomy. BJOG 2001;108:420–2

30. Bakri YN, Amri A, Abdul Jabbar F. Tamponade-balloon for obstetrical bleeding. Int J Gynaecol Obstet 2001;74:139–42

31. Parente JT, Dlugi H, Weingold AB. Pelvic hemostasis: a new technic and pack. Obstet Gynecol 1962;19:218–21

32. Burchell RC. The umbrella pack to control pelvic hemorrhage. Conn Med 1968;32:734–6

33. Cassels JW Jr, Greenberg H, Otterson WN. Pelvic tamponade in puerperal hemorrhage. A case report. J Reprod Med 1985;30:689–92

34. Robie GF, Morgan MA, Payne GG Jr, Wasemiller-Smith L. Logothetopulos pack for the management of uncontrollable postpartum hemorrhage. Am J Perinatol 1990;7:327–8

35. Hallak M, Dildy GA 3rd, Hurley TJ, Moise KJ Jr. Transvaginal pressure pack for life-threatening pelvic hemorrhage secondary to placenta accreta. Obstet Gynecol 1991;78:938–40

36. Howard RJ, Straughn JM Jr, Huh WK, Rouse DJ. Pelvic umbrella pack for refractory obstetric hemorrhage secondary to posterior uterine rupture. Obstet Gynecol 2002;100:1061–3

37. Dildy GA, Scott JR, Saffer CS, Belfort MA. An effective pressure pack for severe pelvic hemorrhage. Obstet Gynecol 2006;108:1222–6

38. Garrison JR, Richardson JD, Hilakos AS, et al. Predicting the need to pack early for severe intra-abdominal hemorrhage. J Trauma 1996;40:923–7; discussion 7–9

39. Abikhaled JA, Granchi TS, Wall MJ, Hirshberg A, Mattox KL. Prolonged abdominal packing for trauma is associated with increased morbidity and mortality. Am Surg 1997;63:1109–12; discussion 12–3

40. FDA. Safety and effectiveness. http://www.accessdata.fda.gov/cdrh_docs/pdf9/K091958.pdf

41. Bouwmeester FW, Jonkhoff AR, Verheijen RH, van Geijn HP. Successful treatment of life-threatening postpartum hemorrhage with recombinant activated factor VII. Obstet Gynecol 2003;101:1174–6

42. Clark SL, Phelan JP, Yeh SY, Bruce SR, Paul RH. Hypogastric artery ligation for obstetric hemorrhage. Obstet Gynecol 1985;66:353–6

43. Vedantham S, Goodwin SC, McLucas B, Mohr G. Uterine artery embolization: an underused method of controlling pelvic hemorrhage. Am J Obstet Gynecol 1997;176:938–48

55

Peripartum Hysterectomy

T. F. Baskett

INTRODUCTION

Emergency peripartum hysterectomy is an unequivocal marker of severe maternal morbidity and, in many respects, the treatment of last resort for severe postpartum hemorrhage (PPH)[1]. Between 2001 and 2010, 32 reports of peripartum hysterectomy have been identified and reviewed[2–33]. Table 1 provides a summary of the maternal outcomes in these reports. A number of consistent factors emerge from this review. There is a preponderance of cesarean deliveries in both the index and previous pregnancies, and this association was established in several studies[3,5–8,10,14,16,19–24,30]. The main indications for hysterectomy were almost evenly divided between abnormal placentation (usually placenta previa and/or accreta) and uterine atony, although two reports from Africa cite uterine rupture as the primary indication[3,33].

The range of prevalence is wide (0.2–5.4/1000), with the higher figures usually found in low-resource countries. Furthermore, most reports were hospital-based and high risk referral patterns were likely to influence this figure. Three population-based studies show prevalence at the lower end of the scale: 0.3/1000 in The Netherlands[19], 0.5/1000 in Israel[10] and 0.5/1000 in one Canadian province[6].

The incidence of peripartum hysterectomy is increasing in some countries, due to higher cesarean delivery rates and concomitant increases in placenta previa and/or accreta in subsequent pregnancies. In Canada from 1991 to 2000, the peripartum hysterectomy rate almost doubled from 0.26/1000 deliveries to 0.46/1000 (RR 1.7, 95% CI 1.48–2.08)[34]. There are reasons to believe that obstetric hysterectomy rates may continue to rise as other factors contribute to the increasing cesarean delivery rate. Multiple pregnancy rates are rising due to assisted reproductive treatments, and the need for critical care and hysterectomy is higher in these women[15,35]. Francois *et al.* found a six-fold increased risk of emergency peripartum hysterectomy in multiple compared with singleton pregnancies, and an almost 24-fold increase in higher order multiple pregnancies[15]. Other changing maternal demographic factors, such as increasing age and obesity also contribute to rising cesarean delivery rates.

The incidence of hysterectomy in women having their first delivery was only recorded in five reports, in which the range was 18–43% and the average 28.4%[5,6,11,22,29]. A study of primigravid women at a teaching hospital in Ghana found an incidence of peripartum hysterectomy of about 1 in 1000 (39 of 36,550) nulliparous deliveries[36].

Maternal mortality in this review was documented to have a wide range, from zero to 23.8%; with deaths tending to occur in, but not limited to, low-resource areas. Severe maternal morbidity was high in all reports and manifest by blood transfusion, disseminated intravascular coagulation (DIC), injury to the bladder and ureter, reoperation, sepsis and the need for intensive care, as outlined in Table 1.

This chapter describes emergency hysterectomy in the immediate postpartum period following vaginal or cesarean delivery.

Table 1 Summary of maternal outcomes in 32 reports of peripartum hysterectomy from 2001 to 2010[2–33]

Outcome	Incidence	
	Mean	*Range*
Prevalence of peripartum hysterectomy (32)*	1.2/1000	0.2–5.4/1000
Primary indication (32)		
Abnormal placentation (16)†		
Atonic PPH (14)		
Uterine rupture (2)		
Primigravid (5)	28.4%	18–43%
Subtotal hysterectomy (9)	57.1%	6–96.5%
Maternal mortality (25)	8.9%	2.8–23.8%
No deaths in (13)		
Deaths in (12)		
Maternal morbidity		
Blood transfusion (7)	90.2%	72–100%
Bladder/ureter injury (7)	10.8%	5.6–21%
Reoperation (3)	23.6%	7.8–38%
Intensive care (7)	41%	17.6–77%

*Number of papers reporting the outcome is in parentheses
†Placenta previa and/or accreta, abruptio placentae

INDICATIONS

By far the most common indication for hysterectomy is hemorrhage associated with the following conditions.

Abnormal placentation

In developed countries, placenta previa, with or without associated accreta, is the most common indication for hysterectomy. This is secondary to the rising incidence of these conditions associated with increasing numbers of women previously delivered by cesarean section. Despite the fact that numerous techniques aimed at preserving the uterus have been proposed and are discussed in this book, hysterectomy is still used in the majority of hospitals to stem the sometimes frightening hemorrhage associated with placenta previa or accreta.

In addition, on rare occasions, concealed abruptio placentae may be associated with extravasation of blood into and through the full thickness of the myometrium (Couvelaire uterus) to such an extent as to make it unresponsive to oxytocic drugs, thus necessitating hysterectomy. It must be emphasized, however, that in the majority of cases of abruptio placentae with Couvelaire uterus, the response to oxytocic drugs is appropriate and the hemorrhage is due to DIC rather than failure of the uterus to contract.

Uterine atony

As outlined elsewhere in this book (see chapters in Section 8), the range of modern oxytocic drugs has greatly improved the management of uterine atony. Nonetheless, there are times when the uterus is refractory to all such agents. This is most commonly present in the prolonged, augmented and/or obstructed labor: simply stated, the exhausted and infected uterus may be unresponsive to oxytocic agents. The majority of these cases are seen at the time of cesarean section for dystocia or cephalopelvic disproportion.

Uterine rupture

The most common cause of complete uterine rupture is a tear within a previous cesarean section scar. If the rupture is extensive and hemorrhage cannot be contained by suture of the lacerated area, hysterectomy may be necessary. In addition, rupture of the intact uterus can occur in multiparous women in response to inappropriate use of oxytocic agents in the first and second stages of labor. In remote areas with limited resources uterine rupture can occur in obstructed, multiparous labor.

Uterine trauma

Traumatic rupture, that is, perforation or laceration of the uterus, can occur with a variety of obstetric manipulations, including internal version and breech extraction, especially in obstructed labor; instrumental manipulation, such as the classical application of the anterior blade of Kielland's forceps; manual exploration of the uterus and manual removal of the placenta or its fragments after obstructed labor with a ballooned and thin lower uterine segment; and during curettage for secondary postpartum hemorrhage.

Cesarean section in the second stage of labor with the fetal head deeply impacted in the vagina may be associated with lateral extension of the lower uterine segment incision into the major vessels[37]. This is more likely if the surgeon has used a straight line as opposed to a curved or 'smile' incision. On rare occasions, the extent of this tear may necessitate hysterectomy, especially if one or both uterine arteries are lacerated and a hematoma obscures the surgical repair. External traumas, such as assault, a fall or motor vehicle accident, are relatively rare causes of uterine perforation and rupture.

Sepsis

In the era of modern antibiotics, sepsis is not a common reason for emergency hysterectomy. However, it still may be necessary in cases with extensive uterine sepsis, particularly with clostridial infections and myometrial abscess formation, in which antibiotic treatment fails to control the infection. Other septic causes of secondary PPH include cesarean scar infection and necrosis, arteriovenous fistula formation secondary to uterine trauma and infection, and endomyometritis associated with retained placental fragments followed by hemorrhage. All may rarely require hysterectomy.

SURGICAL PRINCIPLES

Although the technique of obstetric hysterectomy is similar in principle to that of abdominal hysterectomy in gynecology, numerous anatomical and physiological changes in pregnancy create potential surgical difficulties.

(1) The uterine and ovarian vessels are enlarged and distended, often markedly so, and the adjacent pelvic tissues are edematous and friable.

(2) Abdominal entry may have been via Pfannenstiel or lower midline incision, depending on the urgency and speed required. Many surgeons prefer the midline incision because it provides better exposure.

(3) Maneuvers to obtain hemostasis depend on the cause of the hemorrhage. In cases of uterine rupture, Green-Armytage clamps or sponge forceps can be used to compress the bleeding edges of torn uterine muscle. The uterus should be eventrated from the abdominal wound. The structures of the adnexa on each side are pulled laterally by an assistant, and the surgeon applies straight clamps adjacent to the top sides of the uterus to include the round ligament, the Fallopian tube and the utero-ovarian ligament. This serves to control the collateral blood flow to the uterus from the ovarian arteries. Using transillumination, the avascular spaces in the broad ligament, roughly opposite the level of a transverse lower segment cesarean

incision, should be identified and a catheter passed through on each side to encircle the lower uterine segment just above the cervix. This should be twisted tightly and closed around the lower uterine segment with a clamp, thereby compressing the uterine arteries. These two maneuvers, if properly applied, should occlude the main collateral ovarian and uterine artery supply to the uterus (see Chapter 1).

(4) The vascular pedicles are thick and edematous and should be double clamped. Remove the proximal clamp first and apply a free tie, and then replace the distal clamp with a transfixing suture. The proximal free tie should ensure that there is no hematoma formation in the base of the pedicle.

(5) If the cervix and paracolpos are not involved as the source of hemorrhage, subtotal hysterectomy should be adequate to achieve hemostasis, the objective of the intervention. Additionally it is safer, faster, easier to perform and less likely to injure the bladder or ureters than total hysterectomy. However, if the lower segment and paracolpos are involved in the hemorrhage, such as in cases of placenta previa, total hysterectomy will be necessary for hemostasis.

(6) The ureters should be avoided by placing all clamps medial to those used to secure the uterine arteries.

(7) It may be difficult to identify the cervix, particularly when the hysterectomy is being performed at full cervical dilatation. If a uterine incision has been made, a finger can be placed through this and hooked up to identify the cervical rim. It is safest to enter the vagina posteriorly, identify the rim of the cervix and then proceed anteriorly.

(8) The bladder is particularly vulnerable in cases previously delivered by cesarean section, as it may be adherent to the lower uterine segment and cervix. It is therefore essential to check the integrity of the bladder intraoperatively. This can be done by manipulating the bulb of the Foley catheter to see if it is visible through the bladder wall. The bladder also can be filled with a colored fluid such as methylene blue or sterile milk taken from the neonatal nursery. The latter is preferable as it does not cause permanent staining of the tissues. Accordingly, after repair of any bladder injury, it is easier to check its integrity by instillation of milk into the bladder. Tears in the bladder should be repaired with two layers of 3/0 polyglactin (Vicryl) or equivalent suture. Otherwise, No. 1 polyglactin (Vicryl) or equivalent is used throughout the procedure.

(9) If the integrity of the ureters is in doubt, and after any extensive repair of bladder injury, postoperative cystoscopy can confirm that they are intact by observing urine coming from each ureteric orifice; this test may be facilitated by giving intravenous indigo carmine and waiting 10–15 min.

(10) Within the context of the emergency situation and the available resources, it is best to diagnose and deal with any bladder or ureteric injury at the time of the hysterectomy. If lower urinary tract injuries are not diagnosed until the postoperative period, clinical morbidity is increased, diagnostic and surgical management is more complex, and litigation more likely[38].

(11) In rare cases following hysterectomy traumatized tissues at the base of the pelvis may continue to bleed despite ligation of obvious bleeding pedicles. This bleeding is usually, but not always, associated with DIC. In these cases the application of a pelvic pressure pack can be life-saving and provide hemostasis, either permanent or temporary, until hematological stability and/or vascular embolization is achieved[39]. The details of applying a pelvic pressure pack are described in Chapter 54.

(12) Perioperative antibiotic prophylaxis should be continued for 24–48 hours. Thromboprophylaxis with heparin should be instituted as soon as one is satisfied that hemostasis is secure.

(13) Detailed, timed postoperative notes should be made to include the preoperative events, indications for hysterectomy and the surgical details.

(14) After the initial postoperative recovery, the woman should receive a comprehensive outline of events from an experienced obstetrician. Many women are emotionally traumatized by the rapid sequence of major complications, culminating in the loss of her uterus; a sympathetic explanation and supportive follow-up are necessary.

In a number of series, as many as 25% of women who received an emergency obstetric hysterectomy were primigravid, for whom the fertility-ending nature of the procedure can be devastating. Therefore, particularly in this group of women, obstetricians should be familiar with and be prepared to perform alternative procedures to control the hemorrhage. The application of other techniques to arrest hemorrhage that can be both life-saving and uterus-preserving are outlined in several chapters in this book. When conditions are recognized in the antenatal period that may lead to increased risk of severe obstetric hemorrhage, such as placenta previa and/or accreta, referral of these cases to hospitals with the equipment and personnel to provide the alternative techniques to hysterectomy should be undertaken where feasible.

Ultimately, one has to strike a balance between spending excessive time on alternative techniques that are proving ineffective, leading to delay, further hemorrhage and probably DIC, and moving to the definitive and life-saving hysterectomy. Such is the art of obstetric judgment in trying circumstances.

References

1. Baskett TF. Epidemiology of obstetric critical care. Best Pract Res Clin Obstet Gynaecol 2008;22:763–74
2. Engelsen IB, Albrechsten S, Iverson OE, Peripartum hysterectomy – incidence and maternal morbidity. Acta Obstet Gynaecol Scand 2001;80:409–12
3. Sebitloane MH, Moodley J. Emergency peripartum hysterectomy. East Afr Med J 2001;78:70–4
4. Wenham J, Matijevic R. Post-partum hysterectomies: revisited. J Perinat Med 2001;29:260–5
5. Kastner ES, Figueroa R, Garry D, Maulik D. Emergency peripartum hysterectomy:experience at a community teaching hospital. Obstet Gynecol 2002;99:971–5
6. Baskett TF. Emergency obstetric hysterectomy. J Obstet Gynaecol 2003;23:353–5
7. Bai SW, Lee HJ, Cho JS, Park YW, Kim SK, Park KH. Peripartum hysterectomy and associated factors. J Reprod Med 2003;48:148–52
8. Kacmar J, Bhimani L, Boyd M, Shah-Hosseini R, Peipert J. Route of delivery as a risk for emergent peripartum hysterectomy: a case-control study. Obstet Gynecol 2003;102:141–5
9. Rabenda-Lacka K, Wilczyñski J, Radoch Z, Breborowicz GH. Obstetrical hysterectomy. Ginekol Pol 2003;74:1521–5
10. Sheiner E, Levy A, Katz M, Mazor M. Identifying risk factors for peripartum cesarean hysterectomy. A population-based study. J Reprod Med 2003;48:622–6
11. Yamani Zamzami TY. Indications of emergency peripartum hysterectomy: review of 17 cases. Arch Gynecol Obstet. 2003;268:131–5
12. El-Jallad MF, Zayed F, Al-Rimawi HS. Emergency peripartum hysterectomy in Northern Jordan: indications and obstetric outcome (an 8-year review). Arch Gynecol Obstet 2004;270:271–3
13. Ezech OC, Kalu BK, Njokanma FO, Nwokoro CA, Okeke GC. Emergency peripartum hysterectomy in a Nigerian hospital: a 20-year review. J Obstet Gynaecol 2004;24:372–3
14. Forna F, Miles AM, Jamieson DJ. Emergency peripartum hysterectomy: a comparison of cesarean and postpartum hysterectomy. Am J Obstet Gynecol 2004;190:1440–4
15. Francois K, Ortiz J, Harris C, Foley MR, Elliott JP. Is peripartum hysterectomy more common in multiple gestations? Obstet Gynecol 2005;105:1369–72
16. Eniola OA, Bewley S, Waterstone M, Hooper R, Wolfe CD. Obstetric hysterectomy in a population of South East England. J Obstet Gynaecol 2006;26:104–9
17. Ding DC, Hsu S, Chu TW, Chu TY. Emergency peripartum hysterectomy in a teaching hospital in Eastern Taiwan. J Obstet Gynaecol 2006;26:635–8
18. Katchy KC, Ziad F, Al Nashmi N, Diejomaoh MF. Emergency obstetric hysterectomy in Kuwait: a clinico pathological analysis. Arch Gynecol Obstet 2006;273:360–5
19. Kwee A, Bots ML, Visser GH, Bruinse HW. Emergency peripartum hysterectomy: a prospective study in The Netherlands. Eur J Obstet Gynecol Reprod Biol 2006;124:187–92
20. Whiteman MK, Kuklina E, Hillis SD, Jamieson DJ, Meikle SF, Posner SF. Incidence and determinants of peripartum hysterectomy. Obstet Gynecol 2006;108:1486–92
21. Yoong W, Massish N, Oluwu A. Obstetric hysterectomy: changing trends over 20 years in a multiethnic high risk population. Arch Gynecol Obstet 2006;274:37–40
22. Daskalakis G, Anastasakis E, Papantoniou N, Mesogitis S, Theodora M, Antsaklis A. Emergency obstetric hysterectomy. Acta Obstet Gynecol Scand 2007;86:223–7
23. Habek D, Becareviç R. Emergency peripartum hysterectomy in a tertiary obstetric center: 8-year evaluation. Fetal Diagn Ther 2007;22:139–42
24. Smith J, Mousa HA. Peripartum hysterectomy for primary postpartum haemorrhage: Incidence and maternal morbidity. J Obstet Gynaecol 2007;27:44–7
25. Kayabasoglu F, Guzin K, Aydogdu S, Sezginsoy S, Turkgeldi L, Gunduz G. Emergency peripartum hysterectomy in a tertiary Istanbul hospital. Arch Gynecol Obstet 2008;278:251–6
26. Rahman J, Al-Ali M, Qutub HO, Al-Suleiman SS, Al-Jama FE, Rahman MS. Emergency obstetric hysterectomy in a university hospital: A 25-year review. J Obstet Gynaecol 2008;28:69–72
27. Umezurike CC, Feyi-Waboso PA, Adisa CA. Peripartum hysterectomy in Aba southeastern Nigeria. Aust NZ J Obstet Gynaecol 2008;48:580–2
28. Knight M, Kuriuczuk JJ, Spark P, Brocklehurst P. Cesarean delivery and peripartum hysterectomy. Obstet Gynecol 2008; 111:97–105
29. Glaze S, Ekwalanga P, Roberts G, Lange I, Birch C, Rosengarten A et al. Peripartum hysterectomy, 1999 to 2006. Obstet Gynecol 2008;111:732–8
30. Güngördük K, Yildirim G, Dugan N, Polat I, Sudolmus S, Ark C. Peripartum hysterectomy in Turkey: a case-control study. J Obstet Gynaecol 2009;29:722–8
31. Lone F, Sultan AH, Thakar R, Beggs A. Risk factors and management patterns for emergency obstetric hysterectomy over 2 decades. Int J Gynaecol Obstet 2010;109:12–5
32. Mlyncek M, Kellner M, Uharcek P, Matejka M, Lajtman E, Boledovicová M. Peripartum hysterectomy – an audit in Slovakia in 2007. Ceska Gynekol 2010;75:88–92
33. Rabiu KA, Akinlusi FM, Adewunmi AA, Akinola OI. Emergency peripartum hysterectomy in a tertiary hospital in Lagos, Nigeria: a five-year review. Trop Doct 2010;40:1–4
34. Wen SW, Huang L, Liston RM, Heaman M, Baskett TF, Rusen ID. Severe maternal mortality in Canada, 1991–2001. Can Med Assoc J 2005;173:759–63
35. Baskett TF, O'Connell CM. Maternal critical care in obstetrics. J Obstet Gynaecol Can 2009;31:48–53
36. Seffah JD, Kwame-Aryee RA. Emergency peripartum hysterectomy in the nulliparous patient. Int J Gynaecol Obstet 2007;97:45–6
37. Allen VM, O'Connell CM, Baskett TF. Maternal and perinatal morbidity of caesarean delivery at full cervical dilatation compared with caesarean delivery in the first stage of labour. Br J Obstet Gynaecol 2005;112:986–90
38. Gilmour DT, Baskett TF. Disability and litigation from urinary tract injuries at benign gynaecological surgery in Canada. Obstet Gynecol 2005;105:109–14
39. Dildy GA, Scott JR, Saffer CS, Belfort MA. An effective pressure pack for severe pelvic haemorrhage. Obstet Gynecol 2006;108:1222–6

56

The Management of Secondary Postpartum Hemorrhage

K. M. Groom and T. Z. Jacobson

INTRODUCTION

Secondary postpartum hemorrhage (PPH) is defined as excessive vaginal bleeding from 24 h after delivery up to 6 weeks postpartum[1]. Unlike the definition of primary PPH, there is no clear or standard definition for quantity of the blood loss associated with secondary PPH, and clinical expressions of this definition vary from 'increased lochia' to massive bleeding. The diagnosis is therefore all too often subjective, which may account for the numerous variations in reported incidence. Overall, the reported incidence of secondary PPH in the developed world varies from 0.47% to 1.44%[2,3].

The etiology of secondary PPH is diverse, and management is dependent on identifying the cause and tailoring treatment appropriately (Table 1). In contrast to primary PPH, the published work on the management of secondary PPH is limited[4]. However, with declining maternal mortality rates in many parts of the world, interest in and attention to maternal morbidity and the important topic of management of secondary PPH is increasing. The majority of cases are associated with minor morbidities but may still require re-admission to hospital, use of antibiotics and surgical intervention. In more extreme cases, major morbidity may require hysterectomy, arterial ligation or radiological intervention[5]. Despite the use of all available interventions, maternal death may still result from massive secondary PPH.

ETIOLOGY OF SECONDARY POSTPARTUM HEMORRHAGE

Subinvolution/uterine atony

The major cause of secondary PPH is uterine subinvolution (Table 1). Distinction should be made between the use of this term to describe the finding of a uterine fundus that is not resolving toward its pre-pregnancy size and the histological condition of failure of obliteration of blood vessels underlying the placental site, the latter leading to prolonged bleeding (see Chapter 22)[6]. One recent case report of a maternal death due to hemorrhage 8 days postpartum confirmed a failure of subinvolution of the uteroplacental arteries with large, dilated spiral arteries in the superficial myometrium at the placental implantation site containing partially occluding thrombi[7]. The main causes of this are infection, inflammation (endometritis) and retained placental tissue. Endometritis is more common following prolonged rupture of membranes, prolonged labor, emergency cesarean section or with a retained placenta that had required manual removal. A history of offensive lochia, maternal pyrexia and uterine tenderness is often present, and retained placental tissue is more common in women with a previous history of retained placenta or if there were concerns at the time of delivery of incomplete placenta and/or membranes. The condition is less likely following delivery by cesarean section (Table 2). Differentiation between the two causes is often difficult and both conditions may coexist.

Lower genital tract trauma

Missed vaginal lacerations and hematomas may present as secondary PPH. These are often associated with traumatic deliveries or those requiring ventouse or forceps. Both usually present within the first few days after delivery. Infected suture lines and episiotomy sites may lead to wound breakdown and result in excessive vaginal bleeding.

Placental abnormalities

Placenta accreta, increta and percreta are all known causes of massive primary PPH. When managed conservatively with placental tissue left *in situ* (with or without methotrexate therapy), they can also be associated with delayed bleeding and the need for hysterectomy[8,9] (see Section 5).

Uterine abnormalities

Fibroids usually are associated with primary PPH. They cause uterine enlargement and prevent uterine involution, therefore leading to prolonged bleeding from the placental bed. More rarely, they can be associated with secondary PPH. Fibroids have usually been identified by ultrasound in the antenatal period.

Vascular abnormalities

Abnormalities of uterine vasculature such as arteriovenous malformations and false aneurysms may also lead to secondary PPH. Arteriovenous malformations are due to an abnormal communication between an artery and vein with proliferation of each vessel with interconnecting fistulae. It is believed these malformations may result from venous sinuses becoming incorporated in scars within the myometrium after necrosis of the chorionic villi. The majority are acquired after pregnancy and may result from trophoblastic disease, previous uterine curettage, uterine or cervical malignancy[10,11] or cesarean section[12-15] (see Chapter 26). In particular, there should be a high index of suspicion of uterine artery pseudoaneurysm in women presenting with secondary PPH after cesarean section[16]. Diagnosis can be delayed for a considerable time, with one report describing a case of uterine artery pseudoaneurysm presenting 99 days after cesarean section[17]. Diagnosis is usually made using ultrasound with color Doppler analysis, angiography or computed tomography (CT).

Cesarean section wound dehiscence or surgical injury

Injury to pelvic blood vessels at the time of cesarean section[14] usually presents within 24 h. However, later presentations, in particular those causing broad ligament hematomas, have been described[5] and should be considered in women presenting acutely with signs of intra-abdominal hemorrhage. Delayed presentation of bleeding from non-union/dehiscence of the cesarean section uterine scar has also been described. This is believed to be due to local infection at the site of uterine closure causing erosion of blood vessels. In the cases reported, this led to massive PPH 2–3 weeks after cesarean section and the need for subtotal

Table 1 Causes of secondary PPH

Subinvolution of the uterus – retained placental tissue and/or endometritis, fibroid uterus
Lower genital tract lacerations/hematoma
Surgical injury
Dehiscence of cesarean section scar
Vascular abnormality – arteriovenous malformation
Placental abnormality – placenta accreta, percreta and increta
Choriocarcinoma
Coagulopathies, bleeding disorders, use of anticoagulants

---

hysterectomy[18]. Diagnosis of uterine dehiscence postcesarean section associated with infection has also been made at hysteroscopy[19], although causing less significant PPH and only requiring treatment with antibiotics.

Choriocarcinoma

The majority of cases of choriocarcinoma after a non-molar pregnancy present with secondary PPH or irregular vaginal bleeding[20]. In addition, secondary symptoms of metastatic disease may be present. The diagnosis is made by evaluation of serum human chorionic gonadotropin (hCG) levels, histological findings and radiological imaging including ultrasound, plain film X-ray and CT scan.

Bleeding disorders, coagulopathies and use of anticoagulants

Women with congenital hemorrhagic disorders such as von Willebrand's disease (quantitative or qualitative deficiency of von Willebrand factor), carriers of hemophilia A (factor VIII deficiency), hemophilia B (factor IX deficiency) and factor XI deficiency are at an increased risk of PPH. Often, these abnormalities are undetected until challenged by trauma, surgery or childbirth and thus may be undiagnosed prior to pregnancy. These women are not at increased risk of antepartum hemorrhage[21], but are at significant risk of both primary and secondary PPH with the risk of secondary PPH being greater than primary as the pregnancy-induced rise in maternal clotting factors falls after delivery.

The reported incidence for secondary PPH in these conditions is 20–28% for von Willebrand's disease, 11% for hemophilia carriers and 24% in factor XI deficiency[22-25]. Postpartum acquired hemophilia has also been described. This is a rare condition but can cause severe hemorrhage. It is caused by antibodies to factor VIII which partially or completely suppress factor VIII procoagulant activity in women with previously normal levels and activity of factor VIII. Bleeding usually commences within 3 months of delivery but may be delayed for up to 12 months[21]. The use of anticoagulants in the postpartum period may also cause delayed bleeding. In particular, women using warfarin should be carefully monitored and informed of the risks of hemorrhage.

Table 2 Risk factors for secondary PPH[4]

Pre-existing risk factors	Antepartum risk factors	Intrapartum risk factors	Postpartum risk factors
Maternal smoking at the time the antenatal history is taken	Prelabor rupture of membranes at term	Delivery by cesarean section	Primary postpartum hemorrhage
A previous history of secondary PPH	Threatened miscarriage	Precipitate labor of less than 2 hours	Not breastfeeding
Multiparous women	Multiple pregnancy	Prolonged third stage	Postnatal sepsis
	Antepartum hemorrhage	Incomplete placenta or membranes passed at birth, or both	
	Hospital admission during the third trimester		

MANAGEMENT OF SECONDARY POSTPARTUM HEMORRHAGE

Evidence regarding the management of secondary PPH is limited. A Cochrane review assessed all randomized or quasi-randomized comparisons of drug, surgical and placebo therapies or no treatment for secondary PPH. Forty-five papers were identified, but none met the inclusion criteria, and the review concluded there was no evidence from randomized trials to show the effects of treatments for secondary PPH[4]. The main aims of treatment are to provide basic resuscitation, establish a cause for the bleeding, and tailor the treatment (medical and/or surgical) according to the cause.

Resuscitation

Approximately 10% of cases present with massive hemorrhage[26] and require immediate attention. In these instances, resuscitation should be commenced prior to establishing a cause and should include the involvement of senior staff at the earliest opportunity. Restoration of circulating blood volume should be achieved by gaining intravenous access with two large-bore cannulae and administering intravenous fluids initially with physiological saline (up to 2 liters) and then with plasma expanders until blood is available. *There is considerable discussion in the recent literature that restoration of lost volume with plasma expanders delays the use of blood and that when necessary uncrossmatched blood but preferably type specific (Rh negative) can be used or O negative blood (see Chapter 4).* Blood should be obtained for full blood count, coagulation screen and crossmatch. High concentration oxygen (10–15 l/min) should be administered by a tight-fitting mask[27]. Close observation of vital signs including pulse, blood pressure, oxygen saturation and urine output should be maintained throughout resuscitation. *Blood and blood products should be given according to blood loss, rather than waiting and using the response to initial fluid administration and hemoglobin and coagulation results as the trigger for the infusion of blood.* Identification of the cause of bleeding should then be made and further management planned accordingly. In cases of less significant hemorrhage, basic resuscitation should be instigated as appropriate but blood transfusion should not be delayed whilst establishing a cause for the bleeding.

Clinical presentation

Ninety-five per cent of women with secondary PPH present within the first month after delivery, 19% within 7 days, 41% in 8–14 days, 23% in 15–21 days and 12% in 22–28 days[2]. The amount of blood loss at presentation varies but most patients are hemodynamically stable. A thorough history provides information relating to cause and should include details regarding parity, labor, mode of delivery, third-stage or puerperal complications and any relevant medical and family history.

Clinical signs and symptoms at the time of presentation may include offensive lochia, abdominal cramping, uterine tenderness, pyrexia, enlarged uterus and an open cervical os. Normal postpartum loss may continue beyond 6 weeks in up to 25% of women, especially if breastfeeding[26], and the first period may be heavy, prolonged and painful as a result of an anovulatory cycle. Women should be given this information during normal postpartum care to avoid unnecessary concern and presentation for medical investigation.

Investigations

Baseline blood tests should include full blood count, coagulation studies, C-reactive protein, a group and hold specimen, and serum hCG. Vaginal swabs should be taken at the time of examination for aerobic as well as anaerobic bacterial growth, including swabs from episiotomy or vaginal tear sites. In women with signs of infection, a mid-stream urine specimen should be collected and, if maternal temperature is more than 38°C, blood cultures should be obtained.

Ultrasound imaging of the pelvis should be considered if there are concerns of retained placental tissue. If this is obtained within 7–14 days of delivery, interpretation may be difficult as remaining blood clots may appear as mixed echogenic material in a similar manner to retained tissue. The use of duplex color Doppler helps to improve diagnostic accuracy in differentiating clot and tissue[28], as retained placental tissue will often maintain a blood supply unlike necrotic decidua and clot[29].

The over-diagnosis of retained placental tissue on ultrasound may lead to unnecessary surgical intervention and its potential complications. However, ultrasound does have significant benefits, as it has a good negative predictive value and therefore is helpful in excluding a diagnosis of retained placental tissue. Neill and colleagues assessed 53 women undergoing ultrasound for secondary PPH. Definitive diagnosis of retained placental tissue was made either histologically or, in those women managed conservatively, absence of retained tissue was assumed if bleeding diminished within 1 week. In their hands, ultrasound assessment had a positive predictive value of 46% (95% confidence interval (CI) 31–70%), a negative predictive value of 96% (95% CI 88–100%), with a sensitivity of 93% (95% CI 80–100%) and a specificity of 62% (95% CI 48–79%)[30] (Table 3).

This study also suggested that a standardized approach to reporting an ultrasound investigation of secondary PPH would be helpful. This is shown in Table 3. Additional imaging should also be considered for specific causes of secondary PPH such as plain chest film and CT scanning for metastases in cases of choriocarcinoma, magnetic resonance imaging (MRI) for placenta accreta[31,32] and angiography for intractable bleeding of unknown origin[14].

Treatment

The majority of cases of secondary PPH are due to subinvolution of the uterus caused by uterine infection and/or retained placental tissue. Initial management should include resuscitation as discussed above, the use of uterotonic agents, administration of antibiotics and consideration of surgical evacuation (Table 4).

Uterotonic agents

Syntocinon® can be administered as an intravenous or intramuscular bolus (10 units) or in combination with ergometrine (Syntometrine®) 1 ampoule as an intramuscular injection. This can be followed by a Syntocinon infusion (40 units in 500 ml normal saline at an infusion rate of 125 ml/h). Prostaglandin F2α (Haemabate®/carboprost) can be given by intramuscular injection at a dose of 250 μg every 15 min, up to a total of 2 mg (i.e. 8 doses). Misoprostol can also be given as an alternative prostaglandin (400–800 μg orally or rectally).

Antibiotics

Endometritis is likely to play a significant role in many cases of secondary PPH, and the majority of women are prescribed antibiotics. In a 3-year study of almost 20,000 women, 132 women (0.69%) had a secondary PPH, and 97% of these were treated with antibiotics[2]. However, only 75% of these women had microbiological specimens collected; of these, a positive culture was obtained in only 13.5%. In a similar observational study of 83 women, 45% presented with pyrexia and 64 had bacteriological swabs taken, of which only 12.5% were positive. Organisms identified included group B streptococcus, *Bacteroides sp.*, *Escherichia coli*, *Clostridium perfringens* and group D streptococcus. Despite the lack of evidence to support the presence of a specific bacterial pathogen, 92% of the women received antibiotics[3]. Recommended choices of antibiotic treatment include amoxicillin with clavulanic

acid (Augmentin®)[33] and a combination of amoxycillin, metronidazole and gentamicin[3]. Endometritis is a major contributor to subinvolution of the uterus. Although infection may not be confirmed in a large population of cases, we recommend that antibiotics are always given for secondary PPH.

Uterine evacuation

Examination under anesthetic and surgical evacuation of the uterus should be considered if retained placental tissue is suspected clinically or after ultrasound examination. This intervention has good reported success rates, with bleeding stopping promptly in all 72 women undergoing evacuation of the uterus for secondary PPH in one study, despite only 36% having proven histological evidence of retained tissue[3]. However, this study was unable to find any clear association with presence or absence of retained tissue at the time of evacuation and day of onset of bleeding or other morbidity at the time of secondary PPH. Nonetheless, retained tissue was more likely if membranes were incomplete at delivery, primary PPH had occurred or if secondary PPH was judged to be heavy or moderate (compared with light) in volume.

The use of ultrasound prior to surgical evacuation of the uterus does not appear to significantly alter the chances of histological diagnosis confirming retained tissue. In one study, 33% of those with no preoperative scan had retained placental tissue compared to 37% following a scan[2]. Retained placental tissue is likely to be associated with infection and, therefore, broad spectrum intravenous antibiotics should be given in conjunction with surgical evacuation. As serum concentrations of most antibiotics peak 1 h after intravenous administration, these should be administered just prior to surgery[26]; in women who are hemodynamically stable, however, it may be appropriate to administer 12–24 h of antibiotic cover prior to surgery[1]. At the time of surgery, uterotonic agents such as Syntocinon, ergometrine and prostaglandins may be helpful to aid uterine contractility and control hemorrhage. There is no clear evidence to support which method of evacuation should be used. Manual removal of tissue, use of a suction catheter and sharp curettage with a metal curette have all been described[2]. The risk of uterine perforation is much higher in postpartum uterine evacuation and may be even further increased if associated with endometritis. Hoveyda and colleagues describe uterine perforation in three of 85 women undergoing evacuation for secondary PPH. Procedures were performed from 4 days to 28 days after delivery with both a suction and metal curette. In all cases, operations were performed by senior medical staff. One woman went on to require a hysterectomy, but the two others were managed conservatively[2].

Perforation after cesarean section is more likely and, as these women have a lower risk of retained placental tissue, surgical evacuation in such instances should be considered very carefully. An additional complication

Table 3 A proposed standardized system for reporting postpartum ultrasound scan. Adapted from Neill *et al.*, 2002[30]

1. Normal endometrial cavity
2. Endometrial cavity containing fluid only
3. Endometrial cavity enlarged (anteroposterior (AP) depth >1 cm). Maximum AP dimensions noted
4. Endometrial cavity containing echogenic foci. Dimensions of largest foci noted. Doppler evaluation of blood flow in foci

Table 4 The management of secondary PPH

Medical	Surgical
Oxytocics	Uterine evacuation
Prostaglandins	Uterine tamponade balloon
Antibiotics	Uterine compression sutures
Tranexamic acid	Hysterectomy
Vasopressin	Pelvic arterial ligation
Clotting factor concentrates	
Chemotherapy	*Radiological*
Oral contraceptive pill	Selective arterial embolization

is the risk of Asherman's syndrome. Limited evidence is available to ascertain whether this risk is increased for postpartum uterine evacuation; however, in a large study of intrauterine adhesions, 21.5% of cases had a postpartum curettage as a prior event[34]. The need for a second procedure due to incomplete evacuation of retained tissue may also occur[2]. Hysterectomy may be required to control bleeding in up to 5% of cases[26]. In view of these significant complications, women should always be fully counseled of the risks and informed consent obtained. Surgery should be performed by experienced senior medical staff.

Other surgical procedures

In the event of a large bleed, other surgical procedures should be considered. These include cases of bleeding from an infected placental bed or placental abnormality such as placenta accreta, bleeding from retained placental tissue not controlled with uterine evacuation, non-union/dehiscence of cesarean section scar, bleeding from a surgical injury or uncontrolled bleeding from a lower genital tract laceration. All are discussed in detail in other chapters of this book as is the insertion of an intrauterine tamponade balloon, such as the Bakri[35] or Rüsch balloon[36], which may be considered in cases of secondary PPH due to uterine subinvolution/atony once retained placental tissue has been excluded. Laparotomy may also be required which allows further investigation into the cause of bleeding and treatment by the use of surgical compression sutures, hysterectomy and pelvic arterial ligation as appropriate. The B-Lynch brace suture is well described for the treatment of primary PPH[37] and has now been reported in hundreds of cases of secondary PPH (B-Lynch, personal communication). The use of a surgical compression suture may avoid the need for hysterectomy in women wishing to conserve fertility (see Chapters 44, 47 and 48 for balloons and Chapter 51 for compression sutures).

Within an Australian population with an overall incidence of secondary PPH of 1.44% over 15 years, only nine cases required hysterectomy (0.9%)[3]. However, in a subgroup of women with massive intractable obstetric hemorrhage, two out of seven with secondary PPH required hysterectomy. In one, hysterectomy was performed 7 days after delivery due to intractable bleeding from lower genital tract lacerations but maternal death still resulted. *[Editor's note: It is possible that, as discussed in the first chapter of the book, hysterectomy might not have been the operation of choice given the fact that the bleeding came from vaginal lacerations. L.G.K.]* The second case had further morbidity following her hysterectomy for secondary PPH with bleeding from wound disunion and sepsis; she required bilateral hypogastric artery ligation 14 days after delivery[5].

Hysterectomy in cases of PPH carries significant risks but can be life-saving and should be considered early rather than late in cases of massive hemorrhage, whether primary or secondary. If delayed, patients may already be in shock, have disseminated intravascular coagulopathy (DIC) or acidosis, all of which add significantly to the operation's risk and may contribute to its failure as does its use in patients where the bleeding is not from arteries that perfuse the uterus but rather from those which supply blood to the lower uterine segment and the upper vagina (see Chapter 1).

Pelvic artery ligation may also be considered for cases of massive secondary PPH uncontrolled by medical and simple surgical measures. Lédée and colleagues report the use of bilateral hypogastric artery ligation in 49 of 61 cases of intractable hemorrhage; this includes four out of seven cases of secondary PPH, all of which were successful at arresting bleeding[5] (see Chapter 52) As with primary PPH, arterial ligation should be performed by an experienced surgeon and their involvement should be considered early whilst planning a laparotomy in such cases.

Bilateral uterine artery embolization and selective arterial embolization

Pelvic angiography to assess the internal iliac artery, uterine artery and its vaginal branches is a helpful tool in the assessment of ongoing hemorrhage. It also allows the introduction of embolization agents to arrest bleeding. Pelage and colleagues studied 14 women presenting with uncontrollable secondary PPH at a mean of 16 days after delivery[14]. Six women (43%) had delivered by cesarean section and the remainder by spontaneous vaginal delivery. Eight women exhibited evidence of endometritis (57%), four with histologically proven retained placental tissue; a further four women had genital tract lacerations, and the remaining two had no obvious cause for bleeding. Basic resuscitation with use of medical treatments and/or uterine curettage was performed. Angiography found no extravasation in eight women, active bleeding in three women from uterine and vaginal vessels, a false uterine artery aneurysm in two women, and evidence of an arteriovenous fistula in another. Pledgets of absorbable gelatin sponge were introduced to embolize the uterine arteries bilaterally in 12 women. Unilateral embolization of a false aneurysm and an arteriovenous fistula was performed for the other two women. External bleeding disappeared immediately, and hemodynamic stability and correction of coagulopathy were obtained for all cases. There were no general or local complications[14]. Ganguli et al. reported a clinical success rate for secondary PPH of 88% with uterine artery embolization[16].

One of the authors of this chapter (T.J.) managed a case of massive secondary PPH presenting 4 days after a cesarean section. An emergency subtotal hysterectomy was performed with good initial results. Two hours later, vaginal bleeding restarted. There was no evidence of significant coagulopathy. Pelvic angiography was performed and a bleed from a false aneurysm related to a middle branch of the anterior division of the left internal iliac artery was identified (Figure 1). The vessels were embolized with four coils. There was immediate cessation of bleeding and the patient's vital signs normalized (Figure 2). The patient made a good recovery despite requiring 24 units of blood during the hemorrhage. Subsequent histology of the uterus showed acute inflammation and sub-involution of the placental bed.

Other measures

In cases of massive hemorrhage unsuccessfully treated with surgical measures, the use of intravenous tranexamic acid[38–41], recombinant factor VIIa[42] and local vasopressin[43] have been reported for primary PPH. There are no reports of similar use in secondary PPH but, if available, it may be appropriate to consider their use in combination with other therapies and resuscitative support. A trial currently underway may provide further information in the future[44].

Chemotherapy

The mainstay of treatment for choriocarcinoma is chemotherapy. A low-risk chemotherapy regimen includes the use of methotrexate with folinic acid rescue on a 2-weekly cycle[45]. Medium- and high-risk regimens include the use of etopside, methotrexate, actinomycin, vincristine, cyclophosphomide and 6-mercaptopurine[46,47]. Women with choriocarcinoma are most appropriately treated through specialist trophoblastic disease referral centers[20].

Coagulopathies

Women with inherited coagulation disorders such as von Willebrand's disease and carriers of hemophilia A and B are likely to bleed postpartum if maternal clotting factors are low (<50 IU/dl). Prophylactic administration of desmopressin (DDAVP) and clotting factor concentrates may prevent PPH[21]. The aim is to raise factor levels above 50 IU/dl during labor and delivery, and to maintain these for up to 5 days after delivery. In the event of PPH, replacement of deficient clotting factors should be made and identification and treatment of the cause be instigated. Management should be in close liaison with hematologists and specialist hemophilia centers as available (see Chapter 25). In cases of prolonged or intermittent secondary PPH, the use of tranexamic acid (a fibrinolytic inhibitor)[48] or combined oral contraceptive pill has been reported[22]. Hemorrhage from postpartum acquired hemophilia is treated acutely with factor VIII (human or porcine) or recombinant factor VIIa[21]. Immunosuppressive drugs such as corticosteroids, cyclophosphamide and azathioprine may be used to accelerate the disappearance of factor VIII inhibitors, although complete remission is likely to occur spontaneously with time. Reversal of bleeding due to anticoagulants should follow normal protocols. Vitamin K should be considered in women with uncontrolled bleeding secondary to warfarin use and protamine sulfate may be considered if hemorrhage results from the use of heparin, although this has a much shorter half-life.

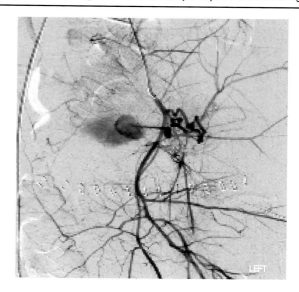

Figure 1 Angiogram demonstrating brisk hemorrhage from false aneurysm prior to embolization

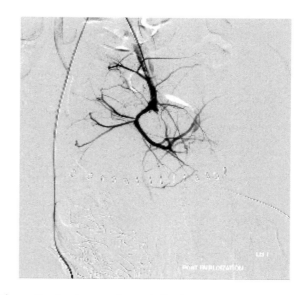

Figure 2 Angiogram after embolization

CONCLUSION

Secondary PPH is an important cause of maternal morbidity and mortality. Basic resuscitation followed by investigation and treatment of the specific cause of hemorrhage are essential. The diverse nature of its etiology and often acute presentation make research in the form of randomized controlled trials difficult. However, particularly for the treatment of hemorrhage due to uterine infection and/or retained placental tissue, this should be achievable and would provide valuable information to further our understanding of the management of secondary PPH.

References

1. Thompson W, Harper M. Postpartum haemorrhage and abnormalities of the third stage of labour. In: Chamberlain G, Steer P, eds. Turnbull's Obstetrics, 3rd edn. Edinburgh: Churchill Livingstone, 2001:619–33

2. Hoveyda F, MacKenzie IZ. Secondary postpartum haemorrhage: incidence, morbidity and current management. BJOG 2001;108:927–30

3. King PA, Duthie SJ, Dong ZG, Ma HK. Secondary postpartum haemorrhage. Aust N Z J Obstet Gynaecol 1989;29:394–8

4. Alexander J, Thomas PW, Sanghera J. Treatments for secondary postpartum haemorrhage (Review). Cochrane Database Syst Rev 2008;(1): http://www.mrw.interscience.wiley.com/cochrane/clsysrev/articles/CD002867/frame.html

5. Ledee N, Ville Y, Musset D, Mercier F, Frydman R, Fernandez H. Management in intractable obstetric haemorrhage: an audit study on 61 cases. Eur J Obstet Gynecol Reprod Biol 2001;94:189–96

6. Babarinsa IA, Hayman RG, Draycott TJ. Secondary postpartum haemorrhage: challenges in evidence-based causes and management. Eur J Obstet Gynecol Reprod Biol 2011;159:255–60

7. Farley NJ. Kohlmeier RE. A death due to subinvolution of the uteroplacental arteries. J Forensic Sci 2011;56:803–5

8. Matthews NM, McCowan LM, Patten P. Placenta praevia accreta with delayed hysterectomy. Aust N Z J Obstet Gynaecol 1996;36:476–9

9. Jaffe R, DuBeshter B, Sherer DM, Thompson EA, Woods JR Jr. Failure of methotrexate treatment for term placenta percreta. Am J Obstet Gynecol 1994;171:558–9

10. Ghosh TK. Arteriovenous malformation of the uterus and pelvis. Obstet Gynecol 1986;68:40S–3S

11. Gaylis H, Levine E, van Dongen LG, Katz I. Arteriovenous fistulas after gynecologic operations. Surg Gynecol Obstet 1973;137:655–8

12. Bardou P, Orabona M, Vincelot A, Maubon A, Nathan N. [Uterine artery false aneurysm after caesarean delivery: an uncommon cause of post-partum haemorrhage]. Ann Fr Anesth Reanim 2010;29:909–12

13. Bhatt A, Odujebe O, Bhatt S, Houry D. Uterine artery pseudoaneurysm rupture: a life-threatening presentation of vaginal bleeding. Ann Emerg Med 2010;55:460–3

14. Pelage JP, Soyer P, Repiquet D, et al. Secondary postpartum hemorrhage: treatment with selective arterial embolization. Radiology 1999;212:385–9

15. Kelly SM, Belli AM, Campbell S. Arteriovenous malformation of the uterus associated with secondary postpartum hemorrhage. Ultrasound Obstet Gynecol 2003;21:602–5

16. Ganguli S, Stecker MS, Pyne D, Baum RA, Fan CM. Uterine artery embolization in the treatment of postpartum uterine hemorrhage. J Vasc Interv Radiol 2011;22:169–76

17. Isono W, Tsutsumi R, Wada-Hiraike O, et al. Uterine artery pseudoaneurysm after cesarean section: case report and literature review. J Minim Invasive Gynecol 2010;17:687–91

18. Nanda S, Singhal S, Sharma D, Sood M, Singhal SK. Nonunion of uterine incision: a rare cause of secondary postpartum haemorrhage: a report of 2 cases. Aust N Z J Obstet Gynaecol 1997;37:475–6

19. Paraskevaides E, Stuart B, Gardeil F. Secondary postpartum haemorrhage from nondehisced lower caesarean section scar: a case for hysteroscopy. Aust N Z J Obstet Gynaecol 1993;33:427

20. Tidy JA, Rustin GJ, Newlands ES, et al. Presentation and management of choriocarcinoma after nonmolar pregnancy. Br J Obstet Gynaecol 1995;102:715–9

21. Economides DL, Kadir RA, Lee CA. Inherited bleeding disorders in obstetrics and gynaecology. Br J Obstet Gynaecol 1999;106:5–13

22. Kadir RA, Economides DL, Braithwaite J, Goldman E, Lee CA. The obstetric experience of carriers of haemophilia. Br J Obstet Gynaecol 1997;104:803–10

23. Greer IA, Lowe GD, Walker JJ, Forbes CD. Haemorrhagic problems in obstetrics and gynaecology in patients with congenital coagulopathies. Br J Obstet Gynaecol 1991;98:909–18

24. Ramsahoye BH, Davies SV, Dasani H, Pearson JF. Obstetric management in von Willebrand's disease: a report of 24 pregnancies and a reivesw of the literature. Haemophilia 1995;1:140–4

25. Kadir RA, Lee CA, Sabin CA, Pollard D, Economides DL. Pregnancy in women with von Willebrand's disease or factor XI deficiency. Br J Obstet Gynaecol 1998;105:314–21

26. Neill A, Thornton S. Secondary postpartum haemorrhage. J Obstet Gynaecol 2002;22:119–22

27. Johanson R, Cox C, O'Donnell E, Grady K, Howell C, Jones P. Managing obstetric emergencies and trauma (MOET): Structured skills training using models and reality-based scenarios. Obstetrician Gynaecologist 1999;1:46–52

28. Achiron R, Goldenberg M, Lipitz S, Mashiach S. Transvaginal duplex Doppler ultrasonography in bleeding patients suspected of having residual trophoblastic tissue. Obstet Gynecol 1993;81:507–11

29. Zuckerman J, Levine D, McNicholas MM, et al. Imaging of pelvic postpartum complications. Am J Roentgenol 1997;168:663–8

30. Neill AC, Nixon RM, Thornton S. A comparison of clinical assessment with ultrasound in the management of secondary postpartum haemorrhage. Eur J Obstet Gynecol Reprod Biol 2002;104:113–5

31. Thorp Jr JM, Wells SR, Wiest HH, Jeffries L, Lyles E. First-trimester diagnosis of placenta previa percreta by magnetic resonance imaging. Am J Obstet Gynecol 1998;178:616–8

32. Levine D, Barnes PD, Edelman RR. Obstetric MR Imaging. Radiology 1999;211:609–17

33. Fernandez H, Claquin C, Guibert M, Papiernik E. Suspected postpartum endometritis: a controlled clinical trial of single-agent antibiotic therapy with Amox-CA (AugmentingR) vs. ampicillin-metronidazole ± aminoglycoside. Eur J Obstet GynecolReprod Biol 1990;36:69–74

34. Schenker JG, Margalioth EJ. Intrauterine adhesions: an updated appraisal. Fertil Steril 1982;37:593–610

35. Bakri YN, Amri A, Abdul Jabbar F. Tamponade-balloon for obstetrical bleeding. Int J Gynecol Obstet 2001;74:139–42

36. Johanson R, Kumar M, Obhrai M, Young P. Management of massive postpartum haemorrhage: use of a hydrostatic balloon catheter to avoid laparotomy. BJOG 2001;108:420–2

37. B-Lynch C, Coker A, Lawal AH, Abu J, Cowen MJ. The B-Lynch surgical technique for the control of massive postpartum haemorrhage: an alternative to hysterectomy? Five cases reported. Br J Obstet Gynaecol 1997;104:372–5

38. Alok K, Hagen P, Webb JB. Tranexamic acid in the management of postpartum haemorrhage. BJOG 1996;103:1250–1

39. Ducloy-Bouthors AS, Jude B, Duhamel A, et al. High-dose tranexamic acid reduces blood loss in postpartum haemorrhage. Crit Care 2011;15:R117

40. Ferrer P, Roberts I, Sydenham E, Blackhall K, Shakur H. Anti-fibrinolytic agents in post partum haemorrhage: a systematic review. BMC Pregnancy Childbirth 2009;9:29

41. Novikova N, Hofmeyr GJ. Tranexamic acid for preventing postpartum haemorrhage. Cochrane Database Syst Rev 2010;(7):CD007872

42. Boehlen F, Morales MA, Fontana P, Ricou B, Irion O, de Moerloose P. Prolonged treatment of massive postpartum haemorrhage with recombinant factor VIIa: case report and review of the literature. BJOG 2004;111:284–7

43. Lurie S, Appleman Z, Katz Z. Subendometrial vasopressin to control intractable placental bleeding. Lancet 1997;349:698

44. Shakur H, Elbourne D, Gulmezoglu M, et al. The WOMAN Trial (World Maternal Antifibrinolytic Trial): tranexamic acid for the treatment of postpartum haemorrhage: an international randomised, double blind placebo controlled trial. Trials 2010;11:40

45. Bagshawe KD, Dent J, Newlands ES, Begent RHJ, Rustin GJS. The role of low-dose methotrexate and folinic acid in gestational trophoblastic tumours (GTT). BJOG 1989;96:795–802

46. Newlands ES, Bagshawe KD, Begent RHJ, Rustin GJS, Holden L. Results with the EMA/CO (etoposide, methotrexate, actinomycin D, cyclophosphamide, vincristine)

regimen in high risk gestational trophoblastic tumours, 1979 to 1989. BJOG 1991;98:550–7

47. Rustin GJ, Newlands ES, Begent RH, Dent J, Bagshawe KD. Weekly alternating etoposide, methotrexate, and actino-mycin/vincristine and cyclophosphamide chemotherapy for the treatment of CNS metastases of choriocarcinoma. J Clin Oncol 1989;7:900–3

48. Bonnar J, Guillebaud J, Kasonde JM, Sheppard BL. Clinical applications of fibrinolytic inhibition in gynaecology. J Clin Pathol Suppl (R Coll Pathol) 1980;14:55–9

57

Use of Fibrin Sealants in Obstetric Hemorrhage

S. Mahmoud and E. El Hamamy

INTRODUCTION

In recent years, a variety of methods have been described to arrest bleeding, including a group of compounds which act as fibrin sealants. In the UK, the Confidential Enquiry into Maternal Deaths recommends that all available interventions should be considered, including hemostatic agents[1]. Topical hemostatic agents have been used with excellent results in other surgical specialities, such as neurosurgery, urology and gynecology. While there is no replacement for meticulous surgical hemostasis, the highly viscous gels have been successfully used in cases of PPH[2]. This chapter reviews their uses and explains how they work.

BACKGROUND AND MECHANISM OF ACTION

Fibrin sealants are biological adhesives that mimic the final step of the coagulation cascade. Main components of sealants include fibrinogen, plasmatic proteins and factor XIII, on the one hand, and thrombin, calcium chloride and an antifibrinolytic agent such as aprotinin, on the other. The first three components are extracted from human plasma, whereas calcium chloride and aprotinin both derive from bovine lungs. Mixing fibrinogen and thrombin simulates the final stages of the natural coagulation cascade to form a structured fibrin clot similar to a physiological clot. This clot is naturally degraded by proteolytic enzymes from the fibrinolytic system, such as plasmin. High concentrations of these enzymes are present in response to tissue inflammation. As a result of their hemostatic and adhesive properties, fibrin sealants have been extensively used in most surgical specialties for over the past two decades[3]. They are used to reduce blood loss and postoperative bleeding. However, their uses in obstetrics are more recent and require further evaluation[4].

Reports published between 2001 and 2003 indicate that fibrin sealants are a safe and highly effective form of surgical adhesive[5]. A survey undertaken in 2000 at the University of Virginia hospital found that over 90% of the surgeons who had used fibrin sealants were pleased with the results[6]. Several studies from the US have reported that fibrin sealants significantly improved surgical outcomes by shortening the time required for operations, lowering the rate of infections and other complications, minimizing blood loss during surgery and reducing the amount of scar tissue formed over incisions. German researchers have found that fibrin sealants containing factor XIII generally give better results than those that do not[7,8]. Fibrin sealants have several advantages over conventional surgical techniques, such as suture, ligation and cautery. These include speeding up the formation of a stable clot, application to very small blood vessels and areas that are difficult to reach with conventional sutures, reducing the amount of blood lost during surgery, lowering the risk of postoperative inflammation or infection and, finally, convenient absorption during the healing process. They are particularly useful for minimally invasive procedures and for treating patients with blood clotting disorders.

PRODUCTS

Fibrin sealants are prepared and sold under many brand names such as TISSEEL® (Baxter Healthcare Corporation), Evicel® (Ethicon, Somerville, NJ), FloSeal® (Baxter Healthcare Corporation), BioGlue® (CryoLife, Kennesaw, GA), Crosseal® (Ethicon, Somerville, NJ) and Hemaseel APR® (Hemacure Corp., Sarasota, FL). The surgeon and operating room staff must be aware that fibrin sealants are not identical in composition or use. For the individual methods of application, please refer to and follow the individual product information leaflet.

PREPARATION

The preparation and application of fibrin sealants are complex. The thrombin and fibrinogen are freeze-dried and packaged in vials that must be warmed before use. These two ingredients are then dissolved in separate amounts of calcium chloride solution. Next, the thrombin and fibrinogen solutions are loaded into a double-barrelled syringe that allows them to mix and combine as they are sprayed on the incision. Pieces of surgical gauze or fleece may be moistened with the sealant solutions to cover large incisions or to stop heavy bleeding[9]. Figure 1 shows the mechanism of action of fibrin sealants.

SAFETY

Because the first commercial fibrin sealants relied on a consistent and concentrated source of human fibrinogen, the Food and Drug Administration in the USA revoked the license for the clinical use of pooled commercial fibrinogen concentrates owing to the high risk of hepatitis transmission with the fibrinogen[10]. In an attempt to resolve this issue, products marketed since that time have adopted various viral inactivation procedures including pasteurization (60°C for 10 h, liquid state), solvent-detergent treatment, steam treatment (60°C for 30 h, dry state), ultraviolet C (UVC) irradiation, nanofiltration (35 nm) and dry heat treatment (100°C for 30 min). Although the risks of viral transmission from fibrin sealants prepared from pooled human plasma are considered to be low, a 'zero' risk cannot be guaranteed[11,12]. Despite their advantages, sealants are not without a major disadvantage in that they must be used topically, as all can cause intravascular thrombosis if injected into the circulation. Furthermore, the risk of air or gas embolism is present when using air- or gas-pressurized spray devices[13]. The following precautions are advised:

- Use the applicator, spray set and pressure control device or regulator as recommended in the labeling or information for use (IFU) of the hemostatic agent

- Use an air or gas pressure setting within the range recommended by the manufacturer of the sprayer

- Ensure that distance between the spray head and the tissue surface is not less than the minimum recommended by the manufacturer of the sprayer

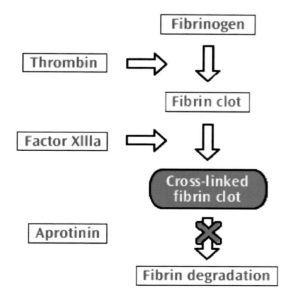

Figure 1 Mechanism of action of fibrin sealant

- Monitor blood pressure, pulse, oxygen saturation and end tidal CO_2 for signs of an air or gas embolism.

USES IN PPH

Although no large trial data are available to date about their safety in obstetric patients using fibrin sealant to deal with PPH is now appearing in the literature. Most of the data come from single case reports with a successful outcome.

Reports of uses of fibrin sealants to manage cases of PPH are shown in Table 1 (see Chapter 58 for discussion of case reports).

Fibrin sealants may be an excellent adjuvant in the Jehovah's Witness patient experiencing PPH, for example, a 30-year-old nulliparous patient underwent cesarean section for dystocia and suspected chorioamnionitis, and subsequently developed PPH that required management with oxytocin, ergometrine, carboprost, uterine artery ligation and Hayman compression sutures. The patient ultimately required two additional visits to the operating room, culminating in hysterectomy. Use of tranexamic acid, recombinant factor VIIa and TISSEEL was instrumental in halting the ongoing hemorrhage[18]. The use of fibrin sealants is a matter of personal choice for Witnesses and should be discussed in the preoperative period as outlined in Chapter 72[19,20].

Palacios-Jaraquemada has written extensively about the uses of fibrin glue with external uterine elastic bandages in patients with severe PPH[21]. After circulatory stabilization by external aortic compression, laparotomy and identification of the source of bleeding, compression sutures were applied and intrauterine fibrin glue was administered; immediately thereafter, an external elastic bandage was wrapped around the uterus to compress it. After hemostasis had persisted for some time, the bandage was removed, and uterus and abdomen were then closed. Application of external uterine elastic bandage resulted in hemostasis within 45 min after aortic compression. Hysteroscopy 6 months after the procedure showed no signs of uterine ischemia or endometrial adhesions. The application of endouterine fibrin provided the placental bed with an excellent hemostatic substrate to avoiding oozing and re-bleeding. Hysteroscopic examination at a later date showed complete recovery of the endometrial cavity without synechiae[21]. This is an important factor as most of the women are young and desire more children. Table 2 shows the risk of developing synechiae after different techniques used to treat PPH.

The procedure for applying the fibrin sealant, FloSeal, is outlined below:

(1) Identify the source of the bleeding at the tissue surface. Apply FloSeal Hemostatic Matrix FAST to the deepest part of the wound or lesion, i.e. the source of bleeding at the tissue surface.

(2) This is the target site for FloSeal Hemostatic Matrix application. Do not inject FloSeal into

Table 1   Reports of uses of fibrin sealants to manage cases of PPH

Report	Year	Sealant	Success rate	Special consideration
Dhulkotia[14]	2009	TISSEEL	1/1	Vulval hematoma and vaginal laceration
Whiteside[15]	2010	TISSEEL	1/1	Vaginal laceration
Law[16]	2010	FloSeal	1/1	Placenta previa
Moriarty[17]	2008	FloSeal	1/1	Vault hematoma
Arab[18]	2010	TISSEEL	1/1	Bleeding in a Jehovah's Witness
Palacios-Jaraquemada[21]	2010	TISSEEL	6/6	External elastic bandages No uterine synechiae

Table 2   Uterine synechiae following different techniques to manage PPH

Report	Year	n	Management of PPH	HSC or HSG	Synechiae	Pregnancy
Poujade[22]	2011	119	Uterine compression sutures	32	18% (6/32)	13
Poujade[22]	2011	33	Uterine compression suture (Hackethal technique)	15	26.7% (4/15)	—
Sentilhes[23]	2010	101	Uterine embolization	8	8% (8/111)	26
Palacios-Jaraquemada[21]	2010	10	Fibrin glue and uterine external elastic bands	8	0% (0/8)	—

HSC, hysteroscopy; HSG, hysterosalpingogram

blood vessels. Do not apply FloSeal in the absence of active bleeding.

(3) The flowable nature of FloSeal allows it to conform to any irregular wound geometries and be applied in difficult-to-reach locations.

(4) After creating a cone-like mound of FloSeal over the bleeding site, immediately gently place FloSeal to the bleeding surface with a moistened gauze sponge for 2 min.

(5) FloSeal granules allow high concentrations of thrombin to react rapidly with the patient's fibrinogen and form a mechanically stable clot.

(6) FloSeal granules have a maximum, controlled swell volume of approximately 20%, which is achieved within about 10 min and physically, restricts the flow of blood.

(7) FloSeal can be reapplied, if necessary. Reapply at the base of the wound and backfill the lesion. Once hemostasis is achieved, gentle irrigation should always occur to remove excess product that has not been incorporated into the clot. Do not disrupt the clot by physical manipulation or suction.

(8) FloSeal allows visualization of the surgical site both during and after application.

(9) FloSeal is biocompatible and fully resorbs within 6–8 weeks, consistent with normal wound healing.

An example of the mechanism of action and usage technique is shown in Addendum A.

CONCLUSION

Fibrin sealants are new tools to arrest bleeding in patients with PPH. Early reports of their use are promising. Fibrin sealants have thrombin and fibrinogen which form a stable clot and arrest bleeding. This is independent of the patient clotting mechanism; hence, they are ideal in the patient with coagulopathy. Fibrin sealants have been called a 'clot in a bottle'. Their use has been reported with traumatic PPH and in patients with placenta previa and Jehovah's Witnesses. Staff need to be trained in its use as well as its preparation. More research is needed to determine its safety and efficiency in managing PPH.

PRACTICE POINTS

- Fibrin sealants are new tools in treating PPH

- Their use mimics the final steps of the physiological clotting cascade, thus achieving hemostasis

- Fibrin sealant produces a fast, effective, clear stable clot

- Sealants function independently of patient's own clotting mechanism

- Early case reports are promising. More studies and training are needed for fibrin sealant evaluation in the management of PPH.

References

1. Confidential Enquiry into Maternal and Child Health, Saving Mothers' Lives, The Seventh Report of the Confidential Enquiries into Maternal Deaths in the United Kingdom, 2005–2007 Triennial Report. London: Royal College of Obstetricians, 2007:78–85
2. Wise A, Clark V. Challenges of major obstetric haemorrhage. Best Pract Res Clin Obstet Gynaecol 2010;24:353–65
3. Bombeli T, Spahn DR. Updates in perioperative coagulation: physiology and management of thromboembolism and haemorrhage. Br J Anaesth 2004;93:275–87
4. Le Guéhennec L, Layrolle P, Daculsi G. A review of bioceramics and fibrin sealant. Eur Cell Mater 2004;8:1–10
5. Beers MH, Berkow R. Haemostasis and Coagulation Disorders. Section 11, Chapter 131. In: The Merck Manual

of Diagnosis and Therapy. Whitehouse Station, NJ: Merck Research Laboratories, 1999–2001

6. Evans LA, Morey AF. Current applications of fibrin sealant in urologic surgery. Int Braz J Urol 2006;.32:131–41

7. Schenk WG III, Burks SG, Gagne PJ. Fibrin sealant improves hemostasis in peripheral vascular surgery: a randomized prospective trial. Ann Surg 2003;237:871–6

8. Dickneite G, Metzner HJ, Kroez M, et al. The importance of factor xiii as a component of fibrin sealants. J Surg Res 2002;107:186–95

9. Virginia R. Sewing wet tissue paper: fibrin sealants in obstetrics. Obstet Gynecol 2010;115:401–2

10. Gibble JW, Ness PM, Fibrin glue: the perfect operative sealant? Transfusion 1990;30:741–7

11. Achneck HE, Sileshi B, Jamiolkowski RM, et al. A comprehensive review of topical haemostatic agents: efficacy and recommendations for use. Ann Surg 2010;251:217–28

12. Radosevich M, Goubran HA, Burnouf T. Fibrin sealant: scientific rationale, production methods, properties, and current clinical use. Vox Sang 1997;72:133–43

13. Risk of Life-Threatening Air or Gas Embolism with the Use of Spray Devices Employing Pressure Regulator to Administer Fibrin Sealants. Baxter Healthcare Corporation, 2009 http://www.fda.gov/BiologicsBloodVaccines/SafetyAvailability/ucm209778.htm

14. Dhulkotia JS, Alazzam M, Galimberti A. Tisseel for management of traumatic postpartum haemorrhage. Arch Gynecol Obstet 2009;279:437–9

15. Whiteside JL, Asif RB, Novello RJ., Fibrin sealant for management of complicated obstetric lacerations. Obstet Gynecol 2010;115:403–4

16. Law LW, Chor CM, Leung TY. Use of haemostatic gel in postpartum hemorrhage due to placenta previa. Obstet Gynecol 2010;116:(Suppl 2):528–30

17. Moriarty KT, Premila S, Bulmer PJ. Use of FloSeal haemostatic gel in massive obstetric haemorrhage: a case report. BJOG 2008;115:793–5

18. Arab TS, Al-Wazzan AB, Maslow K., Postpartum haemorrhage in a Jehovah's Witness patient controlled with Tisseel, tranexamic acid, and recombinant factor VIIa. J Obstet Gynaecol Can 2010;32:984–7

19. Thomas JM. Postpartum hemorrhage in a Jehovah's Witness [Letter]. J Obstet Gynaecol Can 2011;33:897

20. Bodnaruk ZM, Wong CJ, Thomas JM. Meeting the clinical challenge of care for Jehovah's Witnesses. Transfus Med Rev 2004;18:105–16

21. Palacios-Jaraquemada J, Fiorillo A. Conservative approach in heavy postpartum haemorrhage associated with coagulopathy. Acta Obstet Gynaecol Scand 2010;89:1222–5

22. Poujade O, Grossetti A, Mougel L, et al. Risk of synechiae following uterine compression sutures in the management of major postpartum haemorrhage. BJOG 2011;118:433

23. Sentilhes L, Gomez A, Clavier E, et al. Fertility and pregnancy following pelvic arterial embolisation for postpartum haemorrhage. BJOG2010;117:84–93

Addendum A: Example of how to use a fibrin sealant

From Baxter Healthcare Corporation, with permission

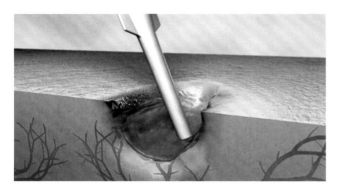

Step 1   Get FloSeal to the site of bleeding. Deliver to base of wound allowing it to conform to the shape of wound

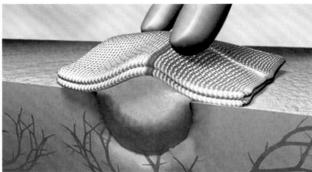

Step 4   Keep FloSeal at the site with a moistened swab, and approximate with fingers to hold in place

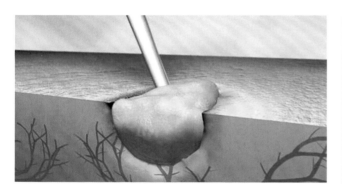

Step 2   Use enough FloSeal to cover the site

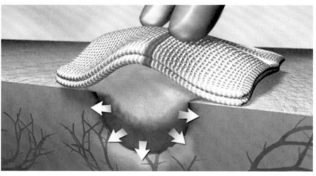

Step 5   Wait 2 min before inspection (brisk bleeding/coagulopathic patients may require longer) to confirm hemostasis. Reapplication may be required

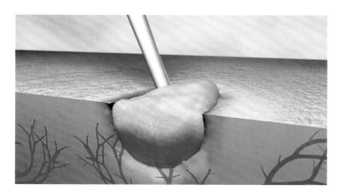

Step 3   Apply sealant quickly. Extrude at a faster rate than the bleeding to prevent product from being washed away by brisk bleeding

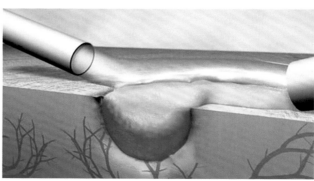

Step 6   Once hemostasis is achieved, gently irrigate excess granules that are not incorporated into the clot.

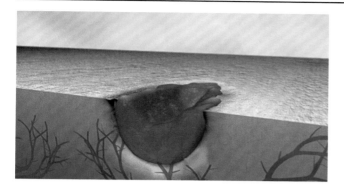

Step 7 FloSeal is reabsorbed by the body within 6–8 weeks, consistent with the time frame of normal wound healing

58

Topical Hemostatic Agents in Obstetric Hemorrhage: International Case Reports

C. Wohlmuth and J. Dela Merced

INTRODUCTION AND BACKGROUND

Topical hemostatic agents are utilized as adjuncts to control intraoperative bleeding when standard surgical techniques (such as suturing, ligature, cautery, or pressure) are insufficient or impractical to implement[1]. Intraoperative scenarios where topical hemostatic agents may serve as adjuncts include bleeding near vital organs or nerves, at needle-holes, from raw surface areas, in friable or attenuated tissue, or in patients who are anticoagulated, have bleeding diatheses, or have platelet dysfunction.

Physical agents and biologically active agents comprise the two main categories of topical hemostatic products. Physical agents promote hemostasis utilizing a passive substrate. Biologically active agents stimulate the coagulation cascade locally at the bleeding site[1].

Biologically active topical hemostatic agents have been marketed in the United States for over 10 years, paralleling the recent advances in biotechnology that resulted in rapid growth of available topical hemostatic agents[2]. Their use for intraoperative hemorrhage control has been described by various surgical specialties, including cardiovascular, otolaryngology, urology, and others[2–6]. Usage in gynecologic surgery has been reported, including laparoscopy, myomectomy, oncologic debulking and inguinal lymphadenectomy[7–11].

In 2007 Moriarty et al.[12] (UK) presented a case report on the use topical hemostatic agents in massive postpartum hemorrhage (PPH) in a patient who underwent emergency cesarean delivery due to placental abruption. Approximately 3 hours after cesarean delivery, the patient underwent laparotomy and total abdominal hysterectomy for life-threatening hemorrhage resulting from uterine atony that was unresponsive to conservative measures. The patient developed disseminated intravascular coagulation, and, after hysterectomy, continued to bleed from vascular venous plexuses at the vaginal vault, as well as from suture holes. The topical hemostatic agent comprised of gelatin–thrombin matrix, FloSeal™ (Baxter Healthcare Corporation, Fremont, California, USA), was applied to the bleeding areas. Thereafter, the authors described rapid achievement of hemostasis.

Subsequently, in 2010, Law et al. (Hong Kong) reported a case of successful control of persistent PPH from the placental implantation site, using FloSeal[13]. Two hours after cesarean delivery for placenta previa, the patient underwent re-laparotomy for persistent vaginal bleeding, where heavy bleeding from the lower uterine segment was noted. The authors described ineffective suturing for controlling bleeding in the deep placental site, and, therefore, FloSeal was applied. Hemorrhage control was achieved with uterine preservation.

In the same year, Fuglsang and Petersen (Denmark) published a series of 15 cases, delivered by cesarean for placenta previa, where excessive or intractable lower uterine segment hemorrhage was successfully controlled with direct local topical application of hemostatic collagen fleece coated with a mixture of human fibrinogen and thrombin (TachoSil™, Nycomed, Denmark), at the time of cesarean section[14].

Subsequently, in 2011, Tinelli (Italy) reported a case where TachoSil application successfully controlled hemorrhage at the uterine incision site. After a scheduled repeat cesarean section, the patient was found in hemorrhagic shock on postoperative day 3. At re-laparotomy, hemoperitoneum was found, resulting from constant oozing from the uterine incision site and bladder vessels. After ineffective hemostatic suturing, TachoSil was applied with successful hemorrhage control[15].

Similarly, in 2011, Wohlmuth and Dela Merced (US) reported a case of placental implantation site hemorrhage, controlled at the time of cesarean delivery, with gelatin–thrombin matrix (FloSeal) in a patient with placenta previa[16].

In the case reports described, topical hemostatic agents were administered after unsuccessful utilization of traditional PPH treatments. These included uterotonic agents, vessel ligation, uterine compression sutures, packing or balloon tamponade, over-sewing placental bed bleeding sites, recombinant activated factor VII and consideration of uterine artery embolization[17]. The ineffectiveness of the traditional methods of hemorrhage control in the cases of placenta previa was attributed to bleeding from the non-contractile lower uterine segment, large surface areas of active bleeding, vascular tissue depth at the placental site and tissue friability[13,14,16]. In the event conservative measures fail to control hemorrhage, hysterectomy, generally, is considered as a life-saving procedure.

Where topical hemostatic agents were used successfully at the time of cesarean delivery, re-laparotomy was avoided and uterine preservation was achieved[14,16]. Additionally, with rapid access and successful application of a topical hemostatic agent, the risks of prolonging bleeding time and associated massive blood transfusion can be decreased.

Topical hemostatic agent use in complicated obstetric genital laceration was reported by Whiteside *et al.* (US), in 2010[18]. A 21-year-old primipara patient was found to have a right labial hematoma that developed 2 hours after spontaneous vaginal delivery of twins with immediate repair of vaginal lacerations. The hematoma disrupted the suture line of the original repair. Despite additional suturing and vaginal packing, the hematoma continued to expand, leading to a 10 cm wide hematoma extending from the superior labia majora to the ischial fossa. At surgical exploration and evacuation, poor tissue quality was encountered, with suturing attempts unsuccessful in the presence of friable tissue. Direct pressure applied to the surgical bed did not control hemorrhage, including pressure applied with adjunctive use of microfibrillar collagen hemostat powder, a non-biologically active topical hemostatic agent. With application of biologically active, prohemostatic fibrin sealant (TISSEEL™, Baxter Healthcare Corporation, Fremont, California,

USA), hemostasis with tissue sealing was promptly achieved.

In 2009, a similar case of TISSEEL use in managing PPH from obstetric trauma was reported by Dhulkotia *et al.*[19] (UK).

BIOLOGICALLY ACTIVE TOPICAL HEMOSTATIC AGENTS

Because the published case reports of successful topical hemostatic agent use in obstetric hemorrhage are of resorbable biologically active products, the focus of discussion in this chapter is on this category of topical hemostatic agents, specific to those agents reported.

Biologically active topical hemostatic agents stimulate the coagulation cascade, primarily through the transformation of fibrinogen to fibrin by thrombin's enzymatic action (Figure 1).

The multitude of topical hemostatic agents available varies in composition, mechanism of action and method of use. The surgeon should be familiar with the various products' similarities and differences before use[2] (Table 1).

Liquid pro-hemostatic fibrin sealant (TISSEEL) was approved by the United States Food and Drug Administration (FDA) in 1998 as an adjunct to hemostasis in cardiopulmonary bypass and splenic injury surgeries. It is comprised of human fibrinogen and human thrombin. At the time of usage, the two components are combined to produce fibrin, mimicking the final stage of the coagulation cascade[20]. The

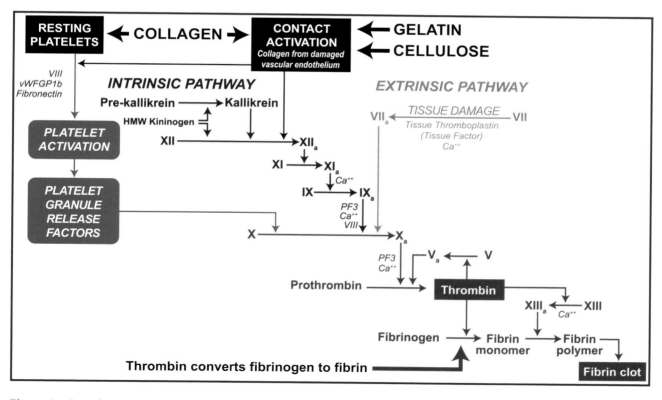

Figure 1 Coagulation cascade. Topical hemostatic agents containing cellulose, collagen, or gelatin stimulate the coagulation cascade through contact activation. Biologically active agents contain, either singly or in combination, thrombin and/or fibrinogen. When combined, thrombin's enzymatic action transforms fibrinogen into fibrin, augmenting the final stages of the coagulation cascade. From Baxter Healthcare Corporation, with permission

Table 1 Topical hemostatic agents in management of postpartum hemorrhage, in published case reports*

Hemostatic agent	Source	Product tradename	FDA† approval	How supplied	Biologically active mechanism	Resorption time	Recommended use	Precautions
Fibrin sealant spray	Human fibrinogen, human thrombin, synthetic aprotinin	TISSEEL™	1998	Liquid spray	When combined, thrombin's enzymatic action transforms fibrinogen into fibrin, augmenting final stages of coagulation cascade	Immediate	Where tissue adherence is desired in addition to hemostasis	Allergic reaction to aprotinin. Do not inject intravascularly. Do not use for severe or brisk bleeding. Made from human plasma and may carry risk of transmitting infectious disease
Gelatin–thrombin matrix	Bovine gelatin, human thrombin	FloSeal™	1999	Viscous gel	Upon contact with blood, the fibrinogen source, concentrated thrombin within the gelatin matrix converts fibrinogen into fibrin	6–8 weeks	Range of degrees of bleeding, from oozing to spurting; Where tissue tamponade effect is desired; Irregular wound surfaces	Swell volume 20%. Allergic reaction to bovine material. Do not inject intravascularly. Made from human plasma and may carry risk of transmitting infectious disease. Excess FloSeal should be removed by gentle irrigation
Fibrin sealant patch	Equine collagen, human thrombin, human fibrinogen	TachoSil®	2010	Fleece patch	An equine collagen sponge is coated on one side with fibrinogen and thrombin, which, upon contact with physiological fluids, form a fibrin sealant patch	13 weeks††	Large bleeding raw surface areas; Where promoting tissue sealing is desired in addition to hemostasis	Allergic reaction to equine proteins. Do not use intravascularly. Do not use for severe or brisk bleeding. Made from human plasma and may carry risk of transmitting infectious disease. Remove unattached pieces

*Off-label use

†Food and Drug Administration, United States.

††TachoSil® Prescribing Information Leaflet, revised: [04/2010]. 12.1 'In animal studies, TachoSil progressively biodegrades with only a few remnants left after 13 weeks. After complete biodegradation, no remnants of the TachoSil patch remained in the body.'

aprotinin component serves as an antifibrinolytic agent. TISSEEL adheres to wound surfaces, achieving hemostasis as well as tissue sealing or gluing. In hemorrhage scenarios, where tissue adherence is desired in addition to hemostasis, liquid fibrin sealant may be preferred.

TISSEEL is supplied as both freeze-dried kits and pre-filled syringes. The freeze-dried kit is stored at 2–25°C. The pre-filled syringe is frozen and stored at −20°C or less. In preparing the freeze-dried kit, to prevent premature clotting, separate syringes are used for reconstituting, as well as applying, the sealer protein and thrombin. In preparing the frozen pre-filled syringe, thawing can be performed at room temperature for up to 48 hours, on the sterile field using 33–37°C sterile water bath, or off the sterile field using water bath or incubator. In geographic regions lacking freezing capabilities, liquid fibrin sealant use is limited to the freeze-dried formulation (Figure 2).

Gelatin–thrombin hemostatic matrix (FloSeal) received FDA approval in 1999 as an adjunct to hemostasis when ligature or conventional procedures are ineffective or impractical. A matrix of bovine gelatin and human thrombin, it provides a concentrated source of thrombin within cross-linked gelatin granules[21] (Figure 3).

To activate the hemostatic matrix coagulation mechanism, blood must be present to provide the fibrinogen source. Upon contact with blood, the concentrated thrombin converts fibrinogen to fibrin. As a high viscosity gel, the gelatin–thrombin matrix fluidity conforms to irregular wound surfaces, thus filling defects and crevices[3,16]. Additionally, gelatin–thrombin matrix provides a tamponade effect, as gelatin granules expand approximately 20% within about 10 minutes of application. Furthermore, FloSeal is described to be 'effective on surgical bleeding, from oozing to spurting'[21]. The combination of fluidity, tamponade and arterial bleed effectiveness deems gelatin–thrombin hemostatic matrix a recommended hemostatic product in cases of irregular wound surfaces or hard-to-reach surfaces and of a range of degrees of bleeding from oozing to spurting[3,21].

Gelatin–thrombin hemostatic matrix is supplied as a freeze-dried kit containing: gelatin matrix in a 10 ml syringe, a vial of human thrombin (lyophilized), a vial of calcium chloride solution, and mixing accessories (bowl for thrombin, two 5 ml syringes, Luer connector and applicator tips). After reconstitution of lyophilized thrombin in calcium chloride solution, gelatin matrix granules are added to the mix by passing thrombin and gelatin between the two syringes. The mixing procedure is reported to take 2 minutes[13] (Figures 4 and 5). FloSeal is stored between 2°C and 25°C (36°F and 77°F), and should not be frozen (see also Chapter 57).

Collagen–thrombin–fibrinogen patch (TachoSil) was granted FDA approval in April 2010 as an adjunct to hemostasis in cardiovascular surgery. An equine collagen sponge is coated on one side with fibrinogen and thrombin[22]. Upon contact with physiological

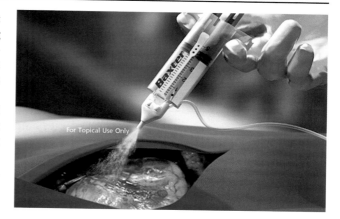

Figure 2 Fibrin sealant liquid spray application. From Baxter Healthcare Corporation, with permission

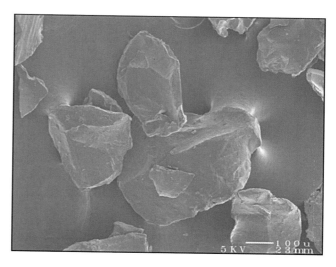

Figure 3 Cross-linked gelatin granules, approximately 0.5 mm diameter, create open spaces that allow high concentrations of thrombin to surround each gelatin particle. From Baxter Healthcare Corporation, with permission

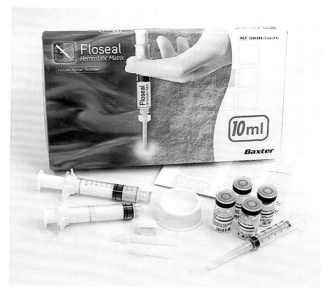

Figure 4 Gelatin–thrombin matrix kit. From Baxter Healthcare Corporation, with permission

fluids or pre-moistening with 0.9% saline solution, the components of the coating dissolve and fibrinogen is converted to fibrin, thus forming a fibrin sealant patch. Supplied in ready-to-use sterile packages, the patch is removed from the blister. The patch can be cut to the appropriate size and shape for the wound, if desired. The patch is applied directly to the bleeding area and pressure applied for at least 3 minutes[22] (Figures 6 and 7). TachoSil should be stored at between 2°C and 25°C (36°F and 77°F). It does not require refrigeration and should not be frozen.

The biologically active topical hemostatic agents discussed contain human plasma, and therefore may carry a risk of transmitting infectious disease despite viral transmission risk reduction procedures applied during manufacturing[20–22]. Hypersensitivity or allergic/anaphylactoid reactions to aprotinin, bovine material and equine material may occur.

Cases of bowel obstruction associated with laparoscopic FloSeal use in gynecologic oncology, urology

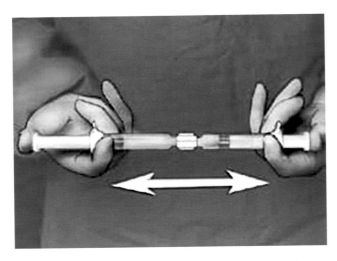

Figure 5 Transfer of gelatin matrix-thrombin solution mixture, back and forth between the syringes. From Baxter Healthcare Corporation, with permission

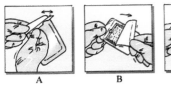
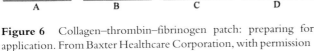

Figure 6 Collagen–thrombin–fibrinogen patch: preparing for application. From Baxter Healthcare Corporation, with permission

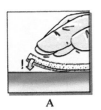
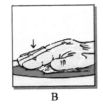
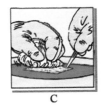

Figure 7 The patch is applied directly to the bleeding area. From Baxter Healthcare Corporation, with permission

and general surgery have been reported[23–25]. The presence of excess FloSeal and local inflammatory reaction were suggested as possible etiologies.

As with all medical agents and devices, sound judgment in evaluating risks and benefits of use is required. Topical hemostatic agents are intended to be adjuncts, not substitutes for, meticulous surgical technique and conventional methods to control bleeding. They are not intended for use as prophylactic hemostatic agents[20–22]. Casual use is not advised. In PPH of uterine origin, where conservative or uterine-sparing measures fail to control hemorrhage, hysterectomy is considered a life-saving procedure.

AN INSTITUTIONAL EXPERIENCE

White Memorial Medical Center (WMMC) is a nonprofit community hospital located just east of downtown Los Angeles, California, USA. Established in 1913 by the Seventh-day Adventist Church, the hospital's mission is to provide quality health services, medical and health education, and outreach services to the Los Angeles community, with care and compassion. With a capacity of 353 beds, WMMC serves a densely populated, low-income region with more than 2 million residents. Average household income is less than $48,000 a year, with 23% earning less than $25,000 per year. Most of this population is dependent on government-sponsored health care programs. Approximately 85% of the hospital's reimbursement comes from government sources.

The obstetric services at WMMC provide a tertiary referral center, with maternal–fetal medicine consultants and level III neonatal intensive care unit. High-risk obstetric patients are transferred to WMMC from local hospitals for the necessary obstetric and neonatal level of care.

In mid-2011, a retrospective chart review of obstetric services at WMMC, from 2004 to 2010, was conducted to identify cases of postpartum hysterectomy at the time of or within 48 hours of delivery. The review included prenatal records, operative reports, discharge summaries and outpatient postpartum visit notes. During the study period, an average of 3652 deliveries was performed per year. The highest number of deliveries performed during the study period was in the final year of chart review, 2010, with 4148 deliveries. From 2004 to 2010, the cesarean delivery rate increased from 28.5% to 35.5% of all deliveries, similar to the national average[26]. Among all cesarean deliveries, the percentage of repeat cesarean sections gradually increased from 42% to 52% between 2004 and 2010. An average of four postpartum hysterectomies were performed each year, with an incidence of 1 per 1000 deliveries. Abnormal placentation was identified as the most common indication for postpartum hysterectomy.

Our findings are consistent with the study by Rossi et al., who reported abnormal placentation to be replacing uterine atony as the most common indicator leading to emergency postpartum hysterectomy[27].

Our institutional experience includes other obstetric hemorrhage cases that were successfully managed with topical hemostatic agents, in addition to our case report of placenta previa hemorrhage[16].

Case 1

A 35-year-old patient, gravidity 2, parity 1, delivered a term male infant by vacuum assisted vaginal delivery. No vaginal or cervical lacerations were noted. Approximately 3 hours after delivery, the patient reported sudden onset profuse vaginal bleeding associated with Valsalva. At examination, a ruptured vaginal hematoma was noted, extending from the rupture site at the 6 o'clock position in the distal vagina at the level of the introitus, to the full length of the vagina with hematoma dissection of the rectovaginal septum and into the right ischial fossa. The depth of the defect was estimated to be 10 cm. Multiple scattered arterial and venous bleeding sites were diffusely distributed over the length of the rectovaginal septum, which was anatomically distorted by the marked distention of the hematoma. An attempt to suture was ineffective in the presence of friable attenuated tissue and large surface area of bleeding. Because the rectal mucosa was in close proximity and at risk when suturing the surrounding poor quality tissue, use of a topical hemostatic agent was chosen. Gelatin–thrombin matrix was preferred due to the presence of arterial bleeding, large hard-to-reach and irregular surface area, tamponade effect feature and desire for a non-adhering agent in order to leave an open drainage site. Bleeding was controlled in less than 2 minutes after one application of hemostatic gel. In the presence of brisk bleeding, a powder form topical hemostatic agent was not chosen due to risk of being washed away in the flow of blood before adequate polymerization of fibrin could occur.

Case 2

A 44-year-old multiparous patient presented with ruptured amniotic membranes in a pre-viable mid-trimester gestation. After passing the fetus vaginally, the patient developed a prolonged prothrombin time, prolonged activated thromboplastin time and thrombocytopenia, with the total clinical picture consistent with coagulopathy of sepsis. Furthermore, the patient continued to have profuse vaginal bleeding, assessed to be from coagulopathy and possibly placenta accreta, as retained placenta was diagnosed in this patient with prior cesarean deliveries. Coordinating the timing for blood replacement to correct the coagulopathy-based source of bleeding, with the timing for prompt surgical removal of the placental-based source of bleeding, is critical in optimizing outcomes. Continued blood loss, whether from coagulopathy of sepsis or from abnormal placentation or both, can exacerbate the underlying condition with the development of hemorrhagic shock and progressive

disseminated intravascular coagulation. As multi-unit blood transfusions were administered, placental delivery was performed by manual removal. Findings were suggestive of placenta accreta. The patient underwent emergency hysterectomy, with intraoperative bleeding consistent with on-going coagulopathy. The pelvic raw surfaces were large, as extensive lysis of adhesions was required in order to complete the hysterectomy. With massive blood transfusion in progress and administration of recombinant activated factor VII[28], control of bleeding at the vaginal cuff and pelvic raw surfaces was achieved with the adjunctive use of gelatin–thrombin hemostatic matrix.

The institutional experience at WMMC is similar to the case reports by Moriarty, Fuglsang and Whiteside[12,14,18].

DISCUSSION

Recent advances in biotechnology have added biologically active features to topical hemostatic agents. These are shown to be effective in controlling intraoperative bleeding in several surgical specialties, including controlled clinical trials of cardiac surgery[3]. In PPH, current literature is comprised of case reports, totaling 20 cases. Seventeen cases were reported for hemorrhage associated with placenta previa[13,14,16]. Two of these were associated with obstetric genital injury[18,19]. One case was associated with disseminated intravascular coagulation at emergency hysterectomy[12].

With a rising cesarean delivery rate[26] and the associated increased risk for placenta previa and placenta accreta[29], the presence of 17 cases in the literature of PPH associated with placenta previa successfully managed with resorbable bioactive topical hemostatic agent invites further investigation and consideration for both adjunct and primary treatment with topical hemostatic agents[13,14,16].

As an adjunct intervention when standard surgical methods fail to control hemorrhage, topical hemostatic agents may have a more primary role where surgical intervention is difficult, such as in under-resourced geographic regions, with limited or no access to emergency surgical facilities, blood banking resources, parenteral administration of medication capabilities and invasive radiology embolization. Availability and accessibility of topical hemostatic agents, with features of quick preparation and easy application, may decrease morbidity and mortality associated with delayed treatment of hemorrhage.

Although the use of topical hemostatic agents in managing PPH in peer-reviewed literature is limited to case reports, further studies may provide information to solidify topical hemostatic agents as an adjunct or primary treatment in PPH.

The authors have no financial interest or other relationship with the manufacturers of the products discussed in this manuscript.

References

1. Peralta E. Overview of topical hemostatic agents used in the operating room. 2011. http://www.uptodate.com/contents/overview-of-topical-hemostatic-agents
2. Achneck HE, Sileshi B, Jamiolkowski RM, et al. A comprehensive review of topical hemostatic agents. Ann Surg 2010; 251:217–28
3. Oz MC, Cosgrove DM 3rd, Badduke BR, et al. Controlled clinical trial of a novel hemostatic agent in cardiac surgery. The Fusion Matrix Study Group. Ann Thorac Surg 2000; 69:1376–82
4. Gall RM, Witterick IJ, Shargill NS, Hawke M. Control of bleeding in endoscopic sinus surgery: use of a novel gelatin-based hemostatic agent. J Otolaryngol 2002;31;5:271–4
5. Hong YM, Loughlin KR. The use of hemostatic agents and sealants in urology. J Urol 2006;176:2367–74
6. Gazzeri R, Galarza M, Neroni M, Alfieri A, Giordano M. Hemostatic matrix sealant in neurosurgery: a clinical and imaging study. Acta Neurochir 2011;153:148–55
7. Angioli R, Ludovico M, Roberto M, et al. Feasibility of the use of novel matrix hemostatic sealant (FloSeal) to achieve hemostasis during laparoscopic excision of endometrioma. J Min Inv Gynecol 2009;16:153–6
8. Ebert AD, Hollauer A, Fuhr N, Langolf O, Papadopoulos T. Laparoscopic ovarian cystectomy without bipolar coagulation or sutures using a gelatin-thrombin matrix sealant (FloSeal): first support of a promising technique. Arch Gynecol Obstet 2009;280:161–5
9. Raga F, Sanz-Cortez M, Bonilla F, et al. Reducing blood loss at myomectomy with use of a gelatin-thrombin matrix hemostatic sealant. Fertil Steril 2009;92:356–60
10. Madhuri TK, Tailor A, Butler-Manuel S. Use of surgical sealant in debulking surgery for advanced ovarian carcinoma – case report. Eur J Gynaecol Oncol 2010;31:582–3
11. Han LY, Schimp V, Oh JC, Ramirez PT. A gelatin matrix-thrombin tissue sealant (FloSeal) application in the management of groin breakdown after inguinal lymphadenectomy for vulvar cancer. Int J Gynecol Cancer 2004;14:621–4
12. Moriarty KT, Premila S, Bulmer PJ. Use of FloSeal haemostatic gel in massive obstetric haemorrhage: a case report. Br J Obstet Gynaecol 2008;115:793–5
13. Law WL, Chor CM, Leung TY. Use of hemostatic gel in postpartum hemorrhage due to placenta previa. Obstet Gynecol 2010;116:528–30
14. Fuglsang K, Petersen LK. New local hemostatic treatment for postpartum hemorrhage caused by placenta previa at cesarean section. Acta Obstet Gynecol 2010;89:1346–9
15. Tinelli A. Post-cesarean section hemorrage treated by a collagen patch coated with the human coagulation factors. J Clinic Case Reports 2011;1:1000e102
16. Wohlmuth C, Dela Merced J. Gelatin-thrombin hemostatic matrix in the management of placental site postpartum hemorrhage, a case report. J Reprod Med 2011;56:271–3
17. Doumouchtsis SK, Papageorghiou AT, Arulkumaran S. Systemic review of conservative management of postpartum hemorrhage: what to do when medical treatment fails. Obstet Gynecol Surv 2007;62:540–7
18. Whiteside J, Asif RB, Novello RJ. Fibrin sealant for management of complicated obstetric lacerations. Obstet Gynecol 2010;115:403–4
19. Dhulkotia JS, Alazzam M, Galimberti A. TISSEEL for management of traumatic postpartum haemorrhage. Arch Gynecol Obstet 2009;279:437–9
20. Baxter Healthcare Corporation. TISSEEL [Fibrin Sealant] Full Prescribing Information. Hayward, California, USA: Baxter Healthcare Corporation, 2010
21. Baxter Healthcare Corporation. FloSeal Hemostatic Matrix Instructions for Use. Hayward, California, USA: Baxter Healthcare Corporation, 2010
22. Baxter Healthcare Corporation. TachoSil® Prescribing Information Leaflet. 2010. www.baxtersurgery.com/resources/pdfs/TachoSil
23. Clapp B, Santillan A. Small bowel obstruction after FloSeal use. JSLS 2011;15:361–4
24. Suzuki Y, Vellinga TT, Istre O, Einarsson JI. Small bowel obstruction associated with use of a gelatin-thrombin matrix sealant (FloSeal) after laparoscopic gynecologic surgery. J Minim Invasive Gynecol 2010;17:641–5
25. Hobday CD, Milam MR, Milam RA, Euscher E, Brown J. Postoperative small bowel obstruction associated with use of hemostatic agents. J Minim Invasive Gynecol 2009;16:224–6
26. Hamilton BE, Martin JA, Ventura SJ. United States Department of Health and Human Services, Centers for Disease Control and Prevention, National Center for Health Statistics, National Vital Statistics Reports 2009;57:12
27. Rossi AC, Lee RH, Chmait RH. Emergency postpartum hysterectomyy for uncontrolled postpartum bleeding, a systematic review. Obstet Gynecol 2010;115:637–44
28. Bouwmeester FW, Jonkhoff AR, Verheijen RH, van Geijn HP. Successful treatment of life-threatening postpartum hemorrhage with recombinant activated factor VII. Obstet Gynecol 2003;101:1174–6
29. Miller DA, Chollet JA, Goodwin TM. Clinical risk factors for placenta previa-placenta accreta. Am J Obstet Gynecol 1997; 177:210–4

Section 10

Consequences of Postpartum Hemorrhage

59

The Normal and Pathologic Postpartum Uterus

P. Kelehan and E. E. Mooney

BACKGROUND AND AIMS

Significant postpartum hemorrhage (PPH) may occur immediately after delivery or may be delayed by weeks or months. In either circumstance, a hysterectomy may be life saving. The uterus normally will be sent for pathologic examination. To facilitate preparation of a useful surgical pathology report, however, the pathologist must be given details of the antepartum course and delivery. Considering how uncommon these specimens are, direct communication between pathologist and clinician is recommended so that the many important details of the case may be fully appreciated. The aim of this chapter is to provide a structured approach to the analysis of the specimen, in order to permit a clinically relevant and pathologically sound diagnosis.

CLINICAL CORRELATION

The patient's parity and gestation should be provided. Any abnormality of the clinical course, in particular pre-eclampsia or polyhydramnios, may be of relevance. Magnetic resonance imaging (MRI) may have been performed for fibroid, placenta creta or congenital abnormality and these images should be available for review. A history of the use of instruments such as forceps is important. The initial clinical appearance of the uterus at the time of operation may provide valuable information on atony. Any therapeutic measures undertaken such as uterine massage or placement of a compression suture(s) should be noted, along with transfusion and fluid replacement. A description of the surgery (ideally a full copy of the operative report) will help the pathologist to interpret tears and sutures that normally characterize these specimens. The patient's postoperative condition will help to guide sampling in the event that amniotic fluid embolism is also a consideration. Finally, the placenta must also be available for examination.

GROSS EXAMINATION

Photography is essential at each step of the dissection, with notes as to what each picture is intended to show. Without a clinical input, however, much effort may be wasted on documenting features of little relevance at the expense of missing more important ones. A detailed macroscopic description of sutures, tears, etc. is important and may be relevant medicolegally. Our approach is to examine the specimen in its fresh state, using photography, and then to open the specimen, avoiding tears and sutures, to permit fixation and further examination. The uterus may be opened laterally, but more information can be gained by complete longitudinal anteroposterior section. This approach should be modified to suit the circumstances as predicted from the clinical information obtained along with the specimen. A useful technique that allows good exposure and photographic demonstration is the placing of two parallel complete longitudinal anteroposterior sections about 2–3 cm apart on either side of the midline. How well the uterine cavity has compressed is immediately apparent, contraction band (if present) formation can be demonstrated, and blood clot and placental tissue fragments can be assessed in the lumen (Figure 1).

In the immediate postpartum period, the uterus is characteristically large. It will weigh 700–900 g on average and will have substantially reduced in size and volume from its antepartum state. Clamp marks on the broad and round ligaments should be inspected for residual hematoma, remembering that the pathology may be outside the clamp. In the fresh specimen with intact vessels, it may be possible to perfuse the vasculature for contrast angiography or vascular casting[1]. In this manner the subplacental vasculature can be demonstrated and the location of any arteriovenous malformations identified (Figures 1 and 2).

UTEROPLACENTAL VASCULATURE

Schapps and Tsatsaris *et al.*[1] have proposed a model of human uteroplacental vascularization. They replace the old concept of maternal blood spurting into the intervillous space from uterine arteries with the blood flowing past fetal chorionic villi in a low-resistance high-flow circuit and behaving as an arteriovenous shunt in the placenta as it flows back into uterine veins. They propose and show evidence for a uterine vascular anastomotic network in the subplacental

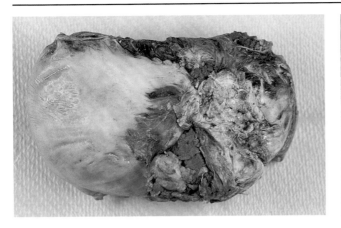

Figure 1 Fixed uterus showing a large anterior and right-sided diverticulum originating in a cesarean section scar. The specimen was sutured at operation, but placental villous tissue can be seen adjacent to the suture

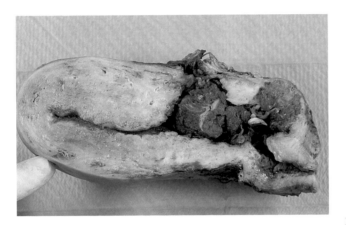

Figure 2 Anteroposterior section of uterus from Figure 1 showing anterior placenta creta

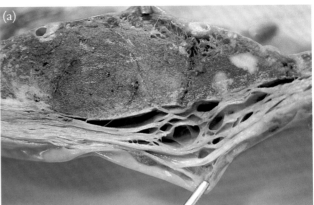

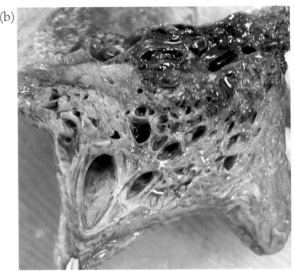

Figure 3 Demonstration of the subplacental uterine vascular anastomotic network described by Schapps and Tsatsaris et al.[1]. (a) Near term undelivered indirect maternal death, flacid myometrium, postmortem allows the dilated vessels beneath the placenta to be easily seen. (b) Postpartum indirect maternal death day 4, vessels remain dilated. There is in addition adherent blood clots associated with subinvolution of the placental site

myometrium, which controls blood flow to the decidual 'spiral arterioles'. Maternofetal exchange occurs within a system in which the uterine vascular network plays an important role, supplying blood to the intervillous space, which is positioned in parallel to the main circuit. In this model, the intervillous space is not a high flow shunt and the fetal circulation is protected from acute maternal hypertensive events. Placental detachment after delivery does not open up high flow vessels, the spiral arterioles are more easily compressible and uterine arterial blood flow is diverted through its anastomoses to the venous system[1]. This concept is of interest in the light of evolving theories of placental mechanical and oxidative stress resulting from pulsatile flow into the intervillous space consequent on inadequate transformation of the spiral arteries[2] (Figure 3). [Editor's note: Interested readers will find more information on this topic in Chapter 24. L.G.K.]

CERVIX

Tears are among the most important pathologies found in the cervix. Small shallow endocervical tears

are almost invariably present in the postpartum state, and may be seen even in those cases where cesarean section has prevailed. In contrast, significant and deep tears tend to be lateral in location, may penetrate through to the serosa (with or without hematoma formation), and may extend up into the lower uterine segment or down into the vagina. If extension is upward, involvement of large uterine arteries is possible and should be sought. As it is common to find meconium staining of the endocervical mucus in the presence of fetal distress, meconium may contaminate the tear. It is axiomatic that cervical tears may have severe consequences; for example, an endocervical tear may cause severe and life-threatening blood loss despite a fully contracted uterus. Tears can be associated with amniotic fluid embolus or with amniotic infusion and local defibrination. Upwardly extending tears may be associated with bleeding into the broad ligament with hematoma formation. Suturing of the cervical tear *per se* without considering the patient's general condition may not prevent a deep hematoma from forming; secondary rupture can result in shock, despite cessation of external vaginal hemorrhage.

In the dilated postpartum cervix, edema, hemorrhage and disarray of the normal architecture of the muscle fibers may make it difficult to identify tears on histologic examination. Torn and contracted muscle fibers and torn arteries with fibrin plugs and tense hematomas provide corroboratory evidence of a tear. Histologic sampling should include blocks from above the apex and from below the tear to identify deep extension and for identification of large torn vessels.

Following amniotic fluid embolism, histologic examination of the uterus will show no evidence of intravascular disease in many cases. Occasionally, however, there may be fibrin clots adherent to vascular endothelium, and squames admixed with fibrin have been found in vessels in the body of the uterus. In some cases of PPH, when there have been no clinical features of acute amniotic infusion but bleeding and unexpected severe onset of consumptive coagulopathy, histological sections of the endocervix will reveal localized areas where amniotic debris fills and expands venules and capillaries. This dramatic appearance is present not only adjacent to the endocervical surface and tears, but also its presence deeper in the stroma distinguishes it from contamination of the surface mucosa by meconium and amniotic fluid at delivery (Figures 4–6).

A subgroup of patients have a lesion of local amniotic infusion associated with disseminated intravascular coagulopathy (DIC) and PPH without systemic collapse. Squamous cells may be present in only one or two sections taken from around the circumference of the cervix. It is usually on one side. Extensive sampling of the cervix may be required to demonstrate amniotic debris in cases of suspected amniotic fluid embolism[3]. It is possible that ongoing blood loss from a tear in this site may occur before the onset of systemic DIC, because the local thromboplastin effect alone of the amniotic debris in the wound may inhibit hemostasis.

LOWER UTERINE SEGMENT

Important pathologies at this location involve placental implantation on a previous cesarean section scar, with abnormal adherence or formation of a diverticulum. A prior cesarean section results in chronic changes in the lower uterine segment, which may include distortion and widening, inflammation, giant cell reaction, implantation endometriosis and adenomyosis[4]. In some instances, a distinctive V-shaped defect of the anterior uterine wall ('tenting') may be present.

Emergency cesarean section in particular may be associated with circumstances that cause the incision repair to be suboptimal. In examining hysterectomy specimens for menorrhagia considerable variation in the morphology of the lower uterine segment repair is seen, sometimes with persistent inflammatory foci many years after the last cesarean section. Approximately one-third of lower segment scars examined

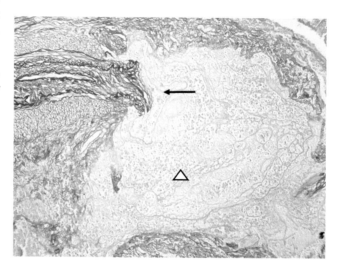

Figure 5 Elastin Van Geisson stain showing torn artery at apex of tear. Arrow, torn elastic artery; arrowhead, thin fibrin blood clot

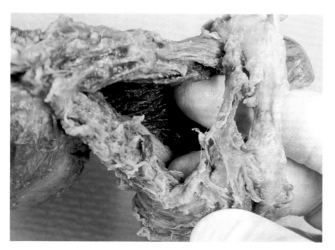

Figure 4 Right lateral endocervical tear at hysterectomy for PPH

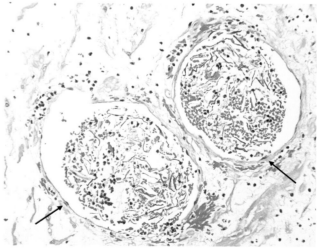

Figure 6 Amniotic debris in venules (arrows) of cervical stroma following a small endocervical tear in labor. PPH and disseminated intravascular coagulopathy necessitated hysterectomy

histologically will show very deficient interweaving or meshing of myometrial fiber bundles. Occasionally they will show only a thin collagen scar or scar and foci of implantation endometriosis which may extend from lumen to serosa.

An important cause of the weakening of any cesarean section scar is infection. Postoperative wound infection (overt and covert) is not uncommon following cesarean section, particularly the emergency variety. Prophylactic antibiotics can modify the extent and rate of infection, as can the quality of closure, the amount of local tissue trauma, the technique used (one- or two-layer), the presence of swelling and/or hematoma and the nature of the organisms infecting the wound. There may be extensive disruption and inflammation in the uterine wound despite a normal healing appearance of the skin wound. Conservative treatment of the skin wound is normal, and surgical debridement the exception. Accordingly, the consequences of infection at the scar site may be only appreciated in a subsequent pregnancy. If the patient does

present before this, hemorrhage and/or vaginal discharge may prompt internal examination. A defect may be identified on palpation. Curettage may be undertaken and may retrieve inflammatory exudate, degenerating decidua, polypoid endometrium or fragments of necrotic myometrium that have prolapsed into the endocervical lumen from the internal edge of the cesarean section scar. Sometimes, quite large pieces of myometrial tissue with edema and coagulative necrosis are obtained. This site related myonecrosis or incisional necrosis is caused by local ischemia[5] (Figures 7–9). Remodeling of blood vessels at the site of the former scar may influence subsequent placental implantation. This is important, because implantation on either a normally healed or a diseased scar will not have the protective effect of the presence of decidua vera (see below), and accordingly postpartum separation at the time of a subsequent pregnancy is less likely to occur. A cesarean section at first birth is associated with increased risks of placenta previa and abruption in second pregnancies[6].

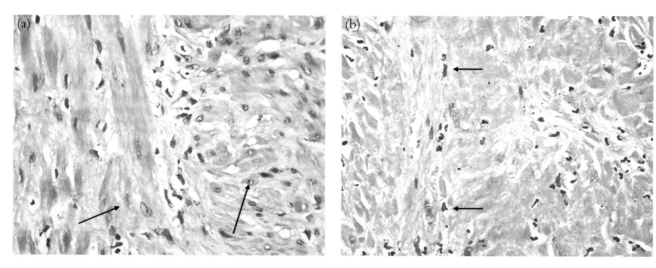

Figure 7   H/E comparison of (a) normal myometrial fibers and (b) myonecrosis in lower uterine segment in hysterectomy specimen for postpartum hemorrhage following cesarean section. Long arrows, normal viable cell nuclei; short arrows, non-viable necrotic cells

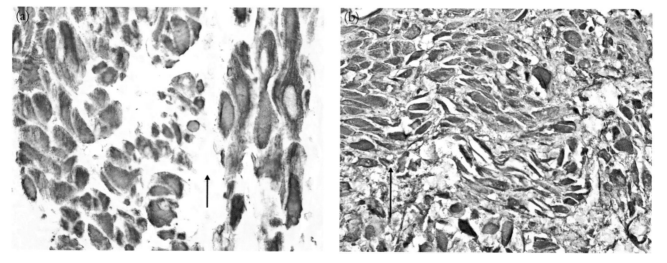

Figure 8   Desmin comparison of same myometrial fibers accentuates the necrosis. (a) Normal; (b) myonecrosis. Long arrow, normal myometrial cells with intercellular edema; short arrow, dense, compacted necrotic myometrial cells at same magnification

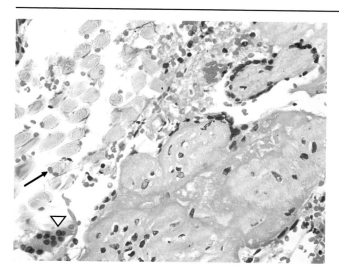

Figure 9 H/E section showing stitch material in uterine curettings following cesarean section. Arrow, absorbable suture; arrowhead, giant cell reaction to suture material

Implantation in the lower segment (adjacent to the defect) can cause expansion of the defect, dehiscence of the wall and the formation of a pulsion diverticulum which will further enlarge and progress with growth of the placenta. If the implantation is fundal, on the other hand, a fortuitous elective section may reveal a thin, almost transparent anterior lower segment wall. This should be more easily resected at the time of closure, as the scar will not be excessively vascular. If implantation is in the lower segment or in the scar, then the potential for catastrophic hemorrhage on attempt at delivery of the placenta is real.

The points noted above should be borne in mind when examining a postpartum hysterectomy specimen where there is a history of previous cesarean section. The recently sutured section incision may be carefully reopened. Following photography, the edges and margins should be inspected for thinning and scar tissue formation. An enlarged, ragged and open defect of the anterior lower uterine segment, now tightly contracted and rigid with formalin fixation, may be all that is left of a huge, thin-walled, placenta-filled diverticulum, the result of scar dehiscence and rupture. It is easy to destroy this thin structure with hurried dissection. Examination of the lateral margins of the defect may indicate left- or more often right-sided extension of the bulging diverticulum into parametrial soft tissue of the pelvis. A complete section through the anterior lower uterine segment can identify previous cesarean section scars with tenting defects and the shape and edges of a recent section. Most importantly, en-face examination of the lateral sides of the lower segment will show the cavity and lateral extension of a dehiscence diverticulum, fresh tears and/or adherent placenta. The issue of abnormal adherence is addressed below.

FUNDUS

Important pathologies include retained products, placenta creta and subinvolution. Placenta creta is the

name given to abnormally adherent or ingrowing placenta that does not detach with full contraction of the uterus after expulsion of the fetus. This term covers placenta accreta (abnormal attachment to the wall), increta (extension of villi into the myometrium) and percreta (extension of villi through to the serosa). The intimate relationship of villous tissue to myometrium, without intervening decidua, is key to the diagnosis. Descriptions of placenta percreta based on illustrations or descriptions of chorionic villi displaced between torn myometrial fibers should be evaluated critically. If MRI has been obtained, views may show the loss of zonation associated with penetration rather than invasion of chorionic villi.

Full-thickness anteroposterior sections of the fundus make it easier to recognize the position of the contracted placental site. It is surprisingly difficult to identify the exact placental site on inspection of the raw decidual surface that is seen if the uterus is opened laterally.

Detachment of the placenta is dependent on the presence of a normal spongy decidua vera, where shearing of the placenta from the myometrium occurs. This soft compressible area is not seen when the postpartum uterine lining is examined histologically, because its many mucous glands are disrupted to facilitate the normal plane of cleavage. It is seen to its full extent in the tragic cases of maternal death prior to labor. Either Alcian blue stain or diastase-PAS can be used to demonstrate mucopolysaccharides in the swollen gland crypts that help to identify this layer. Deficiency of this layer may be focal or, rarely, complete. When it is absent, the thinned Nitabuch's layer with anchoring villi lies in close proximity to muscle fiber bundles or the interstitial fibrous cesarean section scar. An occasional finding is the presence of abundant intermediate trophoblast infiltrating between muscle fibers beneath a firmly adherent Nitabuch's layer. Histological examination of multiple sections can show anchoring villi penetrating Nitabuch's fibrinoid and ghost villi in dense fibrin adherent to muscle. The often described appearance of chorionic villi infiltrating between muscle fibers is characteristic only of invasive mole; the key to the diagnosis of placenta percreta is the absence of decidua. An increased number of implantation site intermediate trophoblasts has been shown in cases of placenta creta compared with controls[7]. Retained placental fragments reflect some degree of placenta creta and are more common in women with a spectrum of changes in previous pregnancies, such as pre-eclamptic toxemia, growth restriction, spontaneous abortion and retained placental fragments. It has been hypothesized that these latter conditions reflect abnormal maternal–trophoblast interaction[8].

Placenta creta is therefore due to a deficiency of the decidua. The end result of penetration of the placenta through a weakened part of the uterine wall includes rupture and secondary changes, including serosal peritoneal reaction. Curette penetration may cause secondary infection or hematoma formation and provide the nidus for dehiscence into the adherent bladder wall, if this had been injured at previous surgery.

Placenta creta is only part of the problem of uncontrolled PPH. The thin myometrium, with little muscle, interstitial fibrosis and increased intermediate trophoblast will contain large dilated arteries of pregnancy and often widespread extrauterine extension of these changes into the parametrium, as demonstrated on Doppler ultrasound. The degree of constriction–contraction of the myometrium is insufficient to close off these vessels. Where there is severe thinning of the muscle of the lower segment with diverticulum formation, abnormal adhesion is not necessary to sustain bleeding (Figures 10 and 11). Conversely, on histological examination of the lining of the postpartum uterus, the finding of chorionic villi in clefts in the placental bed may be an artifact rubbed in following clearance of uterine contents and is of no diagnostic consequence. Smearing of DNA due to crush artifact may be helpful in distinguishing this from true extension.

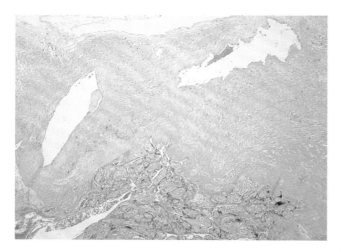

Figure 10 H/E section of lower uterine segment showing placenta creta and large vessels in thin myometrium

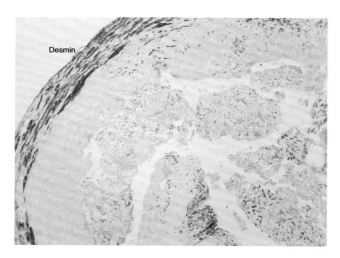

Figure 11 Immunohistochemical stain for desmin accentuates the thin myometrial fibers in scar

RETAINED PLACENTA AND RETAINED PRODUCTS OF CONCEPTION

The failure of total expulsion of the placenta may lead to PPH and attempted removal is a major cause of maternal mortality and morbidity worldwide. Herman and colleagues[9] offer perspectives into third stage mechanisms. They have shown by dynamic ultrasound techniques that the normal third stage has three distinct phases: (1) latent phase – in which the whole uterus can be seen to contract except for the area behind the placenta; (2) contraction phase – the retroplacental myometrium contracts; and (3) detachment and expulsion phase. It is further suggested that an as yet unknown placental factor plays a major part in controlling and inhibiting contraction in the subplacental myometrium[10]. Following delivery of the placenta, fragments that remain in the uterus may be attached or detached. A fragment of placenta remaining attached, assumes a polypoid shape ('placental polyp'), and undergoes compression and some devitalization. Viable trophoblast and villous stromal cells may persist due to continuing uteroplacental perfusion.

Plasma cell infiltrate may be present in the adjacent myometrium; however, this is not always diagnostic of (infective) endometritis in this context. Detached placental fragments are devitalized and along with blood clot form a nidus for delayed involution and ascending infection. The frequency of detection of retained products varies from 27 to 88%[8], but much of this literature is decades old and was obtained before the routine use of ultrasonography. Nevertheless, retained placental fragments are more common in women who have experienced pre-eclampsia or growth restriction in previous pregnancies. This observation has been interpreted as indicative of an abnormal maternal–trophoblast relationship[8].

SUBINVOLUTION

In the absence of retained placental fragments, subinvolution of the blood vessels of the placental bed is an important and distinctive cause of secondary PPH. This important idiopathic and non-iatrogenic condition has been recognized in the pathology literature for more than 50 years, but is rarely mentioned in clinical texts. It is to be distinguished from clinical atony alone, but may also have co-morbidity of retained fragments of placenta or sepsis.

Normal arterial involution involves a decrease in the lumen size, disappearance of trophoblast, thickening of the intima, re-growth of endothelium and regeneration of internal elastic lamina. These changes normally occur within 3 weeks of delivery. With subinvolution, on the other hand, arteries remain distended and contain red cells or fresh thrombus, and trophoblast persists in a perivascular location[11]. In some cases, endovascular trophoblast may be present. Hemorrhage from subinvolution is maximal in the second week postpartum, although it may occur up to several months later. It is commoner in older, multiparous women and may recur in subsequent deliveries.

Subinvolution is not related to the method of delivery and may be regarded as a specific entity, possibly due to an abnormal immunologic relationship between trophoblast and the uterus[11]. Despite this, subinvolution did not show the association with markers of such an abnormal relationship seen with retained placental fragments in another study[8].

Subinvolutionary changes may be recognized on curettage specimens, whereas hysterectomy specimens are characterized by a uterus that is soft and larger than expected[11]. As normally involuted vessels may be present adjacent to subinvoluted ones, multiple blocks of placental bed should be taken to exclude this process (Figure 12).

ATONY

Although this is a well-recognized clinical phenomenon, but there is little to report in the way of pathology. The diagnosis is one of exclusion. The uterus is enlarged, edematous and soft, with edema and hemorrhage apparent microscopically. The diagnosis will depend on clinical information, combined with adequate histologic sampling to exclude other causes.

ARTERIOVENOUS MALFORMATIONS

Uterine arteriovenous malformations (AVMs) are rare and may present with profuse hemorrhage, including hemorrhage in the postpartum period. Congenital AVMs consist of multiple small connections and may enlarge with pregnancy. The more common acquired AVMs are rare in nulliparous women, and are thought to arise following uterine trauma: curettage, myomectomy or even previous uterine rupture (Figure 13). AVMs may co-exist with retained products of conception or trophoblastic proliferation. Pathologically, vessels of arterial and venous caliber are present, along with large vessels of indeterminate nature. It is possible that the special vasculature of the uterus may, in abnormal situations, contribute to the formation of AVMs.

OTHER CAUSES OF POSTPARTUM HEMORRHAGE

Lacerations of the inner myometrium can cause PPH[14]. Women with leiomyomas are at an increased risk of PPH[15]. Less commonly, endometrial carcinomas and congenital anomalies may also result in reduced decidua formation and subsequent PPH. Trophoblastic disease has also been reported in this context.

ENDOMYOMETRITIS

Sepsis causing acute endometritis is reported as a cause of PPH, and hemorrhage may be followed by ascending infection. It is relatively uncommon in modern obstetric practice in the developed world and

may be due to a variety of organisms. Its incidence is increased following emergency cesarean section. It accounted for less than 5% of cases of delayed PPH in one series[8].

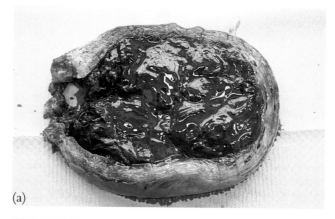

(a)

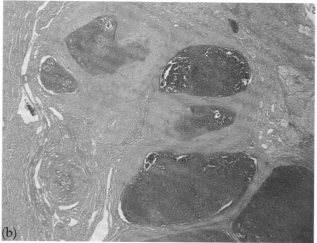

(b)

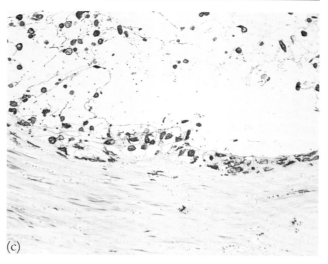

(c)

Figure 12 (a) Anteroposterior section of postpartum uterus 5 days following emergency cesarean section. Secondary PPH with blood filled uterus due to subinvolution of the placental site. Bleeding was from the fundus not the cesarean site. (b) Low power microscopic image of greatly dilated thrombosed subinvoluted blood vessels in the postpartum placental bed. H/E. (c) Cytokeratin staining of endovascular trophoblast

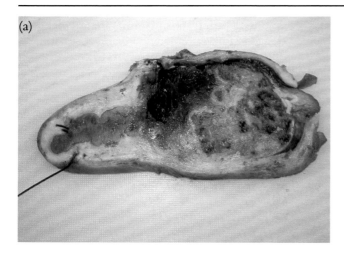
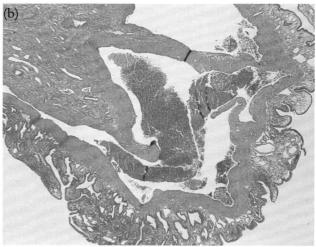

Figure 13 (a) Anteroposterior section of postpartum uterus 2 months following cesarean section for severe placenta accreta with conservative management including uterine artery embolization. Severe bleeding has recurred in association with arteriovenous malformation. (b) Low power microscopic image of part of large arteriovenous malformation which extends to the endocervical mucosa. H/E

PLACENTAL PATHOLOGY

The placenta should be examined wherever possible in cases of PPH. Pre-eclampsia may cause retro-placental hemorrhage: recent and old hemorrhages and infarcts may be seen. The characteristic changes of acute atherosis are only present in 50% of cases of pre-eclamptic toxemia. However, examination of the parenchyma will usually show so-called accelerated villous maturation (distal villous hypoplasia) in response to uteroplacental ischemia. Sampling from the center of the placental disc is important to avoid overinterpretation of physiologic changes[16].

THE AUTOPSY AFTER POSTPARTUM HEMORRHAGE

In data drawn from the Confidential Enquiries into Maternal Deaths in the UK for the period 1970–90, approximately 10% of direct maternal deaths are due to hemorrhage[17]. Roughly half were antepartum and half postpartum. Excess blood loss is more common in older women (>35 or 40 years, depending on the study)[18]. This trend and ratio has continued to the 2006–2008 Confidential Enquiries into Maternal Deaths in the UK report[19].

Before beginning an autopsy in a case of maternal death following postpartum or intrapartum hemorrhage, it is critical to plan the procedure and the sequence of the autopsy in the light of the information received and the suspected cause or causes and mode of death. The autopsy must be unhurried and methodical; it is a fundamental mistake to seek to demonstrate immediately the proposed cause of death. Members of the clinical team should be asked to attend, but it is unwise to have everybody there during what will be a long phase of inspection, measurement and initial systematic dissection. When all is ready, the procedure is stopped and members of the clinical team attend. In this manner, the history can be reviewed, pre-existing

conditions or disease discussed and demonstrated, e.g. chronic pyelonephritis, and the dissection and demonstration of the focus of main clinical interest can commence.

A fundamental aspect of good autopsy practice is the confident exclusion of specific diseases and conditions in a systematic approach. The understandable desire and pressure to skip to the seat of disease must be resisted. The parametrium, pelvic side-walls and vagina are as important objects of attention as is the uterus.

At the time of external inspection of the body, the pathologist must consider in turn each of the major causes of maternal death. Many require modification of routine techniques, e.g. air embolism, amniotic fluid embolism, ruptured aneurysm, and these modifications are detailed elsewhere[20]. Preparation and sampling of blood and fluids for hematology, hemophilia, toxicology and microbiology may be planned, e.g. sample containers should be pre-labeled and set out in sequence. Cardiopulmonary resuscitation attempts most likely preceded death, and therefore the features and sequence of sustained unsuccessful resuscitation must be identified and the complications and accompanying agonal changes interpreted in this context. It is important from a medicolegal aspect not to allow such artifacts to be construed as a major factor in the cause of death, e.g. liver or mesenteric tear, blood in the abdomen, bone marrow embolus.

The traditional Y-shaped autopsy incision should be extended to an abdominal inverted Y with the incision continued to the inguinal femoral triangle on each side. This allows better examination of the ileofemoral vessels and better exposure of the pelvis. Blood and blood clots are removed from the abdomen and the amounts of each measured. The relative size and position of the abdominopelvic organs are assessed. The peritoneal lining of the pelvis is inspected, noting color, texture and degree of congestion. Patches of peritoneal decidual reaction of pregnancy can be identified by their gelatinous appearance.

In traditional autopsy practice, the state of pregnancy can be suspected, even when the uterus is still small, by the characteristic dilated and congested appearance of retroperitoneal veins. The degree of dilation and turgidity of the pelvic veins should be noted early at autopsy as they will be dissected and examined in detail later. Retroperitoneal hematoma and broad ligament hematoma should be identified or excluded at this stage as these may be less easily assessed and measured following organ removal. The uterus may be examined and opened *in situ*, but it is better to remove adrenal, renal and pelvic organs as one complete block.

The traditional method of blunt dissection along the pelvic side-wall and pubis with transection at the mid to upper vagina is extended in the investigation of PPH. Following knife separation of the symphysis pubis, the legs are externally rotated and a knife cut is made along the lower edge of the pubic bone. The pubic bones are forcefully separated by 8–10 cm. This, together with the inguinal femoral incisions, gives good exposure of the paracervical and paravaginal soft tissues. Lateral vaginal wall tears and hemorrhage can be inspected and well demonstrated by this modified technique. The ileofemoral vessels are transected and inspected. The complete urogenital block is placed on a dissection board where it can be opened in layers, beginning with the urethra and bladder, then the vagina and cervix. Alternatively, the block can be placed in formalin and later dissected after short fixation.

The aorta is opened posteriorly and incision is extended into the branches of the iliac arteries for a short distance. The inferior vena cava is opened from the anterior side, probed and dissected into the right and left renal veins; the ovarian veins are identified and opened, and dissection is continued into the branches of the pelvic veins out to the limits of the excised specimen. The intima is examined for evidence of tear or abrasion and for adherent thrombus. Pieces of tissue containing venous plexus from the broad ligament and parametrium are selected for formalin fixation and histological examination.

When the patient has died of hemorrhage and where there has been an attempt to stem the bleeding by hysterectomy and under-sewing of bleeding sites and pedicles, it may be very difficult to identify the exact sites of bleeding, and ancillary techniques may be helpful. Prior to pelvic dissection, an infusion of saline through an intravenous infusion set and cannula into the clamped abdominal aorta may identify a bleeding point. With special preparation and ligation of all peripheral vessels, autopsy specimen angiography may be very valuable in selected cases.

The most useful of all techniques is the histological examination of carefully selected blocks of tissue demonstrating vital reaction to injury and the presence or absence of conditions predisposing to disease.

Detailed histological examination is a prerequisite of good autopsy practice in the investigation of maternal death. Amniotic fluid embolus, pregnancy-induced or essential hypertension, pre-eclampsia and rare conditions such as thrombotic thrombocytopenic purpura or cardiac sarcoidosis always need histological examination for diagnosis or confirmation. A minimum of organs to be sampled and sections taken is recommended in the investigation of all maternal deaths[21].

SUMMARY

In modern obstetrics practice in developed countries, an important cause of life threatening PPH is morbid adhesion of the placenta to a previous cesarean section scar. Recognition of this potential complication is an essential consideration in the investigation and clinical management of the pregnant woman with previous cesarean delivery. Gross and microscopic pathology findings can enhance the interpretation of radiologic images and explain the pathophysiology of this condition. Histological evaluation of poorly appreciated conditions such as subinvolution and arteriovenous malformation are an essential component of the evaluation of PPH.

References

1. Schaaps JP, Tsatsaris V, Goffin F, et al. Shunting the inter-villous space: new concepts in human uteroplacental vascularisation. Am J Obstet Gynecol 2005;192:323–32
2. James JL, Whitley GS, Cartwright JE. Pre-eclampsia – fitting together the placental, immune and cardiovascular pieces. J Pathol 2010;221:363–78
3. Cheung ANY, Luk SC. The importance of extensive sampling and examination of cervix in suspected cases of amniotic fluid embolism. Arch Gynecol Obstet 1994;255:101–5
4. Morris H. Surgical pathology of the lower uterine segment caesarean section scar: is the scar a source of symptoms? Int J Gynecol Pathol 1995;14:16–20
5. Rivilin ME, Carroll CS, Morrison JC. Uterine incisional necrosis complicating caesarean section. J Reprod Med 2003;48:687–91
6. Getahun D, Oyelese Y, Salihu H, Anath CV. Previous caesarean delivery and risks of placenta previa and placental abruption. Obstet Gynecol 2006;107:771–8
7. Kim KR, Jun SY, Kim JY, Ro JY. Implantation site intermediate trophoblasts in placenta cretas. Mod Pathol 2004;17:1483–90
8. Khong TY, Khong TK. Delayed postpartum hemorrhage: a morphologic study of causes and their relation to other pregnancy disorders. Obstet Gynecol 1993;82:17–22
9. Herman A, Weinraub Z, Bukovsky I, et al. Dynamic ultrasonographic imaging of the third stage of labour: new perspectives into third stage mechanism. Am J Obstet Gynecol 1993;168:1496–9
10. Weeks AD, Mirembe FM. The retained placenta – new insights into an old problem. Eur J Obstet Gynecol Reprod Biol 2002;102:109–10
11. Andrew AC, Bulmer JN, Wells M, Morrison L, Buckley CH. Subinvolution of the uteroplacental arteries in the human placental bed. Histopathology 1989;15:395–405
12. Grivell RM, Reid KM, Mellor A. Uterine arteriovenous malformations: a review of the current literature. Obstet Gynecol Surv 2005;60:761–7

13. Ciani S, Merino J, Vijayalakhsmi, Nogales FF. Acquired uterine arteriovenous malformation with massive endometrial stromal component [letter]. Histopathology 2005;46:234–5

14. Hayashi M, Mori Y, Nogami K, Takagi Y, Yaoi M, Ohkura T. A hypothesis to explain the occurrence of inner myometrial laceration causing massive postpartum hemorrhage. Acta Obstet Gynecol Scand 2000;79:99–106

15. Qidwai GI, Caughey AB, Jacoby AF. Obstetric outcomes in women with sonographically identified uterine leiomyomata. Obstet Gynecol 2006;107:376–82

16. Mooney EE, Robboy SJ. Nidation and placenta. In Robboy SJ, Mutter GL, Prat J, Bentley RC, Russell P, Anderson MC, eds. Pathology of the Female Reproductive Tract, 2nd edn. New York: Elsevier, 2009:829–61

17. Toner PG, Crane J. Pathology of death in pregnancy. In Anthony PP, MacSween RNM, eds. Recent Advances in Histopathology. Edinburgh: Churchill Livingstone, 1994; 16:189–212

18. Ohkuchi A, Onagawa T, Usui R, et al. Effect of maternal age on blood loss during parturition: a retrospective multivariate analysis of 10,053 cases. J Perinat Med 2003;31:209–15

19. Cantwell R, Clutton-Brock T, Cooper G, et al. Saving Mothers' Lives: Reviewing Maternal Deaths to Make Motherhood Safer: 2006–2008. The Eighth Report of the Confidential Enquiries into Maternal Deaths in the United Kingdom. BJOG 2011;118 (Suppl 1):1–203

20. Rushton DI, Dawson IMP. The maternal autopsy. J Clin Pathol 1982;35:909–21

21. Royal College of Pathologists. Guidelines on Autopsy Practice. Scenario 5: Maternal Death. London: Royal College of Pathologists, 2010

60

Severe Acute Maternal Morbidity and Postpartum Hemorrhage

A. Vais and S. Bewley

INTRODUCTION

For every woman who dies of postpartum hemorrhage (PPH), many more suffer short- and long-term consequences even when well managed. During the 1990s, the concept of severe adverse maternal morbidity (SAMM) emerged in response to the need for a more sensitive marker of quality of maternity care than maternal death[1,2]. This concept and the accompanying acronym have the advantage of drawing attention to surviving women's health and are applicable in both resource rich and poor countries. As such, SAMM has had increased interest worldwide over the past 5 years, especially in lower income settings such as Brazil[3], Indonesia[4] and several African countries[5,6]; at the same time, it is highlighted in a WHO report aiming to quantify the global problem[7].

The UK is one of the few countries in which every maternal death has been investigated by the Confidential Enquiry into Maternal Death (CEMD) for six decades. In most other developed countries, death from PPH has become too rare for adequate and contemporaneous surveillance of local services. For example, the annual number of maternal deaths from hemorrhage fell from 40 to three in the UK over the past 50 years[8], and only 14 deaths were attributed to hemorrhage in the 2003–2005 CEMD triennium. In the 2006–2008 period which recorded nine deaths, only five were attributable to PPH. Currently, the overall maternal mortality rate in the UK is around 11/100,000 maternities with 0.39 deaths/100,000 attributable to hemorrhage, the lowest since the CEMD began in 1952[9]. Obstetric hemorrhage currently represents the sixth leading cause of direct maternal deaths in the UK. Despite a rising cesarean section rate, the actual number of deaths from hemorrhage and genital tract trauma (including ruptured uterus) has declined slightly (although not statistically so) or is static. Lower death rates may be due to recommendations made in previous reports.

Within the UK, in 2003 Scotland established a national prospective audit of severe morbidity in parallel to the CEMD. The total SAMM rate varied with time, ranging from 4.5/1000 births in 2003 to 6.2/1000 in 2006, with the rate being 5.88/1000 for 2006–2008[10]. This fluctuation is largely due to changes in the rates of major obstetric hemorrhage (MOH, defined as blood loss of more than 2.5 liters), which initially peaked in 2006 (4.9/1000 live births) and has been declining steadily since to 4.3/1000 births. The Scottish authors characterize many cases of severe morbidity as 'great saves' rather than 'near-misses'. Although the audit's threshold for MOH is higher than most other studies, this survey provides a means to monitor trends and is more likely to reflect the burden of severe disease than the extreme 'tip of the iceberg' represented by death.

WHAT IS SEVERE ADVERSE MATERNAL MORBIDITY AS OPPOSED TO A NEAR-MISS?

The term near-miss was previously used to characterize a case where a woman had a near brush with death; in other words, she would have died were good fortune and medical care not on her side. This characterization was also used for women with severe organ dysfunction or organ failure who survived[11,12] whereby, with intensive medical intervention, a maternal death was avoided and a survival ensued[13]. The term SAMM was later introduced to refer to the *morbidity* a woman *actually suffers*, rather than focusing on the fact that she *nearly died* (which may still be more important from a risk management point of view). Recently, the WHO working group on Maternal Mortality and Morbidity recommended a return to the near-miss terminology, referring to the fact that the woman 'nearly died but survived'[7]. Our review for this chapter shows that the two terms, SAMM and near-miss, are currently being used interchangeably in the literature.

Three different definitions for SAMM have been proposed by various authors[7]:

- A severe life-threatening obstetric complication necessitating an urgent medical intervention to prevent the likely death of the mother[14]

- Any pregnant or recently delivered woman, in whom immediate survival is threatened and who survives by chance or due to the hospital care she received[15]

- A very ill woman who would have died had it not been that luck and good care was on her side[11].

Attempting to unify these differences, WHO defines a maternal near-miss as: *a woman who nearly died but survived a complication that occurred during childbirth or within 42 days of termination of pregnancy*[7]. This simplifies the concept and attaches a useful time-frame. However, it excludes complications in pregnancy that do not lead to delivery (such as septicemia, pulmonary embolus or cardiac arrest); moreover, it does not generate a universal system for case identification which would facilitate cross-country comparisons.

The three definitions cited above clearly are similar and illustrate the concept of a continuum of worsening morbidity in the pregnant population, culminating in maternal death. The disease pyramid illustrates this concept (Figure 1) by which the base represents the general pregnant population, and the 'tip of the iceberg' is maternal death with a spectrum of morbidity between[11,12,16]. A clinical insult may be followed by a systemic response and subsequent organ dysfunction, which leads to organ failure and eventual death[2,11]. The figure shows the severity continuum of morbidity as well as factors that move women up and down the pyramid. For example, a faulty ambulance or wrongly cross-matched blood might lead to an anemic woman dying of hemorrhage unnecessarily. If the same patient had been provided iron supplementation antenatally, was well managed and treated promptly, there may be no residual morbidity. On the other hand, pathologies such as placenta previa and uterine rupture would drive women up towards the tip of the pyramid. Interventions such as uterotonics might stop bleeding at an early stage, whereas interventions such as obstetric hysterectomy may be used near the top.

Despite the different definitions of MOH, studies have used three main approaches for case identification (outlined in Table 1). Each approach has advantages and disadvantages:

(1) Specific disease entities (e.g. eclampsia, PPH) allow relatively easy retrospective data collection from case notes or registers. Quality of care and complication rates can be determined for the specific disease and set against standards of care. However, it is difficult to use this for ongoing audits. There may be poor documentation in the worst cases and morbidity criteria may have too low a threshold to be considered a near-miss.

(2) Intervention-based criteria are easily measured and agreed, do not rely on medical diagnosis and coding, but are affected by local units' different facilities, policies, customs and practices, as well as thresholds for transfer (e.g. use and availability of high dependency/intensive-care beds or interventional radiology).

(3) The main advantage of an organ system dysfunction approach is that it allows mortality and morbidity surveys to run in parallel, thus enabling calculations of morbidity : mortality ratios for various disease processes. The Scottish Morbidity Survey is an example, and its findings have been reported in parallel to the CEMD. Trends in diseases can be established. This approach also focuses on diseases which should not cause death if appropriately managed (e.g. PPH). However, cases can only reliably be identified prospectively and depend on investigative test availability.

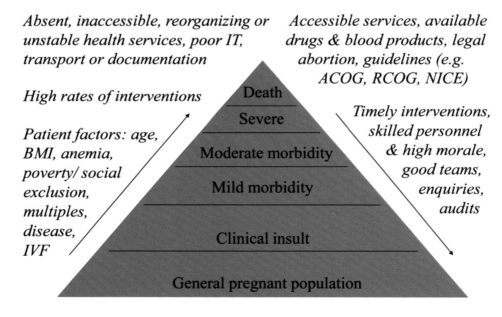

A representation of the morbidity-to-mortality continuum in both resource poor and rich countries

Figure 1 A representation of the morbidity–mortality continuum. ACOG, American College of Obstetricians and Gynecologists; BMI, body mass index; IVF, *in vitro* fertilization; NICE, National Institute for Health and Clinical Excellence; RCOG, Royal College of Obstetricians and Gynaecologists[2,24]

Table 1 Different methodological approaches to the identification of cases of SAMM

Criteria for identification of near-miss	Case definition	Study
Related to specific disease	Starting point is a specific disease and morbidity is defined for each. For example, pre-eclampsia might be the disease with severe morbidity identified by its complications (i.e. renal failure, pulmonary edema, eclampsia, etc.) Can be prospective or retrospective	Waterstone *et al.*, 2001[17] Scottish survey, 2003 ongoing[18,19] LEMMoN, 2008[20] UKOSS, 2005 ongoing[21]
Intervention based	Marker for near-miss is an identifiable event or procedure (e.g. admission to ITU, large blood transfusion or emergency hysterectomy) to save the mother's life Usually retrospective studies	Bewley & Creighton, 1997[13] Killpatrick & Matthay, 2002[22] LEMMoN, 2008[20] UKOSS, 2003 ongoing[21] Obstetric hysterectomy studies[23,24]
Based on organ-system dysfunction	System is based on the concept of the pyramid of disease from good health to death. A clinical insult is followed by a systemic response syndrome, then organ dysfunction, organ failure and death. Near-miss cases are the women with organ dysfunction or failure who survive. Markers for dysfunction for each organ system are specified and criteria for defining a near-miss are given (e.g. cardiovascular shock from hemorrhage) Usually prospective studies	Mantel *et al.*, 1998[11] Pattinson *et al.*, 2003[12] Waterstone *et al.*, 2001[17] Scottish survey, 2003 ongoing[19]
Rare event	A rare event allows large, even national, population estimates. UKOSS, for example, has studied risk factors (e.g. BMI >50), specific diseases (e.g. swine flu, amniotic fluid embolism), complications of obstetric morbidity (e.g. acute fatty liver) or treatment (e.g. extraordinary interventions for massive hemorrhage – hysterectomy, factor VII, intrauterine balloon, brace suture). The disadvantage is the inability to examine common severe morbidities	BEST study, 1995 (eclampsia)[25] Waterstone *et al.*, 2001 (uterine rupture as rare event)[17] UKOSS, 2005 ongoing[21] Obstetric hysterectomy studies[23,24]

BMI, body mass index; UKOSS, UK Obstetric Surveillance System

Rates may be biased if ascertainment problems are present. A diligent unit may report more cases via the organ-system approach, and careful recording could translate into a disproportionately higher rate of SAMM[12]. On the other hand, a poor-quality unit that does not recognize and treat hemorrhage promptly may have more severe sequelae as the natural history progresses. Thus the true incidence of SAMM may be underestimated.

HOW COMMON IS ALL-CAUSE SEVERE ADVERSE MATERNAL MORBIDITY?

Because quantification is problematic, with no international definition and haphazard recording, wide variations are present in incidence estimates (summarized in Table 2).

High income countries

A recent review including studies from Europe, Canada and USA suggested the incidence of SAMM to approximate to 0.5–1% of all deliveries in high income countries (3.3–12/1000)[35]. The rates/1000 births ranged from 3.3 in France, through 3.8 in Scotland, 4.6 in Canada, 7.2 in The Netherlands, 10.9 in South Africa to 12.0 in England.

Low income countries

A 2009 review grouped low income countries into those of Africa, Latin America and Asia[36], and included landmark audits of severe morbidity in South Africa[11,37]. Thirty-seven studies from 24 countries

were examined, ranging from small audits of near-miss morbidity[5,11,37,38] in general and teaching hospitals, to large population based surveys[37,39,40] or surveys of need for life-saving surgery (Tanzania, Guinea, Indonesia)[36]. Comparisons are difficult, however, because all women do not give birth in health facilities and standards vary widely (e.g. availability of ITU beds). African studies exemplified these wide variations. The rate of severe morbidity across several West African states was calculated as 59.8/1000 deliveries (almost 6%)[39], whilst contemporaneous studies in South Africa yielded rates of 1%[11,37], falling to 0.5% in 2004[41], a rate which is similar to that in high income countries.

In low income settings, major surgical interventions such as cesarean section or hysterectomy are likely to be accurately recorded and may be useful markers of severe morbidity. One way to quantify the need for life-saving surgery is by cesarean section for absolute maternal indications (severe antepartum hemorrhage due to placenta previa, major cephalopelvic disproportion, transverse lie or brow presentation). In settings without ITU facilities, a combination of life-saving surgery and organ dysfunction approaches are likely to work best, as evidenced by studies in Brazil[3] and Indonesia[36]. Using transfused blood has limitations as thresholds for transfusion vary, blood may not be available in low income settings or women may refuse transfusion (e.g. Jehovah's Witnesses).

RELATIONSHIP OF SEVERE ADVERSE MATERNAL MORBIDITY TO MORTALITY

Two methods generally are used to address the relationship between severe morbidity and mortality.

Table 2 SAMM studies showing incidence and proportion related to hemorrhage

Study, country and year of publication	Incidence of SAMM per 1000 deliveries (all causes)	Incidence of hemorrhage/ 1000 deliveries (% of total SAMM)	Incidence of hypertension (% of total)	Incidence of severe sepsis (% of total)	Additional comments
Stones et al.[1] UK 1991	8.8	3.23 (36.8%)	2.77 (31.5%)	Not available	SAMM defined as 'potentially life-threatening episodes'. Incidence for total (all) morbidity 267/1000. Incidence of all sepsis 30.5/1000 (severe sepsis not separated). Hemorrhage includes antepartum and PPH if over 2000 ml. One case of secondary PPH due to sepsis
Bouvier-Colle et al.[26] France 1996	3.1	0.62 (20%)	0.81 (26.2%)	0.14 (4.36%)	Third highest cause of morbidity is embolic events at 0.38/1000. Hemorrhage includes uterine rupture. Hypertensive disease includes cerebral hemorrhage
Bewley & Creighton[13] UK 1997	4.97	2.3 (46.7%)	1.98 (40%)	0.49 (10%)	SAMM = ITU admission. Total 30 cases of SAMM. 14 cases classed as hemorrhage (blood loss >2000 ml but a further 2 cases DIC/HELLP so proportion due to hemorrhage could be >50%)
Baskett & Sternadel[27] USA 1998	0.72	0.16 (22%)	0.18 (25%)	0.1 (14.5%)	SAMM = ITU admission
Mantel et al.[11] South Africa 1998	10.9	6.1 (55.8%)	2.82 (25.8%)	2.16 (19.7%)	Sepsis incorporates septic abortion, chorioamnionitis and puerperal sepsis. Hemorrhage incorporates antepartum and PPH and emergency hysterectomy; PPH alone is 1.8/1000
Prual et al.[15] West Africa 2000	50.8	29.6 (49.5%)	6.15 (10.3%)	0.9 (1.5%)	Obstructed labor is significant cause for severe morbidity (20.5/1000 of which 1.2/1000 uterine rupture)
Waterstone et al.[17] UK 2001	12.0	6.7 (55.7%)	4.6 (38%)	0.35 (2.89%)	Clinically based definitions, not including management processes. Estimated blood loss >1500 ml picked up 55% of cases of SAMM due to hemorrhage
Brace et al.[18] Scotland 2004	3.8	1.9 (50%)	1.15 (30%)	0.09 (3%)	Septic shock is the only category for sepsis. Number of SAMM due to hypertensive disease derived by adding the number of cases with eclampsia, renal dysfunction and pulmonary edema. Only one-third of patients with SAMM were admitted to ITU
Zhang[28] MOMS-B Europe 2005	9.48	4.6 (48.8%)	4.33 (45.7%)	0.8 (8.2%)	Multinational study, rates differing widely between countries. Range of SAMM 6–14.7%. Highest rates in Finland, Belgium, UK and lowest rates in Italy, Ireland, France
Minkauskiene et al.[29] Lithuania 2006	7.91	2.83 (35.8%)	4.47 (56.6%)	0.3 (3.8%)	13,399 deliveries, 106 cases SAMM, 1 death 60 cases hypertension (57 severe PET, 3 eclampsia), 38 severe hemorrhage, 4 cases severe sepsis, 3 cases uterine rupture

Study					Comments
Zwart et al.[20] LeMMoN Netherlands 2008	7.1	4.5 (63% of total, 47% of ITU admissions)	0.62 (eclampsia 8.7% of total)	0.23 (3.3% of total, 10% were due to group A streptococcus)	5 categories for SAMM (ITU admission, uterine rupture, needing cesarean/hysterectomy or laparotomy, eclampsia/HELLP, major hemorrhage needing transfusion or hysterectomy and group of others e.g. sepsis, pre-eclampsia). 27% of MOH admitted to ITU. MOH counted as separate group but also a surgery group (some for rupture or hysterectomy, i.e. implies hemorrhage, so rate of MOH may be underestimate)
UKOSS[19,30] UK 2005–2011		0.41 peripartum hysterectomy 0.26 2nd line treatment	0.27 (in 2005)	Not surveyed	National surveillance of rare disorders in pregnancy – system reporting from all consultant-led maternity units in the UK. Different morbidities studied at different times and surveillance is not continuous for all causes. Second-line treatments for MOH are compression sutures, pelvic vessel ligation, embolization or factor VII
Ronsmans et al.[4] Indonesia 2009	141.6	125 (30% of life-saving surgery for placenta previa; 34% of total)	19.3 eclampsia (11.2%)	2.32 (1.35%)	Study in 2 rural and 2 urban areas in West Java; higher incidence of morbidity in urban than rural areas but mortality higher in rural areas. Distinction made between near-miss and life-saving surgery (e.g. labor dystocia is a common cause for life-saving surgery but not for near-miss). Organ dysfunction/management-based criteria (ITU, surgery)/clinical diagnosis. Mortality 42.1/1000 live births
Souza et al.[31] Brazil 2010	21.1	18.4%	0.6%	1%	Near-miss from health records in 5 regions of Brazil over a 5-year period. Questionnaire design, self-reported morbidity. Categories are eclampsia, hysterectomy, transfusion and ITU admission. Validated questionnaire sent to women identified through population database; women more likely to recall procedures than signs and symptoms. Mortality ratio 0.75/1000 live births. Only proportions given without numbers as weighting used
Lawton et al.[32] New Zealand 2010	4	12 (41.4%)	8 (27.6%)	5 septicemia (17.2%)	SAMM = ITU admission. Study during 2005–07 during pregnancy or within 42 days of delivery. Total 29 cases in tertiary center using organ-system dysfunction. 25 postpartum cases, 9 hysterectomies. Hypertension includes high blood pressure and HELLP cases but there are also some CVAs counted separately. Same criteria as Bewley & Creighton[13], cases could have more than one morbidity
Almerie et al.[33] Syria 2010	32.9	11 (34.4%)	17 (52%)	0.9 (2.8%)	Retrospective review of near-miss and maternal mortality in a tertiary hospital in Damascus 2006–2007. 28,025 deliveries, 15 deaths, 901 near-miss cases. MMR = 54.8/100,000 live births, mortality index 1.7%. Most cases referred in critical conditions from other facilities (traditional birth attendants, homes, private practices, primary and secondary care units). 26% of near-miss cases admitted to ITU. Hemorrhage accounted for 60% of mortality cases. Rates are given per 1000 live births rather than deliveries. Sepsis and dystocia are uncommon causes of near-miss but high mortality indices (7.4% and 2.9%, respectively)
Lennox[10] Scotland 2011	5.88	4.51 (76.8%)	0.28 (4.7%)	0.11 (1.85%)	174,430 births in Scotland. Major PPH >2500 ml Mortality: morbidity ratio 1:79. 46.9% of all cases of MOH due to atony. Hypertensive morbidity is eclampsia only. Sepsis = septic shock. Proportions may be slightly different if encompass ICU admission, pulmonary edema, renal or liver dysfunction or CVA
Muthir & Utoo[34] Nigeria 2011	0.27	9.6 (35.4%)	6.8 (24.8%)	4.5 (16.7%)	3 year prospective observational study at a university hospital. 9056 deliveries, 246 SAMM (2.72%). Junior staff supervised almost half of deliveries (43.5%) and this correlated with the degree of morbidity

CVA, cerebrovascular accident; DIC, disseminated intravascular coagulation; HELLP, hemolysis, elevated liver enzymes, low platelets; ICU, intensive care unit; ITU, intensive therapy unit; MOH, massive obstetric hemorrhage (1500 ml in some studies, 2500 ml in others); PET, pre-eclampsia; PPH, postpartum hemorrhage; SAMM, severe adverse maternal morbidity

These are the *mortality-to-morbidity ratio* and the *mortality index*. The mortality-to-morbidity ratio simply describes the number of severe morbidity cases for each maternal death[2,17]. The mortality index, on the other hand, is defined as the number of maternal deaths divided by the sum of women with SAMM and maternal deaths, and is expressed as a percentage[12,37]. Both can be expressed as totals (all-cause) or by condition. Both reflect the fatality of a condition and identify those conditions that are more or less amenable to intervention. Recently WHO have introduced a new set of definitions (see text box below).

In general, the risk of mortality depends on (1) the prior health of the mother, (2) the severity of the particular condition, (3) access to skilled help, and (4) the availability and quality of medical intervention. PPH is the morbidity *par excellence* for assessing these parameters. It is common and has a high morbidity-to-mortality ratio (or low mortality index)[2,12,17,37]. In developed countries, at least, this is because the condition is amenable to treatment. More women's lives can be, and indeed are being, saved daily by the provision of adequate maternity services worldwide. As hemorrhage is largely treatable (and often avoidable), and *because all parturients are at risk*, it is tragic that so many women still die unnecessarily worldwide. The United Nations discusses women's and children's health in terms of fundamental human rights[43]. Progress towards Millennium Development Goal 5 (MDG 5, a 75% reduction in maternal mortality 1990–2015) has been disappointing[44] as only 23/181 (13%) countries analysed are on track to achieve the target[45].

What are the main causes of SAMM?

Most cases of SAMM fall into three major categories of causation:

- Hemorrhage
- Hypertensive diseases of pregnancy (including eclampsia and HELLP syndrome)
- Sepsis.

The incidence of these conditions in European countries appears similar despite the use of different definitions. Regardless of geographical factors, hemorrhage is the largest contributor, accounting for between 20%[26] and 50%[11,18,39] of cases. Hypertensive disease and its consequences account for 10%[39] to 45%[28], whereas morbidity secondary to sepsis is much lower, at 1.5%[39] to 20%[11]. Rarer causes of SAMM include thromboembolic disease and psychiatric illness[46,47].

NEW WHO TERMINOLOGY

WHO has recently published a document aimed at providing a universal framework for defining and counting severe morbidity. The near-miss definition is the same as was used in 2009[7]. New terms which are outlined below have been introduced, with the aim of unifying the near-miss and severe morbidity concepts, whilst recognizing the morbidity ortality continuum as described in Figure 1.

Women with life-threatening conditions (WLTC) = maternal near-misses (MNM) + maternal deaths (MD)

Severe maternal outcome ratio (SMOR) = WLTC (MNM + MD) per 1000 live births; this gives an estimate of the amount of care and facilities that may be needed in an area or facility

MNM ratio (MNMR) = number of near-miss cases per 1000 live births; can also be used to estimate the amount of care or resources needed

Maternal near-miss mortality ratio (MNM : MD) is the ratio of near misses to deaths as MNMR previously described. Higher ratios would indicated better care as more lives are being saved

Whilst the concepts of SMOR and MNMR are useful from a resource planning perspective, comparisons between high and low resource settings remain difficult to make. For example, for PPH the operational definition for severe morbidity is blood loss more than 1000 ml and standard of care implies that all women receive 10 IU Syntocinon for third stage.

In a low-resource setting, a woman with a borderline starting hemoglobin in a facility lacking drugs to manage the third stage and no access to transfusion will create a case of severe morbidity at 1 liter blood loss. Conversely, in a developed country the standard of care would be met simply by the routine use of Syntocinon; a woman with a normal hemoglobin can lose 1000 ml without any significant morbidity. Comparisons based on volume loss alone may encourage complacency in such settings where the minimum intervention set by WHO is already routine and the severe morbidity occurs at bigger volumes of blood loss, increased interventions, ITU care, etc.

The same working party encourages the development of ongoing audit of severe morbidity cases in all health facilities, at local and district level. The aim is mainly for resource planning but also to enable comparisons regarding quality of care. The appendices and checklists provide useful practical tools for implementing an international audit strategy for severe maternal morbidity. They estimate the global prevalence to be around 7.5 per 1000 deliveries, but as shown in Table 2, the worldwide prevalence is more widely spread. Ongoing audit using this universal tool at local and national level would provide valuable information about quality of care and resource planning in different settings, but does not make comparisons across resource brackets (high and low) any easier[42].

WHAT IS THE INCIDENCE OF SEVERE ADVERSE MATERNAL MORBIDITY ATTRIBUTABLE TO HEMORRHAGE?

Hemorrhage illustrates the difficulties faced with defining near-miss or severe morbidity. All women experience some blood loss at delivery. The amount is difficult to measure, and often mixed with amniotic fluid. Hemorrhage is a clinical insult that strikes the general pregnant population, both low and high risk. Whether due to atony, retained placenta or genital tract lacerations it has the potential to cause morbidity ranging from mild to severe or even death (Figure 1). In addition, specific bleeding causes rapidly endanger women (e.g. ruptured ectopic, ruptured or inverted uterus, massive abruption or morbid placental adherence).

Table 2 summarizes some of the landmark studies that have attempted to quantify this problem in developed countries over the past 15 years. Wide variations are present in study settings, definitions and main causes. Some studies use admission to ICU[22,48], others define the actual conditions responsible for the morbidity[11,12], and still others list both[13]. The wide variation in case definition might explain the extreme range of incidence of SAMM (4% in UK to 53% in Hong Kong for studies using retrospective ITU admission to define SAMM; 1–6% incidence in prospective multicenter studies). Regardless of such differences, most studies concluded that up to half of the cases of SAMM were related to hemorrhage, and this continues to be the case in recent investigations (Table 2).

World Health Organization has set some maternal near-miss criteria[7] which aim to incorporate life-threatening clinical signs (e.g. cyanosis, shock, increased respiratory rate) and investigational results (e.g. oxygen saturation, pH, lactate) as well as life-saving interventions (e.g. hysterectomy, transfusion) into an algorithm that ensures severe cases are not missed. Worldwide adoption of this definition would identify all the cases of SAMM regardless of inciting condition but would not facilitate international comparisons between disease processes. This is because different pathologies can lead to the same clinical sign (e.g. raised respiratory rate in shock from hemorrhage as well as pulmonary embolus). A pragmatic proforma for case identification relating to SAMM secondary to hemorrhage would include all aspects shown in Table 3[42].

RISK FACTORS FOR SEVERE ADVERSE MATERNAL MORBIDITY DUE TO HEMORRHAGE

Although it is challenging to define the size of the problem (i.e. the incidence of SAMM as a result of hemorrhage), Table 4 summarizes risk factors identified over the past 10 years that increase the risk of severe hemorrhage.

Some risk factors, such as previous PPH or manual removal of placenta, are intuitive and universal. Induction of labor appears to increase the risk of PPH regardless of the indication[17]. This may relate to an increased duration of labor or risk of sepsis. Anemia is likely to be more prevalent in low income countries as well as in recent immigrants and 'socially excluded' women in high income countries as a reflection of

Table 3 A pragmatic proforma for case identification relating to SAMM secondary to hemorrhage would include all these aspects

Category	Parameters	Advantage	Disadvantage if used alone
Actual blood loss	EBL >1500–2000 ml (or more)	Measured and measurable	Accurate quantification notoriously difficult
Clinical symptoms	Dizziness, faintness Agitation, thirst, collapse Cardiac arrest	Easy to measure Cheap Applicable in low resource settings	Tolerance depends on mother's size, pre-existing total blood volume and pre-delivery hemoglobin Antenatal anemia will cause morbidity out of proportion to actual blood loss
Clinical signs	Pulse >100 or Systolic BP <80 mmHg Respiratory rate Peripartum fall in hemoglobin		May be non-specific to hemorrhage; thus aids recognition but difficult to audit management if used alone
Blood product replacement	Packed red cells >4 or >5 units Use of FFP/clotting factors	Measurable	Product availability Changing guidelines re: ratios of transfusing blood and FFP Jehovah's Witnesses and others who refuse blood
Specific life-threatening conditions	Abruption Uterine rupture Morbid placental adherence Placenta previa Infection	Diagnosis is fixed once made Comparisons of rates can be made	Varying degrees of severity Can have several causes Management and thus degree of morbidity dependent on local resources
Interventions which imply severe hemorrhage	Balloon tamponade Compression sutures Hysterectomy Interventional radiology Use of factor VII	Measurable Easy to identify cases both retrospectively and prospectively	Availability dependent on setting and expertise of personnel Timeliness of intervention decreases severity of morbidity so use itself does not demonstrate standard of care
ITU/HDU admission	Ventilatory support Requirement for inotropes	Auditable Easy case identification	Availability depends on clinical setting

BP, blood pressure; EBL, estimated blood loss; FFP, fresh frozen plasma; HDU, high dependency unit; ITU, intensive therapy unit

Table 4 Risk factors for major obstetric hemorrhage

Risk factor	Odds ratios for SAMM (95% CI)	Study/Country/Year
Age >35 years	1.41 (1.03–1.95)	Waterstone et al./UK/2001[17]
	1.2 (1.1–1.3)/ (1.4 if >40)	Zwart et al./Netherlands/2008[20]
	1.02 (0.96–1.09)	Ford et al./Australia/2007[55]
	1.14 (1.03–1.21)	Al-Zirqi et al./Norway/2008[56]
Hypertension at booking	1.18 (1.06–1.31)	Waterstone et al./UK/2001[17]
	1.33 (1.07–1.66)	Ford et al./Australia/2007[55]
Ethnic minority	1.82 (1.09–3.03)	Waterstone et al./UK/2001[17]
	1.3 (1.2–1.5) non-Western immigrants	Zwart et al./Netherlands/2008[20]
	1.16 (1.1–1.22)	Ford et al./Australia/2007[55]
	1.77 (1.48–2.12)	Al-Zirqi et al./Norway/2008 (SE Asian ethnicity)[56]
Social exclusion	2.91 (1.76–4.82)	Waterstone et al./UK/2001[17]
	2.18 (1.15–4.10)	Souza et al./Brazil/2007[3]
BMI >30	1.5 (1.3–1.7)	Zwart et al./Netherlands/2008[20]
Previous PPH	2.74 (1.69–4.44)	Waterstone et al./UK/2001[17]
Multiple pregnancy	2.29 (1.2–4.37)	Waterstone et al./UK/2001[17]
	4.9 (4.3–5.7)	Zwart et al./Netherlands/2008[20]
	2.34 (2.02–2.7)	Al-Zirqi et al./Norway/2008[56]
Anemia	5.98 (2.28–15.65)	Waterstone et al./UK/2001[17]
	2.2 (1.63–3.15)	Al-Zirqi et al./Norway/2008[56]
Oxytocin augmentation	1.61 (1.2–2.15)	Waterstone et al./UK/2001[17]
IOL	2.45 (1.68–3.57)	Waterstone et al./UK/2001[17]
	3.1 (2.8–3.4)	Zwart et al./Netherlands/2008[20]
	1.5–2.42 (spontaneous vs. instrumental)	Ford et al./Australia/2007[55]
	1.6 (1.46–1.75)	Al-Zirqi et al./Norway/2008[56]
Manual removal of placenta	13.12 (7.72–22.30)	Waterstone et al./UK/2001[17]
Emergency CS	3.09 (2.29–4.17)	Waterstone et al./UK/2001[17]
	5.2 (4.8–5.6) all CSs	Zwart et al./Netherlands/2008[20]
	0.81 (0.7–0.92) CS in spontaneous labor	Ford et al./Australia/2007[55]
	3.61 (3.28–3.95)	Al-Zirqi et al./Norway/2008[56]
Instrumental delivery	1.6 (1.4–1.71)	Zwart et al./Netherlands/2008[20]
	1.87 (1.4–2.42)	Al-Zirqi et al./Norway/2008[56]
	1.25 (1.1–1.42)	Ford et al./Australia/2007[55]
Birth weight >4.5kg	1.93 (1.71–2.17)	Al-Zirqi et al./Norway/2008[56]
	2.55 (2.15–3.03)	Ford et al./Australia/2007[55]

BMI, body mass index; CS, cesarean section; IOL, induction of labor

poorer nutrition. Waterstone et al.[47] defined social exclusion as a composite measure of a woman's social deprivation beyond the traditional use of her marital or partner's employment status or postcode deprivation score. The definition included concealed pregnancy, age less than 16 years, poor housing, 'on income support' (state welfare benefit) written in the notes, previous minor or child in local authority or state care (currently or in the past), in trouble with the law (currently or previously), living alone, unbooked, unwanted pregnancy, currently or previously in foster care, care order being considered on potential child, social worker involved or drug or alcohol dependency.

Other studies in countries such as the USA[49], Brazil[3] and Uganda[50] have found a similar trend. Kaye et al.[50] defined women of 'low status' by a composite of poor education, poverty, low antenatal care attendance, low contraceptive-ever use and little power to make decisions regarding access to health care. Souza et al.[31] referred mainly to the woman's educational achievement, with women educated to high school level having a lower risk of severe morbidity.

IS THE PREVALENCE OF SEVERE ADVERSE MATERNAL MORBIDITY SECONDARY TO HEMORRHAGE RISING?

Health services need to monitor trends of various diseases as well as the actual morbidity suffered or deaths caused. It is plausible that disease burden can be rising or falling at the same time as outcomes are improving which would have implications for service provision. There are only a few register-based studies that track rates of SAMM; these are located in Canada[51], Finland[52] and USA[53].

In 2009 an international group explored trends in PPH in several high-resource countries (Australia, Belgium, Canada, France, UK and USA)[54]. Looking at risk factors for SAMM secondary to hemorrhage (Table 4), it is not surprising that rates of severe PPH are increasing as childbearing women are older and more obese, with more multiple pregnancies and cesareans in high income countries. Maternal mortality rates, however, were largely static in these same settings. However, markers of severe hemorrhage (uterine rupture, hysterectomy) were increased[35]. Knight et al.[54] compared data in several high income countries (Australia, Belgium, Canada, France, UK and USA) from the early 1990s with those of early 21st century and found that rates of hysterectomy for atonic PPH increased from 24/100,000 deliveries in 1991 to 41.7/100,000 deliveries in 2004.

Canada

The rate of SAMM appears similar between the early and late 1990s (4.4/1000 births in 1991–1993 vs. 4.25/1000 births 1998–2000)[35]. However, Sheehan's syndrome increased 4-fold in Canada over the same 10 years, suggesting that the severity of PPH had increased. Also, the rate of peripartum hysterectomy increased by 73% from 24/100,000 births in 1991 to 41.7/100,000 births in 2004[54]. Another retrospective Canadian cohort study[57] looked at all hospital deliveries between 1991 and 2004, identifying a 34% increase in atonic PPH from 29.4/1000 deliveries in 1991 to 39.5/1000 in 2004. The authors could not find a satisfactory explanation for the increased rate.

Finland

The overall rate of severe morbidity increased from 5.9/1000 births in 1997 to 7.6/1000 births in 1999–2002[35].

Scotland

An ongoing prospective audit since 2003 uses the organ-system definitions generated by Mantel *et al.*[11]. The Scottish survey uses a cut-off of 2500 ml or more for defining MOH, which is higher than most other studies, probably for pragmatic reasons and ease of data collection. The mortality : morbidity ratio has improved from 1 : 56 in 2003 to 1 : 79 in 2008; this change reflects an increase in the rate of MOH but no rise in deaths. Over half of the cases of MOH were associated with cesarean section (55.2% for all cesarean sections, 44.3% emergency cesarean sections), of which 20% were deemed of an emergency nature and performed in the second stage. In the same national audits, the rate of peripartum hysterectomy showed a steady decline between 2003 and 2008, as other conservative surgical techniques such as brace sutures and balloon tamponade were increasingly used[10].

Australia

A population-based survey of 752,374 women delivering between 1994 and 2002 in New South Wales, the most populous region in Australia, noted an increased rate of total PPH (defined as 500 ml at vaginal delivery and 750 ml at cesarean section) from 4.7 to 6.0/1000 births. This rate appeared to increase more after vaginal delivery. The authors postulated this may be due to use of Syntocinon rather than Syntometrine for third stage management. It is, however, concerning that PPH increased despite a slight reduction in the delivery rate[55].

USA

Overall morbidity increased from 4.5/1000 deliveries during 1991–1994 to 5.9/1000 in 1999–2003[35]. Another study[58] showed an increase in severe obstetric complications from 0.64% in 1998–1999 to 0.81% in 2004–2005. Amongst causes of severe morbidity there was a 24% increase in cases of shock and 92% increase in transfusion rates. These increases are partly explained by a rising cesarean delivery rate, although adjustment for mode of delivery rendered differences statistically insignificant.

Ireland

A population study based on 649,000 deliveries has found a three-fold increase in PPH rate within a decade in the Republic of Ireland from 1.5% in 1999 to 4.1% in 2009[59]. This trend was observed for both vaginal and cesarean deliveries and was not wholly explicable by demographic changes (i.e. advancing maternal age or multiple birth), or by increased cesarean section rates[59]. The increase was largely related to increased atonic PPH rates, unlike the Australian data[55] where the highest rate was among cesarean section deliveries.

SPECIFIC CAUSES OF SEVERE ADVERSE MATERNAL MORBIDITY RELATED TO HEMORRHAGE

Uterine rupture

Although this diagnosis can be one surrogate measure for SAMM due to hemorrhage, studies report it differently. For example, it has been combined with data for obstructed labor in South Africa[39], and analysed as a cause of hemorrhage in a French study[26]. Waterstone *et al.*[17] in the UK considered uterine rupture as a separate entity, which is a more accurate means of using these data unless there is clear evidence of the blood loss associated with each case. These authors found a rate of 1 : 4000 deliveries (0.025%). Studies in high income countries suggest low rates of uterine rupture causing SAMM which range from 0.002%[60] through 0.017%[21] to 0.06%[20].

A systematic review of the literature published in 2005 examined 83 studies concerning uterine rupture between 1990 and 2005[61]. Prevalence was higher in developing than developed countries. In all countries, rupture affected 1% of women with previous cesarean section. This same trend was found by the UK Obstetric Surveillance Survey (UKOSS) study undertaken in 2010, where 86% of ruptures occurred in women with a previous cesarean section. The 2005 review found variable rates of rupture across the world, especially when studies were conducted in developing countries; in these settings women may die unattended out of hospital, and studies were less likely to distinguish women with scarred and unscarred uteri. Rates of rupture were lowest in developed countries and in women without a uterine scar (0.006%, rising to 1% in women with scarred uteri). In contrast, in the least developed countries rates of rupture could be as high as 25% (one study of 945 women in Ethiopia in the 1990s) and mostly associated with obstructed labor; 75% of cases of uterine rupture in Africa and Asia were found to occur in unscarred uteri. In low-resource settings rupture is associated with a high maternal mortality which ranges from 1 to 13% and a very high perinatal mortality (74–92%)[61]. The WHO review suggests that reducing rupture rates in these populations would require a focus on reducing unwanted pregnancies, especially in women of high parity, accessibility of services and cesarean sections for obstructed labor and adequate guidelines for safe use of misoprostol as an induction agent[61].

Data from Australia and Northern Europe also suggest that rupture is a rare event in developed countries, but the rate is increased by induction of labor[20,56].

Peripartum hysterectomy

Obstetric hysterectomy provides another means of examining SAMM associated with PPH and has the advantage of being more clearly defined, and rare enough for data to be easily collected. The threshold for performing hysterectomy clearly varies with the operator, unit and individual case, but evidence suggests that early hysterectomy decreases both morbidity[62] and mortality[63]. The several studies that have examined the incidence of peripartum hysterectomy as a marker of SAMM from hemorrhage are listed in Table 5. Population studies between 1986 and 2005 yielded rates of 0.3–1.55 hysterectomies/1000 deliveries[23]. More recent rates of 0.33 and 0.77/1000 deliveries have been reported in The Netherlands[20] and the US[64]. The largest population study from the UK showed an incidence of 0.41/1000 deliveries[30].

Table 5 also shows that the main causes of bleeding leading to hysterectomy are atony (30–50%) and adherent placenta (38–40%). Recently, more conservative treatment modalities for PPH have been introduced, but the hysterectomy studies show that even these can fail to arrest bleeding. Failed brace sutures were found in 25% of cases in the UK[30], whilst a Dutch study showed that 9.7% and 13% of cases of hysterectomy followed intrauterine balloon tamponade and uterine artery embolization, respectively[20]. It is difficult to draw meaningful conclusions regarding failed conservative measures as there are no standardized guidelines for use before proceeding to hysterectomy nor are there established guidelines for the timely use of either the brace suture or the balloon. For example, if bleeding has proceeded for a long time prior to institution of therapy, the likelihood that it is accompanied by some degree of coagulopathy (disseminated, dilutional or both) is high (see Chapter 5). Practicing clinicians regularly counsel women regarding the risk of hysterectomy after cesarean section for placenta previa. Studies suggest that the combination of multiparity, history of previous cesarean section and delivery by cesarean section should alert the obstetrician to a significant risk of hysterectomy secondary to placenta accreta/percreta. Combining the odds ratios generated individually by the UKOSS case–control study for these three conditions, the risk could be over 50 times that of the normal pregnant population.

OUTCOMES OF WOMEN WHO SUFFER SEVERE ADVERSE MATERNAL MORBIDITY

Few studies follow up outcomes beyond survival and immediate morbidity. Studies of postnatal morbidity in general populations (low- and high-risk women analysed together) found that problem prevalence is high and persists for a prolonged period of time after delivery[47,65]. Glazener et al.[65] looked at a random sample of deliveries (high and low risk) in a teaching hospital in Scotland and showed that 87% of women suffered at least one health problem after delivery and in 76% problems persisted for 2 months postpartum. Problems ranged from urinary or bowel problems to perineal pain or breakdown, breast problems and persistent vaginal discharge. A case–control study of outcome 6–12 months postpartum compared women who had and had not suffered SAMM[47]. Cases were twice as likely to attend accident and emergency departments, possibly related to the underlying morbidity and its follow-up, but this circumstance clearly points to a continuing burden on health services with

personal, family and economic costs. Cases also suffered slightly more postnatal depression than controls (who were not entirely 'normal' as they included women with operative deliveries and smaller hemorrhages). While this difference was not statistically significant, cases also scored higher on the Edinburgh Postnatal Depression Scale. Significantly more cases than controls (50% vs. 29%, 95% CI for the difference 9.7–33%, $p < 0.001$) were reluctant to re-establish sexual relations with their partners for fear of becoming pregnant, suggesting that a negative experience in one pregnancy may prevent a woman from achieving the family she initially intended[47]. Women with stillbirths are almost always excluded from postnatal studies[65], although a higher proportion of them also suffer SAMM by the nature of underlying conditions (e.g. abruption). Only half of the studies of SAMM quoted give data about perinatal loss. Thus, the figures quoted above are likely underestimates of the true spectrum of postnatal morbidity.

Potential measures to decrease SAMM secondary to PPH

Agreement on definitions and categorizations for comparisons

Before designing studies into effective interventions for reducing SAMM, it is necessary to develop standardized definitions for severe morbidity and its main causes. A pragmatic definition could be based on a mixture of parameters, as outlined in Table 3. Knight et al.[54] also suggest that the ICD classification of PPH should be revised to separate atonic PPH from other causes, particularly due to morbid placental adherence, in order to enable meaningful comparisons to be made between different countries. These authors postulate that the definition should not differ depending on mode of delivery, as the physiological impact of losing blood depends on the volume lost. Obviously, even if there were identical blood losses, the specific morbidity and healing from abdominal or vaginal operations or tears will differ.

Accurate estimation of blood loss

Measuring blood loss accurately is notoriously difficult, but some studies have improved this by using a blood collector bag[66] (see Chapters 9–11). Training programs incorporating clinical reconstructions that include algorithms to facilitate visual estimation of blood loss improved the accuracy of such estimation[67,68]. Routine use of a modified obstetric early warning score (or MEOWS) may aid recognition of hypovolemia where estimated blood loss is inaccurate[69].

Address primary prevention risk factors for PPH

Decreasing major hemorrhage involves trying to reduce all risk factors for PPH (Table 4). In high income countries, increasing age and obesity are contributing to increasing use of oxytocin in labor as well as the

Table 5 A comparison of four recent studies of obstetric hysterectomy

Author, year of publication	Eniola et al.[23] *UK, 2006*	Rossi et al.[24] *USA, 2010*	Zwart et al. (*LeMMoN*)[20] *Netherland, 2008*	Knight et al. (*UKOSS*)[30] *UK, 2007*
Setting type of study number of cases number of deliveries (denominator)	Mar 1997–Feb 1998, SE Thames Population based cohort n = 22 cases 48,865 deliveries >24 weeks	1993–2008 high income countries Systematic review of studies looking at hysterectomies in the first 48 h postpartum (excluded Eniola et al. as that included PPH >24 h) n = 981 cases	Aug 2004–Aug 2006 prospective population cohort study 1606 cases of MOH (defined as 2000 ml) 358,874 deliveries 4.5/1000 n = 107 cases	UK wide Feb 2005–Feb 2006 Case–control reporting n = 318 cases, 614 controls Total no deliveries in UK estimated 775,186 during that period (Office of National Statistics)
Hysterectomy rate	0.45/1000 deliveries	0.8–2.28/1000 deliveries in US 0.2–5/1000 deliveries in the review	0.29/1000 (n = 107) 13% and 10% after failed embolization or intrauterine balloon, respectively	0.41/1000 deliveries
Mortality	4.5% (1 death : 22 hysterectomies)	2.6% (26 deaths : 981 hysterectomies)	Death not reported	0.6% (1 death : 150 hysterectomies)
Risk factors	Multiparity 71% Previous CS 33% CS index pregnancy 68% Placenta previa 24%	Multiparity 78% Previous CS 46% CS in index pregnancy 73% Abnormal placentation Previous gynecological surgery 15.8%	Risk factors for hysterectomy not separated from risk factors for hemorrhage	Age >35 (OR 2.42) Parity >3 (11%) Multiple pregnancy (OR 2.3) Previous CS (28%) (OR 3.52) CS index pregnancy (OR 7.13) Placenta previa (37%) (OR 24 for minor, 232 for major) Placenta accreta (39%)
Cause of bleed leading to hysterectomy	Atony 50% Uterine rupture 0%	Adherent placenta 38% Atony 29% Uterine rupture/dehiscence 12% Placenta previa 7% Abruption 2%	Uterine rupture 0.06% Placenta previa 40% Atony 38.5%	Atony 53% Adherent placenta 39% Uterine rupture 8% Extension of uterine incision at delivery 6% (3 for malignancy)
Long-term morbidity	Transfused 100% Urinary tract injury 21% Repeat surgery 38% Poor health 6–9 months postnatal More than 25% scored >13 on the Edinburgh postnatal depression score (i.e. at risk of significant depression)	Transfused 44% Urinary tract injury 16% Return to theater for bleeding or repeat laparotomy 4.9% 56% of women had conservative management techniques, no detail as to which, 44% went straight to hysterectomy Short-term morbidity similar for total and subtotal hysterectomy	ITU admission 27%	2-day ITU stay 84% Damage to structures 21% Severe morbidity 19% Bladder damage 3 times more likely if accreta than if atonic PPH

CVA, cerebrovascular accident; DIC, disseminated intravascular coagulation; HELLP, hemolysis, elevated liver enzymes, low platelets; ICU, intensive care unit; ITU, intensive therapy unit; MOH, massive obstetric hemorrhage (1500 ml in some studies, 2500 ml in others); PET, pre-eclampsia; PPH, postpartum hemorrhage; SAMM, severe adverse maternal morbidity

rising cesarean section rate[9,54]. Independently of one another, obesity, oxytocin use and cesarean section are risk factors for hemorrhage. The limited length of pregnancy means society-wide public health interventions might be better placed to address obesity.

Multiple pregnancy is another risk factor which, in low income countries, has been more likely to be spontaneous and therefore not preventable. In the UK, however, recent Human Fertilisation and Embryology Authority (HFEA) targets are encouraging greater use of single embryo transfers to reduce the risks associated with IVF multiple pregnancy, including PPH[70,71]. However, there are many countries where larger numbers of embryos are still being transferred (US, Eastern Europe, India), thus contributing to PPH and other obstetric morbidities.

Availability of cheap, effective drugs to use in low resource and out of hospital settings is important. Misoprostol is one such drug which is heat stable and easy to administer in a home birth setting. Studies in Africa have shown reduced rates of PPH when it is used, and its administration does not require trained birth attendants[72,73]. Sublingual administration may be most effective[74,75], and the women can self-administer easily[73], further reducing the cost of an already cheap intervention (see Chapters 32–35).

Basic antenatal care

This cannot be overemphasized, as ample evidence shows that antenatal follow-up decreases a woman's risk at labor and delivery[41,76]. Antenatal screening for complications, treatment and prevention of anemia, cleanliness during delivery, the presence of a skilled birth attendant and active management of the third stage of labor are all basic requirements advocated by WHO[77]. Staff attending deliveries in the primary care sector need to be trained to recognize PPH early and have access to simple drugs to treat it (e.g. misoprostol, ergometrine)[72], as well as to recognize when to refer to a more specialized center[54]. In rural South Africa, health-worker problems were identified as the cause of substandard care in 35–49% of cases[54] out of a total of 65% where substandard care was an issue. Factors identified were delay in diagnosis, treatment, referral and monitoring.

Training, teamwork and skills

Effective teamwork is paramount for timely interventions. Algorithms or diagrams of expected co-ordinated actions may help identify what needs to be done and by whom, especially when several actions need to be undertaken simultaneously as in brisk PPH[78].

Clear management protocols and regular skills-drills training may both contribute to the maintenance of high standards in units[8,27]. Non-adherence to guidelines has been identified as a risk factor for increased maternal morbidity[8,79], whereas dissemination of guidelines and skills-drills are associated with improved adherence to the agreed protocols and reduction in PPH[79]. However, recent research in France has generated conflicting results regarding the efficacy of adherence to guidelines on actual incidence of major PPH. One of the studies involved 19 maternity units within a regional French perinatal network[80] and the other involved 106 units in six regions[81]. Both showed that prompt recognition and aggressive management of PPH improved care, and increased the use of surgery in management, whereas the prevalence of major PPH did not alter. This may be explained by different risk factors dominating the progression from small to large PPH (e.g. previa), and suggests that interventions additional to improved recognition and secondary prevention are necessary to make an impact on PPH rates[81]. Important factors involve multiprofessional training within the local unit and integrating teamwork training within the clinical teaching itself[82].

Access, transport and organizational change

Twenty per cent of avoidable SAMM in rural South Africa is due to organizational or administrative causes such as the shortage of essential drugs, ambulances and recruitment and retention of experienced staff[41]. These factors are less prominent in high income countries. However, implementation of guidelines and issues such as staff training and effective audit usually occur at organizational levels. Geller et al.[49] analysed the 'preventability' of events along the continuum of severe morbidity to near-miss to death and concluded that the same factors contributed to the outcome in all categories (Figure 1). These were patient factors (13–20%), system factors (33–47%) and provider-related factors (90%), mainly incomplete or inappropriate management[49]. Patient factors are potentially the hardest to rectify, especially in low income countries where access to education is limited. System factors figure higher in the US (33–47%)[49] than in South Africa (20%)[41], possibly because failures of well-established systems (as in the US) are likely to have a greater impact than in settings where transport or administrative systems are not established in the first place, e.g. in rural Africa[41]. Provider-related factors have been more prominent as a cause of substandard care in the US (90%)[49] than in primary care settings in South Africa (35–49%)[41]. This is more likely due to the non-availability of specialist staff in the latter, with staff performing to the best of their ability in light of skills they possess. Expected standards change with time, place and facilities, so it is not unsurprising that provider-related factors continue to feature even in low mortality settings.

Health systems

Wider factors relating to health systems can move a woman both up and down the risk pyramid for severity of morbidity. Social exclusion, education and inequality can be tackled at governmental level in both low and high income countries[2,76]. Access to contraception, safe legal abortion and antenatal care can all be addressed. Health service planners may have to provide outreach antenatal services for travelers, teenagers and the mentally ill[2]. The lack of universal coverage for health insurance in the US may play a role, as women most at risk are often not insured[49,83]. The population in major cities is changing, due to increased migration especially from deprived areas or as a result of war and conflict. Access to 24-hour interpreters should become standard and might lead to significant reductions in severe morbidity[2].

CONCLUSION

The UK triennial Confidential Enquiries into Maternal Deaths started in 1952, and the latter part of the 20th century witnessed a gradual decline in maternal mortality. Maternal death is now rare in high income countries, although still prevalent in low income countries. Severe adverse maternal morbidity (SAMM) is prevalent throughout the world, mostly due to treatable conditions. Poor, socially excluded women suffer most, but hemorrhage can strike any woman. For meaningful comparisons to be made, standardized, simple definitions need to be designed and agreed upon as the benchmark for future research.

Hemorrhage accounts for the largest proportion of severe morbidity but is not a major cause of maternal mortality, at least in developed countries[12]. This suggests that registering SAMM would be a valuable way to monitor and improve the quality of maternity services. Several population-based studies in countries such as Scotland, The Netherlands and Australia demonstrate that national morbidity surveys are feasible. Studies are needed at national level as numbers of SAMM cases are relatively small, and trends are easier to analyse. As the causes of maternal deaths can be different from those of SAMM[12], it is most useful to have the two systems running in parallel to aid understanding of the relationship. This has been achieved in Scotland for the past 8 years. The UKOSS rare obstetric register system has been working nationwide in the UK since 2005. The recent study on peripartum hysterectomy showed that there was one death for every 150 hysterectomies performed for hemorrhage, thus reinforcing the value of morbidity and mortality surveys running in parallel.

It is important to continue to monitor trends. In high income countries recognized risk factors for hemorrhage such as age, obesity and cesarean section rates are rising. The current cesarean section rate in the UK is 23%, and it is as high as 50% in Latin America[84,85]. Globally, interventions aimed to reduce a specific morbidity (e.g. cesarean section in obstructed labor to prevent a ruptured uterus) may increase the risk of a different subsequent morbidity (e.g. placenta accreta in previous cesarean section scar or uterine rupture in attempted vaginal birth after cesarean section). Overall, obstetric morbidity may thus rise, fall or remain unchanged, but information to guide high quality practice relies on robust, continuous, population-based SAMM audits.

References

1. Stones W, Lim W, Al-Azzawi F. An investigation of maternal morbidity with identification of life-threatening "near-miss" episodes. Health Trends 1991;23:13–5
2. Bewley S, Wolfe C, Waterstone M. Severe maternal morbidity in the UK. In: Maclean AB, Neilson J, eds. Maternal Morbidity and Mortality. London: RCOG Press, 2002:132–46
3. Souza JP, Cecatti JG, Patrpinelli MA, et al. Appropriate criteria for identification of near-miss maternal morbidity in intensive care facilities: a cross-sectional study. BMC Pregnancy Childbirth 2007;7:20
4. Ronsmans C, Scott S, Adisasmita A, et al. Estimation of population-based incidence of pregnancy-related illness and mortality (PRIAM) in two districts in Java, Indonesia. BJOG 2009;116:82–90
5. Oladapo OT, Sule-Odu AO, Olatunji AO, et al. Near-miss obstetric events and maternal deaths in Sagamu, Nigeria a retrospective study. Reprod Health 2005;2:96
6. Fillipi V, Ganaba R, Baggaley RF, et al. Health of women after severe obstetric complications in Burkina Faso: a longitudinal study. Lancet 2007;370:1329–37
7. Say L, Souza JP, Pattinson RC. Maternal near-miss – towards a standard tool for monitoring quality of maternal health care. Best Pract Res Clin Obstet Gynaecol 2009;23:287–96
8. Hall M. Haemorrhage. In: Department of Health, Welsh Office, Scottish Office Department of Health, Department of Health and Social Services, Northern Ireland, Why Mothers die. Report on Confidential Enquiries into Maternal Deaths in the United Kingdom 2000–2002. London: Her Majesty's Stationery Office, 2004
9. Norman J. Haemorrhage (chapter 4) in CMACE. BJOG 2011;118(Suppl 1):1–203
10. Lennox C. Appendix 2B: summary of Scottish Confidential Audit of Severe Maternal Morbidity Report 2008. CMACE. BJOG 2011;118(Suppl 1):196–8
11. Mantel GD, Buchmann E, Rees H, et al. Severe acute maternal morbidity: a pilot study of a definition for a near-miss. BJOG 1998;105:985–90
12. Pattinson RC, Buchmann E, Mantel G, et al. Can enquiries into severe acute maternal morbidity act as a surrogate for maternal death enquiries? BJOG 2003;110:889–93
13. Bewley S, Creighton S. "Near-miss" obstetric enquiry. J Obstet Gynaecol 1997;17:26–9
14. Fillipi V, Alihonou E, Mukantaganda S, et al. Near-misses: maternal morbidity and mortality. Lancet 1998;351:145–6
15. Prual A, Huguet D, Gabin O, et al. Severe obstetric morbidity of the third trimester, delivery and early puerperium in Niamey (Niger). Afr J Reprod Health 1998;2:10–9
16. Geller SE, Rosenberg D, Cox S, et al. Defining a conceptual framework for near-miss maternal morbidity. J Am Med Women's Assoc 2002;57:135–9
17. Waterstone M, Bewley S, Wolfe C. Incidence and predictors of severe obstetric morbidity: case-control study. Br Med J 2001;322:109–93
18. Brace V, Penney G, Hall M. Quantifying severe maternal morbidity: a Scottish population study. BJOG 2004;111:481–4
19. Penney G, Admason L, Kernaghan D. Scottish confidential audit of severe maternal morbidity second annual report 2004. Scottish Programme for clinical effectiveness in reproductive health. 1–32 www.abdn.ac.uk/specrh
20. Zwart JJ, Richters JM, Ory F, et al. Severe maternal morbidity during pregnancy, delivery and puerperium in the Netherlands: a nationwide population-based study of 371 000 pregnancies. BJOG 2008;115:842–50
21. Knight M, Spark P, Fitzpatrick K, et al. United Kingdom Obstetric Surveillance System (UKOSS) Annual Report 2011. National Perinatal Epidemiology Unit, Oxford 2011. https://www.npeu.ox.ac.uk/files/downloads/ukoss/UKOSS-Annual-Report-2010.pdf
22. Killpatrick SJ, Matthay MA. Obstetric patients requiring critical care. A five-year review. Chest 2002:101:1407–12

23. Eniola OA, Bewley S, Waterstone M, et al. Obstetric hysterectomy in a population of South East England. J Obstet Gynaecol 2006;26:104–9

24. Rossi AC, Richard HL, Chmait RH. Emergency postpartum hysterectomy for uncontrolled postpartum bleeding. Obstet Gynecol 2010;115:637–44

25. The Eclampsia Trial Collaborative Group. Which anticonvulsant for women with eclampsia? Evidence from the collaborative Eclampsia Trial. Lancet 1995;337:1455–63

26. Bouvier-Colle MH, Salanave B, Ancel PY, et al. Obstetric patients treated in intensive care units and maternal mortality. Regional teams for the survey. Eur J Obstet Gynaecol Reprod Biol 1996;65:121–5

27. Baskett TF, Sternadel J. Maternal intensive care and near-miss mortality in obstetrics. BJOG 1998;105:981–4

28. Zhang WH, Alexander S, Bouvier-Colle MH, et al. Incidence of severe pre-eclampsia, post-partum haemorrhage and sepsis as a surrogate marker for severe maternal morbidity in a European population-based study: the MOMS-B survey. BJOG 2005;112:89–96

29. Minkauskiene M, Nadisauskiene RJ, Padaiga Z. Severe and acute maternal morbidity: Lithuanian experience and review. Int J Fertil Womens Med 2006;51:39–46

30. Knight M. Peripartum hysterectomy in the UK: management and outcomes of the associated haemorrhage. BJOG 2007; 114:1380–7

31. Souza JP, Cecatti JG, Parpinelli MA, et al. Maternal morbidity and near-miss in the community: findings from the 2006 Brazilian demographic health survey. BJOG 2010;117: 1586–92

32. Lawton BA, Wilson LF, Dinsdale RA, et al. Audit of severe maternal morbidity describing reasons for transfer and potential preventability of admissions to ICU. Aust N Z J Obstet Gynaecol 2010:50:346–51

33. Almerie Y, Almerie MQ, Matar HE, et al. Obstetric near-miss and maternal mortality in maternity university hospital, Damascus,Syria: a retrospective study. BMC Pregnancy Childbirth 2010;10:65

34. Mutihir JT, Utoo BT. Postpartum maternal morbidity in Jos, north-central Nigeria. Nigerian J Clin Pract 2011;14:38–42

35. Van Roosmalen J, Zwart J. Severe acute maternal morbidity in high income countries. Best Pract Res Clin Obstet Gynaecol 2009;23:297–304

36. Ronsmans C . Severe acute maternal morbidity in low-income countries. Best Pract Res Clin Obstet Gynaecol 2009; 23:305–16

37. Vandecruys H, Pattinson RC, Macdonald A, et al. Severe acute maternal morbidity and mortality in the Pretoria Academic Complex: changing patterns over 4 years. Eur J Obstet Gynaecol Reprod Biol 2002;102:6–10

38. D'Ambruoso L, Achadi E, Adisasmita A, et al. Assessing quality of care provided by Indonesia village midwives: a confidential enquiry. Midwifery 2009;25:528–39

39. Prual A, Bouvier-Colle MH, de Bernis L, et al . Severe maternal morbidity from direct obstetric causes in West Africa: incidence and case-fatality rates. Bull WHO 2000;78: 593–603

40. Fillipi V, Ronsmans C, Gohou V, et al. Maternity wards or obstetric emergency rooms? Incidence of near-miss morbidity in African hospitals. Acta Obstet Gynaecol Scand 2005;84: 11–6

41. Ghandi MN, Welz T, Ronsmans C. Severe acute maternal morbidity in rural South Africa. Int J Gynaecol Obstet 2004; 87:180–7

42. World Health Organization, Department of Reproductive Health and Research. Evaluating the quality of care for severe pregnancy complications: the WHO near-miss approach for maternal health. WHO, 2011 http://www.who.int/reproductivehealth/publications/monitoring/9789241502221/en/index.html

43. Ki-Moon B. Global Strategy for Women's and Children's Health 2009 http://www.un.org/sg/hf/GlobalStategyEN.pdf

44. World Health Organisation Maternal mortality Fact sheet N°348. November 2010 http://www.who.int/mediacentre/factsheets/fs348/en/index.html

45. Hogan M, Foreman KJ, Naghavi M, et al. Maternal mortality for 181 countries, 1980–2008: a systematic analysis of progress towards Millennium Development Goal 5. Lancet 2010;375: 1609–23

46. CMACH 2000–2002. Department of Health, Welsh Office, Scottish Office, Department of Health and Social Services Northern Ireland. Why Mothers Die. Report on Confidential Enquiries into Maternal Deaths in the United Kingdom 2000–2002. London: Her Majesty's Stationery Office, 2004

47. Waterstone M, Wolfe C, Hooper R, et al. Postnatal morbidity after childbirth and severe obstetric morbidity. BJOG 2003;110:128–33

48. Monaco TJ, Spielman FJ, Katz VL. Pregnant patients in the intensive care unit: a descriptive analysis. South Med J 1993; 86:414–7

49. Geller SE, Rosenberg D, Cox SM, et al. The continuum of maternal morbidity and mortality: factors associated with severity. Am J Obstet Gynaecol 2004;191:939–44

50. Kaye D, Mirembe F, Aziga F, et al. Maternal mortality and associated near-misses among emergency intrapartum referrals in Mulago Hospiatl, Kampala, Uganda. East Afr Med J 2003; 80:144–9

51. Wen SW, Huang L, Liston R, et al. Severe maternal morbidity in Canada, 1991–2001. CMAJ 2005;173:759–64

52. Pallasmaa N, Ekblad U, Gissler M. Severe maternal morbidity and the mode of delivery. Acta Obstet Gynaecol Scand 2008; 87:662–8

53. Callaghan WM, Mackay AP, Berg CJ. Identification of severe maternal morbidity during delivery hospitalizations, United States, 1991–2003. Am J Obstet Gynaecol 2008;199:133. e1–133.e8

54. Knight M, Callaghan WM, Berg C, et al. Trends in post-partum haemorrhage in high resource countries: a review and recommendations from the International Postpartum Haemorrhage Collaborative Group. BMC Pregnancy Childbirth 2009;9:55

55. Ford JB, Roberts CL, Simpson JM, et al. Increased postpartum haemorrhage rates in Australia. Int J Gynaecol Obstet 2007;98:237–43

56. Al-Zirqi I, Vangen S, Forsen L, Stray-Pedersen B. Prevalence and risk factors of severe obstetric haemorrhage. BJOG 2008; 115:1265–72

57. Joseph KS, Rouleau J, Kramer MS, et al. Investigation of an increase in post-partum haemorrhage in Canada. BJOG 2007; 114:751–9

58. Kuklina EV, Meikle SF, Jamieson DJ, et al. Severe obstetric morbidity in the United States: 1998–2005. Obstet Gynaecol 2009;113:293–9

59. Lutomski L, Byrne B, Devane D, Greene R. Increasing trends in atonic postpartum haemorrhage in Ireland: an 11-year population based cohort study. BJOG 2012;119:306–14

60. Manoharan M, Wuntakal R, Erskine K. Uterine rupture: a revisit. The Obstetrician Gynaecologist 2010;12:223–30

61. Hofmeyr GJ, Say L, Gulmezoglu AM. WHO systematic review of maternal mortality and morbidity: the prevalence of uterine rupture. BJOG 2005;112:1221–8

62. Al-Nuaim LA, Mustafa MS, Abdel Gader AG. Disseminated intravascular coagulation and obstetric haemorrhage. Management dilemma. Saudi Med J 2002;23;658–62

63. Lewis GE, ed. The Confidential Enquiry into Maternal and Child Health (CEMACH). Saving Mothers Lives: reviewing maternal deaths to make motherhood safer 2003–05. London: CEMACH, 2007

64. Whiteman MK, Kuklina E, Hillis SD, et al. Incidence and determinants of peripartum hysterectomy. Obstet Gynaecol 2006;108:1486–92

65. Glazener CMA, Abdalla M, Stroud P, et al. Postnatal maternal morbidity: extent, causes, prevention and treatment. BJOG 1995;102:282–7

66. Zhang WH, Deneux-Tharaux C, Brocklehurst P, et al. Effect of a collector bag for measurement of postpartum blood loss after vaginal delivery: cluster randomised trial in 13 European countries. BMJ 2010;340:c293

67. Bose P, Regan F, Paterson-Brown S. Improving the accuracy of estimated blood loss at obstetric haemorrhage using clinical reconstructions. BJOG 2006;113:919–24

68. Maslovitz S, Barkai G, Lessing JB, et al. Improved accuracy of post-partum blood loss estimation as assessed by simulation. Acta Obstet Gynaecol Scand 2008; 87:929–34

69. Smith GB, Pryterch DR, Schmidt P, et al. Hospital-wide physiological surveillance – a new approach to the early identification and management of the sick patient. Resuscitation 2006;71:19–28

70. Kjellberg AT, Carlsoon P, Bergh C. Randomized single versus double embryo transfer: obstetric and paediatric outcome and a cost-effectiveness analysis. Hum Reprod 2006;21:210–6

71. Braude P. One Child at a Time 4 One Child at a Time. Report of the Expert Group on Multiple Births after IVF, Oct 2006. http://www.oneatatime.org.uk/images?MBSET_reprt_Final_Dec_06.pdf

72. Prata N, Mbaruku G, Campbell M, et al. Controlling postpartum haemorrhage after home births in Tanzania. Int J Gynaecol Obstet 2005;90:51–5

73. Potts M, Campbell M. Three meetings and fewer funerals – misoprostol in post-partum haemorrhage. Lancet 2004;364: 1110–11

74. Vimala N, Mittal S, Kumar S, et al. Sublingual misoprostol versus methylergometrine for actice management of the third stage of labour. Int J Gynaecol Obstet 2004;87:1–5

75. Hofmeyr GJ, Walraven G, Gulmezoglu AM, et al. Misoprostol to treat post-partum haemorrhage: a systematic review. BJOG 2005;112:547–53

76. World Health Organisation 1994. The mother-baby package: WHO's guide to saving women's and infant's lives. Safe Mother 1994;15:4–7

77. Lazarus JV, Lalonde A. Reducing post-partum haemorrhage in Africa. Int J Gynaecol Obstet 2005;88:89–90

78. Briley A, Bewley S. Management of obstetric haemorrhage: obstetric management. In: Pavord S, Hunt B, eds. The Obstetric Haematology Manual. Cambridge: Cambridge University Press, 2010:151–7

79. Rizvi F, Mackey R, Barett T, et al. Successful reduction of massive post-partum haemorrhage by use of guidelines and staff education. BJOG 2004;111:495–8

80. Audureau E, Deneux-Tharaux C, Lefevre P, et al. practices for prevention, diagnosis and management of postpartum haemorrhage: impact of a regional multifaceted intervention. J Obstet Gynacol 2009;116:1325–33

81. Deneux-Tharaux C, Dupont C, Colin C, et al. Multifaceted intervention to decrease the rate of severe postpartum haemorrhage: the PITHAGORE6 cluster-randomised controlled trial. J Obstet Gynaecol 2010;117:1278–7

82. Siassakos D, Crofts JF, Winter C, et al. The active components of effective training in obstetric emergencies. J Obstet Gynaeol 2009;116:1028–32

83. Deadly Delivery. The Maternal Health Care Crisis in the USA www.amnestyusa.orgIndex AMR 51/007/2010

84. Villar J, Valladares E, Wojdyla D, et al. Caesarean delivery rates and pregnancy outcomes: the 2005 WHO global survey on maternal and perinatal health in Latin America. Lancet 2006;367:1819–29

85. Knight M, Kurinczuk JJ, Spark P. Caesarean delivery and peripartum hysterectomy. Obstet Gynecol 2008;111:97–105

61

Learning to Treat Postpartum Hemorrhage: a Spectrum of Modern Teaching/Learning Modalities

E. El Hamamy and C. B-Lynch

'Medicine is learned by the bedside and not in the classroom.'
William Osler[1]

INTRODUCTION

William Osler (1849–1919) brought forth the concept of bedside teaching/learning in the 19th century[1]. Although more than a century has passed since he first aired this concept, and the practice of medicine both at the bedside and in the office has changed radically, his statement remains entirely true with regard to the management of postpartum hemorrhage (PPH).

Specifically, in recent years training in emergency obstetric skills (including PPH training) has moved from the traditional clinical teaching normally conducted in the labor ward to specific, targeted skills and scenario-based courses that utilize mannequins and simulators most often away from the bedside. Such changes are currently seen as necessary, largely as a result of the limitations of traditional clinical teaching when it comes to genuine patient encounters in an emergency situation[2]. The authors are grateful to Professor Amr El Noury of Cairo University for designing the poster which provides a stepwise guide to the management of PPH (Figure 1).

THE DRIVERS FOR POSTPARTUM HEMORRHAGE TRAINING

The incidence of PPH is increasing in both the developed and developing countries[3,4]. This circumstance preceded increasing demands for training of all caregivers who deal with parturients. Because all staff require regular training to identify and manage maternal collapse, including the identification and management of PPH, different organizations are taking the requisite initiatives to improve the accessibility of training.

The World Health Organization (WHO) set a goal to reduce maternal mortality by 75% by 2015, mainly by reducing maternal deaths related to PPH by training health workers in both developing and developed countries[5]. Recently, further initiatives have been undertaken by WHO in addressing the women's health crisis in Africa by providing a report on women's health in the African Region[6].

Prior to these efforts, the Federation of Gynecology and Obstetrics (FIGO), together with the Confederation of Midwives (ICM) advocated the Global Initiative on the Prevention of Post-partum Hemorrhage in 2004. In addition, both organizations recommend that every skilled attendant (doctors, nurses and midwives) likely to be present at birth have training in uterine massage and bimanual compression. The same document also advises that all skilled birth attendants have access to technical training in administering uterotonics and other techniques such as intravenous infusions and tamponade balloons, and that every doctor who can perform laparotomy be provided with surgical training to perform 'simple conservative surgery' for PPH including compression sutures and sequential devascularization[7].

In the UK, successive Confidential Enquiries into Maternal Deaths have linked the increased numbers of deaths from PPH to recent changes in medical training. Specifically, the reduction in the overall length of obstetric training and in working hours during training may have reduced the amount of experience gained compared with the experiences obtainable in the past. Moreover, these reports have shown a trend towards subspecialization among consultants in the UK, and those with a special interest in obstetrics do not necessarily have highly developed surgical skills. These reports recommend regular 'fire drills' or 'skills drills' for the modern management of PPH for all grades of staff in every obstetric unit. The 2004 and 2007 Confidential Enquiry into Maternal and Child Health (CEMACH) reports repeatedly highlight the role of inadequate clinical care, as well as poor communication and teamwork within labor ward teams and suggest that as many as half of all maternal deaths might be prevented with better care[8,9]. Following this line of thought, the 2011 Confidential Enquiries into Maternal Deaths (CMACE) report recommended that all units should have protocols in place for the identification and management of PPH and that all clinicians responsible for the care of pregnant women,

Postpartum Haemorrhage Guide to Management

| Identify | Risk factors - Blood loss > 1000 ml | or | Hemodynamic compromise: R.R / pulse / systolic / signs of shock |

Known Antenatal Risk			
Substantial risk	**O.R**	**Significant Risk**	**O.R**
Suspected or proven placental abruption	13	Previous PPH	3
Known placenta praevia	12	Asian ethnicity	2
Multiple pregnancy	5	Obesity (BMI >35)	2
Pre-eclampsia/ gestational hypertension	4	Anaemia (<9 g/dl)	2

Intra-partum / postpartum risk			
Substantial risk	**O.R**	**Significant Risk**	**O.R**
Delivery by emergency C.S	4	Operative vaginal delivery	2
Delivery by elective C.S	2	Prolonged labour (> 12 hours)	2
Induction of labour	2	Big baby (> 4 kg)	2
Retained placenta	5	Pyrexia in labour	2
Mediolateral episiotomy	5	Age (> 40 years, not multiparous)	1.4

| Communicate | Resuscitate | Monitor & Investigate | Stop Bleeding |

1 Communicate
Alert all staff

Midwife / Nurse
Senior Obstetrician
Obstetric Anaesthetic staff
Haematologist
Blood Bank
Porters
PPH emergency Box
Member of the team to record events.

2 Resuscitate
A Airway
B Breathing
C Circulation
Oxygen 10—15 L/ min
Position flat
14 G i.v line x2

20 ml blood sample should be taken and sent for diagnostic tests, including full blood count, coagulation screen, urea and electrolytes and cross match (4 units).
Restore circulation
Crystalloid. Hartmann's solution max 2 L
Colloid (e.g. hemacel) max 1.5 L
Improve O2 carrying capacity
Packed Group specific or O Negative Blood
Warm - rapid- no filter

3 Monitor and investigate
Hemoglobin, Ht, platelets
Clotting screen (PT, PTT, Fibrinogen)
Foley's catheter
O2 saturation
Early warning chart
Tone, Tissue, Trauma, Thrombin
Consider ITU (when bleeding is controlled)

4 Stop Bleeding

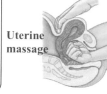

Uterine massage

Syntocinon 5 units by slow intravenous injection (may have repeat dose). (40 units in 500 ml Hartmann's solution at 125 ml/hour)
Ergometrine 0.5 mg by slow I.V or I.M (contraindicated in hypertension).

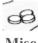

Miso-prostol
Rectal 600—1000 ug

Carboprost
(if available)
0.25 mg by intramuscular injection repeated at intervals of not less than 15 minutes to a maximum of 8 doses (contraindicated in women with asthma).

Fresh Frozen plasma: 4 units for every 6 units of red cells or if relentless bleeding or PT / APTT> 1.5 x normal (12–15 ml/kg or total 1 / L)

Exclude trauma to vulva, vagina, cervix and uterus

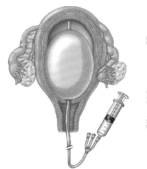
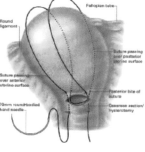
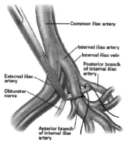

Resort to hysterectomy **SOONER RATHER THAN LATER**

Recombinant Factor VIIa (rFVIIa)

Documentation and debriefing

To woman and family by a senior staff

International training of Postpartum Hemorrhage, Wales, 2011

Prof Amr El Noury & Mr Essam El Hamamy

Figure 1 PPH guide to management poster. Courtesy of Professor Amr El Noury

antenatally, postnatally and intrapartum, including those practicing in the community, should carry out regular skills training for such scenarios[10].

The need for such a recommendation follows the 2007 survey among obstetric trainees in London which documented a reported decline in the numbers of individuals who could manage major PPH. Only 44.6% of respondents felt confident to perform a cesarean hysterectomy; and whereas a similar number (41.7%) could apply a B-Lynch suture, a much smaller number (27.1%) could dissect the ureter if need be. Additionally, a few respondents were less confident in performing any surgical procedure necessary in the management of major obstetric hemorrhage. This finding may have serious implications in the provision of out of hours senior cover for maternity units in the future[11].

The Scottish Confidential Audit of Severe Maternal Morbidity 2008 highlighted errors and substandard care in the management of women who had sustained PPH. These included avoidable delay in diagnosis and treatment, failure to follow protocol/plan, appropriate conclusion/differential diagnosis not made, appropriate tests not performed, inadequate training/supervision of staff, inadequate history/examination, staff practicing beyond their level of competence, inadequate staffing (levels/skill mix), poor communication, inadequate service from other departments such as blood transfusion service and the laboratory, test results not obtained or ignored, lack of team work, defective equipment and inappropriate test performed. All these deficiencies could be improved with adequate and targeted training[12].

The UK Obstetric Surveillance System (UKOSS) publication[13] echoes the growing recognition articulated in numerous chapters of this volume that prompt action is essential in managing PPH. Those who provide care should try to do so within the first 2 hours of the diagnosis and certainly not beyond a delay of 6 hours. Morbidity rises sharply after 2 hours, when it becomes much more likely that hysterectomy will be necessary.

MODALITIES OF TRAINING

Hands-on training

Hands-on training is a simple method for an on-the-job facilitator who works with small numbers of participants to teach them certain procedural applications. The working concept is to prepare the trainee at a workstation to mimic the procedure or scenario, let them practice it, and then review their competency.

This model of training is suitable for teaching practical skills such as the application of bimanual compression of the uterus, the uterine brace suture, uterine tamponade, etc. However, because of the small number of participants, it is not suitable to teach communication skills.

Lecture based training

PPH is one of the catastrophic events where proper management requires a variety of hospital workers with different unique expertise. It is often difficult to get all these people together to arrange a simulation or hands-on training, and lecture based teaching may be more appropriate. All staff should attend; obstetric physicians, midwives, nurses, house staff, anesthesia providers, scrub technicians and unit secretaries participate in the same formal classroom instruction. The purpose is for all team members to hear the same material, to learn the same teamwork language and behaviors, and to feel empowered to flatten hierarchy. The participants from varying disciplines should be allowed ample opportunity for conversation and sharing of varying points of view. It is mandatory that the team should be able to understand each other's roles and competing interests that may not be self-evident.

Classroom based team training allows large numbers of clinical staff to be taught the concepts of teamwork and patient safety. Didactic lectures can be supplemented with clinical scenarios, vignettes, videos and other media to teach both the intellectual concepts and specific behaviors of team based care. The advantages of classroom based training are that it is relatively inexpensive, large numbers of staff can be trained quickly, feedback to and questions from the participants can be included, and multiple specialties can be trained simultaneously. This type of training can highlight patient safety processes that help maintain 'normalcy' on the unit to prevent adverse events (e.g. multidisciplinary meetings, preprocedure briefings, effective handoffs). This helps teach staff techniques to prevent adverse events instead of concentrating on ways to respond to them. Disadvantages include low fidelity training in the teamwork skills, and little or no practice in actual crisis management.

Simulation

Simulation is a learner centered teaching method that mimics real world situations to meet specific learning objectives. A simulator is a generic term referring to a physical object, device, situation, or environment where a task or series of tasks can be realistically and dynamically represented[14].

There are two types of simulators, those with high and low fidelities. The high fidelity type is often used to describe computer driven simulators, whereas the term low fidelity is used to describe simulators that are not computer controlled. High fidelity is desirable in simulation, because the more contextually accurate is the simulation based instruction, the more likely the learning that takes place will transfer to the reality of applied practice. The disadvantages of this type of training include cost, the need to remove clinicians from clinical care and a lack of realism compared with the clinicians' own experience[15].

Simulation based training is an appropriate proactive approach for reducing errors and risk in obstetrics, improving teamwork and communication, and giving students a multiplicity of transferable skills to improve their performances. The drivers for simulation include patient safety, limitation of current educational processes, shortening of the training period, high risk emergencies and the pressure of health care agencies in an attempt to reduce malpractice concerns[16]. A significant portion of hemorrhage-related maternal morbidity may be prevented through early diagnosis and rapid intervention. There is a small but growing body of literature describing the role of patient safety initiatives and simulation training in optimizing outcomes following PPH[17]. Rapid response teams may be used to facilitate coordination between various personnel involved in the management of PPH[18]. Hemorrhage drills and simulation based training may help providers achieve timely and coordinated responses[19]. Protocols may help to standardize management in cases of PPH, thereby minimizing unnecessary errors or delays in care[20].

Only a few models have been used for PPH training. Deering *et al.* used a standard obstetric birthing model equipped with an inflatable uterus to simulate uterine atony. The residents were assessed upon completion of this exercise. The authors found that the majority were unable to correct the hemorrhage within 5 minutes and half made at least one error, either in the dose or the route of administration of medications used to arrest the bleeding[21,22].

Teamwork training in a simulation setting resulted in improvement of knowledge, practical skills, communication and team performance in acute obstetric situations. Training in a simulation center did not further improve outcome compared with training in a local hospital[20].

A simple low fidelity model has been used for the past few years by the authors. It is made of knitted wool and has an incision like opening in the lower part to give the impression of a postpartum uterus after the baby and the placenta have been expelled along with the blood supply of the uterus and the ovaries. It is a useful tool to learn the placement of a B-Lynch or other type of compression suture and it also gives one the ability to practice a form of step-wise devascularization (Figure 2).

INVALUABLE RESOURCES FOR POSTPARTUM HEMORRHAGE TRAINING

(1) PPH hands on training/workshops visit http://www.pphinternationaltraining.org/

(2) A short video demonstration of the B-Lynch suturing technique. This video is presented in real video format. There is a link provided to download, which is available at: www.cblynch.com/index.html

(3) Internet-based training. Visit *The Global Library on Women's Medicine*, launched November 2008, which is available at: www.glowm.com

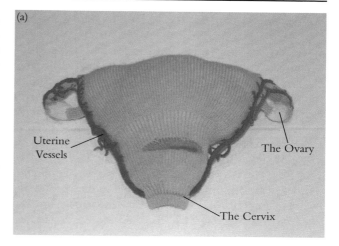
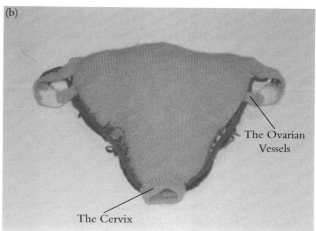

Figure 2 Uterine model (a) front view and (b) rear view

(4) Poster of the B-Lynch suture technique to be displayed in the labor ward. This is available at: www.sapienspublishing.com/pph_pdf/PPH_Poster.pdf

(5) Pocket manual of synopsis of PPH. A special leaflet/wall chart, summarizing the immediate action that needs to be taken when PPH occurs. www.sapienspublishing.com/pph_pdf/PPH-Guidelines.pdf

(6) *A Comprehensive Textbook of Postpartum Hemorrhage*, 2nd edition, 2012. This first stand alone textbook describes a comprehensive guide to evaluation, management and surgical intervention of PPH. Available at: www.sapienspublishing.com and also from www.glowm.com

(7) Postpartum hemorrhage issue of *Best Practice & Research Clinical Obstetrics & Gynaecology*[23]

(8) The California Maternal Quality Care Collaborative Obstetric Hemorrhage Expert Task Force was created with the goal of improving readiness, recognition, response and reporting of maternal hemorrhage. In addition, this task force aimed to collect and publish PPH tools that would aid a broad spectrum of birthing units. A compendium of best practice documents for PPH has been

developed and is available on the California Maternal Quality Care Collaborative website, www.cmqcc.org. A PPH 'tool kit' is included which contains a quick reference checklist, table and flow chart for recognition and clinical management. In this system, hemorrhage is categorized from stage 0 (risk assessment and active management of the third stage) to stage 3 (massive transfusion protocol and invasive surgical approaches for control of bleeding). Collaborative efforts such as this, which incorporate simulation and team training with evidence-based protocols, may be critical in reducing hemorrhage-related maternal morbidity and mortality.

COURSES AND WORKSHOPS

A number of workshops to provide PPH training have been developed. These are available as either separate or part of other obstetric emergencies such as Advanced Life Support in Obstetrics (ALSO)[24], Maternal Obstetrics Emergency Trauma (MOET)[25] and PRactical Obstetric MultiProfessional Training (PROMPT) course[26]. The International Training and Workshop for the Management of Massive PPH Group was set up in 2009 in London with the objective to provide hands on training and workshops in the management of PPH. The group is chaired by the senior author and includes experts who are renowned for their expertise in the management of PPH across the world.

The International Training Group has organized and run regular courses in Milton Keynes and South Wales, UK, all of which were very successful. Recently, the group has run a series of study days and workshops in both Cairo and Alexandria with successful feedback response. It seems that this training program and workshop would be beneficial to other developing countries to reduce maternal mortality rate from PPH.

CONCLUSION

Training in the management of PPH should be mandatory for all clinical staff providing maternity care services. Regular 'fire drills' should also be organized to test the local system in real time. These help to identify problems in the system and generate solutions. Repeat drills should be performed to check the efficacy of solutions. Teams that work together should train together, ideally in their local environment. There is also a need for a nationally approved scenario-based team-training program in the management of massive obstetric hemorrhage, involving not only the obstetric staff, but also the anesthetists, theater, recovery and high-dependency teams. Simulators should be put together to give the candidate and trainees the confidence of feeling a real life situation.

Multiple training modalities are used to accomplish knowledge transfer for modern management of PPH. All are necessary, as it is clear that the traditional methods of reading or attending a lecture are insufficient to prepare the trainee for responsible action when it is needed in an emergency situation. Like many other skills in medicine, the training necessary to attend to a patient who has a life threatening hemorrhage cannot be thought of as 'see one, do one and teach one'.

PRACTICE POINTS

- Regular drills and skills training are essential in the management of PPH

- Trainees should be allowed dedicated and protected time for training

- Simulation of obstetric procedures and emergencies can only augment, not replace, the learning that occurs by caring for actual patients

- In-house training is cheap and associated with improved outcomes

- Funding should be available for training to reduce the cost of medical litigation as a result of substandard care

- Team work is essential for proper coordination of the management

- Above all patients and their relatives must be kept fully informed at all stages of management.

References

1. McCall N, ed. The Portrait Collection of Johns Hopkins Medicine: A Catalog of Paintings and Photographs at The Johns Hopkins University School of Medicine and The Johns Hopkins Hospital. Baltimore: The Johns Hopkins University School of Medicine, 1993
2. To WW. Training in emergency obstetric skills: is it evidence-based? Hong Kong Med J 2011;17:141–6
3. Knight M, Callaghan WM, Berg C, et al. Trends in postpartum hemorrhage in high resource countries: a review and recommendations from the international postpartum hemorrhage collaborative group. BMC Pregnancy Childbirth 2009; 9:55
4. Karoshi M, Keith L. Challenges in managing postpartum hemorrhage in resource-poor countries. Clin Obstet Gynecol 2009;52:285–98
5. World Health Organization. Guidelines for the Management of Postpartum Haemorrhage and Retained Placenta. Geneva: World Health Organization, 2009
6. World Health Organization. Addressing the Challenge of Women's Health in Africa. Report of the Commission on Women's Health in the African Region. Brazzaville, Republic of Congo: WHO, 2011
7. International Federation of Obstetrics and Gynaecology. International Confederation of Midwives. International Joint Policy Statement. FIGO/ICM global initiative to prevent post-partum hemorrhage. J Obstet Gynaecol Can 2004;26: 1100–2
8. Confidential Enquiry into Maternal and Child Health (CEMACH). Why Mothers Die: Report on Confidential Enquiries into Maternal Deaths in the United Kingdom 2002–2004 Triennial Report. London: RCOG Press, 2004: 94–103
9. Confidential Enquiry into Maternal and Child Health. Saving Mothers' Lives. The Seventh Report of the Confidential

Enquiries into Maternal Deaths in the United Kingdom, 2005–2007 Triennial Report. London: RCOG, 2007:78–85

10. Cantwell R, Clutton-Brock T, Cooper G, et al. Saving Mothers' Lives: reviewing maternal deaths to make motherhood safer: 2006–08. The Eighth Report on Confidential Enquiries into Maternal Deaths in the United Kingdom. BJOG 2011;118 (Suppl. 1):71–776

11. Ghaem-Maghami S, Brockbank E, Bridges J. Survey of surgical experience during training in obstetrics and gynaecology in the UK. J Obstet Gynaecol 2006;26:297–301

12. Lennox C, Marr L. Scottish Confidential Audit of Severe Maternal Morbidity 2008: 6th Annual Report. Edinburgh: NHS Quality Improvement Scotland, 2010

13. Kayem G, Kurinczuk JJ, Zarko A, et al. Obstetric Surveillance System (UKOSS), uterine compression sutures for the management of severe postpartum hemorrhage. Obstet Gynecol 2011;117:14–20

14. Gardner R, Raemer DB. Simulation in obstetrics and gynaecology. Obstet Gynecol Clin North Am 2008;35:97–127

15. Fuchs KM, Miller RS, Berkowitz RL. Optimizing outcomes through protocols, multidisciplinary drills, and simulation, Semin Perinatol 2009;33:104–8

16. Clark EA, Fisher JR, Arafeh J, Druzin M. Team training/simulation. Clin Obstet Gynecol 2010;53:265–77

17. Andreatta PB; Bullough AS, Marzano D. simulation and team training, clinical obstetrics and gynecology. Clin Obstet Gynecol 2010;53:532–44

18. Skupski DW, Lowenwirt IP, Weinbaum FI, et al. Improving hospital systems for the care of women with major obstetric hemorrhage. Obstet Gynecol 2006;107:977–83

19. Rizvi F, Mackey R, Barrett T, McKenna P, Geary M. Successful reduction of massive postpartum haemorrhage by use of guidelines and staff education. BJOG 2004;111:495–8

20. Merién AE, Van de Ven BW. Multidisciplinary team training in a simulation setting for acute obstetric emergencies: a systematic review. Obstet Gynecol 2010;115:1021–31

21. Ennen CS, Satin AJ. Training and assessment in obstetrics: the role of simulation. Best Pract Res Clin Obstet Gynaecol, 2010;24:747–58

22. Deering SH, Chinn M, Hoddor J, et al. The use of a postpartum simulator for instruction and evaluation of residents. J Grad Med Educ 2009;1:260–3

23. Alfirevic Z, ed. Postpartum haemorrhage. Best Pract Res Clin Obstet Gynaecol 2010;22:997–1170

24. Advanced life support in obstetrics (ALSO). http://www.also.org.uk/

25. Maternal Obstetrics Emergency Trauma (MOET). http://www.alsg.org/en/?q=moet

26. PRactical Obstetric MultiProfessional Training (PROMPT). http://www.prompt-course.org/

62

Intensive Care Management after Major Postpartum Hemorrhage

R. Hebballi and M. Chauhan

INTRODUCTION

The admission of obstetric patients to the intensive care unit (ICU) is relatively infrequent. Critically ill patients who have sustained postpartum hemorrhage (PPH) are more likely to be sent for after care which involves continuation of resuscitation measures, repetitive and intensive monitoring, and appropriate organ support. Management of this subgroup of obstetric patients must take into account normal physiological changes that occur during pregnancy, the aim being to ensure adequate oxygen delivery and tissue perfusion.

ADMISSION TO INTENSIVE CARE UNIT

Patients should be admitted to ICU before their condition reaches a point from which recovery is impossible. The early detection of the severe physiological changes which may occur in patients with PPH remains a challenge because of the relative rarity of such events and the normal changes in physiology associated with pregnancy and childbirth. The early warning score (EWS)[1] is a tool for bedside evaluation based on physiological parameters. The modified early obstetric warning score (MEOWS) (of the type described in Chapter 10) is another specific tool for bedside evaluation of the obstetric patient based on physiological parameters. The routine use of such charts in patients with PPH assists the prompt and appropriate recognition of the acutely ill woman requiring urgent medical review, thereby preventing further deterioration which can be catastrophic. Patients who trigger a specific score on the MEOWS chart should be referred to intensive care outreach team and intensive care team. The use of MEOWS was recommended in the CEMACH report *Saving Mothers' Lives* (2007)[2]. This is also supported by National Institute for Health and Clinical Excellence (NICE) guidelines for the acutely ill patient[3] and the National Patient Safety Agency (NPSA)[4]. In the ward if there is any concern about the patient's condition, she is admitted to ICU for appropriate organ support. If PPH is diagnosed in the operating theater, then the patient is kept asleep (if already intubated), ventilated and admitted to ICU.

MANAGEMENT

An initial assessment of the patient's condition is made and resuscitation is begun in the labor ward or operating room when the diagnosis of PPH is made. The approach to such an acutely unwell patient is immediate management of airway, breathing and circulation (ABC) with a main aim of supporting the patient's vital functions. At some time after the initial resuscitative and therapeutic efforts have taken place, when the patient is considered to be in a stable or relatively stable condition, the patient is transferred to the ICU with its appropriately trained staff, high intensity nursing and prolonged monitoring capability. These factors act together to prevent further deterioration.

Airway management

The airway is most easily maintained with the patient in the left lateral (recovery) position, thus allowing the tongue, soft palate and any oropharyngeal fluid to move away from the laryngeal inlet. In the supine position, the patent airway is maintained with the head tilt and jaw thrust maneuver. Airway adjuncts such as the oropharyngeal (Guedel) airway also can be used. Any fluid, including vomitus, from the oropharynx must be suctioned. Endotracheal intubation may be indicated to provide airway protection and to institute mechanical ventilation and oxygenation. Rapid sequence induction (RSI) with application of cricoid pressure is necessary to avoid gastroesophageal reflux and aspiration.

Breathing management

Respiratory efforts are assessed for signs of hypoxia by inspecting the patient's color especially around lips, tongue and hands. A dusky, bluish hue may suggest hypoxia. The chest is examined for adequate air entry. Tachypnea may indicate hypovolemia, hypoxia, acidosis or pain. Pulse oximetry is a useful non-invasive method of monitoring the patient's oxygenation. Supplementary high flow oxygen up to 10–15 l/min should be administered to seriously ill patients. Patients may not require mechanical ventilation, but those who do require that their ventilation need be identified as early as possible before they deteriorate further.

Invasive ventilation

Mechanical ventilation is instituted via endotracheal tube when the patient's spontaneous ventilation is inadequate or there is imminent respiratory failure leading to poor gas exchange in the lungs. The underlying condition for respiratory failure (PPH and its complications) should be corrected while the patient is ventilated. Once the underlying condition is treated and the patient is able to support her own ventilation and oxygenation, the ventilatory support is gradually withdrawn (weaning).

Non-invasive ventilation

Non-invasive ventilation (NIV) refers to the provision of ventilatory support through the patient's upper airway using a mask or similar device[5]. Application of non-invasive positive airway pressure may be helpful in some selected patients by both preventing atelectasis and improving oxygenation.

Circulatory management

Acute and continued blood loss leads to hypovolemic shock. The onset of shock is usually secondary to hypovolemia and represents a failure of tissue perfusion. The body responds to an acute hemorrhage by activating various physiological systems. The cardiovascular system responds with tachycardia and compensatory vasoconstriction. In such circumstances, an initially normal blood pressure does not exclude shock, as the blood pressure may be maintained because of vasoconstriction.

The principles of management are to aim for normal tissue oxygen delivery. This is done by adjusting the preload, increasing cardiac contractility and optimizing systemic vascular resistance. The preload is adjusted first to ensure an adequate circulating volume with fluids and then, if necessary, vasoactive drugs are commenced. Increasing the hemoglobin with blood transfusion and good oxygenation optimizes the oxygen content of the blood. The treatment should be aggressive and directed by the response to therapy.

Fluids and bloods

Initially fluids should be infused to compensate for blood loss. However, adequate blood transfusion therapy must be instituted sooner rather than later as discussed elsewhere in this book (see Chapter 4).

Electrolytes

Serum electrolytes such as sodium, potassium, magnesium, calcium and phosphate play important roles in cellular metabolism and regulation of cellular membrane potentials. These should be regularly measured and corrected accordingly.

Monitoring

Physical examination will show the signs and symptoms of hypovolemic shock. Apart from continuous electrocardiogram (ECG), pulse oximetry saturation (SpO_2) and non-invasive blood pressure monitoring, the invasive monitoring should be instituted as soon as possible to guide the therapy.

Invasive blood pressure

Non-invasive blood pressure measurements may not be reliable because of factors such as shock and/or patient restlessness. Arterial cannulation is required for monitoring arterial pressure, arterial blood gas analysis and for frequent blood sampling.

Central venous pressure

A central venous pressure line should be secured at the earliest opportunity and used to guide volume replacement and infusion of vasoactive drugs.

Cardiac output

The measurement of cardiac output constitutes a vital part in the management of critically ill patients. Invasive methods such as the thermodilution technique using a pulmonary artery (Swan-Ganz) catheter are the clinical standard[6]. Despite this, minimally invasive techniques are gaining popularity, as they allow continuous cardiac output monitoring while avoiding the risks associated with invasive procedures[7]. In addition, minimally invasive hemodynamic monitoring provides easier, quicker, cheaper, safer, continuous, on-line, real-time display of the hemodynamics of acutely ill patients compared with invasive monitoring[8]. The minimally invasive cardiac output measurement techniques include esophageal Doppler, arterial pulse contour analysis (LiDCO plus) and thoracic bioimpedance.

Esophageal Doppler The esophageal Doppler technique is based on measurement of blood flow velocity in the descending aorta by means of a Doppler transducer (4 MHz continuous or 5 MHz pulsed wave). In a mechanically ventilated patient, the probe is introduced orally and advanced gently until the tip is located at approximately the mid-thoracic level; it is then rotated so that the transducer faces the aorta and a characteristic aortic velocity signal is obtained. When combined with aortic cross-sectional area, this allows hemodynamic variables including stroke volume and cardiac output to be obtained from interpretation of the size and shape of the waveform (Figures 1 and 2). Probe position is optimized by slow rotation in the long axis and alteration of the depth of insertion to generate a clear signal with the highest possible peak velocity. Gain setting is adjusted to obtain the best outline of the aortic velocity waveform.

The esophageal Doppler cardiac output monitor has undergone significant technological advancement and clinical evaluation[9]. There is good correlation between measures of cardiac output made simultaneously with the esophageal Doppler monitor and conventional thermodilution. Esophageal Doppler ultrasonography has been used for intravascular volume optimization in both the perioperative period and the critical care setting. Its use in cardiac, general and orthopedic surgery has been associated with a reduction in morbidity and hospital stay[10–12].

Arterial pulse contour analysis Arterial pulse contour analysis (PiCCO and LiDCO plus) estimates the left ventricular stroke volume and therefore cardiac output from arterial pulse pressure waveform on a beat to beat basis. This may have advantages over the existing technologies, as the majority of critically ill patients already have the arterial pressure traces transduced, making this technique minimally invasive and providing the ability to monitor changes in stroke volume and cardiac output[13].

The LiDCO plus is based on the lithium bolus indicator dilution method of measuring cardiac output. A small dose of lithium chloride is injected via a central or peripheral venous line; the resulting arterial lithium concentration–time curve is recorded by withdrawing blood past a lithium sensor attached to the patient's existing arterial line. This value is then used to calibrate the LiDCO as well as to give continuous cardiac output and derived variables from arterial waveform analysis. This facilitates patient management by allowing assessment of the immediate response to a fluid challenge, drugs or other therapeutic interventions. In terms of accuracy, clinical studies over a wide range of cardiac outputs demonstrate that the LiDCO method is at least as accurate as thermodilution even in patients with varying cardiac outputs[14]. Having said this, several factors affect the accuracy of cardiac output measurements based on the analysis of arterial waveforms, including damped waveforms and inadequate pulse detection (e.g. severe arrhythmias, catheter dislodgement)[15].

Inotropes and vasopressors

Pharmacologic agents that increase the blood pressure by increasing cardiac contractility are called inotropes, and agents that increase blood pressure by arteriole vasoconstriction are called vasopressors. This group of drugs is useful for resuscitation of seriously ill patients. Inotropes include the catecholamines or phosphodiesterase inhibitors. The catecholamines increase intracellular cAMP levels via adenylate cyclase stimulation; cAMP increases intracellular calcium ion mobilization and force of contraction[16].

These drugs all act directly or indirectly on the sympathetic nervous system, but the effect of each drug varies depending on the sympathetic receptor (Table 1) for which the drug possesses greatest affinity. Direct acting drugs act by stimulating the sympathetic nervous system receptors, whereas indirect acting drugs cause the release of noradrenaline from the receptor which then produces the effect. Some drugs have a mixed effect. Commonly used inotropes

(dopamine, dobutamine and adrenaline) and vasopressors (phenylephrine, noradrenaline and vasopressin) are shown in Table 2.

Dopamine Dopamine acts on D1, D2, β1 and α1 receptors, in a dose dependent manner. At low doses, dopamine causes dopamine receptor (D1, D2) mediated renal and mesenteric vasodilatation and results in diuresis. At an intermediate dose, dopamine increases

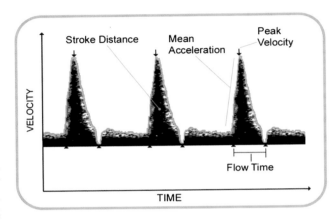

Figure 1 Interpretation of aortic Doppler waveform changes. Image reproduced with kind permission of Deltex Medical© 2012

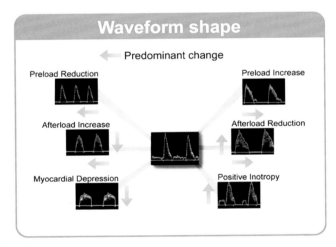

Figure 2 Predictable changes in the shape of the esophageal Doppler waveform occur during changes in the hemodynamic state of an individual. The most common abnormality seen during targeted fluid administration is hypovolemia, which is represented by the narrow triangular waveform 'preload reduction'. Image reproduced with kind permission of Deltex Medical© 2012

Table 1 Noradrenergic receptors and main actions of each receptor subtypes

Receptor	Action
α1	Peripheral arterial vasoconstriction, increases systemic vascular resistance
β1	Increased heart rate, increased atrioventricular conduction velocity, increased ventricular contractility
β2	Vasodilation in skeletal muscle, brochodilatation
DA	Increased renal blood flow

DA, dopaminergic receptors

Table 2 Commonly used inotropes and vasopressors

Drug	Dose range	α1	β1	β2	Other	Major side-effects
Dopamine	2.0–20 μg/kg/min	++	+		DA +++	Ventricular arrhythmias
Dobutamine	2.0–20 μg/kg/min		+++	++	0	Peripheral vasodilator, tachycardia at higher doses
Adrenaline (epinephrine)	0.01–0.1 μg/kg/min	+++	+++	++	0	Ventricular arrhythmias, severe hypertension
Phenylephrine	100 μg/ml at a rate of 30 ml/h	+++			0	Bradycardia, peripheral ischemia
Noradrenaline (norepinephrine)	0.01–3 μg/kg/min	+++	++	+	0	Bradycardia, peripheral ischemia
Vasopressin	0.01–0.1 U/min				V1 +++	Severe peripheral ischemia

DA, dopamine receptors

cardiac output via the β1 receptor. At higher doses, this agent leads to α1 receptor mediated vasoconstriction.

Dobutamine Dobutamine is mainly a β1 receptor agonist with weak β2 receptor agonist properties. It is a potent inotrope with a weaker chronotropic and peripheral vasodilatory effect.

Adrenaline (epinephrine) Adrenaline is a potent β receptor agonist which also has α receptor agonist activity. Adrenaline is useful during resuscitation and maintaining cardiac output during initial stages; however, tachycardia, increased myocardial oxygen demand and arrhythmias are limiting factors in its use.

Phenylephrine Phenylephrine has potent α receptor agonist activity, but virtually no affinity for the β receptor. Phenylephrine is given as a bolus or infusion to increase the mean arterial pressure in the presence of peripheral vasodilatation. It is started as an infusion of 100 μg/ml at a rate of 30 ml/h, but is titrated to keep the blood pressure within 20% of the patient's baseline for as long as it is needed.

Noradrenaline (norephenephrine) Noradrenaline is a potent α1 receptor agonist with some β1 receptor activity leading to potent vasoconstriction, raised blood pressure and compensatory bradycardia. Myocardial oxygen demand is increased markedly after its administration.

Vasopressin Vasopressin or antidiuretic hormone (ADH) has a potent vasoconstriction effect through V1 receptors in the vascular smooth muscle; it causes water retention by the kidney via increased adenylate cyclase activity and cAMP levels. Pressor effects of vasopressin are relatively well-preserved during hypoxic and acidotic conditions, which commonly develop during shock of any origin.

Neurological management

Rapid assessment of global neurological function is achieved using the Glasgow coma scale (GCS). The original GCS[17] has been modified with a maximum score of 15. It is an objective, reliable and accepted

Table 3 The modified Glasgow coma scale (GCS)

	Score
Eye opening response (E)	
Spontaneously	4
To speech	3
To pain	2
None	1
Best verbal response (V)	
Oriented	5
Confused	4
Inappropriate speech	3
Incomprehensible speech	2
None	1
Best motor response (M)	
Obeys command	6
Localizes to painful stimulus	5
Withdrawal to painful stimulus	4
Abnormal flexion to painful stimulus	3
Extension to painful stimulus	2
None	1
Total	15

way of assessing global neurological function. Modification was achieved by adding three components, namely the eye opening response (E, with a maximum score of 4), best verbal response (V, with a maximum score of 5) and best motor response (M, with a maximum score of 6) as shown in Table 3. Although the modified GCS was initially used to assess consciousness level after head trauma, it is a relatively simple and easy to follow neurological assessment tool for most patients, including those who have sustained catastrophic PPH.

Thus GCS = E + V + M

GCS = 15, fully alert and conscious
GCS = 13–14, mild state of unconsciousness
GCS = 9–12, moderate state of unconsciousness
GCS = 3–8, deep state of unconsciousness. The patient needs tracheal intubation and ventilation

Renal management

Acute renal failure (ARF) presenting as oliguria or anurea is one of the commonest complications of acute hypovolemic shock and PPH. Hypovolemia leads to reduced glomerular perfusion, acute tubular necrosis and ultimately renal failure. Patients with pregnancy induced hypertension are more susceptible to ARF following PPH because of decreased intravascular volume and increased vascular response to catecholamines[18,19].

The urinary bladder must be catheterized in all patients with PPH. Hourly recording of urine output provides an early indication of ARF. Management should be aimed at maintaining adequate intravascular volume, supportive care and avoiding nephrotoxic drugs like non-steroidal anti-inflammatory drugs (NSAIDs). Prompt recognition, aggressive resuscitation and intervention may prevent ARF. Traditionally low dose dopamine infusion has been shown to increase renal blood flow; however, current evidence suggests that this does not affect the clinical outcome.

Renal replacement therapy (RRT) in the form of peritoneal dialysis (PD), continuous venovenous hemofiltration (CVVH) or continuous venovenous hemodifiltration (CVVHDF) may be indicated if there is established ARF, not responding to volume replacement and diuretics (Table 4).

Gastrointestinal management

Protein energy malnutrition is a major problem in severely ill hypercatabolic patients in the ICU[21]. Early initiation of enteral nutrition is beneficial, with significant positive effects on septic complications, and improved outcome compared with parenteral nutrition. Enteral nutrition guarantees the preservation of gut mass and prevents increased gut permeability to bacteria and toxins[22].

Hematological management

Blood products and hematological management are discussed in various other chapters of this book (see Chapter 4–6).

Sepsis management

Sepsis is a leading cause of death in critically ill patients despite the aggressive management and use of specific antibiotics. The septic response is an extremely complex chain of events involving both inflammatory and anti-inflammatory processes[23]. Early diagnosis and stratification of the severity of sepsis is very important, thereby increasing the possibility of starting timely and specific treatment[24].

Table 4 Indications for renal replacement therapy in ICU (adapted from Ronco et al.[20])

Oliguria (urine output <0.5 ml/kg/h)
Uncompensated metabolic acidosis (pH <7.1)
Blood urea >30 mmol/l (84 mg/dl)
Serum creatinine >300 μmol/l (3.4 mg/dl)
Serum potassium >6.5 mmol/l or rapidly rising

The Surviving Sepsis Campaign (SSC)[25] is a high profile initiative of the European Society of Intensive Care Medicine, the International Sepsis Forum and the Society of Critical Care Medicine. It was proposed to improve the management, diagnosis and treatment of sepsis. The SSC aims to reduce mortality from sepsis via a multipoint strategy, primarily by:

- Building awareness of sepsis
- Improving diagnosis
- Increasing the use of appropriate treatment
- Educating health-care professionals
- Improving post-ICU care
- Developing guidelines of care
- Facilitating data collection for the purposes of audit and feedback.

Pain relief and sedation

Critical illness can be a frightening experience for the awake and alert patient, and adequate sedation may reduce this. The ideal sedative agent should have minimal cardiovascular effect with rapid onset and offset actions. Commonly used sedatives include benzodiazepines in the form of a midazolam infusion. Midazolam has three metabolites; one of these (1-hydroxymidazolam) can accumulate in the critically ill. The normal elimination half-life is 2 hours, but can be as long as a few days in the long-term sedated, critically ill individual. Shorter acting drugs like propofol infusion can also be used with caution, because it can cause cardiovascular depression in the hypovolemic and septic patient.

Pain is common and may be worsened by invasive and unpleasant procedures that can lead to respiratory and cardiac complications as a result of increased sympathetic activity. Assessment of pain is a vital element in effective pain management. Opioids are the mainstay of treatment and possess sedative, hypnotic effects besides their obvious analgesic effects. They work at the level of the opioid receptors. Morphine sulfate is the most commonly used opioid. Morphine is metabolized primarily in the liver into two main products, morphine-3-glucuronide and morphine-6-glucuronide. Both are excreted renally and accumulate in circumstances of renal dysfunction. Other short acting opioids such as fentanyl or alfentanil infusions can also be used.

Balanced analgesia (multimodal approach) is the method of choice for moderate pain control wherever possible by using other analgesic techniques such as paracetamol, NSAIDs and regional techniques (e.g. epidural infusions for postoperative patients).

General management

General management includes deep vein thrombosis (DVT) prophylaxis, stress ulcer prevention,

prevention of nosocomial pneumonia, line sepsis care and skin care to prevent decubitus ulcerations.

Care bundle

The 'care bundle' is a relatively new concept in intensive care practice. It appears that when several evidence based interventions are grouped together in a single protocol, they result in substantially greater improvement in patient outcome. This concept was developed in the USA by Berenholtz and Pronovost *et al.*[26,27] to eliminate catheter related blood stream infections in the ICU. The care bundle is being promoted by National Health Service Modernisation Agency in UK[28] as it provides a method for establishing best evidence based clinical practice (Table 5).

Various care bundles have been developed all of which can be grouped together under ventilator care bundle. FAST HUG is a mnemonic proposed 5 years ago by Jean-Louis Vincent[29] as a way of assisting health-care workers looking after critically ill patients. The FAST HUG mnemonic has seven basic components (Table 6) that should be considered for every intensive care patient at least once a day: feeding, analgesia, sedation, thromboembolic prophylaxis, head-of-bed elevation, stress ulcer prevention and glucose control. Although all of these elements may not require action as to particular patients each day, it is suggested that considering each of these elements will minimize mistakes, reduce complications and improve positive outcomes and quality of life for ICU patients.

Whenever possible and, if appropriate, the mother should be informed about the baby's health and progress. It is important not to forget that the intensive care patient is not just a series of diseased organs, but a human being with physical, psychological and spiritual needs. Intensive care admission is a stressful event for the patient and her family, and patients recovering from critical illness are at risk of developing post-traumatic stress disorder (PTSD). The provision of an ICU diary is associated with a reduction in the incidence of new-onset PTSD[30]. While the patient is in ICU, the health-care staff and family write about the daily progress of the patient along with photographs in a diary. This diary explains what happened to the patient in the ICU, thus helping fill in significant gaps they have in their memories and putting any delusional memories into context. These efforts aid psychological recovery.

Discharge and follow-up

Once discharged from the ICU, MEOWS charts can be continued in these patients when they return to a step-down unit at which time the intensive care outreach team should provide follow-up on the ward. The intensive care outreach team is a multidisciplinary team comprising senior nurses with a background in intensive care and intensivists. The team works closely with the ICUs. The primary aim is to ensure that these patients receive appropriate and timely treatment after their discharge from the ICU and prevent any readmission.

SUMMARY

The care of the acutely ill PPH patient in the critical care unit is challenging and often requires a multidisciplinary approach. Early recognition and prompt treatment of such patients can help prevent irreversible organ dysfunction.

PRACTICE POINTS

- Management of the PPH patient in the ICU should take into account the normal physiological changes during pregnancy.

- The main aim is to support the patient's vital functions, ensure adequate oxygen delivery and tissue perfusion, thus preventing irreversible organ dysfunction.

- The 'FAST HUG' approach should be considered for every intensive care patient at least once a day.

- Sepsis is a leading cause of death in critically ill patients despite the aggressive management and use of specific antibiotics. The early diagnosis and stratification of the severity of sepsis is important.

Table 5 Central line care bundle[27]

Hand hygiene
Maximum barrier precautions
Chlorhexidine skin antisepsis
Optimal catheter site selection
Daily review of line necessity and prompt removal

Table 6 The seven components of the FAST HUG approach. Reproduced from Vincent, 2005[29], with permission

Component	Consideration for intensive care unit (ICU) team
Feeding	Can the patient be fed orally, if not enterally? If not, should we start parenteral feeding?
Analgesia	The patient should not suffer pain, but excessive analgesia should be avoided
Sedation	The patient should not experience discomfort, but excessive sedation should be avoided; 'calm, comfortable, collaborative'
Thromboembolic prevention	Should we give low-molecular-weight heparin or use mechanical adjuncts?
Head of the bed elevated	Optimally, 30–45°, unless contraindications (e.g. threatened cerebral perfusion pressure)
Stress **U**lcer prophylaxis	Usually H2 antagonists; sometimes proton pump inhibitors
Glucose control	Within limits defined in each ICU

References

1. Morgan RJM, Williams F, Wright MM. An Early Warning Scoring System for detecting developing critical illness. Clin Intensive Care 1997;8:100
2. Confidential Enquiry into Maternal and Child Health (CEMACH). Saving Mothers' Lives. London, UK: Royal College of Obstetricians and Gynaecologists, 2007

3. National Institute for Health and Clinical Excellence (NICE). Clinical guideline 50. Acutely Ill Patients in Hospital: Recognition of And Response to Acute Illness in Adults in Hospital. NICE, 2007 www.nice.org.uk/nicemedia/pdf/CG50FullGuidance.pdf

4. National Patient Safety Agency (NPSA). Recognising and Responding Appropriately to Early Signs of Deterioration in Hospitalised Patients. National Patient Safety Agency, 2007 www.npsa.nhs.uk/search/?q=recognising+and+responding+appropriately

5. British Thoracic Society Standards of Care Committee. Non-invasive ventilation in acute respiratory failure. Thorax 2002;57:192–211

6. Hofer CK, Ganter MT, Zollinger A. What technique should I use to measure cardiac output? Curr Opin Crit Care 2007; 13:308–17

7. Harvey S, Stevens K, Harrison D, et al. An evaluation of the clinical and cost effectiveness of pulmonary artery catheters in patient management in intensive care: a systematic review and a randomized controlled trial. Health Technol Assess 2006; 10:1–152

8. Shoemaker WC, Belzberg H, Wo CC, et al. Multicentre study of non-invasive monitoring systems as alternatives to invasive monitoring of acutely ill emergency patients. Chest 1998;114:1643–52

9. NHS Purchasing and Supply Agency. Evidence Review: Oesophageal Doppler monitoring in patients undergoing high-risk surgery and in Critically Ill Patients. CEP 08012. NHS Purchasing and Supply Agency 2008 www.deltexmedical.com/downloads/CEPreport.pdf

10. Dark PM, Singer M. The validity of trans-oesophageal Doppler ultrasonography as a measure of cardiac output in critically ill adults. Intensive Care Med 2004;30:2060–6

11. Mowatt G, Houston G, Hernández R, et al. Systemic review of the clinical effectiveness and cost effectiveness of oesophageal Doppler monitoring in critically ill and high-risk surgical patients. Health Technol Assess 2009;13:1–118

12. Pearse R, Dawson D, Fawcett J, et al, Early goal-directed therapy after major surgery reduces complications and duration of hospital stay. A randomised, controlled trial. Crit Care 2005;9:R687–93

13. Rhodes A, Sunderland R. Arterial pulse power analysis: the LiDCOplus system. In: Pinsky MR, Payen D, eds. Functional Hemodynamic Monitoring. Update in intensive care and emergency medicine 42. Berlin: Springer–Verlag, 2005: 183–192

14. Pittman J, Bar Yosef S, SumPing J, Sherwood M, Mark J. Continuous cardiac output monitoring with pulse contour analysis: A comparison with lithium indicator dilution cardiac output measurement. Crit Care Med 2005;33:2015–21

15. Van Lieshout JJ, Wesseling KH. Continuous cardiac output by pulse contour analysis? Br J Anaesth 2001;86:467

16. Overgaard CB, Dzavik V. Inotropes and vasopressors, review of physiology and clinical use in cardiovascular disease. Circulation 2008;118:1047–56

17. Teasdale G, Jennett B. Assessment of coma and impaired consciousness. A practical scale. Lancet 1974;2:81–4

18. Grunfeld JP, Ganeval D, Bournerias F. Acute renal failure in pregnancy. Kidney Int 1980:18:179–91

19. Sibai BM, Villar MA, Mabie BC. Acute renal failure in hypertensive disorders of pregnancy. Pregnancy outcome and remote prognosis in thirty one consecutive cases. Am J Obstet Gynecol 1990;126:777–83

20. Ronco C, Bellomo R, Kellum JA. Critical Care Nephrology, 2nd edn. Philadelphia, PA: WB Saunders, 2009

21. Jolliet P, Pichard C, Biolo G, et al. Enteral nutrition in intensive care patients: a practical approach. Working Group on Nutrition and Metabolism, ESICM. Intensive Care Med 1998;24:848–59

22. Kompan L, Kremzar B, Gadzijev E, Prosek M. Effects of early enteral nutrition on intestinal permeability and the development of multiple organ failure after multiple injuries. Intensive Care Med 1999;25:157–61

23. Hotchkiss RS, Karl IE. The pathophysiology and treatment of sepsis. N Engl J Med 2003;348:138–50

24. Kumar A, Roberts D, Wood KE, et al. Duration of hypotension before initiation of effective antimicrobial therapy is the critical determinant of survival in human septic shock. Crit Care Med 2006;34:1589–96

25. Dellinger RP Carlet JM, Masur H, et al. Surviving Sepsis Campaign Management Guidelines Committee. Surviving Sepsis Campaign guidelines for management of severe sepsis and septic shock. Crit Care Med 2004;32:858–73

26. Berenholtz PB, Dorman T, Ngo K, Provonost PJ. Qualitative review of intensive care unit quality indicators. J Crit Care 2002;17:12–5

27. Berenholtz SM, Pronovost PJ, Lipsett PA, et al. Eliminating catheter-related bloodstream infections in the intensive care unit. Crit Care Med 2004;32:2014–20

28. NHS Modernisation Agency. 10 high impact changes, for service improvement and delivery. London: Department of Health, 2004

29. Vincent JL. Give your patient a fast hug (at least) once a day. Crit Care Med 2005;33:1225–9

30. Jones C, Bäckman C, Capuzzo M, et al. Intensive care diaries reduce new onset post-traumatic stress disorder following critical illness: a randomised, controlled trial. Crit Care 2010; 14:R168

63

Litigation: an International Perspective*

K. J. Dalton

INTRODUCTION

The history of litigation after postpartum hemorrhage spans more than 100 years, but only 34 decided cases have been reported in common law jurisdictions.

The LEXIS database includes reported legal cases from the common law jurisdictions, but it does not include civil law jurisdictions such as those that use Napoleonic law. This history was compiled using the following search terms: [(post-partum OR post-partum) AND (haemorrhage OR hemorrhage)]. First, databases of English, Commonwealth and Irish, US Federal and US States case law were searched. Then full-text or abbreviated-text reports of all potential cases were searched visually for key words to determine the relevance of each for inclusion. Most were discarded as irrelevant, for example: 'retinal hemorrhage in the postpartum period'; after this only 34 relevant cases remained. It is possible that some cases from lower courts may have been missed, as no straightforward method exists to retrieve all such cases across all the jurisdictions studied.

FIRST MATERNAL DEATH LITIGATED (1905)

Half (17) of 34 (i.e. 50%) of the litigated cases involved a maternal death. The first of these occurred in the US. On 27 February 1905, Florence Westrup delivered her first child at home outside Newport, Kentucky. She had *'a great aversion to physicians'*, and planned a natural home birth. The birth of the child (at term) went well, but she began to hemorrhage. Despite her protests, her husband called the family physician. He arrived, examined her, and found a retained placenta. He went home to fetch his bag of instruments and returned, but by this time Florence Westrup was dead. The local police charged the husband with involuntary manslaughter, and this was said to have been committed:

'by wilfully neglecting to furnish his wife . . . with such care and attention as were necessary during her confinement in childbirth, thereby causing her death'.

He was tried in Campbell Circuit Court, found guilty and sentenced to 8 months imprisonment. He appealed this decision to the Kentucky Court of Appeals, which expressed its own view of the matter[1]:

'Those of us who reverence the medical profession and implicitly trust the learning and skill of the family physician . . . [take the view that] . . . postpartum hemorrhage is nearly always fatal [and that] . . . the trial judge should have peremptorily instructed the jury to find appellant not guilty'.

Nowadays courts are rarely so deferential to the medical profession or to physicians and, as is shown in numerous other chapters of this book, fatality is less likely if physicians are present and well prepared to treat hemorrhage.

UNLAWFUL PRACTICE OF MEDICINE (1907)

In 1907, Hannah Porn, a diplomate of the Chicago Midwife Institute and a practising midwife of many years experience, was charged with practising medicine unlawfully. Among the reasons cited was the fact that she had used *'formulae'* for treating uterine inertia and postpartum hemorrhage, and also used obstetrical forceps for delivery. These were *'acts confessedly performed by the defendant'* but she did so only rarely, and *'never, if a physician could be called in time'*. Nevertheless, she was convicted, and on appeal the Supreme Court of Massachusetts upheld her conviction on the grounds that:[2]

'The maintenance of a high standard of professional qualifications for physicians is of vital concern to the public health.'

Here, the Kentucky deference to physicians was not afforded to a midwife.

DANGEROUS SIDEWALK (1908)

The second maternal death case was heard in 1908. Mollie Short, the wife of an East St Louis physician, was 36 weeks pregnant. Out shopping on the evening of 17 November 1906, she walked along a wooden sidewalk situated 6 feet above the ground (i.e. a boardwalk). This had been damaged in the cyclone of 1896, but had not been properly repaired. Her left leg slipped down a hole, she dislocated her hip, and

*Reprinted from first edition.

subsequently went into preterm labor. Although the baby survived, she suffered a postpartum hemorrhage from which she died. Her husband sued the city authority for having a dangerous sidewalk, and was awarded damages of $5700. He successfully argued that postpartum hemorrhage was a direct consequence of the preterm labor, which would not have happened had not the sidewalk been dangerous. On appeal, the trial court's verdict was affirmed[3].

TELEPHONE PROBLEM (1909)

At 3 am on an October morning in 1909 in Georgia, Mrs Glawson started bleeding in a pregnancy of unknown gestational age. Her husband telephoned the local physician who was situated 7 miles away. He advised that certain remedies be applied, but these did not ameliorate the situation. The husband repeatedly tried to make telephonic contact again with the physician, but the telephone operator did not answer for over 2 hours. Eventually, connection was re-established with the physician who set off to visit the home immediately. By the time he arrived, Mrs Glawson had miscarried, had a *'postpartum hemorrhage'*, and died. The husband sued the telephone company for gross negligence in not answering his telephone call for 2 hours. His lawyer argued that *'but for this negligence the physician could and would have reached the plaintiff's house in time to save the life of his wife'*. He won his case, and he was awarded $5000 in compensation. The telephone company appealed the decision to the Court of Appeals of Georgia, but their appeal failed[4]. The court held that generally failure of equipment in the telephone exchange would not be negligent, but in this case there was a failure of diligence on the part of the telephone operator in that he did not notice the incoming call.

ROAD TRAFFIC ACCIDENT (1930)

More than 20 years were to pass after the case of Mrs Glawson in 1909 before another postpartum hemorrhage case reached the courts and was reported. This was to be the first road traffic accident in pregnancy that was litigated.

In 1930, only 2 days after Mrs Peterson conceived her second pregnancy, she was involved in a road traffic accident near St Paul, Minnesota. The automobile in which she was travelling overturned. It was said to have been going too fast, but the driver claimed that a tire blew out. By the end of pregnancy, it was recognized that she had a central placenta previa, in which the maternal mortality was known to be *'very high'*. Her doctor consulted with another expert. Rather than carrying out the then relatively rare operation of cesarean section, it was advised that she should be delivered vaginally. Her doctor used what was termed the *'Vorhees bag method'*, and he broke through her placenta by the vaginal route. The child died, the mother had a postpartum hemorrhage and she died too. The driver of the car in which she had been

sitting 9 months previously was sued for negligence. In court, expert medical evidence said the road accident had caused the placenta to be situated in a previa position, and this directly led to the mother's postpartum hemorrhage and death. This evidence did not convince the jury, however, who found in favor of the driver. An appeal to the Supreme Court of Minnesota failed[5].

IATROGENIC OBSTETRIC INJURY (1955)

Occasionally, maternal death has occurred as a result of unusual management of labor. In 1955, Bette Goff had her labor induced by means of pituitrin. During the labor, her doctor diagnosed a constrictive band of cervical muscle, and he incised it just left of the 12 o'clock position. She delivered vaginally, but the cervical incision was not repaired. She had a postpartum hemorrhage over the course of the next few hours, but the two attendant nurses did not recall the doctor until it was too late, and the patient died of blood loss. The family took legal action against the doctor and the hospital as it was vicariously liable for the nurses' omissions. For legal reasons, the case went to retrial[6]. Negligence on the part of the doctor was admitted. As for the nurses, this was evidenced from the records. There was no later report on this case, so presumably it settled.

HEALTH INSURANCE (1956)

Postpartum hemorrhage has occasionally been at issue in insurance matters. The earliest reported case was that of Juanita Whitten in 1956. Her health insurance policy covered hospitalization for any complication of pregnancy. She had had seven pregnancies: two miscarried with severe bleeding, and she had a severe postpartum hemorrhage following the delivery of her last child, after which she was sterilized. Her gynecologist said the sterilization operation was undertaken to prevent further postpartum hemorrhage, a complication of pregnancy that was covered by her insurance policy. However, her insurance company and the Court of Appeals of Alabama disallowed her reimbursement claim, on the grounds that her policy covered only actual complications, and not potential complications that might or might not occur in the future[7].

TRANSFUSION OF THE WRONG BLOOD (1951, 1955, 1972)

Three cases involved allegations that the wrong blood was transfused.

In 1951, Mrs Madison bled heavily postpartum whilst in San Francisco Hospital, a county hospital and a state governmental institution. Unfortunately, she was given a blood transfusion that had been incorrectly cross-matched, and she died as a result. Her husband sued the City and County of San Francisco, but he lost his case as the court held that the state was immune from suit, in a manner akin to sovereign immunity. The appeal court judges said they were unhappy in delivering this decision, but they were bound to follow the precedent of other cases in which state immunity had been the issue, explaining themselves as follows[8]:

> 'This doctrine of non-liability of the state and its agencies for injuries caused by the negligence of an employee engaged in the discharge of a governmental function originated in the fiction that the king can do no wrong.'

[In English law, the Queen is still regarded as above the law, but her ministers of state (i.e. the government) are not above the law, and often a court will find against them.]

In 1955, Josephine Gillen delivered at the Brooke Army Hospital in Texas. She then had a postpartum hemorrhage and she was given a blood transfusion. Her condition deteriorated, and 2 days later she died of renal failure. The family sued the United States of America, alleging negligent military medical care which included the claim that there had been an incompatible transfusion of rhesus O-positive blood into a rhesus O-negative patient, and that this led to her renal problem. In defence, it was claimed that the patient was in fact rhesus O-positive, and she had been given rhesus O-negative blood, which would have been a group-compatible transfusion. The court found that there had been no incorrect blood transfusion, no renal problem arising from this, and no negligence in the medical care. This finding was affirmed on appeal[9].

More than 15 years passed until the case of Theda Parker in 1972. Her third labor was induced at 38 weeks gestation at her request. The birth went well, but she had a postpartum hemorrhage, and her obstetrician had to perform a hysterectomy. During the course of the operation, she needed a blood transfusion, but unfortunately she was given blood that had been cross-matched for another patient. She survived the ordeal, but in the long term she developed hematuria due to cystitis, and her marriage eventually broke down. In 1976, she and her husband sued her obstetrician for inducing her labor too soon (for convenience rather than for medical reasons) which they said led to the postpartum hemorrhage; and for the transfusion error which they claimed had triggered the events that led to their marital breakdown. On appeal, most of their claims were dismissed, except that she was awarded $20 000 compensation to be paid by the hospital for the negligence of its employee in mixing up the bloods[10].

INFECTION FOLLOWING BLOOD TRANSFUSION (1981, 1982, 1985)

Four cases have been litigated where blood-borne infection occurred following transfusion for postpartum hemorrhage. Three cases involved HIV, and one hepatitis C.

HIV

AIDS was recognized in 1982, and the HIV virus was identified in 1983. Shortly thereafter, HIV infection was first reported as a consequence of postpartum hemorrhage. In 1984, the HIV-ELISA test was first marketed as a kit, and the FDA approved it for sale on 2 March 1985. Only 11 days later, on 13 March, the Belle Bonfils Memorial Blood Center in Denver, Colorado took delivery of its first testing kit, but its staff were not yet trained in its use. On that very same day, Mrs KW was admitted to hospital with a secondary postpartum hemorrhage following an apparently uneventful delivery of her baby son 2 weeks earlier. Her bleeding could not be stopped and so a hysterectomy was carried out. Six units of blood were transfused, none of which were tested for HIV. However, by 1986, donor blood was being routinely tested for HIV, and at this time one of her 1985 donors tested positive. All previous recipients of his blood were tracked and tested, and Mrs KW was found to be HIV-positive. She (and her husband and son) sued Belle Bonfils Memorial Blood Center on the grounds that the Center had not appropriately identified and excluded this donor as 'not a suitable person' to donate non-infected blood. (Specific testing for HIV, *per se*, was not an issue in this case.) Most of the legal arguments in the case revolved around confidentiality issues regarding access to the donor's medical records, and so they are not relevant here. The Supreme Court of Colorado ordered limited disclosure of his medical records[11].

In 1981 Matsuko Gaffney, the wife of a US naval man, was booked to deliver at the Long Beach Naval Hospital in California. Her pregnancy went overdue by 4 weeks *(sic)*, but her cervix was judged unfavorable for induction of labor. She was delivered vaginally, but had a postpartum hemorrhage for which she was transfused two units of blood. Various experts later agreed that, if she had had appropriate fetal monitoring, fetal distress would have been recognized, and she would have been delivered by cesarean section, without intrauterine death, infection, postpartum hemorrhage, and blood transfusion, all of which she did have. In 1983, she delivered her next child, a healthy girl, and then in 1985 she delivered a boy. He proved to be a sickly child and was diagnosed with AIDS, from which he died in 1986. Mrs Gaffney and her husband were tested for HIV and both proved positive. She died of AIDS in 1987. After her death, a 1990 Court heard that one of her units of blood came from *'a donor who had engaged in homosexual activity involving the exchange of bodily fluids'*, although he was never actually tested for HIV. The Court found that, as the United States of America was responsible for the military hospital, it was liable for the unfortunate train of events that befell Mrs Gaffney and her family, even though HIV infection had not been discovered at the time. It held that the United States was negligent in the treatment of Mrs Gaffney, that she needed to be transfused as a direct result of that negligence, and that it was foreseeable in 1981 that a communicable disease could be transmitted through blood transfusion[12].

In contrast to this was the case of Sheri Traxler, who delivered her baby in 1982. Two weeks later, she had a major postpartum hemorrhage, for which she was transfused two units of blood. Hysterectomy was considered, but it proved unnecessary. Eight years later, in 1988, it emerged that one of her blood donors had tested positive for HIV, and now she too tested positive. She sued her 1982 obstetrician on two principal grounds: (1) that he had not removed her placenta completely, and (2) that she had not specifically consented to any blood transfusion. His defence was (1) that retention of placental fragments occurs commonly, and (2) that her written general consent to treatment provided sufficient authority for him give blood as she had lost 30–40% of her blood volume. The lower court held that there had been no negligence at the times of delivery or of the postpartum hemorrhage, and that the risk of HIV infection could not be foreseen. This decision was upheld by the Californian Court of Appeal[13].

Hepatitis C

Blood transfusion following postpartum hemorrhage may cause other blood-borne infections, such as hepatitis C. In 1988, Anita Endean delivered vaginally in British Columbia. She had a postpartum hemorrhage, and she was given a transfusion of packed red cells supplied by the Canadian Red Cross (CRC). After she went home, she had a debilitating flu-like illness. Six years later in 1994, she offered to donate blood, but she now tested positive for hepatitis C. Although its short-term effects are transient, hepatitis C carries a long-term risk of cirrhosis (10% per annum) and in those patients a further risk of hepatocellular carcinoma (5% per annum). The CRC carried out a 'traceback' procedure, and found that one of her 1988 blood donors now tested positive for hepatitis C. (Hepatitis C virus (HCV) was first identified in 1988. An antibody test for HCV was soon developed, but British Columbia did not introduce widespread testing until 1990. Nevertheless, surrogate testing for non-A non-B hepatitis had been widely available in 1988.) She took no legal action against her obstetrician, but sued the CRC who supplied the blood transfused in 1988, on the specific grounds that it had neither tested for HCV nor carried out surrogate testing, and thereby failed to prevent hepatitis C contamination of its blood supplies. She also alleged that the CRC had deliberately destroyed some of her medical records, thus disadvantaging her legal action, i.e. a separate tort known as 'spoliation'. Furthermore, together with many other patients infected with hepatitis C from blood transfusions, she joined a class action, or a mass tort action, against the Canadian Red Cross under British Columbia's Class Proceedings Act 1995. Hers proved to be a unique case of postpartum hemorrhage, as she was to become the 'representative plaintiff', or lead case, in this mass tort action. As her case raised novel legal points that were challenged by the CRC, it fell to the Supreme Court of British Columbia to grant her membership of this class action. Because the final outcome of her legal action was not reported, it is possible that the matter was settled out of court[14].

DELAY IN TRANSFUSING BLOOD (1984, 1988, 2000)

In several cases it was alleged that there was unnecessary delay in giving blood after postpartum hemorrhage.

In 1992, a Saskatchewan court considered the dangers of postpartum hemorrhage in a rural setting. In 1984, Corrine Naeth had delivered her baby uneventfully in Hospital A, but her uterus inverted when 'controlled cord traction' was used to deliver the placenta. Before replacing the uterus, the delivering doctor tried to peel the placenta off the inverted uterus, but the placenta was adherent (placenta accreta). Massive hemorrhage ensued, but there was no blood transfusion facility in the hospital. She was then transferred by ambulance to Hospital B, a traveling distance of 90 min, rather than to Hospital C, a traveling distance of only 30 min, but which only had facilities for uncross-matched blood transfusion. During transfer to Hospital B, she lost consciousness in the ambulance, and she was probably brain-dead by the time she arrived there. Hospital B had limited facilities for blood transfusion, but no obstetrician in attendance. Here blood was transfused, and the uterine inversion was corrected using normal saline as in O'Sullivan's method. She was then transferred to University Hospital in Saskatoon (Hospital D) which had full blood transfusion facilities and an obstetrician in attendance. But she was already dead by the time her ambulance arrived at Hospital D. The court recognized the additional hazards of delivery in a remote rural setting but, even so, it held that in a number of respects *'the standard of competency, skill and diligence exercised by the delivering doctor fell below the standard expected of a general practitioner practising in a rural setting'*, and it awarded her estate damages of $343 000[15].

In 2000, a Dr Gabaldoni appeared before the Maryland State Board of Physician Quality Assurance in connection with his management of a patient he had induced at term for pre-eclampsia. The birth went well, but the mother had a postpartum hemorrhage that was thought to be due to retained fragments of placenta. She deteriorated over the next 48 h and her hemoglobin level went as low as 4.7 g/dl. Dr Gabaldoni was said to be leisurely in attendance, and slow to transfuse blood. However, blood transfusion was started at 48 h postpartum, but by this time she was in severe respiratory distress, and her condition continued to deteriorate. She was admitted to the intensive care unit at 72 h postpartum, but she died there 48 h later. Two days later, Dr Gabaldoni was said to have made a series of undated additions to her notes, which suggested that she had received better care than she did. He was said to have made these additional entries in the same color ink as the original progress notes, in such a manner that his alterations to the notes would not readily be apparent. The Maryland Board of Physician Quality Assurance filed charges under the Maryland Medical Practice Act 1995. When this case was considered by the Board, there was dispute about when he had seen the patient, when he had offered a blood transfusion, and whether the medical notes as written were correct. After reviewing the evidence, the Board found he had *'failed to meet the appropriate standard for delivery of medical care'*, and so it issued a reprimand. He appealed, but in a 'deferential review' the Court of Special Appeals of Maryland dismissed his appeal[16].

In 2000, a Malaysian Court of Appeal considered whether a medical center had a duty to keep blood available for transfusion. In 1988, Pearly Choo was booked to deliver her first baby in her local medical center, which carried no stored blood. She was healthy, had an uncomplicated pregnancy, and she was considered to be at low risk. She delivered her baby uneventfully, but she then sustained a major postpartum hemorrhage. In keeping with routine practice, blood was requested from the nearby Kuala Lumpur General Hospital, and her husband was sent to collect it. By the time the husband returned with the blood, his wife had already bled to death. He took legal action against the medical center, on the grounds that it should have carried blood, and it should have transfused blood in a timely fashion. The local Sessions Court found for the defendant hospital. The case was appealed to the High Court, which reversed the decision of the Sessions Court, and it found for the husband. However, the hospital then went to the Court of Appeal, which affirmed the Sessions Court's rejection of expert medical evidence that blood must be stored before any delivery, as this *'would result in an absurd situation when one bears in mind that deliveries are also conducted by midwives in houses of the mothers where blood would not be stored before such deliveries'*. The Court of Appeal thus reversed the High Court's decision, as it held that there was no duty to hold blood for a low-risk patient in case she bled. Further, it held that in this case the postpartum hemorrhage had been managed conventionally[17].

OBSTETRICIAN ON VACATION (1961)

Obstetricians traditionally hand over the management of a complicated case to a colleague when out of town or on vacation. The case may then go wrong due to the colleague's negligence, but the vacationing obstetrician might find himself sued for negligence. In 1961, this happened following death from postpartum hemorrhage. When pregnant with her fifth child, Patricia Sturm told her obstetrician at 33 weeks that she no longer felt fetal movements. He could not detect any fetal heart beat and, as obstetric ultrasound had not yet been invented, he advised a conservative approach. He told her that she would probably deliver normally in due course, but he did discuss the possibility of fetal death. As she was upset, he did not fully

discuss all the possible complications, but he did test her serum fibrinogen levels intermittently. He told her he would be on vacation at the time of her delivery, but would arrange for a colleague to look after her. However, she chose not to attend any further antenatal appointments. At 41 weeks' gestation, when her own obstetrician was away on vacation, she began to bleed vaginally. She was admitted to hospital, and the colleague delivered her of a stillborn infant. A massive postpartum hemorrhage followed for which she had an eight-unit blood transfusion and a hysterectomy. (The court report says it was carried out vaginally, but this may be incorrect.) Unfortunately, she died despite the emergency treatment. The autopsy report attributed her death to postpartum hemorrhage due to a clotting defect that was in turn due to intrauterine death. The family sued both the delivering doctor and the vacationing doctor, on the grounds that he shared in liability for any perinatal negligence on the part of his deputy. The Supreme Court of Oklahoma rejected this argument, and the obstetrician on vacation was exculpated[18].

UNLICENSED PRACTICE OF OBSTETRICS (1963)

Only two cases of postpartum hemorrhage have been litigated where a professional attendant at delivery was not licensed to practise obstetrics. Earlier, the 1907 case of Midwife Porn was discussed. The only other reported case was in 1963. Bernhardt and Lund were two doctors of chiropractic, but they held themselves out as competent in the management of childbirth. They supervised the delivery of Ladean Stojakovich at home, but unfortunately she had a postpartum hemorrhage and she died before she could be transferred to hospital. They were charged and convicted of breach of the Business and Professions Code (for practising medicine) and of manslaughter (for causing a death that was avoidable). Surprisingly, and for complex legal reasons, the Court of Appeals of California reversed both convictions, and it denied a request for retrial[19].

DISCHARGING PATIENT HOME TOO SOON (1977)

In 1977, Patricia Hale (aged 20) delivered vaginally at term at Fannin County Hospital in Texas, under the care of Dr Sheikholeslam. Although she was still bleeding at 30 h after delivery, she was discharged home. At 8 days postpartum, she was readmitted with continued bleeding. She was given a preoperative injection (presumably of ergometrine) to contract her uterus, a blood transfusion and a uterine curettage. After her operation, she was given no injection and no antibiotics. She was discharged home after 36 h, although she felt weak and she was still bleeding. At 20 days, heavy postpartum bleeding restarted. She was then admitted to a different hospital, where a different gynecologist diagnosed an intrauterine infection. Despite a second D&C, her heavy bleeding continued, and a hysterectomy had to be carried out. She sued the first doctor and hospital for negligent care. She won her case in the lower court, which held the doctor and the hospital jointly and severally liable for damages of $100 000. However, the hospital appealed the court's decision on the grounds that the doctor was an independent contractor, and not the hospital's servant or agent and that, as the hospital was a governmental unit, it was immune from tort liability. The Court of Appeals upheld the hospital's appeal, and it reversed the lower court's decision as regards the liability of the hospital. Dr Sheikholeslam did not appeal, and thus the original liability decision against him remained unchallenged[20].

INADEQUATE STAFFING LEVELS (1981)

In 1981, Stephen Martin was born in Ontario by spontaneous vaginal delivery following a labor complicated by fetal distress. He was in poor condition, and later he was diagnosed with cerebral palsy. When the case came to trial 17 years later in 1998, Obstetrical Nurse James was found guilty of negligence in failing to give appropriate care during labor. In her defence, she said she was involved with another patient who was having a postpartum hemorrhage. This was not accepted as a valid excuse as she should have called for help. She and her hospital were each found liable for 25% of the damages of $250 000 awarded to the claimant[21].

NO AUTOPSY (1982)

In 1982, Yong Siew Yin was in labor at term with her first baby. The labor was prolonged and (on one account) she was in labor for over 24 h. She had a small intrapartum hemorrhage. As there was delay in the second stage and fetal distress, urgent delivery was needed. The fetal head was low in the pelvis, and in an occipitoposterior position, so the baby was delivered 'face-to pubes' by Neville Barnes forceps. Following this, she had a postpartum hemorrhage, and this was attributed to vaginal tears. Whilst these were being repaired she collapsed, and a coagulation disorder became manifest. She continued to bleed heavily. An amniotic fluid embolism was suspected, but it was never proved. She was admitted to the intensive care unit where she died. Surprisingly, there was no autopsy. The judge in the lower court found the obstetrician guilty of negligence, and the hospital vicariously liable. This verdict was upheld on appeal[22].

SUING THE WRONG DOCTOR (1982)

Occasionally, a patient may sue the wrong doctor. In 1976, Jean Johnson had a normal vaginal delivery at the Wishard Memorial Hospital in Indiana. This was followed 2 weeks later by a secondary postpartum hemorrhage. She was seen by the Chief Resident, Dr Deaton, who diagnosed retained products of conception, and advised uterine curettage. He checked his diagnosis and treatment plan with Dr Padilla, a staff instructor with the Indiana University Medical School, and the operation was carried out. By 1982, it had become apparent that Jean Johnson was infertile, and this was attributed to over-vigorous curettage of the endometrium in 1976 (Asherman's syndrome). She sued Dr Padilla for negligent performance of the curettage, but did not suggest that the curettage decision itself was negligent. The defence was threefold: (1) Dr Padilla did not carry out the curettage; (2) there was no doctor–patient relationship between Dr Padilla and Jean Johnson; and (3) there was no agency relationship between Dr Padilla and Dr Deaton. The Court of Appeals of Indiana accepted all three lines of defence, and dismissed the case against Dr Padilla[23].

OBSTETRICIAN WITHOUT SUFFICIENT EXPERIENCE (1986)

In 1986, Christine Steinhagen became pregnant for the third time. She had two previous cesarean sections, the second being complicated by 'extreme and profuse bleeding'. In her third pregnancy, she had a sudden vaginal bleed at about 20 weeks' gestation, and an anterior placenta previa was diagnosed. She was kept in hospital for 18 weeks and throughout this time given terbutaline to inhibit uterine contractions. The last dose was given on the morning she was delivered by elective cesarean section. Her obstetrician-gynecologist had recently completed his residency training but was not yet board-certified. Moreover, he had not discussed her management with any board-certified obstetrician-gynecologist, and had no other suitably qualified surgeon in attendance. The cesarean operation was carried out through a low transverse abdominal incision, but surgery proved to be difficult. After the baby was delivered, the uterus failed to contract, and she hemorrhaged profusely. In these circumstances, it would have been usual to give Methergine (methylergonovine) and/or Pitocin (oxytocin) to promote uterine contraction. No Methergine was given; half a dose of Pitocin may have been given, but it was not documented in the medical notes or on the drug chart. A hysterectomy was carried out, but the bleeding continued. Her bladder was damaged and she developed hematuria. A urological surgeon was then called, and he ligated the left internal iliac (or hypogastric) artery. This slowed the bleeding considerably, but it did not stop it completely. The tissues were now friable and so the abdomen was packed and closed, and she was managed overnight in intensive care. The abdomen was reopened the following day as internal bleeding continued. At the second operation, all bleeding was brought under control, but she lost her right ovary. During this episode, she was given a total of 34 units of blood, 14 of fresh frozen plasma and 10 of platelets, but she survived. Postoperatively, she developed a vesico-vaginal fistula, hepatitis, an extremely short vagina that made intercourse impossible, and severe psychological problems. As she was managed and delivered at a naval military hospital in

Illinois, she took legal action against the United States of America. After hearing expert evidence, the trial judge was critical of: an obstetrician-gynecologist who was not board-certified managing this complicated case without more experienced help; his giving terbutaline immediately prior to the cesarean section, thereby inhibiting uterine contraction after delivery; his failure to perform the operation through a midline incision which would have minimized the risk of bladder damage; his failure to give Methergine to contract the uterus; and his failure to ligate both hypogastric arteries which might have avoided the hysterectomy and the loss of an ovary. He awarded her $300 000 in compensation[24].

NO OPERATION NOTE (1992)

In 1992, Mrs Suchorab was delivered in Saskatchewan by cesarean section. Six weeks later, she had a postpartum hemorrhage and was readmitted to hospital. Her obstetrician took her to the operating theater, where he stabilized her condition. The operation log and the anesthetist's note both record that a dilatation and curettage operation was carried out, but no surgical operation note was ever found to confirm this. The following day, she had a further major hemorrhage, and a hysterectomy was carried out. She took legal action against her obstetrician. She argued that his care had been deficient as her bleed was due to retained products of conception, and he had failed to curette her uterus as (she claimed) was evidenced by the absence of any operation note. He claimed that he had curetted her uterus, but he had forgotten to write an operation note. Moreover, he claimed that her bleed was from a *'necrotic cervix'*, and not from the uterine cavity, and so no extra harm would have resulted from failure to curette the uterus. The court rejected her claim[25].

SHEEHAN'S SYNDROME (1977, 1995)

In 1977, Mrs Parker delivered her first child. Her obstetrician delivered the placenta by continuous cord traction. However, she had a uterine inversion and a major postpartum hemorrhage followed. She was taken to the operating theater, and in the operation note it was recorded that her *'uterus had resolved itself'*. Five months later, she was found to have *'an inverted uterus presenting well down in the vagina'*. She had various ongoing symptoms, but it was not until 1991 (14 years later) that Sheehan's syndrome was diagnosed. She then took legal action against her obstetrician of 1977. A four-person jury awarded her $960 000 in damages. Her obstetrician appealed the case on both liability and quantum. The New South Wales Court of Appeal dismissed his appeal on liability, but it ordered a new trial limited to damages, as it considered the jury award excessive[26].

In 1995, Natalie Lomeo was delivered by elective cesarean section at her local Community Medical Center (CMC) in Pennsylvania. She had an extensive blood loss during the operation, and a postpartum hemorrhage followed. Although she exhibited signs of hemorrhagic shock, blood was not transfused until much later in the day. Over the next 3 years, she complained of fatigue, weakness, dizziness, hair loss, amenorrhea, dyspareunia, and vasomotor symptomatology. In 1998, the diagnosis of Sheehan's syndrome was made. She then took legal action against her obstetrician and the CMC. However, the defendants filed for summary judgment, asserting that her claim was time-barred under Pennsylvania law, as it had been filed more than 2 years after the allegedly negligent conduct. The Common Pleas Court denied the motion for dismissal, saying that the litigation clock only started to run when Sheehan's syndrome was diagnosed[27]. What happened next was not reported, so the case was probably settled.

MALIGNANT HYPERTENSION (1993)

In 1993, Evelyn Dybongco-Rimando had an uneventful spontaneous vaginal delivery of a healthy daughter, and she went home shortly afterwards. Some 8 years later, a judge of the Superior Court of Justice of Ontario was to say that her case *'presents a puzzle with a thousand pieces'*. The trial started in 1999, and it lasted for 33 days spread over 3 years. The judge described it as *'a challenge to bench and bar alike'*. Although her delivery was normal, 7 days later she suffered a massive postpartum hemorrhage, and she was readmitted to hospital. Over the next 2 days, she had three operations before her bleeding could be brought under control: uterine exploration, hysterectomy, and then a second-look laparotomy. She was given a large transfusion of blood, and also blood products as she developed a coagulation disorder. She became profoundly hypotensive, and required inotropic agents (principally dopamine) to support her blood pressure. However, her blood pressure then went too high, and within 33 h of readmission to hospital she had developed malignant hypertension. Dopamine was given but discontinued when her pressure reached 237/113 mmHg. However, the maximum level of blood pressure later recorded was 256/126 mmHg. She then had a cerebral hemorrhage, and soon after this she died. Her estate started a legal action against 55 defendants, but only three defendants remained shortly after the trial started in 2000. These were her obstetrician, her internal medicine physician, and her intensivist. In his final judgment, the judge said of the internal medicine physician's testimony *'It reflects a triumph of tactics over truth. He is not credible.'* He found all three defendant doctors guilty of negligence, and he reserved judgment on the amount of damages to be awarded to the deceased patient's estate[28].

NO EXPERT MEDICAL REPORT (1995)

In 1995, Marcia Laidley had a postpartum hemorrhage after delivering her third child. A supracervical hysterectomy was performed. Later, she took legal action against her obstetrician. However, she failed to provide a timely expert medical report in support of her case by the court-imposed deadline, and so summary judgment was awarded against her. She appealed. The Court of Appeals of Ohio held that the trial court had committed a prejudicial error when it granted the defendant's motion for summary judgment without providing the opportunity for sufficient discovery on the issue[29].

POSTPARTUM HEMORRHAGE IN AN AIRCRAFT (1997)

In 1997, Gina Paone delivered her baby in Ontario, but her placenta had to be removed manually. Her uterine cavity was explored and considered to be empty. The placenta was judged to be complete. One month later, she flew to Italy, but she had abdominal pain and heavy vaginal bleeding during the flight. On arrival in Italy, she was admitted to hospital where she had a uterine curettage. She claims she was told there was further placental tissue recovered from the uterus, but there was no written confirmation of this. In 1998, she started legal proceedings in Italy by an Act of Citation naming her obstetrician, two nurses and St Joseph's Health Centre, all of whom were in Ontario. The Italian court refused to hear the case, saying it lacked jurisdiction as the medical treatment had occurred in Ontario. In 2000, she brought a similar legal action in Ontario. However, the defendants prevailed, as Ontario law requires an action against a doctor to be brought within 1 year from when the Plaintiff *'knew or ought to have known'* the material facts on which the malpractice is alleged, and against a hospital or nurse within 2 years of the patient being discharged from hospital or stopping treatment. Furthermore, the Ontario Court of Justice also found that in this case there was no genuine issue for trial as no expert reports were filed[30].

POSTPARTUM HEMORRHAGE INTO THE PLEURAL CAVITY (1997)

In 1997, an unusual case of postpartum hemorrhage occurred in California. Martha Guandique had severe pre-eclampsia at 38 weeks' gestation. Her signs and symptoms included shortness of breath, hypertension, renal malfunction, hepatomegaly and pleural effusion. Labor was induced and she delivered a male infant. She had a postpartum hemorrhage due to uterine atony, so she was given Pitocin. Blood clots were evacuated from her uterus. Shortly after delivery, she had considerable difficulty in breathing, and back pain. Various physicians were called in to see her. Pulmonary embolism and amniotic fluid embolism were in the differential diagnosis. Supportive therapy with oxygen was given and various drugs were used. Her hemoglobin fell at first to 9.5 g/dl, and it continued to fall thereafter. (Subsequent hemoglobin levels were not recorded in the court report.) A blood transfusion was started, but 20 min later she had a cardiopulmonary arrest and then she died. At autopsy, she was found to have suffered a major postpartum hemorrhage (of 1500 ml) into her right pleural cavity. The pathologist reported that *'The mechanism of production of this hemorrhage remains unknown in spite of a careful dissection of the blood vessels in the area. . . . That is why the mode of this death remains undetermined.'* In this case, much of the complicated legal argument before the Court of Appeal of California focused on which doctors might have been liable for her death, but these legal arguments need not concern us here[31].

DISAPPEARING BABY (1999)

This too represents an unusual case, but I have seen something very similar (see below). In 1999, an unmarried mother was having an adulterous affair with a co-worker. He noticed that her abdomen was enlarging, and asked whether she might be pregnant. She said that she could be. The matter was discussed no further, neither with him nor with any other co-workers. A few weeks later, she attended her family doctor complaining of swollen feet. She told him that she was 7 months pregnant. The doctor heard the fetal heart beat and felt fetal movements, and so he pronounced the fetus healthy. This was the only medical care she sought before 12 May 1999, when she was admitted to a Texas hospital with a 2-day history of vaginal bleeding. She was said to be in shock: she was weak and pale, had a low temperature, and a tachycardia. (Her blood pressure was not mentioned in the court report.) She said that she was pregnant, but she did not know the date of her last menstrual period, nor when her baby was due. A blood test showed that she was severely anemic. Her hemoglobin level was not mentioned in the court report, but, from comments in the report, it was probably around 4–5 g/dl. Four units of blood were transfused. An obstetrician was called, and she scanned the uterus with ultrasound. She found no evidence of a baby, but she did find a placenta of a size compatible with a term baby. The placenta was then delivered, but it had no cord attached. Both the patient and her attendant family denied that any baby had been born. Therefore the police were called. They searched her home, and there they found evidence of extensive blood staining of her bed, and of her bathroom – but no baby. A grand jury was convened to determine whether any charge, such as homicide, should be brought. Under oath she said that *'I did not pass a baby'*, and she insisted that she had only passed clots of blood. She was later charged with aggravated perjury before a grand jury, convicted by a jury, and sentenced to 10 years confinement probated for 10 years. She appealed against her conviction on the grounds that the evidence was legally insufficient to support the jury's verdict, and the State had failed to prove the materiality of her alleged false statement. The Court of Appeals of Texas considered her arguments but it dismissed her appeal[32].

[In the late 1970s, I had a similar case in the UK: a 14-year-old girl who presented in shock with heavy vaginal bleeding. She had a perineal midline tear, a widely open cervix, and an enlarged uterus, but there was no baby and no placenta. Her hemoglobin level was only 4 g/dl, so she was transfused with blood. Her presentation was clearly consistent with recent childbirth followed by a major postpartum hemorrhage. Despite the overwhelming evidence, the girl and her parents firmly denied any pregnancy or recent delivery of a baby. The police were duly called in. They investigated the matter and searched the family home, but no baby was ever found. No charges were ever brought.]

ABANDONMENT (2000)

In 2000, the New York Bureau of Professional Medical Conduct considered the case of Dr Wahba, an obstetrician who was charged with professional misconduct in the treatment of seven of his patients. Two of these were at risk of postpartum hemorrhage, and here he was found guilty of negligence and/or incompetence. In both cases, he left the delivery room before the placenta was delivered. The first patient had a stillbirth, and so she was at a higher risk of postpartum hemorrhage. The second was still hemodynamically unstable; she then hemorrhaged but by this time the obstetrician had already left the hospital. Moreover, he refused the nurse supervisor's requests to return. After reviewing his management of all seven patients, the Administrative Review Board for Professional Medical Conduct revoked his licence to practise medicine in the state of New York. He then appealed to the Supreme Court of New York, but his appeal was dismissed[33].

POSTPARTUM HEMORRHAGE IN A FEMALE DOG (2006)

American courts are well known for leading the way into new areas of litigation. Therefore it may come as no surprise to learn that in February 2006 the Court of Appeals of Texas ruled on a case involving the management of postpartum hemorrhage in a female dog in the Bureau of Animal Regulation and Care in Houston in 1999. This facility takes around 20–30 000 animals a year. One of their veterinarians was Dr Levingston. He had made a number of complaints to his employers about the inhumane treatment of animals in their care, but on one particular occasion they accused him of the negligent care of animals, and they terminated his employment. They cited his alleged mismanagement of the care of a female Rottweiler dog who had given birth to nine puppies, and who had a postpartum hemorrhage from which she exsanguinated and died. They said he should have considered the possibilities of hysterectomy or euthanasia. He appealed his termination of employment and won his case. He was awarded damages in the lower court. His employers appealed the decision, and the case went to the Court of Appeals of Texas who dismissed their appeal. The court awarded him a total of

$1.24 million for past and future lost wages and compensatory damages. This amount was to include $194 000 for his lawyers' fees. If the lawyers' fees of his employers, the City of Houston, were of the same order of magnitude, then the legal bill on this case would have been around $400 000. Overall, this case ran for more than 5 years[34].

CONCLUSIONS

This account has been international in its scope, albeit confined to common law jurisdictions. It is clear that the history of litigation following postpartum hemorrhage stretches for over 100 years, from Florence Westrup of Newport, Kentucky in 1905 to the female Rottweiler dog of Houston, Texas in 2006.

In 17 of 34 cases (50%), a maternal death no doubt prompted the litigation, rather than the postpartum hemorrhage itself.

After maternal death, the second most common reason for litigation was a problem with the transfusion of blood, such as infection, delay or possible incompatibility. Such problems occurred in ten of 34 (29%) of the cases.

Equal third reasons for litigation were having a diagnosis made of Sheehan's syndrome after postpartum hemorrhage (only two cases), and having professional birth attendants who were not licensed to practise obstetrics (only two cases, one of which was litigated in 1907).

Apart from the general observation that poor obstetric practice was a typical feature of many of these cases, they were otherwise sporadic in etiology, with no common cause.

Given the millions of women who have delivered over the last 100 years across the English, Commonwealth, Irish, and American jurisdictions studied, given that the incidence of postpartum hemorrhage is around 5–10%, and given that there has been an international increase in litigation for alleged clinical malpractice, it is surprising that there have not been many more cases of postpartum hemorrhage litigated in the courts.

References

1. Westrup v Commonwealth. Court of Appeals of Kentucky. 123 Ky 95; 93 SW 646; 1906 Ky; LEXIS 123
2. Commonwealth v Hanna Porn. Supreme Judicial Court of Massachusetts, Worcester. 196 Mass 326; 82 NE 31; 1907 Mass; LEXIS 1096
3. US Short, Administrator of the Estate of Mollie Short, Deceased v City of East St Louis. Court of Appeals of Illinois. 4d 140 Ill App 173; 1908 Ill App; LEXIS 819
4. Southern Bell Telephone & Telegraph Co v Glawson et al. Court of Appeals of Georgia. 13 Ga App 520; 79 SE 488; 1913 Ga App; LEXIS 247
5. Peterson v Langsten. 28,835; Supreme Court of Minnesota. 186 Minn 101; 242 NW 549; 1932 Minn; LEXIS 844
6. Goff et al. v Doctors General Hospital of San Jose et al. 9408; Court of Appeal of California, Third Appellate District. 166 Cal App 2d 314; 333 P2d 29; 1958 Cal App; LEXIS 1404

7. Reserve Life Insurance Company v Whitten. Court of Appeals of Alabama. 38 Ala App 455; 88 So 2d 573; 1956 Ala App; LEXIS 208

8. Madison et al. v City and County of San Francisco et al. 14410; Court of Appeal of California, First Appellate District, Division One. 106 Cal App 2d 232; 234 P 2d 995; 1951 Cal App; LEXIS 1738

9. Gillen v United States of America. 16584; United States Court of Appeals Ninth Circuit. 281 F2d 425; 1960 US App; LEXIS 4034

10. Parker and Parker v St Paul Fire & Marine Insurance Company et al. Court of Appeal of Louisiana, Second Circuit. 335 So 2d 725; 1976 La App; LEXIS 3976

11. Belle Bonfils Memorial Blood Center v Denver District Court, Judge Phillips, CW, KW and son RW. 88-SA-45; Supreme Court of Colorado. 763 P2d 1003; 1988 Colo; LEXIS 174; 12 BTR 1463

12. Estate of Mutsuko Gaffney; and Gaffney et al. v United States of America. 88-1457-Z; United States District Court for the District of Massachusetts. 1990 US Dist; LEXIS 5184

13. Traxler v Varady. A053098; Court of Appeal of California, First Appellate District, Division One. 12 Cal App 4th 1321; 16 Cal Rptr 2d 297; 1993 Cal App; LEXIS 82; 93 Cal Daily Op Service 747; 93 Daily Journal DAR 1423

14. Endean v Canadian Red Cross Society. British Columbia Supreme Court. 148 DLR (4th) 158; 1997 DLR; LEXIS 1359

15. Naeth Estate v Warburton. Saskatchewan Queen's Bench. 1992 ACWSJ; LEXIS 33936; 1992 ACWSJ 569976; 34 ACWS (3d) 1108

16. Gabaldoni v Board of Physician Quality Assurance. Court of Special Appeals of Maryland. 141 Md App 259; 785 A2d 771; 2001 Md App; LEXIS 180. 'Under Maryland law, the final order of an administrative agency is subject to deferential review by the courts. Deferential review prohibits a court from substituting its judgment for that of the agency if substantial evidence exists to support the agency's decision. The test is 'reasonableness not rightness'.

17. Arayan et al. v Simon et al. Court of Appeal (Kuala Lumpur); Decided 18 April 2000. [2000] 3 MLJ 657; Civil Appeal No W-04-71 of 1996

18. Sturm v Green. 40638; Supreme Court of Oklahoma. 1965 OK 12; 398 P 2d 799; 1965 Okla; LEXIS 364

19. The People v Bernhardt and Lund. Court of Appeal of California, Second Appellate District, Division Three. 222 Cal App 2d 567; 35 Cal Rptr 401; 1963 Cal App; LEXIS 1701

20. Hale v Sheikholeslam and Fannin County Hospital. 83-2047; United States Court of Appeals for the Fifth Circuit. 724 F2d 1205; 1984 US App; LEXIS 25485; 1984 Fed Carr Cas (CCH) P83,141

21. Martin v Listowel Memorial Hospital. Ontario Court (General Division). 1998 ACWSJ; LEXIS 85776; 1998 ACWSJ 523416; 81 ACWS (3d) 548

22. Ping and Anor v Woon Lin Sing et al. Rayuan Sivil No 12-223-92 & 12-225-92. High Court of Shah Alam, Malaysia. 1998 MLJU; LEXIS 1203; [1998] 583 MLJU 1

23. Johnson v Padilla. 2-1280-A-410; Court of Appeals of Indiana, Second District. 433 NE2d 393; 1982 Ind App; LEXIS 1122

24. Steinhagen v United States of America. 89-CV-72453-DT; US District Court for Eastern District of Michigan, Southern Division. 768 F Supp 200; 1991 US Dist; LEXIS 8918

25. Suchorab v Urbanski. Saskatchewan Queen's Bench. 1997 Sask D; LEXIS 744; [1997] Sask D. 610.30.50.70–02

26. Fowkes v Parker [1999]. NSWCA 442; Supreme Court of New South Wales, Court of Appeal. CA 40948/98; 1999 NSW; LEXIS 862; BC9908184

27. Lomeo v Davis. 99-CV-2639; Common Pleas Court of Lackawanna County, Pennsylvania. 53 Pa D & C 4th 49; 2001 Pa D & C; LEXIS 95

28. Dybongco-Rimando Estate et al. v Jackiewicz et al. Court of Ontario: Superior Court of Justice. 2001 OTC; LEXIS 2442; [2001] OTC 682

29. Laidley v St Luke's Medical Center et al. 73553; Court of Appeals of Ohio, Eighth Appellate District, Cuyahoga County. 1999 Ohio App; LEXIS 2567

30. Paone v St Joseph's Health Centre. 00-CV-198822CM; Ontario Superior Court of Justice. 2002 ACWSJ; LEXIS 7091; 2002 ACWSJ 10094; 118 ACWS (3d) 46

31. Guandique et al. v Makabali et al. B157844; Court Of Appeal Of California, Second Appellate District, Division Seven. 2004 Cal App Unpub; LEXIS 6458

32. Steen v State of Texas. 14-00-00429-CR; Court of Appeals of Texas, Fourteenth District, Houston. 78 SW 3d 516; 2002 Tex App; LEXIS 2306

33. Wahba v New York State Department of Health et al. 86017; Supreme Court of New York, Appellate Division, Third Department. 277 AD 2d 634; 716 NYS 2d 443; 2000 N Y App Div; LEXIS 12048

34. City of Houston v Levingston. 01-03-00678-CV; Court of Appeals of Texas, First District, Houston. 2006 Tex App; LEXIS 859

Section 11

How Health Professionals Deal with Postpartum Hemorrhage

64

Management of Postpartum Hemorrhage in Low Resource Settings

V. Walvekar, A. Virkud and R. Majumder

INTRODUCTION

The global rate of maternal mortality is 260/100,000 live births, and approximately 500,000 mothers are lost annually as a result of pregnancy-related issues[1]. Rates of death are disproportionately high in developing countries, where maternal mortality as high as 920/100,000 live births has been recorded in sub-Saharan Africa[2].

Overall, postpartum hemorrhage (PPH) affects 1–5% of all deliveries[3,4], and approximately 30% of maternal deaths are due to hemorrhage, mainly in the postpartum period. Most maternal deaths due to PPH occur in developing countries in settings (both hospital and community) where there are no birth attendants or where birth attendants lack the necessary skills or equipment to prevent and manage PPH and shock[5]. Under such circumstances, it is not surprising that almost 99% of maternal deaths occur in developing countries[6], and 45% of postpartum deaths occur within 1 day of delivery[7]. The Millennium Development Goal of reducing maternal mortality by 75% by 2015[8] will remain beyond our reach unless governments act in partnership with the obstetric community to confront the problem of PPH in the developing world as a priority.

Of deaths due to PPH, 90% occur in women who have none of the so-called classic risk factors, although some conditions do predispose to PPH. It is a preventable cause of death, as evidenced by the decline in hemorrhage-related mortality in the developed world. The maternal mortality rate (MMR) is 35-times lower in the developed world compared with that in developing countries (14 versus 400/100,000 live births)[2].

INDIAN SCENARIO

Rural India is representative of the scope and magnitude of the international problem, where 50% of births occur at home or in rudimentary facilities without a physician in attendance. The MMR in India currently is estimated at 254/100,000 live births with PPH being responsible for 30% of these deaths[9]. This figure mimics that cited above on a worldwide basis.

Although a blood loss of 500 ml of blood following vaginal delivery or 1000 ml following cesarean section represents the standard and accepted definition of PPH, we propose that a more practical definition of PPH in terms of the developing world would be any blood loss that causes a physiological change (e.g. low blood pressure) that threatens the woman's life. Such a definition would also more accurately reflect the fact that anemic women in developing countries are far more susceptible to adverse outcomes as a result of smaller blood losses after delivery. Thus, the addition of 'a 10% drop in hemoglobin level' to the definition would provide an objective laboratory measure for health care providers who may not be able to assess accurately the true quantity of loss. However, such an addition would presume that even this simple test was available and, in reality, it is not.

PREDISPOSING FACTORS

It is very important to evaluate the following issues in the antenatal period, as they significantly affect a parturient's response to a given blood loss.

(1) *Anemia* Iron-deficiency anemia affects 66–80% of the world's population[11]. Anemia, in particular severe anemia, increases the risk of PPH-related maternal morbidity and mortality.

(2) *Maternal depletion syndrome* This is an extremely important consideration in developing countries where mothers have diminished nutritional status due to early marriage and repeated pregnancies[12,13].

(3) *Obstetric conditions* Mothers with pre-eclampsia, multiple pregnancies, retained placenta, abruptio placentae, placenta previa, operative vaginal delivery, prolonged labor, pyrexia in labor, etc. are more prone to PPH.

(4) *Medical infrastructure* In developing countries, significant numbers of deliveries occur in the home or rudimentary health centers, often with minimally skilled birth attendants[14]. This is despite the fact that a critical component of safe delivery practice is to have a competent health worker with at least midwifery skills present at every birth along with plans that provide transport to a referral facility should this be necessary[1,14].

ADEQUACY OF THE DELIVERY SETTING

Countries can be classified in terms of the resources available at the time of delivery.

Low resource settings

Low resource settings are locations where significant numbers of deliveries occur in the home or in rudimentary health centers, often in the presence of minimally skilled birth attendants. Examples of such settings include the developing countries of sub-Saharan Africa such as Nigeria, Senegal and Uganda, while countries in southern Asian are exemplified by India, Bangladesh, Pakistan and Nepal.

High resource settings

High resource settings are locations where most deliveries are conducted in a well-equipped hospital with trained medical and paramedical staff, adequate medications, equipment and space, and facilities to transfer a patient to a center with more complex technology and techniques, as well as a 24-hour power supply and refrigeration facility.

PRINCIPLES OF MANAGEMENT

The principles of management of PPH are outlined below.

(1) Quick and efficient management is extremely important, as a recent Egyptian study showed that 88% of deaths occur in the first 4 hours after onset of PPH[15]. Other data from WHO note that if left untreated, the parturient can die within 2 hours.

(2) Quick assessment of the patient's condition must be made, as well as a decision as to whether she can be treated locally or must be transferred to higher level facility as quickly as possible after initial resuscitation.

(3) Arrangement of adequate manpower is mandatory, as treatment of PPH cannot under any circumstances be considered a one-person show.

(4) Arrangement for adequate fluid replacement and blood products when necessary is a crucial part of the initial resuscitation plan.

(5) Correct estimation of blood loss is essential. In most instances, estimation of blood loss is accomplished visually despite the fact that numerous studies show that this method is up to 50% less accurate than other methods[16–18]. Early and accurate estimation of blood loss is crucial because replacement is so often required. The estimation of blood loss from a cesarean section is generally more accurate than after vaginal delivery, because during vaginal delivery blood is generally mixed with amniotic fluid. Estimation is enhanced using the methods outlined in Table 1 after letting the amniotic fluid drain out as much as possible[19]. Details regarding the use of a drape under the parturient's buttocks to facilitate blood collection are presented in Chapter 11.

Medical management

Table 2 lists the drugs used in the management of PPH.

Misoprostol

In developing countries available medical facilities are often erratic or non-existent. The most important basic facilities required for safe delivery include staff with appropriate training, around the clock availability of the same, and the presence of a 24-hour electricity supply and refrigeration for the maintenance of uterotonic medications. It is this latter requirement that has turned the attention of many caregivers in the developing world to misoprostol. This medication requires no refrigeration, is inexpensive and can be administered by individuals with little or no professional training (see Chapter 42).

Analysis of the cost of misoprostol use in developing countries should not be limited to the cost of the tablets. Costs of misoprostol treatment, trained birth

Table 1 Estimation of blood loss

Methods/materials used	Estimated blood loss (ml)
Small 10 × 10 cm 32-ply swab (max saturated capacity)	60
Medium 30 × 30 cm 12-ply swab (max saturated capacity)	140
Large 45 × 45 cm 12-ply swab (max saturated capacity)	350
1 kg soaked swabs	1000
Kidney dish full of clots	500
50 cm diameter floor spill	500
75 cm diameter floor spill	1000
100 cm diameter floor spill	1500
Vaginal PPH limited to bed only	< 1000
Vaginal PPH spilling over from bed to floor	> 1000

Table 2 Drugs used in the management of postpartum hemorrhage

Drugs	Route of administration	Availability of hospital facility/ skilled staff	Storage	Cost in India
Oxytocin	IV/IM	Skilled staff needed	Refrigeration preferable	Rs 22/amp
Prostodin	IM	Skilled staff needed	Refrigeration needed	Rs 98.42/amp (250 μg)
Methergin	IM/IV	Skilled staff needed	Refrigeration needed	Rs 30.20/amp (0.2 mg)
Misoprostol	Oral/sublingual/PV/PR	Basic skilled person enough	Refrigeration not needed	Rs 72/800 μg

Rs, rupees

attendant (TBA) training, hospital referrals, hospitalization, IV fluids and blood transfusions should be borne in mind. (These data can be derived from the literature and from field data.) Examples of cost models are shown below.

Cost model for misoprostol arm

TBA training cost + TBA time cost + drug cost + cost of side-effects + cost of transport + cost of hospitalization + cost of treatment for PPH

Cost model for standard care arm

Cost of transport + cost of hospitalization + cost of treatment for PPH

Different studies show that more than 80 TBAs are needed to attend 10,000 deliveries and the cost of a 5-day training per TBA including teachers and materials is US dollars 10.05 (Table 3). On average a home delivery costs US dollars 2, while 1000 μg misoprostol costs US dollars 2.75. Cost of hospital stay is US dollars 27.60 per day, patient transportation to a higher referral center is US dollars 5.31 and hydration of a patient is US dollars 4.48. Blood transfusions are generally very expensive and can cost as much as US dollars 63.87. Table 3 shows that the implementation of a comprehensive misoprostol strategy would save US dollars 115,336 per 10,000 births in transport, hospital fees, IV therapy and blood transfusions (range US dollars 13,991–1,563,593 per 10,000 births)[27].

Table 3 Estimation of cost-effectiveness of misoprostol

Parameter	Quantity/cost (US dollars)	References
Number of TBA needed to attend 10,000 deliveries	83	20, 21
Cost of 1 home delivery	$2	22
Cost of 5 day training per TBA, teachers and materials	$10.05	21, 23
Cost of 1000 μg misoprostol	$2.75	24, 25
Cost of hospital bed/day	$27.60	—
Cost of transportation to hospital	$5.31	—
Cost of IV fluids/IV cannula	$4.48	—
Cost of blood transfusion	$63.87	21, 26

TBA, trained birth assistants

A joint statement of the International Confederation of Midwives (ICM) and the International Federation of Gynecology and Obstetrics (FIGO), and a 2007 WHO recommendation for the prevention of PPH advocate the use of misoprostol in situations where no oxytocin is available or the birth attendant's skills are limited. Therefore, misoprostol can play an important part in the strategy to reduce PPH in countries where most births occur in the home (see Chapter 42).

Surgical management

As mentioned previously, and noted in several other chapters of this book, the majority of deaths due to PPH occur in the first few hours after the onset of bleeding. It is also true that most bleeding is due to atony which responds to medical management in most instances. However, medical management alone is not always effective and often must be supported by surgical interventions, some of which can be applied in settings which are not fully equipped for abdominal interventions. Of these more simple techniques, tamponades can be effective because they apply pressure at the site of the placental detachment. Commonly used materials for uterine tamponade and described in other chapters of this book are variable length ribbon gauze, condom catheter, Foley catheter, Sengstaken–Blackmore tube, Bakri balloon, etc. Of these, the use of ribbon gauze, condom catheters and Foley catheters are low cost and very effective in low resource settings. In contrast, the Bakri balloon and Sengstaken–Blakemore tube are expensive and not widely available or affordable in developing countries (Table 4). At the other end of the spectrum, major surgical procedures such as internal iliac artery ligation (see Chapter 52), systemic devascularization or obstetric hysterectomies are not only very expensive, but also accompanied by increases in secondary costs due to prolonged hospital stay. Their widespread application is also hampered by the lack of expertise in performing the operations. Uterine artery embolization (see Chapter 49) can also be an effective procedure, but again it is expensive and needs expert radiology facilities.

Table 4 Cost of surgical equipment and procedures

Method	Material/facility needed	Provider of treatment	Cost in India
Ribbon gauze	Can be done in minor OT	Medical officer	Low cost
Condom catheter	Widely available	Medical officer	Low cost
Foley catheter	Widely available	Medical officer	Low cost
Bakri balloon	Not widely available	Medical officer	Rs 95
Sengstaken–Blakemore tube	Not widely available	Experienced person	Rs 11,000
B-Lynch suture	Major OT set-up	Medical officer	Moderate cost
Uterine artery ligation	Major OT set-up	Medical officer	Moderate cost
Ovarian artery ligation	Major OT set-up	Medical officer	Moderate cost
Internal iliac ligation	Major OT set-up	Experienced person	Expensive
Obstetric hysterectomy	Relatively good hospital set-up	Experienced person	Expensive
Uterine artery embolization	Good hospital set-up with radiology facility in OT	Experienced person	Expensive

OT, operating theater; Rs, rupees

HEALTH CARE INFRASTRUCTURE IN RURAL INDIA

The Indian health care industry (used here as a model of the events occurring in other developing nations) is seen to be growing at a rapid pace and is expected to become a US dollars 280 billion industry by 2020[28]. Even so, the vast majority of the country suffers from a poor standard of health care infrastructure, which has not kept up with the growing economy. Despite having centers of excellence in health care delivery, the numbers of such facilities are limited and they are inadequate in meeting the current health care demands. From a practical point of view, it is important to recognize that 40% of primary health centers in India are understaffed. India also faces a huge needs gap in terms of availability of number of hospital beds per 1000 population. With a world average of 3.96 hospital beds per 1000 population, India has a long way to go to bring its present statistic of 0.7 hospital beds per 1000 population to a more reasonable level.

Types of facilities

Three broad categories of facilities are generally available in developing nations: public, private and traditional. The official Indian policy on public facilities requires that there should be one subcenter, or sometimes an aid-post, staffed by one trained nurse (ANM), for every 3000 individuals. These subcenters provide the first point of care, while the primary health centers or community health centers are the next step, leaving the referral hospitals to deal with the most serious health problems. A primary health center serves 20,000–30,000 individuals and has on average five or six medical personnel appointed, including at least one doctor.

Private facilities include a wide variety of options ranging from facilities run by people who have completed their medical training and have additional postgraduate medical degrees, to traditional birth attendants (Daima's) and pharmacists who in most cases have no formal medical training whatsoever. The degree to which such facilities come under the oversight of any governmental or academic authority is minimal and the quality of care provided varies enormously.

The problem of health care

Delivery of high-quality social services to the poor is never easy, and several factors make it especially difficult. The decision about when and where to seek health care often has very little to do with the nature of the medical condition itself. It often relates to what is available close to a person when help is needed, but it could just as well reflect how the person is feeling about life in general and health in particular. These considerations aside, obtaining health care at any facility depends on a combination of one or more of the following factors: availability or non-availability of doctors at primary health centers; inadequate physical infrastructure and facilities; insufficient quantities of drugs; lack of accountability to the public and lack of community participation; and lack of set standards for monitoring quality care, etc.

STRATEGIES TO PREVENT MATERNAL MORTALITY FROM POSTPARTUM HEMORRHAGE IN LOW RESOURCE SETTINGS

It is important to build strategies to manage preventable causes of maternal death in low resource settings.

Short-term strategies

Prevention where there is a skilled provider

When women give birth with a skilled provider at home or in a hospital facility, up to two-thirds of PPH can be prevented using safe, low-cost, evidence-based practices. Advantages to this set-up are:

(1) Skilled health care providers are able to diagnose the risk factors early and accurately;

(2) Blood loss can be estimated during delivery;

(3) Active management of the third stage of labor (AMTSL) can be provided to all patients in addition to less expensive uterotonics (misoprostol);

(4) Cell phone calls to a more experienced health care provider can be made for advice regarding onsite management or early referral to an institution or center with more advanced therapeutic capabilities.

Prevention where there is no skilled provider

About 66% of births in the least developed countries occur in the home without skilled providers to perform AMTSL. In these low resource settings, use of misoprostol can be a life-saving intervention as it is inexpensive, readily available without refrigeration, can be taken orally without supervision of a medical provider, and provides significant reduction in blood loss from acute PPH and acute severe PPH (see Chapters 13–15)

Community-based emergency care or home-based life-saving skills (HBLSS) can be used in settings where there is no skilled provider. Anyone who attends a delivery can be taught simple home-based life-saving skills.

Community-based obstetric first aid with HBLSS is a family and community focused program that aims to increase access to basic life-saving measures and decrease delays in reaching referral facilities. Family and community members are taught techniques such as uterine fundal massage and emergency preparedness. Field tests suggest that HBLSS can be a useful adjunct in a comprehensive PPH prevention and treatment program[30]. Key to the effectiveness of treatment is the early identification of hemorrhage and prompt initiation of treatment.

Long-term strategies

For long-term efficacy, community involvement and development of political will is important. Aspects of such programs include:

(1) *Education of women* Patients in low resource settings generally have a low socioeconomic status. Many are illiterate or have minimal education. Despite this fact, programs that strive to improve pregnancy related morbidity and mortality must include some discussions related to female health education and PPH. Premarital and periconceptional counseling play a vital role in decreasing pregnancy related complications as well as PPH. Girls and young women should be educated regarding the ideal age at marriage, proper spacing of children and correction of anemia before pregnancy or during the antenatal period well before delivery.

(2) *Awareness* The level of awareness regarding the diagnosis and treatment of PPH must increase among health care workers at all levels, and information must be provided to both male and female health workers as well as health assistants and other paramedic staff. Sometimes, involvement of social workers and/or respected personalities from a given locality may help to increase awareness levels.

(3) *Involvement of specialty in district level* Generally almost all of the facilities required for management of PPH are available at the district level. District health officials should make leaflets for attending mothers in the antenatal clinic about the dangers of PPH, correction of anemia, improving nutrition, etc. There should be regular seminars and continuing medical education programs with emphasis on PPH. There should be regular and repeated PPH drills (see Chapter 36) especially involving junior doctors.

(4) *Availability of tertiary care institution* Excellent co-ordination of different departments, experienced doctors, paramedic staff and relevant facilities is the most important treatment component that is available on a 24-hour basis in a tertiary care unit. Any delay in starting treatment in patients referred from a lower level should be avoided.

(5) *Transport/infrastructure* Treatment of PPH and its sequelae demand very rapid action or intervention. Because so many rural communities are truly isolated, not only in India, but also in other developing countries, the most basic arrangements must be thought of in advance. The use of a cell phone method of triage and referral for local transportation has proved useful in many areas of the world where there is no access to ambulances or a 24-hour flying squad with experienced medical and paramedic personnel with basic life-saving support. The use of the NSAG (Chapter 39) is very helpful when the need arises to transport a patient.

(6) *Involvement of government* Strong political will and strengthening health policy for mothers are very important. At the minimum, governments in developing countries should increase health expenditure, strengthen health policies for mothers along with the health infrastructure, increase health awareness, improve the armamentarium of drugs and equipment, and train birth attendants and people in the community with HBLSS.

(7) *Involvement of non-governmental organizations (NGOs)* Involvement of NGOs is very important when governments fail to take the necessary steps, especially in remote areas of the country. Their roles are to help provide necessary funds for increasing health awareness, training birth attendants and training for HBLSS.

(8) *Involvement of professional societies* Local professional bodies such as the obstetrics and gynecological society or national bodies like the Federation of Obstetric and Gynaecological Societies of India (FOGSI) also can take a very important role in decreasing maternal mortality from PPH. Some of their functions include arranging continuing medical education and seminars on PPH throughout the country, performing medical audits, determining the cost-effectiveness of various training programs and assisting the government to determine whether progress is being made towards decreasing mortality from PPH.

(9) *Involvement of international bodies* Organizations such as WHO, FIGO and ICM can play an important role by improving access to knowledge and guidance, providing support, and advocating/facilitating more investment in management and development.

(10) *Emergency obstetric care (EmOC)* The International Conference on Population and Development[31] led the way to an increased understanding of the pathways to avert maternal deaths and disabilities as well as providing strategies to achieve the most favorable results. Although the provision of EmOC is generally accepted as the corner stone of any successful approach to reduce maternal deaths and disabilities, its integration into existing health services and monitoring of its use remain a challenge to existing health systems in developing countries.

The United Nations process indicators describe the vital elements and performance of health systems for women with obstetric complications[31]. EmOC is one of the three-pronged strategies, taken by United Nations Family Planning Association (UNFPA) in the millennium development goals at the Millennium Summit 2000 to reduce maternal mortality, the other two being family planning and skilled attendance at every birth. EmOC refers to a series of functions performed in health care facilities that can prevent the death of a woman experiencing complications of pregnancy. Used properly and in a timely fashion, it can go a long way to averting death from PPH.

To be qualified as a *basic EmOC* center, the health care provider should be able to administer intravenous or intramuscular antibiotics, uterotonic agents and anticonvulsants. Staff should be able to perform manual removal of placenta, assisted vaginal delivery and removal of retained products of conception. Well-trained nurses and midwives can perform most functions at basic EmOC facilities, and most, if not all, of the requirements can be accomplished in the absence of an operating theater.

Comprehensive EmOC refers to the ability to perform a more complex surgical intervention such as cesarean section to relieve obstructed labor and the ability safely to collect, screen and store blood. In general qualified medical personnel and paramedic staff are required to perform the functions of a comprehensive EmOC facility, as is an operating theater.

CONCLUSION

Considering the magnitude of the problem and the fact that PPH is literally a 'serial killer' responsible for the deaths of thousands of women per year, cost-effective means to combat the problem are of particular importance to developing nations.

These same considerations mean that information directed only towards the medical fraternity and health workers will never be sufficient. A combined effort involving society organizations, NGOs and doctors to create awareness and training will go much further in reducing preventable maternal mortality and preventing the disruption of family fabric.

References

1. Trends in Maternal Mortality: 1990–2008. Estimates Developed by WHO, UNICEF, UNFPA and the World Bank. http://www.data.worldbank.org/indicator/SH.STA.MMRT
2. UNFPA. Reproductive Heath fact sheet. www.unfpa.org/swp/2005/presskit/factsheets/facts_rh.htm
3. Mousa HA, Alfirevic Z. Treatment for primary postpartum haemorrhage. Cochrane Database Syst Rev 2003;(1):CD003249
4. Lu MC, Fridman M, Korst LM, et al. Variations in the incidence of postpartum hemorrhage across hospitals in California. Matern Child Health J 2005;9:297
5. International Confederation of Midwives/International Federation of Gynaecology and Obstetrics. Joint statement: prevention and treatment of postpartum hemorrhage. New advances for low resource settings. The Hague: ICM; London: FIGO, 2006. http://internationalmidwives.org or http://figo.org
6. AbouZahr C. Antepartum and postpartum haemorrhage. In Murray CJL, Lopez AD, eds. Health Dimensions of Sex and Reproduction. Boston, MA: Harvard University Press, 1998: 172–4
7. Li XF, Fortney JA, Kotelchuck M, Glover LH. The postpartum period: the key to maternal mortality. Int J Gynecol Obstet 1996;54:1–10
8. United Nations. Millennium Development Goals. New York (NY): UN; 2000. http://www.un.org/millenniumgoals
9. Registrar General of India. Sample Registration System. Registrar General of India, Special Bulletin on Maternal Mortality in India 2004–06 SRS. New Dehli, India: Office of the Registrar General, SRS Bulletin 2000;33:6
10. POPPHI. Report on postpartum haemorrhage. www.pphprevention.org/pph.php
11. WHO. Micronutrient Deficiencies. www.WHO.int/nut/ida.htm
12. Winkvist A, Rasmussen KM, Habicht JP. A new definition of maternal depletion syndrome. Am J Public Health 1992;82:691–4
13. King J. The risk of maternal nutritional depletion and poor outcomes increases in early or closely spaced pregnancies. J Nutr 2003;133:S1732–6
14. WHO. The role of the health centre in maternal health. www.who.int/reproductive-health/publications/msm_94_2/msm_2_2.html
15. Kane TT, Ei-Kady AA, Saleh S, Hage M, Stanback J, Potter L. Maternal mortality in Giza, Egypt: magnitude, causes and prevention. Stud Fam Plann 1992;23:45–57
16. Chua S, Ho LM, Vanaja K, Nordstrom L, Roy AC, Arulkumaran S. Validation of a laboratory method of measuring postpartum blood loss. Gynecol Obstet Invest 1998;46:31–3
17. Duthie SJ, Ven D, Yung GL, Guang DZ, Chan SY, Ma HK. Discrepancy between laboratory determination and visual estimation of blood loss during normal delivery. Eur J Obstet Gynecol Reprod Biol 1991;38:119–24
18. Pritchard JA. Blood volume changes in pregnancy and puerperium. Am J Obstet Gynecol 1962;84:1271
19. Bose P, Regan F, Paterson-Brown S. Improving the accuracy of estimated blood loss at obstetric haemorrhage using clinical reconstructions. Br J Obstet Gynaecol 2006;113:919–24
20. Hofmeyr GJ, Ferreira S, Nikodem VC, et al. Misoprostol for treating postpartum haemorrhage: a randomized controlled trial [ISRCTN72263357]. BMC Pregnancy Childbirth 2004;4:16
21. WHO. Mother–baby package costing spreadsheet. Geneva: WHO, 1999
22. Assistance Afghanistan. 1999 Appeal for Afghanistan Profile of Submissions under Thematic Group. Assistance Afghanistan, 1999
23. AIM for SEVA. Proposal for maternal and child health care along with mobile dispensary. All Indian movement for Seva, 2005
24. Sanghvi H, Wiknjosastro G, Chanpoing G, Fishel J, Ahmed S. Prevention of postpartum hemorrhage study: West Java, Indonesia. Baltimore, MD: JHPIEGO, 2004
25. Creinin MD, Shore E, Balasubramanian S, Harwood B. The true cost differential between mifepristone and misoprostol and misoprostol- alone regimens for medical abortion. Contraception 2005;71:26–30
26. Hensher M, Jefferys E. Financing blood transfusion services in sub-Saharan Africa: a role for user fees? Health Policy Plan 2000;15:287–95
27. Bradley SEK, Prata N, Young-Lin N, Bishai DM. Cost-effectiveness of misoprostol to control postpartum hemorrhage in low resource settings, international. J Gynaecol Obstet 2007;97:54–5
28. Indian Healthcare. Indian healthcare: the growth story. http://www.indianhealthcare.in/index.php?option=com_content&view=article&catid=131&id=168%3AIndian+Healthcare:+The+Growth+Story
29. Derman RJ, Kodkany BS, Goudar SS, et al. Oral misoprostol in preventing postpartum haemorrhage in resource-poor communities: A randomised controlled trial. Lancet 2006;368:1248–53
30. Sibley L, Buffington ST, Haileyesus D. The American College of Nurse Midwives' Home-based lifesaving skills program: a review of the Ethiopia field test. J Midwifery Womens Health 2004;49:320–8 [Erratum appears in J Midwifery Womens Health 2004;49(6):following table of contents]
31. Oladapo OT, Ariba AJ, Odusoga OL. Changing patterns of emergency obstetric care at a Nigerian University hospital. Int J Gynecol Obstet 2007;98:278–84

65

The Obstetrician Confronts Postpartum Hemorrhage

M. E. Setchell

INTRODUCTION

During the author's career in obstetrics, spanning more than 40 years, one of the most striking changes has been that the individual obstetrician no longer has to deal with the problem of PPH alone, but can call on a sophisticated team of helpers, involving a whole range of other specialists. A mere glance at the contents of this book confirms that the modern management of major PPH now involves a team of anesthetists, hematologists, vascular surgeons, gynecologists and radiologists. Clearly, this change represents an advance which has saved and will continue to save countless lives, not only in the developed world where such teamwork is routine, but also in developing nations that are desperately looking for means to reduce maternal mortality as part of their efforts to comply with the United Nations Millennium Development Goals by the year 2015.

HISTORICAL PERSPECTIVE

In the middle of the 19th century, maternal mortality was around 6 per 1000 live births, and, of those deaths, about one-third were related to puerperal sepsis; the remainder were classified as 'accidents of childbirth', which included ante- and postpartum hemorrhage and deaths from obstructed labor. Table 1 shows birth and death rates in England and Wales from 1847 until 1901[1]. During this period, there was no real improvement in the number of deaths from sepsis in contrast to a relative improvement in deaths from other causes.

The concept of 'lying-in' hospitals was first adopted in the mid-18th century, and by 1904 there were 38 such hospitals in Great Britain. The stated intention was to provide a safer place for delivery and postnatal care, but any purported benefits in better obstetric care were far outweighed by the risks of death from sepsis, which, as seen in Table 2, amounted to 3% in the period of 1838–1860[1]. This appalling figure improved considerably during the latter part of the 19th century, as a result of acceptance of Semmelweis' observations and teachings on hygiene and antisepsis in 1861[2].

Francis Ramsbotham, the first Lecturer and Obstetric Physician to The London Hospital, published *The Principles and Practice of Obstetric Medicine and Surgery in*

Table 2 Number of deliveries, deaths and death rates during different time periods in the General Lying-in Hospital, London[1]

Time period	Deliveries	Deaths	Average death rate from all causes
1838–1860	5833	180	1 in 32.5 or 30.85 per 1000
1861–1879	3773	64	1 in 57.87 or 16.96 per 1000
1880–1887	2585	16	1 in 161.5 or 6.18 per 1000
1888–1892	2364	9	1 in 262.67 or 3.80 per 1000

Table 1 Mortality in childbirth in England and Wales 1847–1901 (a period of 54 years)[1]

Year	Registered births of children born alive	Deaths			Death rate per 1000 children born alive, from		
		Puerperal septic diseases and accidents of childbirth	Puerperal septic diseases	Accidents of childbirth	Puerperal septic diseases and accidents of childbirth	Puerperal septic diseases	Accidents of childbirth
1847	539,965	3226	784	2442	5.97	1.45	4.52
1852	624,012	3247	972	2275	5.20	1.56	3.64
1857	663,071	2787	836	1951	4.20	1.26	2.94
1862	712,684	3077	940	2237	4.32	1.32	3.00
1867	768,349	3412	1066	2346	4.44	1.39	3.05
1872	825,907	3803	1400	2403	4.60	1.70	2.90
1877	888,200	3443	1444	1999	3.88	1.63	2.25
1882	889,014	4524	2564	1960	5.09	2.89	2.20
1887	886,331	4160	2450	1710	4.69	2.80	1.90
1892	897,957	5194	2356	2838	5.78	2.62	3.16
1897	921,693	4250	1836	2414	4.61	1.99	2.62
1901	927,807	4394	2079	2315	4.73	2.24	2.49

Reference to the Process of Parturition in 1841, and provided some poignant case reports describing what the practice of obstetrics was like at that time[3]. The case of a rich patient in the City of London, described below, illustrates how little could really be done for intra- and postpartum hemorrhage in 1841.

'Case CIV

I was summoned to a private patient near the Mansion House, who had been, a few minutes before, attacked with a sudden flooding in the eighth month of pregnancy, while sitting with her family at tea, in the drawing-room. Upon proceeding up stairs, tracks of blood were perceptible upon every step. In the bedroom, I found a neighboring professional gentleman, who had been also called by the servants in their alarm at the state of their mistress; and, although this unfortunate occurrence had not happened a quarter of an hour before, it had already produced such a degree of compression as I have rarely witnessed, with its concomitant symptoms. Upon a vaginal examination a little after six, I detected the Placenta to be placed immediately over the Os Uteri; some discharge was still oozing away, but there was no tendency to pain. The urgency of the hemorrhage appeared therefore to be at present somewhat abating; and the lady for a short time seemed disposed to revive; but presently the flooding returned with its original violence. Anxiously watching its progress for a short time, and observing no diminution in the discharge, I determined on delivery; but previously I requested my professional friend to satisfy himself that the Placenta was presenting. Being answered in the affirmative, I proceeded without further loss of time to empty the Uterus. The Os Uteri was but little opened, yet it was relaxed, and permitted the passage of my hand with ease into the Uterus; but that organ showed at the moment no disposition to active contraction; having brought down the breech, the child was found to be alive; I therefore proceeded gently in its extraction; and after the child was born, the Placenta was thrown off, and was soon withdrawn. The uterine tumor [uterus] proved now to be irregularly contracted, and fell flaccid under the hand. For a short time, this lady appeared comfortable; the discharge ceased, and she expressed her warmest thanks for my prompt assistance; but by-and-by she began to complain of her breath: 'Oh! my breath! my breath!' was her urgent exclamation. My patient continued to sink, and expired soon after seven o'clock; so that in less than two hours, from an apparent state of perfect health, her valuable life was sacrificed to a sudden attack of hemorrhage, in spite of the most prompt assistance. The child was lively, and promised to do well.'

THE LONELINESS OF THE OBSTETRICIAN

Fifty years ago, and for the ensuing 20 years at least, *Practical Obstetric Problems* by the late Professor Ian Donald, Professor of Midwifery in the University of Glasgow, was the essential and valued textbook for all young obstetricians of that day[4]. Nowhere is the famous dedication in the frontispiece more relevant than in relation to PPH:

'To all those who have known doubt, perplexity and fear as I have known them,
To all who have made mistakes as I have,
To all whose humility increases with their knowledge of this most fascinating subject,
This book is dedicated.'

The sense of helplessness, loneliness and fear that Dr Ramsbotham must have felt as he watched his patient expire in spite of all his good work and intentions is something that none of us ever wish to experience in our career.

As modern obstetricians, at least those who are in well or moderately resourced countries, we no longer perform our tasks in isolation. We practice in hospitals which, in the majority of instances, are well or relatively well equipped; we are supported by midwives, junior or senior colleagues, and know that various other skilled specialists can be called in for support. Nevertheless, in dealing with PPH, there comes a moment when our decisions and actions (or lack thereof) determine the sequence of events. Even in complex cases of more prolonged hemorrhage, when all the support of the laboratory hematologists, the blood transfusion service, the anesthetic intensivist and other supporting clinicians has been called in, there comes a time when only the attending obstetrician, using his or her best and most considered judgments, has to make a decision about radical treatments such as hysterectomy, laparotomy and hemostatic suturing, ligation of vessels or embolization.

The author's first 'lone' experience with PPH occurred whilst working as a new registrar at the University Hospital of the West Indies in Jamaica. Having just successfully conducted a very straightforward twin delivery, including completion of the third stage of labor with a standard dose of syntometrine, my state of calm was interrupted by a sudden gush of blood of such proportion that it seemed then (and even now) as if an old-fashioned bath tap had been turned on full force. The sound and sight of that hemorrhage will never leave my memory; it was a moment of absolute panic and helplessness. Miraculously, something took over, and decisions and actions were taken as if they were automatic, probably because Professor Ian Donald had been read, and re-read, in preparation for such an event. Bimanual compression, intravenous ergometrine administered by a much more experienced midwifery sister, who then made up a bottle of intravenous Syntocinon® almost without being asked, and the situation was quickly under control. The young obstetrician grew significantly in maturity and experience in those few minutes, grateful that simple actions had averted what had seemed a potential disaster.

During the remaining years of my training, other dramatic postpartum hemorrhagic situations also occurred, but the range of available interventions was limited. Intravenous or intramuscular ergometrine, intravenous Syntocinon infusions, bimanual compression, or packing the uterus with enormous packs (one teacher described putting a pillow case into the uterus first, and then filling it with as many packs as one could get hold of) were the only effective treatments. One had occasionally seen the need for postpartum hysterectomy and internal iliac artery ligation, but, in those circumstances, there had always been the welcome presence of a more senior colleague.

It is not only the trainee obstetrician who is faced with hard decisions. Sometimes, the presence of a large team leads to confusion of leadership. Whilst protocols, guidelines and practice 'drills' may help to coordinate teamwork and familiarize staff in how to deal with these unusual situations, there remain times when the obstetrician has to take command and make rapid or difficult decisions. Even a very experienced obstetrician may be faced with a situation that is unique and not been met with before. Some memorable and rare such cases which have faced the author are now discussed.

Case number 1

A patient had been admitted at 34 weeks with severe abdominal pain, a tense abdomen and absent fetal heart tones. Signs of shock and the tense, tender abdomen suggested a placental abruption, and the cardiovascular and respiratory collapse was of such severity that she was immediately transferred to the intensive care unit (ITU), with a presumed diagnosis of placental abruption. Despite massive blood transfusion, her condition deteriorated, and, despite ventilation, it was difficult to maintain her pO_2. The ITU team felt that attempts to induce labor needed to be delayed until her condition improved. Eventually, ventilation resistance was so great that the ITU team was of the opinion that death was imminent. The obstetrician was therefore asked to consider carrying out a laparotomy and delivery of the dead baby in the hope that this might improve the situation. As the patient was deemed too ill to leave ITU, the operation was performed on an ITU bed. On entering the abdomen, a massive hemoperitoneum was encountered, and the first thought was of a ruptured uterus. However, the uterus was found to be intact, and after further exploration, it became obvious that the source of the intra-abdominal hemorrhage was a ruptured liver. A general surgeon was called, who then secured hemostasis with several large hemostatic liver sutures, and the patient made a slow recovery. During the postoperative period, however, it became apparent that she developed the HELPP (hemolysis, elevated liver enzymes, low platelets) syndrome. A stormy recovery ensued, but a year later the patient was pregnant again and delivered a healthy baby.

Case number 2

Another once-in-a-lifetime experience concerned a late vaginal termination at 18 weeks for a major chromosomal abnormality. During the procedure, it was apparent that the uterus had been perforated and a laparotomy was therefore carried out. A small tear was found in the cecum and a general surgeon called in. He recommended partial right colectomy, which was elegantly performed, and the perforation of the uterus closed without difficulty. A drain was left in the abdomen. An hour later, it was evident that there was major intra-abdominal hemorrhage. The drainage

bottle had filled and been emptied twice, and the abdomen was distended, tense and tender. Unfortunately, the general surgeon had departed for the weekend and was not contactable. When the obstetrician returned, the patient was in a desperate condition, with major cardiovascular collapse. The anesthetist had inserted a subclavian line in order to obtain good venous access, and in doing so had inadvertently caused a pneumothorax. He was therefore inserting a chest drain. Once this had been accomplished and transfusion had restored the blood pressure, a laparotomy was carried out by the obstetrician. A small arterial bleeder was found at the ileo–colic anastomosis and was easily dealt with. The patient, who was the wife of a solicitor, made an uncomplicated recovery. The obstetrician expected that he might find a legal suit impending, but instead received a case of champagne and letter of thanks from the solicitor husband. This lady also subsequently went on to have a successful pregnancy.

Case number 3

On yet another occasion, the author was called in at 3am by a consultant colleague because a patient who had had a vaginal delivery with a very extensive vaginal and perineal laceration was still bleeding heavily after more than an hour of attempted suturing of the tear, and no fewer than 18 units of blood had been transfused. The operating theater looked like a battlefield theater, and the vaginal tissues appeared like wet blotting paper, with no identifiable anatomical layers. By then, the patient had major clotting deficiencies, and anesthetists and hematologists were busy attempting to correct that. Attempts were made at packing the vagina and applying pressure, but to no avail. A gynecological oncology colleague was contacted to discuss internal iliac artery ligation, and he advised that this should be done forthwith. The author had not participated in such a procedure for something like 20 years, and, although the gynecological oncologist said he would come in, he advised that time should not be wasted in getting on with the procedure. To the author's relief, the requisite details of the anatomy and necessary procedure were retrieved from the cerebral archive almost automatically. By the time the oncologist arrived, the hemorrhage was almost completely under control, and it was then possible to complete hemostasis with a few additional vaginal sutures. After a short period of intensive care, the young woman recovered well, as did the anatomy of the vagina and perineum.

Case number 4

A final case involved a collapse at 36 weeks, with abdominal distension and extreme pain and tenderness. The fetal heart tones were still present, and the presumed diagnosis was placental abruption. The patient was immediately taken to theater for cesarean section. On opening the peritoneum, a massive hemoperitoneum gushed forth, but the uterus was perfectly soft and normal in color. A cesarean section was carried out and a healthy baby delivered. It was first thought that the source of bleeding might be a ruptured splenic arterial aneurysm, and a four-quarter exploration of the abdomen was carried out. However, the upper abdomen revealed no bleeding whatsoever, and eventually an arteriovenous malformation at the brim of the pelvis was found to be bleeding. A vascular surgeon was called in to check that hemostasis was satisfactory. After an 8-unit blood transfusion, the patient and baby did well.

CONCLUSION

The plethora of interventions available to the obstetrician now includes many different drugs to promote uterine contraction and hemostasis, a complex range of hematological products and surgical interventions, including the B-Lynch suture, the use of intrauterine pressure balloons, and early resort to hysterectomy or radiological embolization. All are described in detail in other chapters of this book. However, decisions about which intervention to try, and after how much blood loss, remain difficult, and are influenced by the likely future reproductive wishes of the woman, as well as the facilities or lack thereof available in the particular obstetric unit. Whilst much progress has been achieved in the past few decades, there remain many parts of the world where treatment options either are not much greater than they were 50 or more years ago in more developed countries or are even less, being hampered by the logistic considerations detailed in still other chapters in this volume.

Good maternity departments will ensure that cases of serious hemorrhagic incidents, particularly those with such unusual features, are reviewed at multidisciplinary department meetings to rectify any deficiencies in care, and benefit from the learning points.

The major challenge in the 21st century in this field is to narrow the inequalities of health care provision in childbirth. It is hoped that this textbook, will go a long way in helping health care providers to achieve this goal, for it should be obvious, even to the most neophyte reader, that the problems related to PPH are not confined to one country or to one region. They are indeed worldwide, and their control will be facilitated by collaborations and partnerships, as seen in this textbook in which several chapters present details of what is being done in the developing as well as the developed world.

Developments in digital communication technology, particularly the modern mobile telephone, can provide a means of giving immediate advice and instruction to health care workers in remote areas. The spread of knowledge and skills in this way has huge potential to complement this textbook in reducing the inequities of global health care.

References

1. Williams W. Deaths in Childbed. London: H.K. Lewis, 1904
2. Semmelweis IP. Die Aetiologie, der Begriff und die Prophylaxis des Kindbettfiebers. Hartleben: Pest, Wien & Liepzig, 1861
3. Ramsbotham F. The Principles & Practice of Obstetric Medicine and Surgery in Reference to the Process of Parturition. London: Churchill, 1841
4. Donald I. Practical Obstetric Problems, 4th edn. London: Lloyd Luke Ltd, 1969

66

The Midwife Confronts Postpartum Hemorrhage

A. M. Ward

INTRODUCTION

Midwives practicing in the UK today are fortunate to work in a country with a relatively low maternal mortality rate[1,2] and where there has been a significant reduction in the number of women dying from postpartum hemorrhage (PPH) in the past decade[2]. At first glance, the role of midwives in such circumstances may seem obvious, that is, they should diagnose the bleed, call for help and instigate emergency treatment[3]. However, the reality of the management of PPH is much more complex and involves an ability to work effectively within a multidisciplinary team and to possess in depth knowledge of the social, psychological and physiological processes that surround pregnancy and childbirth. Midwives should be central to the prevention, identification and management of PPH and these precepts form the focus of this chapter. The degree to which midwives can achieve these goals will obviously vary with local customs, resources and practices, but the goals should remain the same regardless.

PREVENTION OF POSTPARTUM HEMORRHAGE

Antenatal prevention

Prevention of PPH should begin in the antenatal period by assessing women's risk factors at every antenatal visit and then, in partnership with the women, planning care that identifies the most appropriate lead health care professional[4]. The antenatal risk factors most commonly reported for PPH are[2,5]:

- Body mass index >30 kg/m^2
- Previous PPH
- Antepartum hemorrhage
- Placental abruption
- Placenta previa
- Multiple pregnancy
- Macrosomic infant
- Previous uterine surgery
- Antenatal anticoagulation.

Other risk factors include anemia, polyhydramnios, maternal age, uterine fibroids and a history of retained placenta[6,7]. Nulliparity has recently been identified as a possible risk factor for PPH, rather than grand multiparity[8]. This is important as this group of women have not previously been identified as being at significant risk of PPH. In the past, the management of such women may have been substandard as PPH was not anticipated[8].

The above-mentioned risk factors focus totally on the physical aspects of pregnancy. To ensure the optimum safety of women and their babies, as well as to ensure provision of holistic care, these factors need to be assessed in conjunction with other risk factors associated with severe maternal morbidity including maternal age more than 34 years, social exclusion and non-white ethnicity[1,2,4,9,10].

Midwives particularly need to focus care on women who book late, are poor attendees, or who do not access antenatal care at all, as these characteristics are key indicators of poorer outcomes[2]. Such an approach requires effective communication links with other groups such as public health nurses, general practitioners and social services, so that these particular women are identified as being pregnant as early as possible and provided care in an appropriate environment tailored to meet their social, cultural and psychological needs[2,11].

Although the National Institute for Clinical Excellence (NICE) has produced guidelines for antenatal care of healthy pregnant women in the UK[4], midwives need to be mindful that the guidelines are intended to guide the care of healthy pregnant women. The NICE document[4] clearly states that women should have a plan of care that is relevant to their individual physical, social and psychological needs, and the World Health Organization (WHO)[11] further indicates that this also needs to be culturally specific to women's backgrounds if it is to be truly effective.

Knowing the risk factors for PPH, and identifying them is not enough if appropriate care is not then instigated[2]. Even where women have strong views about the type of childbirth experience they desire, open, frank discussion of identified risk factors and their implications for women and their babies, with time to assimilate and consider the information provided, leads to stronger relationships between women and midwives, and reduces the potential for conflict when the safest management of care conflicts with women's wishes for their childbirth experience[12–16].

Intrapartum prevention

Intrapartum prevention of PPH should begin antenatally with the aim of helping women to be as healthy as possible, both physically and emotionally, and should include preparation for childbirth, focusing on strategies to keep the process normal[8,16]. Throughout the intrapartum period, midwives need to continually support women, encouraging them to be mobile and offering information on alternative methods of pain relief that are less likely to interrupt the progress of labor[16–18]. As labor causes a great deal of insensible fluid loss, women need to be kept well hydrated to ensure adequate circulating volumes at delivery in the advent of excessive blood loss[16,19]. Women should also be provided with a quiet, private environment where they feel safe and protected, thereby reducing the need for intervention during the process of labor[18,20]. Such practices are even more vital in areas without direct access to intravenous fluids in the event of PPH.

Midwives require an in depth understanding of all intrapartum risk factors for PPH and constantly need to reassess the woman throughout labor[17,21] for the following:

- Prolonged labor >12 h
- Prolonged third stage >30 min
- Retained placenta
- Febrile illness
- Instrumental delivery
- Cesarean section, especially emergencies in late first or second stage of labor
- Amniotic fluid embolism
- Placental abruption.

The first four conditions are most likely to cause uterine atony, whereas operative deliveries are the main cause of uterine, cervical or vaginal trauma; embolisms and abruptions are common causes of coagulopathy, although these causes are the least common reasons for PPH[2,5].

The debate regarding whether to manage the third stage of labor actively could fill an entire text itself, especially when considering practices in the UK and other developed countries. In developing countries, however, this debate takes on a different form, and routine active management of the third stage of labor could and does save many women's lives as well as saving many others from the abject misery of severe morbidity brought about by PPH[1,6,8,9,11].

Table 1 Options for the management of the third stage of labor

Active management	Expectant management
Oxytocic drug given at delivery of anterior shoulder	No oxytocic drug given
Cord clamped and cut immediately	Cord not clamped until pulsation ceased, then only clamped at baby's umbilicus
When uterus is central and well contracted, controlled cord traction applied	No cord traction Signs of separation awaited: • Rise in fundus • Lengthening of cord • Trickle of blood at introitus
Midwife delivers placenta and membranes	Maternal effort delivers placenta and membranes

The type of management used for the third stage of labor may be of no real consequence in a well nourished, healthy population, but it is vitally important that midwives can clearly identify those women at increased risk of PPH, as well as understanding and carrying out expectant and active management of the third stage of labor[22]. Table 1 describes the main components of each management option for the third stage of labor.

DIAGNOSIS AND PREVENTION OF POSTPARTUM HEMORRHAGE

Definitions may not be useful in themselves, as they often involve measurement of blood loss retrospectively[2,23], a task which is notoriously inaccurate and difficult[23] regardless of whether all blood loss is revealed or remains partially concealed (see Chapters 9 and 11). Healthy, young women can compensate for routine postdelivery blood loss very effectively, and this ability is increased even further if there has been a healthy increase in blood volume during pregnancy[19]. Normally, plasma volume increases by 1250 ml and the red cell mass also increases, resulting in women being able to tolerate a drop in their pre-delivery blood volume of up to 25% and remain hemodynamically stable[19]. In practice, however, this means that midwives need to be encouraged to use their clinical observational skills, remaining ever vigilant to signs of the earlier stages of shock – pallor, sweating and muscle weakness characterized by severe and rapid fatigue[19]. When women become restless and confused, shock is advancing rapidly and immediate, aggressive treatment is needed if not already instigated[19] (see also Chapter 13).

PPH is either primary (occurring within the first 24 h after birth) or secondary (occurring after 24 h and before 6 weeks postpartum)[2]. In practice, PPH has three different presentations[23]:

- Rapid loss of blood at or just shortly after delivery
- Constant heavy lochia that persists for a significant length of time after delivery
- Bleeding after the first 24 h following childbirth.

It is the second type of bleeding that can cause problems for health care practitioners, because it is often missed. Women will experience heavy lochia that they report. Their sanitary protection will be changed and then, a little while later, it will happen again and be reported, but this may be to another member of staff who is unaware of the previous loss. Midwives and midwifery assistants should not only quantify the amount of blood lost, but also record this in the maternal notes, keeping a running total of the amount of blood lost to alert them to women who are bleeding significantly but still compensating adequately[19].

MANAGEMENT OF POSTPARTUM HEMORRHAGE

The Royal College of Obstetricians and Gynaecologists[2] discusses how the practical management of PPH can be viewed as having four component considerations:

- Communication
- Resuscitation
- Monitoring and investigations
- Taking measures to arrest the bleeding.

As any PPH has the potential to cause maternal collapse with loss of consciousness, midwives need to be competent with basic life support (ABC algorithm)[19,24,25]. The first principle of which is that a single individual cannot effectively manage an emergency situation, and help must be urgently requested prior to commencing any treatment[25]. Midwives need constantly to ensure that women have patent airways and are breathing adequately; here, expensive technology is not required. If women do not respond when spoken to, then they potentially cannot manage their own airway and an individual with the appropriate skills and training needs to do this. Until the airway and breathing are effectively brought under control, there is little point undertaking any other task, as hypoxia can kill women much faster than hypovolemia[19]. Once sufficient members of the team are present, they can move on to maintaining the circulatory system and determining the cause of the PPH (see Chapter 36).

A major step towards reducing morbidity and mortality in the management of PPH is effective fluid resuscitation[19,23,24] (see also Chapter 10). Midwives may be concerned about which fluids are best, but their focus needs to be on ensuring fluid is administered quickly and is not cold. Where available, fluid warmers and pressure bags must be utilized. Every 1 ml of blood lost needs to be replaced with 3 ml of fluid until blood is available[19,23,24]. To ensure fluid can be delivered as quickly as possible, two wide-bore, short needles should be placed into major veins, as the volume that can be infused through a given cannula is proportional to the diameter and inversely proportional to its length[19]. Midwives justly may be concerned about commencing intravenous fluids without

prescription or written order, but as PPH represents a true emergency situation midwives can administer resuscitative fluids without first obtaining a prescription[3]. Women need to be kept warm as hypothermia is a consequence of hypovolemic shock[19,24]. As the assessment of renal function is an essential part of management, an indwelling urinary catheter should be inserted using strict aseptic techniques to avoid infection in women who are already compromised as a result of the PPH[19].

CARE AFTER POSTPARTUM HEMORRHAGE

Women who have sustained a significant PPH need to receive one-to-one care to facilitate close monitoring[6,8,9,26]. Initially, the focus of care will be on the woman's physical condition, observing and monitoring urinary output, fluid intake, vital signs and subsequent blood loss. Ideally, such care is best provided in an obstetric high-dependency unit if available. On the other hand, any women requiring mechanical ventilation should be cared for in an intensive care unit[6,8,9,26].

Intensive monitoring often means that other aspects of care important to women following childbirth are neglected[27]. Care provided by midwives also needs to include the psychological well-being of women and the integration of the family unit who may be bewildered by the goings-on after the delivery[19,27]. Women who are conscious need to have contact with their babies and feel central in any decision-making around the care of their babies[28]. Skin–skin contact is a simple procedure that can be carried out even for the sickest women and can be beneficial to women as well as their babies; it assists in the effective introduction of breastfeeding and has relaxing properties for women and babies alike[29].

Given the traumatic nature of PPH, women need support for a considerable length of time into the postnatal period as they recover physically and emotionally[30]. Initial debriefing may not be beneficial and may, in fact, be detrimental to these women, as many are too consumed by the rapidity of the ongoing resuscitative efforts to comprehend truly what is being said in an effective manner. Later debriefing may discuss, among other things, the risk of recurrence in a later or subsequent pregnancy. After the initial crisis has passed, these women need effective long-term follow-up. In larger units, it may be appropriate to have a lead midwife and obstetrician to run combined postnatal clinics for the women, where recovery can be monitored and any concerns about subsequent pregnancies can be discussed with relevant health care professionals[30].

DOCUMENTATION

Accurate documentation is crucial during an emergency procedure and the leader of the emergency team needs to designate someone by name to record events as they occur, including the times team members enter and leave the room, as well as the timing of any procedures and drugs administered, including route and dose[31]. Good records are an indication that the quality of care given to women was of an adequate standard[31]. Midwives have a professional duty to ensure records are kept as contemporaneously and accurately as possible[3,31]. Good practice is to ensure that the documentation completed by the named scribe is included in the maternal records and not disposed of once individual health care practitioners have used them to complete their own notes. Accurate record-keeping is vital to reduce the risk of successful litigation, but it is also vital in the active debriefing of all team members[32] (see also Chapter 36). Simple factors dramatically improve the quality of record-keeping and only take seconds[29]. These include:

- Dating and timing all entries

- Printing name and qualification alongside the first signature in any records

- Writing legibly.

Documentation of vital signs and urine output is essential following significant PPH, but documentation itself will not ensure effective management of sick patients. It is vital to ensure that trends in all important physical parameters, especially respiration, are recognized and acted upon, because they indicate the effectiveness of any treatment as well as when women are deteriorating[27,28]. Scoring tools can be developed that assist practitioners to identify women who are not responding to treatment and, therefore, require the expertise of senior obstetricians and anesthetists and admission to an intensive care setting.

COMMUNICATING EFFECTIVELY

In any emergency health care situation, professionals are relieved when help arrives, but the larger the team the more complex the communication process and the more difficult it can be to manage the situation effectively and utilize the team efficiently[32,33]. Someone needs to take charge, stand back, observe and then direct the working of the team[32,34]. The role of this lead individual is also constantly to evaluate the effectiveness of treatments instigated and constantly to be re-thinking the potential causes of PPH when the treatment instigated is not being effective in controlling the bleeding[35]. Historically, this lead person has been the most senior obstetrician on duty in the obstetric maternity unit. Both obstetricians and midwives recognize that the person co-ordinating the team at an emergency should be the most experienced clinician available[32,34]. In some circumstances, however, this may be the senior midwife who will be more experienced than the house officers. An emergency situation is no time for hierarchy to interfere with communication which needs to be precise, with tasks directed to a named individual and feedback requested from that individual at regular intervals. Training of teams, within individual units or the community setting, needs to be multidisciplinary, realistic to the

work environment, scenario-driven and based on real timing and action to make it as realistic as possible[34]. For example, if simulating PPH in a home setting, then paramedics need to be involved and the setting should reflect the equipment that would be available to midwives in those situations. For midwife-led units not attached to obstetric units, the training also should involve paramedics and the ambulance service and not include management regimens using drugs and techniques that are not available to those midwives.

TRAINING

Team sports have recognized for decades that members must train together to ensure that a team functions efficiently and effectively; such training must focus on utilizing individual skills to their greatest potential for the good of the team. In the NHS, individual professional bodies have trained their own practitioners largely in isolation of other health care professionals while, at the same time, expecting them to work as a well-oiled machine in times of great stress with minimal understanding of each others' strengths and weaknesses[32,36]. Happily, this trend is changing and the benefit of multidisciplinary training is now recognized as an essential part of safe maternity services[2].

In the Yorkshire Region (UK), this has been taken one step further with many maternity units adopting a regional training program aimed at managing the first 20–30 min of obstetric emergencies effectively. As medical trainees rotate around the Region, they are expected to complete a systematic approach to the training for management of obstetric emergencies as early as possible in their time in a new unit. Units in the Region that have adopted the training have made it mandatory for anyone involved in the intrapartum care of women, from health care assistants to consultants.

Scenarios are run real-time using mannequins, and participants are expected to carry out procedures as if it were a real emergency. This is then videoed, and the participants debrief themselves, with a facilitator assisting them to focus on issues of breaches of leadership, control and communication, all of which have been highlighted as factors in suboptimal care[2]. Dedicated time is provided for this training, which improves outcomes and can be achieved with effective timing and allocation[37]. Anecdotally, training improves communication and team work, but it also needs to be audited against unit guidelines considering maternal outcomes and focusing on morbidity and mortality rates, as well as adherence to the guidelines themselves.

DEBRIEFING

Part of ensuring a team learns from stressful clinical incidences is a review of their performance as close to the event as possible. The purpose of this 'debriefing' session should be to focus on what was done well and, conversely, to point out those actions that require further attention. Debriefing also can be used to identify what needs to be shared with team members not involved in the emergency, to aid their development and learning, as well as to provide a forum where those involved in the emergency can vocalize how they feel in a protective environment. This will enable learning whilst, at the same time, offering professional and emotional support, recognizing that health care professionals are caring individuals who can be profoundly affected by traumatic situations[38,39].

Finally, debriefing is a useful tool to help team members recognize that they are valued as is the role they play in the effective running of the team, all of which can help increase job satisfaction and reduce the number of professionals leaving midwifery and obstetrics[38,39].

CONCLUSION

Midwives are central to the effective prevention, recognition and treatment of PPH. They need to be aware of the risk factors for this condition and take appropriate action when they are identified. They should also be skilled in basic life support and have an understanding of the pathophysiology of hypovolemic shock. This knowledge must be used in conjunction with an understanding of women's social, cultural and psychological well-being.

Training as multidisciplinary teams can be effective in improving outcomes for women and their families. The Yorkshire model may be beneficial in units that have trainees who rotate throughout the region. Effective communication and leadership are vital in the management of any obstetric emergency and scenario-based training can be used to highlight issues of control and communication.

References

1. Khan SK, Wojdyla D, Say L, Gülmezoglu AM, Van Look P. WHO analysis of causes of maternal death: a systematic review. Lancet 2006;367:1066–74
2. Confidential Enquiry into Maternal and Child Health (CEMACH). Saving Mothers Lives: reviewing maternal deaths to make motherhood safer (2003–2005). London, UK: Royal College of Obstetricians and Gynaecologists, 2010
3. Nursing and Midwifery Council (NMC). Midwives Rules and Standards. London: NMC, 2004
4. National Institute for Health and Clinical Excellence (NICE). Antenatal Care. Routine Care for the Healthy Pregnant Woman. NICE clinical guideline 62, London: NICE, 2008
5. McLintock C. State-of-the-art lectures: Postpartum Haemorrhage. Thrombosis Res 2005;1155:65–8
6. Royal College of Obstetricians and Gynaecologists. Prevention and Management of Postpartum Haemorrhage. Green-top Guideline No. 52. 2009 http://www.rcog.org.uk/files/rcogcorp/GT52PostpartumHaemorrhage0411.pdf. Accessed December 2011
7. Selo-Ojeme DO. Primary postpartum haemorrhage. J Obstet Gynaecol 2002;22:463–9
8. Hazra S, Chilaka VN, Rajendran S, Konje JC. Massive postpartum haemorrhage as a cause of maternal morbidity in a large tertiary hospital. J Obstet Gynaecol 2004;24:519–20
9. Waterstone M, Wolfe C, Hooper R, Bewley S. Postnatal morbidity after childbirth and severe obstetric morbidity. Br J Obstet Gynaecol 2003;110:128–33
10. Doran T, Denver F, Whitehead M. Is there a north-south divide in social class inequalities in health in Great Britain? Cross sectional study using data from 2001 census. Br Med J 2004;328:1043–5
11. World Health Organization. WHO Guidelines for the Management of PPH and Retained Placenta. Geneva, Switzerland: WHO, 2009
12. Graham WJ, Hundley V, McCheyne AL, Hall MH, Gurney E, Milne J. An investigation of women's involvement in the decision to deliver by caesarean section. Br J Obstet Gynaecol 1999;106:213–20
13. Buckley SJ. Undisturbed birth – nature's hormonal blueprint for safety, ease and ecstasy. J Perinatal Psychol Health 2003;17:261–88
14. Guiver D. The epistemological foundation of midwife-led care that facilitates normal birth. Evidence Based Midwifery 2004;2:28–34
15. Hunter B. Conflicting ideologies as a source of emotion work in midwifery. Midwifery 2004;20:261–72
16. National Institute for Health and Clinical Excellence (NICE). Intrapartum care: care of healthy women and their babies during childbirth. NICE clinical guideline 55. London, UK: NICE, 2007
17. Yogev S. Support in labour: a literature review. MIDIRS Midwifery Digest 2004;14:486–92
18. Oudshoorn C. The art of midwifery, past, present and future. MIDIRS Midwifery Digest 2005;15:461–8
19. Stainsby D, MacLennan S, Thomas D, Issac J, Hamilton PJ. Guidelines on the management of massive blood loss. Br J Haematol 2006;135:634–41
20. Ryan M, Roberts C. A retrospective cohort study comparing the clinical outcomes of a birth centre and labour ward in the same hospital. Aust Midwifery J 2005;18:17–21
21. Simpson KR. Failure to rescue: implications for evaluating quality of care during labour and birth. J Perinat Neonat Nursing 2005;19:24–34
22. Prendiville WJP, Elbourne D, McDonald SJ Active versus expected management in the third stage of labour. Cochrane Database Syst Rev 2000;(3):CD000007
23. Mousa HA, Alfirevic Treatment for primary postpartum haemorrhage. Cochrane Database Syst Rev 2007;(1):CD003249
24. Clarke J, Butt M. Maternal collapse. Curr Opin Obstet Gynecol 2005;17:157–60
25. Resuscitation Council (UK). Resuscitation Guidelines 2010 [online]. http://www.resus.org.uk/pages/guide.htm
26. Paruk F, Moodley J. Severe obstetric morbidity. Curr Opin Obstet Gynecol 2001;13:563–8
27. Okafor UV, Aniebu U. Admission pattern and outcome in critical care obstetric patients. Int J Obstet Anesthesia 2004;13:164–6
28. Goebel N. High dependency midwifery care – does it make a difference? MIDIRS Midwifery Digest 2004;14:221–6
29. Carfoot S, Williamson P, Dickson R. A randomised controlled trial in the north of England examining the effects of skin-to-skin contact on breast feeding. Midwifery 2005;21:71–9
30. Kline CR, Martin DP, Deyo RA. Health consequences of pregnancy and childbirth as perceived by women and clinicians. Obstet Gynecol 1998;92:842–8
31. Nursing and Midwifery Council (NMC). Guidelines for Records and Record Keeping. London: NMC, 2009
32. Brownlee M, McIntosh C, Wallace E, Johnston F, Murphy-Black T. A survey of inter-professional communication in a labour suite. Br J Midwifery 1996;4:492–5
33. Duff E. No more 'quarrelling at the mother's bedside': inter-professional approaches can help to stop women dying. MIDIRS Midwifery Digest 2004;14:35–6
34. Cro S, King B, Paine P. Practice makes perfect: maternal emergency training. Br J Midwifery 2001;9:492–6
35. Mousa HA, Walkinshaw S. Major postpartum haemorrhage. Curr Opin Obstet Gynecol 2001;13:595–603

36. Heagerty BV. Reassuring the guilty: the midwives act and the control of English midwives in the early 20th century. In: Kirkham M, ed. Supervision of Midwives. Cheshire: Books for Midwives Press, 1996

37. Sabey A, Jacobs K. Live and learn. Health Service J 2003;16: 32–3

38. Dennis CL, Creedy DK. Psychosocial and psychological interventions for preventing postpartum depression. Cochrane Database Syst Rev 2004;(4):CD001134

39. National Institute for Health and Clinical Excellence (NICE). Antenatal and Postnatal Mental Health: Clinical Management and Service Guidance. NICE clinical guideline 45. London UK: NICE, 2007

67

A Community-Based Continuum of Care Model for the Prevention and Treatment of Postpartum Hemorrhage in Low Resource Settings

C. T. Kapungu, A. Koch, S. Miller and S. E. Geller

World Health Organization (WHO) estimates that 358,000 women died in pregnancy or childbirth in 2008, which is a 34% decline in maternal mortality globally since 1990[1]. Despite this decline, low resource countries, where women deliver at home or in rudimentary health facilities, continue to account for 99% of maternal deaths. The most common cause of preventable maternal mortality and morbidity in these countries is postpartum hemorrhage (PPH)[2].

Numerous challenges to the prevention and treatment of PPH exist in low resource countries. These include unavailability of skilled health care providers, lack of uterotonics and cold storage, minimal or incorrect practice of the principles of active management of the third stage of labor, underestimation of blood loss and, finally, deficiencies in the communication and transportation infrastructure which impede transfer to a higher level of care. In addition, four delays in response to obstetric complications represent key contributors to maternal mortality and inhibit appropriate provision of care in cases of PPH. They are: (1) delay in problem recognition (inability to quantitate accurately the amount of blood loss); (2) delay in deciding to seek assistance from skilled obstetric care providers; (3) delay in reaching a facility that can provide life-saving treatment; and (4) delay at that facility in providing quality emergency treatment[3]. Such delays must be overcome on a regular and continuing basis in order to reduce the burden of morbidity and mortality from PPH that exist in remote settings.

A continuum of care model for PPH (CC-PPH) incorporates multiple strategies to address the full spectrum of clinical, social and system factors related to morbidity and mortality from PPH in low resource settings[4]. The main components of this model (Figure 1) are: (1) community mobilization; (2) the routine use of prophylactic misoprostol or other appropriate uterotonics; (3) early and accurate identification of excessive blood loss; (4) availability of a non-pneumatic anti-shock garment (NASG); (5) systemization of communication, transportation and referral to higher-level facilities; and (6) access to quality, appropriate and timely comprehensive emergency obstetric care (CEmOC). In this chapter, we present a CC-PPH model which can be implemented to address the factors that lead to unnecessary maternal deaths in low resource settings.

IMPLEMENTING CONTINUUM OF CARE MODEL FOR POSTPARTUM HEMORRHAGE IN LOW RESOURCE SETTINGS

Community mobilization

The first component of the CC-PPH model is community mobilization. Community awareness about the four delays and health interventions that can prevent and treat PPH are necessary for women to access life-saving EmOC. Community mobilization is a 'capacity-building process through which community individuals, groups, or organizations plan, carry out, and evaluate activities on a participatory and sustained basis to improve their health and other needs, either on their own initiative or stimulated by others'[5].

Community mobilization/ raising awareness	All births	If excessive bleeding continues	If woman develops signs of shock	Referral
Develop emergency communication/transport referral plan	Administer uterotonics → Measure blood loss	Alert transport → systems and prepare for transport	Apply non-pneumatic → anti-shock garment (NASG)	Refer and transport → to emergency obstetric care

Figure 1 Continuum of care model for postpartum hemorrhage

Community mobilization involves developing an ongoing dialogue between community members about their health issues, empowering the community to address its own health needs, and working in partnership with the health care system to create locally appropriate responses to community health needs[5].

The success of effective and sustainable community-based health interventions is often attributed, at least in part, to an ability to engage and maintain the trust of community members[6–8]. Health providers, non-governmental organizations (NGOs) and ministries of health (MOHs) can provide unique opportunities to identify and build on the assets and resources that already exist in collaboration with communities. Advocacy with government officials and key stake-holders is a necessary step for fostering sustainability and scaling up of community health interventions.

Successful community mobilization requires multiple methods at the community and national level to increase the acceptance and adoption of health interventions. Raising awareness about PPH can promote an understanding of the existing barriers faced in accessing EmOC and mobilize the community to identify strategies that may improve maternal health outcomes. Birth and complication readiness plans can address the first three delays, in recognizing the problem, in deciding to seek care, and in reaching the facility. Community transport plans can be collaboratively developed by community members and health facilities within each neighborhood or village so that families can be prepared when emergencies arise.

One of the authors of this chapter, Stacie Geller, has described the community mobilization activities conducted prior to and throughout the introduction of the use of misoprostol and the blood collection drape for the prevention and early diagnosis of PPH in collaboration with the Millennium Villages Project in rural Ghana. The CC-PPH model was presented to key opinion leaders such as chiefs, religious leaders, senior women, assemblymen, herbalists and traditional birth attendants (TBAs) to establish rapport and obtain community support. Focus group discussions were held with local women's groups such as pregnant and nursing mothers, and those who experienced PPH in their last deliveries. Key opinion leaders developed community sensitization messages to increase awareness of and knowledge about PPH, misoprostol and the blood collection drape (for prompt recognition of excessive bleeding). TBAs, community health educators (CHEWs) and other health providers were also trained on safe delivery and the use of misoprostol and the blood collection drape. Educational materials such as pamphlets, brochures, posters and pictorial flipcharts were developed to provide education about PPH and the danger signs related to hemorrhage. Using these strategies and tools, CHEWs, TBAs and midwives mobilized their communities to make specific plans for emergency response (transport, savings to pay for fuel and facility fees, blood donation) and to take prompt action if PPH were to occur. It is critical to involve the entire community in order to improve individual access to EmOC, and community mobilization should be prioritized as a key strategy in the CC-PPH model. Other components of the model will be more successful if the community is sufficiently engaged early in the process.

Use of misoprostol or other uterotonics

Administration of a uterotonic for prevention of PPH is the next component of the CC-PPH model. Oxytocin, the uterotonic of choice, is often not feasible in community-level settings without skilled attendants, cold storage or sterile equipment. For women delivering outside skilled facilities, misoprostol is accepted to be safe and effective in the prevention of PPH[9–12]. The International Federation of Gynecology and Obstetrics (FIGO) has endorsed misoprostol use for settings in which oxytocin is unavailable or in the absence of active management of the third stage of labor[13]. In such settings, WHO also recommends the administration of 600 μg oral misoprostol by a health worker trained in its use immediately after the birth of the baby[14,15] (see Chapter 42).

Multiple models exist for the distribution of misoprostol in community-level settings, and the appropriate model for each setting depends on the community infrastructure and national policies regarding use of misoprostol, as well as the availability of community-level providers. Misoprostol has been registered for use in PPH in 17 countries in Africa and Asia as of August 2010[16]; however, it has not yet been implemented as the standard of care for all community-level births in any of these countries. Pilot programs of community-based misoprostol distribution are underway, but only a few have been evaluated to date.

Two randomized double-blind placebo-controlled trials of 600 μg oral misoprostol administered by TBAs after delivery showed that misoprostol is associated with a significant reduction in the rate of PPH (blood loss of 500 ml or more)[9,11]. In a remote region of Pakistan, misoprostol was associated with a significant reduction in the rate of PPH in deliveries under the care of TBAs (16.5% vs. 21.9%; RR 0.76, 95% CI 0.59–0.97) compared with placebo. Additionally, significantly fewer women in the misoprostol group experienced a drop of more than 3 g/dl in hemoglobin compared with those in the placebo group (RR 0.53, 95% CI 0.34–0.83)[9]. These findings are consistent with an earlier community-based trial of misoprostol administered by auxiliary nurse-midwives attending births at home or in lower-level facilities in rural India, which showed a nearly 50% reduction in PPH (RR 0.53, 95% CI 0.39–0.74)[11].

In settings where terrain or weather prevents women from delivering in the company of birth attendants or where community-level health providers are barred from distributing medication, direct distribution of misoprostol to pregnant women may be the most feasible model for distribution. Two recent operations research studies of direct provision of misoprostol to pregnant women provide examples for the implementation of this model[17,18]. These studies focused on program effectiveness, the acceptability of misoprostol and adverse effects, but did not aim to prove the efficacy of misoprostol to prevent PPH since it has been previously proven efficacious and safe.

A non-randomized comparative study of women in rural Afghanistan utilized semiliterate community health workers (CHWs) to provide three 200 μg tablets of misoprostol to 2039 women in the 8th month of pregnancy, along with an educational intervention to the women and their household support members on the correct and safe use of misoprostol[17]. In structured interviews conducted 1 week postpartum, all the women who took misoprostol ($n = 1421$) reported taking the drug after delivery of the baby. Women in the intervention group were significantly more likely to have reported experience of no side-effects compared with 1148 women in the control group who received usual care (60.3% vs. 18.6%). The authors stated that the high rate of adverse symptoms in the control groups was likely due to the use of herbal products.

Similarly, female community health volunteers (FCHVs) in rural Nepal distributed three 200 μg tablets of misoprostol to women late in pregnancy for self-administration at home births[18]. Program performance was evaluated through pre- and post-intervention household surveys and data collected by FCHVs and other health providers. The primary outcome was overall coverage with uterotonics among women with vaginal delivery, which significantly increased from 11.6% at baseline to 74.2% at the end of the study (OR 25.0, 95% CI 15.6–40.1). The mortality rate among misoprostol users was 72 per 100,000 compared with 292 per 100,000 among non-users, but the number of deaths by specific causes was too low to evaluate differences statistically. Misoprostol users were more likely to report shivering than non-users, but the difference was not statistically significant.

Administration of a uterotonic for prevention of PPH in a low resource setting is an important component of the CC-PPH model, but even with prophylaxis, some women experience PPH. The next steps in the CC-PPH model address identification of and response to excessive bleeding.

Accurate assessment of blood loss

Visual estimation of blood loss is notoriously inaccurate even among the most skilled health providers[19]. Family members and unskilled birth attendants are believed to perceive the signs of excessive bleeding during labor and postpartum only 11% of the time[20]. To address the delay in problem recognition, community-based health providers and family members need to acquire the necessary skills to recognize danger signs of excessive bleeding. A reliable blood loss detection method assists birth attendants rapidly to recognize excessive bleeding instead of waiting for changes in vital signs (blood pressure, pulse and pallor) and/or unconsciousness.

There are several novel approaches for timely and accurate assessment of PPH in low resource settings. The kanga, a garment used in Tanzania, is a standard sized rectangular cotton cloth used to absorb the blood during delivery. Two kangas have been found to hold slightly more than 500 ml when completely soaked, providing a convenient unit of measure that has been used to recognize PPH[21]. The kanga method can be adapted to other standardized cloths used in other countries such as the sari, dupatta, sarong or to manufactured absorbent pads. However, its utility would always be dependent on the user's judgment of degree of saturation.

The BRASSS-V blood collection drape (Figure 2), a low-cost calibrated and funneled collecting pouch attached to a plastic sheet, was developed to measure accurately postpartum blood loss at the time of deliveries taking place at home and in rudimentary facilities[22,23]. The drape is placed under the woman's buttocks immediately after delivery, and the two strings attached to the upper end of the drape are tied around the woman's abdomen to optimize blood collection. A randomized controlled study found a high level of correlation ($r = 0.928$) between the drape estimate and the 'gold standard' of photospectrometry, demonstrating the accuracy of drape collection[24]. In the same study, visual assessment underestimated postpartum blood loss by 33% compared with drape assessment (203 ml ± 147 ml vs. 304 ml ± 173 ml, $p < 0.001$)[24]. The drape has been used in multiple

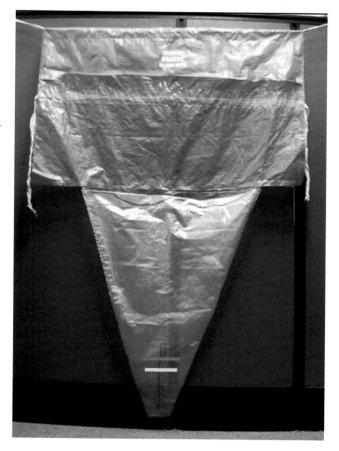

Figure 2   The BRASSS-V blood collection drape

research studies worldwide which have validated its accuracy and ease of use as a practical tool to measure blood loss occurring during the third stage of labor[25,26] (see Chapter 9 and 11).

The blood mat (Figure 3), made of layers of cotton backed by plastic and developed by Dr Abdul Quaiyum, a researcher at the International Centre for Diarrhoeal Disease Research in Bangladesh (ICDDRB), also has been used by families and community health workers to identify hemorrhage in women giving birth at home[27]. Dr Quaiyum received a grant from the Bill and Melinda Gates Foundation in 2010 to develop and test a biodegradable birth mat that can only absorb 500 ml of fluid[28]. Placed under the mother immediately after birth, if the mat stops absorbing blood, it indicates that the mother has bled more than 500 ml, and that she should be referred immediately to a higher-level facility.

Almost any type of fabric or calibrated container can be used to measure blood loss in low resource settings. However, the key factor is standardization and validation of measurement. Regional or local groups of health educators or workers can fashion pads, mats or kangas out of locally acquired materials. They can then take a measured amount of fluid and determine what amount saturates the material. As long as these homemade pads are made of similar materials in absorbency and size, then a somewhat more accurate assessment of blood loss can be made.

Earlier detection of excessive blood loss means earlier action to provide medical management and/or transfer the woman to a higher-level facility. Even with primary prophylaxis and early detection of PPH, however, a woman may continue to bleed and progress into shock. Delayed diagnosis and treatment of continuing blood loss in combination with underestimation may quickly lead to hypovolemic shock, cardiopulmonary arrest and death[29]. The non-pneumatic anti-shock garment (NASG), the fourth component of the CC-PPH model is used to resuscitate and stabilize women in shock until comprehensive care for PPH is available.

Non-pneumatic anti-shock garment

The NASG addresses the delay in reaching the facility by keeping the woman stable long enough to be transported and seek further treatment. It is a lightweight, inexpensive, reusable, first aid device which decreases blood loss and restores vital signs (Figure 4).

When applied in the community or home, it can improve circulation to the core organs and decrease bleeding while the woman is awaiting transport, being transported or during delays in receiving care at higher-level facilities. The NASG is not therapy or treatment for PPH, but it can be used to buy time to obtain definitive treatment. Family members, TBAs, CHWs, rural auxiliary nurses and even ambulance or conveyance drivers can quickly and easily be trained to apply the NASG tightly enough to improve the woman's status without causing harm[30]. The device

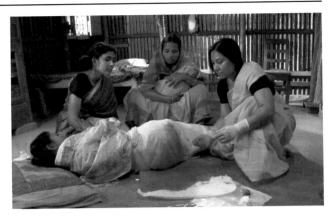

Figure 3 The blood mat in use by Pathfinder International staff in Bangladesh. Photo courtesy of Suellin Miller

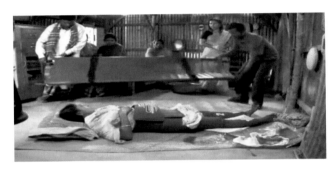

Figure 4 Use of non-pneumatic anti-shock garment. Photo courtesy of Suellen Miller

can be worn over clothing, no inflation is required and it can be re-used up to 40 times (see Chapter 39).

If the NASG has been placed as a first resuscitative measure, the health provider should call for help, assess vital signs and, if possible, find the source of bleeding, and, if the cause is uterine atony, provide uterotonics. The NASG should be removed only under skilled supervision in a facility setting where vital signs can be monitored and there are adequate intravenous fluids and other required treatments. Barriers to implementation include initial skepticism about the NASG's ability to resuscitate women with hypovolemic shock secondary to obstetric hemorrhage, resistance to change and implementation of new behaviors, and lack of knowledge or previous contact with the NASG in medical training[30].

As with any new device or new procedure, the NASG requires training and then modification of use depending on context. However, there are instances where use has been adapted in ways that have not been supported by evidence, and, in fact, may be harmful. For example, after clinical trials were conducted with the NASG following strict protocols in four states in Nigeria, the NASG is now used more widely across the country in the context of Pathfinder International's Clinical and Community Actions to Address PPH. While the protocol for placing a woman in the NASG in Pathfinder training materials is to place the device on a woman with estimated blood loss of at least 500 ml and one sign of hypovolemic shock[31], nurses and midwives in facilities in Nigeria have been seen placing NASGs on women who might be at risk for hemorrhage after the delivery. Instead of using it as a first-aid stabilizing device, it is being used prophylactically. To date, no evidence has been reported on its efficacy for preventing PPH, or whether there are negative effects for women who are not in shock receiving a device intended for shock. Because the NASGs can cause harm to hypovolemic women if removed prematurely or in the wrong sequence, placing the NASG on someone who is not in shock and then removing it rapidly or incorrectly might cause, at the very least, a vagal response. Finally, as the number of NASGs in any facility is limited, using one on a non-shock patient may mean there is none available if a severely shocked patient needed it.

Another potential problem being reported from field work at the time of this writing is the possibility of complacency among providers who, upon seeing the dramatic decrease in bleeding and restoration of vital signs in a woman with hemorrhage/hypovolemic shock, may lose the sense of urgency in referral to a higher level or in providing definitive hemorrhage/shock therapies[32,33]. This must be stressed in training and use. The NASG is not treatment; it only buys time. Transport and obtaining definitive treatment should never be delayed.

Addressing barriers to communication and transportation

Spatial barriers, such as distance or rough terrain, may pose significant obstacles to timely referral of women with PPH to CEmOC facilities[34,35]. Problems related to communication with skilled providers as well as transportation to higher-level facilities must be addressed at both national and local levels. Innovative strategies for addressing delays in communication and transportation have been implemented in several low resource countries.

In 2002, the government of Mali launched a nationwide maternity referral system to improve access to CEmOC through improved radio communications between community and district health facilities, improved ambulance service and community cost-sharing programs[35,36]. In women treated for obstetric emergency, the risk of death was reduced by 50% 2 years after the intervention was implemented, compared with the year before the intervention (OR 0.48, 95% CI 0.30–0.76)[35]. Although the program was national, each region and district developed their own local system through collaborations that ensured broad community support and sustainability.

Four-wheel drive ambulances and a radio communication system in Bo, Sierra Leone, increased the number of obstetric emergency cases transferred to hospitals resulting in the case fatality rate dropping by 50% from 20% (3 of 15) in the 16 months before the intervention to 10% (4 of 41) under the new system[37]. A cluster-randomized study in rural Pakistan examined the impact of a multifaceted intervention to improve education, communication and transportation on maternal and neonatal outcomes. In the intervention areas, local owner/operators of public transport vehicles trained to use stretchers and wireless telecom systems allowed TBAs and drivers to communicate with health facilities. Perinatal mortality among women in the intervention area was half that of women in the control area (adjusted OR 0.5, 95% CI 0.3–0.7)[38]. Other strategies for improving transportation have utilized motorcycles[39], local public bus systems[40], flagging systems along existing truck routes and networks of on-call volunteer drivers from the community[41].

Each local setting has its own unique social, cultural, economic, geographical, political and health systems factors which must be addressed in order to facilitate communication and transportation to facilities that provide higher levels of care. Once a women experiencing excessive bleeding reaches a skilled facility, health care providers must be trained and equipped to provide prompt quality CEmOC. Many countries are also investing in ambulance services; how well they facilitate the transfer and referral of women has not yet been documented.

Comprehensive emergency obstetric care

The final phase of a CC-PPH strategy addresses the delay at the facility in providing quality, definitive emergency treatment. All women need access routes and plans to bring them to EmOC services, because pregnancy complications often cannot be predicted or prevented. A basic EmOC (BEmOC) facility provides six 'signal functions', which are to (1) administer parenteral antibiotics; (2) administer parenteral oxytocics; (3) administer anticonvulsants; (4) perform manual removal of placenta; (5) perform removal of retained products; and (6) conduct assisted vaginal deliveries. A CEmOC facility will offer surgical services, such as cesarean sections, and blood transfusions in addition to the same procedures that are provided at a BEmOC facility.

UNICEF, WHO and UNFPA[42] issued a set of six process indicators to monitor the availability, utilization and quality of EmOC. The six process indicators are: (1) amount of EmOC services available; (2) geographical distribution of EmOC facilities; (3) proportion of all births in EmOC facilities; (4) met need for EmOC services; (5) cesarean sections as a percentage of all births in the population; and (6) case fatality rate. An analysis of 24 national or near-national needs assessments in 2006 showed that all but two countries met the minimum acceptable level of one CEmOC facility per 500,000 population[43]. Despite this progress, quality of care and geographical distribution of EmOC facilities were still a concern. CEmOC facilities were typically located in urban areas and not readily available for women in rural communities. BEmOC facilities were also not consistently available in sufficient numbers in relation to the size of the population and the majority of facilities offering maternity services were not able to provide the full array of signal functions to qualify as EmOC facilities.

Despite the increasing recognition of the importance of EmOC services, several additional challenges exist in accessing quality care in low resource settings, such as overburdened health facilities, shortages of physicians and nurses, poor retention of skilled personnel, lack of operating theaters and emergency equipment, drug shortages, poor sanitation, hospital fees and availability of blood supplies[41,43,44]. If deaths due to pregnancy and delivery are to be substantially reduced, women with complications must have prompt access to quality EmOC. This entails supplying and equipping health facilities appropriately, training health staff to manage obstetric complications and ensuring that a functioning referral system is in place which links peripheral facilities to district health facilities or referral centers that can provide EmOC. Investment by government, ministries of health, NGOs and others in improving access to quality EmOC services has the potential to significantly reduce maternal and child mortality, especially in rural communities that are particularly vulnerable.

CONCLUSION

Many real and perceived barriers hinder accessing medical care, particularly for women in rural areas of low income countries. The high rates of maternal mortality and morbidity in low resource settings are the product of the institutional, environmental, cultural, financial and social barriers to providing skilled care and to preventing, recognizing and managing PPH. No single intervention can prevent PPH-related morbidity and mortality. Having said this, however, we believe a multifaceted, systematic, contextualized PPH continuum of care approach that addresses all factors directly contributing to maternal death from hemorrhage is essential if progress is to be made in this area. Commitment and support from key stakeholders, governmental organizations and policymakers will ensure the feasibility, acceptability and sustainability of evidenced-based interventions, including use of misoprostol, blood collection drape and NASG. Community involvement in developing communication and transportation systems will hopefully address the delays in hemorrhage recognition, stabilization and early management of women with shock and hemorrhage. We believe that the continuum of care model for the prevention and management of PPH may offer promise to improve health care delivery and has the greatest impact for saving women's lives, decreasing maternal morbidity and improving quality of life.

PRACTICE POINTS

- A CC-PPH model is essential to address the spectrum of clinical, social and system factors related to PPH morbidity and mortality in low resource settings

- Community engagement and mobilization can improve access to EmOC and educate the community about birth preparedness

- Use of a prophylactic uterotonic agent such as misoprostol can reduce the incidence of PPH

- Use of a reliable aid to the quantification of blood loss and the NASG can address the delay in recognition of the extent of hemorrhage and subsequent patient stabilization

- A reliable local emergency communication and transport system can facilitate consultation with skilled birth attendants, transfer of a woman to the CEmOC facility and alert staff to the need for prompt care.

References

1. WHO. Trends in maternal mortality: 1990–2008. Estimates developed by WHO, UNICEF, UNFPA, and the World Bank. Geneva: World Health Organization, 2010
2. WHO. Maternal Mortality. Fact Sheet No. 348. Geneva: World Health Organization, 2010
3. Maine D, Rosenfield A, Wallis M, et al. Prevention of maternal deaths in developing countries. New York: Center for Population and Family Health, 1999
4. Geller SE, Adams MG, Miller S. A continuum of care model for postpartum hemorrhage. Int J Fertil Womens Med 2007; 52:97–105
5. Howard-Grabman L, Snetro G. How to mobilize communities for health and social change. 2003. Health Communication Partnership. http://www.hcpartnership.org/Publications/Field_Guides/Mobilize/pdf
6. Fullilove RE, Green L, Fullilove MT. The Family to Family program: a structural intervention with implications for the prevention of HIV/AIDS and other community epidemics. AIDS 2000;14(Suppl 1):S63–7
7. Madison SM, McKay MM, Paikoff R, Bell CC. Basic research and community collaboration: necessary ingredients for the development of a family-based HIV prevention program. AIDS Educ Prev 2000;12:281–98
8. McCormick A, McKay MM, Wilson M, et al. Involving families in an urban HIV preventive intervention: how community collaboration addresses barriers to participation. AIDS Educ Prev 2000;12:299–307
9. Mobeen N, Durocher J, Zuberi N, et al. Administration of misoprostol by trained traditional birth attendants to prevent postpartum haemorrhage in homebirths in Pakistan: a randomised placebo-controlled trial. BJOG 2011;118:353–61
10. Hoj L, Cardoso P, Nielsen BB, Hvidman L, Nielsen J, Aaby P. Effect of sublingual misoprostol on severe postpartum haemorrhage in a primary health centre in Guinea-Bissau: randomised double blind clinical trial. BMJ 2005;331:723
11. Derman RJ, Kodkany BS, Goudar SS, et al. Oral misoprostol in preventing postpartum haemorrhage in resource-poor communities: a randomised controlled trial. Lancet 2006; 368:1248–53
12. Walraven G, Blum J, Dampha Y, et al. Misoprostol in the management of the third stage of labour in the home delivery setting in rural Gambia: a randomised controlled trial. BJOG 2005;112:1277–83
13. ICM/FIGO. Prevention and treatment of post-partum haemorrhage: new advances for low resource settings. ICM/FIGO Joint statement, 2006. www.pphprevention.org/.../FIGO-ICM_Statement_November2006_Final.pdf
14. WHO. WHO Statement regarding the use of misoprostol for postpartum haemorrhage prevention and treatment. Geneva: World Health Organization, 2009

15. WHO. Clarifying WHO position on misoprostol use in the community to reduce maternal death. Geneva: World Health Organization, 2010

16. Venture Strategies Innovations. Global miso map. http://vsinnovations.org/resources.html

17. Sanghvi H, Ansari N, Prata NJ, Gibson H, Ehsan AT, Smith JM. Prevention of postpartum hemorrhage at home birth in Afghanistan. Int J Gynaecol Obstet 2010;108:276–81

18. Rajbhandari S, Hodgins S, Sanghvi H, McPherson R, Pradhan YV, Baqui AH. Expanding uterotonic protection following childbirth through community-based distribution of misoprostol: operations research study in Nepal. Int J Gynaecol Obstet 2010;108:282–8

19. Dildy GA 3rd, Paine AR, George NC, Velasco C. Estimating blood loss: can teaching significantly improve visual estimation? Obstet Gynecol 2004;104:601–6

20. Sibley L, Caleb-Varkey L, Upadhyay J, et al. Recognition of and response to postpartum hemorrhage in rural northern India. J Midwifery Womens Health 2005;50:301–8

21. Prata N, Mbaruku G, Campbell M. Using the kanga to measure postpartum blood loss. Int J Gynaecol Obstet 2005;89:49–50

22. Geller SE, Patel A, Niak VA, et al. Conducting international collaborative research in developing nations. Int J Gynaecol Obstet 2004;87:267–71

23. Kodkany BS, Derman RJ, Goudar SS, et al. Initiating a novel therapy in preventing postpartum hemorrhage in rural India: a joint collaboration between the United States and India. Int J Fertil Womens Med 2004;49:91–6

24. Patel A, Goudar SS, Geller SE, et al. Drape estimation vs. visual assessment for estimating postpartum hemorrhage. Int J Gynaecol Obstet 2006;93:220–4

25. Sloan NL, Durocher J, Aldrich T, Blum J, Winikoff B. What measured blood loss tells us about postpartum bleeding: a systematic review. BJOG 2010;117:788–800

26. Schorn MN. Measurement of blood loss: review of the literature. J Midwifery Womens Health 2010;55:20–7

27. Prata N, Qualyum M, Shahed Hossain S, Azmil A, Bohl D. Community-based prevention of PPH in rural Bangladesh. Presented at the 138th Meeting of the American Public Health Association (APHA), Denver, CO, November 2010

28. Foundation funds 65 novel ideas to improve global health, from vaccines delivered in local cuisine to blankets of light for jaundiced newborns. 2010. Bill & Melinda Gates Foundation. http://www.grandchallenges.org/about/Newsroom/Pages/GCERound5Grants.aspx

29. Dildy GA 3rd. Postpartum Hemorrhage. Washington DC: American College of Obstetricians and Gynecologists, 1998

30. Berdichevsky K, Tucker C, Martinez A, Miller S. Acceptance of a new technology for management of obstetric hemorrhage: a qualitative study from rural Mexico. Health Care Women Int 2010;31:444–57

31. Pathfinder International. Prevention, recognition, and management of postpartum hemorrhage: trainer's guide. 2010. http://www.pathfind.org/site/DocServer/PPH_TG_final.pdf?docID=18682

32. Fathalla M, Mourad M, Meyer C, et al. Non-atonic obstetric hemorrhage: effectiveness of the non-pneumatic anti-shock garment in Egypt. J Obstet Gynaecol 2011; in press

33. Turan J, Ojengbede O, Fathalla M, et al. Positive Effects of the Non-pneumatic Anti-shock Garment on Delays in Accessing Care for Postpartum and Postabortion Hemorrhage in Egypt and Nigeria. J Womens Health (Larchmt) 2011;20:91–8

34. Le Bacq F, Rietsema A. High maternal mortality levels and additional risk from poor accessibility in two districts of northern province, Zambia. Int J Epidemiol 1997;26:357–63

35. Fournier P, Dumont A, Tourigny C, Dunkley G, Drame S. Improved access to comprehensive emergency obstetric care and its effect on institutional maternal mortality in rural Mali. Bull World Health Organ 2009;87:30–8

36. Pirkle CM, Fournier P, Tourigny C, Sangare K, Haddad S. Emergency Obstetrical Complications in a Rural African Setting (Kayes, Mali): The Link Between Travel Time and In-Hospital Maternal Mortality. Matern Child Health J 2010 [Epub ahead of print]

37. Samai O, Sengeh P. Facilitating emergency obstetric care through transportation and communication, Bo, Sierra Leone. The Bo PMM Team. Int J Gynaecol Obstet 1997;59(Suppl 2):S157–64

38. Midhet F, Becker S. Impact of community-based interventions on maternal and neonatal health indicators: Results from a community randomized trial in rural Balochistan, Pakistan. Reprod Health 2010;7:30

39. Hofman JJ, Dzimadzi C, Lungu K, Ratsma EY, Hussein J. Motorcycle ambulances for referral of obstetric emergencies in rural Malawi: do they reduce delay and what do they cost? Int J Gynaecol Obstet 2008;102:191–7

40. Shehu D, Ikeh AT, Kuna MJ. Mobilizing transport for obstetric emergencies in northwestern Nigeria. The Sokoto PMM Team. Int J Gynaecol Obstet 1997;59(Suppl 2):S173–80

41. Lee AC, Lawn JE, Cousens S, et al. Linking families and facilities for care at birth: what works to avert intrapartum-related deaths? Int J Gynaecol Obstet 2009;107(Suppl 1):S65–85, S86–8

42. United Nations Children's Fund. Guidelines for monitoring the availability and use of obstetric services. New York: United Nations Childrens Fund, 1997

43. Paxton A, Bailey P, Lobis S, Fry D. Global patterns in availability of emergency obstetric care. Int J Gynaecol Obstet 2006;93:300–7

44. Hofmeyr GJ, Haws RA, Bergstrom S, et al. Obstetric care in low-resource settings: what, who, and how to overcome challenges to scale up? Int J Gynaecol Obstet 2009;107(Suppl 1):S21–44, S44–5

68

Human Behavior in Medical Emergencies: Learning from Past Mistakes

E. Evans and H. Snelgrove

TEAMWORK MATTERS

Teamwork is increasingly cited by health care organizations in terms of improving patient care and safety. This interest follows decades of investigations into the nature of effective teamwork in aviation, business, military and sport settings[1,2]. More recently, the importance of effective team working for the maintenance of workplace safety has become a special focus for research in health care[3,4].

This chapter highlights key areas from a vast literature; a literature which fails to reach clear conclusions about the extent to which teamwork training is effective, if at all. It presents an overview of teamwork research under three main headings: concepts of teamwork; teamwork training; and, finally, the impact of teamwork training interventions with a particular focus on obstetrics and gynecology. It examines shortcomings in the use of practical models of teamwork training such as crisis resource management to predict patient outcomes in a cause–effect linear way, arguing that this may be reductive. Building effective teamwork requires a broader context of system changes and investment in continuing professional education which should be seen along a learning continuum and within a culture of reiterative training and feedback.

CONCEPTS OF TEAMWORK

Teamwork is commonly defined as 'a distinguishable set of two people who interact, dynamically, interdependently, and adaptively toward a common and valued goal'[5]. Other authors suggest that 'complementary skills' and 'mutual accountability' should also be added[6]. Various conceptual models have evolved to analyse the characteristics of teams which can influence their performance. The basic model from psychological research of what constitutes a high performing team shows that team outputs (e.g. team effectiveness as identified by successful outcomes) is a result of group processes (e.g. leadership, communication, coordination, shared goals, mutual monitoring of performance). These group processes are in turn influenced by a variety of 'inputs' (e.g. work climate, individual task proficiency, attitudes, organizational culture)[5,7,8]. To successfully achieve team goals, Flin *et al.*[8] argue that the 'processes' that teams use to interact with each other are an essential complement to individual team members' abilities and the availability of wider resources. In other words, processes are a mix of systems and methods which combine with a special focus on what the team does to develop the skills and motivation to perform together more effectively. A further level of sophistication has been introduced by research into the causes of error in high-risk organizations[9,10]. According to these latter findings, the basic model of input, throughput and output should not be interpreted as a linear chain but rather in terms of 'causal networks'. Reason[9], for example, describes an accident sequence as a complex interplay of organizational culture, workplace climate, the specific task and the event itself. In other words, rather than isolate the specific components in an error, complexity theorists suggest that the essential way to understand how errors have occurred is embedded not in the single components (e.g. technology failure, individual mistake, team communication) but in their interconnectedness[9,11].

Many of these theoretical insights and much of the impetus for team training and safety in high-risk organizations have arisen from pioneering research in aviation. For instance, aviation accidents have been analysed in terms of 'interconnected' breakdowns in teamwork at various levels[8,9,12,13]. Importantly, also emerging from this research is that safety culture and team processes can be enhanced through specific training interventions[5,14].

TEAMWORK TRAINING: LESSONS FROM AVIATION

The extent to which safety in health care has been influenced by aviation is illustrated by considering how the aviation industry learned to analyse fatal incidents. Half a century ago, root cause analysis of accidents became an established practice in aircraft investigations. The three successive fatal crashes of the first commercial jet liner, a BOAC de Havilland Comet in 1954[9,15], caught the public eye in a similar manner to the Concorde flight 4590 in Paris in 2000[16], the difference being that in 1954 the task of finding out what happened was more difficult. In

1954, the aviation industry did not have black boxes, cockpit voice recorders or flight data recorders. The British Comet investigation thus represented a landmark inquiry into accident investigation[9]. Interestingly, both accidents were either partly or wholly attributable to structural weaknesses in the fuselage of these particular aircraft. In both instances, the remaining aircraft of this specific design were withdrawn from service. In the decades following the Comet tragedies, however, improved aircraft manufacturing, and data collection combined with huge media coverage of air accidents shifted the emphasis to human factors[9,17]. One emblematic case commonly cited by human factor researchers is the Tenerife collision in March 1977 between two jumbo jets. This high profile case brought human factor analysis to a world audience. Along with other high profile disasters, it has also subsequently influenced health care. A total of 583 individuals either died or were mortally wounded in what is still today the worst accident in aviation history. However, using human factor analysis principles, these deaths were entirely avoidable. Briefly, the KLM and Pan AM jets were diverted to the small airport at Tenerife from their scheduled stop in Las Palmas for refueling. This was because of a terrorist bomb scare at Las Palmas. However, the fatal combination of a crowded and unfamiliar landing field, inexperienced control tower operators, crackling audio technology, language problems, fog and poor visibility, flight deck violations, submissive crew members and a dominating senior commander proved to be lethal. Vivid reconstructions based on the official investigation which highlighted the teamwork and human factor contributions to the catastrophe populate the world wide web[18,19].

Flin *et al.*[8] describe many more incidents with strikingly similar dynamics, including the Three Mile Island nuclear accident, and the USS Vincennes and Eastern Airlines flight 401 crash, to name but a few. What emerged from a spate of enquiries into these accidents was a surprisingly short list of critical teamwork problems. These included *poor role clarity; lack of explicit coordination; poor communication between team members; submission to hierarchy; poor situation awareness; poor decision making; failure to assert authority; and workload management.* These were all 'non technical skills'[8,13,20].

In 1979 a reaction to these events led to the development of crew resource management training. Also known as 'human factor training', crew resource management was initially designed to reduce operational errors and improve emergency responses in aircrews. The rationale was that errors are inevitable[21], but that to perform effectively and reduce the risk of making catastrophic mistakes individuals in teams must be proficient in non-technical skills (NTS). The emphasis in aviation, where this training originated, was to shift attitudes among trainees from one of individual autonomy to team centered interdependence. In this new perspective, safety became the binding principle of crew management. Of overriding importance, this

attention to safety has permeated organizational culture in the aviation industry and is no longer confined to crews; rather it is a system philosophy[22]. Crew resource management has now been adapted to other high reliability team settings into other fields such as nuclear power generation, maritime and rail industries, fire services[20,23], the offshore oil industry[24], aviation maintenance[25] and health care[26–28].

In an influential report released in 1999 by the Institute of Medicine *To Err is Human: Building a Better Health Care System*[29] aviation-based crew resource management became crisis resource management and was identified as a key strategy for reducing error in the complex treatment teams that are such a feature in modern health care. Following this report, health care authorities around the world have recommended the implementation of team training to improve teamwork[29,30]. In particular, the need for interprofessional and multidisciplinary team training approaches across the full spectrum of health care education has been included in competency descriptions by European, North American and Australasian medical associations. Communication, partnership and teamwork are identified as core domain competencies by the European General Medical Council (GMC)[31], the Accreditation Council for Graduate Medical Education (ACGME), the Australian Medical Council (AMA), the Medical Council of Canada (MCC) and many others[32–35]. How this evolution of team training in health care has affected obstetric teams is the focus of the next section.

TEAMWORK TRAINING INTERVENTIONS IN OBSTETRICS AND GYNECOLOGY

Effective teams have supported the management of obstetric emergencies for many years; at the same time, when they fail, the results have appeared in many national reports[36]. The ability of functioning obstetric teams to perform in high-stake situations is crucial and forms the basis for widely regarded literature. To be effective, teams require a high degree of technical and non-technical skills, plus the ability to be able to come together in an instant to co-ordinate their diverse members into a rapid response. Teams in obstetrics are multiprofessional and can be extremely fluid. While the static component to any obstetric unit is the midwifery (in the US and many other countries it is nursing) staff, many other members including the trainee obstetricians and anesthetists are mostly temporary. This circumstance makes the ability to implement effective training programs or even to research the effect of interventions on teams challenging, as team members never work together enough to rehearse any new skills learned during training.

Describing those elements which constitute an ideal team has been the basis of research for many years. It starts with identifying what can be replicated from high-risk industries where teams are under scrutiny and trying to apply this information to our own specialty. Several groups have worked with obstetric care givers to define and validate what they feel contributes to successful clinical outcomes within their own practice[37,59]. This has formed a platform from which to measure effectiveness, by setting a standard of teamwork that may have previously been undefined. Of course, good teamwork may mean something different to one profession as compared with another. In their uniprofessional domains, each group experiences a different set of professional boundaries, hierarchies and expectations of themselves and others within an emergency setting. It is the bringing together of these teams that attempts to develop understanding and a common language between them to create superior performance. This is the essence of what Salas describes as 'dynamic interdependence'[5].

Many different approaches can be used to train obstetric teams; these vary from classroom based lectures focusing entirely on obstetric emergencies and/or crisis resource management[38] to simulated emergency scenarios combined either with[39] or without[40] specific teamwork theory to provide a platform from which to discuss team interactions. Each method seeks to develop and incorporate many of the aviation industry principles of crisis resource management which provides the basis for 'portable skills' that can be directly translated into clinical scenarios[41]. Where the training actually takes place can have significant implications for the transfer of these lessons to clinical care. In fact, the location of training is a powerful predictor of transfer[41] and is effective without the time or costs involved in using simulation labs. Local training can improve accessibility, clinical relevance and address system issues unique to a specific obstetric unit[39].

Evaluating the effectiveness of obstetric teamtraining programs has been challenging due to the heterogeneity of interventions, course design and assessment tools[42]. Many interventions, however, can be described in one dimension or another on the Kirkpatrick scale[43]. Kirkpatrick created a framework on which to judge the effectiveness of any educational intervention, extending beyond satisfaction scores used commonly to evaluate training to looking at organizational change and improved patient outcomes that come about.

Level 1: learner reaction

Evaluation limited to participant satisfaction tells us a certain amount about the impact on teams, since team training is not only enjoyed by team participants, but also has the potential to improve knowledge of teamwork and shared decision-making[41]. Even if the impact of clinical outcome is harder to evaluate, participants commonly report improvement in communication and team functioning as a result of training[44].

Level 2a: modification of learner attitudes and perceptions

Attitudes of teams to entering into obstetric emergencies is positively affected by simulation training[45], as is the perception of the importance of communication and the concepts of patient safety particularly in relation to postpartum hemorrhage[46].

Level 2b: learner acquisition of knowledge and skills

Skills and knowledge improve within simulated obstetric emergencies particularly when using high-fidelity models[47]. In addition, using simulation creates the advantageous situation of retained improved knowledge scores for longer times[45]. The benefit of additional specific team training has been questioned by some and is variable[47]. This may in part be due to the way in which these studies sought to evaluate team improvements within simulated emergencies. Others have had more success when team training or crisis resource management principles have been the focus of the training and have not involved simulation[38]. However, Gaba *et al.* support the use of simulation to create a setting for applying the principles[48]. Therefore, there is compelling evidence that even simulation-based training in obstetrics is an appropriate approach to reduce errors and risk in obstetrics.

Level 3: change in learner behavior

In 2007, Birch *et al.*[49] demonstrated that teams trained with simulation sustained their improvement in clinical management, interdisciplinary communication and self-confidence when tested 3 months later compared with their colleagues trained with just lectures or a combined approach. Teams taught with simulation also improved their interdisciplinary communication skills compared with those taught exclusively by lecture.

Level 4: benefits to the organization/patient resulting from learner performance

Of course, the greatest challenge comes to the ability of any form of training, classroom, simulation or otherwise, to transfer its perceived benefits into the clinical environment and ultimately onto patient care. It ultimately comes down to clinical outcomes, and the only real study that has been able to demonstrate a significant impact has done so in perinatal outcomes[50]. Impacts on maternal outcomes have yet to be realized, and this may be, in part, due to the manner in which organizations have approached obstetric team training programs. A recent study suggests that team training without drills with patient simulators have not been shown to lead to improvement in outcome[51]. It is worth questioning, however, whether attempts to apply randomized controlled trial methodologies to multifactorial and complex interactions between team members represents the magic bullet[52] – in other words, whether they can reliably take account of confounding factors or isolate 'interventional' benefits in a convincing way.

Which teams benefit more?

The experience of team members will undoubtedly affect the ability of studies to show improvement in skills or knowledge but also may have positive effects on their behaviors. Most studies on the impact of simulation team training have evaluated midwifery/obstetric teams excluding anesthetists in the structure of the whole team. Anesthetists have historically been familiar with concepts of crisis resource management and simulation based training[53] and thus may be invaluable in disseminating the language of concepts such as situational awareness and 'shared mental models' that are often so unfamiliar in maternity units; basically these terms refer to 'collective wariness' where each member of the team is vigilant and contributing actively to the team's understanding of the clinical situation. Studies which eschew any members of the team run the risk of undermining a key trait of crisis resource management in maintaining safety.

Is it cost-effective?

The cost-effectiveness of such rigorous attention to team work will always be a question for every organization which seeks to invest in it. Litigation within obstetrics sites and poor communication between professions remains a top root cause of error. With bills for organizations in millions of pounds, the relatively small cost of programs targeting team behaviors cannot be ignored as an eminently achievable investment[54].

The location of training has also been evaluated, given the huge potential for unnecessary expense incurred by using simulation centers. No additional benefits to knowledge acquisition are found by training in simulation centers over locally conducted training[40]. Salas finds the same beneficial effect on teams when trained within their clinical environment[39]. This has hugely encouraging implications on the accessibility of simulation-based training in developing countries and has underpinned the success of programs such as PRactical Obstetric MultiProfessional Training (PROMPT)[50].

Although there is evidence suggesting the efficacy, reliability and validity of simulator-based training, its superiority over conventional training with regard to cost-effectiveness has yet to be proven. Because there is a limited amount of high-quality evidence on the effect of simulation-based training, it is important for researchers to reflect carefully on the specific characteristics of the educational environment that may require different approaches to study design and analysis. Studies need to be performed using standardized simulation scenarios to evaluate the fundamental aspects of human performance in health care. In this regard, it is important to keep in mind that it is not randomization *per se* that is critical to the quality of educational experiments, nor is it that the methods of clinical experimental research can and should be adopted wholesale into the educational setting[52].

CONCLUSIONS

Teamwork research is designed to improve workplace training interventions. Few would disagree with the idea that improving teamwork through better communication, clarifying goals, sharing expectations about the task and mutual monitoring of performance are all good things. Equally, it is difficult to deny that programs that encourage these behaviors should have at least some positive benefit on team performance in health care. Despite this, few of the psychological concepts explaining successful teamwork in various high-risk industries such as team situation awareness, shared mental models and adaptive coordination have been investigated systematically in health care. This is borne out in team-based research in obstetrics and gynecology. These conceptual descriptions of good teamwork undoubtedly provide helpful insights and useful analytical traction. However, the findings from these studies are uneven and lack synthesis; for example, they do not make explicit exactly what aspects of teamwork need to be improved. While, on the one hand, it is claimed that many adverse events could have been prevented by improved teamwork, few empirical studies have systematically investigated the role of teamwork in preventing minor problems from escalating into more serious incidents[8,55]. The extent to which this research can influence practice is, as a result, unclear. So why does this training seem less successful than we would like? Is our analytical lens too thick?

Many lessons are available from aviation and research in high risk organizations. Some researchers, however, question whether some of these have been lost in translation into health care[22]. For instance, 'behavioral markers' underlying crisis resource management training refer to explicit, observable behaviors employed by ideal practitioners. The idea has been embraced that if you teach everyone to adopt these and practice them, results will follow that can be measured. As a result, crisis resource management training has directed a growing body of research to identify linear effects of team training on patient outcomes. Interestingly, this is despite the fact that in aviation itself research evidence for the benefits of crisis resource management has been elusive[22,56]. On the other hand, what has been learned from complexity theorists is that factors contributing to patient safety and error are multiple and interdependent; they do not lend themselves exclusively to individual or team analyses[57]. Beneath the behaviors in any specific team are a collection of attitudes and beliefs embedded in the social and work environment and the organizational culture of a workplace[6]. These have been described as the context of teamwork, or what Musson refers to as the 'unobservable ingredients enriching our cognitive processes, and behavior'[22].

What is the implication of all this work? Perhaps there are two. On the one hand, the immense variety of potentially hazardous situations requires that training for safer behavior is delivered at the level of the team. On the other, it is that if team training is not undertaken as part of a wider program to address dysfunctional factors at the organizational level, the work environment level and the individual level, it is difficult to see how behavioral marker-based crisis resource management-oriented team training will be able to fulfil its potential in improving the quality of care in our current systems[22]. Patient safety outcomes as seen through this lens represent an emerging phenomenon arising out of a complex dynamic network which is not amenable to simple causal relations. Nor is it directly attributable to one isolated feature in the system[58]. Most measures of teamwork still focus on individual behaviors. Future evaluation and research of team training will need to be founded on more conceptual clarity as well as wider analytical frames for what constitutes effective teamwork.

References

1. Hackman J. Learning more by crossing levels: Evidence from airplanes, hospitals, and orchestras. J Organ Behav 2003;24: 905–22
2. Hackman J. Leading Teams. Setting the stage for great performance. Harvard: Harvard Business School Press, 2002
3. Awad S. Bridging the communication gap. Am J Surg 2005; 190:770–4
4. Leonard M, Graham S, Bonacum D. The human factor: the critical importance of effective teamwork and communication in providing safe care. Qual Saf Healthcare 2004;13: 85–90
5. Salas E, Dickinson TL, Converse SA. Towards an understanding of team performance and training. In: Swezey RW, Salas E, eds. Teams: their Training and Performance. Norwood, NJ: Ablex Publishing Corporation, 1992:3–29
6. Drinka TJK, Clark P G. Health Care Teamwork: Interdisciplinary Practice And Teaching. Westport, CT: Auburn House/Greenwood, 2000
7. Unsworth K, West M. Teams: the challenges of cooperative work. In: Chimiel N, ed. Work and Organizational Psychology. Oxford: Churchill Livingstone, 2000
8. Flin R, O'Connor P, Crichton M. Safety at the Sharp End. A Guide to Non-technical Skills. Farnham: Ashgate, 2008
9. Reason J. The Human Contribution. Farnham: Ashgate, 2008
10. Hollnagel E. The ETTO Principle: Efficiency Thoroughness Trade-Off. Farnham: Ashgate, 2009
11. Paries J. Complexity, Emergence, Resilience. In: Hollnagel E, Woods D, Leveson N, eds. Resilience Engineering. Concepts and Precepts. Aldershot: Ashgate, 2006
12. Orasanu J. Finding decisions in natural environments: the view from the cockpit. In: Zsambok C, Klein G, eds. Naturalistic Decision Making. Mahwah, NJ: LEA, 1997
13. Weiner E, Kanki B, Helmreich RL. Cockpit Resource Management. San Diego, CA: Academic Press, 1993
14. Salas E, Cooke N, Rosen MA. On teams, teamwork, and team performance: discoveries and developments. Hum Factors 2008;50:540–5
15. de Haviland Comet W. de Havilland Comet. http://en.wikipedia.org/wiki/De_Havilland_Comet. 2011
16. AF 4590 -Wikipedia. Air France Flight 4590. http://en.wikipedia.org/wiki/Air_France_Flight_4590. 2011
17. Reason J, Parker D, Lawton B. Organizational controls and safety: the varieties of rule-related behaviour. J Occup Organ Psychol 1998;71:289–304
18. 1001crash.com. Tenerife crash March 27th, 1977. http://www.1001crash.com/index-page-tenerife-lg-2-numpage-1.html. 2011
19. National Geographic Channel. Air crash investigation videos. http://natgeotv.com/uk/air-crash-investigation/videos?page=7. 2011
20. Salas E. A checklist for crew resource management training. Ergon Design 2006;14:6–15
21. Reason J. Human Error. New York: Cambridge University Press, 1990
22. Musson D. Putting behavioural markers to work. In: Flin R, Mitchell L, eds. Safer Surgery. Analysing Behaviour in the Operating Theatre. Farnham: Ashgate, 2009:430
23. Flin R. Crew resource management. improving teamwork in high reliability industries. Team Perf Man 2002;8:68–78
24. Flin R, Slaven G. Emergency decision making in the offshore oil and gas industry. Hum Factors 1996;38:262–77
25. Max DA, Graeber RC. Human error in maintenance. In: Johnston NM, Fuller R, eds. Aviation Psychology in Practice. London: Ashgate, 1994:87–104
26. Bleakley A, Boyden J, Hobbs A, Walsh L, Allard J. Improving teamwork climate in operating theatres: the shift from multiprofessionalismto interprofessionalism. J Interprof Care 2006;20:461–70
27. Flin R, Fletcher G, McGeorge P, Sutherland A, Patey R. Anaesthetists' attitudes to teamwork and safety. Anaesthesia 2003;58:233–42
28. Baker DP, Salas E, King H, Battles J, Barach P. The role of teamwork in the professional education of physicians: current status and assessment recommendations. Jt Comm J Qual Patient Saf 2005;31:185–202
29. Kohn L. To Err is Human. Institute of Medicine. Washington DC: National Academy Press, 2000
30. Agency for Healthcare Research and Quality. TeamSTEPPS Strategies and tools to enhance Performance and Patient Safety. http://teamstepps.ahrq.gov/abouttoolsmaterials.htm. 2006
31. General Medical Council. http://www.gmc-uk.org.
32. Accreditation Council for Graduate Medical Education. Core Competencies http://www.acgme.org/acWebsite/RRC_280/280_coreComp.asp. 2011
33. Australian Medical Association. Role of the Doctor – 2011. http://ama.com.au/node/65692011
34. General Medical Council. http://www.gmc-uk.org. 2011
35. Medical Counci of Canada. Organisational aspects of the practice of medicine. http://www.mcc.ca/en/exams/objectives/c2leo-e.htm. 2011
36. CEMACH. Saving mothers lives. Reviewing maternal deaths to make motherhood safer. London: RCOG, 2005
37. Guise JM, Deering SH, Kanki BG, et al. Development and validation of the clinical teamwork scale to evaluate teamwork. Simul Healthc 2008;3:217–23
38. Haller G, Garnerin P, Morales MA, et al. Effect of crew resource management training in a multidisciplinary obstetrical setting. Int J Qual Health Care 2008;20:4
39. Salas E, DiazGrandos D, Klein C, et al. Does team training improve team performance? A meta-analysis. Hum Factors 2008;50:903
40. Crofts JF, Ellis D, Draycott TJ, Winter C, Hunt LP, Akande VA. Change in knowledge of midwives and obstetricians following obstetric emergency training: a randomised controlled trial of local hospital, simulation centre and teamwork training. BJOG 2007;114:1534–41
41. Miller KK, Riley W, Davis S, Hansen HE. In situ simulation: a method of experiential learning to promote safety and team behavior. J Perinat Neonat Nurs 2008;22: 105–13
42. Merien AE, van de Ven J, Mol BW, Houterman S, Oei SG. Multidisciplinary team training in a simulation setting for acute obstetric emergencies: A systematic review. Obstet Gynecol 2010;115:1021–31
43. Kirkpatrick D. Evaluating Training Programs: The Four Levels, 2nd edn. San Francisco: CA: Berrett-Kochler Publishers, 1998
44. Clark EA, Fisher J, Arafeh J, Druzin M. Team training/simulation. Clin Obstet Gynecol 2010;53:265–77

45. Robertson B, Gosman G, Kanfer R, et al. Simulation-based crisis team training for multidisciplinary obstetric providers. Simul Healthc 2009;4:77–83

46. Crofts JF, Bartlett C, Ellis D, et al. Patient-actor perception of care: a comparison of obstetric emergency training using manikins and patient-actors. Qual Saf Health Care 2008;17: 20–4

47. Crofts JF, Bartlett C, Ellis D, Hunt LP, Fox R, Draycott TJ. Training for shoulder dystocia: a trial of simulation using low-fidelity and high- fidelity mannequins. Obstet Gynecol 2006;108:1477–85

48. Gaba DM. The future vision of simulation in health care. Qual Saf Health Care 2004;13:2–10

49. Birch L, Doyle PM, Green P, et al. Obstetric skills drills: evaluation of teaching methods. Nurse Educ Today 2007;27: 915–22

50. Draycott T, Owen L, Akande V, et al. Does training in obstetric emergencies improve neonatal outcome? BJOG 2006;113:177–82

51. Nielsen PE, Mann S, Shapiro DE, et al. Effects of teamwork training on adverse outcomes and process of care in labor and delivery: a randomized controlled trial. Obstet Gynecol 2007; 109:48–55

52. Norman G. RCT = results confounded and trivial: the perils of grand educational experiments. Med Ed 2003;37:582–4

53. Fletcher G, McGeorge P, Glavin R, Maran N, Patey R. Anaesthetists Non-technical skills (ANTS): evaluation of a behavioural marker system. Br J Anaesth 2003;5:580–8

54. van de Ven J, Steinweg RA, Scherpbier AJ, Wijers W, Mol BW, Oei SG. Reducing errors in health care: cost-effectiveness of multidisciplinary team training in obstetric emergencies (TOSTI study); a randomised controlled trial. BMC Pregnancy and Childbirth 2010;10:59

55. Reason J. Beyond the organisational accident: the need for "error wisdom" on the frontline. Qual Saf Health Care 2004;13(Suppl 2):ii28–33

56. Salas E, Burke CS, Wilson K. Team training in the skies: Does crew resource management rtraining really work? Hum Factors 2006;43:641–74

57. Woods D, Hollnagel E. Prologue: Resilience Engineering Concepts. In: Hollnagel E, Woods D, Leveson N, eds. Resilience Engineering. Aldershot: Ashgate, 2006:1–6

58. Hollnagel E. Barriers and Accident Prevention. Aldershot: Ashgate, 2004

59. Siassakos D, Bristowe K, Draycott T, Angouri J, Hambly H, Winter C, Crofts J, Hunt L, Fox R. Clinical efficiency in a simulated emergency and relationship to team behaviours: a multisite cross-sectional study. BJOG 2011;118: 596–607

Section 12

Special Circumstances

69

Out-of-Hospital Deliveries

E. Sheiner, I. Ohel and A. Hadar

INTRODUCTION

Out-of-hospital deliveries can be divided into planned and unplanned[1]. The former generally occur in a prepared setting and are attended by medical personnel; the latter generally occur when the woman is entering the active phase of labor rapidly and may take place en route to the hospital or at the home itself. In either event, unplanned out-of-hospital delivery can be a stressful and sometimes even hazardous experience. Unplanned out-of-hospital deliveries carry an increased risk for adverse maternal and perinatal outcomes, specifically hemorrhage and perinatal mortality[2–14].

Out-of-hospital deliveries are not confined to countries with low resources and where home deliveries are the rule rather than the exception. In countries with high resources, specific groups are more likely to experience out-of-hospital deliveries than the general population. For example, Bateman *et al.*[3] reported that patients who delivered out-of-hospital in the USA were more likely to be African-American, multigravid and to have had little or no prenatal care. Similarly, other ethnic minorities such as Asians living a long way from the hospital in Europe are also at risk for out-of-hospital deliveries and for adverse pregnancy outcome[4–6].

In one often-quoted article, albeit written almost 50 years ago and not repeated to our knowledge, approximately 5% of all women who underwent vaginal delivery without complications lost more than 1000 ml of blood[15]. Assuming that this is correct, it has enormous implications for any woman who undergoes an out-of-hospital delivery because the objective evaluation of bleeding after delivery may be difficult in the absence of trained health care providers, especially if bleeding is slow and steady or in the presence of concomitant intra-abdominal bleeding[16]. Of equal importance, the clinical signs of blood loss, such as decrease in blood pressure and increased heart rate, tend to appear late, and only when the amount of blood loss reaches 1500 ml, mainly due to the high blood volume of pregnant women (see Chapters 9–11). Here again, a woman delivering out of hospital would appear to be at greater risk should this occur and not be noticed or monitored.

Our group performed a large population-based study of risk factors for early postpartum hemorrhage (PPH)[17]. Although this was not the first such evaluation[18–21], we were stimulated to characterize women at risk who warrant special attention after birth and, in particular, consultation about the advisability of out-of-hospital delivery. Early PPH complicated 0.43% (n = 666) of all singleton deliveries included in this study (n = 154,311). Independent risk factors for early PPH, which can be of major importance during out-of-hospital deliveries, are presented in Table 1. These risk factors were drawn from a multivariate analysis and included retained placenta, labor dystocia, placenta accreta, severe lacerations, large-for-gestational-age newborn and hypertensive disorders[16].

One of the largest studies regarding out-of-hospital deliveries derives from our hospital, a tertiary medical center located in the Negev region, Israel[12,13]. In this area, most deliveries do occur in the hospital, and virtually all newborns and their mothers are brought to the hospital if delivered outside. This is done mainly because hospital deliveries are entitled to a birth payment from the government, which is also given to newborns who are brought to the hospital within 24 h of birth. The incidence of unplanned, accidental out-of-hospital deliveries in this study was 2% (2328/114,938). These deliveries were described as unattended, as opposed to deliveries that were out-of-hospital but attended by skilled personnel. Perinatal mortality was significantly higher among out-of-hospital deliveries (odds ratio (OR) 2.01, 95% confidence interval (CI) 1.4–2.9), as compared with in-hospital deliveries. In addition, parturients who gave birth out-of-hospital had higher rates of perineal tears and retained placenta, as compared with patients delivered in hospital (Table 2). Finally, patients

Table 1 Independent risk factors for early postpartum hemorrhage, which can be of major importance during out-of-hospital deliveries. Results from a multiple logistic regression model. Adapted from Sheiner *et al.*, 2005[17]

	Odds ratio	95% CI	p Value
Retained placenta	3.5	2.1–5.8	<0.001
Labor dystocia, second stage	3.4	2.4–4.7	<0.001
Placenta accreta	3.3	1.7–6.4	<0.001
Lacerations	2.4	2.0–2.8	<0.001
Large for gestational age	1.9	2.4–1.6	<0.001
Hypertensive disorders	1.6	2.1–1.2	<0.001

delivered out-of-hospital had a higher rate of delayed discharge from hospital as compared with controls.

GLOBAL RATES OF OUT-OF-HOSPITAL DELIVERIES

The number of out-of-hospital deliveries in the world is not well documented (Table 3). It is important to distinguish between *accidental* out-of-hospital deliveries and those intended and planned to take place out-of-hospital, with or without the attendance of medical personnel. In rural and remote regions of developing countries, out-of-hospital deliveries occur mainly due to limited access to health services (see Chapter 64). Often, access to referral health facilities and basic life-saving measures is equally lacking within the home and community. These latter intended out-of-hospital deliveries are associated with high rates of perinatal morbidity and mortality[2–14,22].

Hospital delivery is not a panacea as evidenced by a report from the Pan American Health Organization (PAHO), which documented the fact that 79% of deliveries in the Region of the Americas take place in institutional settings, with only a few countries in the Region reporting institutional deliveries below 50%[23]. Unfortunately, this trend was not accompanied by a corresponding decrease in maternal and perinatal mortality. Rather, even greater variations in neonatal and maternal mortality were seen in countries with high rates of institutional delivery. According to some authors, this may be due to unnecessary interventions, such as cesarean section and episiotomy, which may lead to increased morbidity and even mortality[24,25]. Efforts are being made to promote the use of evidence-based interventions in these countries[23].

In other reports from developed countries, the incidence of accidental out-of-hospital deliveries varied from 0.1 to 2%[7,13,26–28]. Factors associated with accidental out-of-hospital deliveries include multiparity and lack of prenatal care, which by themselves might increase the risk for adverse perinatal outcome[29,30]. A report from a district general hospital in the UK indicated a low incidence of 0.31% of unplanned out-of-hospital deliveries occurring over a 3-year period[26]. Women with unplanned out-of-hospital deliveries were multiparous, and 11 of 14 deliveries (78.6%) occurred during the night, between the hours of 20.00 and 08.00, suggesting difficulties in access to the hospital. In a study from Finland, a trend was found towards a decrease in accidental out-of-hospital deliveries between 1963 and 1973 (from 1.3 to 0.4/1000 births). This trend changed by the 1990s when the rate rose up to 1/1000. This change was attributed to the closing of small hospitals in remote parts of the country, leading to inconvenient access to obstetric facilities[7].

Examples for planned home births are found in two studies. In a prospective study designed to evaluate the safety of home births in North America, all home births involving certified professional midwives across the US and Canada during the year 2000 were assessed. The rate of planned home delivery was 1.6%[28]. A

Table 2 Pregnancy and labor complications of patients delivered out-of-hospital compared with patients delivered in hospital. Adapted from Sheiner *et al.*, 2002[13]

Characteristics	Out-of-hospital (n = 2328)		In hospital (n = 114,938)		
	n	%	n	%	p Value
Lack of prenatal care	809	34.8	10,822	9.4	<0.001
Perineal tear grade 1–2	435	18.7	16,178	14.1	<0.001
Perineal tear grade 3–4	4	0.2	77	0.1	<0.056
Retained placenta	27	1.2	693	0.6	<0.001
Small for gestational age	233	10.0	6809	5.9	<0.001
Large for gestational age	145	6.2	11,774	10.2	<0.001
Perinatal mortality	29	1.2	718	0.6	<0.001
Delayed discharge from hospital	911	39.7	35,343	31.1	<0.001

Table 3 Rates of planned and unplanned out-of-hospital deliveries in the world

Country	Reference	Rate (%)
Planned out-of-hospital deliveries		
United States and Canada	Johnson *et al.*[28]	1
Netherlands	Anthony *et al.*[31]	33
United States	MacDorman *et al.*[32]	0.9
Home births in developing countries		
Ethiopia southern	Sibley *et al.*[33]	90
India	Kodkany *et al.*[34]	50
Nairobi, Kenya	Bazant *et al.*[35]	33
Pakistan	Ayaz *et al.*[36]	44
Unplanned out-of-hospital deliveries		
Israel, Negev region	Sheiner *et al.*[13]	2
UK	Scott *et al.*[26]	0.3
Finland	Viisainen *et al.*[7]	0.1
Scotland catchment	Rodie *et al.*[27]	0.6

statistical report on home births in the US during the years 1990–2006 showed an interesting trend. After a gradual decline from 1990 to 2004, the percentage of out-of-hospital births increased from 0.87% in 2004 to 0.90% in 2005 and 2006. Home birth rates were higher for non-Hispanic white women, married women, women aged 25 and over, women with previous children, and higher in rural counties of less than 100,000 population. Home births were less likely to be preterm, low birth weight, or multiple deliveries.

In The Netherlands, approximately one-third of births are planned home deliveries, attended by midwives. In this cross-sectional study, maternal demographics associated with home birth included multiparity, age above 25 years and living in small as opposed to large cities[31].

The condition is quite different in undeveloped countries. In these areas, home birth with unskilled attendants is the norm, and maternal and neonatal mortality rates are high. Unfortunately, the rates and outcomes of these out-of-hospital births are grossly underreported. The causes for this situation include inadequate emergency care and home-based care by attendants who are poorly equipped or educated to respond to emergencies, leading to inappropriate or delayed action. For example, in rural southern

Ethiopia, over 90% of births take place at home in the presence of unskilled attendants[33].

In conclusion, the number of out-of-hospital deliveries in the world is not well documented. Although it is widely accepted that the quality of maternity care is a main determinant of maternal and fetal morbidity and mortality rates[37], the lack of statistical information on out-of-hospital deliveries is a severe limitation for further evaluation of the relationship between out-of-hospital deliveries and maternal morbidity and mortality in general and specifically PPH. On the other hand, encouraging data now show that simple interventions in community settings can make a change in maternal morbidity, neonatal mortality, stillbirths and perinatal mortality[38].

OUT-OF-HOSPITAL DELIVERY AND POSTPARTUM HEMORRHAGE

Our group[14] compared maternal and neonatal outcomes in out-of-hospital versus in-hospital deliveries in a prospective study. Unplanned out-of-hospital deliveries resulted in a statistically significant higher rate of PPH (OR 8.4, 95% CI 1.1–181.1, $p = 0.018$) (Table 4).

PPH due to uterine atony is the primary direct cause[39] of maternal mortality globally and this statement is equally true for those who deliver out-of-hospital and those who deliver at the most well equipped institute for obstetric care. Management strategies in developed countries involve crystalloid fluid replacement, blood transfusions and surgery. Such definitive therapies are often not accessible in developing countries, particularly in cases of out-of-hospital deliveries. The lack of skilled attendants at delivery who can provide even the minimum of care, long transport times to facilities that can manage uterine atony or severe lacerations of the genital tract, and unattended obstructed labor leading to a ruptured uterus, elevate PPH to its position as the number one killer of women during childbirth[22]. These factors are exacerbated by the prevalence of anemia, estimated to affect half of all pregnant women in the world[40].

Women who deliver out-of-hospital also do not benefit from active management of the third stage of labor, a methodology which clearly is associated with reductions in acute PPH and acute severe PPH (see Chapter 14). A retrospective study from Ghana compared active versus expectant management in a rural setting at Holy Family Hospital in Berekum[41]. The study found that PPH (blood loss = 500 ml) occurred less often in the actively managed group (OR 0.8, 95% CI 0.7–0.9). McCormick and colleagues[42] published a systematic review of studies that assessed the efficacy of active management of the third stage in low-resource settings. Active management of the third stage of labor, especially the administration of uterotonic drugs, reduced the risk of PPH due to uterine atony without increasing the incidence of retained placenta or other serious complications. Oxytocin is preferred over syntometrine, but misoprostol can be used effectively to prevent hemorrhage in situations where parenteral medications are not available (see Chapters 34 and 42). Misoprostol is easily used, effectively administered orally, and can be stored at room temperature for a relatively long period. It is important to keep in mind, however, that uterotonics such as misoprostol can only prevent PPH due to uterine atony; other causes of PPH (such as uterine rupture, cervical tear and vaginal injury, retained placenta, etc.) are unaffected[43]. Misoprostol is currently registered for obstetric and gynecologic use in Brazil, Peru, Egypt, France, Russia, Spain, India, Nepal, Bangladesh, Ghana, Kenya, Nigeria, Sudan, Tanzania, Uganda and Zambia[5,44]. To date, few studies describe misoprostol use at home births other than in the context of an intervention study[45] (see Chapter 42).

A 2003 Cochrane Review of active versus expectant management of the third stage of labor[46] included five randomized, controlled trials and found that, for all women, including women deemed at low risk for PPH, active management decreased the incidence of PPH (both 500–1000 ml and >1000 ml), shortened the third stage of labor, decreased the amount of maternal blood loss and the need for blood transfusion and additional therapeutic uterotonic agents. The incidence of PPH of 500 ml or more was reduced in the actively managed group (relative risk 0.38, 95% CI 0.32–0.46). These figures mean that for every 12 women who are actively rather than expectantly managed, one case of PPH (defined as blood loss of 500 ml) will be averted, whereas the number needed to treat for averting blood loss of greater than 1000 ml would be 57. Actively managed women lost less blood (weighted mean blood loss of 79.33 ml less) than those who managed expectantly. In addition, the third stage was an estimated 9.77 minutes shorter in actively managed women. The authors of this review concluded that the use of routine uterotonic agents to prevent PPH can reduce maternal mortality by 40%[47].

Data on types and incidences of maternal morbidities in communities with limited access to health services are scarce[22]. Bang and colleagues found,

Table 4 Maternal outcomes of patients with unplanned out-of-hospital deliveries and the control group. Adapted from Hadar *et al.*, 2005[14]

| Characteristics | Unplanned out-of-hospital deliveries (n = 151) | | Control group (n = 151) | | |
	n	%	n	%	p Value
Vaginal tears	27	17.9	18	12.0	0.087
Postpartum hemorrhage	8	5.3	1	0.6	0.018
Postpartum endometritis	2	1.3	0	0	0.157
Antibiotic treatment	2	1.3	0	0	0.157
Sutures of vaginal tears	25	16.6	18	12.0	0.249
Revision of uterus cavity	6	4.0	0	0	0.013
Hospitalization (days)	3.2 ± 0.9		2.95 ± 0.6		0.111

in their prospective observational study conducted in Gadchiroli, India, that the incidence of maternal morbidity was 52.6%. The most common intrapartum morbidities were prolonged labor (10.1%), prolonged rupture of membranes (5.7%), abnormal presentation (4.0%) and primary PPH (3.2%)[22]. The postpartum morbidities included secondary PPH (15.2%). In their study, mothers and neonates were prospectively observed at home in 39 villages without interventions. The study included a population of approximately one million parturients. Most deliveries in the area were conducted by traditional birth attendants (TBAs) and family members. This is the first reported study in a rural setting in a developing country where labor and the puerperium were prospectively observed at home in a systematic and objective manner to measure the incidence of maternal morbidities. While it provided interesting information, it also had certain limitations. In particular, the sample may underestimate the incidence of morbidities because many hospital deliveries (which may have a higher proportion of problems) were not studied.

Another randomized, controlled trial was carried out to determine whether suckling immediately after birth reduces the frequency of PPH[48]. Trial participants were attended by TBAs. The TBAs compared blood loss in live born singleton deliveries in the early suckling mothers ($n = 2104$) and in controls ($n = 2123$). The frequency of PPH (loss greater than 500 ml) was similar in both groups, 7.9% in the suckling compared with 8.4% in the controls.

Prual and colleagues reported the frequency of morbidity in a population-based survey of a cohort of 20,326 pregnant women in six West African countries[49]. The main direct cause of severe maternal morbidity was hemorrhage (3.05 per 100 live births); in this report, 23 cases involved uterine rupture (0.12 per 100). Case fatality rates were high for hemorrhage and varied from 1.9% for antepartum or peripartum hemorrhage to 3.7% for placental abruption. The high case fatality rates of several complications reflected a poor quality of obstetric care.

Walraven et al.[50], in a double blind, randomized, controlled trial, sought to evaluate the impact of oral misoprostol on PPH compared with standard treatment in the home birth situation in rural Gambia, with measured blood loss, postpartum hemoglobin, and change in hemoglobin level between the last antenatal care visit and 3–5 days' postpartum as outcome measures. The study was carried out in 26 primary health care villages of the North Bank East Health Division, The Gambia, West Africa. Seventy-two per cent of births occur at home and maternal mortality in the study area was estimated at 424/100,000 live births in a reproductive age mortality survey, with PPH as the most important direct cause of maternal mortality. There were two maternal deaths in the study population (maternal mortality ratio for study population of 163 per 100,000 live births; 95% Poisson CI 20–595), both in the misoprostol group. These deaths were attributed to PPH (measured blood loss 2200 ml) and

Table 5 The risk for postpartum hemorrhage (PPH) in out-of-hospital deliveries

Country	Reference	PPH in out-of-hospital deliveries
West Africa	Prual et al.[49]	3.1%
Malawi	Bullough et al.[48]	8.4%
Ghana	Geelhoed et al.[41]	17.4%
India	Bang et al.[22]	3.2%
Israel	Hadar et al.[14]	5.3%
Israel	Sheiner et al.[13]	3.2%
Scotland	Rodie et al.[51]	0.6%
Mexico (Jalisco)	Avalos-Huizar et al.[52]	12%

disseminated intravascular coagulation due to malaria (measured blood loss 300 ml).

Table 5 summarizes the existing, limited data regarding the association between out-of-hospital deliveries and PPH.

CONCLUSIONS

The fact that so many women deliver in domiciliary conditions clearly affects their risk of PPH. Our research has, for the first time, established an odds ratio of 8.4 for PPH in out-of-hospital deliveries[14]. This number represents an urgent call to the medical community to change this circumstance whenever and wherever possible, as is detailed in other chapters of this book. All births should be attended by adequately trained personnel. Misoprostol has an important role for the prevention of PPH. Misoprostol is a reasonable option where parenteral administration of a uterotonic is not feasible. It is easily used, effectively administered orally, and can be stored at room temperature for a relatively long period. Nevertheless, it is important to keep in mind that misoprostol can only prevent PPH due to uterine atony; other causes of PPH are unaffected. More effective strategies are needed to convince women with high-risk pregnancies to deliver in a hospital which has access to emergency referral services.

References

1. Zur M, Hadar A, Sheiner E, Mazor M. Out-of-hospital deliveries: incidence, obstetrical characteristics and perinatal outcome. Harefuah 2003;142:38–41
2. Burnett CA 3rd, Jones JA, Rooks J, Chen CH, Tyler CW Jr, Miller CA. Home delivery and neonatal mortality in North Carolina. JAMA 1980;244:2741–5
3. Bateman DA, O'Bryan L, Nicholas SW, Heagarty MC. Outcome of unattended out-of-hospital births in Harlem. Arch Pediatr Adolesc Med 1994;148:147–52
4. Hinds MW, Bergeisen GH, Allen DT. Neonatal outcome in planned vs. unplanned out-of-hospital births in Kentucky. JAMA 1985;253:1578–82
5. Goldenberg RL, Hale CB, Houde J, Humphrey JL, Wayne JB, Boyd BW. Neonatal deaths in Alabama. III. Out-of-hospital births, 1940–1980. Am J Obstet Gynecol 1983;147:687–93
6. Bhoopalam PS, Watkinson M. Babies born before arrival at hospital. Br J Obstet Gynecol 1991;98:57–64

7. Viisainen K, Gissler M, Hartikainen AL, Hemminki E. Accidental out-of-hospital births in Finland: incidence and geographical distribution 1963–1995. Acta Obstet Gynecol Scand 1999;78:372–8

8. Moscovitz HC, Magriples U, Keissling M, Schriver JA. Care and outcome of out-of-hospital deliveries. Acad Emerg Med 2000;7:757–61

9. Verdile VP, Tutsock G, Paris PM, Kennedy RA. Out-of-hospital deliveries: a five-year experience. Prehospital Disaster Med 1995;10:10–13

10. Chen CC, Huang CB, Chung MY. Unexpected delivery before arrival at hospital: an observation of 18 cases. Changgeng Yi Xue Za Zhi 2000;23:205–10

11. Walraven GE, Mkanje RJ, Roosmalen J, van Dongen PW, Dolmans WM. Perinatal mortality in home births in rural Tanzania. Eur J Obstet Gynecol Reprod Biol 1995;58:131–4

12. Sheiner E, Hershkovitz R, Shoham-vardi I, Erez O, Hadar A, Mazor M. A retrospective study of unplanned out-of-hospital deliveries. Arch Gynecol Obstet 2004;269:85–8

13. Sheiner E, Shoham-vardi I, Hadar A, Sheiner EK, Hershkovitz R, Mazor M. Accidental out-of-hospital delivery as an independent risk factor for perinatal mortality. J Reprod Med 2002;47:625–30

14. Hadar A, Rabinovich A, Sheiner E, Landau D, Hallak M, Mazor M. Obstetrics characteristics and neonatal outcome of unplanned out-of-hospital term deliveries: a prospective case–control study. J Reprod Med 2005;50:832–6

15. Pritchard JD, Baidwin RM, Dickey JC, Wiggins KM. Blood volume changes in pregnancy and the puerperium. II. Red blood cell loss and changes in apparent blood volume during and following vaginal delivery, cesarean section, and cesarean section plus total hysterectomy. Am J Obstet Gynecol 1962; 84:1271–82

16. Norris CT. Management of postpartum hemorrhage. Am Fam Physician 1997;55:635–40

17. Sheiner E, Sarid L, Levy A, Seidman DS, Hallak M. Obstetric risk factors and outcome of pregnancies complicated with early postpartum hemorrhage: A population-based study. J Matern Fetal Neonatal Med 2005;18:149–54

18. Combs CA, Murphy EL, Laros RK. Factors associated with postpartum hemorrhage with vaginal birth. Obstet Gynecol 1991;77:69–76

19. Combs CA, Murphy EL, Laros RK. Factors associated with hemorrhage in cesarean deliveries. Obstet Gynecol 1991;77: 77–82

20. Magann EF, Evans S, Hutchinson M, Collins R, Howard BC, Morrison JC. Postpartum hemorrhage after vaginal birth: an analysis of risk factors. South Med J 2005;98:419–22

21. Magann EF, Evans S, Chauhan SP, Lanneau G, Fisk AD, Morrison JC. The length of the third stage of labor and the risk of postpartum hemorrhage. Obstet Gynecol 2005;105: 290–3

22. Bang RA, Bang AT, Reddy MH, Deshmukh MD, Baitule SB, Filippi V. Maternal morbidity during labour and the puerperium in rural homes and the need for medical attention: A prospective observational study in Gadchiroli, India. Br J Obstet Gynaecol 2004;111:231–8

23. Pan American Health Organization. Health in the Americas. Pan American Health Organization, 2002;I www.paho.org

24. Lydon-Rochelle M, Holt VL, Martin DP, Easterling TR. Association between method of delivery and maternal rehospitalization. JAMA 2000;283:2411–6

25. Srp B, Velebil P. Proportion of caesarean sections and main causes of maternal mortality during 1978–1997 in the Czech Republic. Ceska Gynekol 1999;64:219–23

26. Scott T, Esen UI. Unplanned out-of-hospital births – who delivers the babies? Ir Med J 2005;98:70–2

27. Rodie VA, Thomson AJ, Norman JE. Accidental out-of-hospital deliveries: an obstetric and neonatal case control study. Acta Obstet Gynecol Scand 2002;81:50–4

28. Johnson KC, Daviss BA. Outcomes of planned home births with certified professional midwives: large prospective study in North America. Br Med J 2005;330:1416

29. Twizer E, Sheiner E, Hallak M, Mazor M, Katz M, Shoham-Vardi I. Lack of prenatal care in a traditional society: is it an obstetrical hazard? J Reprod Med 2001;46:662–8

30. Sheiner E, Hallak M, Twizer E, Mazor M, Katz M, Shoham-Vardi I. Lack of prenatal care in two different societies living in the same region and sharing the same medical facilities. J Obstet Gynaecol 2001;21:453–8

31. Anthony S, Buitendijk SE, Offerhaus PM, Dommelen P, Pal-de Bruin KM. Maternal factors and the probability of a planned home birth. Br J Obstet Gynaecol 2005;112:748–53

32. MacDorman MF, Menacker F, Declercq E. Trends and characteristics of home and other out-of-hospital births in the United States, 1990–2006. Natl Vital Stat Rep 2010;58:1–14, 16

33. Sibley L, Buffington ST, Haileyesus D. The American College of Nurse-Midwives' Home-Based Lifesaving Skills Program: A Review of the Ethiopia Field Test. J Midwifery Womens Health 2004;49:320–8

34. Kodkany BS, Derman RJ, Goudar SS, et al. Initiating a novel therapy in preventing postpartum hemorrhage in rural India: a joint collaboration between the United States and India. Int J Fertil Womens Med 2004;49:91–6

35. Bazant ES, Koenig MA, Fotso JC, Mills S. Women's use of private and government health facilities for childbirth in Nairobi's informal settlements. Stud Fam Plann 2009;40: 39–50

36. Ayaz A, Saleem S. Neonatal mortality and prevalence of practices for newborn care in a squatter settlement of Karachi, Pakistan: a cross-sectional study. PLoS One 2010;5:e13783

37. World Health Organization. Mother–Baby Package (WHO/RHT/MSM/94.11, Rev1). Geneva: World Health Organization, 1998

38. Lassi ZS, Haider BA, Bhutta ZA. Community-based intervention packages for reducing maternal and neonatal morbidity and mortality and improving neonatal outcomes. Cochrane Database Syst Rev 2010;(12):CD005978

39. Miller S, Lester F, Hensleigh P. Prevention and treatment of postpartum hemorrhage: new advances for low-resource settings. J Midwifery Womens Health 2004;49:283–92

40. Levy A, Fraser D, Katz M, Mazor M, Sheiner E. Maternal anemia during pregnancy is an independent risk factor for low birthweight and preterm delivery. Eur J Obstet Gynecol Reprod Biol 2005;122:182–6

41. Geelhoed D, Visser L, Agordzo P, et al. Active versus expectant management of the third stage of labor in rural Ghana. Acta Obstet Gynecol Scand 2002;81:171–3

42. McCormick ML, Sanghvi HC, Kinzie B, McIntosh N. Preventing postpartum hemorrhage in low-resource settings. Int J Gynaecol Obstet 2002;77:267–75

43. Fortney JA. Home use of misoprostol to prevent PPH. Editor's Comment. Int J Gynaecol Obstet 2010;108:268

44. Fernandez M, Coeytaux F, Gomez Ponce de Leon R, Harrison D. Assessing the global availability of misoprostol. Int J Gynecol Obstet 2009;105:180–6

45. Flandermeyer D, Stanton C, Armbruster D. Uterotonic use at home births in low-income countries: a literature review. Int J Gynaecol Obstet 2010;108:269–75

46. Prendiville WJ, Elbourne D, McDonald S. Active versus expectant management in the third stage of labour (Cochrane Review). In The Cochrane Library. Chichester: John Wiley & Sons, 2003, Issue 4

47. Prendiville WJ, Harding JE, Elbourne DR, Stirrat GM. The Bristol third stage trial: active versus physiological management of third stage of labour. Br Med J 1988;297:1295–300

48. Bullough CH, Msuku RS, Karonde L. Early suckling and postpartum hemorrhage: controlled trial in deliveries by traditional birth attendants. Lancet 1989;2:522–5

49. Prual A, Bouvier-Colle MH, de Bernis L, Breart G. Severe maternal morbidity from direct obstetric causes in West Africa: incidence and case fatality rates. Bull WHO 2000; 78:593–602

50. Walraven G, Blum J, Dampha Y, et al. Misoprostol in the management of the third stage of labour in the home delivery

setting in rural Gambia: a randomized controlled trial. Br J Obstet Gynaecol 2005;112:1277–83

51. Rodie VA, Thomson AJ, Norman JE. Accidental out-of-hospital deliveries: an obstetric and neonatal case control study. Acta Obstet Gynecol Scand 2002;81:50–4

52. Avalos-Huízar LM, de la Torre-Gutiérrez M, López-Gallo L, et al. [Out-of-hospital delivery. Experience of ten years in Jalisco, Mexico.] Ginecol Obstet Mex 2010;78:418–22

70

Intraoperative Autologous Blood Transfusion

S. Catling and D. Thomas

INTRODUCTION

Life-saving transfusion using human blood was first described by James Blundell in 1818. He performed ten transfusions, five of which were successful; of these, four were in women suffering postpartum hemorrhage (PPH). He typically used donor blood from the patient's husband, showing that the technique of blood injection with a syringe infusion was safe[1]. In one account, he is credited with the re-infusion of autologous blood[2]. It is entirely appropriate, therefore, that the subject of intraoperative autologous transfusion be described in this textbook on PPH. Blundell's original report described a reasonable outcome considering the crude understanding of blood transfusion techniques in existence almost a century before Landsteiner's identification of the ABO blood groups[3].

Some of the earliest reports of intraoperative blood salvage described the life-saving technique of simply collecting spilt blood from the abdominal cavity, filtering it through a gauze swab, and re-infusing what remained. In the ensuing years, techniques to collect, filter and wash blood lost at the time of surgery have become commonplace, although refinements of the method vary widely and depend not only upon the nature of the surgical procedure, but also the availability of technical resources. As might be expected, expensive apheresis machines are lacking in many, if not most, parts of the world where operative obstetrics are routinely practiced. Nevertheless, the problem of PPH is so common and remains such a clinical challenge that the technique as originally described is still used out of necessity in these circumstances. This chapter describes various methods of autologous blood salvage and, in particular, its evolving use in obstetrics with direct reference to PPH.

DEFINITION

Autologous blood salvage is the collection of spilt blood resulting from surgical or traumatic bleeding that can be undertaken intraoperatively or postoperatively. The collected blood can be filtered and re-infused or filtered, washed and then re-infused.

METHODS

The quality and constitution of re-infused blood vary depending on whether washed or unwashed systems are used. In the absence of automated cell-washing devices, simple collection, filtration and re-infusion during PPH have been described and continue to be used in some areas in the world. However, this technique is not ideal. On the other hand, the use of unwashed blood (particularly for postoperative collection and re-infusion using a sealed postoperative collection unit with a filter) has been used extensively in total knee surgery and appears safe and effective. Interestingly, one report suggested that the use of unwashed blood might have inherent properties that improve the recipient's immune response[4]. The more widely applied intraoperative cell salvage is conducted with apparatus that has the ability to collect spilt blood at the time of the operation and anticoagulate it at the tip of the suction apparatus with citrated solution or heparinized saline (25,000 IU per liter of normal saline) (Figure 1).

Collected blood is then transferred to a centrifugal bowl, where spinning at 5500 revolutions per second moves the heavier red cells to the outer periphery of the bowl. As the bowl fills, the accumulation of red cells forces the plasma, platelets and other cellular debris out of a central exit, discarding waste products of the process. Special sensors identify when the bowl is full of red cells, and the fully automated machine begins to wash the collected and concentrated erythrocytes with normal saline. This process further cleanses the red blood cells. The resultant concentrate is then suspended in normal saline, producing a solution with a hematocrit of 60%. Unfortunately, most of the platelets and clotting factors will have been washed away at this point, and the fluid for re-infusion consists of autologous red cells suspended in normal saline[5]. In the presence of brisk bleeding, any of the commercially available automated cell-washing devices can produce a unit of red cell concentrate in 5–10 min. The volume of lost blood that can be processed is infinite, and reports of cell salvage in major trauma describe its successful use, the process providing approximately 50% of the required red cell transfusion[6]. Of course, in such situations, the use of cell

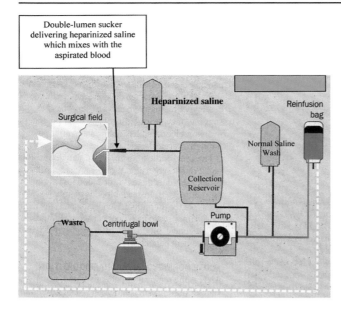

Double-lumen sucker delivering heparinized saline which mixes with the aspirated blood

Figure 1 A diagrammatic representation of intraoperative cell salvage. (Adapted from an original drawing with the kind permission of Haemonetics Inc., Baintree). The dotted line represents infusion sent back to the patient. In the case of a Jehovah's Witness, this is primed with saline before starting to complete continuity of the circuit

salvage only minimizes the demand for allogeneic blood. In cases of massive hemorrhage, cell salvage devices help to recycle transfused allogeneic blood as well as autologous blood. As few platelets and minimal clotting factors are present in these re-infused red cells, careful assessment of coagulation parameters is required, especially in cases of excessive bleeding where massive transfusion is required. Nowadays, this is the case in patients with massive hemorrhage, as the provision of red cells suspended in a mixture of saline, adenine, glucose and mannitol (SAGM) means that only packed allogeneic red cells are being infused, and so similar provisos apply. Under these circumstances, early consideration therefore needs to be given to platelet and fresh frozen plasma administration.

HISTORICAL COMPLICATIONS

Current machines have an extremely good safety record, but it is worthwhile dispelling some misconceptions about the technique that persist. Air embolism is not a problem with modern equipment when it is used correctly. Free hemoglobin is almost completely removed, and the very small amounts that remain have no significant clinical effect. Platelets are activated during salvage, but the majority are removed during the process. Leukocytes, complement and kinins are also activated during salvage, but systemic inflammatory responses have not been reported as clinically relevant.

POTENTIAL CONTRAINDICATIONS

The non-availability of a safe allogeneic blood supply is clearly a situation when the use of cell salvage is justified in an attempt to preserve the patient's own blood and help oxygen carriage. In the UK, current blood conservation recommendations promote the use of cell salvage[7]. The current drive for blood conservation is multifactorial, but the most topical reason is the potential decrease in the availability of donor blood resulting from the introduction of a test for the presence of abnormal prion protein. However, reduced numbers of donors is a problem that had its inception prior to the present testing concerns, as the presence of HIV and other viral pathogens have also restricted the number of potential donors. It is against this backdrop that consideration of cell salvage in PPH was made, and the remainder of this chapter examines the use of intraoperative cell salvage during PPH. Fortunately, the widespread use of such devices has confirmed the safety of this process, providing there is no technical failure and the correct procedure for machine operation is practiced. The use of such devices is endorsed by national guidelines and government directives[8,9].

Following a seminal report[10] supporting this technology, it now is accepted that three areas exist where the process of red cell salvage needs to be used with caution and following a risk–benefit analysis, depending on the clinical urgency of the situation. These involve the use of red cell salvage when spilt operative blood may contain malignant cells, or be heavily contaminated with bowel bacteria. Another area of caution is the use of red cell salvage when contaminated by amniotic fluid. It is accepted that, in the presence of any of these preconditions, cell salvage is not used unless considered necessary.

SAFETY OF CELL SALVAGE IN OBSTETRICS

Two theoretical problems attend the use of cell salvage at the time of cesarean section. First, in an Rh-negative mother, there is a risk of Rh immunization if the fetus is Rh-positive. As the cell saver cannot distinguish fetal from adult red cells, any fetal red cells suctioned from the operative field will be processed and re-infused with the maternal red cells. In practice, studies show that the degree of contamination with fetal red cells during cell salvage at cesarean section is between 1 and 19 ml[11–13]. Applying the standard Kleihauer calculation, this would require between 500 and 2500 units (1–5 ampules) of anti-D to avoid Rh immunization. As all Rh-negative patients require anti-D after cesarean section, patients receiving salvaged blood may simply require an increased dose. Larger doses have been used after mismatched transfusions with no untoward results.

The second theoretical problem is contamination with amniotic fluid, raising the specter of iatrogenic amniotic fluid embolus (AFE). This theoretical complication has been investigated by several workers, and has not been found to be a problem in practice[12–16]. The difficulty is that the precise elements of amniotic fluid which cause the rare and unpredictable 'anaphylactoid syndrome of pregnancy' (as AFE is more correctly called) remain unknown. To conduct a prospective, randomized, controlled trial with an 80% power to demonstrate that cell salvage does not increase the incidence of AFE by five-fold would require up to 275,000 patients, a number so large that the effort is unlikely ever to be undertaken. To demonstrate the absolute safety of a technique without randomized, controlled trials requires careful clinical audit of a large number of cases, supported by robust *in vitro* evidence.

IN VITRO STUDIES OF AMNIOTIC FLUID CLEARANCE

In vitro studies have examined the clearance of α-fetoprotein[14], tissue factor[15], trophoblastic tissue[12], fetal squames and lamellar bodies[13] from maternal blood by the cell salvage process. Small molecules are removed in the plasma fraction by the centrifuge and wash process, whereas particulate material is removed by the use of specialized leukodepletion filters. Using the combination of cell salvage and these specialized filters, every element of amniotic fluid that has been studied so far has been effectively removed from salvaged blood prior to re-transfusion[12–16].

CLINICAL CASES

Prior to 1999, approximately 300 cases in which cell-salvaged blood was administered to patients had been reported worldwide[16]. No obstetric clinical or physiological problems were encountered, despite the fact that filters were not used at this time. This means that each of these patients had some exposure to amniotic fluid, and with no ill effects. Waters and colleagues[13] described not only the complete clearance of squamous cells and phospholipid lamellar bodies from filtered, cell-salvaged blood, but also clearly demonstrated the presence of both these amniotic fluid markers circulating in the maternal central venous blood at the time of placental separation. In 100% of patients in this trial, amniotic fluid was demonstrated in the circulation of healthy parturients undergoing elective cesarean section. It is therefore probable that amniotic fluid routinely enters the maternal circulation and does no harm in the vast majority of cases. This exposure may trigger the syndrome of AFE due to an anaphylactoid reaction to an as-yet unidentified endogenous mediator in a very small number of women, the incidence of which varies between 1 in 8000 and 1 in 80,000 patients[17]. *[Editor's note: As it has never been studied, there is no evidence to state that entry does not occur in an unknown number of cases of vaginal parturition. L.G.K.]* Clearly, reinfusion of cell-salvaged blood, even if contaminated with traces of amniotic fluid, presents no extra risk to the woman from whom that blood has come, as she has already been exposed to it.

In 1999, a single report appeared describing a seriously ill Jehovah's Witness with severe pre-eclampsia complicated by HELLP syndrome who died in Holland after having received cell-salvaged blood[18]. In an oral presentation in London sometime afterward,

one of the speakers referred to this case as a 'death due to obstetric cell salvage'[19]. It should be noted, however, that a patient who is seriously ill with HELLP syndrome and who refuses platelet and coagulation factor transfusion is unlikely to survive. Under such circumstances, it is a mischaracterization to suggest that her death was related to the use of cell salvage rather than to ascribe it to her refusal to accept blood component therapy.

Cell salvage in obstetrics was introduced in the UK in 1999, and its use has grown rapidly, with most major obstetric units now advocating the technique in selected circumstances. The Confidential Enquiry into Maternal and Child Health 2000–2002 (CEMACH)[20] stated that '. . . (cell salvage) may be used in any case of obstetric haemorrhage, not just women who refuse blood transfusion' and described the technique as 'a new development which will prove helpful in the future'. It further stated that 'the risk of causing coagulopathy by returning amniotic fluid to the circulation is thought to be small'. Subsequent to this, the 2005 revised Guidelines for Obstetric Anaesthetic Services were published jointly by the UK Obstetric Anaesthetists Association (OAA) and the Association of Anaesthetists of Great Britain and Ireland (AAGBI)[21], stating that 'an increasing shortage of blood and blood products and growing anxiety about the use of donor blood are leading to an increasing interest in the use of cell salvage in obstetrics. Staff will have to be suitably trained, and equipment obtained and maintained. . .'

In November 2005, the UK National Institute for Clinical Excellence (NICE) reported on Cell Salvage in Obstetrics[22], describing cell salvage as 'an efficacious technique for blood replacement, well established in other areas of medicine' and pointing out the *theoretical* concerns when used in obstetrics. NICE goes on to recommend that clinicians using it in the UK should report any side-effects to the UK Department of Health Regulatory Authority (MHRA), that patients should be fully informed prior to its use, and that cell salvage in obstetrics should be performed by multidisciplinary teams that have developed regular experience in its use.

PRACTICAL USE OF CELL SALVAGE IN OBSTETRICS

The present experience with the use of cell salvage in obstetrics in the UK is substantial; cases include major hemorrhage due to placenta previa, placenta accreta, ruptured uterus, extrauterine placentation, massive fibroids and placental abruption, as well as more routine use in Jehovah's Witnesses to avoid postoperative anemia[14].

The following guidelines used for cell salvage in obstetric use in the Swansea NHS Trust Hospitals, UK are an example:

(1) It may be used for any situation in which allogeneic blood is used, but to date has been confined to cesarean sections and uterine

re-exploration or laparotomy following PPH. In reality, vaginal blood loss can be collected and cell salvaged, as fears about infection have proved unfounded as long as the patients are on antibiotics. The technical problem with physically collecting vaginal blood loss can be addressed with the planned use of the BRASSS drape described in Chapter 11.

(2) The machine is prepared and operated according to standard operating procedure, with an 'in-continuity' set-up for Jehovah's Witnesses (the whole circuit is run through with saline and the re-transfusion bag connected to the intravenous cannula before starting the salvage suction, thereby establishing a continuous circuit between the blood lost and the recipient vein).

(3) In cases where there is doubt about the extent of expected blood loss, it is economical to set up the aspiration and reservoir kit only – the decision to process and re-transfuse can be made when the degree of hemorrhage becomes clear (e.g. 'expected' bleeding from placenta previa).

(4) Where practicable, amniotic fluid should be removed by separate suction prior to starting cell salvage. However, some authors suggest that this is not necessary and that the quality of the washing procedure is sufficient to remove fetal contaminants[23].

(5) Suction should be via the wide-bore suction nozzle already supplied in the kit, and the surgeon should try to suction blood from 'pools' rather than 'dabbing' tissue surfaces with the suction tip, as this minimizes erythrocyte damage.

(6) Blood from swabs can be gently washed with saline and salvaged from a sterile bowl into the main reservoir.

(7) Suction pressure should be kept as low as practicable (less than 300 mmHg) to avoid red cell damage, although higher vacuum can be safely used if necessary with only a minimum increase in red cell damage.

(8) It is advisable to use a leukocyte depletion filter (Leukoguard® RS Pall) in the retransfusion circuit if there is any risk of amniotic fluid contamination. This is currently the only filter that removes all particulate elements of amniotic fluid (fetal squames, lamellar bodies). Such a filtration process will necessarily slow down the rate at which blood can be infused, but it is permissible to pressurize the bag of salvaged red cells up to 200 mmHg after having ensured there is no air in the bag (otherwise it may burst!). In situations when hemorrhage is rapid, it is possible to connect more than one suction nozzle to the reservoir, and two filters and a dual line to the re-infusion bag.

(9) As with any transfusion, the patient should be carefully monitored, preferably in an obstetric 'critical care' facility for 24 h. Coagulation tests should be obtained post-transfusion, and repeated if abnormal or if clinically indicated. If the patient is Rh-negative, a Kleihauer–Braun–Betke test should be performed and appropriate quantities of anti-D administered within 72 h.

Obstetric units that use cell salvage should keep a careful records for audit reporting in due course – with any problems also being reported to SHOT (Serious Hazards of Transfusion) (UK) as per NICE guidelines. Since the original edition of this textbook was published in 2006, no instances of AFE have been reported as a result of cell salvage use in the area of obstetrics. However, there have been reports of adverse events when leukodepletion filters (LDF) are used to improve the quality of the returned red cells.

LEUKOCYTE DEPLETION FILTERS: PAST AND CURRENT ISSUES

Concern regarding AFE led to the introduction of LDFs (Pall Medical, Pall Europe Ltd, Portsmouth, England). These filters have two mechanisms of action. First, they act as a passive sieve when blood passes through a microfiber web and there is active adhesion to a negative surface charge[24]. The original *in vitro* studies all used an LDF of some kind[12,13], and therefore, the use of an LDF was advocated in composing guidelines. Such filters are not without their own problems. In May 1999, the US FDA reported that in the preceding 5 years significant hypotensive events had occurred in over 80 patients receiving blood products transfused through a bedside LDF[25]. During the same time period, however, it was estimated that approximately 20 million bedside LDFs had been used. Given the rarity of this reaction, a recommendation was made that should a patient develop signs of an 'LDF reaction', the transfusion should be stopped immediately and the symptoms should resolve rapidly. Of interest, this reaction occurred only with bedside leukodepletion, and not with blood that had been stored after filtration, suggesting that the act of leukodepletion pre-storage altered the quality of the blood being returned.

In January 2011 the FDA repeated its concerns regarding LDFs stating that 'bedside filtration has been associated with precipitous hypotension in the transfusion recipient, an infrequent yet serious adverse effect not associated with pre-storage leukocyte reduction. Patients on ACE [angiotensin converting enzyme] inhibitors appeared to be particularly susceptible'[26]. It is possible that there is something present in filtered blood following the passage through an LDF that is transient and is removed or disappears following a period of storage at 4°C.

All blood in the UK has been LD filtered prior to storage since 1999. Following the NICE recommendations that cell salvage with LDFs for obstetrics and malignancy seemed a safe process to manage troublesome hemorrhage and provide a source of autologous blood, 13 reports of hypotension have been made to SHOT. Reporting of adverse events related to autologous techniques was commenced with a pilot scheme in 2007[27–29]. The 2007 report does not state whether a filter was used, but the other 12 cases from 2008 to 2010 all have LDF and acid-citrate-dextrose (ACD) anticoagulant use as common factors. Two case reports were published in 2010 describing severe hypotension occurring in relation to cell salvaged blood transfusion in obstetrics[30,31]. In both instances, the hypotension resolved on cessation of the infusion. As discussed in the accompanying editorial, it could not be determined with absolute certainty that the LDF was responsible as in neither case was transfusion attempted without filtration[32]. SHOT have analysed these reactions in detail and have not identified any other drug or agent as a precipitant (personal communication – Sue Catling).

These rare events have been studied by SHOT and by the UK Cell Salvage Action Group (Better Blood Transfusion – NHS Blood and Transfusion (NHSBT)) who are also aware of other cases that have been informally discussed and do not yet appear in the SHOT statistics. One case reported the use of heparin as anticoagulant compared with all others that had used ACD. Some cases are complex and multifactorial with massive hemorrhage in sick individuals, where it is difficult to ascertain the precise cause of the hypotension; in others there is a clear time relationship between the onset of sudden hypotension and infusion of cell salvaged, LD filtered blood. The other common factor is the use of ACD anticoagulant, rather than heparin. At present there is no UK national database on cell salvage, so it is not known how many patients received cell salvaged blood during these years, nor how many times the LDF was used.

Bradykinin has been suggested as one possible cause of the LDF related hypotension. It is a potent vasodilator with a short plasma half-life of 15 seconds due to its breakdown by ACE in the lungs. Evidence already exists in the dialysis population that filter membranes can cause hypotension as a result of bradykinin release[33,34]. Iwama investigated the effect of these negatively charged membranes on whole autologous blood *in vitro*[35]. He showed that passing whole blood through a negatively charged membrane at room temperature caused massive release of bradykinin, the concentration of which increased 4000 fold from 13 pg/ml to 55,933 pg/ml. These levels are capable of causing significant hypotension on re-infusion, and Iwama confirmed this point by giving such blood to six patients which resulted in a greater than 20% reduction in blood pressure. The proposed mechanism is that the negatively charged non-biologic filter surface activates coagulation factor XII. This activation process then triggers formation of the enzyme kallikrein from pre-kallikrein, resulting in cleavage of bradykinin from its high molecular weight precursor kininogen. The role of bradykinin is also supported by the clinical reports that patients on ACE inhibitors appear to be particularly susceptible[26].

Nevertheless, some uncertainty still exists as to whether bradykinin is responsible. To date, only whole blood has been studied, and cell salvaged blood consists of red cells suspended in saline with minimal plasma remaining; as such, it lacks a plasma source of bradykinin. Other potential mechanisms are that bradykinin is generated on the negative membrane from a non-plasma source, such as the white cells themselves, or that an entirely different mediator is involved. Cysteinyl leukotrienes can cause bronchoconstriction via the leukotriene (LT)1 receptor and can increase vascular permeability and inflammation via receptor pathway LT2. However, currently these substances have no identified role in acute vasodilation.

Further doubts exist in relation to LDFs being responsible for the observed hypotension. For example, if exposure to a negative membrane consistently causes vasoactive mediator release, then why is this reaction not seen consistently with every cell salvaged transfusion that uses a LDF? Potentially such reactions may only be occurring in individuals who are either constitutionally or therapeutically ACE deficient. Studies to investigate the bradykinin and leukotriene concentration in cell salvaged blood before and after passage across the LDF in normal clinical conditions are about to start in the UK, and the results should help to answer these questions.

In the meantime, the MHRA[36], the AAGBI[37] and SHOT[29] have issued statements warning clinicians to be aware of this possible adverse reaction, which has in every case been rapidly and effectively treated by stopping the transfusion and the appropriate use of fluids and vasopressors. In some cases, the cell salvage transfusion has then been completed without the LDF[38]. This raises the issue as to the necessity of the LDF in obstetric practice.

Before the introduction of LDFs, unfiltered cell salvaged blood was re-infused in almost 400 cases without the development of AFE or any other adverse effect[39–41]. Indeed, parturients who were completely well have been shown to have unequivocal evidence of amniotic fluid in their circulation[13]. In addition, very early studies from Peru suggested that deliberate infusion of amniotic fluid is not harmful[42], and this is consistent with the animal studies that have failed to replicate human AFE[43–46].

A technical problem with using an LDF is that it significantly reduces the rate at which salvaged blood can be given. This should not be circumvented by pressurizing the blood, and thus it severely restricts transfusion in a torrential hemorrhage. In practice, where rapid transfusion is required, or hypotension due to the filter is suspected, it can be removed and transfusion continued without it. As highlighted in the introduction to this chapter, anecdotal reporting from many countries where LDFs are not available describes the life-saving use of red cell salvage often undertaken with the most rudimentary equipment. The use of citrate as an anticoagulant and simple gauze filtration has been reported as a useful source of red cells for transfusion in the emergency situation.

SUMMARY

The use of intraoperative cell salvage is a safe method of conserving operative blood loss and minimizing the need for allogeneic transfusion. In an environment where allogeneic blood is in limited supply or the demands for blood transfusion are great, as in the case of massive PPH, the use of intraoperative cell salvage may be life-saving. Its use in this area continues to gain clinical acceptance.

References

1. Blundell J. Experiments on the transfusion of blood by the syringe. Med Chirg Trans 1818;9:57–92
2. Allen JG. Discussion. Ann Surg 1963;158:137
3. Landsteiner K. Ueber Agglutinationserscheinungen normalen menschlichen Blutes. Wien Klin Wochenschr 1901;14:1132–4
4. Gharehbaghian A, Haque KM, Truman C, et al. Effect of autologous blood on postoperative natural killer cell precursor frequency. Lancet 2004;363:1025–30
5. Tawes RL, Duvall TB. The basic concepts of an auto-transfusor: the cell saver. In: Tawes RL, ed. Autotransfusion. Michigan: Gregory Appleton, 1997
6. Hughes LG, Thomas DW, Wareham K, et al. Intra-operative blood salvage in abdominal trauma: a review of 5 years' experience. Anaesthesia 2001;56:217–20
7. A National Blood Conservation Strategy for NBTC and NBS. Compiled by Virge James on behalf of the NBS Sub-Group 'Appropriate Use of Blood', January 2004
8. NHS Executive. Better Blood Transfusion: Appropriate Use of Blood. London: Department of Health, 2002 (Health Service Circular 2002/009)
9. Peri-operative Blood Transfusion for Elective Surgery. http://www.sign.ac.uk
10. Council on Scientific Affairs. Autologous blood transfusions. JAMA 1986;256:2378–80
11. Fong J, Gurewitsch ED, Kump L, Klein R. Clearance of fetal products and subsequent immunoreactivity of blood salvaged at Cesarean delivery. Obstet Gynecol 1999;93:968–72
12. Catling SJ, Williams S, Fielding AM. Cell salvage in obstetrics: an evaluation of the ability of cell salvage combined with leucocyte depletion filtration to remove amniotic fluid from operative blood loss at caesarean section. Int J Obstet Anesth 1999;8:79–84
13. Waters JH, Biscotti C, Potter PS, Phillipson E. Amniotic fluid removal during cell salvage in the Cesarean section patient. Anaesthesiology 2000;92:1531–6
14. Thornhill MI, O'Leary AJ, Lussos SA, Rutherford C, Johnson MD. An in vitro assessment of amniotic fluid removal from human blood through cell saver processing. Anaesthesiology 1991;75:A830
15. Bernstein HH, Rosenblatt MA, Gettes M, Lockwood C. The ability of the Haemonetics 4 cell saver to remove tissue factor from blood contaminated with amniotic fluid. Anesth Analgesia 1997;85:831–3
16. Catling SJ, Freites O, Krishnan S, Gibbs R. Clinical experience with cell salvage in obstetrics: 4 cases from one UK centre. Int J Obstet Anesthes 2002;11:128–34
17. Morgan M. Amniotic fluid embolism. Anaesthesia 1979;34:20–32
18. Oei SG, Wingen CBM, Kerkkamp HEM [letter]. Int J Obstet Anesth 2000;9:143
19. Controversies in Obstetric Anaesthesia Meeting. London, UK, March 2004
20. Confidential Enquiry into Maternal and Child Health (CEMACH) 2000–2002. The 6th Report of the Confidential Enquiries into Maternal Deaths in the UK. London, UK: RCOG,
21. AAGBI Guidelines for Obstetric Anaesthetic Services, revised edn. 2005. www.aagbi.org/sites/default/files/obstetric05.pdf
22. National Institute for Health and Clinical Excellence. Intra-operative blood cell salvage in obstetrics. November 2005. www.nice.org.uk/nicemedia/live/11038/30691/30691.pdf
23. Sullivan I, Faulds J, Ralph C. Contamination of salvaged blood by amniotic fluid and fetal red cells during elective Caesarean section. Br J Anaes 2008;101:225–9
24. Dzik S. Leukodepletion blood filters: Filter design and mechanisms of leukocyte removal. Transfus Med Rev 1993;7:65–77
25. US Food and Drink Administration. Hypotension and bedside leukocyte reduction filters. 1999. www.fda.gov/medicaldevices/safety/alertsandnotices/publichealthnotificati ons/ucm062284.htm
26. US Food and Drug Administration. Pre-Storage Leukocyte Reduction of Whole Blood and Blood Components Intended for Transfusion http//www.fda.gov/downloads/BiologicsBloodVaccines/GuidanceComplianceRegulatoryInf ormation/Guidances/Blood/UCM241461.pdf
27. SHOT. Annual Report 2007. www.shotuk.org/wp-content/uploads/2010/03/SHOT-Report-2007.pdf
28. SHOT. Annual Report 2008. www.shotuk.org/wp-content/uploads/2010/03/SHOT-Report-2008.pdf.
29. SHOT. Annual Report 2010. www.shotuk.org/wp-content/uploads/2011/07/SHOT-2010-Report1.pdf
30. Kessack LK, Hawkins N. Severe hypotension related to cell salvaged blood transfusion in obstetrics. Anaesthesia 2010;65:745–8
31. Sreelakshmi TR, Eldridge J. Acute hypotension associated with leucocyte depletion filters during cell salvaged blood transfusion. Anaesthesia 2010;65:742–4
32. Hussain S. Cell salvage-induced hypotension and London buses. Anaesthesia 2010;65:659–63
33. Stoves J, Goode NP, Visvanathan R, et al. Bradykinin response and early hypotension. Artificial Organs 2001;25:1009–21
34. Schulman G. Bradykinin generation by dialysis membranes: possible role in anaphylaxis. J Am Soc Nephrol 1993;3:1563–9
35. Iwama H. Bradykinin-associated reactions in white cell-reduction filter. J Crit Care 2001;16:74–81
36. MHRA. One liners issue 82. http://www.mhra.gov.uk/Publications/Safetyguidance/OneLiners/CON105973
37. AAGBI Safety Guideline. Blood transfusion and the Anaesthetist – intra-operative cell salvage. London, UK: The Association of Anaesthetists of Great Britain and Ireland, 2009
38. Waldron S. Hypotension associated with leucocyte depletion filters following cell salvage in obstetrics. Anaesthesia 2011;66:133–4
39. Rainaldi MP, Tazzari PL, Scagliarini G, Borghi B, Conte R. Blood salvage during caesarean section. Br J Anaesth 1998;80:195–8
40. Grimes DA. A simplified device for intraoperative autotransfusion. Obstet Gynecol 1988;72:947–50
41. Jackson SH, Lonser RE. Safety and effectiveness of intra-caesarean blood salvage. Transfusion 1993;33:181
42. Tio AG, quoted in letters. JAMA July 1956:996
43. Spence MR, Mason KG. Experimental amniotic fluid embolism in rabbits. Am J Obstet Gynecol 1974;119:1073–8
44. Stolte L, van Kessel H, Seelen J, Eskes T, Wagatsuma T. Failure to produce the syndrome of amniotic fluid embolism by infusion of amniotic fluid and meconium into monkeys. Am J Obstet Gynecol 1967;98:694–7
45. Petroianu GA, Altmannsberger SH, Maleck WH, et al. Meconium and amniotic fluid embolism: effects on coagulation in pregnant mini-pigs. Crit Care Med 1999;27:348–55
46. Hankins GD, Snyder RR, Clark SL, Schwartz L, Patterson WR, Butzin CA. Acute hemodynamic and respiratory effects of amniotic fluid embolism in the pregnant goat model. Am J Obstet Gynecol 1993;168:1113–29

71

Treating Hemorrhage from Secondary Abdominal Pregnancy: Then and Now

N. A. Dastur, A. E. Dastur and P. D. Tank

INTRODUCTION

Abdominal pregnancy is an unusual but real cause of postpartum hemorrhage (PPH). The high maternal morbidity and mortality associated with abdominal pregnancy is a function of abnormal placentation, which leads to intra-abdominal hemorrhage or the aftermath of retention of large amounts of dead tissue. To date, no evidence based guidelines have been published on this subject. The chapter begins with a series of four cases treated at the Nowrosjee Wadia Maternity Hospital in Mumbai, India, which are illustrative of the available treatment options. Wadia Hospital is a tertiary care center with a wide referral base, both inside the city and throughout the surrounding areas. This is followed by a discussion on the technical aspects of the surgical intervention and a review of the literature on modern treatment options.

CASE 1

In 1970, a primigravida aged 24 years was referred to the hospital with an abnormal presentation. The senior author (NAD) was practicing as a junior trainee. At that time, it was routine to confirm the diagnosis of abnormal presentation with abdominal radiography. Because the radiograph was suspicious of an abdominal pregnancy, the senior consultant planned an exploratory laparotomy to deliver the woman. A male child weighing 2700 g was delivered in good condition. However, the placenta was attached to the mesentery, and an attempt to separate it set off massive hemorrhage. Local measures such as ligation of vessels and compression failed to reduce the hemorrhage, so the peritoneal cavity was packed under pressure with a large bed sheet as a last resort. The patient was stable for the first 6 hours postoperatively, but then developed hypovolemic shock from intraperitoneal hemorrhage and died on the first postoperative day.

CASE 2

The second case occurred 4 years later at the same institute. A cesarean delivery was undertaken to deliver a 30-year-old multiparous woman with no progress in labor. On opening the peritoneum, the amniotic sac was encountered directly. A 2400 g female child was delivered. The placenta covered the lateral pelvic wall and posterior surface of the uterus. The senior consultant was called and an attempt at placental separation was made. This effort was soon abandoned in view of the difficulty in separation and ensuing hemorrhage. The cord was then cut short and tied, the placenta left *in situ* and the abdomen closed. The abdomen was packed under pressure with large abdominal packs for control of the hemorrhage. However, the patient developed a disseminated intravascular coagulopathy and died within 48 hours of the surgery.

CASE 3

In 1980, the senior author was involved in a third case of abdominal pregnancy. A 20-year-old primigravida was referred to the hospital at full term with abdominal pain thought to be of a surgical cause. There was a strong clinical suspicion of acute appendicitis which did not respond to conservative treatment. A laparotomy was performed. A full term abdominal pregnancy was found with the sac just below the peritoneum. A female child weighing 2600 g was delivered in good condition. The placenta was firmly adherent to the right pelvic sidewall. No attempt was made to remove it. The cord was cut short and tied and the abdomen was closed with a pelvic drain. The postoperative course was complicated by fever for the first 10 days despite treatment with antibiotics. The patient continued to have abdominal pain for 6 months after delivery. She had sequelae of a retained placenta but survived the pregnancy.

CASE 4

Although this is not a case of an abdominal pregnancy, it is used to illustrate the management of abnormal placentation. In 2001, the senior author performed a cesarean section for a 25-year-old primigravida at term. She was diagnosed to have an anterior placenta previa with accreta. Blood vessels were seen invading into the bladder wall on color Doppler. After delivering a 2.5 kg male child in good condition, no attempt at placental separation was initiated. Rather, a decision was made to leave the placenta *in situ* followed by methotrexate therapy. The woman was monitored in hospital for 3 weeks after delivery and administered a prolonged course of antibiotics. She had an uneventful course. Further follow-up was provided on an out-patient basis with color Doppler and serum β-human chorionic gonadotropin (hCG) levels. The placental mass underwent gradual involution over a period of 5 months, and the patient resumed menstruation 7 months after delivery.

INCIDENCE

Abdominal pregnancies are rare events. In the US, it is estimated that it occurs once in 10,000 live births and once for every 1000 ectopic pregnancies[1]. A more recent African report provides a much higher estimate of 4.3% of ectopic pregnancies, which is probably a reflection of the referral patterns in that region as well as a higher baseline rate of inherent tubal disease in the patient base of the hospital catchment area[2]. However, it also may be reasonable to assume that the incidence of abdominal pregnancies may have risen over the years, considering that the risk factors such as ectopic pregnancy, infertility from tuberculosis and endometriosis, pelvic infections and infertility treatments are more common today. Regardless, an obstetrician practicing alone may never come across an abdominal pregnancy in a career spanning decades. In the singular instance where he/she does have the need to treat such a patient, it may be in circumstances far from ideal. Although unusual, obstetricians should be aware of this potentially fatal condition, a circumstance which is amply illustrated by the first two cases described above.

DIAGNOSIS

A primary abdominal pregnancy presents in the first trimester in much the same fashion as an ectopic pregnancy. An advanced secondary abdominal pregnancy, on the other hand, is much more difficult to diagnose. Presenting complaints may include abdominal pain (ranging from mild discomfort to unbearable pain), painful or absent fetal movements, nausea, vomiting, abdominal fullness, flatulence, diarrhea and general malaise. On examination, there may be an abnormal lie (15–20% of cases), easily palpable fetal parts, a closed uneffaced cervix on vaginal examination and the failure to stimulate contractions with oxytocin or prostaglandins on attempting induction of labor[3]. Obviously, these symptoms and circumstances are far from specific. Taken together, however, they may (and should) raise a question about the location of the pregnancy. On reviewing the laboratory findings, one may also find an unexplained transient anemia in early pregnancy corresponding to the time of tubal rupture or abortion. The serum α fetoprotein value may be abnormally elevated without explanation. Early

diagnosis has been described in response to evaluation of abnormal biochemical screening results[4].

The diagnosis can be established with far greater certainty by imaging studies. Ultrasound is ubiquitously used in pregnancy, but does not always provide an unequivocal diagnosis. Even under ideal conditions, the diagnosis is missed on ultrasound in more than half of cases[3]. Akhan *et al.*[5] report the following criteria as suggestive of abdominal pregnancy:

- Visualization of the fetus separate from the uterus
- Failure to visualize the uterine wall between the fetus and the maternal urinary bladder
- Close approximation of fetal parts to the maternal abdominal wall
- Eccentric position (relation of fetus to uterus) or abnormal fetal attitude (relation of fetal parts to one another) and visualization of extrauterine placental tissue.

Unusual maternal vasculature in the placental periphery on Doppler examination may provide a clue to the diagnosis of an abdominal pregnancy[6]. In the past, radiography was commonly used to establish or at least point to this diagnosis. Features such as absence of uterine shadow around the fetus, maternal intestinal shadow intermingling with fetal parts on anteroposterior view and overlapping of the maternal spine by fetal small parts in a lateral view were all described. Today, however, radiography has largely been supplanted by magnetic resonance imaging (MRI) and computed tomography. Both these techniques, with their ability to produce images in different planes, have much greater accuracy and specificity than ultrasound. There is little to choose between the two imaging modalities in cases of fetal demise. If the fetus is alive, MRI may be preferable since ionizing radiation is avoided.

TIMING OF INTERVENTION

Maternal mortality is about 7.7 times higher with an abdominal pregnancy compared with a tubal ectopic pregnancy and 90 times higher compared with an intrauterine pregnancy[1]. These risks are thought to be chiefly related to the delay in diagnosis and mismanagement of the placenta. To minimize the risk from sudden, life-threatening intra-abdominal bleeding, it seems prudent to time intervention as soon as feasible after the diagnosis is confirmed. There is no controversy if there is maternal hemodynamic instability, the fetus is dead or pre-viable (less than 24 weeks' pregnancy), or has oligohydramnios or gross abnormalities on ultrasound. The hypothesis that fetal death will bring about placental involution and hence reduced bleeding at laparotomy is not substantiated. Surgical intervention is mandated if any of the above conditions are present.

Some clinicians argue that if there is an ongoing abdominal pregnancy greater than 24 weeks, a conservative approach should be taken to allow fetal maturity and improve chances of survival[7]. However, even after 30 weeks, fetal survival is only 63%, and 20% of fetuses have deformations (craniofacial and various joint abnormalities) and malformations (central nervous system and limb deficiencies)[8]. With advancing gestation, one also has to contend with the growing placenta and greater risk of bleeding. In our opinion, it would very rarely be justified to manage an abdominal pregnancy conservatively.

PREOPERATIVE PREPARATIONS

The major risk with surgery is torrential hemorrhage. When a diagnosis of abdominal pregnancy is established in advance, the opportunity to be prepared should not be lost. At least six units of blood should be cross matched and ready to transfuse in the operating room and other blood products should also be available. Two intravenous infusion systems capable of delivering large volumes of fluids rapidly should be established. A mechanical bowel preparation should be effected if time permits. A MAST (medical antishock garment) suit has been utilized successfully in controlling intractable hemorrhage with an abdominal pregnancy[9], but these garments are not always available (see Chapter 39 for a full discussion). Kerr *et al.*[10] have advocated preoperative transfemoral catheterization and embolization of selective vessels before surgical intervention. This intervention was used successfully in three cases, and the catheters can be left in place for their potential to assist in treating postoperative bleeding as well. The operating team should be experienced, and preferably should include a general, vascular and genitourinary surgeon. The anesthesia team should comprise senior consultants and their assistants. The operating room and nursing staffs should be fully aware of the nature of the diagnosis and its implications and schedule extra personnel in the room and as 'runners'.

SURGICAL APPROACH

A midline vertical approach is preferential, as it can easily be extended above the umbilicus if necessary. The amniotic sac may be adherent to the abdominal wall and viscera. It should be dissected free and opened in an avascular area away from the placenta. The fetus should be removed in such a way as to minimize placental manipulation and avoid bleeding. If the pregnancy has been retained for a long period after fetal death, the fetus will have undergone suppuration. Bacterial contamination and abscess formation are highly likely, especially if the placenta is adherent to the intestines. There may be frank pus upon entering the peritoneal cavity. Rarely, the fetus may be mummified and calcified into a lithopedion or have been converted into a yellow greasy mass called adipocere formation.

MANAGEMENT OF THE PLACENTA

The torrential hemorrhage that often ensues with surgery for abdominal pregnancy is related to the lack of constriction of the hypertrophied opened blood vessels after placental separation. Usually, the placenta is firmly attached to the parietal peritoneum, mesentery and bowel and *there is no bleeding if it is left alone*. The umbilical cord should be ligated close to the placenta, excess membranes trimmed away and the abdomen closed with drainage. Only very rarely is the placental implantation limited to the reproductive organs by a single pedicle, so that it can be easily removed[11].

In some instances, the placenta may separate spontaneously simulating an abruption, but the situation in which hemorrhage becomes uncontrollable is more likely to arise from failed attempts at placental removal. Some clinicians advocate routine placental removal[3,9], but these papers were written before the obstetrics community appreciated the value of methotrexate in such cases. Placental separation requires complete ligation of the blood vessels supplying the placenta and manipulating it at its insertion. More importantly, placental separation is not always straightforward and fails in 40% of cases[3]. This is where the blood supply cannot be completely ligated resulting in massive hemorrhage and shock[2]. The hemorrhage from the placenta is torrential and rapid surgical action is essential. Various local techniques such as compression of the bleeding site, ligating the vascular pedicles, lavage with cold saline and local and/or systemic coagulation promoting agents (tranexamic acid, plasminogen derivatives, absorbable gelatin sponge, etc.) have been described. Repair of placental lacerations may need to be performed. The removal of the organ to which the placenta is adherent (hysterectomy and/or salpingoophrectomy, resection of the bowel and/or bladder) may be justified to control the hemorrhage. If a hysterectomy has been performed and bleeding continues, a Logothetopulos pack brought out through the vaginal cuff can be used to exert pressure on the pelvic sidewalls and bleeding vessels (see Chapter 54 for complete details). As a last resort, the abdomen may be packed tight with abdominal sponges and closed partially. The packs can be removed 48 hours postoperatively or sooner if directed by hemodynamic instability.

POSTOPERATIVE CARE

Even when the placenta is left *in situ*, complications such as infection, abscesses, bowel obstruction secondary to adhesions or wound dehiscence occur in about half of the patients[12,13]. Although the problems associated with an abdominally retained placenta may be distressing and lead to subsequent repeat laparotomy, they are potentially less disastrous than an ill-advised attempt at removing the placenta. Prophylactic antibiotics should be administered so as to cover a substantial part of the postoperative course. Less common complications of the retained placenta include reversible maternal hydronephrosis[14] and prolonged persistent postpartum pre-eclampsia[15].

To hasten resorption, methotrexate as a single dose of 50 mg/m^2 can be used. However, this too is not without its specific problems. In a series of 10 cases, accelerated placental destruction led to accumulation of necrotic tissue and abscess formation[16]. It is difficult to attribute this to methotrexate therapy alone, as these complications arise even without administration of methotrexate.

The patient with a retained placenta is monitored with clinical evaluation, ultrasound, color Doppler and serum β-hCG levels. Hormonal parameters drop rapidly in the postoperative period as most live cells will be destroyed early. The physical mass of the placenta is resorbed slowly over an average period of 6 months. A resorption period of 5 years has been reported[17], although this is highly unusual.

NEW APPROACHES

First trimester ultrasound is a norm today. Imaging technology is more sophisticated and awareness higher than in the past. Recently, abdominal pregnancies have even been diagnosed in the first trimester. These pregnancies are small, less vascular and can be treated with a minimally invasive approach. Although laparotomy remains a valid option even in these circumstances, there are reports of abdominal pregnancies being managed by laparoscopy. These pregnancies are small, but there is a potential for substantial hemorrhage. Bleeding may be managed by excision, coagulation, injection of vasopressin or suturing of the implantation site[18,19]. Laparoscopic management requires an advanced degree of skill and preparation. Another possibility that may be explored is interventional ultrasound. At present, there are no reported cases, but one could inject potassium chloride into the fetal heart to stop cardiac activity and hasten placental resolution by a local or systemic injection of methotrexate.

CONCLUSION

Secondary abdominal pregnancy is an uncommon and exceedingly dangerous variant of ectopic pregnancy. It is usually not diagnosed until laparotomy which leaves the obstetrician little preparation to face the prospect of torrential PPH, albeit not from the usual sources. In this situation, minimizing placental handling and leaving it in the abdominal cavity can be life saving.

References

1. Atrash HK, Friede A, Hogue CJR. Abdominal pregnancy in the United Status: frequency and maternal mortality. Obstet Gynecol 1987;69:633–7
2. Ayinde OA, Aimakhu CO, Adeyanju OA, Omigbodun AO. Abdominal pregnancy at the University College Hospital, Ibadan: a ten-year review. Afr J Reprod Health 2005;9:123–7
3. Costa SD, Presley J, Bastert G. Advanced abdominal pregnancy. Obstet Gynecol Surv 1991;46:515–25
4. Bombard AT, Nakagawa S, Runowicz CD, Cohen BL, Mikhail MS, Nitowsky HM. Early detection of abdominal pregnancy by maternal serum AFP+ screening. Prenat Diag 1994;14:1155–7
5. Akhan O, Cekirge S, Senaati S, Besim A. Sonographic diagnosis of an abdominal ectopic pregnancy. AJR Am J Radiol 1990;155:197–8
6. Sherrer DM, Daloul M, Gorelick C, et al. Unusual maternal vasculature in the placental periphery leading to the diagnosis of abdominal pregnancy at 25 weeks gestation. J Clin Ultrasound 2007;35:268–73
7. Hage ML, Wall LL, Killam A. Expectant management of abdominal pregnancy. A report of two cases. J Reprod Med 1988;33:407–10
8. Stevens CA. Malformations and deformations in abdominal pregnancy. Am J Med Genet 1993;47:1189–95
9. Sandberg EC, Pelligra R. The medical antigravity suit for management of surgically uncontrollable bleeding associated with abdominal pregnancy. Am J Obstet Gynecol 1983;146:519–25
10. Kerr A, Trambert J, Mikhail M, Hodges L, Runowicz C. Preoperative transcatheter embolization of abdominal pregnancy: Report of three cases. J Vasc Interv Radiol 1993;4:733–5
11. Noren H, Lindblom B. A unique case of abdominal pregnancy: what are the minimal requirements for placental contact with the maternal vascular bed? Am J Obstet Gynecol 1986;155:394–6
12. Bergstrom R, Mueller G, Yankowitz J. A case illustrating the continued dilemmas in treating abdominal pregnancy and a potential explanation for the high rate of postsurgical febrile morbidity. Gynecol Obstet Invest 1998;46:268–70
13. Martin JN Jr, McCaul JF 4th. Emergent management of abdominal pregnancy. Clin Obstet Gynecol 1990;33:438–47
14. Weiss RE, Stone NN. Persistent maternal hydronephrosis after intra-abdominal pregnancy. J Urol 1994;152:1196–8
15. Piering WF, Garancis JG, Becker CG, Beres JA, Lemann J Jr. Preeclampsia related to a functioning extrauterine placenta: Report of a case and 25-year follow-up. Am J Kidney Dis 1993;21:310–3
16. Rahman MS, Al-Suleiman SA, Rahman J, Al-Sibai MH. Advanced abdominal pregnancy – observations in 10 cases. Obstet Gynecol 1982;59:366–72
17. Belfar HL, Kurtz AB, Wapner RJ. Long-term follow-up after removal of an abdominal pregnancy: Ultrasound evaluation of the involuting placenta. J Ultrasound Med 1986;5:521–3
18. Hong JH, Shin JH, Song KH, et al. Laparoscopic management of primary omental pregnancy. J Min Invas Gynecol 2008;15:640–1
19. Kar S. Primary abdominal pregnancy following intrauterine insemination. J Hum Reprod Sci 2011;4:95–9

72

Jehovah's Witnesses and Those Who Refuse Blood Transfusion

E. El-Hamamy and D. S. Newman

The management of postpartum hemorrhage (PPH) is particularly challenging when a pregnant woman refuses transfusion of primary blood products for religious or personal reasons. This chapter outlines strategies and techniques that can be used in such a situation or when the blood supply is limited or unsafe because of lack of testing (see Addendum A)[1].

INTRODUCTION

According to World Health Organization (WHO), approximately 92 million blood donations are collected every year[2]. Of these, 50% take place in low- and middle-resource countries where 85% of the world's population lives[2]. In many such nations, blood is not available for treatment of PPH (or anything else, for that matter) because effective blood collection programs do not exist[3]. According to WHO, donated blood 'should always be screened for HIV, hepatitis B, hepatitis C and syphilis prior to transfusion, but in 39 countries (out of 164 reporting in 2008), not all donated blood is tested for one or more of these infections. Testing is not reliable in other countries because of staff shortages, poor quality test kits, irregular supplies, or lack of basic laboratory services'[4].

Even in middle- and high-resource countries, where donated blood is screened for these conditions, patients are concerned about the transmission of variant Creutzfeld-Jakob disease (vCJD) as well as other side-effects such as transfusion related acute lung injury (TRALI), transfusion related immunomodulation (TRIM) and the administration of the wrong blood to the wrong patient. A 2002 survey in the UK of 228 pregnant women determined that 8% of respondents would not accept a blood transfusion for either religious reasons (4%) or no stated reason (4%)[5]. Regardless of the patient's preferences, the cost of a transfusion is significant. A 2010 investigation into the actual cost of blood in surgical patients found that when direct and indirect costs were included, costs per red blood cell unit varied between $522 and $1183[6].

Prominent among those individuals refusing transfusion of primary blood components are members of the Jehovah's Witness faith. A growing number of physicians and surgeons have developed techniques and strategies for providing appropriate medical and surgical management for members of this group without the use of blood. These techniques and strategies can also be adopted in situations where there are acute blood shortages or where the blood supply is not tested for HIV, hepatitis B, hepatitis C and syphilis.

As many readers of this volume do not understand why Jehovah's Witnesses refuse the transfusion of primary blood components, this chapter begins with a discussion of this topic and proceeds to describe an overview of how PPH may be avoided or treated in this group.

JEHOVAH'S WITNESSES AND THEIR VIEW OF MEDICINE AND BLOOD

Modern day Jehovah's Witnesses descend from an informal Bible Study Group that began in Allegheny, Pennsylvania, USA, in the early 1870s. The aim of the group was to try, by means of Bible study, to determine the original teachings of Jesus Christ and the first century Christians, unfettered by the traditions and teachings of other denominations. The results of their deliberations were eventually published in *Zion's Watch Tower and Herald of Christ's Presence*, the first issue of which appeared in July 1879. In 1881, the Zion's Watch Tower Tract Society was formed. Ultimately, the Society's name was changed to The Watch Tower Bible and Tract Society, but it did not adopt its present title, 'Jehovah's Witnesses', until 1931.

Jehovah's Witnesses believe that the Bible is the inspired Word of God, accepting both the Old and New Testaments. During the First World War, the practice of blood transfusion became established. The 1 July 1945 issue of *The Watchtower* magazine[7] advised Jehovah's Witnesses that this practice was contrary to scriptural passages such as:

> 'Everything that lives and moves will be food for you. Just as I gave you the green plants, I now give you everything. But you must not eat meat that has its lifeblood still in it.' *New International Bible, Genesis 9:3–4*

> '. . . because the life of every creature is its blood. That is why I have said to the Israelites, "You must not eat the blood of any creature, because the life of every creature is its blood;

anyone who eats it must be cut off.'" *New International Bible, Leviticus 17:14*

'It seemed good to the Holy Spirit and to us not to burden you with anything beyond the following requirements: You are to abstain from food sacrificed to idols, from blood, from the meat of strangled animals and from sexual immorality. You will do well to avoid these things.' *New International Bible, Acts 15:28–29*

Jehovah's Witnesses are not antimedicine or antisurgery; many are doctors and nurses. They view life as sacred and as a gift from God and therefore seek medical attention for themselves and their families. Their stance on medical/surgical treatment is summarized in Table 1. Although Jehovah's Witnesses refuse blood components, plasma derivatives are a matter of personal choice. Table 2 summarizes the Witness position in these areas.

In the final analysis, the decision to abstain from blood transfusion is a personal one and not, as commonly portrayed, a dictate from the world headquarters in the USA. The depth of belief of each individual Witness is well summarized in the booklet *Management of Anaesthesia for Jehovah's Witnesses*, published by the Association of Anaesthetists of Great Britain and Ireland: 'Administration of blood to a competent patient, against their will and in conflict with their genuinely held beliefs, has been likened by the Witnesses to rape. It will not result in expulsion from the community if it was carried out against the expressed wishes of the patient but may have as deep a psychological effect as forceful sexual interference'[8].

In the UK, the General Medical Council has issued guidance about personal beliefs of patients with special reference to the treatment of Jehovah's Witnesses[9]: 'You should not make assumptions about the decisions that a Jehovah's Witness patient might make about treatment with blood or blood products. You should

Table 1 The Jehovah's Witness position on medical treatment

Accept all forms of medical treatment except blood transfusions
Are not exercising a right to die
Are keen to cooperate with medical professionals

Table 2 The Jehovah's Witness position on blood

Unacceptable
Whole blood
Red cells
White cells
Platelets
Plasma (fresh frozen plasma)
Preoperative autologous donation (PAD)

Personal choice
Derivatives from red cells
Derivatives from white cells (e.g. interferons)
Derivatives from platelets (e.g. autologous platelet gel or glue)
Derivatives from plasma
    Fibrin glues/sealants
    Clotting factors
    Prothrombin complex concentrates
    Immunoglobulins (e.g. anti-D)

ask for and respect their views and answer their questions honestly and to the best of your ability. You may also wish to contact the hospital liaison committees established by the Watch Tower Society (the governing body of Jehovah's Witnesses) to support Jehovah's Witnesses faced with treatment decisions involving blood. These committees can advise on current Society policy regarding the acceptability or otherwise of particular blood products. They also keep details of hospitals and doctors who are experienced in 'bloodless' medical procedures.'

ARE PREGNANT JEHOVAH'S WITNESSES AT HIGHER RISK OF MORTALITY AND MORBIDITY?

Although several studies describe the risks of refusal of primary blood components in major surgery and trauma[10–12], the data estimating the increased risk due to PPH in Jehovah's Witnesses are limited. Mostafa et al.[13] in 1982 concluded that 'major operative procedures can be carried out on Jehovah's Witness patients without blood transfusions or blood products.' However, these authors also stated, 'The most dreaded problem a Jehovah's Witness could face is a hemorrhagic complication of pregnancy. Specifically, severe disseminated intravascular coagulation, placental abruption, or placenta accreta often results in substantial blood loss that is unmanageable without transfusions. When these complications arise, little can be done with currently available blood substitutes.'

A 2001 study by Singla et al.[14] concluded that 'Women who are Jehovah's Witnesses are at a 44-fold increased risk of maternal death, which is due to obstetric hemorrhage.' Massiah et al.[15] in 2007 published a study of 116 deliveries over a period of 14 years amongst Jehovah's Witnesses and reported one maternal death due to PPH, leading them to conclude that there was a 65-fold increase of maternal death amongst this cohort of patients. A more recent (2009) study from The Netherlands[16] concluded that: 'Women who are Jehovah's Witnesses are at a six times increased risk for maternal death, at a 130 times increased risk for maternal death because of major obstetric hemorrhage and at a 3.1 times increased risk for serious maternal morbidity because of obstetric hemorrhage, compared to the general Dutch population.' A comparison of these three studies is shown in Table 3.

In the UK, statistics on PPH are collected and published triennially by the Centre for Maternal and Child Enquiries (CMACE). The report for 2000–2002 identified ten deaths due to PPH; two were in women who declined blood transfusion[17]. Commenting on these deaths, the report stated: 'Both were delivered by elective section, for reasons which were not clearly documented, and both subsequently required hysterectomy. Delay in carrying out the subsequent hysterectomy in one case may have been due to difficulty in obtaining consent.' The report continued: 'There have only been six cases of death in women refusing blood transfusion in the last 21 years (1982–2002), so

Table 3 Comparison of studies reporting morbidity and mortality rate in Jehovah's Witness patients

	Singla et al.[14]	*Massiah et al.*[15]	*Van Wolfswinkel et al.*[16]
No. of deliveries	391	116	8850 (estimated)
% Cesarean section	16%	24%	Not given
No deaths	2	1	6 (3 substandard care)
% PPH	6%	6%	Not given
Increased risk of maternal death	44 fold	65 fold	130 fold

it is a very uncommon event, although it may well be that those women are over-represented among deaths.'

The Eighth Report of the Confidential Enquiries into Maternal Deaths in the United Kingdom reports five deaths due to PPH during the period 2006–2008, one of which occurred in a woman refusing blood transfusion[18].

Even with the paucity of data regarding the increased risk of mortality and morbidity during pregnancy, Jehovah's Witnesses accept the fact that obstetricians and midwives classify them as high risk. As a result, they seek to be as cooperative as possible in minimizing the consequences that their conscientiously held beliefs impose.

MANAGING THE JEHOVAH'S WITNESS IN THE ANTENATAL PERIOD

Pregnant Jehovah's Witnesses are encouraged to make their position on blood transfusion known early during their antenatal visits. This is in harmony with the recommendation of the 2003–2005 Confidential Enquiry into Maternal and Child Health report *Saving Mothers' Lives*[19], which says with respect to those who refuse blood transfusion: 'Consultant obstetric and anaesthetic involvement is necessary during the antenatal period in order to develop a care plan together with the woman, her husband and family, and, if necessary, religious advisors, should any difficulty occur.' In some countries, the patient will bring a copy of *Care Plan for Women in Labor Refusing a Blood Transfusion*[20] as the basis for discussion and the formulation of a treatment plan Addendum B.

Blood samples should be taken and checked for anemia and any coagulation abnormalities. Correction of anemia can be accomplished by the use of oral or intravenous iron[21–23], folic acid, vitamin B_{12} and erythropoietin[24]. Hemoglobin (Hb) levels should be monitored monthly throughout the pregnancy. Although oral iron is prescribed to most pregnant women, a not insignificant proportion of women arrive at term with a Hb level of less than 10 g/dl. A Hb level of 11 g/dl in the first and third trimesters, and 10.5 g/dl in the second, is often regarded as the lowest

acceptable level during pregnancy. A Hb level of less than 10.5 g/dl is considered anemia[25]. For women who will refuse blood transfusion, it is appropriate to maintain Hb at a target level of 12 g/dl or higher.

Coagulation abnormalities should be investigated and corrected wherever possible. A review of all medications that the patient may be taking including non-steroidal anti-inflammatory drugs (NSAIDs), warfarin, antibiotics, etc. should be undertaken. Where there may be a risk of a thromboembolic event if anticoagulants are withdrawn, these should be changed for agents with a shorter half-life, such as low molecular weight heparin, allowing for perioperative correction in the event of hemorrhage. Where indicated, the administration of vitamin K should be considered. During the antenatal period, it is important to ascertain the woman's views on intraoperative cell salvage (ICS), acute normovolemic hemodilution (ANH) and total or subtotal hysterectomy.

As previously mentioned, Jehovah's Witnesses have differing, albeit conscientiously held views about the use of plasma derivatives. It is therefore essential that a member of the anesthetic team meets with the patient during the antenatal period to ascertain whether cryoprecipitate, fibrin glues and sealants, prothrombin complex concentrate or other clotting factors would be acceptable in the event of major hemorrhage[8]. (A suggested checklist for this purpose also is included in the Addendum C.)

During late pregnancy ultrasound should be used to determine the location of the placental site in order to ascertain whether there is the risk of placenta previa or accreta so that strategies may be formulated for delivery by high-risk cesarean section.

Jehovah's Witnesses are encouraged to complete an advance decision document[26] or durable power of attorney (DPA) declining the administration of blood and blood products. The document also serves as a release for the hospital and obstetric team in the event that the woman dies. An example of such a document is shown in Addendum D. The woman also may wish to wear a 'no blood' wristband to make it clear to all members of the care team that blood transfusion is not to be used[26].

MANAGING THE JEHOVAH'S WITNESS IN LABOR

The Annexe to the 2002 CEMACH report[17] recommends: 'The consultant obstetrician and anaesthetist should be informed when a woman who will decline transfusion is admitted in labour or for delivery. Vaginal delivery is usually associated with lower blood loss than caesarean section, and caesarean section should be performed only if there is a clear medical indication. In that case it should be performed by a consultant obstetrician.'

The third stage of labor should be actively managed using intramuscular or intravenous oxytocin with the delivery of the anterior shoulder and slow delivery of the posterior shoulder and body[27]. The placenta should be delivered using controlled cord traction, while displacing the uterus upwards by suprapubic pressure[28]. The placenta should be checked for completeness and the uterus inspected for any retained products of conception or trauma. The prophylactic administration of Syntometrine® marginally decreases the risk of PPH compared with oxytocin alone[29]. At the completion of the delivery, the obstetrician should arrange for close observation, uterine palpation, assessment of bleeding and monitoring vital signs for at least 1 hour.

MANAGING THE HEMORRHAGING JEHOVAH'S WITNESS

In the event of PPH, obstetric, anesthetic and hematology consultants should be immediately involved. Colloid such as Gelofusine® or Haemacel® should be infused using two large bore needles. However, in the actively bleeding patient, aggressive fluid resuscitation may inhibit hemostasis, disrupt clot stability or exacerbate hemorrhage as well as dilute coagulation factors. Published data suggest that adequate tissue oxygenation can be maintained by moderate under-resuscitation and mild hypotension[30].

After administering uterotonic agents and ensuring that retained products of conception or trauma are not the cause of the bleeding, it is appropriate to proceed with bimanual uterine compression. Oxygen should be administered; 100% oxygen has been shown to improve systemic oxygen transport[31]. An indwelling catheter allows monitoring of urine output. Insertion of a central venous pressure (CVP) line may be of value in certain patients, and aortic compression against the spine, using a fist just above the umbilicus, may buy time in an emergency.

PROMOTION OF HEMOSTASIS

In addition to the administration of drugs to correct uterine atony, the use of specific hemostatic agents may also be effective in the management of PPH. The antifibrinolytic agent tranexamic acid controls hemorrhage in a number of situations, including PPH[32–34]. The use of recombinant factor VIIa (rFVIIa; Novo-Seven®) to arrest uncontrolled hemorrhage is well described in Chapter 50 of this volume. A 2010 paper by Franchini et al.[35] contains a useful flow diagram for the administration of factor VIIa (Figure 1) and recommends an initial intravenous bolus of 90 μg/kg over a period of 3–5 min. Because of its expense, the administration of factor VIIa is often recommended as a last resort. However, in the bleeding Jehovah's Witness patient, where the administration of fresh frozen plasma and platelets is not an option, it may be advisable to administer the drug at an earlier stage before the depletion of the clotting factors. Factor VIIa has also been found to be of value in dealing with hemorrhage in placenta accreta/percreta, ruptured uterus and HELLP (hemolysis, elevated liver enzymes, low platelets) syndrome. Consideration should also be given to the intravenous administration of vitamin K.

When a Witness patient indicates during antenatal discussions that she is willing to accept derivatives from blood plasma, therapeutics such as fibrin sealants containing fibrin and thrombin (e.g. Evicel® and FloSeal®) assist in arresting bleeding[36] (see Chapters 57 and 58). Again, where acceptable to the patient, cryoprecipitate, prothrombin complex concentrate may be administered in order to promote coagulation.

SURGICAL AND OTHER INTERVENTIONS

In addition to uterine packing[37], intrauterine balloon tamponade has successfully controlled PPH (see Chapters 46–48 and 54)[38]. Application of the B-Lynch brace suture is a well established, simple, cheap and effective technique for controlling PPH, with a high success rate (see Chapter 51)[39,40]. The suture can be combined with an intrauterine balloon tamponade if bleeding persists[41]. The successful application of the B-Lynch brace suture as a prophylactic measure in a high-risk cesarean section in a Jehovah's Witness patient is also possible[42].

Where available, radiological embolization of the internal iliac arteries effectively treats active hemorrhage[37,43] and prophylactic placement of catheters may be considered in cases where there is a high risk of bleeding (see Chapter 49). The same may be said of ligation of the internal iliac artery or bilateral mass ligation of uterine vessels (see Chapters 52 and 53)[44].

In the event of intractable hemorrhage, then hysterectomy may be the only life-preserving alternative. Subtotal hysterectomy can be quicker and safer (see Chapter 55). The uterine arteries should be clamped as early as possible. The possibility of hysterectomy should have been discussed with the patient during the antenatal period and permission, as a life-saving option, given prior to the onset of labor when there is no question of duress.

The non-pneumatic antishock garment has been successful in the treatment of PPH in that it allows transfer of a patient to a facility with more therapeutic options or buys time till help arrives[45,46]. This neoprene Velcro-fastened garment can be applied in approximately 2 min and redirects blood from the lower body and abdomen to the vital organs by as much as 0.5–1.5 liters (see Chapters 38 and 39).

USE OF AUTOLOGOUS BLOOD

Intraoperative cell salvage

Many Jehovah's Witness patients are willing to accept intraoperative cell salvage (ICS) if the equipment is set up in such a manner that they can perceive it to be an extension of their own circulatory system. One such set-up, suggested by the UK Cell Salvage Action Group[47] is shown in Figure 2. Many obstetricians are reluctant to consider cell salvage as an option for fear of the possible risk of amniotic fluid embolism. However, it has been safely used in a large number of cases with separate suction devices, one for the amniotic

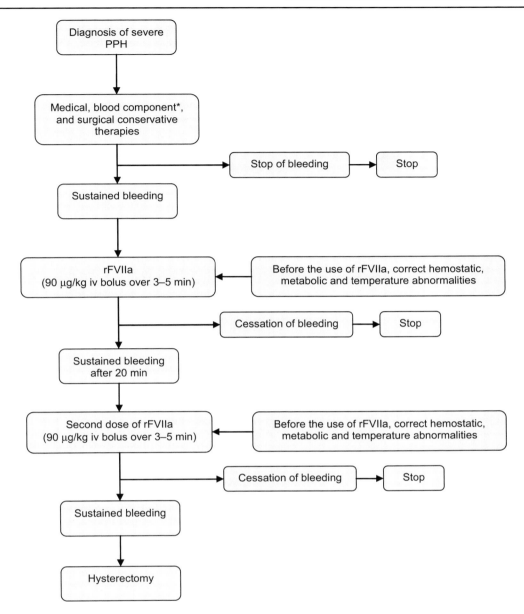

Figure 1 Flow diagram on the potential role of recombinant activated factor VII (rFVIIa) in the treatment of postpartum hemorrhage. *Note blood derivatives should only be used if acceptable to the Jehovah's Witness patient. From Franchini *et al.*[35], with permission

fluid and one for blood, with blood returned to the patient via a leucodepletion filter[48,49].

Acute normovolemic hemodilution

Acute normovolemic hemodilution (ANH) has been used with success in high-risk situations such as cesarean section for placenta percreta[50–52]. Hemodilution involves attaching blood bags to the patient and drawing off a calculated volume of blood while replacing it with an asanguinous fluid such as crystalloid or colloid (Figure 2). If bleeding occurs, then effectively, it is diluted blood that is being shed.

The amount of blood that can be drawn off is calculated using the equation[53]:

$$ABV = \frac{EBV \times (H_o - H_T)}{\dfrac{H_o + H_T}{2}}$$

Where ABV is the autologous blood volume to be withdrawn, H_o the prehemodilution Hb, H_T the target Hb, and EBV the estimated blood volume of the patient.

In the event that ANH is viewed as part of the management plan in a high-risk procedure, then it is essential to optimize antenatal hemoglobin. Although the amount of blood which can be drawn off is limited, it does have the advantage of retaining coagulation factors and platelets which can be returned to the patient. ANH will be acceptable to many Jehovah's Witnesses if the withdrawn blood is left connected to their circulatory system during the procedure. Again, this should be discussed with the patient at the antenatal stage.

Managing postpartum anemia

In the event that a major hemorrhage results in severe anemia, several innovative therapeutic possibilities

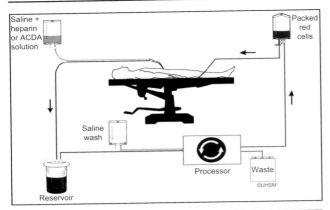

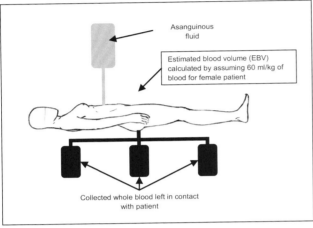

Figure 2 Diagrams illustrating intraoperative cell salvage (upper) and acute normovolemic hemodilution (lower). ACDA, acid citrate dextrose solution A

exist. First, where available, hyperoxic ventilation is more effective in improving tissue oxygenation than red cell transfusions[31]. Second, hematopoiesis can be stimulated using recombinant human erythropoietin (rHuEPO), dosage 300 IU/kg, three times weekly subcutaneously[54,55]. In order for the EPO to be effective, however, it should be supplemented with IV iron, such as low molecular weight iron sucrose (e.g. Venofer®). Other hematinics such as vitamin B$_{12}$ and folic acid should also be administered. Oral iron supplementation by itself is slow and unreliable[18]. Subsequent patient monitoring should limit blood sampling by phlebotomy with the use of micro-sampling or pediatric techniques. Where available, hyperbaric oxygen therapy has been shown to be effective in the treatment of a Jehovah's Witness patient whose hemoglobin fell to 2.0 g/dl[56]. This is interesting but needs amplification; what else did she get in terms of medication, how long was the treatment and how long did it take for her to recover?

Where problems may arise

The appropriate care of a pregnant woman refusing blood transfusion for religious or other reasons relies heavily on pre-planning and a multidisciplinary approach. Difficulties may arise when someone has

been brought up as a Jehovah's Witness but has then not gone on to follow the faith. Despite this, their personal decision not to have blood products often represents the last vestige of their previous religious conviction to which they still cling. In this event they may well advise the midwife or obstetrician of their refusal to receive blood products when they have actually commenced labor. In order to prevent such a situation, it would be wise to ask all pregnant women on their initial antenatal visit whether they have any objection to transfusion of primary blood products.

SUMMARY

The care of Jehovah's Witnesses and others who refuse blood transfusion requires a multidisciplinary approach, which includes the preparation of a management plan in the event of major PPH.

PRACTICE POINTS

- Antenatally ascertain women's acceptability/refusal of red blood cells/platelet transfusion/plasma derivatives
- Check Hb in last 3 months of pregnancy and correct if necessary
- Plan for active management of third stage of labor
- Plan for B-Lynch suture technique/hysterectomy if all else fails
- Manage postpartum anemia with hyperoxic ventilation/IV iron support.

References

1. Map of Medicine. Blood transfusion refusal care pathway. International View. London: Map of Medicine, 2011. http://healthguides.mapofmedicine.com/choices/map/blood_transfusion6.html
2. World Health Organization. http://www.who.int/features/factfiles/blood_transfusion/blood_transfusion/en/index4.html
3. Improving blood safety worldwide. Lancet 2007;370:361
4. World Health Organization. Ten Facts on Blood. 2008 www.who.int/features/factfiles/blood_transfusion/blood_transfusion/en/index7.html
5. Khadra M, Rigby C, Warren P, Leighton N, Johanson R. A criterion audit of women's awareness of blood transfusion in pregnancy. BMC Pregnancy and Childbirth 2002;2:7
6. Shander A, Hofmann A, Ozawa S, et al. from the Society for the Advancement of Blood Management (SABM) and the Medical Society for Blood Management (MSBM). Activity-based costs of blood transfusions in surgical patients at four hospitals. Transfusion 2010;50:753–65
7. The Watchtower. Published by the Watchtower Bible and Tract Society, 1 July 1945:200–1
8. Ward ME, Dick J, Greenwell S, et al. Management of Anaesthesia for Jehovah's Witnesses, 2nd edn. London: Association of Anaesthetists of Great Britain and Ireland, 2005:6 www.aagbi.org/sites/default/files/Jehovah's Witnesses_0.pdf
9. General Medical Council. Personal Beliefs and Medical Practice. 2008. www.gmc-uk.org/static/documents/content/Personal_Beliefs.pdf
10. Kitchens CS. Are transfusions overrated? Surgical outcome of Jehovah's Witnesses. Am J Med 1993;94:117–9

11. Varela JE, Gomez-Marin O, Fleming LE, Cohn SM. The risk of death for Jehovah's Witnesses after major trauma. J Trauma 2003;54:967–72

12. Bodnaruk Z, Wong CJ, Thomas MJ. Meeting the clinical challenge of care for Jehovah's Witnesses. Transfus Med Rev 2004;18:105–16

13. Mostafa I, Bonakdar MI, Eckhous AW, Bacher BJ, Tabbilos RH, Peisner DB. Major gynecologic and obstetric surgery in Jehovah's Witnesses. Obstet Gynecol 1982;60:587

14. Singla AK, Lapinski RH, Berkowitz RL, Saphier CJ. Are women who are Jehovah's Witnesses at risk of maternal death? Am J Obstet Gynecol 2001;185:893–5

15. Massiah N, Athimulam S, Loo C, Okolo S, Yoong W. Obstetric care of Jehovah's Witnesses: a 14-year observational study. Arch Gynecol Obstet 2007;276:339–43

16. Van Wolfswinkel ME, Zwart JJ, Schutte JM, et al. Maternal mortality and serious maternal morbidity in Jehovah's witnesses in the Netherlands. BJOG 2009;116:1103–10

17. Hall MH. Haemorrhage. In: Why Mothers Die 2000–2002. The Sixth Report of the Confidential Enquiries into Maternal Deaths in the UK. London: RCOG, 2004:86–93

18. Centre for Maternal and Child Enquiries (CMACE). Saving mothers' lives: reviewing maternal deaths to make motherhood safer: 2006–2008. BJOG 2011;118(Suppl 1):72–75 http://onlinelibrary.wiley.com/doi/10.1111/j.1471-0528.2010.02847.x/pdf

19. Confidential Enquiry into. Maternal and Child Health (CEMACH). Saving Mothers' Lives 2003–2005. London: RCOG, 2007

20. UK Blood Transfusion and Tissue Transplantation Services. Care Plan for Women in labour refusing a blood transfusion, Hospital information services for Jehovah's witnesses, 2005. http://www.transfusionguidelines.org.uk/docs/pdfs/bbt-04_care-plan.pdf

21. Bayoumeua F, Subiran-Buisseta C, Bakaa N, et al. Iron therapy in iron deficiency anemia in pregnancy: Intravenous route versus oral route. Eur J Obstet Gynecol Reprod Biol 2005;123:S15–S19

22. Al RA, Unlubilgin E, Kandemir O, Yalvac S, Cakir L, Haberal A. Intravenous versus oral iron for treatment of anemia in pregnancy: a randomized trial. Obstet Gynecol 2005;106:1335–40

23. Kalu E, Wayne C, Croucher C, Findley I, Manyonda I. Triplet pregnancy in a Jehovah's witness: recombinant human erythropoietin and iron supplementation for minimising the risks of excessive blood loss. BJOG 2002;109:723–25

24. Sifakis S, Angelakis E, Vardaki E, et al. Erythropoietin in the treatment of iron deficiency anemia during pregnancy. Gynecol Obstet Invest 2001;51:150–6

25. Auerbach M, Goodnough LT, Picard D, Maniatis A. The role of intravenous iron in anemia management and transfusion avoidance. Transfusion 2008;48:988–1000

26. Royal College of Obstetricians and Gynaecologists. Blood Transfusion in Obstetrics. Green-top Guideline No. 47. London: RCOG, 2008:8

27. Thomas JM. The world need for education in nonblood management in obstetrics and gynaecology. J SOCG 1994;16:1483–7

28. Khan GQ, John IS, Wani S, Doherty T, Sibai BM. Controlled cord traction versus minimal intervention techniques in delivery of the placenta: a randomized controlled trial. Am J Obstet Gynecol 1997;177:770–4

29. McDonald S, Prendiville WJ, Elbourne D. Prophylactic syntometrine versus oxytocin for delivery of the placenta. Cochrane Database Syst Rev 2000;(2):CD000201

30. Bickell WH, Wall MJ, Pepe PE, et al. Immediate versus delayed fluid resuscitation for hypotensive patients with penetrating torso injuries. N Engl J Med 1994;331:1105–9

31. Suttner S, Piper SN, Kumle B, et al. The influence of allogeneic red blood cell transfusion compared with 100% oxygen ventilation on systemic oxygen transport and skeletal muscle oxygen tension after cardiac surgery. Anesth Analg 2004;99:2–11

32. Ducloy-Bouthors A, Broisin F, Keita H, et al. Tranexamic acid reduces blood loss in postpartum haemorrhage. Critical Care 2010;14(Suppl 1):370

33. CRASH-2 trial collaborators, Shakur H, Roberts I, Bautista R, et al. Effects of tranexamic acid on death, vascular occlusive events, and blood transfusion in trauma patients with significant haemorrhage (CRASH-2): a randomised, placebo-controlled trial CRASH-2 trial collaborators. Lancet 2010;376:23–32

34. As K, Hagen P, Webb JB. Tranexamic acid in the management of postpartum haemorrhage. Br J Obstet Gynaecol 1996;103:1250–1

35. Franchini M, Bergamini V, Montagnana M, et al. The use of recombinant activated FV11 in postpartum haemorrhage. Clin Obstet Gynecol 2010;53:219–27

36. Moriarty K, Premila S, Bulmer P. Use of FloSeal haemostatic gel in massive obstetric haemorrhage: a case report. BJOG 2008;115:793–5

37. Dildy III GA. Postpartum hemorrhage: New management options. Clin Obstet Gynecol 2002;45:330–44

38. Condous, G. Arulkumaran, S, Symond I, Chapman R, Sinha A, Razvi K. the "tamponade test" in the management of massive postpartum hemorrhage. Obstet Gynecol 2003;101:767–72

39. B-Lynch C, Coker A, Lawal AH, Abu J, Cowen MJ. The B-Lynch surgical technique for the control of massive postpartum haemorrhage: an alternative to hysterectomy? Five cases reported. BJOG 1997;104:372–5

40. El-Hamamy, Wright, B-Lynch. The B-Lynch suture technique for postpartum haemorrhage: A decade of experience and outcome. J Obstet Gynaecol 2009;29:278–83

41. Danso D, Reginald P. Combined B-Lynch suture with intrauterine balloon catheter triumphs over massive postpartum haemorrhage. BJOG 2002;109:963

42. Kalu E, Wayne C, Croucher C, Findley I, Manyonda I. Triplet pregnancy in a Jehovah's witness: recombinant human erythropoietin and iron supplementation for minimising the risks of excessive blood loss. BJOG 2002;109:723–25

43. Drife J. Management of primary postpartum haemorrhage. BJOG 1997;104:275–7

44. Joshi V, Otiv S, Majumder R, Nikam Y, Shrivastava M. Internal iliac artery ligation for arresting postpartum haemorrhage. BJOG 2007;114:356–361

45. Miller S, Hamza S, Bray E, et al. First aid for obstetric haemorrhage: the pilot study of the non-pneumatic anti-shock garment in Egypt. BJOG 2006;113:424–9

46. Mourad-Youssif M, Ojengbede O, Meyer C, et al. Can the non-pneumatic anti-shock garment (NASG) reduce adverse maternal outcomes from postpartum hemorrhage? Evidence from Egypt and Nigeria. Reprod Health 2010;7:24

47. UK Blood Transfusion and Tissue Transplantation Services. Transfusion guidelines. http://www.transfusionguidelines.org.uk/index.aspx?Publication=BBT&Section=22&pageid=1459

48. Catling S. Blood conservation techniques in obstetrics: a UK perspectiveInt J Obstet Anesth 2007;16:241–9

49. King M, Wrench I, Galimberti A, Spray R. Introduction of cell salvage to a large obstetric unit: the first. Int J Obstet Anesth 2009;18:111

50. Estella NM, Berry DL, Baker BW, Wali AT, Belfort MA. Normovolemic hemodilution before cesarean hysterectomy for placenta percreta. Obstet Gynecol 1997;90:669–770

51. Nagy C. Acute normovolemic haemodilution, intraoperative cell salvage and PulseCO hemodynamic monitoring in a Jehovah's Witness with placenta percreta. Int J Obstet Anesth 2008;17:159–63

52. Grange C, Douglas MJ, Adams TJ, Wadsworth LD. The use of acute hemodilution in parturients undergoing cesarean section. Am J Obstet Gynecol 1998;178:156–60

53. Seeber P, Shander A. Basics of Blood Management. Malden, MA: Blackwell Publishing, 2007:204

54. Breyman C. The use of iron sucrose complex for anemia in pregnancy and the postpartum period. Semin Hematol 2006; 43(Suppl 6):S28–S31

55. Breymann C, Zimmermann R, Huch R, Huch A. Use of recombinant human erythropoietin in combination with parenteral iron in the treatment of postpartum anaemia. Eur J Clin Invest 1996;26:123–30

56. McLoughlin PL, Cope TM, Harrison JC. Hyperbaric oxygen therapy in the management of severe acute anaemia in a Jehovah's Witness. Anaesthesia 1999;54:891–5

Addendum A: Map of Medicine 'Blood transfusion refusal care pathway'

From Map of Medicine, London, UK, with permission[1]

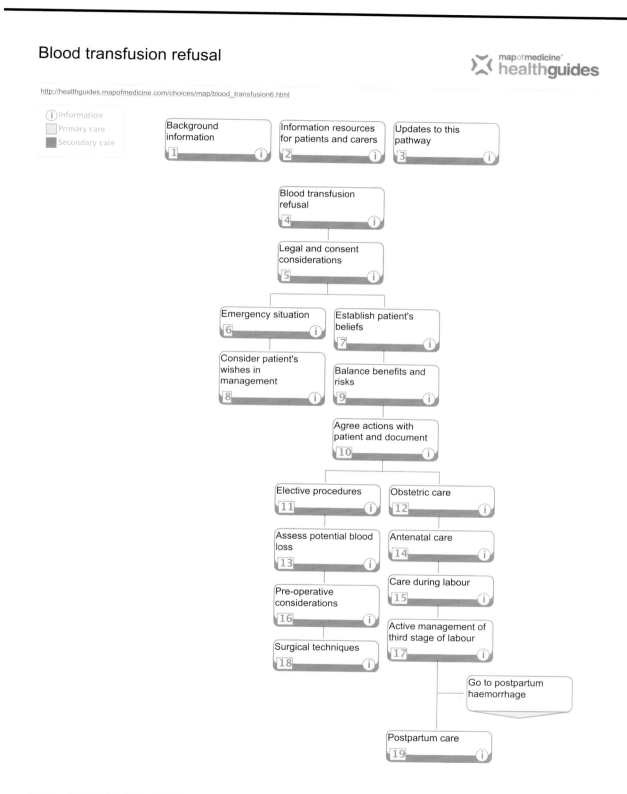

Postpartum haemorrhage (PPH)

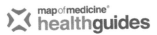

http://healthguides.mapofmedicine.com/choices/map/postpartum_haemorrhage1.html

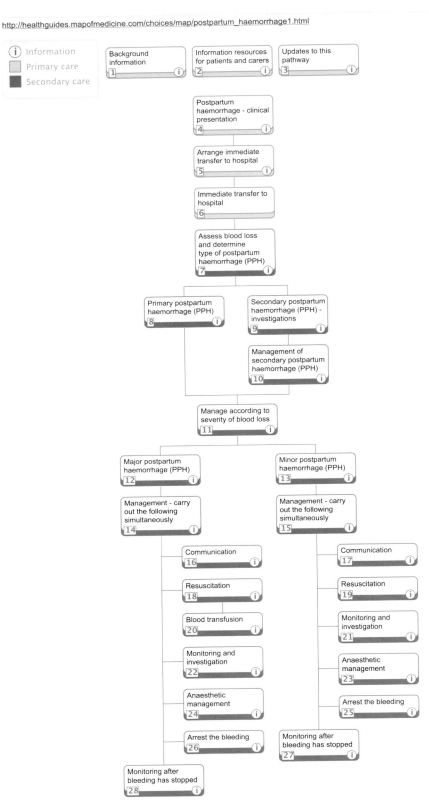

Published: 29-Jul-2010   Valid until: 31-May-2012 © Map of Medicine Ltd   All rights reserved

This care map was published by International. A printed version of this document is not controlled so may not be up-to-date with the latest clinical information.

Addendum B: Care plan for women in labor refusing a blood transfusion

From Hospital Information Services for Jehovah's Witnesses http://transfusionguidelines.org/docs/pdfs/bbt-04_care-plan-v2.pdf, with permission

---

CARE PLAN FOR WOMEN IN LABOUR REFUSING A BLOOD TRANSFUSION
(As referred to in the *RCOG News* of the Royal College of Obstetricians & Gynaecologists)

This document is an aid for medical staff and midwives managing a Jehovah's Witness or other patient who declines blood. Autologous procedures such as **blood salvage** and the use of **plasma-derived products** such as clotting agents are a **matter of personal choice for each Witness**. Most will carry an advance decision document expressing their wishes. Please check with the patient.

Risk management

- All Jehovah's Witnesses or those declining a blood transfusion should be seen in a consultant clinic.
- Clinicians should **plan in advance for blood loss**. If the Hb is ≤ 10.5g/dl use **ferrous sulphate 200mg tds and folic acid**–with acidic fruit juice or 100mg ascorbic acid to aid absorption. If unresponsive to oral iron, use **IV iron** which replenishes iron stores faster and more effectively than oral iron[1,2]. A single total-dose IV iron preparation may be more acceptable to the patient than repeat infusions. Addition of **recombinant human erythropoietin (EPO)**, which does not cross the placenta and is reportedly safely used in pregnancy, enhances Hb response[3,4].
- High-risk patients should be booked into a unit with **facilities such as interventional radiology, blood salvage and surgical expertise**. All elective surgery must be planned as far ahead as possible.
- For **high-risk caesarean section**, e.g. abnormal placentation, consider with the interventional radiologist elective insertion of catheters for **uterine artery embolisation** immediately pre-operatively and arrange **blood salvage**.
- At the time of labour ensure the **consultant obstetrician and anaesthetist are aware a Jehovah's Witness has been admitted**.
- The **third stage of labour should be actively managed** with oxytocics with consideration of **prophylactic syntocinon** infusion.
- Consider **delayed cord clamping 1-2 min for pre-term infants** to maximise Hb, with controlled cord traction after placental separation[5].
- Check patient's **vital signs and evidence of uterine contraction** every 15 min for 1 to 2 hours after delivery.
- Contact the **Hospital Liaison Committee for Jehovah's Witnesses** in an emergency (contact details over page).

Management of active haemorrhage

First steps: AVOID DELAY. Involve obstetric, anaesthetic and haematology consultants. Establish IV infusion, along with **uterine massage** (every 10 min for 1 hour can reduce blood loss[6]). **Give oxytocic drugs first, then exclude retained products of conception or trauma** (this could save time). Proceed with **bimanual uterine compression**. Give oxygen. Catheterise and monitor urine output. Consider CVP line. **Slow, but persistent blood loss requires action**. Anticipate coagulation problems. Keep patient fully informed. Proceed with following strategies if bleeding continues:

Oxytocic agents: Ergometrine with oxytocin (**Syntometrine**): Marginally more effective than oxytocin alone. If patient is hypertensive, use **oxytocin** 10U (not 5U) by **slow** IV injection (in serious PPH the benefits of higher dose outweigh the risks)[7,8]. **Carboprost (Hemabate)** 250μg/ml IM, can be repeated after 15 min. Direct intra-myometrial injection is faster (less hazardous at open operation).

Misoprostol (Cytotec): Useful option in atonic PPH where first-line treatment has failed. Can be given either by **sub-lingual** (600-800μg), **rectal** (800-1000μg) or **intrauterine route** (800μg)[9,10,11]. Control of haemorrhage reported for rectal and intrauterine routes when unresponsive to oxytocin, ergometrine and carboprost[10,11].

Intrauterine balloon tamponade: Have available purpose-designed 500 ml **Bakri tamponade balloon** (Cookmedical). Drainage of blood and cessation of bleeding can be observed via the catheter drainage shaft. Continue oxytocin. Expulsion of balloon can be prevented by vaginal packing. To minimise bleeding risk during removal, use graduated deflation or slowly deflate to half volume and observe; if no bleeding, continue deflation; if bleeding starts, reinflate[12,13]. Alternatively, stomach balloon of **Sengstaken-Blakemore oesophageal catheter** has controlled haemorrhage in 84% of 43 cases (in 2 studies), in the majority of successful cases bleeding was due to uterine atony[12,14]. Distal end of tube beyond balloon should be cut off to reduce risk of occlusion or perforation. Indwell time of balloon averaged 24 hours[14]. **Bakri balloon also used to control PPH due to vaginal lacerations**[15].

Non-inflatable anti-shock garment: Recently developed neoprene Velcro-fastened garment (zoexniasg.com) can be applied in 2 minutes and allows perineal access for obstetric procedures. Can reduce blood loss and reverse hypovolaemic shock within minutes by the transfer of 0.5 to 1.5 litres of blood from the lower body and abdomen to the vital organs. This can stabilise the patient and gain time while awaiting senior staff input. Successful trials have been conducted with >400 women experiencing PPH in developing countries[16].

Recombinant factor VIIa (NovoSeven): Increasing evidence of effectiveness for control of PPH unresponsive to standard therapies. This product and the following haemostatic agents should be used under consultant guidance. 90 μg/kg provide site-specific thrombin generation, repeat if unresponsive. Successfully used to stop or reduce bleeding in 88% of 118 massive PPH cases[17]. Also to control bleeding in 17 anecdotal PPH cases complicated by DIC[18]. (Novo Nordisk have 24-hour emergency distribution for UK-wide delivery [01889 565652] or a small stock can be held to avoid delivery delay.) Occasional failure of FVIIa has been attributed to a low fibrinogen level[19]. The **fibrinogen concentrate Haemocomplettan** (a plasma-derived **alternative to cryoprecipitate;** available on a named-patient basis within 24 hours from CSL Behring; 01444 447400) can enhance clot strength and normalise clotting in the presence of FVIIa[20,21].

Other haemostatic agents: Prothrombin complex concentrates (PCCs) such as **Beriplex** and **Octaplex** (plasma-derived), are proposed as substitutes for fresh frozen plasma and are widely prescribed as such in Europe. Beriplex reported to achieve control of bleeding in cardiac and other surgery[22]. **Tranexamic acid (Cyklokapron)**: anti-fibrinolytic agent well established for controlling haemorrhage, use 1gm IV x tds, slowly[23]. **Fibrin sealants: Flowseal** used to arrest massive bleeding in surgical bed following hysterectomy[24]; **Tisseel** has controlled bleeding of complicated vulval and vaginal lacerations when suture haemostasis failed due to tissue friability[25]. Also consider IV **vitamin K**.

B-Lynch uterine compression suture: The B-Lynch brace suture can also be **combined with intrauterine balloon catheter** if bleeding persists[26]. **Prophylactic insertion of this suture** has been used in high-risk caesarean section[4]. The **Hayman suture technique** may be a simpler procedure and quicker to apply as the lower uterine segment is not opened[27].

Embolisation/ligation of internal iliac arteries or embolisation/bilateral mass ligation of uterine vessels: Angioplasty balloon catheters can be used for emergency temporary occlusion in theatre, with transfer to the angiography suite for definitive embolisation[28].

Hysterectomy and care in theatre: Subtotal hysterectomy can be just as effective, also quicker and safer. Use Flowtrons Excell to decrease risk of DVTs. Avoid hypothermia (impairs coagulation), use fluid warmer, bair hugger, hats etc. Avoid unnecessary over-dilution. Have blood salvage and experienced operator on hand (see below).

Intraoperative blood salvage: Endorsed by NICE (2005) and RCOG (2008) guidelines. Should be set up whenever possible (check if acceptable to the patient). Either single or double suction methods can be used for collection. However, to maximise blood recovery, there is good evidence that single suction is a safe procedure[29]. Swab washing also increases RBC recovery. A 'collect only' set-up of the anticoagulation/suction tubing will enable blood salvage to begin within minutes[30]. Conventionally, a leukocyte filter has been used when reinfusing, though in an emergency situation the filter may be removed completely to maximise the flow rate, as prior to availability of filters no adverse events were reported. These are clinical decisions based on the balance of benefit/risk.

Management of postpartum anaemia—continued over page

597

Management of postpartum anaemia

IV iron should be considered for severe anaemia as oral iron is known to be slow and unreliable. In a randomised controlled study of 44 women with postpartum anaemia, significantly higher mean haemoglobin and ferritin levels from baseline were achieved for patients on **IV iron sucrose** (200 mg x 2, 48 hours apart) in comparison to those on oral iron (mean Hb day 5: IV vs oral iron, 2.5 vs 0.7gm/dl - day 14 Hb: 3.8 vs 1.5gm/dl, p = <0.01 for both periods)[31]. Comparable results for IV iron sucrose were reported in 2 similar trials (mean Hb 2.8 & 3.1, both day 14)[32,33]. These increases in Hb from baseline with IV iron exceed the expected rise after a 2U blood transfusion[32]. The level of life-threatening adverse drug events of IV iron preparations is now very low, varying from 0.6 to 3.3 per million, depending on the iron preparation (FDA data)[34].

Erythropoiesis-stimulating agents (ESAs) should be administered **together with IV iron** in life-threatening anaemia to further accelerate erythropoiesis. A **once weekly EPO dosage of 600 IU/kg subcutaneously** (**e.g. 40,000IU for a 66kg patient**) is being increasingly used and found to be satisfactory in critically ill anaemic patients[35,36]. An **EPO dosage of 300 IU/kg x 3 weekly together with IV iron (200mg x 3 weekly)** has also proved efficacious for postpartum anaemia[37]. Augment with **vitamin B-12 and folic acid**.

Check oxygen saturations: Give **100% oxygen** if necessary (no contraindications for 48-72 hrs of use). Use **microsampling techniques** to conserve blood (e.g. HemoCue), as well as **paediatric sample tubes**. If bleeding continues consider reinfusing washed drain fluid.

Hyperbaric oxygen therapy: Option in life-threatening anaemia[38]. (0151 648 8000 [24 hrs] for suitable and available centres.)

References:

1. Al RA, Unlubilgin E, Kandemir O, Yalvac S, Cakir L, Haberal A. Intravenous versus oral iron for treatment of anemia in pregnancy: a randomized trial. *Obstet Gynecol* 2005; 106: 1335-40.
2. al-Momen AK, al-Meshari A, al-Nuaim L, Saddique A, Abotalib Z, Khashogji T, Abbas M Intravenous iron sucrose complex in the treatment of iron deficiency anemia during pregnancy. *Eur J Obstet Gynecol Reprod Biol* 1996; 69: 121-4.
3. Breymann C, Visca E, Huch R, Huch A. Efficacy and safety of intravenously administered iron sucrose with and without adjuvant recombinant human erythropoietin for the treatment of resistant iron-deficiency anemia during pregnancy. *Am J Obstet Gynecol* 2001; 184: 662-667.
4. Kalu E, Wayne C, Croucher C, Findley I, Manyonda I. Triplet pregnancy in a Jehovah's Witness: recombinant human erythropoietin and iron supplementation for minimising the risks of excessive blood loss. *BJOG* 2002; 109: 723-725.
5. McDonald SJ, Middleton P. Effect of timing of umbilical cord clamping of term infants on maternal and neonatal outcomes. *Cochrane Database Syst Rev* 2008 Apr 23; (2): CD004074.
6. Hofmeyr GJ, Abdel-Aleem H, Abdel-Aleem MA. Uterine massage for preventing postpartum haemorrhage. *Cochrane Database Syst Rev* 2008 Jul 16; (3): CD006431.
7. Davies GA, Tessier JL, Woodman MC, Lipson A, Hahn PM. Maternal hemodynamics after oxytocin bolus compared with infusion in the third stage of labor: a randomized controlled trial. *Obstet Gynecol* 2005; 105: 294-9.
8. Choy CMY, Lau WC, Tam WH, Yuen PM. A randomised controlled trial of intramuscular syntometrine and intravenous oxytocin in the management of the third stage of labour. *BJOG* 2002; 109: 173-177.
9. Blum J, Winikoff B, Raghavan S, Dabash R, Ramadan MC, Dilbaz B, Dao B, Durocher J et al. Treatment of post-partum haemorrhage with sublingual misoprostol versus oxytocin in women receiving prophylactic oxytocin: a double-blind, randomised, non-inferiority trial. *Lancet* 2010; 375: 217-23.
10. O'Brien P P, El-Refaey H, Gordon A, Geary M, Rodeck CH. Rectally administered misoprostol for the treatment of postpartum hemorrhage unresponsive to oxytocin and ergometrine: a descriptive study. *Obstet Gynecol* 1998; 92: 212-214.
11. Adekanmi OA, Purmessur S, Edwards G, Barrington JW. Intrauterine misoprostol for the treatment of severe recurrent atonic secondary postpartum haemorrhage. *BJOG* 2001; 108: 541-542.
12. Condous GS, Arulkumaran S, Symonds I, Chapman R, Sinha A, Razvi K. The "tamponade test" in the management of massive postpartum hemorrhage. *Obstet Gynecol* 2003; 101: 767-772.
13. Danso D, Reginald PW. Internal Uterine Tamponade. In: A Textbook of Postpartum Haemorrage. Ch 28, p 263-67. Ed Christopher B-Lynch et al. Sapiens Publishing. 2006.
14. Doumouchtsis SK, Papageorghiou AT, Vernier C, Arulkumaran S. Management of postpartum hemorrhage by uterine balloon tamponade: prospective evaluation of effectiveness. *Acta Obstet Gynecol Scand* 2008; 87: 849-55.
15. Yoong W, Ray A, Phillip SA. Balloon tamponade for postpartum vaginal lacerations in a woman refusing blood transfusion. *Int J Gynaecol Obstet* 2009; 106: 261.
16. Miller S, Hamza S, Bray EH, Lester F, Nada K, Gibson R, Fathalla M, Mourad M, Fathy A, Turan JM, Dau KQ, Nasshar I, Elshair I, Hensleigh P. First aid for obstetric haemorrhage: the pilot study of the non-pneumatic anti-shock garment in Egypt. *BJOG* 2006; 113: 424-29.
17. Franchini M, Franchi M, Bergamini V, Salvagno GL, Montagnana M, Lippi G. A critical review on the use of recombinant factor VIIa in life-threatening obstetric postpartum hemorrhage. *Semin Thromb Hemost* 2008; 34: 104-12.
18. Pepas LP, Arif-Adib M, Kadir RA. Factor VIIa in puerperal hemorrhage with disseminated intravascular coagulation. *Obstet Gynecol* 2006; 108: 757-61.
19. Lewis NR, Brunker P, Lemire SJ, Kaufman RM. Failure of recombinant factor VIIa to correct the coagulopathy in a case of severe postpartum hemorrhage. *Transfusion* 2009; 49: 689-95.
20. Weinkove R, Rangarajan S. Fibrinogen concentrate for acquired hypofibrinogenaemic states. *Transfus Med* 2008; 18: 151-57
21. Tanaka KA, Taketomi T, Szlam F, Calatzis A, Levy JH. Improved clot formation by combined administration of activated factor VII (NovoSeven) and fibrinogen (Haemocomplettan P). *Anesth Analg* 2008; 106: 732-8.
22. Bruce D, Nokes TJ. Prothrombin complex concentrate (Beriplex P/N) in severe bleeding: experience in a large tertiary hospital. *Crit Care* 2008; 12: R105.
23. Gai M-y, Wu L-f, Su Q-f, Tatsumoto K. Clinical observation of blood loss reduced by tranexamic acid during and after caesarian section: A multi-center, randomized trial. *Eur J Obstet Gynecol Reprod Biol* 2004; 112: 154-157.
24. Moriarty KT, Premila S, Bulmer PJ. Use of FloSeal haemostatic gel in massive obstetric haemorrhage: a case report. *BJOG* 2008; 115: 793-95.
25. Whiteside JL, Asif RB, Novello RJ. Fibrin Sealant for Management of Complicated Obstetric Lacerations. Case Reports. *Obstet & Gynecol* 2010: 115; 403-404
26. Danso D, Reginald P. Combined B-Lynch suture with intrauterine balloon catheter triumphs over massive postpartum haemorrhage. *BJOG* 2002; 109: 963.
27. Ghezzi F, Cromi A, Uccella S, Raio L, Bolis P, Surbek D. The Hayman technique: a simple method to treat postpartum haemorrhage. *BJOG* 2007; 114: 362-5.
28. Choji K, Shimizu T. Embolization. In: A Textbook of Postpartum Haemorrage. Ch 30, p 277-85. Ed Christopher B-Lynch et al.. Sapiens Publishing. 2006.
29. Sullivan I, Faulds J, Ralph C. Contamination of salvaged maternal blood by amniotic fluid and fetal red cells during elective Caesarean section. *Br J Anaesth* 2008; 101: 225-9.
30. Catling S. Blood conservation techniques in obstetrics: a UK perspective. *Int J Obstet Anesth* 2007; 16: 241-49.
31. Bhandal N, Russell R. Intravenous versus oral iron therapy for postpartum anaemia *BJOG*. 2006; 113: 1248-52.
32. Wågström E, Akesson A, Van Rooijen M, Larson B, Bremme K. Erythropoietin and intravenous iron therapy in postpartum anaemia *Acta Obstet Gynecol Scand* 2007; 86: 957-62.
33. Broche DE, Gay C, Armand-Branger S, Grangeasse L, Terzibachian JJ. Acute postpartum anaemia. Clinical practice and interest of intravenous iron. *Gynécol Obstét Fertil* 2004; 32: 613-19.
34. Chertow GM, Mason PD, Vaage-Nilsen O, Ahlmén J. Update on adverse drug events associated with parenteral iron. *Nephrol Dial Transplant* 2006; 21: 378-82.
35. Corwin HL, Gettinger A, Pearl RG, Fink MP, Levy MM, Shapiro MJ, Corwin MJ, Colton T. Efficacy of recombinant human erythropoietin in critically ill patients: a randomized controlled trial. *JAMA* 2002; 288: 2827-35.
36. Georgopoulos D, Matamis D, Routsi C, Michalopoulos A, Maggina N, Dimopoulos G, et al. Recombinant human erythropoietin therapy in critically ill patients: a dose-response study *Crit Care* 2005; 9: R508-15.
37. Breymann C, Richter C, Hüttner C, Huch R, Huch A. Effectiveness of recombinant erythropoietin and iron sucrose vs. iron therapy only, in patients with postpartum anaemia and blunted erythropoiesis. *Eur J Clin Invest* 2000; 30: 154-161.
38. McLoughlin PL, Cope TM, Harrison JC. Hyperbaric oxygen therapy in the management of severe acute anaemia in a Jehovah's Witness. *Anaesthesia* 1999; 54: 891-895.

Hospital Information Services for Jehovah's Witnesses (020 8906 2211 (24 hrs); his@uk.jw.org)

cpw Jan 2011

Addendum C: Antenatal checklist for women refusing blood transfusion

Patient Name and Address	
Date of Birth	
Hospital Number	
Telephone Number(s)	
Consultant Surgeon	
Consultant Anesthetist	
Sp Registrar (and Bleep Number)	

Statement: I, the above-named patient, am prepared to accept the following treatments, before, during or after my operation:—

TREATMENT	WILLING TO ACCEPT
Recombinant Erythropoietin$^{\boxtimes}$	Yes/No
Hematinics (e.g. Intravenous/Oral Iron, Folic Acid, Vitamin B_{12}) $^{\boxtimes}$	Yes/No
Acute Normovolaemic Hemodilution*	Yes/No
Intraoperative Cell Salvage*	Yes/No
Fresh Frozen Plasma$^{\#}$	Yes/No
Cryoprecipitate*	Yes/No
Immunoglobulins, Anti-D*	Yes/No
Prothrombin Complex Concentrate (PCCs, e.g. Beriplex)*	Yes/No
Fibrinogen, Fibrin Glues and Sealants (Human and Non-Human)*	Yes/No
Recombinant Clotting Factors (e.g. Factor VIIa) $^{\boxtimes}$	Yes/No
DDAVP (Desmopressin), Tranexamic Acid (TXA), Aprotinin$^{\boxtimes}$	Yes/No
Packed Red Cells, Plasma, Platelets if required to save life$^{\#}$	Yes/No

_____   Date: __/__/__
Signature of Patient

Addendum D: Example of document serving as a release for hospital in the event that a woman dies after declining administration of blood and blood products

Advance Decision to Refuse Specified Medical Treatment

1. I, _____ (print or type full name), born _____ (date) complete this document to set forth my treatment instructions in case of my incapacity. **The refusal of specified treatment(s) contained herein continues to apply even if those medically responsible for my welfare and/or any other persons believe that such treatments are necessary to sustain my life.**

2. I am one of Jehovah's Witnesses with firm religious convictions. With full realization of the implications of this position I direct that **NO TRANSFUSIONS OF BLOOD or primary blood components (red cells, white cells, plasma or platelets)** be administered to me in any circumstances. I also refuse to predonate my blood for later infusion.

3. **Regarding minor fractions of blood** (for example: albumin, coagulation factors, immunoglobulins): [Initial **one** of the three choices below.]

   (a) _____ I refuse all

   (b) _____ I accept all

   (c) _____ I want to qualify either (3a) or (3b) above and my treatment choices are as follows:

   _____

   _____

4. **Regarding autologous procedures** (involving my own blood, for example: haemodilution, heart bypass, dialysis, intra-operative and post-operative blood salvage):
   [Initial **one** of the three choices below.]

   (a) _____ I refuse all such procedures or therapies

   (b) _____ I am prepared to accept any such procedure

   (c) _____ I accept only the following procedures:

   _____

   _____

   I am prepared to accept diagnostic procedures, such as blood samples for testing.

5. **Regarding other welfare instructions** (such as current medications, allergies, and medical problems):

   _____

   _____

   _____

6. I consent to my medical records and the details of my condition being shared with the Emergency Contact below and/or with member(s) of the Hospital Liaison Committee for Jehovah's Witnesses.

7. _____   _____
   Signature   Date

   _____
   Address

8. **STATEMENT OF WITNESSES:** The person who signed this document did so in my presence. He or she appears to be of sound mind and free from duress, fraud, or undue influence. I am 18 years of age or older.

   _____   _____
   Signature of witness   Signature of witness

   _____   _____
   Name   Occupation   Name   Occupation

   _____   _____
   Address   Address

   _____   _____
   Telephone   Telephone

   _____   _____
   Mobile   Mobile

9. **EMERGENCY CONTACT:**

   _____
   Name

   _____
   Address

   _____
   Telephone   Mobile

10. **GENERAL PRACTITIONER CONTACT DETAILS:** A copy of this document is lodged with the Registered General Medical Practitioner whose details appear below.

    _____
    Name

    _____
    Address

    _____
    Telephone Number(s)

Page 2 of 2

Advance Decision to Refuse Specified Medical Treatment
(signed document inside)

NO BLOOD

73

MamaNatalie®: a Birthing Simulator for Realistic Training to Control Postpartum Hemorrhage

I. Neuman and A. B. Lalonde

Skilled care at birth can save the lives of women and their babies[1]. Of the approximately 1000 maternal deaths that occur each day, 800 could be saved if a birth attendant with appropriate skills was present during delivery[2]. In order to prevent these unnecessary deaths, there is an urgent need to train a large number of birth attendants in how to master simple yet life-saving techniques before, during and after delivery[3].

Implementing programs to reduce maternal mortality and morbidity due to postpartum hemorrhage (PPH) requires not only guidelines, but also continuous training and evaluation of health care workers at all levels. The International Federation of Gynecology and Obstetrics (FIGO) committee on safe motherhood and newborn care has seen new developments in this area, and we bring information on the Mama-Natalie® birthing simulator that provides realistic life-like situations to train health care workers on a continuous basis.

The MamaNatalie birthing simulator was developed in response to the action call for 'significantly lower cost, durable, easy-to-disassemble and sanitize, high-fidelity mannequins with culturally appropriate features'[4]. This birthing simulator is an easy-to-use 'pregnant belly' that is strapped on the instructor, allowing the instructor – by only using his/her hands – to simulate birth scenarios (Figure 1).

Scenarios include fetal heart sounds, delivery of placenta, baby positions in birth tract and uterine firmness. The birthing simulator can also be used to train students on how to manage and detect more complicated situations, such as incomplete/retained placenta, atonic uterus, breech/shoulder dystocia, cord prolapse, vacuum assisted delivery and catheterization.

More importantly, MamaNatalie provides a realistic training tool to simulate PPH, the number one cause of maternal death during childbirth[3]. By wearing the MamaNatalie, the instructor takes the role of the mother and can control the intensity of bleeding and volume of blood loss as well as simulate a mother suffering from severe blood loss or shock. This teaches the students not only how to manage correctly PPH during and after delivery, but also how to

communicate with the mother and other team members during such a critical and stressful situation (Figures 2 and 3).

In 2010–2011, MamaNatalie underwent extensive field testing in developing and developed countries, showing excellent applicability as a simulator for both pre- and in-service courses in emergency obstetric and newborn care. The birthing simulator is currently being evaluated in a large prospective cohort study with over 6000 births in a rural hospital in Tanzania. The focus of this study is to look at behavior change and maternal survival outcomes in relation to training and use of MamaNatalie[6]. The birthing simulator is expected to have a particular impact when implemented through 'Helping Mothers Survive'. This is a new program led by Jhpiego which is based on the educational principles of effective hands-on simulation training, and focusing on basic skills with major life-saving potential. The first module, 'Bleeding after

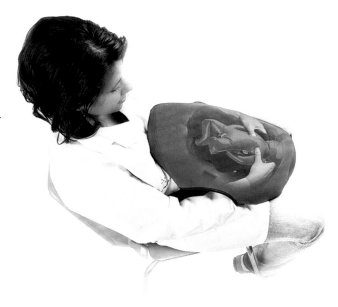

Figure 1 The instructor wears MamaNatalie and controls all the features of the birthing simulator with his/her hands. Reproduced with kind permission of Laerdal Global Health

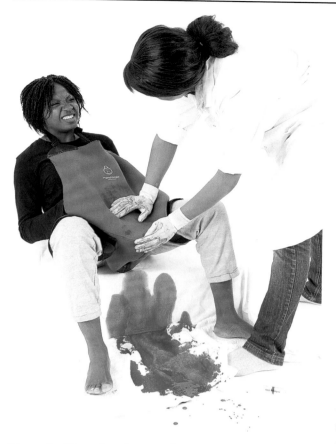

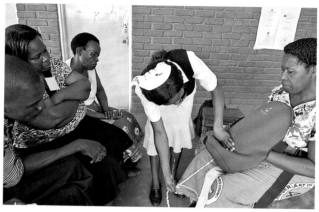

Figure 4 As MamaNatalie does not require electricity and the model fits in a backpack, it can be used in any setting. Here it is used in an in-service training at Mitundu Community Hospital in Malawi, April, 2012

Figure 2 The unique features of MamaNatalie train students to control PPH and develop communication skills with the mother. Reproduced with kind permission of Laerdal Global Health

Birth', is currently being field tested using the MamaNatalie in India, Tanzania, Malawi and Zanzibar[6] (Figure 4). The principles of risk management and adult education are embodied in this training module and accompanying instruction/ participant manual.

MamaNatalie is an innovative low-cost solution that has the potential to improve the confidence and skills of health workers in how to handle normal and complex birthing scenarios, in particular, controlling PPH in developing countries where currently 99% of all the maternal deaths occur[7]. It is therefore fitting that *A Comprehensive Textbook of Postpartum Hemorrhage* highlights educational materials that enable simulation of PPH in a low-cost effective teaching environment.

Video demonstrations are available on www.laerdalglobalhealth.com/mamanatalie.html.

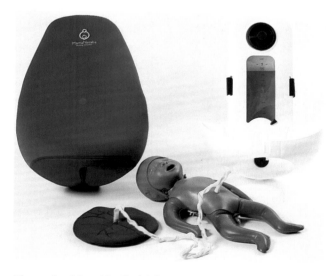

Figure 3 MamaNatalie birthing simulator comes with uterine bladder, umbilical cord, placenta, uterus and blood tank with a capacity of 1.5 liters. MamaNatalie also gives birth to NeoNatalie, a realistic newborn simulator that can be used to train management of birth asphyxia and essential newborn care. Reproduced with kind permission of Laerdal Global Health

References

1. World Health Organization, Maternal mortality Fact sheet No348, May 2012 http://www.who.int/mediacentre/factsheets/fs348/en/index.html
2. UNICEF. The State of the World's Children. 2009:2; and The Lancet 2010;375:1609–23
3. UNFPA, The State of the World's Midwifery 2011. Delivering Health, Saving Lives 2011 http://www.unfpa.org/sowmy/resources/docs/main_report/en_SOWMR_Full.pdf
4. Hofmeyr GJ, Haws RA, Bergström S, et al. Obstetric care in low-resource settings: what, who, and how to overcome challenges to scale up? Int J Gynecol Obstet 2009;107:s21–s45
5. Nelissen E. Helping Mothers Deliver – an assessment of the quality of the impact of simulation based training in emergency obstetric care in a resource-limited rural hospital in Tanzania. Research Protocol, 2010
6. Jhpiego. http://www.jhpiego.org/en/content/maternal-newborn-and-child-health
7. World Health Organization, Maternal mortality Fact sheet No348, May 2012 http://www.who.int/mediacentre/factsheets/fs348/en/index.html

Appendix

Appendix

FIGO Guidelines: Prevention and Treatment of Postpartum Hemorrhage in Low-Resource Settings*

Board and Safe Motherhood and Newborn Health Committee (SMNHC) members: *A. Lalonde, Canada (Chair); P. Okong, Uganda (Co-Chair); S. Zulfigar Bhutta, Pakistan; L. Adrien, Haiti; W. Stones, Kenya; C. Fuchtner, Bolivia; A. A. Wahed, Jordan; C. Hanson, Germany; and P. von Dadelszen, Canada*

Corresponding members: *B. Carbonne, France; J. Liljestrand, Cambodia; S. Arulkumaran, UK; D. Taylor, UK; P. Delorme, UK; S. Miller, USA; and C. Waite, UK*

Ex officio: *G. Serour, FIGO President; H. Rushwan, FIGO Chief Executive; and C. Montpetit, SMNHC Coordinator*

These guidelines were reviewed and approved in June 2011 by the International Federation of Gynecology and Obstetrics (FIGO) Executive Board and SMNHC.

INTRODUCTION

This statement does not change the two previous statements on management of the third stage of labor (both available at http://www.figo.org/projects/prevent/pph): ICM/FIGO Joint Statement − Prevention and Treatment of Post-partum Haemorrhage: New Advances for Low Resource Settings (November 2006); and ICM/FIGO Joint Statement − Management of the Third Stage of Labour to Prevent Postpartum Haemorrhage (November 2003)[1,2].

The following guideline provides a comprehensive document regarding best practice for the prevention and treatment of postpartum hemorrhage (PPH) in low-resource settings.

FIGO is actively contributing to the global effort to reduce maternal death and disability around the world. Its mission statement reflects a commitment to the promotion of health, human rights, and well-being of all women − most especially those at greatest risk for death and disability associated with childbearing. FIGO promotes evidence-based interventions that, when applied with informed consent, can reduce the incidence of maternal morbidity and mortality.

This statement reflects the best available evidence, drawn from scientific literature and expert opinion, on the prevention and treatment of PPH in low-resource settings.

Approximately 30% (in some countries, over 50%) of direct maternal deaths worldwide are due to hemorrhage, mostly in the postpartum period[3]. Most maternal deaths due to PPH occur in low-income countries in settings (both hospital and community) where there are no birth attendants or where birth attendants lack the necessary skills or equipment to prevent and manage PPH and shock. The Millennium Development Goal of reducing the maternal mortality ratio by 75% by 2015 will remain beyond our reach unless we prioritize the prevention and treatment of PPH in low-resource areas[4].

FIGO endorses international recommendations that emphasize the provision of skilled birth attendants and improved obstetric services as central to efforts to reduce maternal and neonatal mortality. Such policies reflect what should be a basic right for every woman. Addressing PPH will require a combination of approaches to expand access to skilled care and, at the same time, extend life-saving interventions along a continuum of care from community to hospital[1,2]. The different settings where women deliver along this continuum require different approaches to PPH prevention and treatment.

CALL TO ACTION

Despite Safe Motherhood activities since 1987, women are still dying in childbirth. Women living in low-resource settings are most vulnerable owing to concurrent disease, poverty, discrimination, and limited access to health care. FIGO has a central role to play in improving the capacity of national obstetric and midwifery associations to reduce maternal death and disability through safe, effective, feasible, and

*Reproduced, with permission granted by FIGO, from Lalonde A. Prevention and treatment of postpartum hemorrhage in low-resource settings. *Int J Gynaecol Obstet* 2012;117:108−18

sustainable strategies to prevent and treat PPH. In turn, national obstetric and midwifery associations must lead the effort to implement the approaches described in this statement.

Professional associations can mobilize to:

- Lobby governments to ensure health care for all women.

- Advocate for every woman to have a midwife, doctor, or other skilled attendant at birth.

- Disseminate this statement to all members through all available means, including publication in national newsletters or professional journals.

- Educate their members, other health care providers, policy makers, and the public about the approaches described in this statement and about the need for skilled care during childbirth.

- Address legislative and regulatory barriers that impede access to life-saving care, especially policy barriers that currently prohibit midwives and other birth attendants from administering uterotonic drugs.

- Ensure that all birth attendants have the necessary training – appropriate to the settings where they work – to administer uterotonic drugs safely and implement other approaches described in this statement, and ensure that uterotonics are available in sufficient quantity to meet the need.

- Call upon national regulatory agencies and policy makers to approve misoprostol for PPH prevention and treatment and to ensure that current best evidence regimens are adopted.

- Incorporate the recommendations from this statement into current guidelines, competencies and curricula.

We also call upon funding agencies to help underwrite initiatives aimed at reducing PPH through the use of cost-effective, resource-appropriate interventions.

POSTPARTUM HEMORRHAGE DEFINITION

Postpartum hemorrhage has been defined as blood loss in excess of 500 ml in a vaginal birth and in excess of 1000 ml in a cesarean delivery[5]. For clinical purposes, any blood loss that has the potential to produce hemodynamic instability should be considered a PPH. Clinical estimates of blood loss are often inaccurate.

Primary postpartum hemorrhage

Primary (immediate) PPH occurs within the first 24 hours after delivery. Approximately 70% of immediate PPH cases are due to uterine atony. Atony of the uterus is defined as the failure of the uterus to contract adequately after the child is born.

Secondary postpartum hemorrhage

Secondary (late) PPH occurs between 24 hours after delivery of the infant and 6 weeks postpartum. Most late PPH is due to retained products of conception, infection, or both.

Etiology

It may be helpful to think of the causes of PPH in terms of the 4 'T's:

- Tone: uterine atony, distended bladder.

- Trauma: uterine, cervical, or vaginal injury.

- Tissue: retained placenta or clots.

- Thrombin: pre-existing or acquired coagulopathy.

The most common and important cause of PPH is uterine atony. Myometrial blood vessels pass between the muscle cells of the uterus; the primary mechanism of immediate hemostasis following delivery is myometrial contraction causing occlusion of uterine blood vessels – the so-called 'living ligatures' of the uterus (Figure 1).

PREVENTION OF POSTPARTUM HEMORRHAGE

Pregnant women may face life-threatening blood loss at the time of birth. Anemic women are more vulnerable to even moderate amounts of blood loss. Most PPH can be prevented. Different approaches may be employed, depending on the setting and the availability of skilled birth attendants and supplies.

Active management of the third stage of labor

Data support the routine use of active management of the third stage of labor (AMTSL) by all skilled birth attendants, regardless of where they practice; AMTSL reduces the incidence of PPH, the quantity of blood loss, and the need for blood transfusion, and thus should be included in any program of intervention aimed at reducing death from PPH[7].

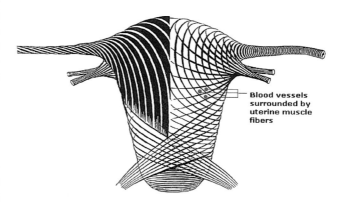

Figure 1 Muscle fibers of the uterus. Image reproduced, with permission, from reference 6

The usual components of AMTSL include:

- Administration of oxytocin (the preferred storage of oxytocin is refrigeration but it may be stored at temperatures up to 30°C for up to 3 months without significant loss of potency) or another uterotonic drug within 1 minute after birth of the infant.

- Controlled cord traction.

- Uterine massage after delivery of the placenta.

The Bristol[8] and Hinchingbrooke[9] studies compared active versus expectant (physiologic) management of the third stage of labor. Both studies clearly demonstrated that, when active management was applied, the incidence of PPH was significantly lower (5.9% with AMTSL vs 17.9% with expectant management[8]; and 6.8% with AMTSL vs 16.5% without[9]) (Table 1).

Step 1: How to use uterotonic agents

- Within 1 minute of delivery of the infant, palpate the abdomen to rule out the presence of an additional infant(s) and give oxytocin 10 units intramuscularly (IM). Oxytocin is preferred over other uterotonic drugs because it is effective 2–3 minutes after injection, has minimal adverse effects, and can be used in all women.

- If oxytocin is not available, other uterotonics can be used, such as: ergometrine or methylergometrine 0.2 mg IM; syntometrine (a combination of oxytocin 5 IU and ergometrine 0.5 mg per ampoule IM[10]); or misoprostol 600 μg orally. Uterotonics require proper storage:

  ○ Ergometrine or methylergometrine: 2–8°C and protect from light and from freezing.

  ○ Misoprostol: in aluminum blister pack, room temperature, in a closed container.

  ○ Oxytocin: 15–30°C, protect from freezing.

- Counseling on the adverse effects and contraindications of these drugs should be given.

- Uterine massage after delivery of the placenta.

Warning! Do not give ergometrine, methylergometrine, or syntometrine (because it contains ergot alkaloids) to women with heart disease, pre-eclampsia, eclampsia, or high blood pressure.

Misoprostol and the prevention of postpartum hemorrhage

The 18th Expert Committee on the Selection and Use of Essential Medicines met in March 2011, and approved the addition of misoprostol for the prevention of PPH to the WHO Model List of Essential Medicines. It reported that misoprostol 600 μg orally can be used for the prevention of PPH where oxytocin is not available or cannot be safely used. Misoprostol should be administered by health care workers trained in its use during the third stage of labor, soon after birth of the infant, to reduce the occurrence of PPH[11,12]. The most common adverse effects are transient shivering and pyrexia. Education of women and birth attendants in the proper use of misoprostol is essential. Recent studies in Afghanistan and Nepal demonstrate that community-based distribution of misoprostol can be successfully implemented under government health services in a low-resource setting, and, accompanied by education can be a safe, acceptable, feasible, and effective way to prevent PPH[13,14].

The usual components of management of the third stage of labor with misoprostol include:

- A single dose of 600 μg administered orally (data from two trials comparing misoprostol with placebo show that misoprostol 600 μg given orally reduces PPH with or without controlled cord traction or use of uterine massage[8]).

- Controlled cord traction only when a skilled attendant is present at the birth.

- Uterine massage after delivery of the placenta, as appropriate.

Step 2: How to do controlled cord traction (Figure 2)

- If the newborn is healthy, you can clamp the cord close to the perineum once cord pulsations stop or after approximately 2 minutes and hold the cord in one hand (immediate cord clamping may be necessary if the newborn requires resuscitation)[15,16].

- Place the other hand just above the woman's pubic bone and stabilize the uterus by applying counter-pressure during controlled cord traction.

Table 1 Active versus physiologic management of postpartum hemorrhage

	When active management of the third stage was applied	When expectant management of the third stage was applied	Odds ratio (95% confidence interval)
Bristol trial[8]	50 PPH cases/ 846 women (5.9%)	152 PPH cases/ 849 women (17.9%)	3.13 (2.3–4.2)
Hinchingbrooke trial[9]	51 PPH cases/ 748 women (6.8%)	126 PPH cases/ 764 women (16.5%)	2.42 (1.78–3.3)

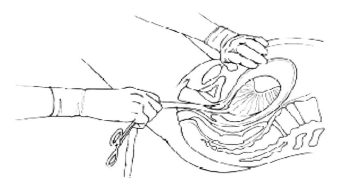

Figure 2 Controlled cord traction

- Keep slight tension on the cord and await a strong uterine contraction (2–3 minutes).

- With the strong uterine contraction, encourage the mother to push and very gently pull downward on the cord to deliver the placenta. Continue to apply counter-pressure to the uterus.

- If the placenta does not descend during 30–40 seconds of controlled cord traction, do not continue to pull on the cord:

  › Gently hold the cord and wait until the uterus is well contracted again.

  › With the next contraction, repeat controlled cord traction with counter-pressure.

Never apply cord traction (gentle pull) without applying counter-traction (push) above the pubic bone on a well-contracted uterus.

- As the placenta delivers, hold the placenta in two hands and gently turn it until the membranes are twisted. Slowly pull to complete the delivery.

- If the membranes tear, gently examine the upper vagina and cervix wearing sterile/disinfected gloves and use a sponge forceps to remove any pieces of membrane that are present.

- Look carefully at the placenta to be sure none of it is missing (Figures 3 and 4). If a portion of the maternal surface is missing or there are torn membranes with vessels, suspect retained placenta fragments and take appropriate action[17].

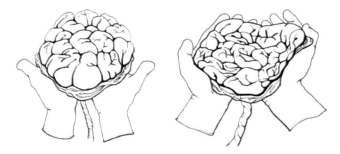

Figure 3 Examining the maternal side of the placenta. Reproduced with permission from reference 18

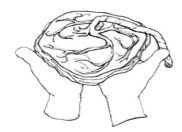

Figure 4 Examining the fetal side of the placenta. Reproduced with permission from reference 19

Step 3: How to do uterine massage

- Immediately after expulsion of the placenta, massage the fundus of the uterus through the abdomen until the uterus is contracted.

- Palpate for a contracted uterus every 15 minutes and repeat uterine massage as needed during the first 2 hours.

- Ensure that the uterus does not become relaxed (soft) after you stop uterine massage.

In all of the above actions, explain the procedures and actions to the woman and her family. Continue to provide support and reassurance throughout.

Management of the third stage of labor in the absence of uterotonic drugs

FIGO promotes the routine use of AMTSL as the best, evidence-based approach for the prevention of PPH and emphasizes that every effort should be made to ensure that AMTSL is used at every vaginal birth where there is a skilled birth attendant. However, FIGO recognizes that there may be circumstances where the accessibility or the supply of uterotonics may be sporadic owing to interruptions in the supply chain, or it may be nonexistent in a country because it is not part of the approved list of essential medicines or included in the national guidelines/protocols. It is in this context that the birth attendant must know how to provide safe care (physiologic management) to prevent PPH in the absence of uterotonic drugs (Table 2).

The following guide reflects the best practice, drawn from scientific literature and expert opinion, in the management of the third stage when uterotonics are not available.

Physiology of the third stage

Excerpt from *Williams Obstetrics*[19]:

'Near term, it is estimated that at least 600 ml/min of blood flows through the intervillous space. This flow is carried by spiral arteries and accompanying veins. With separation of the placenta, these vessels are avulsed. Hemostasis at the placenta site is achieved first by contraction of the myometrium that compresses the blood vessels followed by subsequent clotting and obliteration of their lumens. Thus, adhered pieces of placenta or large blood clots that prevent effective myometrium contraction can impair hemostasis at the implantation site.

Fatal post partum haemorrhage can result from uterine atony despite normal coagulation however conversely, if the myometrium within and adjacent to the denuded implantation site contracts vigorously, fatal hemorrhage from the placenta implantation site is unlikely, even in circumstances when coagulation may be severely impaired.'

Immediately following the birth and while awaiting delivery of the placenta

The birth attendant:

- Ensures the birth will be conducted in a semi-sitting position and/or position of comfort for the mother,

Table 2 Comparison of expectant (physiologic) versus AMTSL. Reproduced from reference 6 with permission

	Physiologic (expectant) management	*Active management*
Uterotonic	Uterotonic is not given before the placenta delivered	Uterotonic is given within one minute of the baby's birth (after ruling out the presence of a second baby)
Signs of placental separation	Wait for signs of separation: Gush of blood Lengthening of cord Uterus becomes rounder and smaller as the placenta descends	Do not wait for signs of placental separation. Instead: palpate the uterus for a contraction Wait for the uterus to contract Apply CCT with counter traction
Delivery of the placenta	Placenta delivered by gravity assisted by maternal effort	Placenta delivered by CCT while supporting and stabilizing the uterus by applying counter traction
Uterine massage	Massage the uterus after the placenta is delivered	Massage the uterus after the placenta is delivered
Advantages	Does not interfere with normal labor process Does not require special drugs/supplies May be appropriate when immediate care is needed for the baby (such as resuscitation) and no trained assistant is available May not require a birth attendant with injection skills	Decreases length of third stage Decrease likelihood of prolonged third stage Decreases average blood loss Decreases the number of PPH cases Decreases need for blood transfusion
Disadvantages	Length of third stage is longer compared to AMTSL	Requires uterotonic and items needed for injection safety

CCT, controlled cord traction

and places the infant on the mother's thorax/chest to provide skin-to-skin contact for warmth and to encourage breast feeding as soon as possible.

- Monitors both the mother's and the infant's vital signs (see below).

In the case where the birth attendant needs to care for another woman in labor/delivery, she needs to find help to observe vital signs and/or bleeding. In this case, the person who takes over monitoring of vital signs needs to report back to the primary birth attendant.

Umbilical cord management

The cord is left alone until either it has stopped pulsating or the placenta has been delivered, at which point the cord is then clamped or tied and cut.

Physiologic signs of placental separation

The birth attendant visually observes for the following signs:

- A change in the size, shape, and position of the uterus; palpating the uterus should be avoided.

- A small gush of blood.

- The cord lengthens at the vaginal introitus.

- The woman may become uncomfortable, experience contractions, or feel that she wants to change position. She may also indicate heaviness in the vagina and a desire to bear down.

Most placentas will be delivered within 1 hour; if this does not occur, the attendant must seek further assistance. If there is presence of excessive bleeding at any time, further assistance and/or transfer needs to be effected and treatment of PPH initiated.

Facilitating delivery of the placenta

Upon observation of the signs of placental separation, the birth attendant:

- Encourages the woman into an upright position.

- Either waits for the placenta to be expelled spontaneously or encourages the woman to push or bear down with contractions to deliver the placenta (which should be encouraged only after signs of separation have been noted).

- Catches the placenta in cupped hands or a bowl. If the membranes are slow to deliver, the birth attendant can assist by holding the placenta in two hands and gently turning it until the membranes are twisted, then exerting gentle tension to complete the delivery. Alternatively, the attendant can grasp the membranes gently and ease them from the vagina with an up-and-down motion of the hand.

Controlled cord traction is not recommended in the absence of uterotonic drugs or prior to signs of separation of the placenta because this can cause partial placental separation, a ruptured cord, excessive bleeding, and/or uterine inversion.

POSTPARTUM CARE REGARDLESS OF THIRD-STAGE MANAGEMENT

Immediately following the birth of the placenta

The birth attendant:

- Monitors the mother's vital signs every 5–10 minutes during the first 30 minutes, then every 15 minutes for the next 30 minutes, and then every 30 minutes for the next 2 hours:

  - Blood pressure, pulse, level of the uterine fundus.

    ○ Massages the uterus, looks for bleeding, and makes sure the uterus is contracted (the uterus will be found in the area around the navel and should feel firm to the touch).

- Observes the infant's color, respirations, and heart rate every 15 minutes for the first 2 hours.

- Examines the placenta for completeness.

Treatment of postpartum hemorrhage

Even with major advances in prevention of PPH, some women will still require treatment for excessive bleeding. Timely interventions and appropriate access, or referral and transfer to basic or comprehensive emergency obstetric care (EmOC) facilities for treatment are essential to saving the lives of women.

All health care professionals should be trained to prevent PPH, to recognize the early signs of PPH, and to be able to treat PPH. Health care professionals should refresh their knowledge and skills in emergency obstetrics on a regular basis through workshops that include didactic practical exercises and evaluations. There exist several in-service emergency obstetric courses developed to provide skill in this area, which are offered globally, such as ALSO, MOET, ALARM, MORE[OB], and JHPIEGO. It is also recommended that obstetric units in hospitals introduce regular emergency drills for care of PPH. Once introduced, such emergency drills are invaluable for keeping all staff updated and alert to the emergency treatment of PPH, eclampsia, and other major obstetric emergencies.

Community-based emergency care: home-based life-saving skills[12]

Anyone who attends a birth can be taught simple home-based life-saving skills (HBLSS). Community-based obstetric first aid with HBLSS is a family- and community-focused program that aims to increase access to basic life-saving measures and decrease delays in reaching referral facilities. Family and community members are taught techniques such as uterine fundal massage and emergency preparedness. Field tests suggest that HBLSS can be a useful adjunct in a comprehensive PPH prevention and treatment program[20]. Key to the effectiveness of treatment is early identification of hemorrhage and prompt initiation of treatment.

Clinical management of postpartum hemorrhage

Currently, the standard of care in basic EmOC facilities includes administration of intravenous (IV)/IM uterotonic drugs and manual removal of the placenta/retained products of conception; comprehensive EmOC facilities would also include blood transfusion and/or surgery[21].

Oxytocin

Oxytocin is the preferred uterotonic. It stimulates the smooth-muscle tissue of the upper segment of the uterus – causing it to contract rhythmically, constricting blood vessels, and decreasing blood flow through the uterus. It is a safe and effective first choice for treatment of PPH. For a sustained effect, IV infusion is preferred because it provides a steady flow of the drug. Uterine response subsides within 1 hour of cessation of IV administration[1,19].

Ergot alkaloids

Ergot alkaloids such as ergometrine, methylergometrine, and syntometrine cause the smooth muscle of both the upper and the lower uterus to contract tetanically. Although the ampoules can be found in different concentrations (either 0.2 mg/ml or 0.5 mg/ml), the recommended dose of ergometrine or methylergometrine is 0.2 mg IM, which can be repeated every 2–4 hours for a maximum of 5 doses (1 mg) in a 24-hour period. Ergot alkaloids are contraindicated in women with hypertension, cardiac disease, or pre-eclampsia because they can cause hypertension.

Misoprostol

Research has shown that a single dose of 800 μg (4 × 200-μg tablets) misoprostol administered sublingually is a safe and effective treatment of PPH due to uterine atony in women who have received oxytocin prophylaxis as well as those who have received no oxytocin prophylaxis during the third stage of labor[22,23]. In home births without a skilled attendant, misoprostol may be the only technology available to control PPH. Studies on treatment of PPH found that misoprostol significantly reduces the need for additional interventions[24]. Rarely, non-fatal hyperpyrexia has been reported after 800 μg of oral misoprostol[25]. There is no evidence about the safety and efficacy of the 800-μg dose for treatment of PPH when given to women who have already received 600 μg of prophylactic misoprostol orally. There is evidence that misoprostol provides no added benefit when given simultaneously with other injectable uterotonic drugs for the treatment of PPH, and therefore adjunct treatment of misoprostol simultaneously with oxytocin for PPH treatment is not recommended[26].

Management of postpartum hemorrhage

Definition of postpartum hemorrhage:

- Blood loss is more than 500 ml or two cups after a vaginal delivery, or in excess of 1000 ml after a cesarean delivery.

Maternal signs and symptoms of hypovolemia:

- A rising pulse rate is an early indicator, followed later by a drop in blood pressure, pallor, sweating, poor capillary refill, and cold extremities.

- Symptoms may include faintness/dizziness, nausea, and thirst.

If excessive blood loss occurs:

- Call for help and set up an IV infusion using a large-bore cannula, and consider opening a second IV infusion.

- Place the woman on a flat surface, such as a delivery table or birthing bed, with her feet higher than her head.

- The birth attendant places a hand on the fundus of the uterus and gently massages until it is firm and contracted. This helps express out blood clots and allows the uterus to contract.

- Empty the bladder. The woman may be able to void on her own or she may need to be catheterized.

- Start oxygen, if available.

- Give uterotonic as soon as possible:

  ○ Oxytocin

    ○ 10 units IM

      Or

    ○ 20–40 IU in 1 L of normal saline at 60 drops per minute

    ○ Continue oxytocin infusion (20 IU in 1 L of IV fluid at 40 drops per minute) until hemorrhage stops

      Or

  ○ Ergometrine or methylergometrine (used if oxytocin is not available or if bleeding continues despite having used oxytocin)

    ○ 0.2 mg (formulation may differ from country to country [ergometrine 0.2 or 0.5 mg]) IM or can be given slowly IV

    ○ If bleeding persists, 0.2 mg IM can be repeated every 2–4 hours for a maximum of 5 doses (1 mg) in a 24-hour period

    ○ Do not exceed 1 mg (or 5 0.2-mg doses) in a 24-hour period

    ○ Hypertension is a relative contraindication because of the risk of stroke and/or hypertensive crisis

    ○ Contraindicated with concomitant use of certain drugs used to treat HIV (HIV protease inhibitor, efavirenz, or delavirdine). If there is no alternate treatment available to control the hemorrhage, use the lowest dosage/shortest duration. Use it only if the benefits of ergometrine outweigh the risks

      Or

  ○ Syntometrine (combination of oxytocin 5 units and ergometrine 0.5 mg)

    ○ 1 ampoule IM (warning, IV could cause hypotension)

      Or

  ○ Misoprostol (if oxytocin is not available or where administration is not feasible)

    ○ A single dose of 800 µg sublingually (4 × 200-µg tablets).

For management of PPH, oxytocin should be preferred over ergometrine or methylergometrine alone, a fixed-dose combination of ergometrine and oxytocin, carbetocin, and/or prostaglandins such as misoprostol. If oxytocin is not available, or if the bleeding does not respond to oxytocin or ergometrine, an oxytocin–ergometrine fixed-dose combination, carbetocin, or misoprostol should be offered as second-line treatment. If these second-line treatments are not available or if the bleeding does not respond to the second-line treatment, a prostaglandin such as carboprost (Hemabate tromethamine; Pfizer, NY, NY, USA) should be offered as the third line of treatment, if available[27].

If bleeding persists after administration of uterotonics, consider these potentially life-saving procedures:

- Bimanual compression of the uterus (external or internal) (Figures 6 and 7).

- Aortic compression.

- Hydrostatic intrauterine balloon tamponade.

- Use of an anti-shock garment for the treatment of shock or transfer to another level of care, or while waiting for a cesarean.

- Laparotomy to apply compression sutures using B-Lynch or Cho techniques.

Although uterine atony is the cause of PPH in the majority of cases, the birth attendant should also exclude retained products of conception (check the placenta again), vaginal or cervical tears, uterine rupture, uterine inversion, and coagulation disorders (bedside clotting test).

Internal bimanual compression to stop excessive blood loss[28]

- Explain to the woman and family the need to do bimanual compression and that it may be painful.

- Ensure clean hands and use sterile gloves, if possible.

- Place one hand in the vagina and clench hand into a fist.

- Place other hand on the fundus of the uterus.

- Bring the two hands together to squeeze the uterus between them, applying pressure to stop or slow the bleeding.

FIGO recommendations
Drug regimens for the prevention and the treatment of PPH

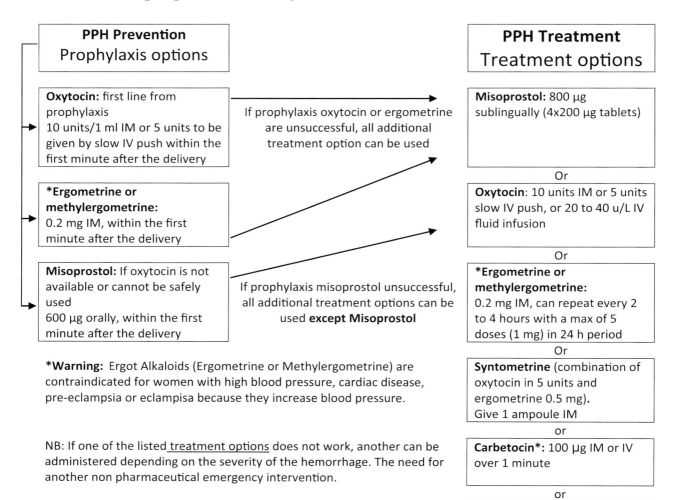

PPH Prevention Prophylaxis options		**PPH Treatment** Treatment options
Oxytocin: first line from prophylaxis 10 units/1 ml IM or 5 units to be given by slow IV push within the first minute after the delivery	If prophylaxis oxytocin or ergometrine are unsuccessful, all additional treatment option can be used	**Misoprostol:** 800 µg sublingually (4x200 µg tablets)
		Or
*Ergometrine or methylergometrine: 0.2 mg IM, within the first minute after the delivery		**Oxytocin:** 10 units IM or 5 units slow IV push, or 20 to 40 u/L IV fluid infusion
		Or
Misoprostol: If oxytocin is not available or cannot be safely used 600 µg orally, within the first minute after the delivery	If prophylaxis misoprostol unsuccessful, all additional treatment options can be used **except Misoprostol**	***Ergometrine or methylergometrine:** 0.2 mg IM, can repeat every 2 to 4 hours with a max of 5 doses (1 mg) in 24 h period
		Or
		Syntometrine (combination of oxytocin in 5 units and ergometrine 0.5 mg). Give 1 ampoule IM
		or
		Carbetocin*: 100 µg IM or IV over 1 minute
		or
		Carboprost*: 0.25 mg IM or IMM q15 minutes (max 2 mg)

*Warning: Ergot Alkaloids (Ergometrine or Methylergometrine) are contraindicated for women with high blood pressure, cardiac disease, pre-eclampsia or eclampisa because they increase blood pressure.

NB: If one of the listed treatment options does not work, another can be administered depending on the severity of the hemorrhage. The need for another non pharmaceutical emergency intervention.

Figure 5 FIGO recommendations for drug regimens for the prevention and treatment of PPH

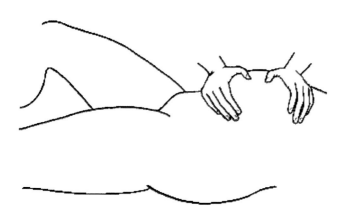

Figure 6 External bimanual massage

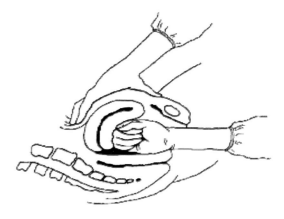

Figure 7 Internal bimanual compression of the uterus. Reproduced with permission from reference 29

- Keep the uterus compressed until able to gain medical support.

Aortic compression

Aortic compression (Figure 8) is a life-saving intervention when there is a heavy postpartum bleeding, whatever the cause. It may be considered at several different points during management of PPH. Aortic compression does not prevent or delay any of the other steps to be taken to clarify the cause of PPH and remedy it. Circulating blood volume is restricted to the upper part of the body and, thereby, to the vital organs. Blood pressure is kept higher, blood is prevented from reaching the bleeding area in the pelvis, and volume is conserved. Initially, the most qualified person at hand may have to carry out the compression to stop massive bleeding. As soon as possible, this technique is assigned to a helper so that the most qualified person is not tied up and interventions delayed. While preparing for a necessary intervention, blood is conserved by cutting off the blood supply to the pelvis via compression.

Step-by-step technique:

(1) Explain the procedure to the woman, if she is conscious, and reassure her.

(2) Stand on the right side of the woman.

(3) Place left fist just above and to the left of the woman's umbilicus (the abdominal aorta passes slightly to the left of the midline [umbilicus]).

(4) Lean over the woman so that your weight increases the pressure on the aorta. You should be able to feel the aorta against your knuckles. Do not use your arm muscles; this is very tiring.

(5) Before exerting aortic compression, feel the femoral artery for a pulse using the index and third fingers of the right hand.

(6) Once the aorta and femoral pulse have been identified, slowly lean over the woman and increase the pressure over the aorta to seal it off. To confirm proper sealing of the aorta, check the femoral pulse.

(7) There must be no palpable pulse in the femoral artery if the compression is effective. Should the pulse become palpable, adjust the left fist and the pressure until the pulse is gone again.

(8) The fingers should be kept on the femoral artery as long as the aorta is compressed to make sure that the compression is efficient at all times.

Note 1: Aortic compression may be used to stop bleeding at any stage. It is a simple life-saving skill to learn.

Note 2: Ideally, the birth attendant should accompany the woman during transfer.

Hydrostatic intrauterine balloon tamponade

"This is a 'balloon' usually made of synthetic rubber balloon catheters such as Foley catheters, Rusch catheters, SOS Bakri catheters, Sengstaken-Blakemore and even using sterile rubber glove, condom, or other device that is attached to a rubber urinary catheter and is then inserted into the uterus under aseptic conditions. This device is attached to a syringe and filled with sufficient saline solution, usually 300 ml to 500 ml, to exert enough counter-pressure to stop bleeding. When the bleeding stops, the care provider folds and ties the outer end of the catheter to maintain pressure. An oxytocin infusion is continued for 24 hours. If bleeding persists, add more saline solution. If bleeding has stopped and the woman is in constant pain, remove 50 ml to 100 ml of the saline solution. The 'balloon' is left in place for up to 24 hours; it is gradually deflated over two hours, and then removed. If bleeding starts again during the deflating period, re-inflate the balloon tamponade and wait another 24 hours before trying to deflate a second time. A balloon tamponade may arrest or stop bleeding in 77.5% to 88.8% or more cases without any further need for surgical treatment"[31]. Other reviews state that the balloon tamponade (Figure 9) is effective in 91.5% of cases and recommend that this relatively simple technology be part of existing protocols in the management of PPH[32]. Further, the balloon tamponade can test if the bleeding is uterine or from another source. If the bleeding does not stop with inflation, it is likely to be coming from a laceration or cause other than uterine atony.

Both aorta compression and balloon tamponade are illustrated by teaching videos available at www.glowm.com.

Non-pneumatic anti-shock garment

The non-pneumatic anti-shock garment (NASG) is a first-aid compression garment device made of neoprene and hook-and-loop fastener (Velcro; Zoex Niasg, Stork Medical, Coloma, CA, USA) comprising lower-extremity segments, a pelvic segment, and an abdominal segment, which includes a foam compression ball that goes over the uterus[33]. The NASG reverses shock by compressing the lower-body vessels, decreasing the container size of the body, so circulating blood is mainly directed to the core organs: heart; lungs; and brain. It also compresses the diameter of pelvic blood vessels, thus decreasing blood flow[34]. In preliminary pre-intervention/intervention trials in

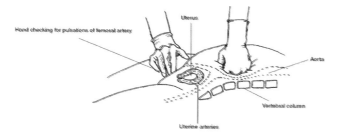

Figure 8 Compression of abdominal aorta and palpation of femoral pulse. Adapted from reference 30

(a) 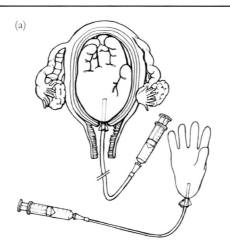 (b)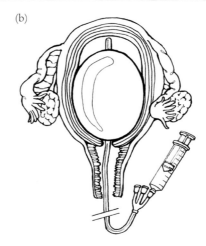

Figure 9 Types of intrauterine tamponade devices. (a) Hydrostatic intrauterine balloon tamponade and glove[9]. (b) Hydrostatic intrauterine balloon tamponade and Bakri SOS balloon[19]

tertiary facilities in Egypt and Nigeria, the NASG was shown to significantly improve shock[35], decrease blood loss, reduce emergency hysterectomy for atony, and decrease maternal mortality and severe maternal morbidities associated with obstetric hemorrhage[36,37]. A definitive trial of the NASG for use prior to transport from lower-level facilities to tertiary facilities is currently underway in Zambia and Zimbabwe. The NASG is applied to women experiencing hypovolemic shock secondary to obstetric hemorrhage, starting with the ankle segments and rapidly closing the other segments until the abdominal segment is closed (Figure 10). The woman can then be transported to a higher-level facility or, if already in such a facility, survive delays in obtaining blood and surgery. The NASG is not a definitive treatment – the woman will still need to have the source of bleeding found and definitive therapy performed. The NASG can remain in place during any vaginal procedure; the abdominal segment can be opened for surgery. Removal of the NASG occurs only when the source of bleeding is treated, the woman has been hemodynamically stable for at least 2 hours, and blood loss is less than 50 ml/hour. Removal begins at the ankles and proceeds slowly, waiting 15 minutes between opening each segment, and taking vital signs (blood pressure and pulse) before opening the next segment[37].

Laparotomy to apply compression sutures using B-Lynch or Cho techniques

If bleeding does not stop despite treatment with uterotonics, other conservative interventions (e.g. uterine massage), and external or internal pressure on the uterus, surgical interventions should be initiated. The first priority is to stop the bleeding before the patient develops coagulation problems and organ damage from underperfusion. Conservative approaches should be tried first, rapidly moving if these do not work to more invasive procedures. Compression sutures and uterine, utero-ovarian, and hypogastric vessel ligation may be tried, but in cases of life-threatening bleeding

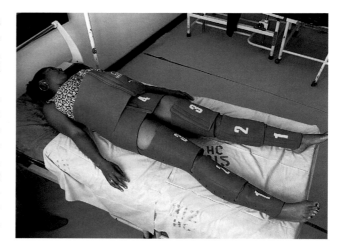

Figure 10 Anti-shock garments work through the application of counter-pressure to the lower body, which may reverse shock by returning blood to the vital organs. The garment is applied first to the lowest possible extremity (the ankles), then upwards. Reproduced with permission from reference 38

subtotal (also called supracervical) or total hysterectomy should be performed without delay[39]. More information about these techniques is available in Section 9 of *A Comprehensive Textbook of Postpartum Hemorrhage*, 2nd edition. The full text of this book can be downloaded for free at: http://www.sapiens-publishing.com/medical-publications.php?view=1.

Other innovative techniques

Other promising techniques appropriate for low-resource settings for assessment and treatment of PPH include easy and accurate blood loss measurement[40,41], oxytocin in Uniject (Becton Dickinson & Company (BD), Franklin Lakes, NJ, USA)[42], and the anti-shock garment[37]. These innovations are still under investigation for use in low-resource settings but may prove programmatically important, especially for women living far from skilled care.

Continued care of the woman

Once the bleeding has been controlled and the woman is stable, careful monitoring over the next 24–48 hours is required. Signs that the woman is stabilizing include a rising blood pressure (aim for a systolic blood pressure of at least 100 mmHg) and a stabilizing heart rate (aim for a pulse under 90)[19].

Adequate monitoring includes:

- Checking that the uterus is firm and well contracted, and remains contracted.

- Estimating ongoing blood loss: to estimate bleeding accurately, put a sanitary napkin or other clean material under the woman's buttocks and ask her to extend her legs and cross them at the ankles for about 20–30 minutes. The blood will then collect in the area of the pubic triangle.

- Assessment of her vital signs:
  - Temperature
  - Pulse
  - Respiration
  - Blood pressure
  - General condition (e.g. color, level of consciousness)

- Ensuring adequate fluid intake:
  - After the woman has stabilized, IV fluids should be given at a rate of 1 L in 4–6 hours.
  - If IV access is not available or not possible, give oral rehydration salts (ORS) by mouth if able to drink, or by nasogastric tube. Quantity of ORS: 300–500 ml in 1 hour.
  - Monitoring blood transfusion, including the volume of blood and other fluids that have been transfused. The transfused amount is recorded as part of the fluid intake.

- Monitoring urinary output.

- Keeping accurate records of the woman's conditions and any further interventions needed.

- Ensuring the continuous presence of a skilled attendant until bleeding is controlled and the woman's general condition is good.

Before the woman is discharged from the health care facility, consider these interventions:

- Check her hemoglobin.

- Give iron and folate supplementation as indicated by the woman's condition.

Research needs

Important strides have been made in identifying life-saving approaches and interventions appropriate for PPH prevention and treatment in low-resource settings. The field is rapidly evolving and the following issues have been identified as priorities for further research in low-resource settings:

- Assess the impact of better measurement of blood loss (e.g. with a calibrated drape or other means) on birth attendants' delivery practices.

- Further assess options for treatment of PPH in lower-level (basic EmOC) facilities – in particular, uterine tamponade and the anti-shock garment.

- Identify the most efficient and effective means of teaching and supporting the skills needed by birth attendants and for community empowerment to address PPH.

- Investigate how PPH can be managed effectively at the community level.

Key actions to reduce postpartum hemorrhage

(1) Disseminate this clinical guideline to all national associations of midwives, nurses, medical offices, and obstetrician–gynecologists, and ask them to implement the guideline at the national, district, and community level.

(2) Obtain support for this statement from agencies in the field of maternal and neonatal health care, such as UN agencies, donors, governments, and others.

(3) Recommend that this guideline become a Global Initiative to be adopted by health policy makers and politicians.

(4) Recommend that this Global Initiative on the prevention of PPH be integrated into the curricula of midwifery, medical, and nursing schools.

FIGO will work toward ensuring that:

(1) Every mother giving birth anywhere in the world will be offered AMTSL for the prevention of PPH.

(2) Every skilled attendant will have training in AMTSL and in techniques for the treatment of PPH.

(3) Every health facility where births take place will have adequate supplies of uterotonic drugs, equipment, and protocols for both the prevention and the treatment of PPH.

(4) Blood transfusion facilities are available in centers that provide comprehensive health care (secondary and tertiary levels of care).

(5) Physicians are trained in simple conservative techniques such as uterine tamponade, compression sutures, and devascularization.

(6) The study of promising new drugs and technologies to prevent and treat PPH is supported by donors and governments.

(7) Member countries are surveyed to evaluate the uptake of recommendations.

FIGO Recommendations
Prevention and Treatment of Post-Partum Hemorrhage (PPH)

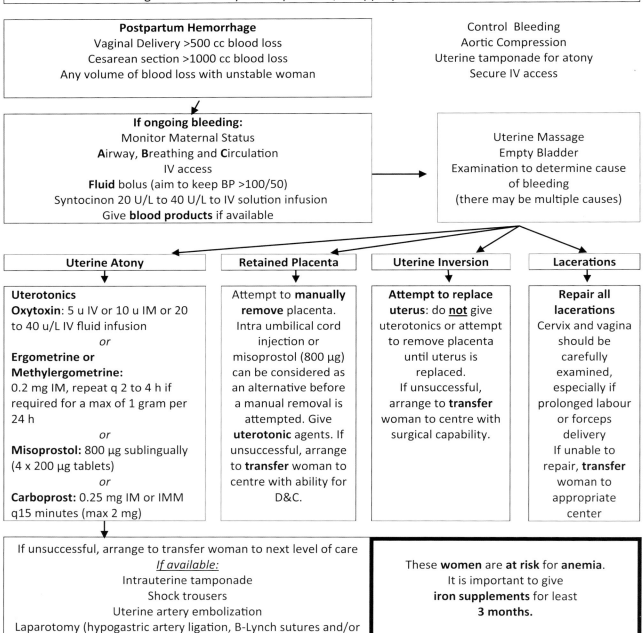

Prevention
Active Management of the Third Stage of Labor
- Administration of uterotonic agents (Oxytocin 10 iu IM or Misoprostol 600 µg po if Oxytocin is neither available nor feasible)
- Controlled cord traction
- Uterine massage after delivery of the placenta, as appropriate

Postpartum Hemorrhage
Vaginal Delivery >500 cc blood loss
Cesarean section >1000 cc blood loss
Any volume of blood loss with unstable woman

Control Bleeding
Aortic Compression
Uterine tamponade for atony
Secure IV access

If ongoing bleeding:
Monitor Maternal Status
Airway, **B**reathing and **C**irculation
IV access
Fluid bolus (aim to keep BP >100/50)
Syntocinon 20 U/L to 40 U/L to IV solution infusion
Give **blood products** if available

Uterine Massage
Empty Bladder
Examination to determine cause
of bleeding
(there may be multiple causes)

Uterine Atony	**Retained Placenta**	**Uterine Inversion**	**Lacerations**
Uterotonics **Oxytoxin**: 5 u IV or 10 u IM or 20 to 40 u/L IV fluid infusion *or* **Ergometrine or Methylergometrine:** 0.2 mg IM, repeat q 2 to 4 h if required for a max of 1 gram per 24 h *or* **Misoprostol:** 800 µg sublingually (4 x 200 µg tablets) *or* **Carboprost:** 0.25 mg IM or IMM q15 minutes (max 2 mg)	Attempt to **manually remove** placenta. Intra umbilical cord injection or misoprostol (800 µg) can be considered as an alternative before a manual removal is attempted. Give **uterotonic** agents. If unsuccessful, arrange to **transfer** woman to centre with ability for D&C.	**Attempt to replace uterus:** do **not** give uterotonics or attempt to remove placenta until uterus is replaced. If unsuccessful, arrange to **transfer** woman to centre with surgical capability.	**Repair all lacerations** Cervix and vagina should be carefully examined, especially if prolonged labour or forceps delivery If unable to repair, **transfer** woman to appropriate center

If unsuccessful, arrange to transfer woman to next level of care
If available:
Intrauterine tamponade
Shock trousers
Uterine artery embolization
Laparotomy (hypogastric artery ligation, B-Lynch sutures and/or hysterectomy)

These **women** are **at risk** for **anemia**.
It is important to give
iron supplements for least
3 months.

Figure 11 FIGO recommendations for the prevention and treatment of postpartum hemorrhage

CONCLUSION

(1) Ensure pre- and in-service training to health care providers to practice AMTSL. Promote and reinforce the value and effectiveness of this intervention as a best practice standard.

(2) All health care providers/professionals and/or birth attendants need to continue advocating for a secure continuous supply of oxytocics.

(3) Health care professionals need to be knowledgeable about physiologic management because they may practice in an environment where AMTSL may not be feasible. Training of all health care providers/professionals and/or birth attendants in the practice of physiologic management, AMTSL, diagnosis, and management of PPH.

(4) Prepare and disseminate PPH prevention and treatment protocols (Figure 11).

(5) Monitor the incidence of PPH and ensure quality assurance at local, regional, and national levels.

ACKNOWLEDGMENTS

FIGO and its SMNHC members would like to thank the Society of Obstetricians and Gynaecologists of Canada (SOGC), especially its staff Christine Nadori RN and Moya Crangle RM, who worked substantially in the creation of this document. In addition, we recognize Caroline Montpetit (SMNH Coordinator) and Becky Skidmore (Medical Research Analyst) for their contributions.

References

1. International Confederation of Midwives and International Federation of Gynaecology and Obstetrics, Joint statement: Management of the Third Stage of Labour to Prevent Post-partum Haemorrhage. London: FIGO, 2003

2. International Confederation of Midwives and International Federation of Gynaecology and Obstetrics, Prevention and Treatment of Post-partum Haemorrhage New Advances for Low Resource Settings: Joint Statement. Int J Gynecol Obstet 2007;97:160–3

3. Khan KD, Wojdyla L, Say A, et al. WHO analysis of causes of maternal death: a systematic review. Lancet 2006;1066:74

4. United Nations. United Nations Millennium Development Goals 2000 http://www.un.org/millenniumgoals.

5. Smith JR, Brennan BG. Postpartum hemorrhage. In: eMedicine clinical knowledge base [database online]. Omaha (NE): eMedicine, Inc., 2006. http://www.emedicine.com/med/topic3568.htm

6. POPPHI. Prevention of Postpartum Hemorrhage: Implementing Active Management of the Third Stage of Labor (AMTSL): A Reference Manual for Health Care Providers. Seattle: PATH, 2007

7. Prendiville W, Elbourne D, McDonald S, Active versus expectant management in the third stage of labour, Cochrane Database Syst Rev 2009;(3):CD000007

8. Prendiville W, Harding J, Elbourne D, Stirrat G. The Bristol third stage trial: active versus physiological management of the third stage of labour. BMJ 1988;297:1295–300

9. Rogers J, Wood J, McCandlish R, Ayers S, Trusdale A, Elbourne D. Active versus expectant management of third stage of labour: the Hinchingbrooke randomised controlled trial. Lancet 1998;351:693–9

10. Mousa HA, Alfirevic Z. Treatment for primary postpartum haemorrhage. Cochrane Database Syst Rev 2007;(1): CD003249

11. World Health Organization, Unedited Report of the 18th Committee on the Selection and Use of Essential Medicines. 2011 [cited 9th May, 2011]; http://www.who.int/selection_medicines/Complete_UNEDITED_TRS_18th.pdf.

12. Mobeen N, Durocher J, Zuberi N, et al. Administration of misoprostol by trained traditional birth attendants to prevent postpartum haemorrhage in homebirths in Pakistan: a randomised placebo-controlled trial. BJOG 2011;118:353–61

13. Sanghvi H, Ansari N, Prata NJ, et al. Prevention of postpartum hemorrhage at home birth in Afghanistan. Int J Gynecol Obstet 2010;108:276–81

14. Rajbhandari S, Hodgins S, Sanghvi H, McPherson R, Pradhan YV, Baqui AH. Expanding uterotonic protection following childbirth through community-based distribution of misoprostol: Operations research study in Nepal. Int J Gynecol Obstet, 2010;108:282–8

15. Rabe H, Reynolds G, az-Rossello J. Early versus delayed umbilical cord clamping in preterm infants [Cochrane review]. In: Cochrane Database of Systematic Reviews 2004 Issue 4. Chichester (UK): John Wiley & Sons, Ltd, 2004

16. Hutton EK, Hassan ES. Late vs early clamping of the umbilical cord in full-term neonates: systematic review and meta-analysis of controlled trials. JAMA 2007;297:1241–52

17. Managing Complications in Pregnancy and Childbirth: WHO, UNFPA, UNICEF, World Bank. Managing Complications in Pregnancy and Childbirth. WHO/RHR/00.7, 2000

18. Society of Obstetricians and Gynaecologists of Canada. ALARM International Program, 4th edn. Chapter 6. Ottawa: SOGC, 2008

19. Cunningham F, Leveno K, Bloom S, Hauth J, Rouse D, Spong C. Obstetrical hemorrhage. In: Williams Obsterics, 23rd edn. 2010; US: McGraw-Hill Professional 2010:760

20. Sibley L, Buffington S, Haileyesus D, The American College of Nurse Midwives' Home-based lifesaving skills program: a review of the Ethiopia field test (published erratum appears following table of contents). J Midwif Womens Health 2004; 49:320–8

21. United Nations Population Fund. Emergency obstetric care: checklist for planners. 2003 12 October 2006, http://www.unfpa.org-pload.lib_pub_file/150_filename_checklist_MMU.pdf

22. Blum J, Winikoff B, Raghavan S, et al. Treatment of postpartum haemorrhage with sublingual misoprostol versus oxytocin in women receiving prophylactic oxytocin: a double-blind, randomised, non-inferiority trial. Lancet 2010; 375:217–23

23. Winikoff B, Dabash R, Durocher J, et al. Treatment of postpartum haemorrhage with sublingual misoprostol versus oxytocin in women not exposed to oxytocin during labour: a double-blind, randomised, non-inferiority trial. Lancet 2010; 375:210–6

24. Prata N, Mbaruku G, Campbell M, Potts M, Vahidnia E. Controlling postpartum hemorrhage after home births in Tanzania. Int J Gynaecol Obstet 2005;90:51–5

25. Chong Y, Chua S, Arulkumaran S. Severe hyperthermia following oral misoprostol in the immediate postpartum period. Obstet Gynecol 1997;90:703–4

26. Widmer M, Blum J, Hofmeyr GJ, et al. Misoprostol as an adjunct to standard uterotonics for treatment of post-partum haemorrhage: a multicentre, double-blind randomised trial. Lancet 2010;375:1808–13

27. World Health Organization, guidelines for the management of postpartum haemorrhage and retained placenta, 2009; http://whqlibdoc.who.int/publications/2009/9789241598514_eng.pdf

28. Crafter H. Intrapartum and primary postpartum heamorrhage. In: Boyle M, ed. Emergencies Around Childbirth: a

Handbook for Midwives. UK: Radcliffe Medical Press Ltd, 2002

29. World Health Organization (WHO). Managing complications in pregnancy and childbirth: a guide for doctors and midwives. Geneva: World Health Organization, 2003. http://www.who.int/reproductive-health/impac/mcpc.pdf

30. World Health Organization (WHO). Managing Postpartum Haemorrhage: Education Mterial for Teachers of Midwifery, Second Edition. Geneva: World Health Organization, 2006:173. http://whqlibdoc.who.int/publications/2006/9241546662_5_eng.pdf

31. Lalonde AB, Daviss BA, Acosta A, Herschderfer K. Postpartim hemorrhage today: ICM/FIGO intiative 2004–2006. Int J Obstet 2006;94:243–53

32. Georgiou C. Balloon tamponade in the management of postpartum haemorrhage: a review. BJOG 2009;116:748–55

33. Miller S, Fathalla MMF, Ojengbede OA, et al. Obstetric hemorrhage and shock management: using the low technology Non-pneumatic Anti-Shock Garment in Nigerian and Egyptian tertiary care facilities. BMC Pregnancy Childbirth 2010;10:64

34. Lester F, Stenson A, Meyer C, Morris J, Vargas J, Miller S. Impact of the non-pneumatic antishock garment on pelvic blood flow in health postpartum women. Am J Obstet Gynecol 2011;204:409

35. Miller S, Turan JM, Dau K, et al. Use of the non-pneumatic anti-shock garment (NASG) to reduce blood loss and time to recovery from shock for women with obstetric haemorrhage in Egypt. Global Public Health J 2007;2:110–24

36. Turan J, Ojengbede O, Fathalla M, et al. Positive Effects of the Non-pneumatic Anti-shock Garment on Delays in Accessing Care for Postpartum and Postabortion Hemorrhage in Egypt and Nigeria. J Womens Health 2011;20:1

37. Miller S, Hensleigh P. Non-pneumatic Anti-shock Garment for Obstetric Hemorrhage. In: B-Lynch C, Keith LG, Lalonde A, Karoshi M, eds. A Textbook of Postpartum Hemorrhage. UK: Sapiens Publications, 2006

38. Miller S, Martin HB, Morris JL. Anti-shock garment in postpartum haemorrhage. Best Pract Res Clin Obstet Gynaecol 2008;22:1057–74

39. B-Lynch C. Conservative Surgical Management. In: B-Lynch C, Keith L, Lalonde A, Karoshi M, eds. A Textbook of Postpartum Hemorrhage. UK: Sapiens Publishing, 2006

40. Tourne G, Collet F, Lasnier P, Seffert P. Usefulness of a collecting bag for the diagnosis of postpartum haemorrhage (French). J Gynecol Obstet Biol Reprod (Paris) 2004;33:229–34

41. Prata N, Mbaruku G, Campbell M. Using the kanga to measure post-partum blood loss. Int J Gynaecol Obstet 2005;89:49–50

42. Tsu V, Sutanto A, Vaidya K, Coffey P, Widjaya A. Oxytocin in prefilled Uniject injection devices for managing third-stage labor in Indonesia. Int J Gynaecol Obstet 2003;83:103–11

Index